FOGSI's
POSTGRADUATE
OBSTETRICS
A TEXTBOOK

FOGSI's POSTGRADUATE OBSTETRICS
A TEXTBOOK

Volume 1

Editor-in-Chief

Alpesh Gandhi
MBBS DGO FICOG FRCOG Post PG (Hospital Management)
Senior Consultant, Obstetrics and Gynecology
Critical Care in Obstetrics and
High-risk Pregnancy Expert
Arihant Women's Hospital, Ahmedabad, Gujarat
President, The Federation of Obstetric and Gynaecological Societies of India (FOGSI), 2020

Editors

Parikshit Tank
MD DNB DGO DFP MNAMS FICOG FRCOG
Senior Consultant Obstetrician and Gynecologist
Ashwini Maternity and Surgical Hospital
Jupiter Hospital, Mumbai, Maharashtra, India
Honorary Professor, Assisted Reproduction
Pacific Medical College and Hospital
Udaipur, Rajasthan, India
Treasurer, The Federation of Obstetric and Gynaecological
Societies of India (FOGSI), 2021-2024
Joint Secretary, FOGSI, 2012
Joint Treasurer, FOGSI, 2018-2020
Chairperson, Safe Motherhood
FOGSI, 2014-2017

Ameya Purandare
MD DNB FCPS DGO DFP MNAMS FICMCH FICOG Fellowship in Gyne
Endoscopy (Germany)
Senior Consultant Obstetrician and Gynecologist
Purandare Hospital, KJ Somaiya Medical College and Hospital
Sir HN Reliance Foundation Hospital and Research Centre
Bhatia Hospital, Masina Hospital, Mumbai Police Hospital
Mumbai, Maharashtra, India
2nd Vice President Elect, The Association of Maharashtra Obstetric
and Gynaecological Societies (AMOGS), 2022-2024
Joint Secretary, FOGSI, 2019
Chairperson, Food, Drugs and Medical and Surgical Equipments
Committee, FOGSI, 2015-2017
Assistant Administrator, FOGSI Manyata Project

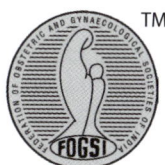

An Official Publication of
The Federation of Obstetric and Gynaecological Societies of India

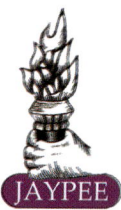

JAYPEE BROTHERS MEDICAL PUBLISHERS
The Health Sciences Publisher
New Delhi | London

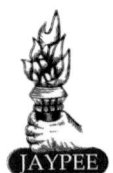
Jaypee Brothers Medical Publishers (P) Ltd

Headquarters
Jaypee Brothers Medical Publishers (P) Ltd
EMCA House, 23/23-B
Ansari Road, Daryaganj
New Delhi 110 002, India
Landline: +91-11-23272143, +91-11-23272703
+91-11-23282021, +91-11-23245672
Email: jaypee@jaypeebrothers.com

Corporate Office
Jaypee Brothers Medical Publishers (P) Ltd
4838/24, Ansari Road, Daryaganj
New Delhi 110 002, India
Phone: +91-11-43574357
Fax: +91-11-43574314
Email: jaypee@jaypeebrothers.com

Overseas Office
JP Medical Ltd
83 Victoria Street, London
SW1H 0HW (UK)
Phone: +44 20 3170 8910
Fax: +44 (0)20 3008 6180
Email: info@jpmedpub.com

Website: www.jaypeebrothers.com
Website: www.jaypeedigital.com

© 2022, Jaypee Brothers Medical Publishers

The views and opinions expressed in this book are solely those of the original contributor(s)/author(s) and do not necessarily represent those of editor(s) of the book.

All rights reserved. No part of this publication may be reproduced, stored or transmitted in any form or by any means, electronic, mechanical, photocopying, recording or otherwise, without the prior permission in writing of the publishers.

All brand names and product names used in this book are trade names, service marks, trademarks or registered trademarks of their respective owners. The publisher is not associated with any product or vendor mentioned in this book.

Medical knowledge and practice change constantly. This book is designed to provide accurate, authoritative information about the subject matter in question. However, readers are advised to check the most current information available on procedures included and check information from the manufacturer of each product to be administered, to verify the recommended dose, formula, method and duration of administration, adverse effects and contraindications. It is the responsibility of the practitioner to take all appropriate safety precautions. Neither the publisher nor the author(s)/editor(s) assume any liability for any injury and/or damage to persons or property arising from or related to use of material in this book.

This book is sold on the understanding that the publisher is not engaged in providing professional medical services. If such advice or services are required, the services of a competent medical professional should be sought.

Every effort has been made where necessary to contact holders of copyright to obtain permission to reproduce copyright material. If any have been inadvertently overlooked, the publisher will be pleased to make the necessary arrangements at the first opportunity. The **CD/DVD-ROM** (if any) provided in the sealed envelope with this book is complimentary and free of cost. **Not meant for sale.**

Inquiries for bulk sales may be solicited at: jaypee@jaypeebrothers.com

FOGSI's Postgraduate Obstetrics: A Textbook

First Edition: **2022**

ISBN: 978-93-5465-385-8

Printed at: Samrat Offset Pvt. Ltd.

Dedicated to

The students of Obstetrics and Gynecology, especially the postgraduates and their teachers
And
The girls and women of our country whom they are privileged to take care of

Section Editors

Amita Maheshwari MD
Professor and Head
Department of Gynecologic Oncology
Tata Memorial Centre
Mumbai, Maharashtra, India
President Elect
Association of Gynaecologic Oncologists of India

Anuradha Khanna MD FAMS FAICOG FUICC MANAMS FICS FUWAI
Former Professor and Head
Department of Obstetrics and Gynecology
Institute of Medical Sciences
Banaras Hindu University
Varanasi, Uttar Pradesh, India

Gokul Das MD FICOG FICMCH
Former Professor and Head
Department of Obstetrics and Gynecology
Gauhati Medical College Guwahati
Founder Professor and Head
Department of Obstetrics and Gynecology
Tomo Riba Institute of Health and Medical Sciences
Nagarlagun, Arunachal Pradesh
Senior Consultant and Head
Department of Obstetrics and Gynecology
Health City Hospital, Guwahati
Vice President FOGSI 2014

JB Sharma MD FRCOG FAMS PhD FICOG DNB
Professor, Department of Obstetrics and Gynecology
All India Institute of Medical Sciences
New Delhi, India

PK Shah MD DGO DFP FCPS
Former Professor and Unit Head
Department of Obstetrics and Gynecology
Seth GS Medical College and KEM Hospital
Mumbai, Maharashtra, India
President, FOGSI 2012

Pratima Mittal MD FICOG FICMCH PGDHHM FRCOG (Hon)
Former Professor and Head
Department of Obstetrics and Gynecology
Vardhman Mahavir Medical College and Safdarjung Hospital
New Delhi, India

Pushpa Junghare MD
Professor and Head
Department of Obstetrics and Gynecology
Dr Panjabrao Deshmukh Memorial Medical College
Amravati, Maharashtra, India

Suyajna Joshi MD (OBG) DNB
Head, Department of Obstetrics and Gynecology
District Hospital, Ballari
Consultant
Geetha Medical Center
Ballari, Karnataka, India

Contributors

Aanya Sharma MS (Obs & Gynec)
Resident
Department of Obstetrics and
Gynecology
Indira Gandhi Medical College
Shimla, Himachal Pradesh, India

Abha Rani Sinha MBBS MD DGO
Professor
Department of Obstetrics and
Gynecology
Sri Krishna Medical College and
Hospital (SKMCH)
Muzzafarpur, Bihar, India

Ajit C Rawal MBBS MD DGO
Consultant Obstetrician and
Gynecologist, Micro-Surgeon
Endoscopic Gynecologic Surgeon
Ex-Professor and Head
Department of Endoscopy and
Microsurgery
Sheth VS General Hospital
Ahmedabad, Gujarat, India

Ajith S MD DGO DNB FRCOG (UK)
Professor and Head
Department of Obstetrics and
Gynecology
Pariyaram Medical College
Kannur, Kerala, India

Alka Pandey MBBS MD FICOG
Associate Professor
Department of Obstetrics and
Gynecology
Patna Medical College and Hospital
Patna, Bihar, India

Alok Sharma MBBS MD (Obs & Gynec) DHA
MICOG
Assistant Professor
Department of Obstetrics and
Gynecology
Dr Rajendra Prasad Government
Medical College
Kangra, Himachal Pradesh, India

Alpesh Gandhi MBBS DGO FICOG FRCOG
Senior Consultant, Obstetrics and
Gynecology
Critical Care Obstetrics and
High Risk Pregnancy Expert
Arihant Women's Hospital
Ahmedabad, Gujarat, India
President, The Federation of Obstetrics
and Gynaecological Societies of India
(FOGSI), 2020

Amarjeet Kaur MBBS MD
Senior Resident
Department of Obstetrics and
Gynecology
Government Medical College
Amritsar, Punjab, India

Ami Surti MD
Consultant
Department of Obstetrics and
Gynecology
Surya Hospitals
Mumbai, Maharashtra, India

Amita Gandhi MD (Medicine)
Associate Professor
Department of Medicine
Sola GMERS Medical College
Ahmedabad, Gujarat, India

Amita Maheshwari MD
Professor and Head
Division of Gynecologic Oncology
Tata Memorial Centre
Mumbai, Maharashtra, India

Anahita Chauhan MD DGO DFP FICOG
Honorary Consultant
Saifee Hospital, Mumbai
Former Professor and Unit Head
Seth GS Medical College and KEM
Hospital, Mumbai, Maharashtra, India
Vice President, Mumbai Obstetric and
Gynaecological Society, 2021-22
First Joint Assistant Editor, Journal of
Obstetrics and Gynaecology of India

Ananth K MBBS MD
Consultant
Department of Anesthesia
Fernandez Hospitals
Hyderabad, Telangana, India

Anjali Otiv MBBS MD (Ped)
Pediatrician, Associate Professor
Terna Medical College
Apollo Hospitals
Navi Mumbai, Maharashtra, India

Ankita Rajesh Shah MD
Assistant Professor
Department of Obstetrics and
Gynecology
Government Medical College and
Hospital
Aurangabad, Maharashtra, India

Ankita Srivastava MBBS MS DNB MRCOG
Clinical Assistant
Institute of Obstetrics and Gynecology
Sir Ganga Ram Hospital
New Delhi, India

Aparna Setia MS
Fellow
Division of Maternal Fetal Medicine
Bhagwan Mahaveer Jain Hospital
Bengaluru, Karnataka, India

Arati Shah MD MICOG
Consultant
Department of Obstetrics and
Gynecology
Pulse Clinic
Ahmedabad, Gujarat, India

Archana Kumari MBBS MD
Assistant Professor
Department of Obstetrics and
Gynecology
All India Institute of Medical Sciences
New Delhi, India

Contributors

Arindam Halder MD
Associate Professor
Chittaranajn Seva Sadan for Maternal and Child Health
Kolkata, West Bengal, India

Arulmozhi Ramarajan MBBS MD (Obs & Gynec) PGD-Medical Law
Consultant Gynecologist-Obstetrician
Bhagwan Mahaveer Jain Hospital
Bengaluru, Karnataka, India

Ashis Kumar Mukhopadhyay MBBS DNB (Obs & Gynec)
Principal, Professor and Unit Chief
Chittaranajn Seva Sadan for Maternal and Child Health
Kolkata, West Bengal, India
GC Member, ICOG, 2021-22
Scientific Chair, AICOG 2022
Kolkata, WHO Fellow, Maternal Health

Ashish Mehta MBBS MD
Director and Consultant Neonatologist
Department of Pediatrics
Wadia Hospital
Ahmedabad, Gujarat, India

Ashvin Vachhani MD DNB
Medical Specialist
Department of Obstetrics and Gynecology
Atmiya Hospital
Surat, Gujarat, India

Ashwini Kale DGO DNB FICMCH
IVF Consultant
Ashakiran Hospital
Pune, Maharashtra, India

Aswath Kumar MBBS MD (Obs & Gynec)
Gynec-oncology Fellowship
Professor
Department of Obstetrics and Gynecology
Jubilee Mission Medical College and Research Institute
Thrissur, Kerala, India

Ayesha Ahmad DGO DNB MNAMS MRCOG
Fellow in Advanced Gynecology Laparoscopy
Associate Professor
Department of Obstetrics and Gynecology
Era's Lucknow Medical College and Hospital
Lucknow, Uttar Pradesh, India

Bakul Jayant Parekh MD
Consultant Pediatrician
Bakul Children's Hospital
Mumbai, Maharashtra, India

Bharathi KR MBBS MD
Associate Professor
Department of Obstetrics and Gynecology
Adichunchangiri Institute of Medical Sciences
Mandya, Karnataka, India

Bharti Sharma MD
Assistant Professor
Department of Obstetrics and Gynecology
Postgraduate Institute of Medical Education and Researh
Chandigarh, India

Bhavik Doshi MS
Associate Professor (Anatomy)
Sola GMERS Medical College
Ahmedabad, Gujarat, India

Bhawana Tiwary MD
Assistant Professor
Department of Reproductive Medicine
Indira Gandhi Institute of Medical Sciences
Patna, Bihar, India

Bhawna Garg MBBS
Junior Resident
Department of Obstetrics and Gynecology
Jawaharlal Nehru Medical College
Belgaum, Karnataka, India

Brig Sanjay Singh MD
Professor
Department of Urogynecology
Obstetrics and Gynecology
Armed Forces Medical College
Pune, Maharashtra, India

BS Jodha MBBS MS DGES
Senior Professor
Department of Obstetrrics and Gynecology
Dr SN Medical College
Jodhpur, Rajasthan, India

Chinmayee Ratha MS (Obs & Gynec)
MRCOG(UK) FIMSA FICOG
Director – Resolution Fetal Medicine Centre, Hyderabad
Consultant – Yashoda Hospitals
Hyderabad, Telangana, India

Dilip Kumar Dutta MD PHD FRCOG FIAOG
Senior Consultant
GICE Nursing Home and Diagnostic Centre
Kalyani, West Bengal, India

Dilip Walke MD (Obs & Gynec) MBBS
Consultant Gynecologist
Jupiter Hospital and Aster Medipoint
Pune, Maharashtra, India

Divya Pandey MBBS MS (Obs & Gynec)
Associate Professor
Department of Obstetrics and Gynecology
Vardhman Mahavir Medical College and Safdarjung Hospital
New Delhi, India

Evita Fernandez MBBS DGO MRCOG (UK) FRCOG (UK)
Gynecologist, General Physician
Obstetrician
Managing Director
Fernandez Hospital
Senior Consultant Obstetrician at Stork Home
Hyderabad, Telangana, India

Ganpat Sawant MD DNB FCPS DGO DFP DICOG
Former Professor and Head
DY Patil Medical College, Navi Mumbai
Director, Noble Hospital and
Noble Plus Hospital, Mumbai
Committee Member of MOGS and IAGE

Gaurav S Desai MS FCPS
Pelvic Surgeon
Assistant Professor
Department of Obstetrics and Gynecology
Seth GS Medical College and
KEM Hospital
Mumbai, Maharashtra, India

Geetha Balsarkar MBBS MD (Obs & Gynec)
DGO DNB (Obs & Gynec)
Consultant
Department of Obstetrics and Gynecology
Maniben Jamnadas Memorial Clinic
Mumbai, Maharashtra, India

Girija Wagh MD (Obs & Gynec) Diploma in Endoscopy FICOG
Gynecologist, Obstetrician and Infertility Specialist
CloudNine Hospital
Pune, Maharashtra, India

Halvi Ediger Ramaraju MBBS DGO
Associate Professor
Department of Obstetrics and Gynecology
Vijaynagar Institute of Medical Sciences
Ballari, Karnataka, India

Haresh Doshi PhD MD (Obs & Gynec) MBBS
Professor and Head
Department of
Obstetrics and Gynecology
GCS Medical College
Ahmedabad, Gujarat, India

Hema Divakar MBBS MD DGO FICOG
FICMCH
Consultant and Managing Director
Divakar's Specialty Hospital
Bengaluru, Karnataka, India

Hema J Shobhane MBBS MD FICMCH
Professor
Department of Obstetrics and
Gynecology
Government Medical College
Azamgarh, Uttar Pradesh, India

Hemant Deshpande MD
Professor and Head
Department of Obstetrics and
Gynecology
Dr DY Patil Medical College and Hospital
Pune, Maharashtra, India

Hemraj R Narkhede MBBS MD
Former Assistant Professor
Department of Obstetrics and
Gynecology
N Wadia Maternity Hospital and
Seth GS Medical College
Mumbai, Maharashtra, India

Hiralal Konar MD DNB MRCOG MNAMS
FRCOG FACS
Professor and Head
Department of Obstetrics and
Gynecology
Agartala Government Medical College
and GB Pant Hospital
Agartala, Tripura, India

Indrani Roy MS
Senior Consultant and Head
Department of Obstetrics and
Gynecology
Nazareth Hospital
Shillong, Meghalaya, India

Indranil Dutta MS PGDHHM PGDMLS
FIAOG
Professor
Department of Obstetrics and
Gynecology
IQ City Medical College
Durgapur, West Bengal, India

Jaideep Malhotra MD FICMCH FICOG FICS
FMAS FIAJAGO FRCOG FRCPI
Managing Director ART Rainbow IVF, Agra
Professor Dubrovnik International
University, Croatia
Immediate Past President IMS
President Elect SAFOMS 2019-2021
President Elect ISPAT
Editor in Chief SAFOMS & SAFOG Journal
Member FIGO – Reproductive
Endocrinology and Infertility
Member FIGO – RDEH
Regional Director of South Asia Ian
Donald School of Ultrasound
Vice President ISAR

Janki Pandya MS (Obs & Gynec)
Assistant Professor
Department of Obstetrics and
Gynecology
AMC MET Medical College
Sheth LG Hospital
Ahmedabad, Gujarat, India

Jayam Kannan MD DGO
Emeritus Professor
Tamil Nadu Dr MGR Medical University
Consultant
Gharbbha Rakshambigai Fertility Centre
Chennai, Tamil Nadu, India

Jayprakash Shah MD FICOG
Chairman – Imaging Science Committee
FOGSI
Fetal Medicine Expert
Rajni Hospital, Ahmedabad
Ex Sonologist, Sheth VS General Hospital
and Smt NHL Municipal Medical College
CIMS Hospital, Ahmedabad
Akar IVF Center, Anand, Gujarat, India

Jyothika Desai MBBS MD (Obs & Gynec)
DGO
Gynecologist
Dr PR Desai Hospital
Bengaluru, Karnataka, India

Jyoti Bindal MBBS MS
Obstetrician and Gynecologist
Gajra Raja Medical College
Gwalior, Madhya Pradesh, India

Jyotsna Suri MD
Professor
Department of Obstetrics and
Gynecology
Vardhman Mahavir Medical College and
Safdarjung Hospital
New Delhi, India

K Aparna Sharma MD
Additional Professor
Department of Obstetrics and
Gynecology
All India Institute of Medical Sciences
New Delhi, India

Kaizad R Damania MD DGO DNB FCPS
DFP (Obs & Gynec)
Professor and Unit Head
Department of Obstetrics and
Gynecology
Nowrosjee Wadia Maternity Hospital
Mumbai, Maharashtra, India

Kanan Yelikar MD
Dean
Government Medical College and
Hospital
Aurangabad, Maharashtra, India

Kanika Chopra MBBS MS
Assistant Professor
Department of Obstetrics and
Gynecology
Lady Hardinge Medical College
New Delhi, India

Kasturi Donimath MBBS MD
Consultant Gynecologist-Obstetrician
Tatwadarsha Hospital
Hubli, Karnataka, India

Krishnendu Gupta DGO MD
Professor and Unit Head
Department of Obstetrics and
Gynecology
Vivekananda Institute of Medical Sciences
Kolkata, West Bengal, India

M Krishna Kumari MBBS MD (Obs & Gynec) DGO FICOG
Consultant
Senior Gynecologist and Obstetrician,
Laparoscopic Surgeon
Medicover Woman and Child Hospitals
Hyderabad, Telangana, India

Madhuri Arvind Patel MBBS MD DGO
FICOG
Hon Clinical Associate, N Wadia Hospital,
Mumbai
Ex Professor and Head OBGY
ESIC-PGIMSR, MGMH, Mumbai
Ex Associate Professor, GMC, Mumbai
Deputy Secretary General, FOGSI
Joint Secretary, FOGSI – 2009
Former Committee Member, FIGO
Preterm Birth
Associate Editor, Journal of Obstetrics and
Gynaecology of India (JOGI)

Madhuri Chandra MD (Obs & Gynec) DNB (Obs & Gynec) FICOG CMCL FAIMER Fellow
Former Professor and Unit Head
Department of Obstetrics and Gynecology
Gandhi Medical College
Bhopal, Madhya Pradesh, India
Member ICOG Governing Council 2017-19
President Bhopal Menopause Society 2018-2020

Madhva Prasad S MS DNB PGDMLS PGDCR
Associate Professor
Department of Obstetrics and Gynecology
Vydehi Institute of Medical Sciences and Research Centre, Bengaluru
National Corresponding Editor, Journal of Obstetrics and Gynaecology of India
Bengaluru, Karnataka, India

Mala Srivastava MBBS DGO DNB FICOG
Senior Consultant and Robotic Surgeon
Institute of Obstetrics and Gynecology
Sir Ganga Ram Hospital
New Delhi, India

Manasi Venkatraman DGO DNB
Obstetrician, Gynecologist and Infertility Specialist
Siddhi Nursing Home
Mumbai, Maharashtra, India

Mandakini Pradhan MBBS MD DNB DM
Professor and Head
Department of Obstetrics and Gynecology
Sanjay Gandhi Postgraduate Institute of Medical Sciences
Lucknow, Uttar Pradesh, India

Manisha Madhai Beck MD
Professor and Unit Head
Department of Obstetrics and Gynecology
Christian Medical College and Hospital
Vellore, Tamil Nadu, India

Manju Puri MD FICOG
Head and Director-Professor
Department of Obstetrics and Gynecology
Lady Hardinge Medical College
New Delhi, India

Manjula Patil MBBS DGO DNS
Consultant
Department of Obstetrics and Gynecology
Motherhood Hospital, HRBR Lay out
Bengaluru, Karnataka, India

Mansi Medhekar MS DNB FICOG Diploma in Gynecological Endoscopy (Germany)
Consultant Obstetrician and Gynecologist
SL Raheja Hospital, Hinduja Healthcare, Ramkrishna Mission Hospital and Surya Hospital, Mumbai, Maharashtra, India
Member of Managing Council- MOGS

Maya Mukhopadhyay MD
Consultant
Department of Gynecologist and Obstetrician
Kolkata, West Bengal, India

MB Bellad MBBS MD (Obs & Gynec)
Professor
Department of Obstetrics and Gynecology
KAHER's JN Medical College
Belagavi, Karnataka India

MC Patel MD
Consultant Gynecologist Obstetrician and Medicolegal Adviser
Niru Maternity and Nursing Home
Ahmedabad, Gujarat, India

Megha Chauhan MD
Gynecologist and Obstetrician
Bengaluru, Karnataka, India

Milind R Shah MD DGO DFP FICOG FIAOG
Professor and Head
Department of Obstetrics and Gynecology
Gandhi Natha H Medical College
Solapur, Maharashtra, India
Peer Reviewer for Journal of Obstetrics and Gynecology of India

Monika Anant MD
Additional Professor
Department of Obstetrics and Gynecology
All India Institute of Medical Sciences
Patna, Bihar, India

Monika Maan Sharma MBBS MS FIMSA FICMCH
Assistant Professor
Department of Obstetrics and Gynecology
Dr DY Patil Medical College and Hospital
Pune, Maharashtra, India

Muralidhar V Pai MBBS DGO MD (Obs & Gynec) FICOG FICMCH
Professor and Head
Department of Obstetrics and Gynecology, Kasturba Medical College
Manipal, Karnataka, India

N Palaniappan MBBS DNB MNAMS FICS
Professor and Unit Head
Department of Obstetrics and Gynecology
Sri Ramachandra Medical College, Chennai
President Obstetric and Gynecological Society of Southern India (OGSSI) 2020
Chairperson of Safe Motherhood Committee FOGSI 2017- 2019

Nanak Bhagat MBBS
Specialty Trainee
Department of Obstetrics and Gynecology, UK

Narendra Malhotra MD FICOG FICMCH FRCOG FICS FMAS AFIAP
Managing Director
Global Rainbow Healthcare, Agra
Prof. Dubrovnick International University
Vie President WAPM (World Association of Prenatal Medicine)
President ISPAT (2017-2019)

Navin Srinivasan MBBS MS (Obs & Gynec)
Assistant Professor
Department of Obstetrics and Gynecology
Seth GS Medical College and KEM Hospital
Mumbai, Maharashtra, India

Neharika Malhotra MD (Obs & Gynec) FICMCH FMAS DRM (Germany) Fellowship in Reproductive Medicine Fellowship in Ultrasound
Infertility Consultant at Rainbow IVF Hospital
Agra, Uttar Pradesh, India

Nitin Agrawal MBBS MD
Consultant
Department of Obstetrics and Gynecology
Global Rainbow Healthcare
Agra, Uttar Pradesh, India

Nuzhat Aziz MBBS DGO DNB
Consultant and Head
Department of Obstetrics and Gynecology
Fernandez Hospitals
Hyderabad, Telangana, India

Parag Biniwale MBBS DGO MD FICOG FICMCH
Consultant
Department of Obstetrics and Gynecology
Pune, Maharashtra, India

Contributors **xiii**

Parikshit Tank MD DNB FCPS DGO DFP MNAMS FICOG FRCOG
Senior Consultant Obstetrician and Gynecologist
Ashwini Maternity and Surgical Hospital
Jupiter Hospital
Mumbai, Maharashtra, India
Honorary Professor
Assisted Reproduction
Pacific Medical College and Hospital
Udaipur, Rajasthan, India
Treasurer, Federation of Obstetrics and Gynecological
Societies of India (FOGSI), 2021-2024
Joint Secretary, FOGSI, 2012
Joint Treasurer, FOGSI, 2018-2020
Chairperson, Safe Motherhood, FOGSI, 2014-2017

Parth Shah MD DGO FIGE
Laproscopist and Fetal Medicine Expert
Rajni Hospital
Ahmedabad, Gujarat, India

Parul J Kotdawala MD FICOG FICMCH
MAMS Diploma in Celioscopy (Germany)
Consultant
Kotdawala Women's Clinic
Ahmedabad, Gujarat, India

Parul P Tank MD DNB DPM MRC (Psych)
Honorary Head
Department of Psychiatry
Rajawadi Hospital, MCGM
Consultant Psychiatrist
Nimai Healthcare, Ashwini Maternity and Surgical Hospital, Fortis Hospital
Asian Heart Hospital
Mumbai, Maharashtra, India

Picklu Chaudhuri MD
Professor and Head
Department of Obstetrics and Gynecology
Rampurhat Medical College
Rampurhat, West Bengal, India

PK Sekharan MD
Former Professor
Department of Obstetrics and Gynecology
Government Medical College
Calicut, Kerala, India

PK Shah MD DGO DFP FCPS
Former Professor and Unit Head
Department of Obstetrics and Gynecology
Seth GS Medical College and KEM Hospital
Mumbai, Maharashtra, India
President, FOGSI 2012

Pooja Bhat MBBS MD
Assistant Professor
Department of Obstetrics and Gynecology
Adichunchangiri Institute of Medical Sciences
Mandya, Karnataka, India

Pooja Lodha MBBS DNB (Obs & Gynec)
Gynecologist
Ruby Hall Clinic
Pune, Maharashtra, India

Pragya Mishra Choudhary MRCOG FRCOG PhD DFFP FICOG
Consultant Infertility Specialist and Colposcopist with Special Interest in Genetics and Fetal Medicine
Chairperson, Genetic and Fetal Medicine Committee, FOGSI 2016-2018

Prakash K Mehta MBBS MD DGO DNB
Chief
Division of Maternal Fetal Medicine
Bhagwan Mahaveer Jain Hospital
Bengaluru, Karnataka, India

Pralhad Kushtagi MD DNB FICOG
Consultant
Department of Obstetrics and Gynecology
Bengaluru, Karnataka, India

Pratik Tambe MD FICOG
Chairperson, AMOGS Endocrinology Committee (2020-22)
Governing Council member, ICOG (2021-22)
Chairperson, FOGSI Endocrinology Committee (2017-19)
Managing Council member, MOGS and ISAR

Pratima Mittal MD
Former Professor and Head
Department of Obstetrics and Gynecology
Vardhman Mahavir Medical College and Safdarjung Hospital
New Delhi, India

Priyanka S Deshpande MS EFOG
Clinical Fellow Cambridge University
NHS Teaching Hospital
United Kingdom

Purnima Satoskar MD DNB FRCOG
Senior Consultant
Department of Obstetrics and Gynecology
Jaslok Hospital and Research Centre
Mumbai, Maharashtra, India

Ragini Verma MBBS MD (Obs & Gynec)
Professor and Head
Department of Obstetrics and Gynecology
Government Medical College
Surat, Gujarat, India

Rahul Gupta MBBS
Consultant
Global Rainbow Healthcare
Agra, Uttar Pradesh, India

Rajesh V Darade MBBS DNB DGO DFP FICS(USA) FCPS FICMCH FICOG
Associate Professor and Head of Unit
Department of Obstetrics and Gynecology
Government Medical College
Endoscopic Surgeon, Vaishnavi Hospital
Latur, Maharashtra, India

Rajeshwari G MBBS MRCOG
Senior Resident
Department of Obstetrics and Gynecology
All India Institute of Medical Sciences
Raipur, Chhattisgarh, India

Rakhee R Sahu MBBS MD
Consultant Gynecologist and Obstetrician
Dr LH Hiranandani Hospital, Mumbai
Ex Associate Professor, Nowrosjee Wadia Maternity Hospital
Mumbai, Maharashtra, India

Ramalingappa C Antaratani MBBS MD DNB FICOG
Director, Professor and Unit Chief
Department of Obstetrics and Gynecology
Karnataka Institute of Medical Sciences
Hubli, Karnataka, India

Ranjana Desai MD
Professor
Department of Obstetrics and Gynecology
Dr SN Medical College
Jodhpur, Rajasthan, India

Ravindra Rupwate MD DNBE
Consultant Chest Physician
Fortis Hospital
Mumbai, Maharashtra, India

Rekha Bharti MD FICOG
Associate Professor
Department of Obstetrics and Gynecology
Vardhman Mahavir Medical College and Safdarjung Hospital
New Delhi, India

Contributors

Ruchi Nimish Nanavati MBBS MD
Professor and Head
Department of Neonatology
Seth GS Medical College and KEM Hospital
Mumbai, Maharashtra, India

Sabnam Nambiar MD
Associate Professor
Department of Obstetrics and Gynecology, Pariyaram Medical College
Kannur, Kerala, India

Sachin Ajmera MD DNB MNAMS FICMCH FCPS DGO DFP
Consultant Gynecologist
Disha Hospital
Mumbai, Maharashtra, India

Sadhana Gupta MBBS MS FICOG FICMU FICMCH
Director and Senior Consultant
Department of Obstetrics and Gynecology
Jeevan Jyoti Hospital and Medical Research Centre, Gorakhpur
FOGSI representative to SAFOG 2018-21
FOGSI Vice President 2016
ICOG governing council member (2015-2021)
Corresponding National Editor JOGI (2017-2020)

Saloni Suchak MBBS MS (Obs & Gynec) TDD DGO
Gynecologist, Obstetrician and Infertility Specialist
Department of Obstetrics and Gynecology, CloudNine Hospitals
Mumbai, Maharashtra, India

Sanjana K MBBS
Department of Obstetrics and Gynecology
Karnataka Institute of Medical Sciences
Hubli, Karnataka, India

Sanjay Gupte MD DGO FICOG FRCOG
Consultant
Gupte Hospital and Centre for Research in Reproduction
Pune, Maharashtra, India

Sapana Shah MD
Professor
Department of Obstetrics and Gynecology
Sardar Vallabhbhai Patel Institute of Medical Sciences and Research and NHL Municipal Medical College
Ahmedabad, Gujarat, India

Sareena Gilvaz MD
Professor and Head
Department of Obstetrics and Gynecology
Jubilee Mission Medical College
Thrissur, Kerala, India

Sarita Agrawal MBBS DGO
Professor and Head
Department of Obstetrics and Gynecology
Associate Dean, Student Welfare
All India Institute of Medical Sciences
Raipur, Chhattisgarh, India

Sarita Bhalerao MD DGO FCPS DNB FRCOG DFP
Consultant Obstetrician and Gynecologist
Breach Candy, Bhatia, Saifee and Wadia Hospitals, Mumbai
Vice President, MOGS
Governing Council Member, ICOG
Joint Secretary FOGSI 2017

Sasikala Kola MBBS MD (Obs & Gynec) DGO
Gynecologist
Department of Obstetrics and Gynecology
Lakshmi Clinic
Hyderabad, Telangana, India

Savitri Verma MBBS MD
Gynecologist and Obstetrician
Dharamhla MB Government Hospital
Udaipur, Rajasthan, India

Shailesh Kore MD DNB FCPS DGO DFP DICOG
Professor and Unit Head
Department of Obstetrics and Gynecology
TN Medical College and BYL Nair Charitable Hospital
Clinical Secretary, MOGS
Past Chairperson, Genetic and Fetal Medicine Committee, FOGSI

Shanthakumari S MD DNB FICOG FRCPI (Ireland) FRCOG (UK)
Senior Consultant
Department of Obstetrics and Gynecology
Yashoda Hospital
Hyderabad, Telangana, India

Shashank Parulekar MD
Professor and Head
Department of Obstetrics and Gynecology
KEM Hospital
Mumbai, Maharashtra, India

Shilpa Agrawal DGO FCPS DNB FNB
Director, Department of Obstetrics and Gynecology
Jaslok Hospital and Research Centre
Mumbai, Maharashtra, India

Shirish N Daftary MBBS MD (Obs & Gynec) MD FICOG
Consultant Gynecologist
Dr Daftary's Total Care Clinic
Mumbai, Maharashtra, India

Shraddha Paliwal MBBS MS
Senior Resident
Department of Obstetrics and Gynecology
MGMMC and MYH group of Hospitals
Indore, Madhya Pradesh, India

Shrinivas N Gadappa MBBS MD (Obs & Gynec)
Professor and Head
Department of Obstetrics and Gynecology
Government Medical College and Hospital
Aurangabad, Maharashtra, India

Shruti Panchbudhe MS DNB DGO MRCOG
Assistant Professor
Department of Obstetrics and Gynecology
Seth GS Medical College and KEM Hospital
Mumbai, Maharashtra, India

Shyam V Desai MD (Obs & Gynec) MBBS
Gynecologist, Obstetrician, Infertility Specialist, Laparoscopic Surgeon
Reproductive Endocrinologist (Infertility)
CloudNine Hospital
Mumbai, Maharashtra, India

Siddesh Iyer MRCOG (UK) MBBS DGO DNB (Obs & Gynec)
Consultant Obstetrician and Gynecologist
Apex Hospitals
Mumbai, Maharashtra, India

Siri Yerubandi MD
Consultant, Department of Obstetrics and Gynecology, Fernandez Hospitals
Hyderabad, Telangana, India

Smriti Agrawal MBBS MD DNB
Additional Professor
Department of Obstetrics and Gynecology
King George's Medical University
Lucknow, Uttar Pradesh, India

Sonal Kumta MD DNBE FCPS DGODHA
Diploma in Pelvic Endoscopy (Germany)
Consultant Obstetrician and Gynecologist
Fortis Hospital
Mumbai, Maharashtra, India

Sonali Deshpande MD
Academic Professor
Department of Obstetrics and Gynecology
Government Medical College andHospital
Aurangabad, Maharashtra, India

Sonali Tank MBBS Diploma in Child Health (DCH) DNB (Ped)
Pediatrician and Consultant Physician
Dr Sonali Tank Clinic
Mumbai, Maharashtra, India

Suchitra N Pandit MD DNB FRCOG (UK) FICOG DFP MNAMS B Pharm
Specialist in High Risk Pregnancy Adolescent and Menopausal Problems Nondescent Vaginal Hysterectomy and Pelvic Floor Surgery
Director, Department of Obstetrics and Gynecology
Surya Group of Hospitals, Mumbai
Chair, AICC RCOG (2017- 20)
President, ISOPARB (2018-19)
Chairperson, Medical Education SAFOG

Sudeep Gupta MBBS MD
Professor
Department of Medical Oncology
Director, Advanced Centre for Treatment, Research and Education in Cancer
Tata Memorial Centre
Mumbai, Maharashtra, India

Sudha Gandhi MBBS MS (Obs & Gynec)
Consultant Obstetrician and Gynecologist
Maharana Bhupal Hospital
Udaipur, Rajasthan, India

Sudhakshi Kinger MBBS MS (Obs & Gynec)
Senior Professor
Department of Obstetrics and Gynecology, Dr SN Medical College
Jodhpur, Rajasthan, India

Sujata A Dalvi MD DGO FCPS FICOG
Hon Clinical Associate, Nowrosjee Wadia Hospital, Jag Jeevan Ram Railway Hospital, Mumbai
Consultant Obstetrician and Gynecologist
Global, Saifee, Bhatia, St Elizabeth, Ruxmani Jain Group of Hospitals, Mumbai
Assistant Editor of Journal of Obstetrics and Gynaecology of India (JOGI)
Member of Managing Council of The Mumbai Obstetrics and Gynaecological Society

Sujata Misra MD FICOG
Professor and Head
Department of Obstetrics and Gynecology
FM Medical College
Balasore, Odisha, India

Sujata Sharma MBBS MD DGO FICOG
Professor and Head
Department of Obstetrics and Gynecology
Government Medical College
Amritsar, Punjab, India

Suman Rao PN MBBS MD DM (Neonatology)
Professor
Department of Neonatology
St John's Medical College Hospital
Bengaluru, Karnataka, India

Sumitra Yadav MS DNB FICOG MNAMS
Professor
Department of Obstetrics and Gynecology
MGMMC and MYH Group of Hospitals
Indore, Madhya Pradesh, India

Sunil Shah MBBS MS FICOG
Consultant Gynecologist and IVF Specialist
Sarvamangal Hospital
Ahmedabad, Gujarat, India

Surya Malik MD MRCOG
Specialist Obstetrician and Gynecologist
King Khalid Hospital
Riyadh, Saudi Arabia

Suyajna Joshi D MD DNB
Senior Consultant and Head
Department of Obstetrics and Gynecology
District Hospital
Ballari, Karnataka, India

Tamkin Khan MD DNB MNAMS FICOG
Professor and Head
Department of Obstetrics and Gynecology
Jawaharlal Nehru Medical College
Aligarh, Uttar Pradesh, India

Tripti Nagaria MD FICOG
Director Professor and Dean
Chhattisgarh Institute of Medical Science
Bilaspur, Chhattisgarh, India

Uday Thanawala MD DGO FCPS DNB
Consultant
Department of Obstetrics and Gynecology
Fortis Hiranandani Hospital
Navi Mumbai, Maharashtra, India

Upendra Kinjawadekar MBBS MD (Obs & Gynec)
Pediatrician
Kamlesh Mother and Child Hospital
Navi Mumbai, Maharashtra, India

Usha Krishna MD DGO FICS FICOG
Consultant Obstetrician and Gynecologist
Breach Candy, Bhatia Hospital
Past President, MOGS and FOGSI
Ex Professor, Seth GS Medical College and KEM Hospital
Mumbai, Maharashtra, India

Vandana Bansal MD DGO DNB MNAMS MRCOG (Obs & Gynec) FICOG FNB (High Risk Pregnancy and Perinatology)
Associate Professor
Nowrosjee Wadia Maternity Hospital
Director, Fetal Medicine
Surya Mother and Child Hospital
Mumbai, Maharashtra, India

Vanita Raut MD DGO
Consultant
Department of Obstetrics and Gynecology
Dr LH Hiranandani Hospital
Mumbai, Maharashtra, India

Vanita Suri MBBS MD
Professor and Head
Department of Obstetrics and Gynecology
Postgraduate Institute of Medical Education and Research
Chandigarh, India

Vidya M Ranga Rao MBBS DGO MD (Obs & Gynec)
Consultant Gynecologist
Kavya Nursing Home
Hyderabad, Telangana, India

Vidya Thobbi MD FICOG
Professor and Head
Department of Obstetrics and Gynecology
Al Ameen Medical College
Vijayapur, Karnataka, India
Chairperson, Food and Drug Medico-Surgical Equipment Committee, FOGSI 2018-2020

Vijeta Jagtap MBBS MD (Obs & Gynec)
Assistant Professor
Department of Obstetrics and
Gynecology
Government Medical college
Surat, Gujarat, India

Vikash K Chatrani DM (Obs & Gynec)
Head
Department of Obstetrics and
Gynecology
Queen Elizabeth Hospital
Consultant Obstetrician, Gynecologist
and Gyne-Oncologist
Associate Lecturer University of the West
Indies

Vinita Das MD
Professor and Head
Department of Obstetrics and
Gynecology
Chhatrapati Sahu Ji Maharaj Medical
University
Lucknow, Uttar Pradesh, India

Vinita Salvi MBBS MD DNBE FCPS DGO DFP
(Obs & Gynec) MPhil (Sports Science)
Consultant Obstetrician and Gynecologist
Professor and Head
Department of Obstetrics and Gynecology
Seth GS Medical College and KEM
Hospital
Mumbai, Maharashtra, India

VP Radhadevi MD
Former Associate Professor
Department of Obstetrics and
Gynecology
Government Medical College
Calicut, Kerala, India

Preface

It is with great pride that I present to you the *FOGSI's Postgraduate Obstetrics: A Textbook*.

At the beginning of the year, we declared our wish to compile a detailed textbook that will comprehensively, yet in a concise manner, cover all the topics with the latest scientific evidences that a postgraduate student requires to thoroughly understand this subject. We believe that FOGSI being such a large and responsible federation should have its significant contribution in the curriculum for undergraduate and postgraduate education in Obstetrics and Gynecology. The content of such a curriculum should be scientifically and ethically sound, and useful in our Indian scenario.

This textbook has been a labor of love. At FOGSI, we have always believed that an investment in training and guiding future clinicians will reap the best rewards. With this in mind, we have made PG students our primary focus this whole year. This includes initiatives like the PG Forum, the PG Training Program, and the UG-PG Curriculum. This textbook is the crowning glory of the PG activities. The idea behind these activities was to promote respect and brotherhood among colleagues, to provide them with training, education and research opportunities, facilitate interactions between PG teachers and students from all over the country, to provide a mentor-mentee type experience and enable better learning; in short, to help them to become well-rounded practitioners once they go out into the world. This book is a continuation of that theme.

It is a source of great pride to have our FOGSI research and guidelines on many topics highlighted in this book. It gives our future clinicians a straightforward perspective when it comes to making decisions. It also provides a sense of uniformity to have students across the country referencing the same guidelines.

This is an exhaustive compendium, divided into 2 volumes with a total of 207 chapters, encompassing every aspect of our ever-changing and evolving field. We start with the basics of Obstetrics, where we discuss anatomy, communication, counseling, and good clinical practices. We then cover normal pregnancy and fetal evaluation, stressing on newer concepts like genetics and genomics, noninvasive prenatal testing, as well as covering the gold standards like antenatal assessment and laboratory evaluation. We have five separate sections dedicated to complications in early and late pregnancy, preexisting medical conditions, and their management. We then move on to labor, its mechanisms and management, as well as its complications, anesthesia and analgesia, and rounding up with postpartum issues. We have separate sections dedicated to social obstetrics, to enlighten our readers about the steps that are being taken to tackle public health issues like maternal mortality and perinatal deaths. There is also a section on critical care, to make our future obstetricians capable of managing emergency situations with confidence.

The second volume is on Gynaecology. We begin with contraception and pregnancy termination, to highlight the importance of a woman's choice to motherhood. The next sections cover the basics of the reproductive cycle, including chapters on neuroendocrine development, puberty and adolescence going on to menopause. We then cover basic ultrasound and diagnostic techniques. There are three dedicated sections on the care, management and operative aspects in general gynecological conditions. We then move on to specialized topics like infertility, endoscopy, urogynecology and oncology, giving our readers a 360-degree viewpoint of every aspect of gynecology.

It was a Herculean task, which could not have been completed successfully without the wholehearted support of the editors, Dr Parikshit Tank and Dr Ameya Purandare.

A special thanks to my amazing, energetic and efficient section editors, who worked quickly and competently to follow-up on authors, validate data, and compile this manuscript into the version you see today.

The final result is this magnum opus. We sincerely hope that it proves to be of value, not just to PG students, but to clinicians and academicians all across the country and beyond.

To quote Carl Jung, "Medicines can treat diseases, but only doctors can treat patients."

We aim to create such doctors.

We look forward to your feedback.

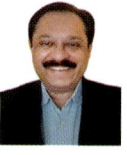

Alpesh Gandhi
President, FOGSI, 2020

FOGSI Office Bearers 2020

Dr Alpesh Gandhi
President FOGSI

Dr Jaydeep Tank
Secretary General FOGSI

Dr Anita Singh
Vice President

Dr Archana Baser
Vice President

Dr Atul Ganatra
Vice President

Dr Ragini Agrawal
Vice President

Dr T Ramani Devi
Vice President

Dr Madhuri Patel
Deputy Secretary General

Dr Suvarna Khadilkar
Treasurer

Dr Parikshit Tank
Joint Treasurer

Dr Sunil Shah
Joint Secretary

Dr Nandita Palshetkar
Immediate Past President

Dr Shantha Kumari
Incoming President Elect

Acknowledgments

We thank the office bearer of FOGSI 2020. We are thankful to them for their wholehearted motivation and support throughout the year for this initiative. The entire FOGSI family has been a source of strength.

We are thankful to all the medical colleges and teachers across India for inspiring us for this useful initiative.

This book comprises 207 chapters and we had to work closely with more than 400 amazing authors for the last one and a half years. They are the experts in the subjects that they have written on. We would like to personally thank each of these brilliant authors who contributed high quality chapters for this project.

We are thankful for the immense work of editing and compilation of the chapters by our team of experienced section editors—Dr Pratima Mittal, Dr Suyajna Joshi, Dr PK Shah, Dr Pushpa Junghare, Dr Gokul Das, Dr Anuradha Khanna, Dr JB Sharma, and Dr Amita Maheshwari. It was a huge task. They worked day and night with great care and expertise to make this a high-quality textbook. We sincerely appreciate their invaluable contribution. The section editors have been helped in this work by the ablest doctors in their departments. We place on record our thanks in particular to Dr Jyotsna Suri and Dr Rekha Bharati (both Professors in the Department of Obstetrics and Gynecology, Vardhman Mahavir Medical College and Safdarjung Hospital, New Delhi, Dr Priya Ballal (Professor and Head, Department of Obstetrics and Gynecology at the KMC, Mangaluru), Dr Shweta Tahlan from Tata Memorial Hospital, Mumbai and Dr Shikha Sachan (Associate Professor, Department of Obstetrics and Gynecology, IMS, BHU, Varanasi).

We thank Jaypee Brothers Medical Publishers (P) Ltd, New Delhi, India. They are one of the most reputed and largest medical publishing houses in the world. They have been instrumental in giving us insights into the publishing process and giving much sought suggestions throughout the project.

Mr Jitendar P Vij (Group Chairman) took great personal interest and care of this project. His patience and trust was a great support. Ms Chetna Malhotra (Associate Director–Content Strategy) played the role of a seasoned and experienced facilitator. Ms Saima Rashid, Ms Kritika Dua and other team members were thorough professionals and pure perfectionists. They provided amazing support with their personal care. We sincerely appreciate their support.

TEAMWORK MAKES THE DREAM WORK.

Contents

Volume 1

PART 1: Obstetrics and Perinatology

Section 1: Introduction to Obstetrics

1.1. A Brief History of Women's Health 3
Parikshit Tank

1.2. Communication and Counseling 10
Tripti Nagaria

1.3. Evidence-Based Medicine and Medical Informatics 22
Anahita Chauhan, Madhva Prasad S

1.4. Good Clinical Practice and Research Methodology for Obstetricians 31
Ramalingappa C Antaratani, Sanjana K

1.5. Pelvic Anatomy for the Obstetrician and Gynaecologist 37
Bhavik Doshi, Ashvin Vachhani

1.6. Violence against Healthcare Professionals 46
MC Patel, Dilip Walke

Section 2: Normal Pregnancy

2.1. Fertilization, Implantation, and Placental Development 53
Milind R Shah, Rajesh V Darade

2.2. Fetal Physiology: Growth and Development 61
Halvi Ediger Ramaraju, Surya Malik

2.3. Clinically Relevant Embryology for Obstetricians 65
Madhuri Arvind Patel, Hemraj R Narkhede, Navin Srinivasan

2.4. Maternal Adaptations in Normal Pregnancy 80
Sadhana Gupta, Hema J Shobhane

2.5. Preconception and Routine Antenatal Care 88
Vanita Suri, Bharti Sharma

2.6. Minor Ailments in Pregnancy and Care 98
Aswath Kumar

2.7. Normal Laboratory Values in Pregnancy 104
Sumitra Yadav, Shraddha Paliwal

Section 3: Fetal Evaluation

3.1. Genetics and Genomics for the Obstetrician 113
Pragya Mishra Choudhary, Manisha Madhai Beck

3.2. Fetal Abnormalities: Definitions, Etiology, and Pathophysiology 122
Mandakini Pradhan

3.3. Ultrasound in First Trimester: Milestones and Pathology 126
PK Shah, Pooja Lodha

3.4. Biochemical Test for Fetal Screening 133
Vinita Das, Smriti Agrawal

3.5. Second-trimester Anatomy Scan 138
Narendra Malhotra, Neharika Malhotra, Jaideep Malhotra, Rahul Gupta, Nitin Agrawal

3.6. Invasive Tests for Fetal Diagnosis 149
Purnima Satoskar, Shilpa Agrawal

3.7. Antepartum Fetal Surveillance Tests in Third Trimester 157
Shailesh Kore, Mansi Medhekar

3.8. Color Doppler in Obstetrics 165
Chinmayee Ratha

3.9. Fetal Echocardiography 174
Jayprakash Shah, Parth Shah

3.10. Noninvasive Prenatal Test 186
Hemant Deshpande, Monika Maan Sharma

Section 4: Early Pregnancy Complications

4.1. Abortion 193
Ranjana Desai

4.2. Ectopic Pregnancy 202
K Aparna Sharma, Archana Kumari

4.3. Gestational Trophoblastic Disease 210
VP Radhadevi, PK Sekharan

4.4. Pregnancy after Previous Fetal Loss 227
Sudha Gandhi, Savitri Verma

Section 5: Pregnancy with Pre-existing Morbidities

5.1. Chronic Hypertension in Pregnancy 233
Ragini Verma, Vijeta Jagtap

5.2. Heart Disease in Pregnancy 243
Vanita Raut, Shruti Panchbudhe, Anahita Chauhan

5.3. Diabetes Mellitus 258
Sujata Misra

5.4. Thyroid Disorders in Pregnancy 266
Kanan Yelikar, Sonali Deshpande, Ashwini Kale

5.5. Anemia 273
Hema Divakar, Arulmozhi Ramarajan

5.6. Other Anemias in Pregnancy 279
    Jyothika Desai, Megha Chauhan

5.7. Renal Disease and Pregnancy 291
    Pralhad Kushtagi

5.8. Liver and Gastrointestinal Disease: Abnormal Pregnancy with Pre-existing Conditions 301
    Sujata A Dalvi

5.9. Autoimmune Disorders of Pregnancy 308
    Vinita Salvi, Ami Surti

5.10. Respiratory Conditions, the Lung and Pregnancy 318
    Ravindra Rupwate, Sonal Kumta

5.11. Neurological Conditions 327
    Jyoti Bindal

5.12. Dermatological Disorders in Pregnancy 335
    Bharathi KR, Pooja Bhat

5.13. Mental Health Issues and Substance Use in Pregnancy and Puerperium 340
    Parul P Tank

5.14. Obesity 347
    Ashis Kumar Mukhopadhyay, Maya Mukhopadhyay

5.15. Cancer in Pregnancy 356
    Amita Maheshwari, Vikash K Chatrani, Sudeep Gupta

5.16. HIV/AIDS and Other Sexually Transmitted Infections 367
    Archana Kumari, Monika Anant

5.17. Infections in Pregnancy 378
    Prakash K Mehta, Aparna Setia

5.18. COVID–19 in Pregnancy 393
    Ajith S, Kasturi Donimath, Sabnam Nambiar

Section 6: Maternal Complications Arising in Pregnancy

6.1. Hypertensive Disorders in Pregnancy (Gestosis) 398
    Sanjay Gupte, Arati Shah

6.2. Liver Diseases in Pregnancy: (HELLP, IHCP, AFLP, HELLP and Infective Hepatitis) 408
    Suyajna Joshi D, Manjula Patil

6.3. Gestational Diabetes 420
    Girija Wagh

6.4. The Surgical Abdomen in Pregnancy 428
    Shashank Parulekar

6.5. Trauma in Pregnancy 434
    Alok Sharma, Aanya Sharma

6.6. Poisoning in Pregnancy 442
    Sujata Sharma, Amarjeet Kaur

Section 7: Fetal Complications

7.1. Fetal Infections 450
    Geetha Balsarkar

7.2. Multiple Pregnancy 457
    Sanjay Singh, Parag Biniwale

7.3. Abnormalities of Amniotic Fluid Volume 470
    Sasikala Kola, Vidya M Ranga Rao

7.4. Abnormalities of the Placenta and Cord 478
    Tamkin Khan, Ayesha Ahmad

7.5. Fetal Growth Restriction 485
    Pratik Tambe, Sarita Bhalerao, Usha Krishna

7.6. Fetal Hydrops 495
    Muralidhar V Pai, Krishnendu Gupta

Section 8: Late Pregnancy Complications

8.1. Antenatal Care: Malpresentations 499
    N Palaniappan

8.2. Preterm Labor 503
    MB Bellad, Bhawna Garg

8.3. Preterm Premature Rupture of Membranes 512
    Shyam V Desai, Gaurav S Desai

8.4. Antepartum Hemorrhage 518
    Madhuri Chandra

8.5. Placenta Accreta Spectrum Disorders 528
    Shrinivas N Gadappa, Ankita Rajesh Shah

8.6. Post-term Pregnancy 535
    Mala Srivastava, Ankita Srivastava

8.7. Intrauterine Fetal Demise 539
    Vandana Bansal, Kaizad R Damania

Section 9: Labor

9.1. Mechanism of Labor 550
    Shirish N Daftary, Gaurav S Desai

9.2. Labor in Malposition and Malpresentations 555
    Sareena Gilvaz

9.3. Routine Intrapartum Care and Intrapartum Tests ..567
    Ganpat Sawant, Sachin Ajmera

9.4. Induction of Labor 577
    Uday Thanawala, Manasi Venkatraman, Saloni Suchak, Nanak Bhagat

9.5. Labor in Special Situations (Previous Cesarean Birth, Poor Progress in Labor, Fetal Compromise in Labor, Meconium Stained Amniotic Fluid) 585
    BS Jodha, Sudhakshi Kinger

9.6. Instrumental Vaginal Delivery 595
    Haresh Doshi

9.7. Shoulder Dystocia 604
    Abha Rani Sinha, Bhawana Tiwary

9.8. Cesarean Section 609
    Suchitra N Pandit, Rakhee R Sahu

9.9. Rupture Uterus 616
    Vidya Thobbi, Priyanka S Deshpande

9.10. Obstetric Analgesia and Anesthesia 621
    Siddesh Iyer, Shanthakumari S, M Krishna Kumari

Section 10: Postpartum Issues: Maternal and Neonatal

10.1. Normal Puerperium 628
Indrani Roy

10.2. Episiotomy and Perineal Trauma 635
Picklu Chaudhuri, Arindam Halder, Hiralal Konar

10.3. Postpartum Hemorrhage and its Management....641
Parul J Kotdawala, Sapana Shah, Sunil Shah

10.4. Obstetric Hysterectomy 652
Ajit C Rawal, Janki Pandya

10.5. Postpartum Pyrexia 663
Indranil Dutta, Dilip Kumar Dutta

10.6. Problems with Breastfeeding 670
Sarita Agrawal, Rajeshwari G

10.7. Neonatal Adaption to Extrauterine Life 682
Ruchi Nimish Nanavati, Suman Rao PN

10.8. Neonatal Resuscitation 688
Sonali Tank

10.9. Perinatal Asphyxia 696
Ashish Mehta

10.10. Birth Injuries 704
Upendra Kinjawadekar, Anjali Otiv

10.11. Common Neonatal Problems 710
Bakul Jayant Parekh

Section 11: Social Obstetrics

11.1. Perinatal Mortality, Surveillance and Response ...720
Manju Puri, Kanika Chopra

11.2. Safe Motherhood Initiative 725
Alka Pandey

11.3. Maternal Death: Surveillance and Response.........733
Jayam Kannan

11.4. Role of Midwifery in Obstetrics 736
Evita Fernandez

Section 12: Critical Care in Obstetrics

12.1. Role of HDU/ICU in Obstetrics 743
Pratima Mittal, Rekha Bharti

12.2. Monitoring in Obstetric HDU and ICU 749
Nuzhat Aziz, Siri Yerubandi, Ananth K

12.3. Fluid and Blood Therapy in Obstetric Shock 762
Jyotsna Suri, Divya Pandey

12.4. Sudden Obstetric Collapse 770
Alpesh Gandhi, Amita Gandhi

Index 783

Volume 2

PART 1: Contraception and Termination of Pregnancy

Section 1: General

1.1. Population Dynamics: The Indian Perspective.......... 3
Anita Soni, Seeru Garg, Ruchi Shah

1.2. Government Policies and Population Stabilization.. 7
Mandakini Megh, Bhumika Kotecha Mundhe

1.3. Legal Aspects in Medical Termination of Pregnancy and Contraception 12
Nikhil Datar, Meghana Shedge

Section 2: Contraception: Spacing Methods

2.1. Natural and Behavioral Methods of Contraception.. 16
Vijyalakshmi Pillai

2.2. Male Barrier Methods 22
Rujuta Fuke

2.3. Female Barrier Methods 27
Shobha Gudi

2.4. Vaginal Spermicides 31
Gorakh Mandrupkar

2.5. Combined Oral Contraceptive Pills 33
Poonam Varma Shivkumar, Darshana Legha

2.6. Progesterone-only Pills 38
Nalini Anand

2.7. Injectable Contraceptives 41
Mukta Jain

2.8. Newer Routes for Contraceptions: Implants, Rings and Patches.. 47
Ashwini Bhalerao-Gandhi, Sanket Pisat, Minal Dhanvij

2.9. Intrauterine Contraception (Including PPIUCD): Copper Devices 54
Pushpa Junghare, Sayali Jahagirdar

2.10. Levonorgestrel Intrauterine System 60
Priya Ballal K, Nikhil Shetty

2.11. Emergency Contraception 68
Lila Vyas, Preeti Sharma

Section 3: Termination of Pregnancy

3.1. Termination of Pregnancy: Counseling and Evaluation 75
Chandravati, Priti Kumar, Bhawna Khera

3.2. Choices and Methods of Procedures in Pregnancy Termination in First and Second Trimesters 81
Suma Natarajan, Gayathri V, Jayashree Natarajan

3.3. Difficult Situations in Pregnancy Termination 90
Jaydeep Tank, Kunal Doshi

3.4. Complications of Termination of Pregnancy 96
Bharti Maheshwari

3.5. Counseling after Pregnancy Termination 104
Basab Mukherjee

3.6. Access to Safe Pregnancy Termination 107
Atul Ganatra, Freni Shah

Section 4: Permanent Contraception

4.1. Male Sterlization including Nonscalpel Vasectomy: Methods and Strategies to Improve Acceptance 112
Phiroze Soonawala

4.2. Female Sterilization: Standards, Surgical Approaches, and Techniques 116
Madhuri Mehendale, Shraddha Mevada

4.3. Sterilization Failure 121
Kiran Pandey, Pavika Lal

4.4. Reversal of Sterilization 126
Abha Singh, Prabha Lal

Section 5: Contraception and Pregnancy Termination for Special Groups

5.1. Contraception in Adolescents 136
Sucheta Kinjawadekar, Unmesh Santpur

5.2. Perimenopausal Women 143
Nisha Rani, Shikha Sachan

5.3. Contraception and Pregnancy Termination for Women with Medical Disorders 150
Ashok Kumar, Sai Charisma

5.4. Contraception and Pregnancy Termination in the Postabortal Period 157
Trupti Nadkarni

5.5. Contraception in Postdelivery and Lactation 161
Kavita Singh, Deepti Gupta

PART 2: Gynaecology

Section 6: Reproductive Physiology and Basic Sciences

6.1. Embryonic Development and Sexual Differentiation 171
Madhu Nagpal, Manjitkaur Mohi

6.2. Neuroendocrinology and Reproductive Cycle 193
Kamini A Rao, Vyshnavi A Rao

6.3. Normal Menstrual Cycle: Physiology and Care 213
Ameya Purandare, Ritu Hinduja

6.4. Normal Puberty and Adolescence: Physiology and Care 221
Maya Padhi, Lucy Das

Section 7: Basic Aspects of Gynaecological Care

7.1. Eliciting History and Examining Gynaecological Patients 229
S Sampathkumari

7.2. Cytology: Cervicovaginal Smear and Endometrial Biopsy 236
Anita Singh, Richa Jha

7.3. Ultrasound in Gynaecology: Uterine Disease 251
Sonal Panchal, Chaitanya Nagori

7.4. Ultrasound in Gynaecology: Adnexal Disease 267
Archana Baser, Anshu Baser

7.5. CT and MRI in Gynaecology 276
Jyoti Jaiswal, Anand Kumar Jaiswal

7.6. Hormone Assays: Indications, Techniques, and Interpretation 295
Anuradha Ridhorkar

7.7. Preoperative Care and Preparation 304
Gokul Das, Shehla Jamal

7.8. Postoperative Care in Obstetrics and Gynaecology 311
Kavita V Kapadia, Vaibhav V Kapadia

Section 8: Puberty and Adolescence

8.1. Amenorrhea: Evaluation and Management 320
Rajrani Sharma, Ameya Purandare, Parikshit Tank

8.2. PCOS in Adolescence 329
Ameet Patki, Mrinmayi Dharmadhikari

8.3. Developmental Abnormalities of Genital Tract 337
Ragini Agrawal, KV Divya

8.4. Disorder of Sex Development in an Adolescent Girl 342
Kunal Thakkar, Vijaya Sarthi, Nalini Shah

8.5. Body Issue Images in Adolescents 351
Reeti Dutta Mehra

8.6. Eating Disorders in Adolescence 357
Nirmala Sharma, Anand Sharma, Neha Seehara

8.7. Precocious Puberty 364
Surveen Ghumman, Rajal Thaker

Section 9: General Gynaecology

9.1. Premenstrual Syndrome 371
Abha Singh

9.2. Dysmenorrhea...377
    PB Hiremath
9.3. Chronic Pelvic Pain 380
    Anupam Gupta, Shikha Singh
9.4. Heavy Menstrual Bleeding: Approach to
    Evaluation and Treatment............................387
    Amala Khopkar Nazareth, Gillian Ryan,
    Alka Kriplani, CN Purandare
9.5. Heavy Menstrual Bleeding: Uterine
    Conservative Surgery....................................404
    Anuradha Khanna, Shikha Sachan
9.6. Fibroid Uterus..413
    PC Mahapatra, Nitin Raithatha
9.7. Adenomyosis 427
    N Sanjeeva Reddy, Radha Vembu
9.8. Endometriosis..437
    Kanthi Bansal, Anu Agarwal, Shweta Shah
9.9. Hysterectomy: Choice of Surgical Approach.........450
    Shirish S Sheth, Kurush P Paghdiwalla
9.10. Technical Aspects of Abdominal and Vaginal
    Hysterectomy 457
    VP Paily, Raji Raj
9.11. Technical Aspects of Laparoscopic
    Hysterectomy 465
    PG Paul, George Paul, Sanghamitra Thakur

Section 10: Benign Gynaecological Conditions

10.1. Vaginal Discharge 473
    Sheela Mane
10.2. Sexually Transmitted Infections and
    HIV in Women 489
    Atul Munshi, Munjal Pandya
10.3. Pelvic Inflammatory Disease 497
    Kusum Lata Singhal, Uma Jain
10.4. Female Genital Tuberculosis........................510
    Jai Bhagwan Sharma, Eshani Sharma,
    Sona Dharmendra
10.5. Benign Diseases of Ovary and Fallopian Tube 516
    Shobhana Mohandas, Haritha C
10.6. Benign Lesions of Vulva and Vagina 525
    Rajashree Dayanand Katke, Deepti Prasad
10.7. Genital Tract Trauma and Sexual Assault..............529
    Saroj Singh, Neha Agarwal
10.8. Dyspareunia and Vaginismus 537
    Shantanu Abhyankar
10.9. Premature Ovarian Insufficiency 545
    Duru Shah, Vishesha Yadav
10.10. Menopause: Physiology and Adaptations 554
    Sheela HS, Ashwini Neelakanthi

10.11. Implications of Menopause on Cardiovascular
    and Bone Health 561
    Revathy Janakiram, Krithika Meenakshi
10.12. Hormone Therapy in Menopause 568
    Suvarna Khadilkar, Madhva Prasad S
10.13. Non-hormonal Therapy at Menopause 576
    Meeta, Akanshi Madan, Tanvir

Section 11: Endoscopy

11.1. Laparoscopy: Safe Entry Technique and
    Instrumentation..584
    Rajendra Sankpal, Damodar Rao
11.2. Hysteroscopy: Instrumentation and
    Distension Media 592
    Subash Mallya
11.3. Robotic Surgery in Gynaecology 596
    Seema Singhal, Alka Kriplani
11.4. Complications of Gynaecological Laparoscopy.....603
    Sunita Tandulwadkar, Abhishek Chandavarkar,
    Rohan Krishnakumar
11.5. Surgical Training in Gynaecological
    Endoscopic Surgery..613
    Pragnesh Shah, Foram Vora
11.6. Energy Sources in Endoscopic Surgery 623
    Prakash Trivedi, Soumil Trivedi

Section 12: Reproductive Endocrinology and Infertility

12.1. Infertility: Etiology and Clinical Evaluation 631
    Charmila Ayyavoo, Sunil Shah
12.2. Investigations for the Male Partner............638
    Fessy Louis T, Parvathy T
12.3. Investigations for the Female Partner 645
    Rishma Dhillon Pai, Meenu Handa
12.4. Male Infertility: Etiology and Management............652
    Ajay S Shetty, Rupin Shah
12.5. Anovulation: Etiology and Management 662
    Manish Banker, Jwal Banker
12.6. Hormonal Issues and Infertility:
    Thyroid, Prolactin and Androgens 669
    Krishnendu Gupta, Muralidhar V Pai
12.7. Tubal Factor Infertility: Etiology and
    Management 672
    Pratap Kumar, Aswathy Kumaran
12.8. Uterine Factor in Infertility: Etiology and
    Management 682
    Laxmi Shrikhande
12.9. Unexplained Infertility: Treatment Approach........690
    Rohan Palshetkar, Nandita Palshetkar
12.10. Intrauterine Insemination 693
    Sudha Prasad, Aswathy Kumaran, Saumya Prasad

12.11. Assisted Reproductive Technology 699
   Jaideep Malhotra, Shally Gupta, Neharika Malhotra,
   Neerja Sachdev, Narendra Malhotra, Keshav Malhotra

12.12. Assisted Reproductive Technologies:
   New Techniques and Research 712
   Hrishikesh Pai, Sunita Arora, Nandan Roongta,
   Rishma Dhillon Pai, Nandita Palshetkar

12.13. Recurrent Pregnancy Loss 721
   Mala Arora

12.14. Third Party Reproduction 727
   Nayana Patel, Molina Patel, Niket Patel,
   Yuvraj Jadeja, Harmi Thakkar

12.15. Adoption 735
   T Ramani Devi, D Gayathri

PART 3: Urogynaecology and Gynaecological Oncology

Section 13: Urogynaecology

13.1. Assessment of Lower Urinary Tract
   Complaints and Function 743
   Achla Batra, Karishma Thariani

13.2. Nonsurgical and Surgical Treatment of
   Stress Urinary Incontinence 747
   N Rajamaheswari, Vaishnavy

13.3. Overactive Bladder 755
   Subhash Ch Biswas, Ramprasad Dey

13.4. Urinary Tract infections 760
   Susheela Rani BS

13.5. Urogenital Prolapse: Assessment and
   Treatment Approaches 767
   RM Saraogi, Chirag Patel

13.6. Posthysterectomy Vaginal Vault Prolapse 780
   L Krishna, N Shailaja

13.7. Anal Incontinence 785
   Pranav Mandovra, Roy Patankar

13.8. Fistulas in Obstetrics and Gynaecology 791
   Manu Sobti

Section 14: Gynaecological Oncology

14.1. Neoplastic Diseases of Vulva 796
   Niranjan Chavan, Dinesh Wade,
   Prathamesh Kane, Richa Deshmukh

14.2. Vulval Carcinoma 799
   SP Somashekhar

14.3. Intraepithelial Disease of the Cervix 810
   Nikhil Parwate, Sabina Hasan Ali Moman

14.4. Malignant Diseases of Vagina 829
   Shalini Rajaram, Bindiya Gupta

14.5. Malignant Disease of Vagina 834
   Saritha Shamsunder

14.6. Premalignant and Malignant
   Diseases of the Uterus 844
   SK Giri, BL Nayak

14.7. Benign Ovarian Neoplasia 861
   Neerja Bhatla, Anju Singh, Seema Singhal

14.8. Malignant Ovarian Neoplasia 872
   Harshad Parasnis, Suchita Dabhadkar

14.9. Neoplastic Diseases of Fallopian Tube 883
   Uma Singh, Manjulata Verma

14.10. Principles of Radiation Therapy 889
   Umesh Mahantshetty, Gargee Mulye, Lavanya Gurram

14.11. Principles of Chemotherapy 902
   Anant Ramaswamy, Sudeep Gupta

14.12. Palliative Care in Gynaecologic Oncology 909
   Jayaraman Nambiar M, Thiencherry Rema

14.13. Screening for Ovarian Cancer
   Current Perspective 914
   Usha B Saraiya, Nidhi Shah Gandhi

Index 921

Obstetrics and Perinatology

- Introduction to Obstetrics
- Normal Pregnancy
- Fetal Evaluation
- Early Pregnancy Complications
- Pregnancy with Pre-existing Morbidities
- Maternal Complications Arising in Pregnancy
- Fetal Complications
- Late Pregnancy Complications
- Labor
- Postpartum Issues: Maternal and Neonatal
- Social Obstetrics
- Critical Care in Obstetrics

SECTION 1

Introduction to Obstetrics

1.1 A BRIEF HISTORY OF WOMEN'S HEALTH

Parikshit Tank

■ HISTORY IS HERSTORY TOO

The study of history is a window into the minds of the thinkers and influences that have brought science to the current state. It is not merely a collection of facts or a source of trivia, but an evolution of thought and attitude that determines history in any field. History is the witness that testifies to the passing of time; it illuminates reality, vitalizes memory, provides guidance in daily life and brings us tidings of antiquity.[1] The history of women's health is very broad. There are fragments of the history of evolution, humanity, medicine, and specific techniques. But it is also a history of the place of women, their achievements and the attitudes toward them with the passage of time.

■ TIMELINES

To set the context in terms of evolutionary history, **Figure 1** is a broad timeline of the universe, which is believed to be 14 billion years old. *Homo sapiens* or modern man has existed for about 200,000 years which is a tiny fraction of the age of the universe. Modern history is then, just a blink of an eye in such a large timeframe. **Table 1** indicates the division of the more recent timeline into historical ages. Though this construct is simplistic, it helps to describe and structure the discussion on historical evolution.

■ PREHISTORY (FIRST HUMANS: 200,000 YEARS AGO TILL BEFORE CHRIST ERA)

The earliest representations of the female form date back to about 20,000 years BCE. This was in the form of cave drawings and stone figures. One of the oldest preserved statuettes is the Venus of Willendorf from the Middle Aurignacian period somewhere in Western Europe. The statuette probably represents a fertility goddess.[2]

There are scattered instances of cave drawings, figurines, statuettes and representations of the female form till about 2,000 BCE when the Indus valley came into existence. As we explore the origins of recorded and credible medical history and science, a central theme which emerges is that much of medicine seems to have evolved in the Indus valley. There are some records that the uterus was identified as a separate

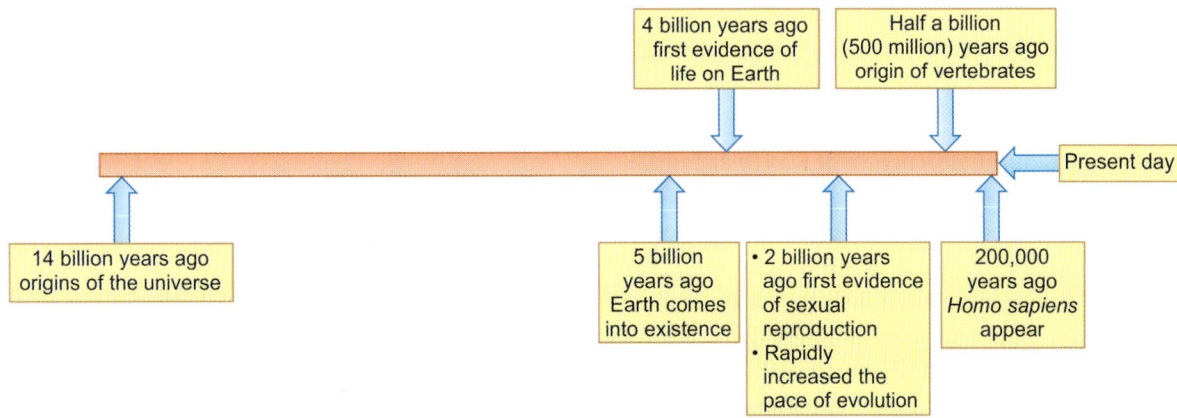

Fig. 1: Broad timelines of the universe.

PART 1: Obstetrics and Perinatology

TABLE 1: Historical ages and women's health.

Time	Nomenclature	Important events related to women's health
200,000 years ago till Before Christ Era (BCE)	Prehistory	• Earliest references to women's bodies, their anatomy in recorded history • Indus valley civilization, Upanishads (Garbha Upanishad) and Ayurveda addresses women's health and science
After Christ Era to 5th century Anno Domini (AD)	Ancient history	Greek, Egyptian and Middle Eastern science predominate the world
5th–15th century AD	Dark ages	Older Roman and European literature on women's health and the misconceptions
1500–1700s	Renaissance	Initiation of scientific study of human anatomy and health in Europe
1700–1850s	Early modern history	Rudimentary surgery and medicinal cures
1850s onward	Late modern history	Rapid revolutionary strides in all aspects of health and those pertaining to women's health
Current times	Contemporary history	Subspecialization and evolution of molecular technology

organ with a study of its function as early as 900 years BCE. The Hindus (in this context, it means people of the Indus valley) recorded this in the Rigveda. The Garbha Upanishad describes the formation of the embryo, its growth in the uterus, the time of pregnancy at which it can be deemed viable and the process of labor. These observations are in line with the knowledge we have today. It also contains spiritual and philosophical discussions which are not possible to substantiate even with the current state of knowledge as these deal with fundamental questions such as the origins of life and the place of self in the cosmos.[3] Much of this knowledge remained mysterious and inaccessible to the rest of the world for centuries to follow.

ANCIENT HISTORY (AFTER CHRIST ERA TILL 5TH CENTURY AD)

In this period, the study of human beings, medicine, and philosophy was largely in the Greek, Roman, and Middle Eastern empires. Hippocrates, Heraclides and a number of Greek and Roman physicians wrote about birth and diseases of women in general. However, the authoritative treatise on the subject of women's disease in those times came from Soranus. He was a Greek scholar born in the city of Ephesus. The city was a seat of learning and housed the great library of Celsus. In the first century AD, Soranus published on the diseases in women: De Morbis Mulierum. He gave an accurate description of the human uterus, correctly describing the size, position, layers, and internal structure. It was clear from his descriptions that he had access to studying human cadavers. Soranus is also credited with performing the first recorded hysterectomy for prolapse, which was more of an amputation than a surgery.[4] Another figure of note is Agnocide. There is debate about the veracity of her story and her origins. She was an exception to the gender rule and is perhaps the first woman midwife of record. She had to dress herself up as a man to render her services and was so popular among women that she was accused of seducing them. In court, she was exonerated when she revealed her gender.[5] A better documented history belongs to the Roman midwife Scribonia Attica whose tomb in Ostia, near Rome is maintained even today. It has bas-relief of her at work in a special birthing chair. Incidentally, she married an equally illustrious surgeon of the times, Marcus Ulpius.[6]

DARK AGES (5TH–15TH CENTURY AD)

For religious and political reasons, cadaver study was banned in much of the Western world after the second century. Cadavers were difficult to obtain, their study was strictly regulated and performing dissection was punishable by law. Autopsies were meant only for the clergy and royalty. This inhibition of exploration and knowledge led to the Dark Ages. Myths abounded. One of the enduring myths which originated at this time was that the uterus was responsible for hysteria. The uterus was depicted as a separate animal, a parasite in the woman's body. The anatomy of the female body was represented wrongly with many descriptions being far removed from reality in Arabic, European, and Persian texts. Anatomical descriptions ranged from the simplistic to the ridiculous. One of the most popular ones was that the uterus was made up of two compartments, separate for male and female fetuses. A seven compartment model was also proposed. The fetus would occupy a different compartment based on the day of the week it was conceived. Science stagnated and knowledge from the ages before was drowned in a pool of ignorance and myth.[7]

RENAISSANCE AND WOMEN'S HEALTH (1500–1700s)

In the West, in the 1600s, the change in the political climate saw a change in the mindset of the leading thinkers—scientists, artists, and scholars. Anatomical dissection and study of the human body resumed in the 16th century. A notable figure in this context is Andreas Vesalius from Belgium. Much of the knowledge and detailed description from this time comes from his treatise, De Humani Corporis Fabrica. It had the first good illustrations and descriptions of the uterus in modern times.[8]

In women's health, perhaps the most significant change was the scientific understanding of the process of vaginal delivery. The accurate description of the cardinal movements of the fetal head through the maternal pelvis was given by a Scottish obstetrician, William Smellie. But even more significant was the discovery of the obstetric forceps. Before the obstetric forceps came into being, obstructed labor was dealt with by destructive operations. The history of this instrument is one filled with myth and wonder. The Chamberlen family of French Huguenots from Normandy is credited with this invention in the 1570s, more specifically, Peter (the Elder) Chamberlen. He was appointed as the royal obstetrician to the English and French courts. The forceps was a secret instrument which only the members of the Chamberlen family used. It remained hidden for about 150 years after its invention. Much later, in 1813, Peter Chamberlen's tools were discovered in an attic of a house in Mortimer Hall in Oxford, United Kingdom. The forceps is an instrument that has undergone innumerable iterations and will forever be in a state of evolution. Notable Indian contributions to the field were from Sir Kedarnath Das (modification of the Simpson's forceps making it lighter and more friendly to the maternal pelvis) and Dr Aroo Mulgaonkar (modification of the Kielland's forceps). James Young Simpson made a significant contribution to the advancement of the forceps and also described the use of the first vacuum device—the suction tractor—to facilitate delivery.[9]

An important event in women's health in this period was the first recorded intentional cesarean birth where the mother and the child survived. There are anecdotal reports dated before this where babies have been delivered by cesarean performed by mothers themselves or accidentally by injuries from horns of livestock. But these are to be considered with due skepticism. In 1500, Jacob Nufer, a gelder in Switzerland recorded this event. His wife was in labor for days and despite help from a number of midwives, could not be delivered. He sought permission from the authorities and with his rudimentary knowledge of animal husbandry, performed a cesarean birth for his wife. The mother and child survived. The couple had five more children.[10]

■ EARLY MODERN HISTORY (1700–1850s)

The early modern history of women's health is marked by a number of innovations from "medicine men". These were times of great advancements in chemistry and experimentations with newly discovered elements and compounds on the human body. There were also some attempts at characterization of herbal and vegetable products by their chemical composition.

In women's health, surgery made some progress. Before the 19th century, vaginal hysterectomies were largely palliative procedures for cervical cancer. The first planned, successful vaginal hysterectomy is credited to JCM (Conrad) Langenbeck in 1813. Around the same time, other surgeons such as Osiander, Dupuytren and Hatin had also performed vaginal hysterectomies but these were either accidental or emergencies (for severe hemorrhage in cervical cancer or uterine inversion) or resulted in the woman's death. Langenbeck operated on a 50-year-old woman with cervical cancer. There was alarming hemorrhage toward the end of the surgery. Working without an assistant, anesthesia, or a hemostatic forceps, Langenbeck heroically compressed the bleeding part with his left hand and managed to throw the last hemostatic suture with his right hand, holding the other end between his teeth. The woman survived—almost miraculously.[11]

Another advance in surgery on women was made in deliberately opening the abdomen to remove an ovarian cyst by Ephraim McDowell in Kentucky in 1809. The first abdominal hysterectomy was performed by Charles Clay in Manchester, England in 1843; unfortunately the diagnosis was wrong and the patient died in the immediate postoperative period. The following year, Charles Clay was almost the first to claim a surviving patient; however, she died postoperatively and it was not until 1853 that Ellis Burnham from Lowell, Massachusetts achieved the first successful abdominal hysterectomy although again the diagnosis was wrong. He was performing exploratory surgery for what he believed to be an enlarged ovarian tumor. During the procedure, the patient vomited, pushing an enlarged uterus through the abdominal incision. Burnham was unable to reduce it into the abdominal cavity, and had no alternative but to remove it. The woman survived the procedure.[12]

■ LATER MODERN HISTORY (1850s ONWARD)

Medical science as we know it today had its Big Bang moment in the early 1900s. There were rapid strides in every field of science. The cross applications into medicine significantly improved safety and technique in medical practice and surgery. The most significant strides are outlined in **Table 2**. These are general advances but had an important role to play in women's health, just as for everyone else.[6]

This period of history saw some events in medical history specific to women which form the basis of care even in modern times. These advances and discoveries have shaped women's health in the most significant of ways. Some of these are highlighted here.

Childbirth fever was recognized as a ruthless killer since 3,000 years. Various myths surrounded its causation including remorse, possession by spirits, seduction, and fretting. The institutionalization of obstetrics in the 18th century brought a keen focus on the problem. Oliver Wendell Holmes, though

TABLE 2: Significant strides in general medical practice in the 1800s onward.

Field	Year	Scientist	Background and comments
Anesthesia	1846	Francis Bott (USA), Robert Liston (UK)	Started consistently using ether for anesthesia in surgery
	1850s	James Young Simpson (UK)	Advocated the use of ether inhalation as an analgesic in labor
	1850s	John Snow (UK)	Replaced ether with chloroform, which was safer. Administered analgesia to Queen Victoria during childbirth and gained royal backing and widespread approval for anesthesia by chloroform
Antisepsis	1890s	Louis Pasteur (France)	Proposed the germ theory, mechanisms of infection and decay and possible methods to avoid the effects of microbes
	Early 1900s	Joseph Lister (UK)	Applied the principles of germ theory to surgical practice and devised the antisepsis system which forms the basis of infection control till date
Blood transfusion	1900	Karl Landsteiner (Austria)	Described the ABO system of blood groups and the technique of crossmatching, making transfusions compatible
Radiology	1895	Wilhelm Röntgen (The Netherlands)	Röntgen was studying the effect of passing electricity through a gas at very low pressures and noticed the effect on a plate. He took an impression of his wife's hand and this was the first Roentgenogram (X-ray)
Radiation	1903	Marie Curie, Pierre Curie, Henri Becquerel (France)	Jointly, these three scientists described the theory of radioactivity. Marie Curie further went on to discover two elements—radium and polonium. She also described isotopes which are important tools in the treatment of cancers
Insulin	1922	Frederick Banting and Charles Best (Canada)	Banting, an orthopedic surgeon and Best, a research assistant studied glucose metabolism in dogs who had been subjected to removal of the pancreas and developed diabetes. John Macleod was instrumental in purifying the extract called "isletin" for human use
Antibiotics	1928	Alexander Fleming (UK)	Serendipitous observation of elimination of bacterial growth due to the growth of a mold (fungus) identified as *Penicillium*
	1938	Various scientists working in the United Kingdom	Various scientists working in Oxford—Howard Florey (Australia), Ernst Chain (German), and Dorothy Hodgkin (UK)—worked out the chemical structure of penicillin and mass produced it for clinical use

not an obstetrician, was an astute clinician and hypothesized that childbirth fever was contagious and could possibly be prevented. It was Ignaz Philipp Semmelweis, a Hungarian physician working at the University of Pest who took a keen interest and studied this subject. He observed that units where care was provided by midwives had a tenfold lower rate of puerperal fever than where care was provided by medical students and doctors. This difference was that midwives did not conduct autopsies. He further studied the autopsy findings of women who died of puerperal fever and concluded that they arose due to "toxins". To perform detoxification, he advocated washing hands, and later instruments and the entire ward with a chlorinated solution of lime. This nearly eliminated mortality from puerperal fever. However, his findings were treated with scorn and he was dismissed from his professional position. Ironically, he died of sepsis himself, in a mental asylum. It was only later that the value of his observations was realized and he was feted.[13]

Surgery became safer with the practice of anesthesia, antisepsis, blood transfusions, and antibiotics. Performing an operation was not looked upon as a death sentence anymore and it became a reasonable option for treating certain conditions. The rapid evolution of safe surgery had a major impact on the practice of cesarean birth. From the practice of leaving the uterine wound open, to exteriorizing or cauterizing it to finally, suturing it the cesarean operation was largely an upper segment procedure. It was the untiring advocacy and practice in the 1920s of John Munro Kerr in Britain and Joseph B DeLee in the United States that the operation became a lower segment procedure. Munro Kerr is said to have exclaimed "Hallelujah! The battle's o'er; the victory's won" when the Royal College accepted that the lower segment procedure was the superior one.[14]

Around the same time, Professor Henry Dale, a British pharmacologist described the uterotonic actions of oxytocin in 1906. Oxytocin was also the first ever polypeptide hormone to be sequenced and synthesized. This of course was much later in 1953 by the French chemist, Vincent du Vigneaud.[15]

A pioneer who was inspired by personal tragedy was Victor Bonney. His wife had large fibroids causing intractable symptoms which resulted in a hysterectomy. The couple was left childless. Working at the Chelsea Hospital for Women in London, Bonney refined the myomectomy and ovarian cystectomy in the 1920s. He is looked upon as a major influence in propagating the concept of organ preservation in gynecological surgery.[16]

As with conservative gynecological surgery, the hysterectomy operation was also progressing in technique.

The mortality rates of the 1880s in the range of 75% were down to 2–3% by the 1920s. This was keeping in line with the general improvements in surgical outcomes. In the 1920s, two important advancements were the development of the total hysterectomy with the removal of the cervix by Richardson in United States of America and the use of the lower transverse abdominal incision by Johannes Pfannenstiel in Austria.[17]

The field of contraception saw some great improvements moving away from the myth-bound traditional techniques which were marred by risk and dubious efficacy. The intrauterine device is a classic example of a technique that has had a long evolution. From the legends of pebbles being inserted into the wombs of camels in the Middle East centuries ago, we know that the concept of a foreign body in the uterus providing contraception is not a new one. In modern history, the first intrauterine device that was published and invented in 1909 by Richard Richter in Germany. It was made of two strands of silkworm gut with a bronze filament thread to diagnose expulsion and retrieve it. Some early devices were the Grafenberg ring (Germany) and the Ota device (Japan). The devices evolved in term of design (rings, coils, loops, T-shaped frames) and content (nonmedicated, silver, copper and hormones) and have reached a point where low-dose hormones can be delivered directly into the uterine cavity.[18]

Perhaps the single most important change in women's health which empowered women to a greater extent than any other came with the evolution of hormones and the oral contraceptive pill. Oral contraception was practiced with herbs, roots, minerals, and oils. However, a reliable method did not exist. Edgar Allen and Edward Doisy published about the hormonal activity of the "ovarian hormone"; this was estrogen. Early work on the extraction of progesterone was being done in the 1930s by Russell Marker and Carl Djerassi which was important for the mass production of the hormone. It was the passion of Margaret Sanger, the capital of Katherine McCormick, the pharmacological genius of Gregory Pincus and the clinical responsibility of John Rock that saw the birth of the pill.[19] It was introduced in the United States of America in 1955 under the guise of regularizing the menstrual period and ironically, to promote fertility. However, further trials in Latin America proved its efficacy as a contraceptive. The pill has undergone generations of changes and today, more than a 100 million women use it.

CONTEMPORARY HISTORY AND EMERGENCE OF SUBSPECIALTIES

Women's health, just like all other medical fields, has diversified vastly in contemporary history. This has come about through an amalgamation of various medical and nonmedical specialties especially genetics, molecular biology, radiology, and engineering in various contexts (mechanical, electrical, and lenses). Over and above all these are the overarching influence of an exponential rise in the computing power that is available for research and day-to-day clinical practice. These have changed the way medicine in general and women's health in particular is practiced.

The treatment of cervical cancer had been proposed, studied, and practiced with varying degrees of success and safety. The early 1900s saw the emergence of the "radical hysterectomy" under the surgical expertise of surgeons such as John Clark in the United States of America and the Austrian teacher-pupil team of Friedrich Schauta and Ernst Wertheim. The technique was refined to a great degree in the 1940s by Joe Vincent Meigs in the United States of America.[17] These techniques along with radiotherapy had reduced mortality from cervical cancer to some extent. However, in terms of public health, the big breakthrough in women's cancer care came from early detection by a cervicovaginal smear. Since the 1960s, this is arguably the most successful preventive health program in any form of medicine. The success stories have been resounding and repeated across geographies. The credit goes to a Greek military doctor, George Papanicolaou, who migrated to the United States of America. His wife, Andromache (Mary) Mavroyeni, whom he met on the ferry crossing, was an equal contributor to the research.[20] In the 1940s, they teamed up with Herbert Taut, a gynecological pathologist at the Cornell University and published on the early detection of uterine cancer by vaginal smear.[21] The practice was adopted gradually and is a routine test in modern times.

The Second World War brought great tragedy but also saw advancement in technology. One such instance was the use of SONAR (sound navigation and ranging) for submarines. Later, the same technology was extrapolated to medical imaging. Ian Donald was the epitome of a modern day renaissance man for obstetrics. He was born in Cornwall, United Kingdom and after spending his childhood in South Africa, returned to practice in the United Kingdom in the 1930s. After his wartime assignment as a Royal Air Force pilot, he specialized in obstetrics and published the treatise on Practical Obstetric Problems, which has undergone a number of editions and is still in circulation. But his most significant work came through his curiosity about imaging. He worked with Tom Brown, an engineer at the Babcock and Wilcox factory at Renfrew and devised the first contact scanner. They published their work and laid emphasis on the instant feedback that the technique provided.[22] Ultrasound has become a specialty in its own right and has made it possible to treat the fetus as a patient in today's world.

Just as the imaging, the field of endoscopy has evolved from a similar curiosity to understand the internal structure and function of human beings. The revolution of endoscopy had begun in the early 1800s, with the work of Philipp Bozzini. In 1869, Pantaleoni from Ireland looking into the uterine cavity of a postmenopausal woman with a modified cystoscope and candlelight. This was the first hysteroscopy and he even went on to operate on the uterine polyps by cauterizing them with silver nitrate. It was only in the 1970s that hysteroscopy progressed from being a novelty to a reasonable treatment option. Neuwirth and Amin reported the first series of hysteroscopic submucous fibroids excision in 1976. In 1987, Alan DeCherney at the University of California, Los Angeles (UCLA) described the use of a urological resectoscope to treat intractable uterine bleeding.[23] Similarly, by the 1900s, various surgeons had described laparoscopy but it was Harry Reich, who first published about laparoscopically assisted vaginal hysterectomy in 1989 and Kurt Semm described the classic intrafascial serrated edged macro-morcellator (SEMM) hysterectomy in the early 1990s. This has paved the way for innumerable innovations and changed the approach to surgery in the pelvis. Today, we are looking at the frontiers in the form of robotic surgery.[17]

In 1978, one of the most revolutionary events occurred with the birth of Louise Brown. Ordinarily, the birth of a girl in a remote English town would not have been newsworthy, but she was on the front page of every newspaper in the world, for she was conceived outside a human body. Apart from her parents and nature, she was as much a creation of Patrick Steptoe and Robert Edwards. Patrick Steptoe was a naval surgeon and after the war, his career interest was in laparoscopic surgery. He published on the detection of ovulation in women by laparoscopy. This caught the attention of Robert Edwards, who was studying oocytes maturation in mammals. His work was facilitated by Molly Rose, who provided him with ovarian tissue resected from women with Stein–Leventhal syndrome (modern day polycystic ovarian syndrome). The partnership between Edwards and Steptoe began with a phone call and flourished at the Oldham and District General Hospital. The first attempts were futile and in fact, the first in vitro fertilization pregnancy was an ectopic. Working against the odds and with courageous and persistent patients, the field of assisted reproduction was born with success in the form of Louise Brown's birth. Since then, various technological advances such as intracytoplasmic sperm injection, culture systems and robust equipment, and drug protocols have changed the face of human reproduction forever.

■ A DISREPUTABLE HISTORY

Human attitude and behavior is a product of the times and what is deemed to be acceptable in those times and circumstances. There could be a lot said and criticisms leveled about each and every advance of science in terms of the documentation, consent, and safety standards when compared to current ones. However, these criticisms could be dismissed as hindsight. But there are certain events in medical history which are unacceptable by any set of standard scientific or human behavior.

James Marion Sims is a classic example of such a revised view of historical events.[24] He was arguably the greatest American gynecological surgeon and was regarded as the "Father of Gynaecology" in the United States of America. His fame grew from the surgical technique for the repair of vesicovaginal fistulae. Even though he eventually perfected the technique and the principles are in use even today, it is the way in which he conducted the surgical experiments that has changed modern views about him. The criticisms that have been leveled against him are that he experimented on African slaves without their consent. The surgeries were repeated over and over again on the same individual. Among the first women who had the surgeries were Anarcha, Betsy, and Lucy. It is estimated that there were forty surgeries conducted on them before a successful result was achieved. More disturbingly, Sims would not use anesthesia for these women, even though ether anesthesia was established practice. This was a racist attitude as he would perform the same procedures under anesthesia for white women. The changed views on Sims have led to a fall from grace as was witnessed by the removal of several of his statues in American cities.[25]

Scientific knowledge has advanced in subhuman conditions at times. War, genocide and unethical acts have been involved in the advancement of scientific knowledge and knowledge about women's health care. Some examples are the knowledge about the timing of Anti-D administration from the work of Nazi physicians in the Second World War, the use of cervical cancer cells from Henrietta Lacks without her consent or even acknowledgment and so many others. As history evolves, there is bound to be revisionism and changes in our view of events of the past.

■ INDIAN CONTRIBUTION IN MODERN TIMES

Indian gynecologists have in the large part embraced modern practice and have contributed to scientific advances with some important works. One name that stands out is that of Professor VN Shirodkar. In the 1950s, second trimester abortions were a mysterious entity. He studied the cervix in the nonpregnant and pregnant states, understanding the changes in anatomy and physiology. He was particularly interested in the changing nature of the cervix in normal pregnancy from a fibrous one to a dynamic muscular organ. His answer to the problem of habitual second trimester abortion was a surgery which put India firmly on the map of operative obstetrics and gynaecology. In 1955, Shirodkar described the cervical cerclage operation. Over time, it has been modified by many surgeons, most notably by McDonald, but the original surgery is a masterpiece. Through his illustrious career, he developed various gynecological surgical techniques for tuboplasty, vaginoplasty, and sling surgery for conservative repair of prolapse.[26]

The problem—genital prolapse and its conservative repair—has been addressed by doyens of Indian gynaecology including VN Purandare, RP Soonawala, Brigadier SD Khanna, and Ajit Virkud. These surgeries have been innovative and scientific. They are being modified to suit the laparoscopic route.[27]

Professor VB Patwardhan is credited with describing formally, the technique of delivering the fetal head that is impacted into the pelvis in the second stage of labor.[28] This technique is now accepted to be a better alternative to pushing the head up in terms of reducing maternal and fetal injury and morbidity.

One of the tragic events in Indian gynecological history is the life and death of Professor Subhas Mukhopadhyay. He created history in India working with Sunit Mukherji, a cryobiologist and gynecologist Dr Saroj Kanti Bhattacharya. This team was responsible for the birth of Durga (Kanupriya Agarwal) in October 1978, just a few months after Louise Brown. However, Mukhopadhyay faced criticism, ostracism and was driven to suicide by the hostility of the bureaucracy and the state government of the day. It was only later that his contributions were acknowledged and accepted.[29]

■ CONCLUSION

The history of medicine is impossible to encapsulate completely in a text of any length. This chapter is a bird's eye view of the important events and milestones that have shaped how we care for women in today's time. It is hoped that it serves as a stimulus for the interested reader to delve deeper into history and to reflect on the road ahead.

■ REFERENCES

1. Cicero MT, Grant M. Selected Works. New York: Penguin Classics; 1962.
2. Witcombe CL. Venus of Willendorf. Art History and Image Studies—Essay 1. Cambridge: Cambridge University Press; 1995. [online] Available from: http://arthistoryresources.net/willendorf/ [Last accessed September, 2021].
3. Kak S. (2019). The Garbha Upanishad: How Life Begins. [online] Available from: https://subhashkak.medium.com/the-garbha-upanishad-how-life-begins-76e25d68da45. [Last accessed September, 2021].
4. Drabkin IE. Soranus and his system of medicine. Bull Hist Med. 1951;25:503-18.
5. Fluff35. (2017). Agnodice: reading the story. Mistaking histories. [online] Available from: https://mistakinghistories.wordpress.com/2017/10/18/agnodice-reading-the-story/ [Last accessed September, 2021]
6. British Broadcasting Corporation (BBC). The Story of Medicine. London: Immediate Media Company; 2017.
7. Green MH. The Trotula: An English Translation of the Medieval Compendium of Women's Medicine. Pennsylvania: University of Pennsylvania Press; 2010.
8. Fulton JF. Logan Clendening Lectures on the History and Philosophy of Medicine. Vesalius Four Centuries Later. Lawrence, Kansas: University of Kansas Press; 1950. [online] Available from: https://kuscholarworks.ku.edu/bitstream/handle/1808/6347/upk.vesalius_four_centuries_later.pdf?sequence=1&isAllowed=y [Last accessed September, 2021].
9. Drife J. The start of life: a history of obstetrics. Postgrad Med J. 2002;78:311-5.
10. US National Library of Medicine. (1993). Cesarean section - a brief history. [online] Available from: https://www.nlm.nih.gov/exhibition/cesarean/part1.html [Last accessed September, 2021].
11. Senn N. The Early History of Vaginal Hysterectomy. Chicago: American Medical Association Press; 1895.
12. Sutton C. Hysterectomy: a historical perspective. Baillieres Clin Obstet Gynaecol. 1997;1:1-22.
13. Dastur AE, Tank PD. Milestones: Ignaz Philipp Semmelweis and puerperal fever. J Obstet Gynecol India. 2008;58:206-7.
14. Baskett, T. On the Shoulders of Giants: Eponyms and Names in Obstetrics and Gynaecology, 2nd edition. London: Royal College of Obstetricians and Gynaecologists; 2010. p. 214.
15. Magon N, Kalra S. The orgasmic history of oxytocin: love, lust, and labor. Indian J Endocrinol Metab. 2011;15:S156-61.
16. Chamberlain G. Victor Bonney: The Gynaecological Surgeon of the Twentieth Century, 1st edition. London: CRC Press; 2000.
17. Sparic R, Hudelist G, Berisava M, Gudović A, Buzadzić S. Hysterectomy throughout history. Acta Chir Iugosl. 2011;54:9-14.
18. Thiery M. Pioneers of the intrauterine device. Eur J Contracept Reprod Health Care. 1997;2:15-23.
19. Dastur AE, Tank PD. The oral contraceptive pill: the early days of a 50-year old legend. J Obstet Gynecol India. 2010;60:207-9.
20. Dastur AE, Tank PD. George Papanicolaou and the cervicovaginal smear. J Obstet Gynecol India. 2009;59:299-300.
21. Papanicolaou GN, Traut HF. The diagnostic value of vaginal smears in carcinoma of the uterus. Am J Obstet Gynecol. 1941;42:193-206.
22. Donald I, MacVicar J, Brown TG. Investigation of abdominal masses by pulsed ultrasound. Lancet. 1958;1:1188-95.
23. Tarneja P, Duggal BS. Hysteroscopy: past, present and future. Med J Armed Forces India. 2002;58:293-4.
24. Wall LL. The medical ethics of Dr J Marion Sims: a fresh look at the historical record. J Med Ethics. 2006;32:346-50.
25. BBC News. New York: James Marion Sims statue removed from Central Park. BBC Online. April 17, 2018.
26. Shirodkar VN. Contributions to Obstetrics and Gynaecology. London: E and S Livingstone Ltd.; 1960.
27. Virkud A. Conservative operations in genital prolapse. J Obstet Gynecol India. 2016;66:144-8.
28. Patwardhan BD, Motashaw ND. Caesarean section. J Obstet Gynecol India. 1957;8:1-15.
29. Mukherjee S, Mehta RH. Dr. Subhas Mukherjee: A Visionary and Pioneer of IVF. Mumbai: ICMR-National Institute for Research in Reproductive Health; 2020.

■ LONG QUESTIONS

1. What are the important events in the 1800s that contributed to safety of surgery on women and in general?
2. Write an overview of the important contributions of Indian obstetrician and gynecologists in modern practice.
3. Write a critique the statement "James Marion Sims as the father of modern gynaecology".

■ SHORT QUESTIONS

1. Write a short note on the history of the obstetric forceps.
2. Why was puerperal sepsis a deadly disease and how did Semmelweis deal with it?
3. Ian Donald is looked upon as the modern day legend in obstetrics. Mention his stellar contributions.
4. How has the history of assisted reproduction been rewritten in India in recent times?

MULTIPLE CHOICE QUESTIONS

1. What is the estimated age of the universe?
   a. 34 billion years
   b. 14 billion years
   c. 4 billion years
   d. 1 billion years
2. From how long ago are the oldest representations of the female form and anatomy?
   a. 50,000 years BCE
   b. 40,000 years BCE
   c. 20,000 years BCE
   d. 2,000 years BCE
3. The following Indian text has the earliest scientific description about embryology:
   a. Govind Upanishad
   b. Yuga Upanishad
   c. Rig Upanishad
   d. Garbha Upanishad
4. The landmark textbook of women's health and disease published by Soranus of Ephesus was:
   a. De Morbis Mulierum
   b. De Humani Corporis Fabrica
   c. Historia Plantarum
   d. Hippocratic Corpus
5. The accurate description of human anatomy from dissection of cadavers was published by:
   a. Andreas Vesalius
   b. William Smellie
   c. Marcus Ulpius
   d. Agnocide
6. The first vaginal hysterectomy that was conducted successfully in modern times is credited to:
   a. Ephraim McDowell
   b. JCM (Conrad) Langenbeck
   c. Charles Clay
   d. James Marion Sims
7. Professor Henry Dale described the action of which commonly used drug?
   a. Methergin
   b. Prostaglandin F2 alpha
   c. Oxytocin
   d. Misoprostol
8. The following are considered as the pioneers of radical hysterectomy, except:
   a. Joe Vincent Meigs
   b. James Young Simpson
   c. Friedrich Schauta
   d. John Clark
9. All the following played a vital role in the development of the cervicovaginal smear technique for early detection of cervical cancer, except:
   a. Ernst Wertheim
   b. Herbert Taut
   c. Andromache (Mary) Mavroyeni
   d. George Papanicolaou
10. The first baby by the in vitro fertilization technique was born in:
    a. 1968
    b. 1975
    c. 1978
    d. 1982

Answers
1. b 2. c 3. d 4. a 5. a 6. b
7. c 8. b 9. a 10. c

1.2 COMMUNICATION AND COUNSELING

Tripti Nagaria

"Extensive research has shown that no matter how knowledgeable a clinician might be, if he or she is not able to open good communication with the patient, he or she may be of no help".

Healthcare system is dependent upon the effective communication between the healthcare provider and the receiver, i.e., the patient and the community. Communication should not be considered as simple interaction or process of exchange of information, it is an important and powerful tool in bringing about change in existing human behavior and attitude increasing the knowledge and acquiring skill.

WHAT IS COMMUNICATION?

"Communicate", a Latin word from which the word communication is derived, means to share. Communication is defined as the process of transmission of information from one individual to another individual or group of people or from one organization to another by using any suitable medium like speaking, writing, or any other.

COMMUNICATION PROCESS

The key elements in the communication process **(Fig. 1)** are:[1,2]
1. Sender (source of generation of information)
2. Receiver (recipient of information)
3. Message (content of information)
4. Channel (medium of communication)
5. Feedback (effect of communication)

Sender

The sender or the communicator is the one who originates the message or information and sends it to other individual/individuals or organization/organizations.

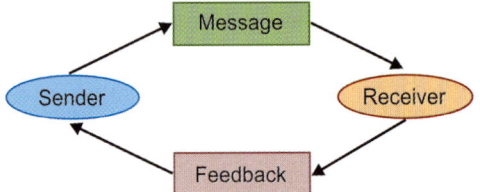

Fig. 1: Key elements in the communication process.

For effective communication sender must have the knowledge of:
- Objective of communication—clearly defined
- Receiver—about their type, interest and abilities
- Message—must have accurate, useful contents
- Channel(s) of communication—medium of transmitting information written, spoken or otherwise
- Professional limitations and abilities as sender.

Status and the knowledge of the communicator also influence the impact of the communication.

Receiver

The receiver is the individual/organization or a group of the individuals/organizations whom the message is directed. The group can be homogeneous means a group having common interest or heterogeneous having varying interests. Communication of message in a homogeneous group is more effective as compared to heterogeneous one. The extent of comprehension of the message by the receiver depends on their receptivity or readiness to accept the message, prior knowledge about the topic and the relationship and trust that exists between sender and receiver.

Message

It is the information the sender wishes to deliver to the receiver to understand, accept or act upon. It may be in form of words, spoken or written, in form of signs, symbols, audio or video, drawing, pictures, placards.
- The key to success of communication is transmission of right message at right time to right audience in right way.

Channels of Communication

Channel is the media of communication between the sender and the receiver(s).

Media systems which can be used:
1. *For interpersonal communication:*
   - Verbal both oral and written, or sign language
2. *For mass communication:*
   - Television (TV), radio, printed media, etc.
   - Traditional folk media—folk dances, drama, singing, Nautanki, etc.

Considering the advantages and limitations of every channel, many a time one may use more than one medium for effective communication. Selection of the right media whether oral or written is very important for effective delivery of message. It depends upon several factors like:
- Urgency
- Need of feedback
- Need of documentation or a permanent record
- Complexity of message
- In case of organization—whether the message will be delivered to individual/s or department/s of the organization or outside the organization
- The skill of the receiver to understand the verbal or written communication
- The audience whether a person, a small group or large group or population.

Feedback

Feedback is the response of the receiver to the message transmitted. It may be again verbal or nonverbal like a spoken or written comment, a gesture, facial expression, nonverbal behavior, a smile, or some other action. "No response is also a form of response".

Feedback is of paramount importance in communication as it allows evaluation of the effectiveness of the message and provides an opportunity to modify or clarify a misunderstood message, rectify the transmission errors, and make it acceptable. Feedback can be immediate as in interpersonal communication or can take some time as in mass media communication. Feedback is the key component of the communication to confirm that the receiver has interpreted the message correctly.

In healthcare settings, all these elements of the communication are affected by various factors particularly in an understaffed setting.

In such setup, the healthcare personnel have to do many works or perform duties at multiple sites. The pressure of working result in fatigue, less concentration, distractions, lapses in memory, stress, frustrations, etc., these can lead to errors, misunderstanding of messages, miscommunication, poorer responses and can affect the patient care.

■ COMMUNICATION SKILLS

In a healthcare system, knowledge of the processes of communication and communication skill play a very vital role. From the very first contact with, till discharge from the healthcare system the patient and their relative/caretakers need to know various information essential for the management of the case, may it be information about disease, diagnosis, how to and where to get admitted, for making decision for various intervention, medicines, follow-up, etc. Thus, interaction with various persons of different cadres in the system is a routine in hospital setting. Different patients and relatives have different ability to transmit, receive and understand the message, as well as to react based upon their age, literacy skills, language, social and cultural background, disabilities, etc.

Similarly in the system not all the personnel have similar efficiencies in communication and various factors apart from above mentioned other factors like pressure of the work, multitasking, background noises, interruptions, fatigue, lack of sleep, etc., may affect their ability.

Discharge summary or transfer tickets at the time of shifting to another care system is another very essential and important written document which conveys the essential features of condition of intervention done and the treatment and follow-up instructions. Improperly made or communicated notes can lead to errors in the further understanding and management of the patient.

At various points of contact and stages of care, the communication method may change in terms of senders, messages need to be given, means or channels used, receivers may be patient himself or family members and expected feedback. Therefore, ultimate outcome depends upon both how efficiently message is conveyed as well how efficiently the receiver has perceived and understood it. Thus, a deep understanding and knowledge of communication skill is essential for success and failure of the system.

■ METHODS OF COMMUNICATION

Broad categories of communication are:
1. One-way communication (Didactic method)
2. Two-way communication (Socratic method)
   The characteristics of two methods are as shown in **Table 1**.
   Communication can also be categorized as follows **(Table 2)**:
1. Based on communication channels
2. Based on style and purpose

Verbal Communication

Verbal literally means spoken, oral, vocal or unwritten; therefore, verbal communication in general gives an impression of spoken communication. However, in communication, verbal includes use of language and words in both spoken and written forms and for those who are with hearing impairment sign language as well.

Examples of two methods are as shown in **Table 3**.

Nonverbal Communication

Nonverbal communication is "Wordless communication", where no words whether spoken or written are used still it is a powerful tool of conveying message and feedback. It is often complementary to verbal communication and if used properly aids to its effectiveness. It usually expresses the mood, opinion, reluctance, and reaction to the message received.

Some of the modes of nonverbal communication are:
- *Physical nonverbal communication*: Bodily physical movements can be most expressive observable way of nonverbal communication. In day-to-day practices and routine life, it comprises more than half of the communication. Some of the common examples are facial expressions, body language, hand movements, gestures, posture, walk, touch, gaze, etc. these are the common way of expressing reactions to the messages received.
- *Paralanguage*: Nonverbal aids to spoken communication are by changes in the tone, pitch and quality of voice, and style of speaking. It conveys the mood of the sender as well as the receiver, reaction of the receiver, expresses the emotions in more or less 36% of communications are supported or aided with these paralanguages to convey the feelings.

Major differences between verbal and nonverbal communication are as shown in **Table 4**.

Nonverbal communication by patient: Nonverbal communication plays a vital role in the healthcare delivery system as it may be more important feedback from the patient than any verbal one. It provides a reliable indicator about the condition of the patient.

TABLE 1: Characteristics of one-way and two-way communication.

	One-way communication	Two-way communication
Flow of transmission of information	One-way from sender to receiver	Two-way both take part
Active participation of receiver	No	Yes
Feedback generation	No	Yes
Place for clarification	No	Yes
Learning	Passive, authoritative	Active, democrative
Influence on human behavior	No	Yes
Complex message	Difficult to transmit	Easier, more effective
Examples	Classroom lecture, notice, advertisement	Discussion, interpersonal communication

TABLE 2: Categories of communication.

Communication			
Based on communication channel		Based on style and purpose	
Nonverbal	Verbal	Formal	Nonformal

	• Oral
	  – Face-to-face
	  – Distance		

	Written		
	Visual		

TABLE 3: Examples of verbal communication.

Written	Oral	
Exchange of information in written form	Exchange in spoken words	
	Direct, face-to-face	Indirect, distance
Examples: • Emails • Letters • Reports • Consent • Discharge papers • Posters, flyers • Documents • Handbooks • Posts on social media, etc.	Examples: • Face-to-face communication, Counseling • Personal communication • Presentation • Meetings • Lectures • Discussions • Conferences • Interviews	Examples: • Telephonic conversation • Chat talk • Voice message

TABLE 4: Differences between verbal and nonverbal communication.

	Verbal communication	*Nonverbal communication*
Based upon	Use of language, words	Use of signs, body language, and others
Chances of confusion in understanding the message	Very few as language is used	High as no language is used
Time taken in interchanging the message between the receiver and sender	Fast hence feedback is also rapid	Takes time to understand hence slow
Location of both the parties	May or may not be at same location	Needed for effective communication

TABLE 5: Examples of nonverbal behavior.

Nonverbal behavior

Body language	*Paralanguage*
• Gestures • Facial expressions • Postures • Body orientations • Body proximity/distance • Eye contact • Mirroring • Remove the barriers (e.g., desks, keeping the mobiles off/silent)	• Sighs • Grunts • Groans • Voice volume • Voice pitch alteration • Voice fluency • Nervous giggles

- While examining, interacting with the patient, observation of the nonverbal communication of like facial expression is informative. However, while examining a patient, one should watch for the comfort zone of the patient, sometimes closeness may disturb and make the patient uncomfortable.
- *Body language*: Various body languages of the patient can express the emotional response like anger, depression, frustration, feeling good, greeting, etc., For example, avoiding of eye contact, silence, various gestures, hand movements, eye movements, clinching of jaw, fist, etc.
- *Paralanguage*: Pauses, changes or variations in voices during communication again give important clue of the emotional status of the patient.

Some of the nonverbal behaviors are as shown in **Table 5**.

Both verbal and nonverbal forms of communication are complementary to each other. Whereas the verbal form is the face-to-face communication and better way of understanding the message, the nonverbal form satisfies the emotional understanding.

Other ways of nonverbal communication: Following are some of other ways particularly in group or mass communication.

- *Visual communication*: Communication through visual aids like drawings, placards, tables, maps, charts, graphs, pictogram, poster presentations, illustrations, etc.
- *Esthetic communication*: Various types of art forms like drawing, sketches, and paintings are also powerful means of transmitting the message.
- *Appearance*: The appearance, clothes, and the color of the fabrics, etc., also have important impact on the reaction of audience.

Formal and Informal Communication

Written verbal communication using scientific and official language, observing systematic policies, and procedures is formal communication. In healthcare system, this form of communication is done with following objectives:

- Patients' education and counseling to ensure their safety
- Information or documents on medical policies, rules and regulations, guidelines, notifications, publications, instructions, etc.
- Formal records system and prescription, etc.

Informal communication is casual nonspecific or common communication between members of the organizations (gossips). However, health information internet has expanded this form of communication. Various healthcare-related advertisements and information are now available on healthcare media. Exchange of information between patients and their healthcare providers related to patients' illness is another example of it.

Both formal and informal communication play vital role in improving the quality of healthcare, patient safety, and behavior of patients.

CHARACTERISTICS OF EFFECTIVE COMMUNICATION

Effective communication is one which end with transmission of message or feeling from the sender and perceived by the receiver.

There is a concept of "7Cs" or characteristics that must qualify the communicating activities and processes to make it effective **(Box 1)**.

1. *Clear*: The message being transmitted must be very clear and easily understandable with simple and short sentences. In written documentation, one should use active voice over the passive voice and if multiple messages are to be conveyed separate bulleted points must be used.
2. *Concise*: Any attention span is just a few minutes long; therefore, to be effective the message should be short and concise.
3. *Concrete*: Whatever message or information or data is present in the communication, it should be suitably backed up. A tangible argument is always easy to understand.
4. *Coherent*: For written documentation, coherence is very essential. It should be well planned, the information should be in sequential manner, follow each other. The main ideas should be well-differentiated.
5. *Courteous*: The information or the communication whether written or verbal must not hurt the feelings of

> **BOX 1: Characteristics ("7Cs") of effective communication.**
> - Concise
> - Concrete
> - Coherent
> - Courteous
> - Consideration
> - Consistent/correctness
> - Complete

the receiver, it should be respectful, polite, thoughtful, with proper care and kindness. Language used must not be offensive, insensitive or awful to the receiver.

6. *Consideration*: For effective communication, one must get connected to and involved with the target audience. Hence, the presenter must know/assess the background knowledge on the topic, level of literacy, age, and interests of the receiver/s before start of communication.
7. *Consistent*: Consistency in the information given adds to clarity of communication. Various statements or facts must be systematically presented to avoid any confusion.

WHAT ARE THE BARRIERS OF COMMUNICATION? (BOX 2)

Any parameter that limits the purpose or channel of communication between the transmitter and the receiver is a barrier to communication. It may limit or reduce the ease at which one communicates and the intended message will often be disturbed and distorted leading to a condition of misunderstanding and failure of communication.

Although the barriers to effective communication may be different for different situations, the following are some of the main barriers as shown in **Table 6**.

APPLICATIONS OF HEALTH COMMUNICATION

1. IEC—information, education, and communication—aims to generate specific awareness in targeted population.
2. BCC—behavior change communication—aims to generate awareness in the targeted population with an aim to change the behavior.
3. SBCC—social behavior change communication—aims to change the social condition and individual behavior.

Health education can be defined as the principle by which individuals and groups of people learn to behave in a manner conducive to the promotion, maintenance, or restoration of health, e.g., information and awareness about various national programs, immunization program, antenatal intranatal and postnatal care services, family planning services, safe abortion services, breastfeeding awareness, cancer awareness, etc.

This can be done using all the methods of communication:
1. *Individual method:* Counseling and interview
2. *Group method:* Group discussion, role play, brainstorming, workshop/seminar, demonstration, mini-lecture, symposium. problem solving, panel discussion, field trip/educational tour, etc.
3. *Mass media method:* Using visual aids—posters, video, paintings, etc.

> **BOX 2: Barriers of communication.**
> - Linguistic barriers
> - Psychological barriers
> - Emotional barriers
> - Physical barriers
> - Cultural barriers
> - Attitude barriers
> - Perception barriers
> - Physiological barriers
> - Technological barriers
> - Socioreligious barriers

TABLE 6: Barriers of communication.

S. No.	Barriers	Factors causing difficulties in communication
1.	Linguistic barriers	Difference in language or dialects between the providers and receiver
2.	Psychological barriers	Mental issues like fear, speech disorder, depression, etc.
3.	Emotional barrier	Emotional IQ of persons, anger, frustration, humor, etc.
4.	Physical barrier	Noise, closed doors, faulty equipment used for communication, etc.
5.	Cultural barriers	Differences in cultural values of the society
6.	Attitude barriers	Ego, inconsiderate behavior, etc.
7.	Perception barrier	Differences in ability to perceive, understand the messages, literacy, previous knowledge, age, prolong ill health, etc.
8.	Physiological barrier	Disorder like shrillness of voice, dyslexia, etc.
9.	Socioreligious barrier	Woman, transgender may face difficulty in certain community

COUNSELING

Counseling is a bidirectional interpersonal communication to analyze the feelings, opinion, believes, thoughts, and problems of a person and helps him to take sensible decision. Herein two unrelated persons meet to discuss and find out the ways to conquer the crisis or problem in an atmosphere which is supportive to let the person define the situation, build up self-confidence and respect and readiness to bring about lifestyle modifications to reduce the brunt of the problem on himself and on their close ones.

Counseling is not about taking the decision for the person/client and also not about judging, cross-examining, disagreeing with what the client is speaking or instructing the client but it is a process by which the client is conversed in such a way that he himself becomes confident enough to take suitable decision, it can only be done when the counselor though working very closely is not emotionally attached to the client. This approach aims to help the clients in developing the skills to solve the problems and to cope up better with the situations they are facing. This engrosses the individual to handle with their emotions and feelings and to help them make positive choices and decisions.

BASIC COMMUNICATION QUALITIES OF A COUNSELOR

1. *Focus and attention*: While receiving or transmitting information, focus and attention are very important. Any mislaid communication could be unsuccessful as if one loses attention, important part of the information may be overlooked or failed to notice altogether.
   Attending: It refers to the way the counselor is connected to the patient both physically and psychologically, i.e., how does he position himself to listen to the client carefully. Gerard Egan defined SOLER as a part of his "Skilled Helper" staged approach to counseling. It is a nonverbal listening process used in communication and is stand for:
   - S: Squarely face your patient
   - O: Open posture
   - L: Lean toward the patient
   - E: Eye contact with the patient
   - R: Try to be Relaxed or natural with the patient
2. *Listening for understanding*: It refers to capturing and understanding the message, the patient wants to give irrespective of the way verbal or nonverbal.
   Four skills are involved in active listening:
   i. Listening to understand the verbal message of the client
   ii. Listening to and interpreting the nonverbal message of the client such as bodily posture, gestures, groaning, facial expression, voice-related behavior, psychological reactions, general appearance, etc.
   iii. Listening to and considering the client in perspective of her social background
   iv. Listening with empathy.
3. *Basic empathy*: Basic empathy involves active listening skill of the counselor to appreciate and consider the concerns of clients as best as he can. The understanding should then be communicated back to the clients in such a manner that help them to comprehend themselves more fully and act thoughtful. In other words, it is the skill to be acquainted with and acknowledge the reaction or emotions of another person with experiencing those same emotions. These feelings then must be communicated to the client in either verbal or nonverbal way.
4. *Questioning*: It makes the counselor to get more issues from the clients. It also helps keeping the client more focused on main issues describing at large. Care must be taken to ask open-ended questions to let client describe the problem.
5. *Use silence effectively*; do not interrupt unless necessary.
6. *Reflection and echoing*: The provider observes the clients emotions and reflects them back. This helps provider to check whether his/her observations are correct. It also reflects the empathy and respect toward clients feeling.
7. *Praise and encouragement*: The provider uses gestures and words to encourage and motivate the client and ensure his/her approval.
8. *Give information* to the client clearly.
9. Being nonjudgmental
10. *Emotional awareness and control*: Remain emotionally stable to accept or reject any message with the intention, it is being relayed.
11. *Summarizing and paraphrasing*: At the end, the counselor must summarize what the client had described; it provides an opportunity to the client to clarify.

The counseling is intended to help the patient to understand and develop the capability to cope up with his or her condition/disease, so as to promote a better quality of life.

IMPACT OF COMMUNICATION IN HEALTH CARE

Success of integrated healthcare delivery system to provide quality care to the patients and good outcome is founded in effective communication. Apart from providing better working environment with increased job satisfaction, it is the key to better patient outcomes with higher rates of patient satisfaction and continuation of treatment and reduced adverse events, hospital stay, and readmission rates.[3-8] Several researchers have observed communication failure as the main factor contributing to the just the contrary outcomes.[9-15]

CHALLENGES IN COMMUNICATION IN DIFFERENT SITUATIONS

There are many models of communication and every healthcare provider has his or her own style. Certain principles from different sources may be followed for effective communication as discussed here.

In Outpatient Department

From the very first contact to start of the treatment by the patient communication is the constant and most essential aspect of the medical practice involved right from getting the history of illness to explaining the treatment plan. Effective communication not only builds up good physician patient relationship but also leaves therapeutic effect on the patient.[3]

Steps to be followed:
1. Greet the patient and know the problem he/she had
2. Interview the patient:[16]
   - Focus and attention
   - Discover the understanding and knowledge the patient is already having about her illness
   - Evaluate or assess what does she want to know, before starting to inform
   - Be empathetic

- Give information slowly
- Keep it simple
- Tell the truth
- Observe nonverbal behavior of patient
- Be prepared for reaction

3. *Closing:*
   - Use name of patient
   - Make positive statement.

A number of factors may affect the outcome like a busy outpatient department (OPD), short of time, noises, multitasking situation, mobile phone, etc. only by careful and effective handling of barriers and following principles of effective communication a trust and rapport can be build up.

During Transition of Care

Throughout the continuum of care, patients need to be transferred to different locations of varying levels, and to various healthcare providers for management as their condition demands, this needs movements of patients and their family members and/caretakers to different places within and sometimes to different hospitals. It involves multiple other persons too like medical, paramedical, and ancillary staff of healthcare delivery system.[17] As with this transfer or relocation of the patient, the healthcare providers, decision taker, and the setup changes, a clear communication of the patient status regarding disease is necessary to make sure the quality of care.[18] For effective transition, care apt and precise communication of information between providers, patients, and family caregivers are decisive. Any failure in execution of this safety measure leads to uncertainty about the care the patient is receiving, therefore, delay in care, improper monitoring, roughly one-half of all hospital-related medication errors and one-fifth of all adverse drug events, adverse outcomes, rehospitalization, and increased healthcare expenditures.[3,19-21]

Inadequate Handovers

During hospital stay, the patient has to come across many medical and paramedical staff in each shift of duty, intradepartmental or interdepartmental shifting to different location, for consultations, checkups, investigations and interventions, discharge, etc. For continuity of care and safety of patient during these shifting and change of heathcare providers, proper handovers are of paramount importance.[22] Effective communication is therefore fundamental to safe and effective patient care.[23] Failure of proper communication is identified as the one of the main root causes of serious medical errors.[24] Penalty of such failure during handovers is in the form of medication errors, erroneous patient plans, delay in discharge or transfer to critical care, or/and repetitive tests among others.[25]

Lack of proper communication can occur at multiple levels; between physicians, physician and nurses, between nurses, between medical and paramedical staff, and between members of team involved in providing health care and the patients and the caretakers, relatives, etc. These can result in delay in start of treatment, wrong treatment, medication error and sometime wrong surgical invention and even fatalities.

This can be avoided by following measures during handing over:

- Bedside handovers at all the levels should be done.
- Properly written records should be provided.
- Instructions must be clear.
- Recent updates of the condition and treatment must be provided.
- Using SBAR structured format[26] to transfer the information.
  S—Situation: Why the information is being communicated? What updating the patient's condition, clarifying orders, alerting regarding emergency developed, etc.
  B—Background: What is the background information? (History or complaints or diagnosis with which patient was admitted/referred, treatment being given, change in condition of case, any new development of sign or symptom or emergency).
  A—Assessment: What is the assessment of problem at that moment of time? (Clinical examination finding) what appears to be the problem based upon clinical examination finding?
  R—Recommendation: What is needed to be done for solving the problem at that moment of time? How should the problem be corrected?

The use of SBAR tool in clinical setting has been endorsed by many healthcare organizations including WHO for improving the verbal communication among healthcare providers for handover.[27-31]

I-PASS is another strong tool for communication for handovers during shift change and other transition care by healthcare providers, physician and nursing staff, to cut down the miscommunication and adverse outcomes. I-PASS is a mnemonic for: Illness severity (I), Patient summary (P), Action list (A), Situation awareness and contingency planning (S), and Synthesis by receiver (S).[32] Facilities can adapt to ensure all the following information is communicated when providers perform handoffs **(Table 7)**.

Inadequate Discharge

In a meta-analysis, Kripalani et al. observed discharge summaries often lacked important information such as main diagnosis (13–17.5%), diagnostic test results (missing from 33 to 63%), treatment or hospital course (7–22%), discharge medications (2–40%), test results pending at discharge (65%), patient or family counseling (90–92%), and follow-up plans (2–43%).[33]

To avoid this, few points should be kept in mind:

- Discharge must be well-planned.
- Computer-generated discharge summaries or standardized format must be used to emphasize the most important information to improve the quality of documents.

SECTION 1: Introduction to Obstetrics

TABLE 7: I-PASS tool for handover.

I	Illness severity	Current status of the patient: OK/under observation/stable/unstable/to be discharged
P	Patient summary	*At admission:* • History, physical finding, test results • During the course of stay in the hospital • Ongoing assessment • Plan for further management
A	Action list	To do list—includes: • Actions to complete, e.g., diagnostic tests, consultations, procedures • Timeline and ownership
S	Situational awareness and contingency planning	• Know what is going on and • Plan for what might happen, e.g., if the condition deteriorates, what is to be done immediately to address the change
S	Synthesis (by the receiver)	• The receiver summarizes what was heard • Clarifies any doubt, asks questions • Repeats the key actions/to do list

TABLE 8: 5Ds of discharge.

Element	Points to be discussed and ensured
Diagnosis	Why was he admitted and given care?
Drugs	Medicines—need for taking them How to take—dose, route, time, in relation to meals. etc.
Diet	Any dietary restriction, consultation with nutrition specialist if suggested
Doctor follow-up	Plan for next visit/s, name of doctor and place where to visit for further continuum of care
Directions	• Any other direction for achieving optimal health, e.g., exercise • Warning signs of urgency/emergency • If emergency arise whom to contact and/where to report for care

- Sufficient time must be given to explain the contents of discharge summary, i.e., about the condition of the patient at the time of discharge, plan for follow-up and treatment in simple language in a way which is easily understandable and to make sure that the patient and their relatives have understood.
- "5Ds of discharge" is one important tool which can be stressed in communication at the time of discharge to make sure the patient understands the information given and to do list.[34] Following are the elements of 5Ds—Diagnosis, Drugs, Diet, Doctor follow-up plan, and Directions for any emergent situation **(Table 8)**.

Handling Difficult Patient

Many a times certain difficulties to handle patients are encountered by healthcare providers, if not properly handled frustrations are likely to develop in both the parties. Prevention of difficult interaction is best approach.

- Recognize and concentrate on the psychological issues of the patient.
- Listen to them with great attention and empathy as the feeling that "they are not heard" or "they are not worth" is the greatest cause of dissatisfaction of most of the patients.
- Body language should be appropriate, should not be a cause of displeasure to patient.
- Be careful of your own emotional state.

If encounter becomes tense, follow the following points:
- Remain professional
- Do not let your emotion overcome you
- Active listening with summarizing
- Acknowledging the emotions they are expressing.[16]

COMMUNICATING WITH SERIOUSLY ILL PATIENTS

Special care and attention is required while communicating with seriously ill patients and to improve it various principles have been recommended, as follows:[35]

1. Before starting the interaction specific to her illness, spend a few moments giving the patient completely focused attention.
2. Start with what the patient wants to discuss or know.
3. Observe and follow the emotional feedback from the patient.
4. Move the conversation forward slowly, one step at a time.
5. Express empathy overtly.
6. Start with positive information like what can be done before informing what cannot be.
7. Start with ultimate big goals before talking about specific medical interventions.

Age-related Challenges

There are particularly unique challenges associated with communicating with extremes of age, adolescents as well as elderly people.

Communication with Adolescent

Adolescents may get engage in high-risk behavior and require medical advices or care. However, to get the information from them is not always easy as they are afraid of being assessed.

1. Greet them
2. Break the ice by asking few general questions not related to health
3. Give privacy
4. Avoid distractions while interactions
5. Listen with concentration, observe, and understand the nonverbal communications of the patient
6. Allow her to speak, too many interruptions may let them feel being judged
7. Mind your body language while interacting
8. Show concern
9. Give information in simple language, allow questioning.

If given appropriate friendly atmosphere, appreciated as adult and opportunity to discuss, they may disclose their information. Confidentiality is the foundation of building up of healthy relationship with youth. With proper communication/counseling, adolescents can be helped to take sensible decision to overcome the situations or the problems they are facing.

At the other extreme end of the age range, the elderly patients also present challenges in different ways. Multiple age-related and psychological issues make the communications challenging for the healthcare workers. Physical disabilities like visual and hearing impairment, medical disorder or comorbidities and medications for chronic disease, along with memory lapses and lack of psychological, social support put them at higher risk for adverse outcome, suboptimal care and medications particularly at the transition of care.

- Spare more time for older patients; do not appear hurried or uninterested[36]
- Avoid or reduce visual and auditory distractions[37,38]
- Assess and compensate for any visual or auditory impairment
- Ascertain respect from the beginning
- Maintain eye contact[4]
- Begin conversation with questions about family members or other interests rather than illness to decrease the anxiety
- Go slow—speak slowly, in a clear and loud voice and give patient sufficient time to understand the information
- Do not interrupt—listen till she completes
- Use simple, common words.
- Summarize repeatedly the most salient points
- Discuss only one topic at a time, inform the patients at the time of changing the subject
- Give clue to help her understand what is being said—such as brief pause, speaking a little louder, indicating or making gestures to make her understand topic to be discussed, asking questions to lead to the topic, etc.
- Think about use of alternatives to printed materials for visually impaired patients or patients with low literacy skill—such as vocal instructions, e.g., recorded instructions, visual large pictures or diagrams, or other aids.

Cultural Difference

It must be addressed while providing health care. Providing efficient and effective care requires having conversations in which the provider and patient both understand the meaning of words, concepts, and metaphors. Cultural differences also affect the working relationships between providers, as physicians and nurses, for example, sometimes have different value systems relating to how patients are cared for and treated.

Errors in Medical Orders and Test Results

Errors in medication in healthcare system can also be due to the verbal communication of the orders and test reports to the comembers of the team, patient or their caretakers, especially over phone.

- Difficulty can arise in understanding the message or the order due to difference in language, tone of voice and pronunciation or articulations.
- Another error prone verbal communication is giving instruction about sound alike drug name, number as this may affect the accuracy of the order and thereby the end result.
- Distracters like background noise, any break in continuity of speech due to other involvement, and use of unusual or new drug names and terminology often accentuate the magnitude the problem.
- Verbal and vague orders often end up with mismanagement, delay in treatment, over treatment or even omissions of medication treatment jeopardizing the patient safety.

To avoid this type of error, the healthcare system should develop a standardized protocol of communicating the order and test reports. Orders, prescription, reports should be properly written rather than verbally communicated. Healthcare providers must use of specific rather than uncommon terms for the intervention.[39]

During Treatment/Intervention

Communication failures during health care can be of multiple types viz. too late to be effective, not communicated to all the members of the team involved in the particular health care, incomplete and inaccurate transmission of information and not ending with fulfillment of the purpose until emergent situation arises.[38] Such failures are responsible for poor outcome and need to be addressed.

Also, throughout the continuum of care of a patient a number of procedures are needed and carried out which require adequate and effective communication to explain the procedure, need and related risk and benefits. Any deficient communication or no communication can end up in patients or relative's dissatisfaction and professional liability. Therefore, a defined procedure must be developed by every hospital to obtain an informed patient consent for various procedures being carried out during the inpatient care like any high-risk treatment, blood or blood product transfusion, surgical intervention, anesthesia, investigative procedures requiring anesthesia or sedation or carrying inherent risk, etc., in a manner and language the patient can understand.

Errors likely to Occur during Surgical Procedure in Operation Theater

Analysis of 421 communication events in the operating room (OR) found communication failures in approximately 30% of team exchanges; one-third of these jeopardized patient safety by increasing cognitive load, interrupting routine, and increasing tension in the OR setting.[40]

The most dreaded adverse event that can occur is a wrong operation carried out on a wrong person or wrong site. To prevent errors during surgery (wrong site, procedure, and

person), a universal protocol is designed.[41] One must check for the following before start of the surgery.
- Preprocedure verification process of the correct patient, procedure, and site
- Surgical site marking
- Ensuring the availability of all relevant documents and studies of the patients
- Images are properly labeled and displayed
- Verifying the availability of any required blood products grouped and crossed matched
- Special medical equipment if needed are present[42]
- To ascertain the site, patient must be actively involved in marking whenever possible and having the mark be visible after the patient is prepared and draped.

Obtaining a Consent for Surgical Treatment

- Obtaining an informed consent for surgical treatment is the need and also a challenge for the treating doctor/surgeon. It is not merely asking the patient and/their relatives sign the form. It requires surgeon to have good rapport with the patient and their relative or their caretakers so that necessary information can be transmitted to help them to decide to undergo surgical treatment. There should be clarity of explanation that leads to informed and deliberate consent.
- There must be a discussion on the various options of the management.
- Outcomes if the patient does not opt for surgery.
- Discussion on the need of procedure, the expected benefits, chances of success or failure, risks involved and complications that may develop.
- Need of additional management should the need arise.
- Type of anesthesia and related information.
- Follow-up plans and further additional management if needed.
- Surgeons involved in the intervention.
- The patient and relative/caretaker should be given time to think over, discuss and to ask any question or more information if they want.
- Consequences of nonoperative alternatives should also be explained.
- Consent should be in the language they understand.
- It must be read, understood and signed by the patient, relative or guardian and witnessed with a mention of time.

Consent should be looked as a procedure of shared decision making with patient and their relative/guardian. Informed consent as the one where the treating physician has explained the patient and their relative and they understood diagnosis, treatment options, the risk and benefits involved therein, chances of success and failure of the procedure, immediate and delayed complication if any and also of no treatment if they opt for and finally came to the decision.[43]

Thus, obtaining informed consent challenges professional competence. It is a time taking process of communication involving education, patient sympathetic listening and satisfying the queries of the patient, relatives/caregivers that continues through the continuum of care. It requires good patient-surgeon communication and lack of which may lead to professional liability.[44]

CONCLUSION

Effective communication and counseling play a very vital role in improving the health outcomes in healthcare system resulting in better management, patients' satisfaction, and higher chances of continuation of treatment and follow up and building up of trust in the system. It is the responsibility of not only the doctors and nursing staff but of every member of the team involved in the management of patient including the paramedical and the ancillary staff to develop the skill of effective communication and counseling for achieving the ultimate goal of health care.

FURTHER READING

1. AIPC's Counsellor Skills Series. [online] Available from: https://www.aipc.net.au/articles/; https//www.counsellingconnection.com/ [Last accessed September, 2021].
2. Joint Commission International. Communicating Clearly and Effectively to Patients: How to Overcome Common Communication Challenges in Health Care. A white paper by Joint Commission International. 2018.
3. Kabir SM. Essentials of Counseling. Banglabazar, Dhaka: Abosar Prokashana Sangstha; 2017.
4. Kadri AM, Kundapur R, Khan AM, Kakkar R. IAPSM'S Textbook of Community Medicine, 1st edition. New Delhi: Jaypee Brothers Medical Publishers Pvt. Ltd.; 2019.
5. Park K. Park's Textbook of Preventive and Social Medicine, 25th edition. Jabalpur, Madhya Pradesh: Banarasidas Bhanot Publishers; 2019.
6. The Naz Foundation (India) Trust. Guide to Communication and Counseling: A Training Manual for Trainers. [online] Available from: https://www.who.int/hiv/topics/vct/sw_toolkit/guide_communication_counseling_naz.pdf [Last accessed September, 2021].

REFERENCES

1. Kadri AM, Kundapur R, Khan AM, Kakkar R. IAPSM'S Textbook of Community Medicine, 1st edition. New Delhi: Jaypee Brothers Medical Publishers Pvt. Ltd.; 2019.
2. Park K. Park's Textbook of Preventive and Social Medicine, 25th edition. Jabalpur, Madhya Pradesh: Banarasidas Bhanot Publishers; 2019.
3. Travaline JM, Ruchinskas R, D'Alonzo GE. Patient-physician communication: why and how. J Am Osteopath Assoc. 2005;105(1):13-8.
4. Institute for Healthcare Communication. (2011). Impact of communication in healthcare. [online] Available from: http://healthcarecomm.org/about-us/impact-of-communication-in-healthcare/ [Last accessed September, 2021].
5. Senot C, Chandrasekaran A, Ward PT, Tucker AL, Moffatt-Bruce S. The impact of combining conformance and experiential quality on hospitals' readmissions and cost performance. Manage Sci. 2015;62(3):829-48.

6. Baggs JG, Schmitt MH, Mushlin AI, Mitchell PH, Eldredge DH, Oakes D, et al. Association between nurse-physician collaboration and patient outcomes in three intensive care units. Crit Care Med. 1999;27:1991-8.
7. Baggs JG, Ryan SA, Phelps CE, Richeson JF, Johnson JE. The association between interdisciplinary collaboration and patient outcomes in a medical intensive care unit. Heart Lung. 1992;21:18-24.
8. Mitchell PH, Armstrong S, Simpson TF, Lentz M. American Association of Critical-Care Nurses demonstration project: profile of excellence in critical care nursing. Heart Lung. 1989;18:219-37.
9. Zwarenstein M, Reeves S. Working together but apart: barriers and routes to nurse—physician collaboration. Jt Comm J Qual Improv. 2002;28:242-7.
10. Fagin C. Collaboration between nurses and physician: no longer a choice. Acad Med. 1992;67:295-303.
11. Woolf SH, Kuzel AJ, Dovey SM, Phillips RL Jr. A string of mistakes: the important of cascade analysis in describing, counting, and preventing medical errors. Ann Fam Med. 2004; 2(4):317-26.
12. Balogh EP, Miller BT, Ball JR. Improving Diagnosis in Health Care. Washington (DC): National Academies Press (US); 2015.
13. Larson E. The impact of physician-nurse interaction on patient care. Holist Nurs Prac. 1999;13:38-47.
14. Sexton J, Thomas EJ, Helmreich RL. Error, stress, and teamwork in medicine and aviation: cross sectional surveys. Br Med J. 2000;320:745-9.
15. Vermeir P, Vandijck D, Degroote S, Peleman R, Verhaeghe R, Mortier E, et al. Communication in healthcare: a narrative review of the literature and practical recommendations. Int J Clin Pract. 2015;69:1257-67.
16. State of Washington Medical Quality Assurance Commission Guideline. Communication with patients, family, and health care team. MD2016-04.
17. National Transitions of Care Coalition. (2016). Improving transitions of care: findings and considerations of the "Vision of the National Transitions of Care Coalition. [online] Available from: http://www.ntocc.org/portals/0/pdf/resources/ntoccissuebriefs.pdf [Last accessed September, 2021].
18. Wittkowsky AK. Impact of target-specific oral anticoagulants on transitions of care and outpatient care models. J Thromb Thrombolysis. 2013;35(3):304-11.
19. The Joint Commission. Hot topics in health care: transitions of care: the need for a more effective approach to continuing patient care. [online] Available from: http://www.jointcommission.org/assets/1/18/hot_topics_transitions_of_care.pdf [Last accessed September, 2021].
20. American Pharmacists Association, American Society of Health-System Pharmacists, Steeb D, Webster L. Improving care transitions: optimizing medication reconciliation. J Am Pharm Assoc. 2012;52(4):e43-52.
21. American College of Clinical Pharmacy, Kirwin J, Canales AE, Bentley ML, Bungay K, Chan T, et al. Process indicators of quality clinical pharmacy services during transitions of care. Pharmacotherapy. 2012;32(11):e338-47.
22. Edwards C, Woodard EK. SBAR for maternal transports: going the extra mile. Nurs Womens Health. 2008;12(6):515-20.
23. Riesenberg LA, Leitzsch J, Little BW. Systematic review of handoff mnemonics literature. Am J Med Qual. 2009;24(3):196-204.
24. The Joint Commission. Sentinel event statistics released for 2014. [online] Available from: http://www.jointcommission.org/sentinel_event.aspx.last [Last accessed September, 2021].
25. Flemming D, Hübner U. How to improve change of shift handovers and collaborative grounding and what role does the electronic patient record system play? Results of a systematic literature review. Int J Med Inform. 2013;82(7):580-92.
26. Shahid S, Thomas S. Situation, background, assessment, recommendation (SBAR) communication tool for handoff in health care—a narrative review. Saf Health. 2018;4:7.
27. Von Dossow V, Zwissler B. Recommendations of the German Association of Anesthesiology and Intensive Care Medicine (DGAI) on structured patient handover in the perioperative setting: The SBAR concept. Anaesthesist. 2016;65(1):1-4.
28. Agency for Health care Research and Quality. [online] Available from: https://psnet.ahrq.gov/search?topic=SBAR&f_topicIDs=680,711 [Last accessed September, 2021].
29. Australian Commission for Safety and Quality in Health Care. ISBAR revisited: identifying and solving barriers to effective handover in inter-hospital transfer. [online] https://www.safetyandquality.gov.au/sites/default/files/migrated/ISBAR-toolkit.pdf
30. Institute of Health Care improvement, Tools. [online] Available from: http://www.ihi.org/resources/Pages/Tools/SBARToolkit.aspx [Last accessed September, 2021].
31. WHO Collaborating Centre for Patient Safety Solutions. (2007). Patient safety solutions. [online] Available from: www.who.int/patientsafety/solutions/patientsafety/PS-Solution3.pdf [Last accessed September, 2021].
32. Starmer AJ, Spector ND, Srivastava R, Allen AD, Landrigan CP, Sectish TC, et al. I-PASS, a mnemonic to standardize verbal handoffs. Pediatrics. 2012;129:201-4.
33. Kripalani S, LeFevre F, Phillips CO, Williams MV, Basaviah P, Baker DW. Deficits in communication and information transfer between hospital-based and primary care physicians: implications for patient safety and continuity of care. JAMA. 2007;297:831-41.
34. Joint Commission International. Communicating Clearly and Effectively to Patients: How to Overcome Common Communication Challenges in Health Care. A white paper by Joint Commission international. 2018.
35. Back A, Arnold R, Tulsky J. Mastering Communication with Seriously Ill Patients: Balancing Honesty with Empathy and Hope. New York, NY: Cambridge Univ Press; 2009.
36. Robinson TE 2nd, White GL Jr, Houchins JC. Improving communication with older patients: tips from the literature. Fam Pract Manag. 2006;13(8):73-8.
37. Dreher BB. Communication Skills for Working with Elders. New York: Springer; 1987.
38. Osborne H. Communicating with clients in person and over the phone. Issue Brief Cent Medicare Educ. 2003;4(8):1-8.
39. Kaufmann J, Laschat M, Wappler F. Medication errors in pediatric emergencies: a systematic analysis. Dtsch Arztebl Int. 2012;109:609-16.
40. Lingard L, Espin S, Whyte S, Regehr G, Baker GR, Reznick R, et al. Communication failures in the operating room: an observational classification of recurrent types and effects. Qual Saf Health Care. 2004;13:330-4.
41. The Joint Commission. Universal protocol. [online] Available from: https://www.jointcommission.org/standard/universal-protocol/ [Last accessed September, 2021].

42. Stahel PF, Mehler PS, Clarke TJ, Varnell J. The 5th anniversary of the "Universal Protocol": pitfalls and pearls revisited. Patient Saf Surg. 2009;3:14.
43. Hall DE, Prochazka AV, Fink AS. Informed consent for clinical treatment. CMAJ. 2012;184(5):533-40.
44. Bernat JL, Peterson LM. Patient-centered informed consent in surgical practice. Arch Surg. 2006;141(1):86-92.

LONG QUESTIONS

1. What are the characteristics of effective communications?
2. Discuss the barriers to good communication and modalities to overcome them.

SHORT QUESTIONS

1. What are the key elements of the communication process.
2. What are the broad methods of communication?
3. What are the characteristics of one-way and two-way communications?
4. What are the differences between verbal and nonverbal communication?

MULTIPLE CHOICE QUESTIONS

1. Sign language is an example of:
   a. Nonverbal communication
   b. Verbal communication
   c. Formal communication
   d. Paralanguage
   e. None of the above
2. Feedback allows the sender:
   a. To evaluate the effectiveness of message
   b. To clarify the message
   c. To confirm whether it is interpreted correctly by the receiver
   d. To rectify transmission error
   e. All of the above
3. SOLER is a:
   a. Method of questioning
   b. Method of listening and attending the patient
   c. Method of giving information
   d. Method of judging the patient
   e. Method of taking informed consent
4. In counseling, all are true, except:
   a. Listening   b. Summarizing
   c. Being judgmental   d. Questioning
   e. Giving information
5. Effective communication is helpful in all, except:
   a. Reducing readmission rate
   b. Reducing hospital stay
   c. Reducing patient satisfaction
   d. Reducing unnecessary investigation
   e. Reducing adverse events
6. Transition of care is movement of patient between:
   a. One location to another in same hospital
   b. One hospital to another
   c. Health care providers
   d. Hospital and home setting at the time of discharge
   e. All of the above
7. SBAR structured format comprises of:
   a. Safety, background, assessment, recommendation
   b. Situation, background, assessment, rationale
   c. Safety, background, awareness, recommendation
   d. Situation, background, assessment, recommendation
   e. Situation, barriers, awareness, review
8. 5Ds are used for:
   a. Disabilities   b. Diseases
   c. Difficulties   d. Discharge
   e. Dilemmas
9. While communicating with adolescents which one is most important:
   a. Confidentiality   b. Concise
   c. Consistency   d. Clarity
   e. None of the above
10. Current evidences suggest for better management of patient with effective communication skill, the approach should be:
    a. Disease-centered approach
    b. Treatment-centered approach
    c. Outcome-centered approach
    d. Patient-centered approach
    e. None of the above
11. Informed consent for surgery should include:
    a. Purpose of intervention   b. Expected benefit
    c. Follow-up plans   d. Complications
    e. All of the above
12. Communication is a responsibility of:
    a. Doctors and nurses only
    b. Doctors only
    c. Nurses only
    d. Paramedical staff and doctors only
    e. Whole health care team
13. All except one are not an example of verbal communication:
    a. Informed consent   b. Discharge ticket
    c. Hospital policy document
    d. Groan   e. History taking
14. Medication error can occur:
    a. Sound alike drug   b. Sound like number
    c. Inadequate handovers d. Illegible handwriting
    e. All of the above
15. IEC means:
    a. Information, education, and communication
    b. Information, education, and compliance
    c. In house, education center
    d. Individual education chart
    e. None of the above

Answers

1. a   2. e   3. b   4. c   5. c   6. e
7. d   8. d   9. a   10. d   11. e   12. e
13. d   14. e   15. a

1.3 EVIDENCE-BASED MEDICINE AND MEDICAL INFORMATICS

Anahita Chauhan, Madhva Prasad S

INTRODUCTION

Medical textbooks usually begin with the disclaimer "Medicine is an ever-changing science, with new information being added on a regular basis. The reader is advised to verify the validity of the information provided in light of constant changes." This oft-neglected guidance is extremely important as there is now a steady and sure movement away from traditional repositories of knowledge (such as physical/paper books and journals), toward an increasingly electronic interface. Textbooks undergo revisions and updating once in a few years, and serve only as a starting point for information; hence online resources are relied upon and encouraged by many institutions. In-person seminars are also being replaced by internet-based webinars, as are in-patient consultations. These changes in our understanding of the subject and our practice can be overwhelming for the student and the reader.

This chapter aims to decode EBM and stimulate the student to pose the inquisitive question "Is this evidence-based?" while reading any medical text. Exciting changes occurring at the intersection between information technology and medicine are also addressed in Medical Informatics. We hope this chapter provides the student "a lens" through which the rest of this textbook can be viewed.

EVIDENCE-BASED MEDICINE

Definitions

Evidence-based medicine has been defined as *"the use of scientific methods to organize and apply current data to improve health care decisions. Thus, the best available science is combined with the healthcare professional's clinical experience and the patient's values to arrive at the best medical decision for the patient".*[1]

Evidence-based medicine can also be defined as *"the conscientious, explicit, judicious and reasonable use of modern, best evidence in making decisions about the care of individual patients".*[2]

The three key elements of an EBM approach are shown in **Figure 1**.

1. *Good clinical expertise*: This refers to "what the clinician knows". This mainly relates to the competency of each individual clinician, which is irreplaceable and is learnt over years of practice.
2. *Patient preferences and values*: This refers to "what the patient is desirous of". Consenting to the type of the treatment forms the crux of the matter.
   While these two concepts are being learned constantly, the third concept is a relatively new one.

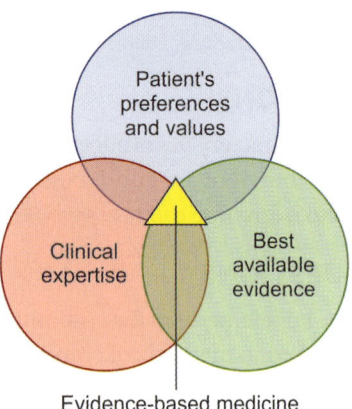

Fig. 1: Evidence-based medicine (EBM) triad.

3. *Best available evidence from research*: This is the major addition to the field and refers to how the healthcare provider can utilize constantly evolving data and information to best serve the patient.

The term "evidence-based medicine" was first introduced by the pioneering clinician epidemiologist David Sackett, at the McMaster Medical School, Canada.[3] It was a gradual movement which attempted to increase the quality of clinical research and help in better decision making. For most of the 20th century, medicine "trusted in the experts". The EBM movement helped in changing the mindset toward "trust in the numbers". The biggest change is the introduction of systematic reviews, with the ability to identify individual studies which are similar and of good quality, and interpret them after combining them. Thus, the conclusions are drawn from a larger number.

Levels of Evidence

The level of evidence, which is now a standard nomenclature, is available as an essential information in most guideline documents/textbooks and is summarized in **Table 1**.[4]

There is a clear hierarchy among the different types of studies **(Fig. 2)** and their corresponding levels of EBM. Individual case reports and case series of a few patients do not help in drawing any particular conclusions. These form the bottom of the pyramid. Next are case-control studies and cohort studies. While they answer questions pertaining to the epidemiology, risk factors and associations of a condition, they cannot provide specific clinical guidance, and may in fact, be biased in study design and methodology. A correctly conducted randomized controlled trial (RCT) is the gold standard of EBM. A group of patients having a particular clinical condition are subjected to two different management modalities, in a systematic manner. The data of the clinical outcomes are analyzed by an impartial observer,

TABLE 1: Levels of evidence.

Level	Components	Comments
1++	Meta-analysis of high quality, systematic reviews of RCTs or RCTs with a very low risk of bias	• Properly-conducted RCTs when repeated and combined in meta-analysis yield the strongest results • *The properly-conducted RCT is considered the gold standard in medicine*
1+	Meta-analysis, systematic reviews of RCTs or RCTs with a low risk of bias	
1–	Meta-analysis, systematic reviews of RCTs or RCTs with a high risk of bias	
Level 2++	High-quality systematic reviews of case-control or cohort studies or high-quality case-control or cohort studies with a very low risk of confounding, bias or chance and a high probability that the relationship is causal	• Introduction of bias is possible when there is no randomization • Some topics in medicine cannot be addressed ethically or effectively by randomization (inability to take a control group)
Level 2+	Well-conducted case-control or cohort studies with a low risk of confounding, bias or chance and a moderate probability that the relationship is causal	
Level 2–	Case-control or cohort studies with a high risk of confounding, bias or chance and a significant risk that the relationship is not causal	
Level 3	Nonanalytical; nonexperimental study such as case-series. A poorly-designed case-control or cohort study also features here	Control groups or cohorts are not possible in some rare diseases or occasional occurrences
Level 4	Expert opinion from respected authorities on the subject	Extreme level of inter-expert heterogeneity is possible

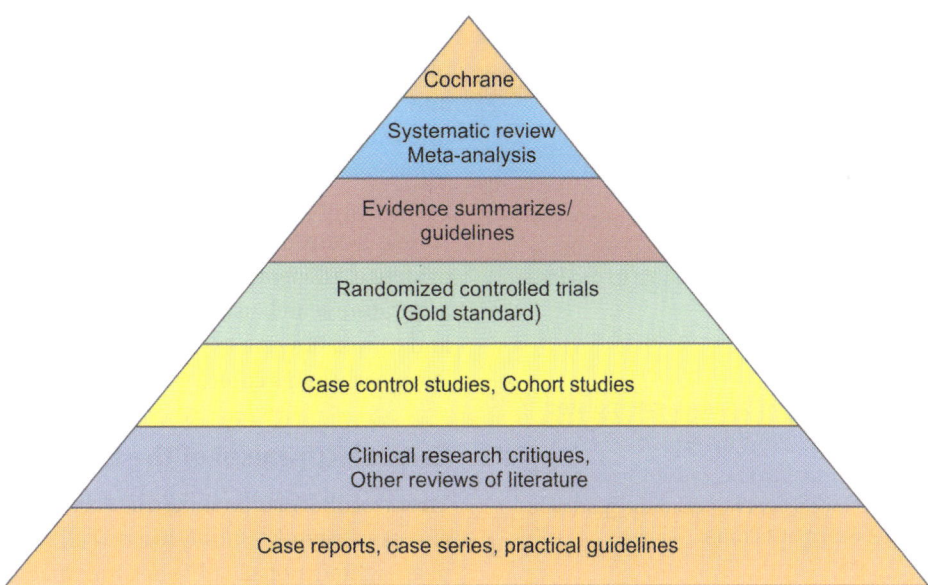

Fig. 2: Evidence pyramid (types of research).

and the results of such a study are considered to be "Level 1 evidence" **(Table 1)**. A nonstatistical collation of the results of various RCTs presented as evidence summaries and clinical guidelines are inferior to systematic reviews. Meta-analysis and systematic reviews, which bring all available information on the subject together, form the apex of the pyramid or the highest level of evidence.

Grading of Recommendations

In any particular subject, each recommendation is assigned a particular grade based on the level of evidence available. The higher the grade of recommendation, the stronger is the support given by the body of evidence available. Grading of evidence is shown in **Table 2**. Various international bodies and institutions develop guidelines systematically using standardized methodology after reviewing all the available literature. For example, the Royal College of Obstetricians and Gynaecologists (RCOG) defines "clinical guidelines" as *"systematically developed statements which assist clinicians and patients in making decisions about appropriate treatment for specific conditions"*. Details about how these guidelines are developed and kept transparent are also published.

Effective Utilization of Evidence-based Medicine

Incorporating EBM is a lifelong process, which is self-directed, and is a problem-based approach while caring for one's patients. An effective method of utilizing EBM in practice is summarized in **Figure 3**. Apart from the clinical skills that are acquired to manage patients, the EBM movement requires the clinician to be able to:

- Use summary of evidence in clinical practice
- Help in development and updating of systematic reviews or guidelines in their specific areas
- Enrol patients in studies to eventually help in generation of better evidence.

TABLE 2: Grades of recommendation.

Grade of recommendation	Interpretation
A	At least one meta-analysis, systematic review or randomized controlled trial rated as 1++. A systematic review of RCTs or a group of evidence composed of studies rated as 1+. These should be applicable to the population concerned. There should be overall consistency of results
B	• Evidence from studies which are 2++ with overall consistency of results. This should be applicable to the population concerned • Evidence extrapolated from studies ranked as 1++ or 1+
C	• Evidence from studies which are 2+ with overall consistency of results. This should be applicable to the target population • Extrapolated evidence from studies rated as 2++
D	Evidence level 3 or 4; or extrapolated evidence from studies rated as 2+
Good practice point (GPP)	Recommended best practice based on the clinical experience of the guideline development group

Types of Questions Answered by Evidence-based Medicine

- *Therapy question*: In pregnant women with hypertension of 160/110 mm Hg, is labetalol a better choice than nifedipine?
- *Prognosis question*: Does the use of alpha methyldopa among preeclamptic women have any implication on postpartum psychosis?
- *Diagnosis question*: Is 24-hour urine albumin mandatory to achieve a diagnosis of preeclampsia?
- *Harm question*: Does preconceptional smoking increase the risk of development of preeclampsia?

It is advisable to fit any clinical question into a PICO (patient/population, intervention, comparison/control, and outcome) format, which is illustrated with examples in **Table 3**.[5]

Acquisition of Best Evidence

While textbooks form the best source of consolidated evidence, by the time they are published, medical science may already be outdated. Hence, an electronic search of available literature is the preferred method for the latest updated evidence. Cochrane review, disseminated by Cochrane Database, is a charitable independent group which focuses on systematically reviewing the available health care information and facilitating evidence-based health interventions. Scores of health care scientists and volunteers contribute to the evidence generation in an impartial manner. The motto of Cochrane, "*Trusted Evidence, Informed Decisions, Better Health*" is the embodiment of EBM. For any particular subject or intervention, a Cochrane review is considered equivalent to the highest possible level of evidence. Efficient and correct use of search engines to perform a literature search using resources such as PubMed, UpToDate, and ClinicalKey are essential skills which the clinician should learn early in his career.

Critical Appraisal of the Evidence

The ideal information should be valid, relevant, comprehensive, and user-friendly. Blindly trusting all published information is near-sighted; not all published material is of equal importance or value.

Ensuring the Correct Perspective of Evidence-based Medicine

The intention of clinical recommendations is *not* to "dictate" a singular course of treatment or management. However, these recommendations should be utilized after a critical evaluation with special reference to each individual patient's needs and resources. The clinician should exercise judgment and understanding of the limitations which prevail in their respective institution(s) and local population variations. It is important to explain to the patient the evidence-based rationale behind a particular treatment modality.[6]

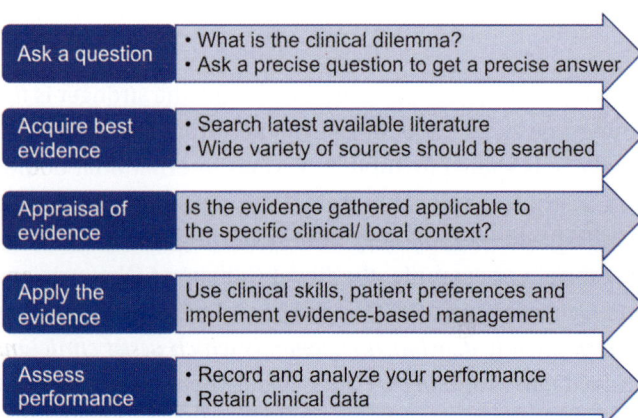

Fig. 3: Steps in utilizing evidence-based medicine.

TABLE 3: Constructing a question using the PICO format.

P—Patient/Population	I—Intervention	C—Comparison	O—Outcome
Who?	What?	Alternative intervention?	Outcomes
To which group would this patient be described as belonging to?	Which treatment, test or other intervention is being considered for this patient/group	• Is there an existing gold standard? • What other treatment or test exists or perhaps to doing nothing	What are the patient-oriented outcomes? Better survival? Better prognosis? Higher rate of cure? etc.
Examples			
Patients with preeclampsia beyond 37 weeks of gestation	Induction of labor	Watchful expectancy	Occurrence of eclampsia/maternal morbidity/maternal mortality
Patients with polycystic ovary syndrome (PCOS) with infertility	Ovulation induction with letrozole	Ovulation induction with clomiphene	Documentation of ovulation, chemical pregnancy rate, clinical pregnancy rate, live birth
Patients with stage III epithelial ovarian cancer	Neoadjuvant chemotherapy followed by operative procedure	Operative procedure	Success at debulking, residual disease, 1-year survival, 5-year survival

Challenges in the Everyday Application of Evidence-based Medicine[7]

Inability to Subject Every Aspect of Medicine to an RCT

"If truth speaks for itself, why do you have to test it with the nontruth?"

Though RCT is the gold standard, no formal RCT has been conducted to prove the efficacy of Pap smear in preventing cancer cervix. Subjecting patients who have an open wound to an RCT comparing suturing and nonsuturing is never possible. Clinical medicine offers many such scenarios. It is absurd to say that the level of evidence and grade of recommendation regarding such "obvious" clinical practice are "poor".

Statistical Jingo, Mathematical Absurdity, and Extrapolative Fallacies

"I chose to study biology and medicine, because I knew I was weak in Math."

"If there is indeed a difference between the two groups, no statistical test should be required to prove the difference."

In most higher levels of evidence, there is a definite reliance on statistical formula and tests of significance, proving either difference or similarity. However, one should refrain from blindly trusting any result as "the absolute proof" if the statistical cutoff p value < 0.05 is reached.

There are a few infamous and controversial examples of how even a statistically significant yet realistically small difference has been blown out of proportion and brought in rather major changes in clinical practice. For example, use of tamoxifen and aromatase inhibitors in breast cancer was found to have similar survival rates. However, the disease-free survival period was slightly better with aromatase inhibitors. Though this is an unmissable statistical derivation, it means little to the patient. Notwithstanding this, multiple publications favored the replacement of tamoxifen by aromatase inhibitor, which is considered unjustified, in retrospect.

Publication Bias

"We do not know what we do not see."

The process involved from the generation of data up to appearance in scientific literature leads to a host of possibilities of bias. Once analysis is done, if the result is "positive", there is a tendency to hasten its submission. Upon submission, "positive" results have higher chance of acceptance by journals. On the contrary, "negative" results tend to be abandoned, and not worked upon further for publication. Even if it is eventually submitted to journals, a lot of time has elapsed. Even after submission, the chance of acceptance is diminished. All these constitute "publication bias".

"In Situ" Publication Bias

"If I choose not to show, you do not get to see."

Researchers are free to analyze the specific parameters that they wish to analyze, and hence this leads to writing up of only that data which the researcher feels relevant and important. The overall picture tends to be narrow-visioned, because a lot of what has to be presented lies shelved in the researcher's drawers.

Many initiatives have been taken to reduce such publication bias. This includes mandatory registration of clinical trial protocols with trial registries. This ensures that every protocol which is registered is analyzed and the details published within a given time frame.

■ MEDICAL INFORMATICS

The standard dictionary definition of "informatics" is *"the sciences concerned with gathering and manipulating and storing and retrieving and classifying recorded information"*. Hence, medical informatics can be regarded as "an interdisciplinary field combining systematic processing of data, information and knowledge in medicine and health care".

The definitions can vary and depend on the specific subfield they relate to. For example, clinical informatics will refer to the activities pertaining to clinical information; "pathology informatics" referring to pathological laboratory data, etc.[8]

Types of Data

Before we can make sense of what informatics systems can do with data, it is important to identify what types of data can be collected. **Table 4** lists the various types of data, which we clinicians are otherwise familiar with.[9] **Figure 4** shows the differences between the traditional model and the "informatics" model of medical data handing.

Advantages of Electronic Health Informatics

The health informatics evolution promises changes such as efficiency, EBM, enhancement of quality of care, etc. which are summarized in **Figure 5**.[10]

■ ARTIFICIAL INTELLIGENCE

Artificial intelligence is simply defined as "*the ability of machines to learn and display intelligence*". Such intelligence may be in stark contrast to the "natural" intelligence which is demonstrated by humans and animals.

The rise of artificial intelligence is supported by the rise of computer power, vast amounts of memory, ability to store data securely; this has led to the successful handling of increasingly complex learning tasks. Speech recognition, face recognition, advanced gaming, voice assistants, and self-driving vehicles are some examples.

The exponential rise in the volume of biomedical data generated has led to clinicians grappling with how to make sense of this vast data; the best way to deal with this is to automatism it using artificial intelligence systems.[11]

Computer Calculations versus Artificial Intelligence

The difference between simple use of mathematical calculators and artificial intelligence is vast. Mathematical

TABLE 4: Types of clinical data.

Type of data	Brief description
Survey	• Includes questionnaires or survey tools • It may be target-specific or population-specific
Admission data/Discharge data	Includes the demographic and treatment details of patients admitted in a healthcare facility
Administrative data/Claims data	Includes the details of patients who have submitted their records for the purpose of reimbursement or otherwise
Registries	Includes details of patients suffering from a particular condition, e.g., cancer registry
Population data	• Includes (basic) information about the entire population • Birth and Death registration is one example
Electronic medical record	Includes the details of all complaints, evaluation, consultations, advice, interventions and improvement of individuals involved in one particular institution

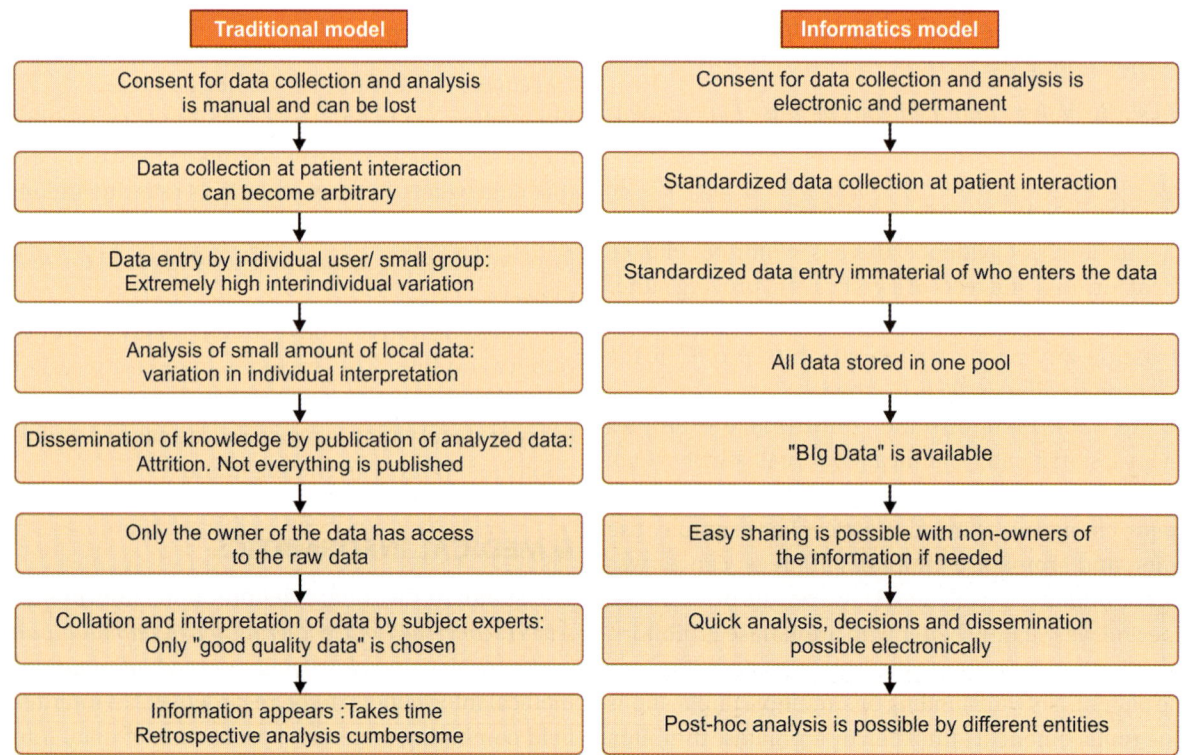

Fig. 4: Traditional and informatics model of healthcare information processing.

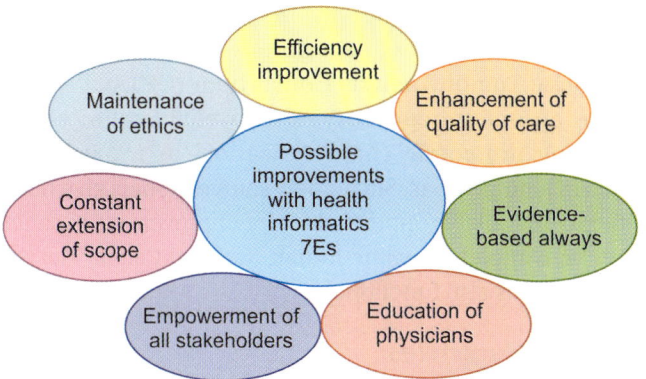

Fig. 5: Possible improvements with health informatics.

models enable computerized programs to identify patterns which are present in voluminous and complex data entities automatically. These are then used to make predictions and prognostications, important for clinicians. In traditional computer-based statistics, the main objective is to merely estimate the disease condition and score the severity or classify the disease conditions. However, machine learning has the ability to build on automated clinical decisions for the optimal management of conditions. This assists doctors to solve clinical problems. The accuracy of the model improves when more data is inputted. Supervised learning, unsupervised learning, self-learning, artificial neural networks, decision trees, and support vector machines are some examples of machine learning modes.

■ MEDICAL SIMULATION TECHNOLOGY

Simulation technology development is an important offshoot of medical informatics. The Medical Council of India (MCI) is also promoting and emphasizing the use of simulation technology for teaching undergraduates and postgraduates. The steady advances in patient activism and unfavorable teacher:patient:student ratios make simulation-based teaching imperative. Readers are encouraged to get accustomed to this exciting field of medical education. The flipside of utilization of applications such as YouTube, where vast amount of material may be available, is that there may be loss of authenticity and accuracy.

■ ELECTRONIC HEALTH RECORD

Though not exhaustive, a list of the components of an electronic health record (EHR) is mentioned in **Figure 6**. The ideal EHR allows for flexibility and inclusion of information pertaining to specific problems such as maternal conditions, neonatal outcomes, etc. Since pregnancy has both a discrete starting and ending point, obstetrics is one field where accuracy of EHR can be easily achieved.[12]

Ensuring Uniformity and Interuser Portability of Health Information and the Indian Perspective

One of the major disadvantages of the traditional method of health information process is the arbitrary manner in which

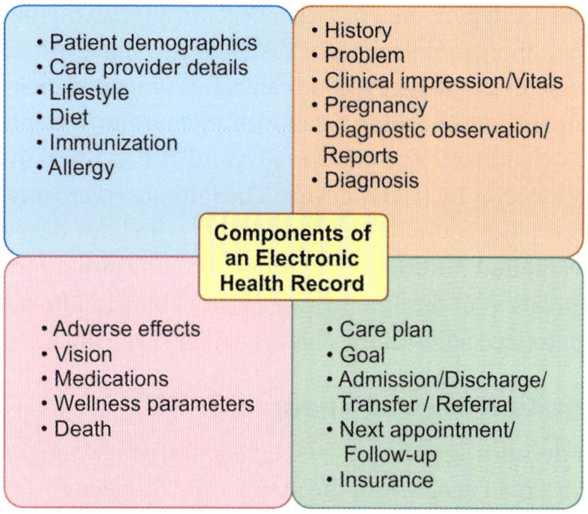

Fig. 6: Components of an electronic health record.

TABLE 5: Data sets and suggested standards.

Data gathered	Suggested standard
Structured clinical information exchange	Fast Healthcare Interoperability Resources® (FHIR 4)
Clinical terminology	SNOMED CT
Coding system for diseases	ICD-10
Laboratory measurements, test-panels, etc.	LOINC
Still images	JPEG
Documents	PDF
Audio/Video	MP3 (OGG)/MP4 (MOV)
Radiological investigations	DICOM

data is collected. However, the informatics approach can also be plagued by arbitrariness if uniformity is not maintained. Successfully classifying "cause of death" was one of the initial successes of medical informatics. The use of the International Classification of Diseases (ICD), with its regular modifications, greatly helped in ensuring uniformity.

Now, each and every data set of health care informatics should undergo standardization **(Table 5)**, as promulgated by the Ministry of Health and Family Welfare's (MoHFW) National Digital Health Blueprint 2017. This blueprint envisages "creation of a national digital health ecosystem that supports universal health coverage in an efficient, accessible, inclusive, affordable, timely, and safe manner, through provision of a wide-range of data, information and infrastructure services, duly leveraging open, interoperable, standards-based digital systems, and ensuring the security, confidentiality and privacy of health-related personal information".[13]

■ POSITIVE IMPACT BY INFORMATICS ON OBSTETRIC AND GYNAECOLOGICAL PRACTICE

Cardiotocography/Electronic Fetal Monitoring

Conventional electronic fetal monitoring uses paper tracings and human visual interpretation.

Can the dependence on paper be reduced? Can this be done on a handheld mobile device? Yes. Das et al.[14] have proved in a Indian setting that there is good clinical accuracy and inter-rater agreement between interpretation of antepartum/intrapartum traces visualized conventionally and those on a mobile cardiotocography (CTG) device. The interobserver variability has been overcome by Sbrollini et al.,[15] who have developed and validated automatic identification, interpretation, and classification of fetal heart rate (FHR) abnormalities using computerized algorithms. This is a rapidly evolving field.

Estimation of Fetal Aneuploidy Risk

A few decades ago, the only risk estimation of fetal aneuploidy was based on age. One of the major areas of success of health informatics is in the prediction of fetal aneuploidy risk. Using demographic, physical (examination), ultrasonographic, and biochemical parameters, multiple statistical analytics are done to determine risk ratios. However, it should be noted that machine learning approaches are likely to be even better than the conventional informatics approach.[16]

Cervical Cancer Screening

Cervical cancer screening has moved on from conventional smears to liquid-based cytology (LBC). Lack of skilled manpower has been cited as a major reason for inadequate coverage of screening. Feasibility of screening of patients at remote locations using smartphones by nurses has been demonstrated by Sharma et al.[17] One skilled cytologist using a centralized computer can analyze thousands of images generated at different locations, enabling better coverage. Machine learning approaches are being studied and have been proven to be more accurate in Indian settings.[18]

Male Infertility

For over half a century, diagnosis has relied upon manual visual counting of spermatozoa of semen smeared over a slide. Computer-assisted analysis has helped recreate the volumetric three-dimensional spaces similar to the intrauterine milieu. This method has much higher accuracy than conventional analysis.[19] Here again, machine learning models are in the nascent stage and further expansion is expected in the subject.[20]

Carcinoma Ovary

The development of a vast database of the molecular and genomic variations in serous ovarian cancer is a major contribution of medical informatics to our field. "Individuals with similarities in genetic makeup tend to respond better with some specific chemotherapeutic agents than the others"—is the simple principle applied. This is an example for "personalized medicine" or "precision medicine".[21] This individualization of treatment based on patient characteristics not only helps in improving accuracy, prevention of side effects but also in reduction of economic burden.

The application of "big data" in this context is exemplified by the establishment of data portals such as the "Clinical Proteomic Tumor Analysis Consortium (CPTAC)" portal. This is an online repository of all available clinical data including proteomic characterization, as a part of the Cancer Genome Atlas. Such open-source models give rise to hitherto unavailable opportunities for improvement of patient care.[22] A completely online Indian National Cancer Registry Programme is also functional.[23]

National Registries

A contemporary example of the use of informatics in developing good data is the barrage of minute-by-minute facts and figures available online about the coronavirus disease 2019 (COVID-19) pandemic. To this end, FOGSI's National Registry on COVID-19 Infection in Pregnancy is an excellent tool which could be developed rapidly only due to informatics.[24]

■ TELEMEDICINE

Telemedicine can be defined as the "healthcare service delivery, distance being a critical factor, provided by healthcare professionals by utilizing information and communication technologies for the exchange of reliable information for diagnosis, management, and prevention of disease". Telemedicine is the result of enhanced penetration of informatics into both the medical field and ease of availability by the population. The obvious advantages are quicker access to services, better healthcare delivery in remote areas, and feasible option during accidents, epidemics, and disasters. While in some situations like chronic diseases, long-term dependence on telemedicine is possible by interlinking patients, physicians, laboratories, and pharmacies; in some situations, like hypoglycemic episodes, short-term usage is appropriate. Telemedicine can be administered using short messaging services (SMS), voice messages over the phone, livestreaming over internet or suitable application platforms, or via email.

The National Medical Commission (erstwhile MCI) have published the "*Telemedicine Practice Guidelines: Enabling Registered Medical Practitioners to Provide Healthcare Using Telemedicine*" in March 2020.[25]

In this elaborate document, detailed definitions of the terms "telemedicine" and "telehealth" are provided. It is summarized that most consultations are in the form of:
- Providing health education as appropriate in the case; and/or
- Providing counseling related to specific clinical condition; and/or
- Prescription of medicines

The various tools for telemedicine are enumerated and a classification is provided:
- Based on the mode of communication (video/audio/text based)

- Timing of transmission of information [real-time (immediate)/asynchronous (late)]
- The purpose of the consultation (emergency/nonemergency)
- Interaction between the individuals [patient to Registered Medical Practitioner (RMP)/RMP to RMP/caregiver to RMP, etc.)].

Some salient principles that are to be kept in mind when using telemedicine are listed:

- Accurate identification of the patient using digital information like phone number/email ID is needed.
- Accurate verification of the doctors' details such as qualifications and registration number is needed.
- Ascertaining that the patient is willing to abide for advice suggesting an in-person referral if the doctor deems fit, and in situations such as life-threatening emergencies, in-person consultation is needed.
- An appropriate form of consent (implied if patient initiates the consultation) has to be ensured.
- Adherence to the explicit details regarding medicine prescription should be ensured.
- Adherence to the tenets regarding medical ethics, data privacy (with respect to images and videos) and confidentiality should hold importance.

The strengths and limitations based on technical, financial, and feasibility issues are explained in the guideline. The commission has also proposed a compulsory training in telemedicine for all RMPs. Immaterial of which technological platform is used for communicating with the patient, the basic tenets of medical ethics which govern in-patient consultations, should be adhered to at all times. All RMPs are encouraged to familiarize themselves with this important document.[25]

CONCLUSION

Understanding the levels of EBM and learning how to utilize the available information is an essential skill set which should be learned by every practicing clinician. As the world uses digital platforms for more and more aspects of daily life, advances in information technology should also be assimilated and incorporated by every practitioner.

KEY MESSAGES

The singular aim of clinicians is to offer the best care to their patients. Evidence-based medicine (EBM) is a systematic collation and rational presentation of clinical information gathered in settings all over the world. Simply put, it aims at answering questions like "In this patient, what works; what does not work?" EBM is "a lens" through which all medical information should be viewed. The use of modern advances in information technology in the improvement of patient care is "medical informatics". The modern doctor should acquaint himself and embrace the exciting changes in this field.

REFERENCES

1. Tenny S, Varacallo M. Evidence Based Medicine. In: StatPearls [Internet]. Treasure Island (FL): StatPearls Publishing; 2021.
2. Masic I, Miokovic M, Muhamedagic B. Evidence-based medicine—new approaches and challenges. Acta Inform Med. 2008;16(4):219-25.
3. Thoma A, Eaves FF 3rd. A brief history of evidence-based medicine (EBM) and the contributions of Dr David Sackett. Aesthet Surg J. 2015;35(8):NP261-3.
4. Royal College of Obstetricians and Gynaecologists. Green-top guideline development. [online] Available from: http://www.rcog.org.uk/green-top-development [Last accessed September, 2021].
5. Ford LG. Melnyk BM. The underappreciated and misunderstood PICOT question: a critical step in the EBP process. Worldviews Evid Based Nurs. 2019;16(6):422-3.
6. Jassem J. Bright and dark sides of evidence-based Medicine. Pol Arch Med Wewn. 2016;126(5):347-52.
7. Braithwaite RS. Evidence-based medicine: clinicians are taught to say it but not taught to think it. BMJ Evid Based Med. 2019;24(5):165-7.
8. Medical informatics. [online] Available from: https://www.wikilectures.eu/w/Medical_Informatics [Last accessed September, 2021].
9. Goodin A, Delcher C, Valenzuela C, Wang X, Zhu Y, Roussos-Ross D, et al. The power and pitfalls of big data research in obstetrics and gynecology: a consumer's guide. Obstet Gynecol Surv. 2017;72(11):669-82.
10. Emerging into E-health information management. [online] Available from: https://www.slideshare.net/katnick56/emerging-into-ehealth-information-management [Last accessed September, 2021].
11. Wang R, Pan W, Jin L, Li Y, Geng Y, Gao C, et al. Artificial intelligence in reproductive medicine. Reproduction. 2019;158:R139-54.
12. Ministry of Electronics and Information Technology, Government of India. National digital health blueprint. [online] Available from: https://www.meity.gov.in/DeitY_e-book/e-gov_policy/download/Policy%20Document.pdf [Last accessed September, 2021].
13. Ministry of Health and Family Welfare, Government of India. Electronic health record standards - 2016 for India. [online] Available from: https://www.nhp.gov.in/NHPfiles/EHR-Standards-2016-MoHFW.pdf [Last accessed September, 2021].
14. Das MK, Tripathi R, Kashyap NK, Fotedar S, Bisht SS, Rathore AM, et al. Clinical validation of mobile cardiotocograph device for intrapartum and antepartum monitoring compared to standard cardiotocograph: an Inter-Rater Agreement Study. J Family Reprod Health. 2019;13(2):109-15.
15. Sbrollini A, Carnicelli A, Massacci A, Tomaiuolo L, Zara T, Marcantoni I, et al. Automatic identification and classification of fetal heart rate decelerations from cardiotocographic recordings. Annu Int Conf IEEE Eng Med Biol Soc. 2018;2018:474-7.
16. Yang J, Ding X, Zhu W. Improving the calling of non-invasive prenatal testing on 13-/18-/21-trisomy by support vector machine discrimination. PLoS One. 2018;13(12):e0207840.
17. Sharma D, Rohilla L, Bagga R, Srinivasan R, Jindal HA, Sharma N, et al. Feasibility of implementing cervical cancer screening program using smartphone imaging as a training aid for nurses in rural India. Public Health Nurs. 2018;35(6):526-33.

18. Kudva V, Prasad K, Guruvare S. Automation of detection of cervical cancer using convolutional neural networks. Crit Rev Biomed Eng. 2018;46(2):135-45.
19. Talarczyk-Desole J, Berger A, Taszarek-Hauke G, Hauke J, Pawelczyk L, Jedrzejczak P. Manual vs. computer-assisted sperm analysis: can CASA replace manual assessment of human semen in clinical practice? Ginekol Pol. 2017;88(2):56-60.
20. Goodson SG, White S, Stevans AM, Bhat S, Kao CY, Jaworski S, et al. CASAnova: a multiclass support vector machine model for the classification of human sperm motility patterns. Biol Reprod. 2017;97(5):698-708.
21. Cojocaru E, Parkinson CA, Brenton JD. Personalising treatment for high-grade serous ovarian carcinoma. Clin Oncol (R Coll Radiol). 2018;30(8):515-24.
22. Edwards NJ, Oberti M, Thangudu RR, Cai S, McGarvey PB, Jacob S, et al. The CPTAC data portal: a resource for cancer proteomics research. J Proteome Res. 2015;14(6):2707-13.
23. National Cancer Registry Programme (Indian Council of Medical Research). Development of an Atlas of Cancer in India. [online] Available from: http://www.ncdirindia.org/ncrp/ca/about.aspx. [Last accessed September, 2021].
24. FOGSI's National Registry on COVID-19 Infection in Pregnancy. [online] Available from: https://www.fogsi.org/fogsi-national-registry-on-covid-19-infection-in-pregnancy/ [Last accessed September, 2021].
25. Ministry of Health and Family Welfare, Government of India. Telemedicine Practice Guidelines: Enabling Registered Medical Practitioners to Provide Healthcare Using Telemedicine. [online] Available from: https://www.mohfw.gov.in/pdf/Telemedicine.pdf [Last accessed September, 2021].

■ LONG QUESTIONS

1. What is evidence based medicine? What is meant by Levels of Evidence? Discuss the advantages, disadvantages and problems in applications of evidence based medicine in daily clinical practice.
2. What is a Randomized Controlled Trial? What are the features of a well-conducted Randomized Controlled Trial? Explain using practical clinical examples.

■ SHORT QUESTIONS

1. Discuss the role of information technology in medicine, with specific reference to obstetrics and gynaecology.
2. Evidence pyramid.
3. Publication bias.

■ MULTIPLE CHOICE QUESTIONS

1. The following are components of the Evidence Based Medicine Triad, except:
   a. Good Clinical Expertise
   b. Patient preferences and values
   c. Availability of medico-legal consultant
   d. Best available evidence from research
2. All statements about EBM are true, except:
   a. Introduced by Prof David Sackett in Canada
   b. Focusses on "trusting the experts"
   c. Focusses on "trusting the numbers"
   d. Is a gradual movement rather than a revolutionary change
3. Which of the following is true?
   a. Case series provide a good guide to clinical management of common conditions
   b. Case control studies are appropriate for rare diseases
   c. Retrospective study designs are equivalent to prospective study designs
   d. Expert opinions are usually consistent and homogenous
4. Which of the following is false?
   a. Randomized controlled trials form the "gold standard" in Evidence Based Medicine
   b. All topics in medicine can be resolved by Randomized Controlled Trials
   c. Systematic review of RCTs form the highest level of evidence available
   d. It is possible to classify different RCTs as having high probability of bias or lesser probability of bias
5. While obtaining the best evidence all these steps should be followed, except:
   a. Narrow down the clinical dilemmas into precise questions
   b. Fit the question into a PICOT format
   c. Search for evidence from the single best source
   d. Check for applicability of evidence obtained in the local setting
6. A clinician wants to check the usefulness of a new antihypertensive drug for management of preeclampsia. Regarding generation of good quality evidence, which one of the following statements is appropriate?
   a. Interviewing of many experts and noting their views and opinions about how the drug has performed in their patients is likely to yield good quality evidence
   b. Analysis of the clinical records of patients who have used the drug in the past one year is likely to yield the best evidence
   c. It would be acceptable to start the new antihypertensive drug for all forthcoming patients to generate good quality evidence
   d. Allocating few patients to the new drug and other patients to the existing gold standard drug is likely to generate good quality evidence
7. Artificial Intelligence/Machine Learning. Find the false statement:
   a. They can analyze patterns, predict and prognosticate clinical conditions
   b. There is standardization in data entry and data output.
   c. Data access is possible at locations by multiple individuals
   d. Providing more data reduces the accuracy of the machine learning process
8. All are true about Telemedicine, except:
   a. It ensures accessibility to remote areas also
   b. It should be preferred during epidemic

c. The usual tenets of ethical practice in medicine are applicable
d. It should not be used for chronic diseases.
9. While reading and evaluating a published scientific medical article, which is appropriate:
    a. All published material should be given equal merit and accepted unconditionally
    b. It is acceptable to skip reading the analysis and look into only the conclusions
    c. Evidence generated on patients of different population groups should be extrapolated to local population with utmost caution
    d. A statistical significance of p<0.05 is considered absolute mathematical proof
10. With respect to the PICO methodology of forming a research question, choose the correct combination:
    a. P-Population, I-Information, C-Comparison, O-Outcome
    b. P-Population, I-Intervention, C-Comparison, O-Outcome
    c. P-Population, I-Information, C-Complication, O-Outcome
    d. P-Population, I-Intervention, C-Complication, O-Outcome

Answers
1. c 2. b 3. b 4. b 5. c 6. d
7. d 8. d 9. c 10. b

1.4 GOOD CLINICAL PRACTICE AND RESEARCH METHODOLOGY FOR OBSTETRICIANS

Ramalingappa C Antaratani, Sanjana K

■ INTRODUCTION

Today, clinical research is a necessity to establish the safety and efficacy of medical products and practices. All that we have known about the medical products or treatments have come from randomized control clinical trials. A general definition of human research is—"Any proposal related to human subjects including healthy volunteers that cannot be considered as a part of accepted clinical management or public health practice and the one that involves either physical or psychological intervention or observation; or collection, storage or dissemination of information related to individuals".[1] Before medical products are introduced to the market or to public health programs, they must undergo a series of investigations designed to evaluate the safety and efficacy and detailed information on the method of administration, dosage, contraindications, warnings, precautions, interactions, and safely information has to be documented.

The research work can be relied upon only if they have been conducted as per the principles and standards collectively known as "Good clinical research practice" (GCP). The responsibility of GCP is to be shared by the sponsors, investigators, site staff, contract research organizations (CROs), ethical committees, regulatory authorities, and the research subjects.

■ DEFINITION OF GOOD CLINICAL PRACTICE

Good clinical practice is an international ethical and scientific quality standard for designing, conduct, performance, monitoring, recording, auditing, analysis, and reporting of clinical trials. GCP assures that data and reported results are credible, accurate and that the rights, integrity, and confidentiality of trial subjects are respected and protected.[2]

■ HISTORY

It is interesting to know why and how the GCP were put forward. Like it is said "curiosity is the mother of discoveries", many curious and enthusiastic researchers since a very long time carried out experiments on humans and animals. On a negative note, this led to disastrous effects on mankind including death due to unregulated and unlawful research activities. This made laws for carrying out research very much necessary. The events that led to the acts and the acts perse have been chronologically tabulated in **Table 1**.

■ INTERNATIONAL COUNCIL FOR HARMONISATION-GOOD CLINICAL PRACTICE

The International Council for Harmonisation-Good Clinical Practice (ICH-GCP) is defined as a harmonized standard that protects the rights, safety, and welfare of human subjects, minimizes the exposure of human beings to investigational products, improves the quality of data, speeds up marketing of new drugs and decreases the cost to sponsors as well as to the public.

■ REASONS FOR GOOD CLINICAL PRACTICE

- Increase in ethical awareness among the people
- Improved methods of clinical trials
- Better understanding of concept of clinical trial
- Public or political concern over the aspects of safety
- Frauds and accidents during the clinical trials
- Increasing research and development costs
- Increasing competition
- Mutual recognition of data
- New market structure.

TABLE 1: History of good clinical practice (GCP) recommendations.

S. No	Year	Landmark act/declaration	Events that forced the act	Laws laid down by the act
1.	460 BC	The Hippocratic oath		Brought out the concept of "Good physician"
2.	1906	Food and drugs act	Over the counter sale of harmful and lethal drugs in the United States	
3.	1930	US Food, Drugs, And Cosmetic Act		Compulsory testing of drugs for safety before marketing
4.	1947	Nuremberg code[3]	Unethical and horrific experiments conducted during World War II at Nazi war camps	Need for scientific basis in research on human subjects and voluntary consent
5.	1948	Declaration of Human Rights	Atrocities of World War II	Further reiterated the human factor involved in medical experiments
6.	1962	Kefauver–Harris amendment	Severe fetal limb deformities linked to the use of maternal thalidomide	Required the Food and Drug Administration (FDA) to evaluate all new drugs for safety and efficacy
7.	1964	Declaration of Helsinki by the World Medical Association[4]		Statement of ethical principles to provide guidance to physicians and participants in Human Research Forms
8.	1979	The Belmont report[5]	For the protection of human subjects of biomedical research	Laid down principles of respect for people, beneficence, and justice
9.	1982	International guidelines for biomedical research involving human subjects by the World Health Organization (WHO) and the Council for International Organizations of Medical Sciences (CIOMS)		Issued a document entitled "International guidelines for biomedical research involving human subjects"
10.	1996	ICH-GCP guidelines[6]	International GCP inconsistencies	Standards to protect the rights, safety, and welfare of human subjects

PRINCIPLES OF ICH-GCP[6]

- Clinical trials should be conducted in accordance with ethical principles that have their origin from the declaration of Helsinki, and are consistent with GCP.
- Before a trial is initiated, probable risks and inconveniences should be weighed against anticipated benefit for the individual trial subject and society. A trial should be initiated and continued only if the anticipated benefits outweigh the risks.
- The rights, safety, and well-being of the trial subjects are the most important considerations and should be considered over the interest of science and society.
- The available nonclinical as well as clinical information on a particular investigational product should be adequate to support the proposed clinical trial.
- Clinical trials must be scientifically sound, and need to be described in a clear and detailed protocol.
- A trial should be conducted according to the protocol that has received prior institutional review board (IRB)/independent ethics committee (IEC) approval/favorable opinion.
- The medical care that is given the subjects and medical decisions made on behalf of subjects should always be the responsibility of a qualified physician.
- Each individual involved in conducting a particular trial should be qualified by education, training, and experience to perform his or her respective tasks.
- Freely given informed consent from every subject is a must prior to participation in clinical trials.
- The clinical trial information should be recorded, handled, and stored in a way that helps its accurate reporting, interpretation, and verification.
- The confidentiality of records which identify the subjects should be protected hence respecting the privacy and confidentiality of the subjects.
- Investigational products must be manufactured, handled, and stored in accordance with good manufacturing practice (GMP). They must be used in accordance with the approved protocol.
- Systems with procedures that can assure the quality of the trial should be implemented.

Ethical Principles of GCP

The ICH-GCP guidelines are considered the "Bible" of clinical trials and have become a global law which safeguards humanity, it has three basic ethical principles being:

1. Respect for persons
2. Beneficence
3. Justice.

OVERVIEW OF THE CLINICAL RESEARCH PROCESS

The process of clinical research is guided by a sequence of activities for which the sponsors, investigators, ethics committees, and regulatory authorities are collectively responsible. **Table 2** briefly describes the key activities involved in the conduct of a clinical trial and the individuals responsible for each of them.

TRIALS IN OBSTETRICS

Research in pregnant women is associated with scientific, legal, and ethical problems. The physiology of pregnancy changes drastically over weeks, months, and trimesters within and between the maternal body, placenta, and fetus. Attitudes of researchers toward inclusion of women in trials have changed grossly over the past few decades although a gap still exists in the available data on health and disease in pregnant women.

Pregnancy Research: Historical Background of Exclusion

Pregnant women have often been kept away from trials, possible reasons include:
- Fear of harm to the fetus
- Concern about the complicated physiology of pregnant women
- Uncertainty whether pregnant women will consent to participate
- Labeling pregnant women as the "vulnerable" population[7]
- Unfortunately, exclusion of women from clinical trials will perpetuate the paucity of applicable data and force the

TABLE 2: Key activities in conducting a clinical trial.

S. No.	Key trial activity	Responsibility	Details of the activity
1.	Development of trial protocol	Sponsor in consultation with clinical investigators	Risk identification, study design, statistical methodology
2.	Development of standard operating procedures (SOPs)	Sponsors, clinical investigators, ethics committees, institutional review boards, contract research organizations (CROs)	Develop SOPs that define responsibilities, records, and methods to be used for study-related activities
3.	Development of support systems and tools	Sponsor	Tools to facilitate the conduct of the study and collection of data required by the protocol
4.	Generation and approval of trial-related documents	Sponsor	Provision of standardized forms and checklists to assist the clinical investigator to capture and report data
5.	Selection properly qualified, trained, and experienced investigators and study personnel	Sponsor	Sponsors should review the requirements of the study protocol and recruit appropriate staff who are qualified
6.	Ethics committees review and approval of the protocol	Investigator	Study to be reviewed by ethics committee or institutional review board
7.	Review by regulatory authorities	Sponsor	To ensure that the study is appropriately designed to meet its stated objectives
8.	Enrollment of subjects into the study: recruitment, eligibility, and informed consent	Clinical investigator	Eligible subjects are enrolled in the study after taking an informed consent
9.	The investigational product—quality, handling, and accounting	Sponsors	Assured by good manufacturing practices
10.	Trial data acquisition: conducting the trial	Clinical investigator	Research to be conducted according to the approved protocol and regulatory requirements
11.	Safety management and reporting	Clinical investigator Sponsor	Identifying and reporting any adverse events during the trial
12.	Monitoring the trial	Sponsors	Verify adherence to the protocol, ensure ongoing implementation of appropriate data entry, adherence to good clinical practice (GCP)
13.	Managing trial data	Sponsor Investigator	Ensuring the data is complete, reliable, processed correctly and that data integrity is preserved
14.	Quality assurance of the trial performance and data	Sponsors	Verified through systematic, independent audits
15.	Reporting the trial	Sponsors	The results should be summarized and described in an integrated clinical study report

application of male-derived research results to women's health.

Pregnant Women in Clinical Trials

- *Problems with excluding women from research trials*: Though there is concern that including pregnant women in the study of new drugs could harm the fetus, it is also true that excluding pregnant women from research also can lead to considerable harm. The best example that can be quoted in this context is teratogenicity due to thalidomide leading to >10,000 adverse pregnancy outcomes; had it been studied in pregnant women before it was released in the market, the disaster would not have occurred.[8]
Another apt example that can be quoted in the current scenario is the "the exclusion of pregnant and lactating women from coronavirus disease 2019 (COVID-19) vaccine". This represents a missed opportunity for the protection of a huge group at risk for COVID-19 that is—pregnant and puerperal women. This exclusion cannot be justified as Pfizer and Moderna excluded pregnant and lactating women from their mRNA COVID-19 vaccine trial with no evidence to suggest that the vaccine could be teratogenic or could be secreted in breast milk.[9]
- *Nonpregnancy-related interventions that benefit a woman during pregnancy*: With increasing number of pregnancies in old age, there has been a proportionate increase in the incidence of medical disorders in pregnancy. A significant proportion of the pregnant women undergo therapies aimed at managing nonobstetrics medical conditions most of which have not be studied specifically in pregnancy.[10] Had these drugs been adequately studied in pregnant women, we would have an opportunity to balance the risks and benefits of their use.
- *Interventions directly related to pregnancy*: Pregnancy is the only opportunity to conduct studies related to interventions in pregnancy like tocolysis, prevention on preterm birth, and so on. Research during pregnancy and labor is the only way to improve care for women and their newborns.
- *Paternal consent issues*: Consent of the pregnant woman alone is sufficient in most cases whereas, consent of the father is also required in cases where there is a chance of significant benefit or harm to the fetus. However, the regulations regarding this are controversial.[11]
- *Trials on lactating women*: When we consider exposure of a breastfed infant to a risk, the research must not involve "greater than minimal risk" unless the research would provide generalizable knowledge about the child's disorder or condition. All clinical lactational studies should define the risks to the breastfed infant that occur only as a result of the research and obtain informed consent from the lactating woman.

During the Office of Research on Women's Health (ORWH) workshop in 2010, the present status of research involving pregnant women and its future needs were discussed and a few recommendations were put forward:[12]

Recommendation 1: Define Pregnant Women as a Scientifically Complex and Change the Presumption of Exclusion

- Pregnant women should be reclassified from their present status as "vulnerable group" to that as a medically complex population necessitating special scientific and ethical considerations.
- Pregnant women are a dynamic subset of women in whom as physiological changes of pregnancy can alter a drug's pharmacokinetics and efficacy. Treatment of conditions in pregnant women has to optimize results for the maternal-fetal pair.

Recommendation 2: Clarify Existing Regulations and Focus on IRB as it Facilitates or Impedes Pregnancy Research

There is a need for clarifying the regulations governing the inclusion of pregnant women and fetuses in clinical research and for increasing the consistency among IRBs in decision-making procedures.

Recommendation 3: Develop a Pregnancy Research Agenda

- A pregnancy research agenda should include the following: research to promote evidence-based clinical practice, identification of questions that can be addressed with existing data and through ongoing studies, identification of new studies in high scientific impact areas
- Promotion of evidence-based clinical practice
- Capitalizing on existing studies and resources.

LANDMARK TRIALS IN OBSTETRICS

What is a Landmark Trial?

- A trial which has made an impact on our understanding of a disease.
- A trial which has caused a dramatic change in our approach to a clinical condition.
- A trial which has changed our management of a disease.
- A trial which has changed our clinical practice.

The following is a list of some of the landmark trials in obstetrics:

- *Antenatal steroid trial*: A controlled trial of antepartum glucocorticoid treatment for prevention of the respiratory distress syndrome in premature infants (Liggins GC, Howie RN. Pediatrics. 1972;50(4):515-25.) → Early neonatal mortality was found to be 3.2% in the steroid-treated group compared to 15% in the control group.
- *Folic acid supplementation trial*: Prevention of neural tube defects: results of the Medical Research Council

Vitamin Study. MRC Vitamin Study Research Group (Lancet. 1991;338(8760):131-7.) → Concluded that folic acid gives 72% protection against neural tube defects.
- *The eclampsia trial*: Study on the choice of anticonvulsant for women with eclampsia: evidence from the Collaborative Eclampsia Trial. The Eclampsia Trial Collaborative Group (Lancet. 1995:345(8963);1455-63.) → There is compelling evidence for the use of magnesium sulfate over phenytoin or diazepam for eclampsia.
- *MAGPIE trial*: Do women with pre-eclampsia, and their babies, benefit from magnesium sulphate? The Magpie trial: a randomized placebo-controlled trial (Altman D, Carroli G, Duley L, Farrell B, Moodley J, Neilson J, et al. Lancet. 2002;359(9321):1877-90.) → Concluded that magnesium sulfate halves the risk of eclampsia and probably reduces the risk of maternal death.
- *Term breech trial*: Planned cesarean section compared to planned vaginal birth for breech presentation at term: a randomised multicentre trial (Hannah ME, Hannah WJ, Hewson SA, Hodnett ED, Saigal S, Willan AR. Lancet. 2000;356(9239):1375-83.) → Concluded that planned C-section is better than planned vaginal delivery for a term fetus in breech presentation.
- *ASPRE trial*: Combined multimarker screening and randomized patient treatment with low-dose aspirin: evidence-based preeclampsia prevention trial (Rolnik DL, Wright D, Poon LC, Syngelaki A, O'Gorman N, de Paco Matallana C, et al. Ultrasound Obstet Gynecol. 2017;50(4):492-5.) → Estimated detection rate of screening using the stated factors was 77% for preterm preeclampsia and administration of aspirin 150 mg to high-risk group resulted in 62% decrease in the incidence of preterm preeclampsia.

KEY MESSAGES

- Clinical research is a necessity to establish the safety and efficacy of medical products and practices.
- Good clinical practice (GCP) is an international ethical and scientific quality standard for designing, conduct, performance, monitoring, auditing, recording, analysis, and reporting of clinical trials.
- GCP assures that the data and reported results are credible, accurate and that the rights, integrity, and confidentiality of trial subjects are respected and protected.
- The ICH-GCP guidelines have become a global law which safeguards humanity, it has three basic ethical principles being: (1) respect for persons, (2) beneficence, and (3) justice.
- Pregnant women should be reclassified from their present status as "vulnerable group" to that as a medically complex population necessitating special scientific and ethical considerations—research in pregnancy to be encouraged.

REFERENCES

1. World Health Organization. Handbook for Good Clinical Research Practice (GCP): Guidance for Implementation. Geneva: World Health Organization; 2005.
2. Malaysian Guidelines for Good Clinical Practice, 2nd edition. Ministry of Health Malaysia: National Committee for Clinical Research (NCCR); 2004.
3. Nuremberg Code. Trials of War Criminals before the Nuremberg Military Tribunals under Control Council Law No. 10, Vol. 2, pp. 181-2. Washington DC: U.S. Government Printing Office; 1949. [online] Available from: https://www.loc.gov/rr/frd/Military_Law/pdf/NT_war-criminals_Vol-II.pdf [Last accessed September, 2021].
4. World Medical Association. (2004). Declaration of Helsinki 2004; [online] Available from: https://www.wma.net/what-we-do/medical-ethics/declaration-of-helsinki/doh-oct2004/ [Last accessed September, 2021].
5. The National Commission for the Protection of Human Subjects of Biomedical and Behavioral Research. The Belmont Report: Ethical Principles and Guidelines for the Protection of Human Subjects of Research. 1979.
6. European Medicines Agency. ICH Harmonised Tripartite Guideline E6: Note for Guidance on Good Clinical Practice (PMP/ICH/135/95). London: European Medicines Agency; 2002.
7. Blehar MC, Spong C, Grady C, Goldkind SF, Sahin L, Clayton JA. Enrolling pregnant women: issues in clinical research. Womens Health Issues. 2013;23(1):e39-45.
8. Kim JH, Scialli AR. Thalidomide: the tragedy of birth defects and the effective treatment of disease. Toxicol Sci. 2011;122:1-6.
9. Van Spall HG. Exclusion of pregnant and lactating women from COVID-19 vaccine trials: a missed opportunity. Eur Heart J. 2021;42(28):2724-6.
10. Daw JR, Mintzes B, Law MR, Hanley GE, Morgan SG. Prescription drug use in pregnancy: a retrospective, population-based study in British Columbia, Canada (2001–2006). Clin Ther. 2012;34:239-49.e2.
11. US Department of Health and Human Services. Protection of human subjects. 45 CFR part 46. 2014.
12. US Department of Health and Human Services, Public Health Service, National Institutes of Health, Office of Research on Women's Health. Enrolling Pregnant Women: Issues in Clinical Research. Bethesda, MD: National Institutes of Health; 2011.

LONG QUESTIONS

1. Describe in detail the history, reasons for recommendation, and the basic ethical principles of ICH-GCP.
2. Explain the key activities in the conduct of a clinical trial.
3. Define ICH-GCP. Add a note on the recommendations for research in obstetrics and the challenges faced in obstetric trials.

SHORT QUESTIONS

1. Define GCP recommendations. Why are they required?
2. What are the three basic ethical principles of ICH-GCP?
3. Name three landmark trials in obstetrics and their conclusions.

4. State three reasons why pregnant and lactating women have been excluded from most trials.
5. What are the challenges faced by the researcher in obstetric trials?
6. What are landmark trials? Name a few landmark trials in obstetrics.
7. Why are GCP recommendations necessary?
8. Write a brief note on the history and evolution of the GCP recommendations.
9. Write a note on recommendations for research in obstetrics.

■ MULTIPLE CHOICE QUESTIONS

1. A clinical trial refers to experiments on:
   a. Animals
   b. Healthy human volunteers
   c. Humans with disease
   d. Both healthy and diseased human beings
2. The current GCP guidelines have been derived from:
   a. The Hippocratic oath
   b. Kefauver–Harris amendment
   c. Declaration of Helsinki
   d. The Belmont report
3. Which of the following is false regarding the reasons for GCP?
   a. Increased ethical awareness
   b. Improved clinical trial methods
   c. Better understanding of clinical trial concept
   d. Decreasing competition
4. Which of the following is false regarding the Kefauver–Harris amendment?
   a. It was passed in 1962
   b. It was done in response to severe fetal limb deformities linked to the use of maternal thalidomide
   c. It forms the basis of the current GCP recommendations
   d. It requires the FDA to evaluate all new drugs for safety and efficacy
5. Development of standard operating procedures (SOPs) for a clinical trial is done by:
   a. Sponsors   b. Clinical investigators
   c. Ethics committees   d. All of the above
6. In a clinical trial, which of the following is not a responsibility of the sponsors?
   a. Ethics committee review and approval of the protocol
   b. Development of support systems and tools
   c. Generation and approval of trial-related documents
   d. Selection of properly qualified, trained, and experienced investigators and study personnel
7. The term breech trial compared:
   a. Planned vaginal delivery and planned cesarean section (C-section) in term pregnant women with fetus in breech presentation
   b. Planned vaginal delivery versus emergency C-section in term pregnant women with fetus in breech presentation
   c. Spontaneous unplanned vaginal delivery versus emergency C-section in term pregnant women with fetus in breech presentation
   d. Spontaneous unplanned vaginal delivery versus planned C-section in term pregnant women with fetus in breech presentation
8. Which of these is the right description of a landmark trial?
   a. A trial which has made an impact on our understanding of a disease
   b. A trial which has caused a dramatic change in our approach to a clinical condition
   c. A trial which has changed our management of a disease
   d. All of the above
9. Which of these is not a basic ethical principle of ICH-GCP?
   a. Respect for persons   b. Confidentiality
   c. Beneficence   d. Justice
10. Which of the following is not a recommendation for clinical trials in pregnant women?
    a. Define pregnant women as a scientifically complex and change the presumption of exclusion
    b. Clarify existing regulations and focus on IRB as it facilitates or impedes pregnancy research
    c. Consider the pregnant as "vulnerable" group and avoid clinical trials on them
    d. Develop a pregnancy research agenda
11. What are the challenges in obstetric trials?
    a. Dynamic physiology of pregnancy
    b. Possibility of teratogenicity to the fetus
    c. Less cooperation and consent by the women
    d. All of the above
12. Which of the following is false as per the ICH-GCP?
    a. The medical care given to the subjects and medical decisions made on behalf of subjects should always be the responsibility of a qualified physician.
    b. Each individual involved in conducting a particular trial should be qualified by education, training, and experience.
    c. Informed consent from subjects is not necessary prior to participation in clinical trials.
    d. All clinical trial information should be recorded, handled, and stored in a way that helps its accurate reporting, interpretation, and verification.

Answers

1. d 2. c 3. d 4. c 5. d 6. a
7. a 8. d 9. b 10. c 11. d 12. c

1.5 PELVIC ANATOMY FOR THE OBSTETRICIAN AND GYNAECOLOGIST

Bhavik Doshi, Ashvin Vachhani

INTRODUCTION

Female reproductive tract can be divided into external genitalia and internal genitalia. The external genitalia **(Fig. 1)** include labia minora, labia majora, clitoris, vestibule, greater vestibular glands, and bulbs of vestibule. Internal organs include uterus, cervix, fallopian tubes, and ovary.

Vulva includes mons pubis, labia majora and minora, clitoris, hymen, and vestibule. Blood is supplied from branches of internal pudendal artery and superficial external pudendal artery. Venous return is internal pudendal vein and long saphenous vein. Lymphatic is drained from vulva into superficial inguinal nodes, deeper tissues to internal iliac nodes. Nerve supply to vulva is anteriorly ilioinguinal and genital branch of genitofemoral nerve (L1–L2), posteriorly pudendal branches of posterior cutaneous nerve of thigh (S1–S3), and pudendal nerve (S2–S4).

Mons pubis: It is fibrofatty tissue that produces the rounded elevation just in front of pubic symphysis. The pubic hair grows over the mons pubis at the onset of puberty.

Labia majora: It is homologous with scrotum in male. It is rounded fold of skin, narrow behind where it reaches to anus, but as it passes forward, becomes increasing in size. Anteriorly it meets in midline at anterior commissure and ends in median elevation as mons pubis. Laterally it contains numerous sebaceous glands and medially it is smooth and covered by delicate cutaneous covering. It does not contain any muscle fiber as we found in scrotum. Posteriorly it is connected across the midline in front of anus, by the posterior commissure.

Labia majora hide the pudendal cleft and opening of urethra and vagina are in cleft. The round ligament of uterus is attached to skin and fibrofatty tissue of labium majus.

It develops from genital swellings. The ilioinguinal nerve supplies anterior part of majora and pudendal nerve supplies posteriorly.

Labia minora: They are a pair of fat-free narrower longitudinal folds of skin usually completely hidden in between the cleft of labia majora. When traced it forward, it splits into two parts upper and lower in relation to clitoris. The upper layer of both sides covers the upper surface of glans clitoris is known as prepuce of clitoris. The lower layer of both sides covers the lower surface of glans is known as frenulum of clitoris. Frenulum of vestibule is a fold which lies posteriorly where two sides of labia minora meet.

Developmentally, it resembles fused ventral surface of the penis and the floor of the spongy urethra.

Vestibule: It is a space between two labia minora where opening of urethra and vagina lies. The urethral opening has a vertical slit or inverted V-shaped appearance situated 2.5 cm behind the glans. The vaginal opening is H-shaped and covered by hymen. Hymen is a muscular fold projecting into vaginal opening and its margin is smooth in outline. But when margin is fissured during sexual act, it is known as caruncula hymenalis. The greater vestibular gland opens on either side of opening of vagina in vestibule.

Clitoris: It resembles the penis of male only difference is that it is not traversed by urethra. The body of clitoris is made up of erectile tissue and tapering anteriorly. It is made up

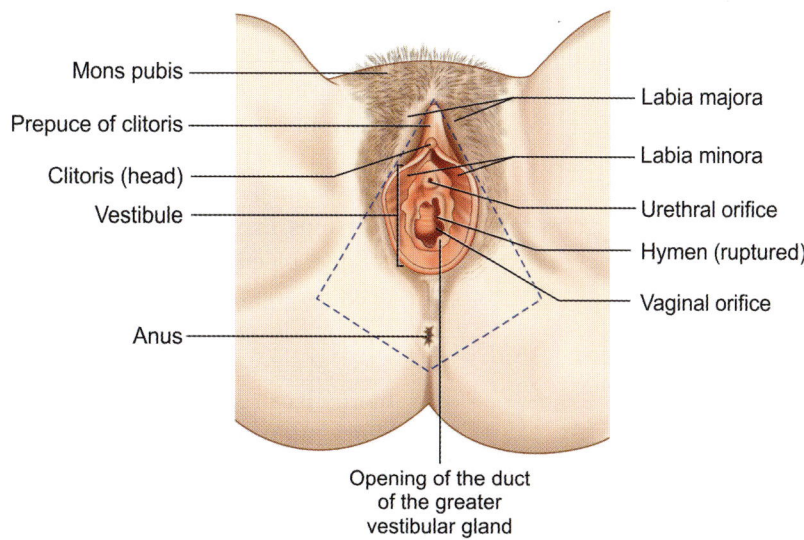

Fig. 1: Female external genitalia.

of pair of corpora cavernosa which form crura near the root of clitoris. A glans is mass of erectile tissue present over the pointed end of the body and covered by sensitive epithelium. The crus is attached to pubic arch. Each crus is continuous with firm fibrous fascia which is covered by corresponding ischiocavernosus muscle.

The crus is supplied by deep artery of the clitoris, a branch of internal pudendal artery. The dorsal arteries of clitoris supply the glans. The nerve supply is from inferior hypogastric plexuses and partly from dorsal nerves of clitoris which are branches from pudendal nerves.

Bulbs of vestibule: They are a pair of erectile tissue which lies in the lateral wall of the vagina and lower surface of perineum. They are elongated masses which are pointed anteriorly and separated by vaginal and urethral opening anteriorly. They are covered by bulbospongiosus superficially.

Greater vestibular glands (Bartholin's glands) **(Fig. 2)**: They are a pair of mucus-secreting tubule—alveolar glands similar to bulbourethral gland situated in superficial perineal pouch and its ducts open into each side of vaginal orifice below the hymen. Each is about size of small bean and having long slender ducts which pierce the perineal membrane. It is involved in acute gonorrhea. Blockage of its duct due to recurrent infection can lead to Bartholin's cyst/abscess.

Hymen: It is a delicate incomplete membrane at the entrance of vagina. It has one or more apertures for blood flow. It is generally avascular. Imperforate hymen can lead to cryptomenorrhea and requires surgical incision.

Vagina: It is a highly distensible muscular passage of about 9 cm size. It is directed upward and backward having slight convex curve forward. It makes 90° angle with uterus. The cervix enters vagina through its upper part in anterior wall. The more posterior portion of cervix is inserted in vagina then its anterior portion, so recess (fornix) between vaginal wall and cervix is deep in posterior part. This is anterior recess, posterior recess, and lateral recess in relation to cervix and vagina. The anterior wall of vagina is about 7.5 cm, whereas the posterior wall is about 9 cm.

Anteriorly vagina is related from above downward to cervix, base of urinary bladder, and terminal parts of ureters separated by loose areolar tissue. It is also related anteriorly to urethra.

Posteriorly vagina is related from above downward to rectouterine peritoneal pouch for upper one-third part then to ampulla of rectum which is separated from vagina by rectovaginal fascia. In lower one-third part, it is related posteriorly to perineal body.

Laterally, it is related to root of broad ligament, and crossing of ureter by uterine vessels. Levator ani muscle forms slings surrounding vagina and forms the sphincter vaginae. Still lower it is related to greater vestibular gland, bulb of vestibule, and bulbospongiosus muscle **(Fig. 3)**.

It is made up of serous coat derived from peritoneum on its outward aspect, then fascial coat derived from endopelvic fascia and inner muscular coat. There are two muscle layers—outer longitudinal and inner circular layer of smooth muscle. Still internally it is lined by nonkeratinized stratified squamous epithelium and is devoid of mucus glands.

The Doderlein's bacilli are normal inherent of vagina and produce lactic acid so vaginal fluid is acidic in reaction having pH 4–5.

The arterial supply is from vaginal artery, vaginal branches from uterine artery, the vaginal branches of the middle rectal artery, and the branch of internal pudendal artery.

The lymphatic from upper two-thirds drains into internal iliac nodes and lower one-third drains into upper superficial inguinal nodes in the groin.

Defects in the supports of vagina can lead to anterior and posterior vaginal wall prolapsed, stress incontinence, and vault prolapsed after hysterectomy.

Pelvic hematoma: Collection of blood anywhere between pelvic peritoneum and perineal skin is known as pelvic hematoma. It may be infralevator or supralevator hematomas. Infralevator is common.

Vulval hematoma is the common infralevator hematoma which may be due to vaginal tears, episiotomy (apex not sutured), and rupture of paravaginal venous plexus during instrumental delivery. It can cause pain, swelling, and rectal tenesmus. Exploration in operation theater under anesthesia is done, bleeders are secured, dead space is obliterated by deep mattress sutures.

Supralevator hematoma can occur due to extension of cervical tears, colporrhexis, and rupture of lower segment of uterus. It can cause pain late, bladder tenesmus, unexplained shock, uterus pushed to contralateral side, boggy swelling in **Figures 4 and 5**. Laparotomy is performed to treat it, anterior leaf of broad ligament is opened and then bleeders are sutured. If needed, anterior division of internal iliac artery is ligated.

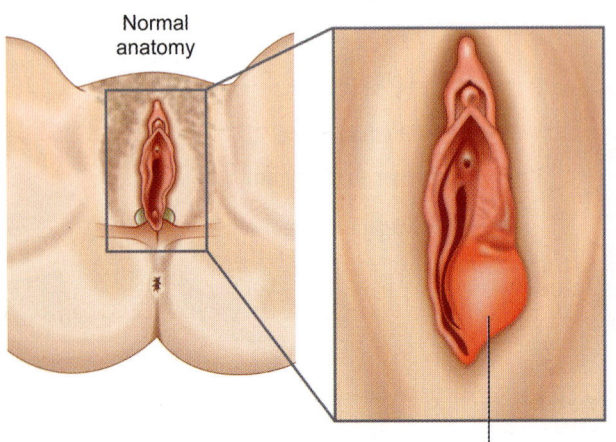

Fig. 2: Bartholin's gland.

SECTION 1: Introduction to Obstetrics

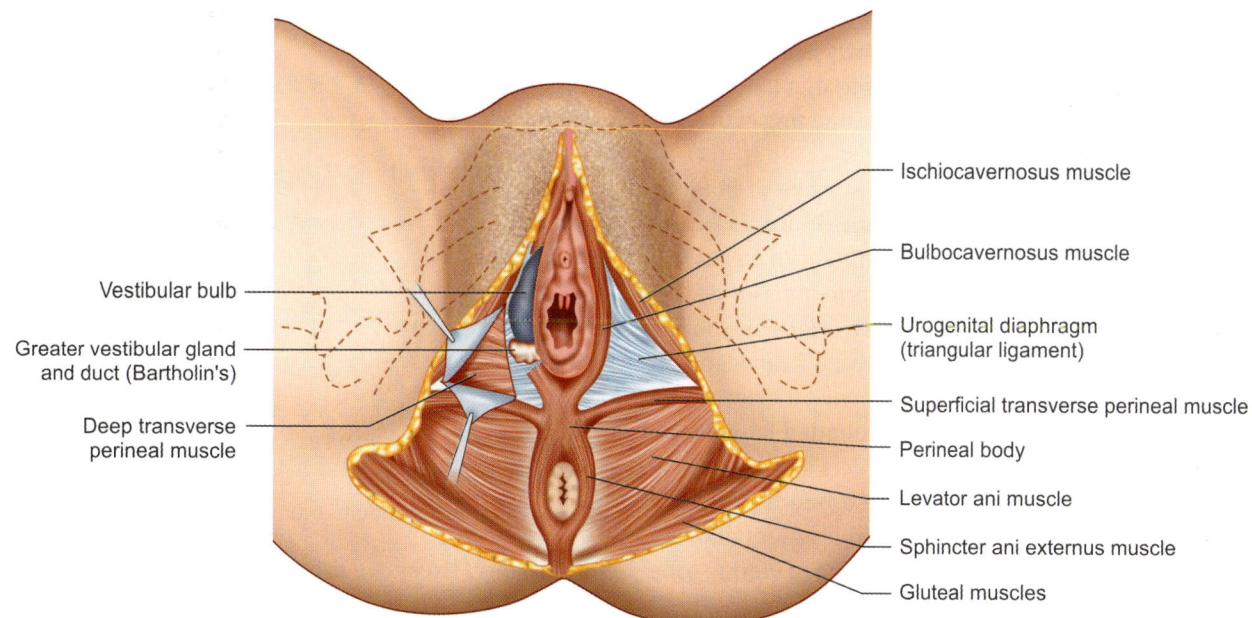

Fig. 3: Pelvic floor muscles.

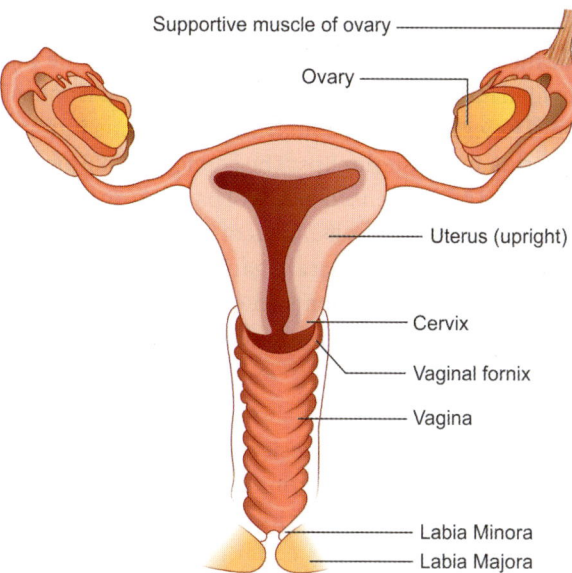

Fig. 4: Internal reproductive tract.

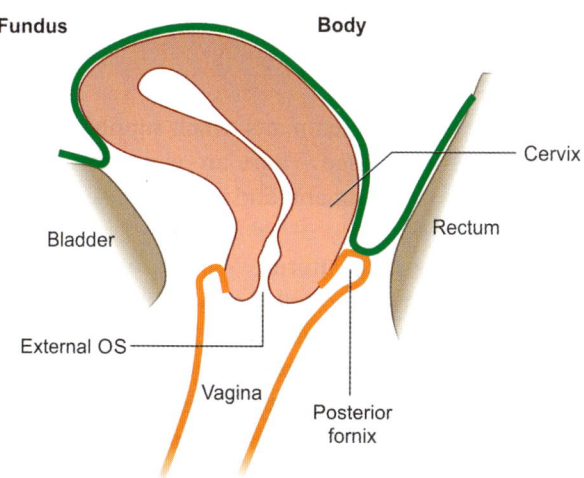

Fig. 5: Reflections of the peritoneum.

■ UTERUS

It is a pyriform-shaped hollow muscular organ situated in lesser pelvis and projects upward and forward above the bladder. In nulliparous uterus, the length of the uterus is about 7.5 cm. It divided into fundus, body, and cervix. The ratio of body, fundus with cervix is 2:1 in adults and 1:2 in children. The uterine cavity is about 6 cm long and weight of the uterus is 30–40 g.

The axis between the cervix and that of vagina measuring about 90° is called anteversion. The normal uterus lies in pelvic cavity and slightly inclines laterally frequently on left side. The uterus corresponds with the axis of pelvic inlet and vagina corresponds with the axis of the pelvic outlet. This position (anteversion) is maintained by forward pull of round ligament and backward pull of the cervix by uterosacral ligament.

The cervix is continuous with the wall of vagina and makes 125° angle with that of body of uterus is called anteflexion. The transverse axis passes through internal os.

Lower segment of the uterus: Anatomically, it is a part which lies below the uterovesical fold of the peritoneum. Physiologically, it is a part which passively stretches in labor and takes hardly any active contractile part in expulsion of fetus. Taking up of lower segment of uterus is a very important event during progress of labor. It facilitates labor process.

Parts of the Uterus

Fundus: The expanded upper part of uterus lying above the opening of uterine tube is called fundus.

Body or corpus: It is a triangular part which lies between fundus above and isthmus below. Body has anteroinferior or vesical surface and posterosuperior or intestinal surface and these two surfaces are separated by right and left borders.

The length, breadth, and thickness of body are 5 cm, 5 cm, and 2.5 cm, respectively. The uterine cavity is a vertical slit on sagittal section. The cavity of body is triangular on cross section, the base is formed by line joining opening of uterine tube and apex is by internal os.

The peritoneum from the superior surface of bladder is reflected posteriorly on vesical surface of uterus (up to isthmus) and then covers the intestinal surface of uterus (up to posterior fornix of vagina) and projects to anterior wall of rectum. The vesicouterine pouch and the rectouterine pouch are formed by above reflections, respectively. The deepness of rectouterine pouch is 7.5 cm or just above the anus. The peritoneum reflections on uterus are extended laterally on the lateral pelvic wall from its lateral borders as an extensive peritoneal fold which is known as the broad ligament of uterus. The round ligament of uterus and ligament of ovary are attached to uterus just below the opening of uterine tube anteroinferiorly and posterosuperiorly, respectively. These three structures are all enclosed in broad ligament near its upper free end.

The anterior part of broad ligament is drawn forward by the round ligament of uterus, which is a narrow flat band of fibrous tissue, extending from lateral border of uterus, crossing the obliterated umbilical artery and external iliac vessels, and reaches to deep inguinal ring. Here, it hooks around the lateral side of inferior epigastric artery and traversing the inguinal canal and ends in subcutaneous tissue of the labium majus. The ligament of ovary is a round fibrous band extending from uterus to ovary.

The part of broad ligament between the ligament of ovary, the ovary and uterine tube is known as mesosalpinx. The lateral part of mesosalpinx is freer and permits posterior curve of lateral end of uterine tube around the ovary. The mesosalpinx contains epoophoron and paroophoron and the anastomosis between the uterine and ovarian arteries. The ovary is attached to posterior layer of broad ligament by mesovarium.

Layers of the uterus: Uterus has mainly three layers: (1) serous, (2) muscular, and (3) endometrium. Serous is formed by the peritoneum which covers the anterior two-thirds and whole of posterior surface.

Muscular is middle layer which consists of smooth muscle cells, arranged in three layers—outer in longitudinal, inner in circular, and middle interlacing muscles.

Endometrium is a mucosal layer lining uterus cavity. Endometrium is directly apposed to the muscle coat. It is the inner most layer with thickness of 1–10 mm based on different days of menstrual cycle. Thickness varies due to repetitive cyclic changes **(Fig. 6)**. It has two layers: (1) functional and (2) basal. It consists of surface epithelium glands and interglandular tissue, columnar epithelium dips to form tubular or spiral glands. Basal one-third of it is supplied by small straight and short artery and superficial two-thirds by

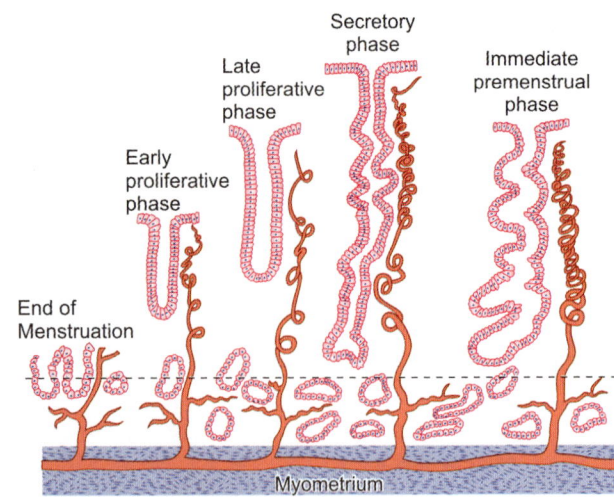

Fig. 6: Thickness of endometrium in different menstrual phases.

coiled artery. Excessive thin endometrium compare to the day of menstrual cycle can cause problem with implantation of fertilized ovum and can cause infertility.

Cervix: It is a part below the internal os and separated from body of uterus by constriction, isthmus. It contains the cervical canal which communicates the uterine cavity with the vagina. It is divided into supravaginal and vaginal parts as it opens into vagina. The external os through which it opens into vagina has anterior and posterior lips. The cervicovaginal junction is strengthened by condensed bands of parametric tissue which extends to lateral pelvic walls. A pair of Mackenrodt's ligaments laterally, a pair of uterosacral ligaments posteriorly, and a pair of bulbocervical ligaments anteriorly help in positioning of cervix and prevent downward displacement of the uterus through the vagina.

Relations of uterus: Anteriorly above the internal os, the body forms the posterior wall of vesicouterine pouch and below the internal os, it separates from the base of the bladder by the loose areolar tissue. Posteriorly, it forms anterior wall of pouch of Douglas containing coils of intestine. Laterally, it is related to broad ligament of uterus with its contents. Laterally, cervix is also related to ureter where it is crossed superiorly by uterine arteries.

Ligaments of Uterus

They are true and false ligaments which support the uterus and prevent its prolapsed. There are eight fibromuscular bands which are true ligaments and six peritoneal folds which are false ligaments.

Round ligaments of uterus, Mackenrodt's ligaments, uterosacral ligaments, and pubocervical ligaments are true ligaments in which round ligaments discussed earlier.

The Mackenrodt's or transverse cervical ligaments form a fan-shaped fibromuscular band extending from cervicovaginal junction to the fascia covering the levator ani muscle. It is related above with the broad ligament and crossing of uterine artery over ureter.

The uterosacral ligaments extend from the cervix to the 3rd sacral vertebra and help in anteversion and anteflexion position of uterus.

The pubocervical ligaments extend from the cervix to pubic bone and pull the uterus forward.

The levator ani muscle, urogenital diaphragm, perineal body, and superior surface of urinary bladder give support to uterus from below.

■ FALLOPIAN TUBE

It is a hollow tube, two in number transporting ova from ovary and sperm from uterus for fertilization. It is about 10 cm in length, extending from lateral angle of uterus to ovary in upper part of broad ligament of uterus. It is more or less transversely placed in upper free margin of broad ligament having curve in lateral part.

It has four parts from lateral to medial: (1) infundibulum, (2) ampulla, (3) isthmus, and (4) intramural part.

The infundibulum is lateral end of fallopian tube around 1 cm in length and 3 mm in diameter. It is in contact with ovary through its fimbriae. One of the fimbriae is long enough to reach the surface of ovary which is known as ovarian fimbriae.

The ampulla is thin-walled, dilated, and tortuous 5 cm long part of fallopian tube having 4 mm diameter. Fertilization takes place in ampulla. The isthmus is about 3 cm in length and 2 mm in diameter. It is succeeded by intramural part which is 1 cm in length, 1 mm in diameter and passes through the muscle layer of uterus.

Microscopically, from outside to inside, it is made up of parietal layer, muscle layer, and inner mucous membrane. The muscle layer consists of outer longitudinal and inner circular smooth muscle. Mucous layer is made up of ciliated columnar cell showing primary, secondary and tertiary longitudinal folding.

It is supplied by uterine and ovarian artery which forms anastomoses below the fallopian tube in broad ligament of uterus.

Lymphatics drain into preaortic and lateral aortic group of lymph node except that of intramural part which drains into superficial inguinal group of lymph node.

Developmentally, it is derived from upper vertical part of paramesonephric or Müllerian duct.

Clinical importance: Acute infection of fallopian tube is known as salpingitis and it is responsible for most common cause for tubal block and subsequent infertility. Fallopian tube is the most common site for ectopic pregnancy. Tubectomy/tubal ligation is the permanent method of female contraception.

■ OVARY

It is a pair of female reproductive glands situated in lesser pelvis in ovarian fossa. Ovarian fossa is bounded anteriorly by obliterated umbilical artery, behind by ureter and internal iliac artery.

Dimensions: 3 cm vertical, 2 cm transverse, and 1.5 cm anteroposterior diameter.

External features: It is almond-shaped. In nulliparous women, it is vertically situated. Each ovary has two ends (tubal and uterine), two borders (mesovarium or anterior and free or posterior), two surfaces (medial and lateral). The upper end is in relation with fallopian tube which arches over the ovary. The upper end of ovary and infundibulum is attached to lateral pelvic wall by double fold of peritoneum known as infundibulopelvic ligament or suspensory ligament of ovary. The lower end of ovary is attached to uterus by ligament of ovary. The anterior border is attached to posterior layer of broad ligament through peritoneal fold which acts as a hilum through which ovarian vessels and nerves pass. Free posterior border is in relation with fallopian tube in its upper part. Medial surface is convex and related in its upper part with ovarian fimbriae. The lateral surface lies in ovarian fossa.

The blood supply of ovary is by ovarian artery which is a branch of abdominal aorta. It runs into suspensory ligament of ovary then into mesovarium and then it reaches to ovary.

Lymphatics drain into lateral and preaortic group of lymph node.

Structure of Ovary (Fig. 7)

Its surface is covered by a single layer of cubical cells that constitute the germinal epithelium. But it does not produce germ cells. The substance is divided into cortex and medulla. In cortex, it contains various stages of development of ovarian follicles. Each follicle contains developing ovum. The medulla consists of connective tissue in which numerous blood vessels, elastic fibers, and smooth muscles are seen. It contains the Graafian follicle, which undergoes ovulation.

Developmentally, the ovary is developed from the middle part of the genital ridge. It is bulging of coelomic mesothelium covering the medial surface of the mesonephric ridge. The primitive sex cells derived from the dorsal wall of hindgut by the proliferation of the endodermal cells.

Clinical importance: Ovulation study is important clinical aspect in infertile women and usually done by transvaginal ultrasonography (USG). Various drugs are used for ovulation induction. Abnormal ovarian function can lead to various types of functional ovarian cysts like follicular cyst, corpus luteal cyst, theca-lutein cysts, etc. Many types of benign and malignant tumors may arise from ovary.

Muscles of pelvic region: The piriformis and obturator internus form part of lateral wall of pelvis and they are considered as muscles of lower limb. The levator ani and coccygeus muscles form pelvic diaphragm which in turn forms the floor of true pelvis. It forms partition between the pelvic cavity and perineum.

Pelvic diaphragm: It is a pair of two muscles and forms the gutter-shaped floor of pelvic cavity. Two muscles are levator

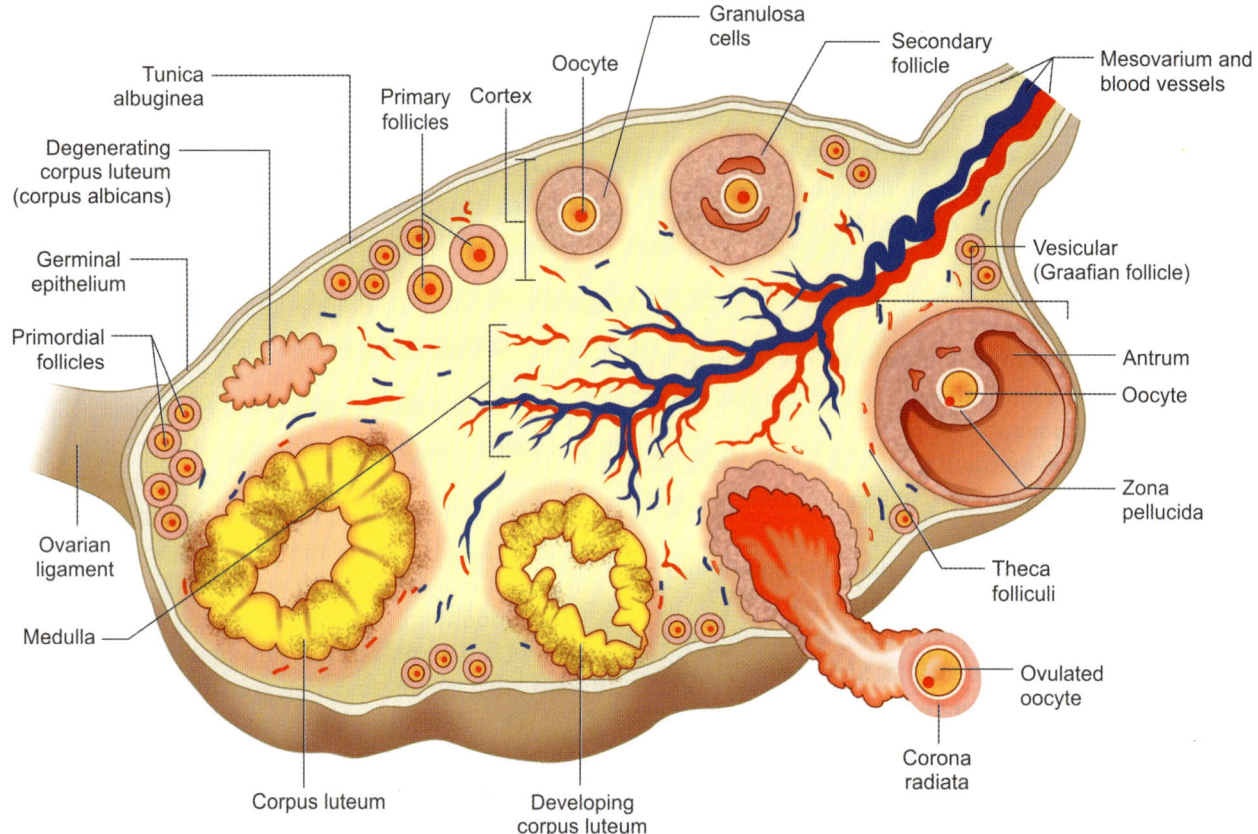

Fig. 7: Structure of ovary.

ani and coccygeus. Morphologically, they are considered as single muscular unit and divided into three parts: (1) pubococcygeus, (2) iliococcygeus, and (3) ischiococcygeus from before backward.

Pubococcygeus arises from posterior surface of body of pubis and anterior part of white line. It passes backward, downward and medially, and anterior most fibers form sling around the posterior wall of vagina and inserted on perineal body. Some fibers are inserted in wall of anal canal and called puboanalis. Puborectalis fibers wind the posterior part of anorectal junction and form puborectal sling and continue with deep part of external anal sphincter.

The iliococcygeus arises from the posterior part of the white line on the obturator fascia and from ischial spine and inserts into anorectal raphe and side of lower two pieces of coccyx.

The ischiococcygeus arises from ischial spine and sacrospinous ligament and inserts into side of upper two pieces of coccyx and last piece of sacrum.

Pubococcygeus and iliococcygeus are supplied by 4th sacral nerve and perineal branch of pudendal nerve and ischiococcygeus is supplied by 4th and 5th sacral nerves.

Pelvic fascia: There are two types of pelvic fascia: (1) parietal fascia and (2) visceral fascia.

The parietal fascia covers the lateral pelvic wall to form strong membrane. Here, it forms obturator fascia over obturator internus muscle. Obturator fascia shows linear thickening for the origin of levator ani muscle. The fascia covering piriformis is thin and beyond the muscle it attaches to periosteum.

The parietal fascia covers the both superior and inferior layer of pelvic diaphragm.

The visceral layer surrounds the pelvic viscera loosely and allows the distention of bladder, rectum, and vagina.

Perineal body: It is a fibromuscular node situated about 1.25 cm in front of the anal margin. Most of muscles of perineum converge to insert on it.

Clinical importance: Injury to perineal body, pelvic fascia and/or pelvic diaphragm may occur during difficult childbirth, which may lead to uterine prolapsed, vaginal prolapsed, rectal prolapsed, stress urinary incontinence or fecal incontinence.

INTERNAL ILIAC ARTERY (FIG. 8)

The internal iliac artery is the smaller terminal branch of the common iliac artery which supplies all pelvic organs except those supplied by superior rectal, ovarian and median sacral arteries.

Course: It begins in front of the sacroiliac joint where it lies medial to the psoas muscle. The artery runs downward and backward, and ends near the upper margin of the greater sciatic notch, by dividing into anterior and posterior divisions.

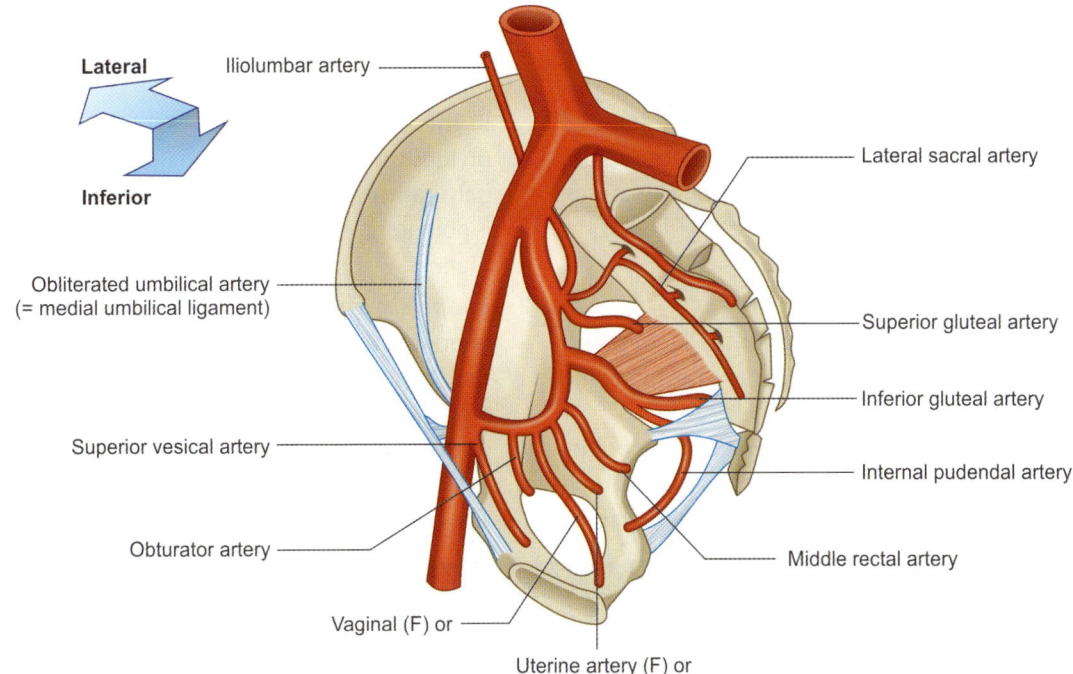

Fig. 8: Branches of internal iliac artery.

Branches of anterior division: (1) superior vesical, (2) obturator, (3) middle rectal, (4) vaginal artery, (5) inferior gluteal, (6) internal pudendal, and (7) uterine artery.

Branches of posterior division: (1) iliolumbar, (2) two lateral sacral, and (3) superior gluteal.

Clinical importance: Bilateral or unilateral ligation of the IIA is a lifesaving surgical procedure to stop pelvic hemorrhage **(Fig. 9)**. Bilateral ligation of IIA reduces the pelvic arterial blood flow by 49% and pulse pressure by 85% which allows clot formation at bleeding site. After bilateral IIA ligation in a long-term period, the collateral circulation will maintain the refunctioning of the IIA. This procedure is commonly used for stoppage of bleeding in case of uncontrolled atonic postpartum hemorrhage (PPH), broad ligament hematoma, advance cervical cancer with intractable bleeding, and uncontrolled intraoperative or postoperative bleeding.

■ PELVIC URETERS

Anatomy: The ureter is a tubular viscus about 25 cm long, divided into abdominal and pelvic portion of equal length, made up of inner longitudinal and outer circular muscle layers. It enters in pelvis by passing over the bifurcation of the internal and external iliac arteries **(Fig. 10)**, just medial to the ovarian vessels. During in its course through the cardinal ligaments, ureter crosses under the uterine artery ("water under bridge"). At this point, it lies along the anterolateral surface of the cervix, about 1 cm from it. Then it passes to lie on the anterior vaginal wall and enters into the bladder.

During its pelvic course, the ureter receives blood from the common iliac, internal iliac, uterine, and vesical arteries.

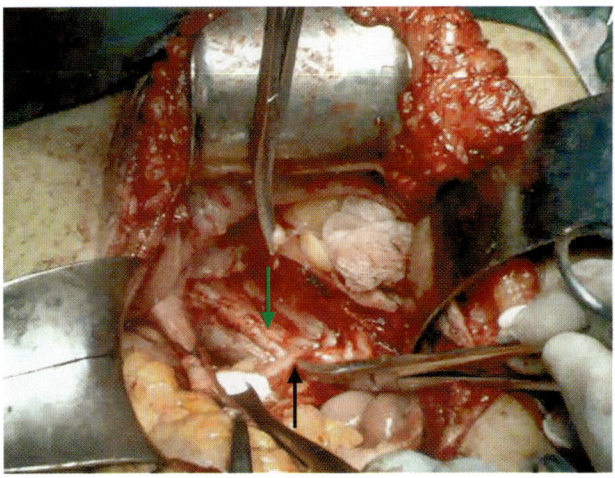

Fig. 9: Ureter (lifted with artery forceps, black arrow) crossing the internal iliac artery (green arrow).

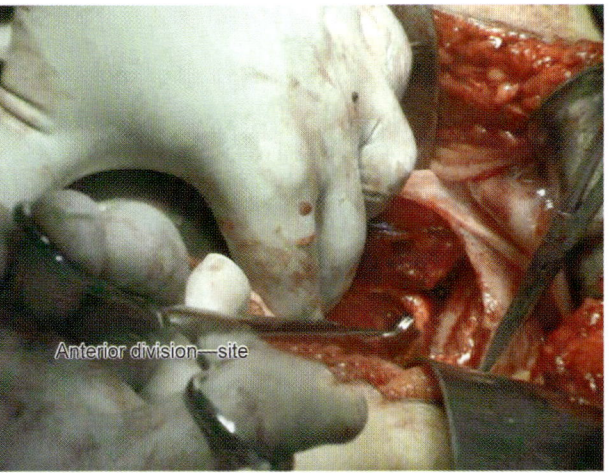

Fig. 10: Anterior division of the internal iliac artery being isolated with a mixter.

Clinical importance: Ureteric injuries have been recognized as potential complications of gynecologic surgery in nearly 1–2% of cases. It can occur during many gynecological surgeries like total laparoscopic hysterectomy (TLH), total abdominal hysterectomy (TAH), adnexal surgery, retropubic surgery, radical pelvic surgery. Sound knowledge of ureteral anatomy is crucial to the avoidance of injury.

■ BONY PELVIS (TABLES 1 AND 2)

Bony pelvis: It is formed by two hip bones: (1) sacrum and (2) coccyx. The pelvis can be described to have the following three major planes:

1. *Pelvic inlet*: The line between the narrowest bony points formed by the *sacral promontory* and the inner *pubic arch* is termed *obstetrical conjugate*. It should be 11.5 cm or more. This anteroposterior line at the inlet is 2 cm less than the *diagonal conjugate* (distance from undersurface of *pubic arch* to sacral promontory). The transverse diameter of the pelvic inlet measures 13.5 cm. The pelvic inlet divides the pelvic cavity into upper part—greater or false pelvis and lower part—lesser or true pelvis. The pelvic inlet is obliquely placed and makes 50–60° angle with horizontal plane.

2. *Midpelvis*: The line between the narrowest bone points connects the *ischial spines*; it typically exceeds 12 cm. The importance of the *ischial spine known as obstetric plane is manifold*. Plane at this level is of the least pelvic dimensions. The levator ani muscles are situated at this level. The obstetric axis of the pelvis changes its direction. The head is considered engaged when it is felt at or below

TABLE 1: The bony pelvis.

Plane	Diameter	Description	Typical measurement
Pelvic inlet	*Anteroposterior* or true *conjugate*	From midpoint of sacral promontory to upper border of pubic symphysis	11 cm
	Transverse diameter	Extends across the greatest width of the superior aperture, from the middle of the brim on one side to the same point on the opposite	13 cm
	Oblique diameter	Extends from the iliopectineal eminence of one side to the sacroiliac articulation of the opposite side	12 cm
Midpelvis	*Anteroposterior* diameter	From midpoint of vertebra S3 to the posterior surface of the pubic symphysis	12 cm
	Transverse diameter	Greatest width of the midpelvis	12 cm
	Oblique diameter	From the lowest point of one sacroiliac joint to the midpoint of the opposite obturator membrane	12 cm
Pelvic outlet	*Anteroposterior diameter*	From the tip of the coccyx to the inferior margin of the pubic symphysis	13 cm
	Transverse diameter or bituberous diameter	Between ischial tuberosities	11 cm
	Oblique diameter	From midpoint of the sacrotuberous ligament on one side to the junction of the ischiopubic rami on the other side	12 cm

TABLE 2: Classification of the bony pelvis.

	Gynecoid	Anthropoid	Android	Platypelloid
Shape	Round	Anteroposteriorly oval	Triangular	Transversely oval
Anterior and posterior segment	Almost equal and spacious	Both increased with slight anterior narrowing	Posterior segment short and anterior segment narrow	Both reduced; flat
Sacrum	• Sacral angle (SA) > 90% inclined backward. Well curved • From above down and side to side	SA > 90% inclined posteriorly. Long and narrow. Usual curve	SA < 90% inclined forward and straight	SA > 90% inclined posteriorly and straight
Sacrosciatic notch	Wide and shallow	More wide and shallow	Narrow and deep	Slightly narrow and small
Side walls	Straight or slightly divergent	Straight or divergent	Convergent	Divergent
Ischial spines	Not prominent	Not prominent	Prominent	Not prominent
Pubic arch	Curved	Long and curved	Long and straight	Short and curved
Subpubic angle	Wide (85%)	Slightly narrow	Narrow	Very wide (>90%)
Bituberous diameter	Normal	Normal or short	Short	Wide

this level. Internal rotation of the head occurs when the occiput is at this level. Forceps is applied only when the head is below it. Pudendal nerve block is carried out at this level.
3. *Pelvic outlet*: The distance between the *ischial tuberosities* (normally > 10 cm), and the angulation of the pubic arch.

The conjugate diameter is distance from midpoint of sacral promontory to upper margin of pubic symphysis. It is about 11 cm in female. The transverse diameter is widest measurement of inlet.

So, according to pelvic brim index that is conjugate diameter of brim × 100/widest transverse diameter, we divide the pelvis into four types.

Dolichopellic or anthropoid, when the conjugate diameter is greater than the transverse diameter. *Platypellic*, when the transverse diameter is much greater than the conjugate diameter. *Mesatipellic or gynecoid,* when the transverse diameter is slightly greater than the conjugate diameter as in normal female. *Brachypellic or android* type which resembles to male pelvis. In all above types, only mesatipellic permits normal delivery and others are considered as contracted pelvis.

CLINICAL PELVIMETRY

- It is also known as internal pelvimetry and it is done by digital examination per vaginum.
- The diagonal conjugate is the distance between midpoint of promontory and lower border of anterior surface of pubic symphysis. By deducting 1.5–2 cm from diagonal conjugate, we can know true conjugate.
- Try to touch both ischial spines during digital examination to measure interischial spinous diameter which is difficult to touch normally.
- Also assess the curvature of the sacrum, the mobility of the coccyx, length of the sacrospinous ligament, and pelvic sidewalls for any conversion inside.
- Disproportion in the size of fetal head and maternal pelvis leads to cephalopelvic disproportion or contracted pelvis, which requires delivery of fetus by cesarean section.

CONCLUSION

Understanding of basic anatomy and physiological functions are very much important in management of obstetrics and gynecological conditions. Surgical procedure can be learned easily if knowledge of reproductive anatomy is clear. Prevention of surgical complication and their management require sound knowledge of pelvic anatomy.

FURTHER READING

1. Garg K. BD Chaurasia's Human Anatomy, 8th edition, Vol. 2. India: CBS Publishers and Distributors Pvt Ltd; 2021.
2. Jones HW, Rock JA. Te Linde's Operative Gynecology, 11th edition. Philadelphia: Wolters Kluwer Health; 2015.
3. Singh V. Textbook of Anatomy: Abdomen and Lower Limb, 3rd edition, Vol. 2. India: Elsevier Health Science; 2020.

LONG QUESTIONS

1. Discuss the muscular and ligamentous supports of the uterus.
2. What are the branches of the internal iliac artery and discuss the applied surgical anatomy of internal iliac artery ligation.

SHORT QUESTIONS

1. What are the important characteristics of the vaginal epithelium?
2. Name the parts of the fallopian tube and their importance in pelvic pathology.
3. What are the types of pelvis based on bony characteristics?

MULTIPLE CHOICE QUESTIONS

1. Nerve supply to the vulva anteriorly is by:
    a. Pudendal branches of cutaneous nerves
    b. Pudendal nerves
    c. Ilioinguinal and genitofemoral nerves
    d. Sciatic nerve
2. Regarding the Bartholin's glands the following is false:
    a. They are tubuloalveolar glands
    b. They are located in the deep perineal pouch
    c. It is involved in acute gonorrhea
    d. Blockage of the duct leads to a cyst or abscess
3. The arterial supply of the vagina include all the following, except:
    a. Vaginal artery
    b. Branches of the inferior rectal artery
    c. Branches of the uterine artery
    d. Branches of the internal pudendal artery
4. The following statement of the bony pelvis is true:
    a. AP diameter of inlet is usually 11 cm
    b. AP diameter of the outlet is the widest diameter of the pelvis
    c. Gynecoid pelvis is flat and narrow
    d. Subpubic angle is narrow in platypeloid pelvis
5. The following is NOT a branch of the anterior division of the internal iliac artery:
    a. Middle rectal   b. Uterine
    c. Internal pudendal d. Inferior rectal

Answers
1. c   2. b   3. b   4. a   5. d

1.6 VIOLENCE AGAINST HEALTHCARE PROFESSIONALS

MC Patel, Dilip Walke

■ INTRODUCTION

The medical profession is considered the noblest profession but dealing with the most complicated science of human life which is very precious. It is an unpredictable science. Even in common clinical situations, there are plenty of variables such as a person's individual biology, disease stage and process, drugs, doses, and surgical techniques. To say the least, medicine is not exact science.

One would expect that violence would become uncommon as the population becomes literate. However, this has not been the case in the real world. One may also believe that violence against doctors would be restricted to a particular type of patient population based on socioeconomic status, religion, or occupation. However, global and local experience tells us that these notions do not always hold true.

■ HISTORY

Violence against physicians and healthcare professionals is not a new phenomenon. The oldest of ethical and moral codes, the one established by Hammurabi is based on the principle of "an eye for an eye" and it was particularly severe on physicians. If a patient lost his life the physician may be sentenced to have his hand cutoff, if the patient was a nobleman. If the patient happened to be a slave, the physician was expected to pay the price of the slave to his master.[1]

Even in more recent history, a paper from 1892 can be quoted below:

"No physician, however conscientious or careful, can tell what day or hour he may not be the object of some undeserved attack, malicious accusation, black mail or suit for damages...."[2]

In recent times, one could argue, that the frequency of such incidents is increasing. However, this could simply be from more visibility due to media and social media.

■ INCIDENCE

Violence against doctors is a common problem in India. It is only recently being highlighted in media and coming into public attention. It is estimated that nearly three-fourths of all doctors face some form of violence during their careers.[3] The survey was carried out by the Indian Medical Association and further stated that a majority of incidents of violence are related to emergency care, intensive care, and postsurgical situations. This is a startlingly high number. There are numerous news articles and publications which bear witness to the incidents in recent times.[4] Such incidents are often followed by doctors' strikes in the public and private sector. Even in the times of the coronavirus disease (COVID) pandemic, when there has been a new awareness and positive media portrayal of healthcare workers (HCWs), attacks on doctors have not stopped.

Violence against doctors is not unique to India. It is seen with a similar frequency in the South East Asian Region. Israel, Pakistan, and Bangladesh have all reported similar incidents of violence.[4] Even in the Western countries, violence against doctors is a well-documented phenomenon.

A global review of 253 eligible studies (with a total of 331,544 participants) showed that 61.9% of the participants reported exposure to any form of workplace violence, 42.5% reported exposure to nonphysical violence, and 24.4% experienced physical violence. The form of violence was most commonly verbal, but also included threats, physical violence, and sexual harassment. The prevalence of violence against HCWs was particularly high in Asian and North American countries, in Psychiatric and Emergency departments, and among nurses and physicians.[5]

In the United States of America, the rates are similar to those in India. Chinese doctors also face violence at the workplace just as commonly. It appears that the frequency of serious attacks on doctors may be higher in these two countries resulting in more severe physical damage, deaths, loss of professional ability, and forced retirement.[6]

■ WHO IS AT RISK?

Every doctor and HCW can be at risk of violence. This includes doctors of all cadres (from duty doctors to consultants), paramedical workers (nurses, physiotherapists, ward boys, ayahs, and cleaners), and personnel who do not have any medical context (receptionists, security staff, etc.).

The risk level could be graded according to the likelihood of violent incidents. The highest risk is faced by doctors on duty in the casualty or emergency departments. Physical violence is usually first directed towards the on-duty doctor in these departments. In these settings, the male doctor is more likely to face violence than females.[4] Other studies have shown a substantial risk for younger doctors as compared to more senior ones. Nonphysical violence is more likely to be directed towards female doctors and nurses in the obstetrics and gynaecology department.[7]

■ HIGH-RISK SITUATIONS

Work place violence often takes place during times of high activity, at the time of hurried and emergent interaction with patients, such as admission in emergency ward, at the time of patient transportation, or when patient is involuntarily admitted. The risk in these situations gets magnified at times of negative outcomes. Other situations where violence may occur is when hospital rules are enforced such as on number of visitors, use of certain facilities, and at the time of billing and clearing financial dues.

TYPES OF VIOLENCE

Violence does not only mean a physical attack. It encompasses a range of negative behaviors exhibited by the patient and/or attendants against HCWs. By legal definition, "violence" means an act, which causes or may cause any harm, injury or endangering the life of, or intimidation, obstruction or hindrance to, any Medicare Service Person in discharging his duty in a Medicare Service Institution or causing damage or loss to the property in a Medicare Service Institution.[8]

The gamut of violence against doctors and HCWs is depicted in **Figure 1**. A grading system of violence against HCWs has been proposed. This is useful for a quick assessment of a situation and statistical comparisons.[9] Such systems are useful but may not encompass all the permutations in a given situation. Nonpersonal violence could be a damage or loss of property in terms of breaking furniture, furnishings, nonmedical machinery, and medical equipment. Nonphysical violence includes a large range including remotely directed or in-person violence. Remotely directed violence could be threatening or intimidating electronic messages or pictures and telephonic conversations which are abusive or repeated phone calls. In-person nonphysical violence includes the above behaviours and also staring, abusive gestures, and threats. Physical violence could result in minor injuries such as cuts and bruises, grievous injuries such as loss of an eye, hearing or limb, and even murder. Sexual violence is almost entirely directed towards female HCWs and could range from insulting the modesty of a woman to assault and rape.

A particular situation that occurs in some settings is the violent mob. This is considered more in detail as it represents a high-risk situation for the physical health of the doctor, other HCWs, and the facility. The genesis and inciting factors leading to mob violence are illustrated in **Figure 2**. It is observed that in a mob, there are only a handful of people who actually take part in the violence, while a majority may encourage the violent ones or will only stand by silently, take pictures or videos. The typical distribution of a mob is illustrated in **Figure 3**.[10]

WHAT CONTRIBUTES TO VIOLENCE AGAINST DOCTORS AND HEALTHCARE PERSONNEL?

Various other factors also play a role in the general situation of causing dissatisfaction and possible violence against HCWs.

With advancements in science in general and medicine in particular, there is a dramatic shift in the expectation with which patients and their attendants view doctors, HCWs, and the therapeutic process. The expectation of a "guaranteed result" is altogether misplaced, yet these expectations are commonplace.

The world in general has become a faster and more impulsive place to be in over the last few decades marked by "on touch technology" and this has fuelled expectations further with a very small tolerance for unfavorable outcomes.

When there is an unexpected or unfavorable outcome in a given clinical situation, it becomes a trigger for the patient and/or attendants to be dissatisfied or aggrieved at best and violent at worst.

Some contributory factors are highlighted in **Table 1**.

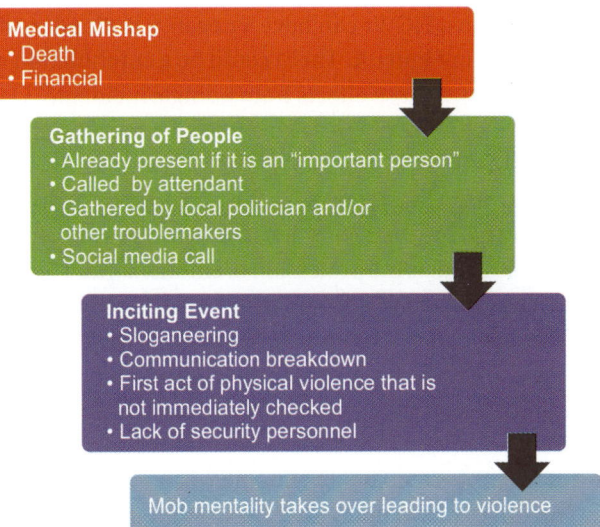

Fig. 2: Genesis of mob violence in healthcare settings.

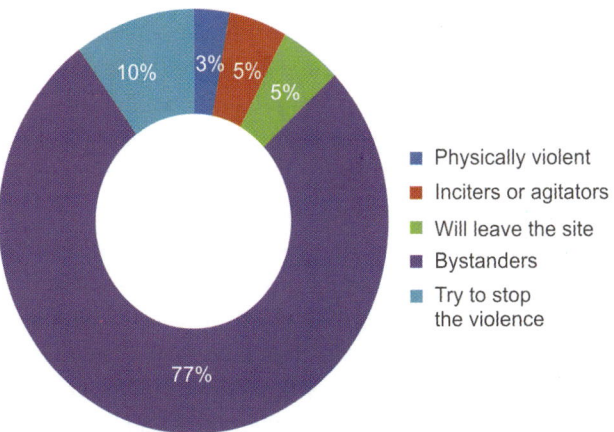

Fig. 3: What comprises a mob in violent situations?

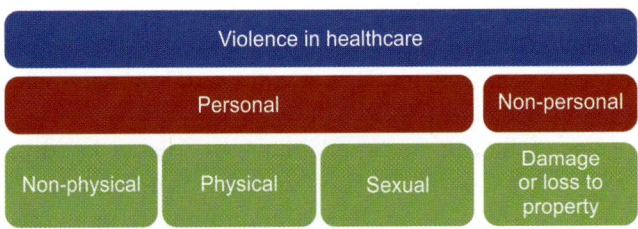

Fig. 1: Types of violence in healthcare.

TABLE 1: Contributors to healthcare personnel violence.

Unrealistic expectations	Changes in society	Role of doctors	Doctors as a soft target	Media fueling	Inadequate deterrents
Incomplete knowledge leading to a belief that medical science is above nature	Greater impulsivity from touch technology and instant gratification becoming the norm and low tolerance in general	Unrealistic counseling or offering guaranteed results	Usually isolated, not in a team or a group, without security	Highlighting medical mishaps	Law is not applied or does not run the full course to justice
Low health literacy	Frustration with existing public health facilities making non-affording people also seek private care	Not highlighting complications and negative outcomes	Corporate hospitals may present doctors as scapegoats	Sensationalizing incidents for viewership	Perpetrators get away scot free to repeat the actions
Doctors are placed on a pedestal till the treatment is completed	Medical profession is no longer viewed in the same esteem as earlier and may be looked down upon or even envied	Inadequate information about finanacial implications of a condition	Succum easily to external pressures (police, political, and antisocial elements)		Other people are emboldened to be violent

■ EFFECTS OF VIOLENCE AGAINST DOCTORS

Violence against HCWs can have a negative multiplier effect as illustrated in **Figure 4**. There could be a combination and compounding of these effects from a single incident.

Doctors who face physical violence suffer from the physical impact of the injuries which could be minor or serious ones. They could result in temporary or long-term physical disability leading to a loss of ability to work at all or to one's full capacity. In turn, this impacts the professional, emotional, and financial wellbeing of a doctor.[9]

Violence can also result in a range of mental health problems including anxiety, agoraphobia, panic attacks, posttraumatic stress disorder, and depression. It could lead to absenteeism as a mechanism to avoid the workplace and the loss of profession and livelihood.[11]

The effect of violence is not restricted only to doctors, but also translates to other patients and the society at large. When a doctor faces violence, it immediately hampers her ability to provide good quality care or any care to the patients who are in her charge. Incidents of physical violence are often followed by strikes or periods of limited medical service provision, which further affect medical care delivery. In the long term, violence or even the threat of violence leads to more defensive medical practice and therefore, more medical tests, investigations, interventions, and costs.[9,11]

Incidents of violence and their reporting results in young people and doctors from getting disheartened and disillusioned with regards to the profession. Fewer young people may opt for medicine as a profession. Fewer doctors would accept challenging assignments such as emergency care or the high-risk settings mentioned above or would agree to work in remote rural areas where this is isolation.

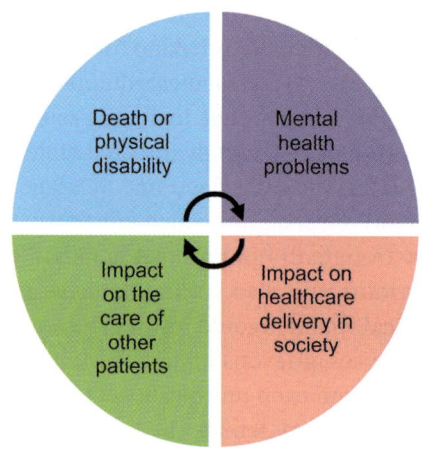

Fig. 4: Impact of violence on healthcare workers.

Ultimately, this could result in fewer available doctors where they are needed the most and could have a long-term negative impact to society.[11]

■ MEASURES TO MITIGATE VIOLENCE IN HEALTH CARE

All HCWs, doctors, and facilities should do their utmost to prevent violence towards themselves. Some measures can be taken to reduce the risk as discussed in **Table 2**. Ultimately, the situation has to be addressed at the level of the establishment and the society. All incidents of violence may not be preventable. However, the goal is to reduce their frequency and intensity and the risk of physical injury.

One of the common spark points in violence is a death. Every hospital or facility should have a protocol or drill to handle these situation. Death should not be announced casually or abruptly. It should be done in a gradual manner

TABLE 2: Mitigating violence in healthcare.

Individual level	Team and ward level	Facility or hospital level	Establishment level
Good communication skills for doctors of all cadres and other healthcare workers	Documentation of counseling with acknowledgement of the patient and attendant for all important condition and care aspects	Closed-circuit television cameras with notices stating that recording is on	Zero tolerance policy for violence against healthcare workers
Avoid loose talk	Empathetic approach	Large notices in public places stating that violence will not be tolerated and will have legal implications	Laws that address healthcare violence specifically should be in place
Dignified conduct and polite behaviour	Dedicated space for counseling with privacy and allowing informed video recording	Transparent and simplified processes for admission, billing, and discharge	Application of law and proper carriage of justice against perpetrators to send a message to violent and antisocial members of society
Follow ethical and professional standards	Senior team members should be available in crisis situations and should be visible	Crowd management with limitation on number of visitors	
	Formation and activation of rush teams	Security personnel—stationed in the hospital and those available from other private agencies as a backup at short notice	

with information being conveyed about the deteriorating condition of the patient. Death should be announced in the presence of a rush team or other doctors and if thought necessary, in the presence of security personnel.

When a death occurs, there are plenty of questions surrounding issuing the death certificate and the cause of death. In case of a postoperative or maternity death, this has important legal ramifications. No law in our country prevents doctors from giving a death certificate, if the cause of death is known. However, in case of intraoperative or maternal death which is generally not expected to occur, it is better to get the postmortem examination done. Hence even if the relatives (or even at time the police) are forcing the doctors to give a death certificate, it is prudent to convince the police to take away the body for a medicolegal postmortem examination.

THE RUSH TEAM

This is a measure that should be in place in every hospital, locality, and geographical setting. It is a group of geographically accessible and closeby doctors.
- The team should comprise of senior, well-known and familiar, respectable practitioners such as general practitioners, anesthetists, surgeons, gynecologists, and physicians.
- A group such as this should be only a phone call away to other doctors working in the geographical location. It is useful to have a social media group which is used only as an SOS call in distress situations.
- The team should be called in situations of distress when there is impending violence or when violence has occurred.
- The team's responsibility is to ease the situation that a doctor may be faced with by opening rational channels of communication with the attendants. If there has been a death, it should preferably be declared only when the team has arrived on site.
- The team should assess the situation and mobilize other resources in the background.
- The treating doctor is stabilized and encouraged to communicate with a small group of three to four attendants. The team members should support this process and not have an interfering attitude. They should contribute by their presence and occasional inputs to cool down flared tempers and if the communication is being derailed.

ACTION IN SITUATIONS WHERE VIOLENCE IS OCCURRING OR LIKELY

The doctor and other HCWs when faced with a situation where violence is likely or is occurring should do their best to protect their own physical condition. The most important and protective measure in these situation is to leave the site as soon as possible. Even though, this may appear like cowardice, it drastically reduces the chance of physical harm and may actually diffuse the situation.

In the meantime, other team members can take over the medical duties of the doctor. The hospital establishment and/or the rush team should be activated and they should swing into action. Locally stationed security personnel should be summoned, but it may be possible that they may flee looking at a mob.

The police should be immediately informed in situations where there is violence likely occur or is occurring. This in fact is the first step that has to be taken, when mob violence is even suspected. Presence of police usually averts any law and order problem.

The role of politicians during the incident and in the wake of violence is debatable. It could be a double-edged sword. In case of physical risk which the doctor may think could be averted by a politician's intervention, the help should be sought without hesitation. However, the downside to their routine involvement could be that:

- They may side with the mob who could be their "vote bank"
- Erasing of evidence or influencing police work negatively
- Pressurizing the doctor to withdraw the complaint.

There is a raging debate about whether doctors and other HCWs should bear arms legally to protect themselves. This gains ground when one hears about violent attacks resulting in loss of life and limb. However, violence may beget more violence and accidental events from arms are a huge risk to be considered.

ACTIONS AFTER THE INCIDENT OF VIOLENCE IN HEALTH CARE

The following are the important aspects to bear in mind when violent incidents have occurred in a healthcare setting.

- Physical condition of doctors and healthcare personnel should be assessed and appropriate care should be administered.
- Injury certificate should be obtained from the closest government hospital to document the injuries to any doctor or HCW. This is important for the further legal process.
- The doctor and other team members may be in a state of mental shock. Early intervention with mental health professionals at an appropriate time can reduce the long-term impact.
- Documentation and recording of the events is a vital step. The doctor and healthcare team should collectively list out the events in a chronological manner at the earliest opportunity. The paperwork related to patient care should be completed. The conversations, events, and incidents leading to the violence should be documented separately.
- Photographs, video footage from mobile phones of bystanders, and other hospital personnel should be collated. The closed-circuit television (CCTV) footage should be downloaded. All these should be secured in an electronic format. These are important for the police enquiry and insurance claim.
- The police should be informed in case they have not been informed earlier. They will then conduct a "panchanama" or enquiry. It is imperative that the doctor and healthcare team should cooperate with the police. The evidence in the form of papers, notes, documents, and the electronic evidence as outlined above should be made available to them. They may take the originals with them, so a copy should be made without fail before handing over.
- The police are obliged to register an first information report (FIR) in these circumstances. They may avoid or delay in doing this to prevent a backlash from a violent crowd or in fact take the doctor into protective custody. However, the doctor should insist on an FIR. If there is a delay or denial, the doctor should bring this to the notice of the supervising officer at the local police station. Further actions include filing an right to information (RTI) or a writ petition in case of inaction. Occasionally, the police personnel who are attending the situation may not be aware of the available laws on violence against HCWs. They may be gently reminded of the same.
- The further legal process usually takes its own time. The doctor and other HCWs may not wish to pursue the same under pressure or of their own will. However, they should be encouraged strongly to do so. They should be supported by the hospital that they are working in and local professional bodies. This is important to ensure the full carriage of justice.

THE LAW AND HEALTHCARE-RELATED VIOLENCE

The Protection of Medicare Service Persons and Medicare Service Institutions (Prevention of Violence and Damage to Property) Act, also known as the Medical Protection Act (MPA), has currently been implemented in about 23 states in India.[8,12]

Some of the key points of MPA are as follows:
- Any act of violence against a "Medicare Service Person" or damage or loss to the property of a "Medicare Service Institution" is prohibited.
- Any offender who commits or attempts to commit or abets or incites the commission of any act of violence shall be punished with imprisonment, which may extend to 3 years and with a fine, which may extend to Rs 50,000 and compensation double the amount of loss or as judged by the court.
- Any offense committed under this act shall be cognizable and nonbailable and triable by the Court of Judicial Magistrate of the First Class.

The Epidemic Diseases (Amendment) Ordinance, 2020 was promulgated on April 22, 2020. The Ordinance amends the earlier Epidemic Diseases Act of 1897. The Ordinance provides for the prevention of the spread of dangerous epidemic diseases. The key point is that this Ordinance amends the Act to include protections for the healthcare personnel combatting epidemic diseases such as COVID-19 and expands the powers of the central government to prevent the spread of such diseases.[13] The text of key provisions of the Ordinance is set out below:

- "Healthcare service personnel" as a person who is at risk of contracting the epidemic disease while carrying out

duties related to the epidemic. They include: (1) public and clinical healthcare providers such as doctors and nurses, (2) any person empowered under the Act to take measures to prevent the outbreak of the disease, and (3) other persons designated as such by the state government.
- An "act of violence" includes any of the following acts committed against a healthcare service personnel: (1) harassment impacting living or working conditions, (2) harm, injury, hurt, or danger to life, (3) obstruction in the discharge of his duties, and (4) loss or damage to the property or documents of the healthcare service personnel. Property is defined to include a: (1) clinical establishment, (2) quarantine facility, (3) mobile medical unit, and (4) other property in which a healthcare service personnel has a direct interest, in relation to the epidemic.
- The Ordinance specifies that no person can: (1) commit or abet the commission of an act of violence against a healthcare service personnel, or (2) abet or cause damage or loss to any property during an epidemic. Contravention of this provision is punishable with imprisonment between 3 months and 5 years, and a fine between ₹ 50,000 and 2 lakh. This offense may be compounded by the victim with the permission of the Court. If an act of violence against a healthcare service personnel causes grievous harm, the person committing offense will be punishable with imprisonment between 6 months and 7 years, and a fine between ₹ 1 lakh and 5 lakh. These offenses are cognizable and nonbailable.

■ CONCLUSION

Violence against doctors is not always avoidable. Until there is a sociological gap, economic rift and frustration, this phenomenon will be there. It is imperative that every effort should be made to curb violence. These measures should be institutionalized. Violence against HCWs should be curbed with a firm hand. The doctor who is assaulted is not in the same position as a lay person. He is discharging his duty while being assaulted. The full force of justice should be faced by the perpetrators of such incidents.

■ REFERENCES

1. Halwani T, Takrouri M. Medical laws and ethics of Babylon as read in Hammurabi's code (History). Internet J Law Healthc Ethics. 2006;4:1-8.
2. Assaults on Medical Men. JAMA. 1892;18:399-400.
3. S, Dey. Over 75% of doctors have faced violence at work, study finds. Mumbai: Times of India; 2015.
4. Dora SK, Batool H, Nishu RI, Hamid P. Workplace Violence Against Doctors in India: A Traditional Review. 2020;12: e8706.
5. Liu J, Gan Y, Jiang H, Li L, Dwyer R, Lu K, et al. Prevalence of workplace violence against healthcare workers: a systematic review and meta-analysis. Occup Environ Med. 2019;76:927-37.
6. Yang SZ, Wu D, Wang N, Hesketh T, Sun KS, Li L, et al. Workplace violence and its aftermath in China's health sector: implications from a cross-sectional survey across three tiers of the health system. BMJ Open. 2019;9: e031513.
7. Kumar M, Verma M, Das T, Pardeshi G, Kishore J, Padmanandan A. A study of workplace violence experienced by doctors and associated risk factors in a Tertiary care hospital of South Delhi, India. J Clin Diagn Res, 2016;10:LC06-10.
8. Government of Maharashtra. (2010). The Maharasthra Medicare Service Persons and Medicare Service Institutions (Prevention of Violence and Damage or Loss of Property) Act 2010. [Online] Available from https://lj.maharashtra.gov.in/Site/Upload/Acts/H-75%20Act%20PDF.pdf. [Last accessed October, 2021].
9. Kumari A, Kaur T, Ranjan P, Chopra S, Sarkar S, Baitha U. Workplace violence against doctors: Characteristics, risk factors, and mitigation strategies. J Postgrad Med. 2020;66:149-54.
10. Russel GW. Aggression in the Sports World: A Social Psychological Perspective. Oxford: Oxford University Press; 2008.
11. Sun T, Gao L, Li F, Shi Y, Xie J, Wang S, et al Workplace violence, psychological stress, sleep quality and subjective health in Chinese doctors: a large cross-sectional study. BMJ Open. 2017;7:e017182.
12. Indian Medical Association (IMA). (2018). States Acts and Ordinance on Violence Against Doctors and Medical Insitutions. [Online] Available from: https://ima-india.org/windata/ccima/Legal/17.pdf. [Last accessed October, 2021].
13. Ministry of Health and Family Welfare, Government of India. (2020). The Epidemic Diseases (Amendment) Ordinance, 2020. [Online] Available from: https://prsindia.org/billtrack/the-epidemic-diseases-amendment-ordinance-2020. [Last accessed October, 2021].

■ LONG QUESTIONS

1. What is the broad meaning of the term violence against doctors? What are the types of violence that healthcare workers face?
2. Discuss the short- and long-term impact of violence against doctors.
3. Discuss the short- and long-term strategies to mitigate violence against healthcare workers.
4. How should the aftermath of a violent incident against healthcare workers and facilities be managed?

■ SHORT QUESTIONS

1. What is Hammurabi's code? What does it say about punishment of doctors?
2. Which medical personnel are considered as high risk for violence in healthcare?
3. What are high-risk situations for violence in healthcare?
4. What are the usual inciting factors for mob violence?
5. What is a rush team? What is its role in healthcare-related violence?

6. What are the vital steps that a doctor should take when faced with a situation that has potential for violence or when violence is occurring?

MULTIPLE CHOICE QUESTIONS

1. Which of the following about violence against doctors is true?
    a. It occurs only in illiterate sections of society
    b. Violence is a problem seen in public hospitals only
    c. It is an ancient phenomenon
    d. Violence is only communal in origin
2. What proportion of doctors have faced violence in some form in India?
    a. 10%
    b. 50%
    c. 75%
    d. 95%
3. Of the following who are considered not to be at a high risk of violence in healthcare?
    a. Gynecologists
    b. Casualty doctors
    c. Women doctors
    d. Pathologists
4. The majority of people who gather in a mob violence situation will be:
    a. Physically assaulting doctors
    b. Will be shouting slogans
    c. Bystanders
    d. Trying to prevent violence
5. Which of the following is true about impact of violence against doctors?
    a. Most doctors stop working after one episode of violence
    b. Doctors are financially compensated by the state when faced with violence
    c. Doctors who face violence encourage young people to take up medicine as a profession
    d. Absenteeism is common in doctors who face violence
6. Under the Medical Protection Act a violent incident against healthcare is:
    a. Bailable
    b. To be tried in the High Court
    c. Punishable by imprisonment up to 3 years
    d. A fine of ₹ 5,000,000 can be levied

Answers
1. c 2. c 3. d 4. c 5. d 6. c

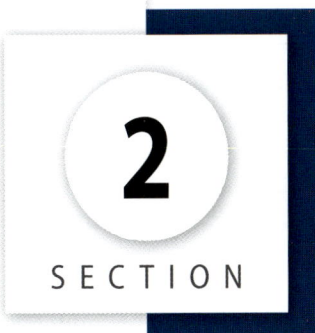

SECTION 2

Normal Pregnancy

2.1 FERTILIZATION, IMPLANTATION, AND PLACENTAL DEVELOPMENT

Milind R Shah, Rajesh V Darade

■ INTRODUCTION

It is essential that human species should pass on genetic material from generation to generation for existence. It is possible if adults are capable of producing fertile offspring. Then only this chain continues.[1] Scientists discovered the dynamics of human fertilization in the 19th century.[2]

As ovarian follicle grows in ovary in first half of menstrual cycle, oogonium in the follicle also grows and undergoes maturation. It becomes primary oocyte and undergoes first meiotic division to shed the first polar body. Second meiotic division is also in progress at the time of ovulation but not complete unless spermatozoon enters ovum. When ovulation occurs, ovum is released from Graafian follicle and enters infundibulum of fallopian tube, spindle is already formed for separation of second polar body.

Fertilization occurs in ampulla of fallopian tube. As spermatozoon enters ovum, completion of second meiotic division takes place, which is already in progress, and second polar body is shed. Now nucleus of the ovum becomes female pronucleus and gets ready to unite with male pronucleus, which is transformed from head of spermatozoon. Both these pronuclei loss their membranes, there is mixing of 23 chromosomes from either of these pronuclei to form new 23 pairs. These 46 chromosomes undergo changes leading to formation of embryo with two cell stage. So one can see that there is no one cell stage of the embryo.

Now as this zygote travels towards uterus it undergoes segmentation and still surrounded by zona pellucida which has very important function of preventing zygote getting attached to tubal epithelium. By the time it enters uterus, zygote has already reached the stage of morula that is 16 cell stage and looks like mulberry because of cleavage which is still in process. The outer layer of morula, which constitutes now trophoblast which has property to get attached and invade tissues it comes in contact, leads to sticking of zygote to uterine endometrium which is called as implantation. Approximate time period from fertilization to implantation is 6 days in human being. Another peculiarity of implantation in humans is invasion of trophoblast continues till entire blastocyst gets buried in thickness of endometrium which is called as interstitial implantation.

After implantation of embryo to uterine endometrium, which is now called as decidua, it gets discriminated into various parts according to its position in relation to embryo. The part, which separates embryo from uterine lumen, is called as decidua capsularis, part which covers rest of the uterine cavity is called as decidua parietalis, and part which is deeper to embryo is called decidua basalis which forms placenta eventually.

■ BIOCHEMICAL CHANGES

There are many biochemical changes, which occur during these events:

- Glycoprotein of the zona pellucida induces acrosomal reaction which releases acrosomal enzymes which helps sperms to penetrate ovum.
- Plasma membranes of sperm and ovum fuse together at specific receptor sites which are species specific.
- There are certain alterations in zona and plasma membrane after fertilization to prevent entry of other spermatozoa.
- Plasma membrane of ovum has also some role in entry of sperm as it releases lysosomal enzymes which are called as zonal reaction.
- The process of restoration of diploid chromosomes is again very complicated. Chromosomes of both pronuclei have single chromatid which undergoes deoxyribonucleic acid (DNA) replication to form second chromatids. Meanwhile spindle is formed and one chromosome of each pair moves to end of spindle. This leads to formation of two cells with 46 chromosomes.

- Now here onwards, two daughter cells which are smaller in size than ovum undergo continuous cleavage to form more cells and size also gets smaller and smaller to reach the size of most cells of our body.

PROCESS OF FERTILIZATION

There are many steps in process of fertilization. These are as follows:
- Sperm transport
- Capacitation
- Egg transport
- Oocyte maturation
- Fusion of gametes
- Acrosome reaction
- Cortical reaction
- Zona reaction
- Cell division.

Sperm Transport

Spermatogenesis is a complex process where spermatozoa are formed within seminiferous tubules of human testes. This process is possible because of androgens, which are secreted mainly by testicular Leydig cells located in the interstitial tissue outside the seminiferous tubules. After production, it also needs to undergo maturation in epididymis which is again dependent on androgens. This maturation is essential for mobility of sperms and also to gain fertility potential. So sperms when produced in the seminiferous tubules which are immotile are released into luminal fluid and transported to the epididymis. As they do not have motility they are transported passively to the rete testis. Rete testis is a branched reservoir of the openings of the seminiferous tubules. There are efferent ducts between rete testis and epididymis whose number varies in different individuals. The epididymis can be divided into three parts, called caput, corpus, and cauda. The transit of spermatozoa through the epididymis in humans usually takes 2–6 days. The proximal cauda is a segment of epididymis where most spermatozoa attain their full fertilizing capacity. Now after this process of maturation the spermatozoa are capable of moving progressively. This characteristic of spermatozoa is must before fertilization. Transportation of spermatozoa from the vagina is active process because of mobility of sperms and is via the cervical canal and the uterine cavity to reach the ampulla of the fallopian ducts, where fertilization occurs. In fact, the ejaculated semen is deposited near the external cervical opening where the environment is very acidic due to lactic acid and thus hostile to spermatozoa. The alkaline pH of the ejaculate protects spermatozoa in this acidic environment. This protection is temporary and that is why only few spermatozoa remain motile in the vagina and that too for few hours.

This process of transportation of sperms from vagina into the cervical canal is supported by the pressure alterations in the vagina due to the female orgasm. Once transported in cervical canal, the spermatozoa are stored in cervical crypts. Again here this transport is cumulative effect by the muscle contractions of the reproductive tract wall and motility of sperms. It is also essential to have harmony between sperms and cervical mucus and the motility of spermatozoa during the transport are important, and if it is lacking can cause infertility. The change in the composition of cervical mucus at midcycle also affects the passage. The transportation further of spermatozoa through the fallopian tubes is a cumulative effect of sperm motility, fluid flow, and contractive movements of the tubal walls.

Capacitation

This is again a process dependent on many enzymes where removal of adherent seminal plasma proteins and reorganization of plasma membrane lipids and proteins takes place to make them able to complete process of fertilization. It involves an influx of extracellular calcium, increase in cyclic adenosine monophosphate (AMP), and decrease in intracellular pH. Capacitation occurs while sperm reside in the female reproductive tract. Capacitation is now commonly regarded as the reversible, prefertilization activation process of sperm which results in the spermatozoa gaining the ability to:
- Develop hyperactivated motility, with vigorous nonlinear flagellar motion
- Bind to the zona pellucida
- Undergo the acrosome reaction
- Proceed eventually to fusion with the oolemma and egg fertilization.

Ovum Transport

Now ovum also needs to get transported from process of ovulation and also even after fertilization to enter in uterine cavity as morula. Ovulated eggs adhere to the surface of the ovary. The fimbrial end of the tube picks up those eggs which is similar like sweeping and possible because of fimbrial process. Once captures by fimbria, muscular movements of tubes help for further transport towards ampulla of tubes. Total time spent by oocyte in tubes is about 80 hours. Out of this, the oocyte and its surrounding cumulus are in the ampulla of fallopian tube within 15–20 minutes. Remaining time is basically to allow time for the endometrium to become receptive and the blastocyst to become capable of implantation **(Fig. 1)**.

Oocyte Maturation

Oocyte also needs to undergo maturation which is affected and regulated by the sex hormones. There is interaction of growth factors and cytokines in the follicular fluid.

Acrosome Reaction

Binding of sperm to the zona pellucida is the easy part of fertilization. But next challenge is more important, which

SECTION 2: Normal Pregnancy

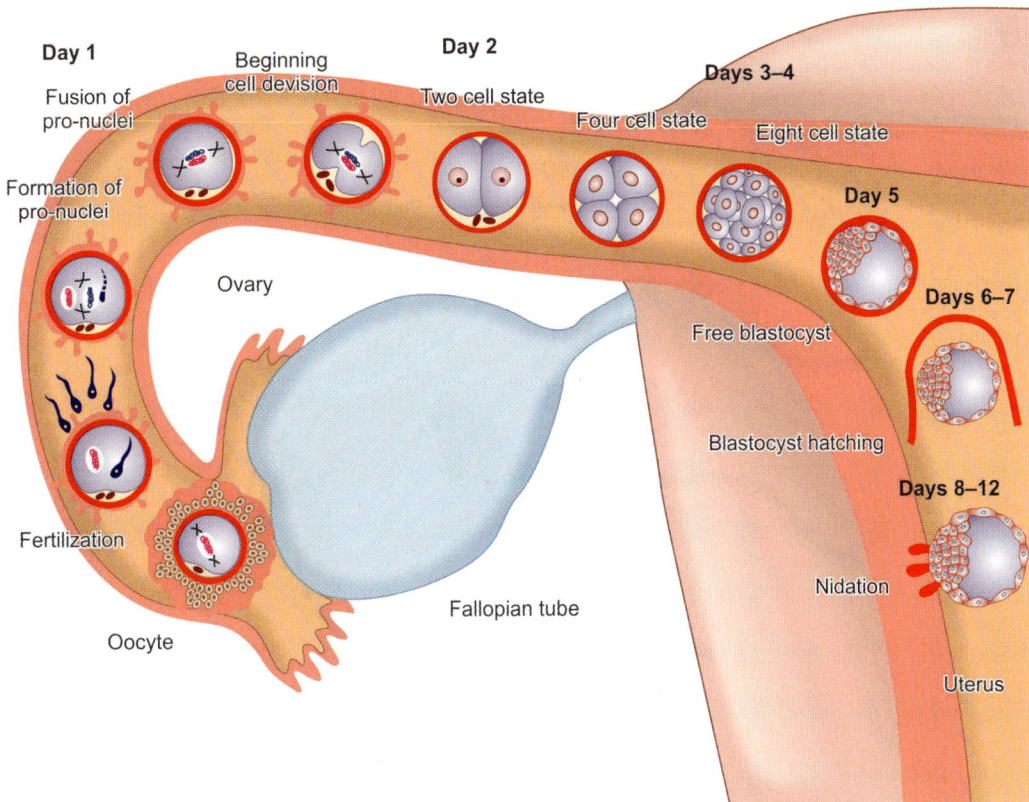

Fig. 1: Fertilization and implantation.

is penetration of zona pellucida to reach to the oocyte. This challenge is possible because of the acrosome. Acrosome is modified lysosome that is packed with zona-digesting enzymes and located around the anterior part of the sperm's head **(Fig. 2)**.

The acrosome reaction is like a drill, which is enzymatic drill to the zona pellucida. The same zona pellucida protein that serves as a sperm receptor also stimulates a series of events that lead to many areas of fusion between the plasma membrane and outer acrosomal membrane. Membrane fusion and vesiculation denudes the acrosomal contents and leads to release of acrosomal enzymes from the head of sperm.

This denuding is continuous process, as sperm passes through the zona pellucida and also leads to more loosing of the plasma membrane and acrosomal contents. So as an end entire anterior surface of its head, down to the inner acrosomal membrane, is denuded **(Fig. 3)**.

As we understand importance of these acrosomes, it explains if sperm lose their acrosomes before encountering the oocyte are unable to bind to the zona pellucida and thereby unable to fertilize. So in semen analysis and sperm function tests, assessment of acrosomal integrity of ejaculated sperm is very important.

Penetration of the Zona Pellucida

This penetration is like knife cutting and even shape of human sperm head is like knife and it is also supported by constant

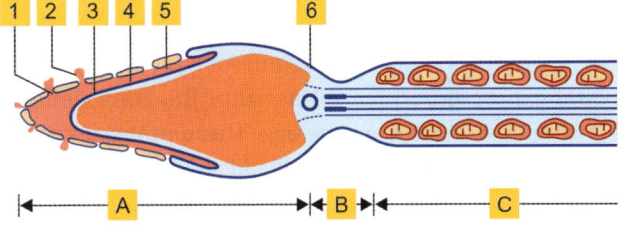

Fig. 2: Sperm acrosome reaction.

propulsive force from tail of sperms. So its combination with acrosomal enzymes, allows the sperm to create a tract through the zona pellucida **(Fig. 4)**.

Sperm-Oocyte Binding

Once a sperm penetration is complete through zona pellucida, it binds to and fuses with the plasma membrane of the oocyte. Naturally as acrosomes are utilized, binding occurs at the posterior region of the head of sperm.

It is mediated by specific proteins:
- PH-20 also called SPAM1
- PH 30 also called fertilin.

Egg Activation and Cortical Reaction

Egg is very silent prior to fertilization and is arrested in metaphase of the second meiotic division. Binding of a sperm initiates a number of metabolic and physical changes

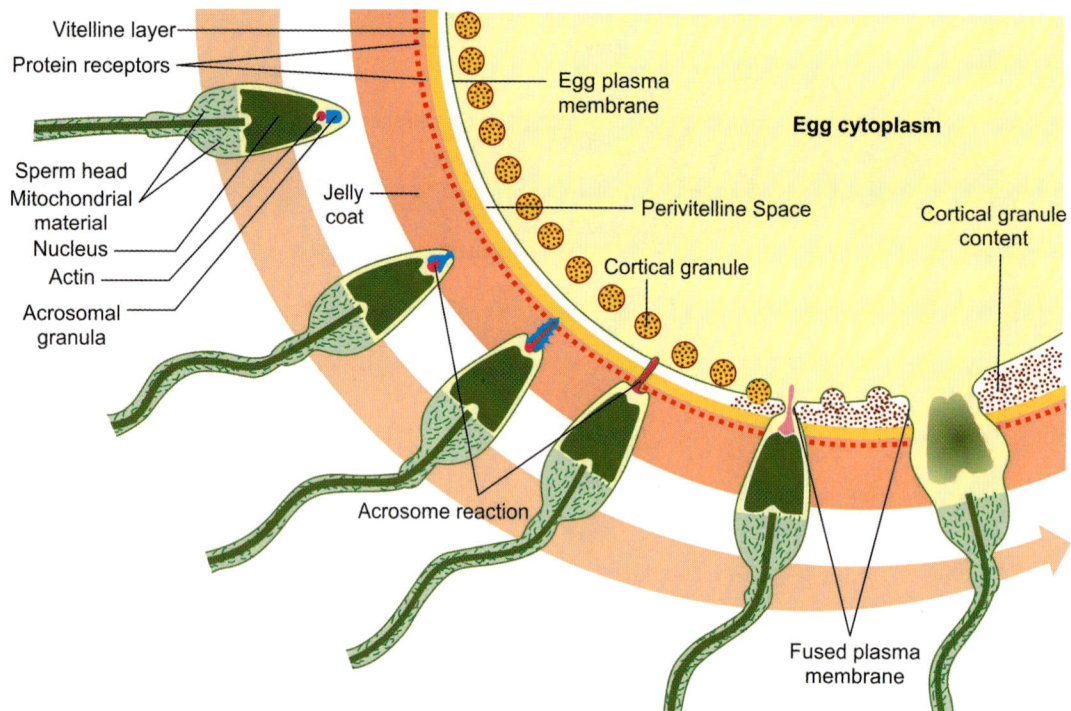

Fig. 3: Oocyte denudation.

that is called as egg activation. Main changes are rise in the intracellular concentration of calcium, completion of the second meiotic division, and also cortical reaction.

The cortical reaction means large exocytosis of cortical granules which are seen after sperm-oocyte fusion. These cortical granules contain a mixture of enzymes, including several proteases, which diffuse into the zona pellucida following exocytosis from the egg. These proteases help to alter the structure of the zona pellucida which we call as zona reaction. There is also interaction between components of cortical granules and the oocyte plasma membrane.

Zona Reaction

The importance of the zona reaction is that it causes inhibition to polyspermy in most mammals. This effect is due to two important changes in the zona pellucida:
1. The zona pellucida becomes hard like concrete. Sperm which are following successful sperm are stopped in their tracks.
2. Also there is destruction of sperm receptors in the zona pellucida. Therefore, there is no chance to all those sperms that have not yet bound to the zona pellucida to bind and they lose the race of fertilization.[3]

■ DEFECTS IN FERTILIZATION

Now anything we saw above can go wrong and leads to some defects in the fertilization process leading to some disorders like polyspermy. That leads to multiple sperm fertilizing an egg.

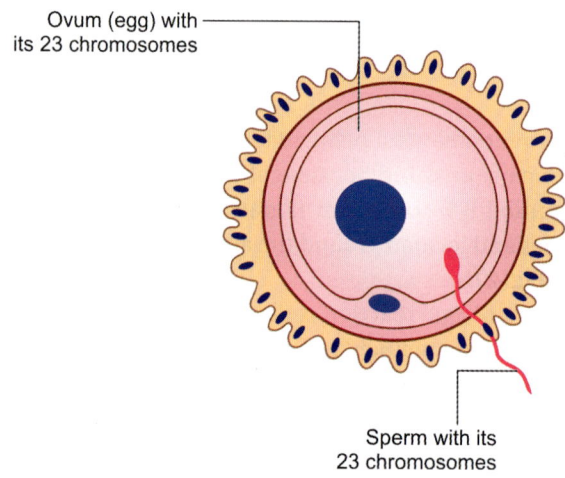

Fig. 4: Penetration of the zona pellucida.

■ IMPLANTATION

In human being, implantation of a fertilized ovum is most commonly occurs about 9 days after ovulation, which varies between 6 and 12 days.[4]

Implantation of the human embryo is a complex process. It involves several steps such as embryo apposition and attachment to the epithelium, traversing the epithelium and invasion of the epithelial stroma (*see* **Fig. 1**).[5]

The reception-ready phase of the endometrium of the uterus is usually termed as the "implantation window" and lasts about 4 days. There is every probability of oocyte getting flushed from uterine cavity in this time. There is hypothesis that the hormones cause a swelling and causes filling of uterine cavity which is otherwise flattened, which may also help to press the blastocyst against the endometrium.[6]

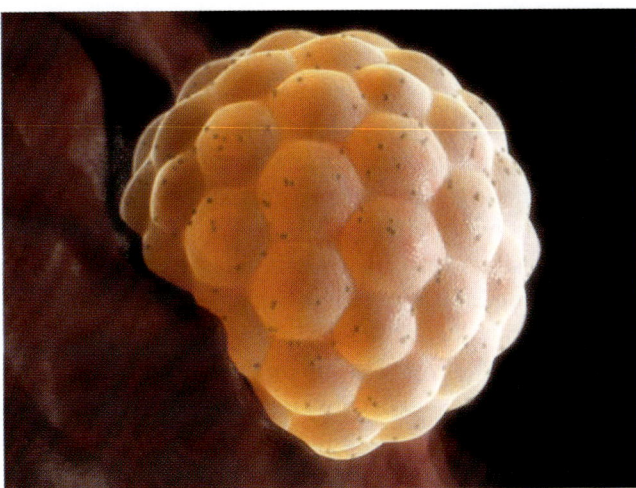

Fig. 5: Morula stage embryo.

Implantation can be studied under following headings:
- The embryo at implantation
- Endometrium at implantation
- Embryo-endometrial interaction.

The Embryo at Implantation

Four days after fertilization and after a series of mitotic division the zygote reaches the uterus at the morula stage **(Fig. 5)**.[7,8] On the fifth day, a blastocyst is formed in the uterus and on day 6 it sheds its zona pellucida and starts to implant in the endometrium. The blastocyst at this stage consists of an inner cell mass, which forms the fetus and outer cells, the trophectoderm that ultimately form the trophoblast, and then placenta. The zona pellucida is shed as the embryo hatches just before implantation. This occurs as a result of the direct effect of the uterine fluid on the zona as well as the penetration of the zona by the trophectoderm of the embryo. Hatching apparently starts in the anembryonic pole. Implantation starts at the embryonic pole of the blastocyst. Size of cells at embryonic pole is larger apparently syncytial, while cells at anembryonic pole are smaller. The specific embryonic anembryonic axis of the blastocyst is an essential component of implantation. Human embryos attach through the trophectoderm overlying the inner cell mass. Trophectoderm differentiates rapidly during this stage. Leptin receptors are present in endometrial tissue during midluteal phase. Various cytokines and galectins become expressed in trophectoderm. Leukemia inhibitory factor (LIF) has a significant role in implantation.

Endometrium at Implantation

Establishment of uterine receptivity is still a great biological mystery. Endometrium undergoes cyclical development with the sole purpose of establishing a pregnancy. In normal 28 days cycle, the maximal receptivity is between days 20 and 24 and is effected by the many different endometrial products. These proteins can be used as markers of uterine receptivity, especially to identify women at risk for implantation failure.

At this phase, very important morphological change occurs in the endometrium. That is formation of uterine pinopodes. Pinopodes are small, finger-like protrusions from the endometrium. They appear between day 19 and day 21 of gestational age. This corresponds to a fertilization age of approximately 5–7 days, which corresponds well with the time of implantation. They only persist for 2–3 days.[9] Pinopodes are ultramicroscopic club-shaped structure that appears at the edges of the gland openings. Their appearance is progesterone dependent. They absorb the uterine fluid and help in the process of apposition of the embryo to the endometrium. Their presence is associated with loosening of the intraepithelial cell bridges, which help in invasion. During the window of implantation, screening for a number of protein products may help to assess receptivity of the endometrium. Some of these products are:

- Cell adhesion molecules such as mucins, integrins, and trophinin
- Growth factors such as cytokines, epidermal growth factor (EGF), LIF, colony-stimulating factor-1 (CSF-1), and transforming growth factor-beta (TGF-beta)
- Enzyme inhibitors such as tissue inhibitors of metalloproteinase (TIMP), esophageal cancer (EC), etc.

Embryo-endometrial Interaction

The embryo-endometrial dialogue is characterized by three essential events:
1. Apposition
2. Adhesion
3. Invasion.

Apposition

Apposition occurs when the embryo comes in contact with the endometrium. This is facilitated by the absorption of the uterine fluid by the pinopodes.[10] In the apposition-phase, the presence of blastocyst causes inhibition of apoptotic pathway, which saves endometrial epithelial cells (EEC), maintaining more EEC prepared for the initial contact. This suggests the existence of an antiapoptotic effect exerted by a soluble factors secreted by the human embryos for a few days. This process continued by induction of a juxtacrine apoptotic reaction that is maximal in the EEC in close contact with the blastocyst. Apoptotic death of EEC induced by the embryos is an important mechanism to allow the blastocyst to invade and breach the luminal epithelial barrier and as a consequence its trophectoderm comes in contact with the basement membrane and stromal invasion can proceed **(Fig. 6)**.

Adhesion

Adhesion is influenced by various cytokines and adhesion molecules. The cytokines include CSF-1, LIF, interleukin-1 (IL1), and ECF-1.

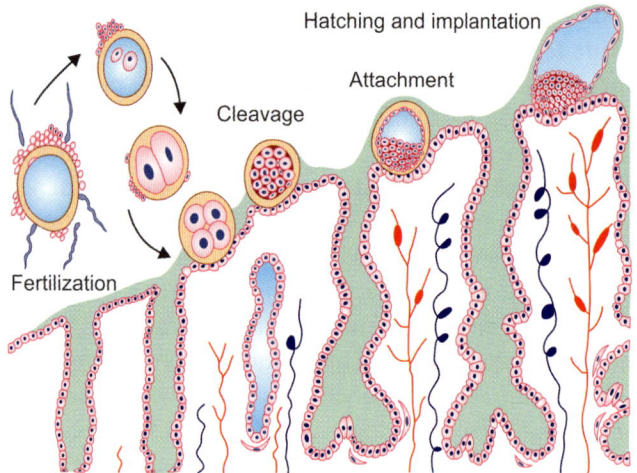

Fig. 6: Apposition.

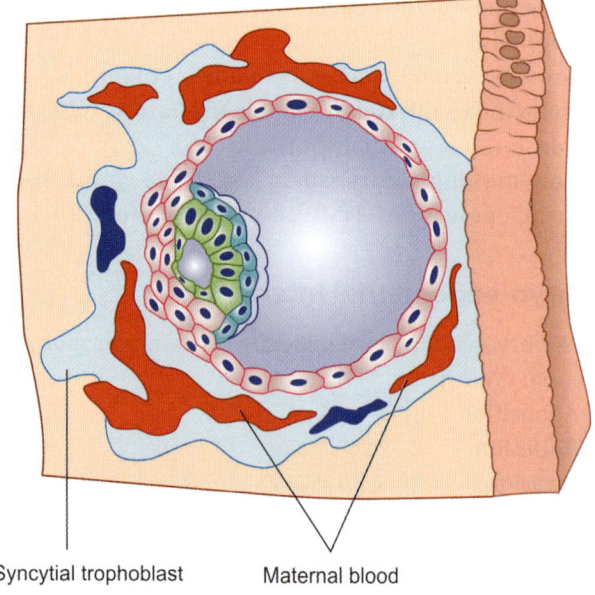

Fig. 7: Invasion.

Adhesion molecules including integrin and selectin family, fibronectin and laminin also help in adhesion. Integrins are transmembrane receptor, which helps connect cell to cell or cell to ground matrix. Fibronectin acts as a bridge in connecting the integrin molecules.

Invasion

The trophectoderm after adhesion invades the endometrium, basement membrane, and enter the stroma **(Fig. 7)**.[11]

The process of invasion involves minimal destruction of endometrial cells. The trophoblasts edge their way in between the endometrial cells, lift the basement membrane, and enter the decidua. Once the blastocyst enters the stroma, the decidual cells make way for it by property of contact inhibition. The trophoblasts produce enzymes such as serine proteases and matrix metalloproteinases (MMPs) which help to digest the matrix and help in invasion. Once implantation has proceeded sufficiently, the production of MMP ceases. This is under the influence of TIMP (inhibitors of MMP) and certain other proteins such as "*jun*" and "*fos*" gene products which bind to the promoter region of the *MMP* gene and prevent its transcription. The trophoblastic cells have receptors for plasminogen is converted to plasmin which in turn activates metalloproteinases like collagenase, gelatinase, and stromelysins.

Now the hydrolytic enzymes secreted by trophoblast digest the extracellular matrix between the endothelial cells to allow the embryo to penetrate completely into the decidua. There is morphological change in inner cell mass to form the primitive ectoderm and primitive endoderm. This contact of polar trophoblast to decidua is crucial factor in induction of proliferation of the trophoblast at the embryonic pole. A space appears between the ectoderm and trophoblast is the amniotic cavity.

Failure

Implantation failure has diverse causes, including abnormal cytokine and hormonal signals as well as epigenetic alterations. In cases of repeated early pregnancy loss, pregnancy rates can be improved by optimizing endometrial receptivity for implantation. Evaluation of implantation markers may help to predict pregnancy outcome and detect occult implantation deficiency.[12] One of the means by which this can be achieved by luteal support with progesterone which supports function of corpus luteum.

DEVELOPMENT OF PLACENTA

The fetomaternal organ, which we call as placenta, has two components: the *fetal placenta*, or chorion frondosum, which develops from the same sperm and egg cells that form the fetus; and the *maternal placenta*, or decidua basalis, which develops from the maternal uterine tissue **(Fig. 8)**.[13]

The trophoblasts which are precursor cells of the human placenta appear 4 days after fertilization as the outer layer of cells of the blastocyst. These early blastocyst trophoblasts differentiate into all the other cell types found in the human placenta. When fully developed, the placenta serves as the interface between the mother and the developing fetus. The placental trophoblasts perform many functions for a successful pregnancy by mediating such critical steps as implantation, pregnancy hormone production, immune protection of the fetus, increase in maternal vascular blood flow into the placenta, and delivery. For almost 9 days the embryo is surrounded by two layers of trophoblasts: the inner mononuclear cytotrophoblast and the outer multinucleated syncytiotrophoblast layer. This arrangement of embryo, trophoblasts, and maternal tissue remains the paradigm throughout gestation. This trophoblast interface not only serves as the means to extract nutrients from the mother, but protects the embryo and fetus from maternal immunologic attack.

The placental growth continues throughout pregnancy. However, development of the maternal blood supply to the placenta is complete by the end of the first trimester of pregnancy that is approximately 12–13 weeks **(Fig. 9)**.

After the Fourth Month[14]

The cytotrophoblast slowly disappears from the walls of the tertiary villi. Therefore, the distance between the maternal and fetal vessels diminishes. Cytotrophoblast also disappears from the chorionic plate. In the basal plate, the cytotrophoblast remains mainly at the level of the cytotrophoblast layer. Together with the decidua and fibrin deposits, they form protrusions which are intercotyledon septa that project into the intervillous space to form cotyledons. The formative mechanism of these intercotyledon septa remains speculative and probably depends on the folding together of the basal plate which, for its part, has resulted from the proliferation of the stem villi. They push the basal plate back. In addition, the spread of the placenta into the uterine cavity also appears to contribute to the creation of the septa **(Fig. 10)**.

Though these septa form the cotyledons but never go deep in the chorionic plate. This arrangement is basically for circulation of maternal blood which can circulate freely between cotyledons.[15] Towards end of pregnancy, villous stems of the placenta increase in length and the fibrinoid deposits such as extracellular substance made up of fibrin, placental secretions, and dead trophoblast cells, accumulate in the placenta. This happens to form the subchorial Langhans' layer, as well as at the level of the basal plate beneath the stem villi and the cytotrophoblast layer, where the fibrin deposits form Rohr's layer. Still deeper in the decidua basalis these deposits form Nitabuch's layer. This is where the placenta detaches itself from the uterus at birth.

Pathologies Related to Placental Development

- Placenta accreta, when the placenta implants too deep into actual muscle of uterus
- Placenta previa, when the placement of the placenta is closer to or covers the cervix
- Placental abruption where it separates before third stage.

Infections which can involve the placenta are:
- Placentitis, due to the toxoplasmosis, rubella, cytomegalovirus, herpes simplex, and herpes simplex virus (TORCH) infections
- Chorioamnionitis.

■ KEY MESSAGES

- Fertilization and implantation is useful to maintain the continuity of species and to pass the genetic information from generation to generation.

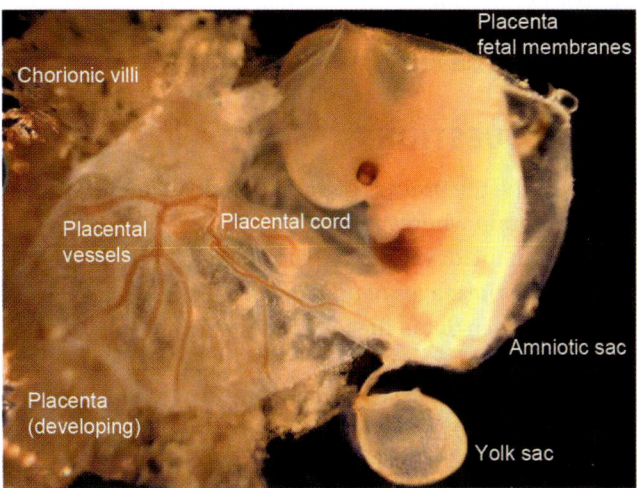

Fig. 8: Development of placenta.

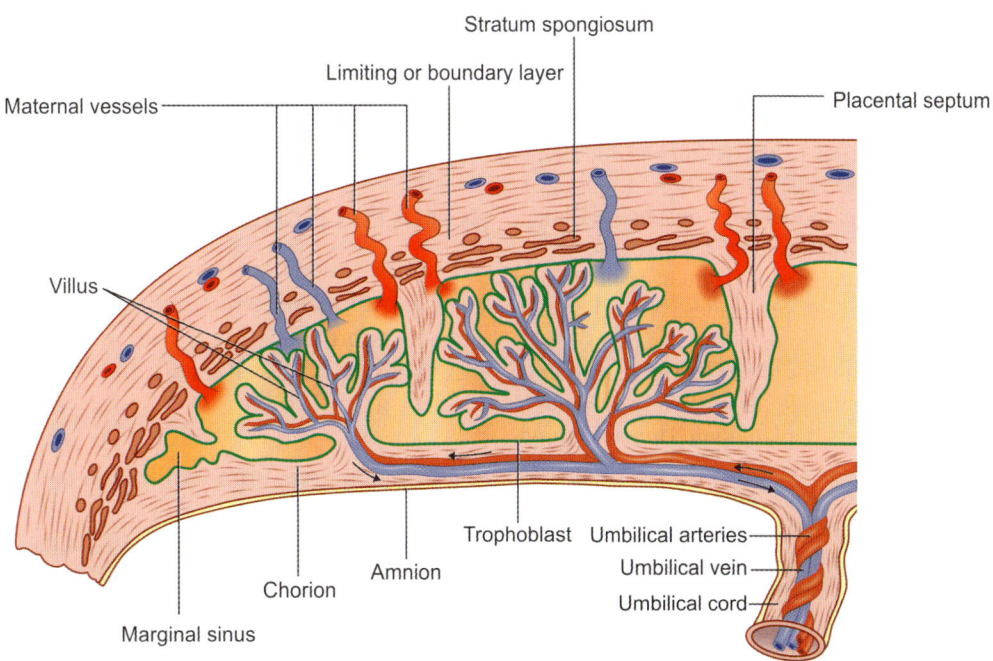

Fig. 9: Development of the maternal blood supply to the placenta.

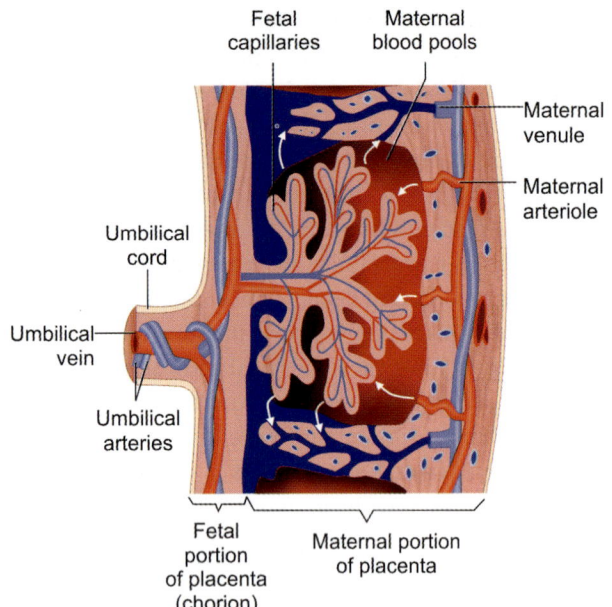

Fig. 10: Placental circulation and septation.

- There are lots of biochemical changes occur from fertilization to implantation.
- Two daughter cells continuously cleavage to form more cells and size also gets smaller and smaller to reach the size of most cells of our body.
- Some defects in the fertilization process can cause some disorders.
- Fertilization involves multiple steps.
- The embryo-endometrial dialogue is characterized by three essential events; apposition, adhesion, and invasion.
- Implantation failure has diverse causes.
- After full development, placenta serves as the interface between the mother and the developing fetus.

REFERENCES

1. Fritz MA, Speroff L. Clinical Gynecologic Endocrinology and Infertility, 9th edition. Netherlands: Wolters Kluwer; 2019.
2. Fielding G. An Introduction to the History of Medicine. Philadelphia: Saunders; 1921. pp. 566-7.
3. Simon C, Pellicer A, Remohi J. Emerging Concepts on Human implantation. Oxford: Oxford University Press; 1999.
4. Wilcox AJ, Baird DD, Weinberg CR. Time of implantation of the Conceptus and loss of pregnancy. N Engl J Med. 1999;340(23):1796-9.
5. Scott L, Alvero R, Leondires M, Miller B. The morphology of human pronuclear embryos is positively related to blastocyst development and implantation. Human Reprod. 2000;15:2394-403.
6. "Implantation stages" (http://www.embryology.ch/anglais/gnidation/etape 02. html). *Human Embryology*
7. Hansotia M, Desai S, Parihar M. Advanced Infertility Management. New Delhi: Jaypee Brothers Medical Publishers (P) Ltd.; 2002. pp. 338-40.
8. Tucker MJ, Morton PC, Wright G, Ingargiola PE, Sweitzer CL, Elsner CW, et al. Enhancement of outcome from intracytoplasmic sperm injection: does co-culture or assisted hatching improve implantation rates? Human Reprod. 1996;11:2434-7.
9. Walter B, Boulpaep E. Medical Physiology: A Cellular and Molecular Approach. Oxford: Elsevier; 2004.
10. Bentin-Ley U, Sjögren A, Nilsson L, Hamberger L, Larsen JF, Horn T. Presence of uterine pinopodes at the embryo-endometrial interface during human implantation in vitro. Human Reprod. 1999;14:515-20.
11. Aplin JD. The cell biology of human implantation. Placenta. 1996;17:269-75.
12. Cakmak H, Taylor HS. Implantation failure: molecular mechanisms and clinical treatment. Hum Reprod Update. 2011;17(2):242-53.
13. The Free Dictionary. Maternal Placenta. [online] Available from: https://medical-dictionary.thefreedictionary.com/maternal+placenta. [Last accessed October, 2021].
14. Ecker JJ, Laufer MR, Hill JA. Measurement of embryonic factors predictive of pregnancy outcome in women with a history of recurrent abortion. Obstet Gynecol. 1993;81:84-7.
15. Wilcox AJ, Weinberg CR, O'Connor JF, Baird DD, Schlatterer JP, Canfield RE, et al. Incidence of early loss of pregnancy. N Engl J Med. 1988;319:189-94.

LONG QUESTIONS

1. Describe the process of implantation in detail with help of diagram wherever necessary.
2. Explain the development of placenta.
3. Explain the stages of oogenesis.
4. Describe in detail the journey of sperm from tubules till fertilization.
5. Explain the various biochemical changes that take place in process of fertilization.

SHORT QUESTIONS

1. What is capacitation?
2. Describe acrosome reaction in detail with diagram.
3. What is sperm transport?
4. What are causes of failure of fertilization?
5. What is embryo-endometrial reaction?

MULTIPLE CHOICE QUESTIONS

1. Fertilization occurs in........portion of fallopian tube.
   a. Ampullary   b. Fimbrial
   c. Isthmic   d. Infundibulum
2. Morula is........cell stage.
   a. 8   b. 16
   c. 32   d. 4
3. Time interval from fertilization to implantation is........days.
   a. 8 days   b. 4 days
   c. 6 days   d. 10 days
4. All are parts of epididymis, except:
   a. Caput   b. Corpus
   c. Cauda   d. Zona

5. Time spent by the egg in tube is:
   a. 80 hours   b. 24 hours
   c. 60 hours   d. 48 hours
6. Binding of sperm to oocyte is by:
   a. Acrosome   b. Post acrosomal region
   c. Body   d. Tail
7. Fertilin protein is:
   a. PH20   b. PH10
   c. PH30   d. PH40
8. Zona pellucida (reaction) is catalyzed by:
   a. Kinase   b. Dehydrogenase
   c. Reductase   d. Protease
9. Implantation window lasts for about........days.
   a. 4   b. 6
   c. 8   d. 10
10. Precursor of human placenta is:
    a. Zona pellucida   b. Trophoblast
    c. Theca cells   d. Granulosa cells
11. Following are the changes in embryo-endometrial interaction, except:
    a. Apposition   b. Adhesion
    c. Invasion   d. Implantation
12. Multiple sperm fertilizing an egg is called as:
    a. Polyspermy   b. Oligospermy
    c. Azoospermy   d. Asthenospermy
13. Prior to fertilization egg is arrested in...........stage of second meiotic division.
    a. Metaphase   b. Anaphase
    c. Telophase   c. None
14. Spermatozoa are formed in:
    a. Epididymis   b. Seminiferous tubules
    c. Rete testis   d. None
15. Factors responsible for penetration of zona pellucida are:
    a. Motility   b. Zona digestive enzymes
    c. Both   d. None
16. Leptin receptors are present in endometrium during:
    a. Luteal phase   b. Proliferative
    c. Secretary phase d. None
17. Steps in process of fertilization are:
    a. Sperm transport   b. Capacitation
    c. Oocyte maturation d. All
18. Ovarian follicle grows in ovary in:
    a. First half of menstrual cycle
    b. Second half
    c. Both
    d. None
19. During acrosomal reaction sperm passes through which layer of oocyte:
    a. Zona pellucida   b. Granulosa cells
    c. Theca cells   d. None
20. Constant propulsive force for sperm is from:
    a. Tail   b. Head
    c. Body   d. None

Answers											
1. a	2. b	3. c	4. d	5. a	6. b
7. c	8. d	9. a	10. b	11. d	12. a
13. a	14. b	15. c	16. a	17. d	18. a
19. a	20. b

2.2 FETAL PHYSIOLOGY: GROWTH AND DEVELOPMENT

Halvi Ediger Ramaraju, Surya Malik

INTRODUCTION

Growth is a crucial characteristic of a child that differentiates child from an adult. This process of growth begins from the time of conception and continues till adulthood.

Fetal growth is categorized into three stages:
1. *Ovular stage*: From the time of fertilization to blastocyst formation—duration 3 weeks (5 weeks of amenorrhea)
2. *Embryonic stage*: From 3 to 8 weeks—formation of an embryo
3. *Fetal stage*: From 8 weeks (10 weeks of amenorrhea) fetal development.

FETAL DEVELOPMENT

By the 8th week after fertilization or 10th week after last menstrual period (LMP), the embryo develops into a fetus which has identifiable human characteristics. Thereafter, the fetus continues to grow in both length and weight.

Length

The length of the fetus, measurement is usually taken from the vertex to the coccyx (crown-rump length) in earlier weeks. While from the end of 20th week onwards, it is measured from vertex to the heel [crown-heel length (CHL)].

By the 11th week, CHL measures 8–9 cm. During the 4th and 5th month, the CH is gauged by Haase rule, i.e., CHL equals square of the lunar month (at the 4th lunar month. CH length is 4 × 4 = 16 cm).

From the 7th lunar month onwards the CHL in centimeter is the number of lunar months multiplied by 5.

Weight

The fetal weight increases in a linear fashion up to about 20 weeks. It is controlled by genetic factor in the first half and by extraneous environmental factors in the second half.

Factors influencing fetal weight are:
- Race (European babies are heavier than Indian)
- Gender (male > female)
- Height and weight of parents (tall and heavier mother have heavier babies)
- Birth order (weight rises from first to second pregnancy) and
- Social factors (heavier babies in social class I and II).

Fetal growth is predominantly controlled by insulin-like growth factor 1 (IGF-1), insulin, and growth factors. Growth hormone is essential for postnatal growth. The average fetal weight at term varies between 2.5 kg and 3.5 kg and increases with the maternal age and parity.

Age of the Fetus

It can be measured by gestational age. Gestational age is measured from the first day of last LMP, it indicates how far along the pregnancy is.

The length is more reliable criterion than weight to calculate the age of the fetus. In the first trimester, CRL (mm) + 6.5 = gestational age in weeks.

Morphological Growth

After ovulation in the first 2 weeks, development phases include:
- Fertilization
- Blastocyst formation
- Blastocyst implantation.

Primitive chorionic villi are formed soon after implantation of the fertilized ovum. With the development of chorionic villi, the products of conception are conventionally referred to as an embryo. The early stages of preplacental development and formation of the placenta are described in another chapter of the textbook.

Embryonic Period

With respect to human embryology, the term embryo means "an unborn human in the first 8 weeks" from fertilization.

At the beginning of the third week after ovulation and fertilization the embryonic period commences, which coincides with the time of beginning of next menstrual cycle. This embryonic period lasts for about 6 weeks, this is when organogenesis take place.

These 8 weeks of embryonic period are divided into 23 developmental stages (Carnegie stages).

■ FETAL GROWTH AND DEVELOPMENT

During the first 8 weeks, the term embryo is used to denote the developing organism because it is the time when organogenesis takes place. The "fetal period" is marked by rapid growth in length and weight of the conceptus as a whole, which influences growth in each organ system. A term fetus arbitrarily is defined as one which has attained 37 weeks of gestational age.

Fetal Period (Epochs)

Transition from the embryonic period to the fetal period occurs at 7 weeks after fertilization, corresponding to 9 weeks after onset of the last menses. At this time, the fetus approximates 24 mm in length, most organ systems have developed.

12 Weeks

The fetus is 7–9 cm long and weighs 12–15 g. The fingers and toes have nails, and the external genitalia begin to differentiate as male or female. The volume of amniotic fluid is about 30 mL. The intestine undergo peristalsis and are capable of absorbing glucose. At this time fetus makes spontaneous movements.

16 Weeks

The length is 14–17 cm and weight about 100 g. The gender is determined by experienced observer by 14 weeks. In addition to hemoglobin F, formation of hemoglobin A begins.

20 Weeks

The fetus weighs 300 g. Fetus moves about every minute and is active 10–30% of time (DiPietro, 2005). The fetal skin has become less transparent; a downy lanugo covers its entire surface.

24 Weeks

The fetus weight is about 600 g. Some fat is beginning to be deposited beneath the wrinkled skin. Survival at this stage would be extremely rare, because though canalicular growth of lungs have occurred, alveoli for gas exchange have not yet formed.

28 Weeks

The fetus weight is about 1,050 g. Length is about 37 cm. The skin covered with vernix caseosa, pupillary membrane from eyes has disappeared. Normal neonate born at this gestational age has 90% survival without physical and neurological impairment.

32 Weeks

The fetus weight is about 1,700 g and length is 42 cm. Skin is still red and wrinkled.

36 Weeks

The fetus weight is about 2,500 g and length is about 47 cm. Because of deposition of subcutaneous fat, body become more rounded, previously wrinkled appearance of the face has been lost.

40 Weeks

The term fetus averages about 50 cm in length and 3,200–3,500 g in weight.

Placenta and Fetal Growth

The placenta is the organ of transfer between mother and fetus. At the maternal fetal interface, there is transfer of oxygen and nutrients from mother to fetus and carbon dioxide and metabolic waste from the fetus to mother. There is no direct communication between fetal blood circulation and maternal blood circulation as fetal blood stays in fetal capillaries and maternal blood in sinusoids. Bidirectional transfer depends on the processes that permit or aid the transport through the syncytiotrophoblast of the intact chorionic villi.

FETAL NUTRITION

Glucose and Fetal Growth

Glucose is an important nutrient for fetal growth and energy. This mechanism exists during pregnancy so that to minimize maternal glucose use so that the limited maternal supply is available to the fetus.

Glucose Metabolism and Transport

There is a significant correlation between maternal arterialized venous blood glucose and fetal umbilical venous glucose concentrations in 14 fetuses examined between 17 and 21 weeks of gestation, with the fetal glucose concentration lower than in mother. These investigators found that at maternal glucose concentrations <4.4 mmol/L, fetal umbilical venous glucose may excess with maternal glucose concentration and may be independent of it and later in gestation there is a close linear relationship between maternal and fetal glucose.

FETAL CIRCULATION

Environmental changes occurring in the abrupt transition from intrauterine life to an independent existence necessitate certain circulatory adaptations in the newborn. These include diversion of blood flow through the lungs, closure of ductus arteriosus and foramen ovale, and obliteration of the ductus venosus and umbilical vessels.

Infant circulation has three phases: (1) The predelivery phase, in which the fetus depends upon the placenta; (2) the intermediate phase, which begins immediately after delivery with the infant's first breath; and (3) the adult phase which is normally completed during the first few weeks of life.

Predelivery Phase

The umbilical vein carrying the oxygenated blood (80% saturated) from the placenta enters the fetus at the umbilicus and runs along the free margin of the falciform ligament of liver. In liver, it gives off branches to the left lobe of the liver and receives the deoxygenated blood from the portal vein. The greater portion of the oxygenated blood, mixed with some portal venous blood, short circuits the liver through the ductus venosus to enter the inferior vena cava (IVC) and hence to right atrium of the heart. The O_2 content of this mixed blood is thus reduced. The terminal part of IVC receives blood from the right hepatic vein.

In the right atrium, most of the well oxygenated (75%) ductus venous blood is preferentially directed into the foramen ovale by the valve of the IVC and crista dividens and passes into the left atrium. Here it is mixed with small amount of venous blood returning from the lungs through pulmonary veins. This left atrial blood is passed on through the mitral opening into the left ventricle.

During ventricular systole, the left ventricular blood is pumped into the ascending arch of aorta and distributed by their branches to the heart, neck, brain, and arms. The right ventricular blood with low oxygen content is discharged into the pulmonary trunk. Since the resistance in the pulmonary arteries during fetal life is very high, the main portion of the blood passes directly through the ductus arteriosus into the descending aorta by passing the lungs where it mixes with the blood from the proximal aorta. The deoxygenated blood leaves the body by way of two umbilical arteries to reach the placenta where it is oxygenated and gets ready for recirculation.

Adult Phase

The ductus arteriosus usually is obliterated in the early postnatal period, probably reflex action secondary to an elevated oxygen tension and the interaction of some prostaglandins. If the ductus remains open, a systolic crescendo murmur, which diminishes during diastole (machinery murmur), is often/ heard over the second left interspace.

Obliteration of the foramen ovate is usually complete in 6–8 weeks as pressure in right atrium drops with fusion of its valve to the left interatrial septum. The foramen may remain patent in some of the newborns.

FURTHER READING

1. Barclay AEJ, Barcroft J, Barron DA, Franklin KJ, Pritchard MML. Studies of the fetal circulation and of certain changes that takes place after birth. Am J Anat. 1941;69:383.
2. Boddy K, Dawes GS. Fetal breathing. Br Med Bull. 1975;31:3.
3. Brace RA, Wolf EJ. Normal amniotic fluid volume changes throughout pregnancy. Am Obstet Gynecol. 1989;161:382.
4. Chez RA, Mintz DH, Reynolds WA, et al. Maternal-fetal plasma glucose relationships in late monkey pregnancy. Am J Obstet Gynecol. 1975;121:938.
5. Clymann RI, Heymann MA. Pharmacology of the ductus arteriosus. Pediatr Clin North Am. 1981;28:77.
6. Comline RS, Cross KW, Dawes GS, Nathanielsz PW. Fetal and neonatal physiology: proceedings of Sir Joseph Barcroft Symposium Cambridge,1973.
7. Dawes GS. The umbilical circulation. Am J Obstet Gynecol. 1962;84:1634.

8. DiPietro JA. Neurobehavioral assessment before birth. MRDD Res Rev. 2005;11:4.
9. Gilbert WM, Brace RA. Amniotic fluid volume and normal flows to and from the amniotic cavity. Semin Perinatol. 1993;17:150.
10. Grisaru-Granovsy S, Samueloff A, Elstein D. The role of leptin in fetal growth: a short review from conception to delivery. Eur J Obstet Gynecol Reprod Biol. 2008;136(2):146.
11. Gruenwald P. Growth of the human foetus. In: McLaren A (ed): Advances in Reproductive Physiology. New York, Academic Press, 1967.
12. Jansson T, Powell TL. Human placental transport in altered fetal growth: does the placenta function as a nutrient sensor? A review. Placenta. 2006;27:S91.
13. Liggins GC. Fetal lung maturation. Aust NZ J Obstet Gynaecol. 1994;34:247.
14. Lissauer D, Piper KP, Moss PA, et al. Persistence of fetal cells in the mother: friend or foe? BJOG. 2007;114:1321-5.
15. Manganaro L, Perrone A, Savelli S, et al. Evaluation of normal brain development by prenatal MR imaging. Radiol Med. 2007; 112:444.
16. Moore KL. The Developing Human: Clinically Oriented Embryology, 4th edition. Philadelphia, Saunders, 1988.
17. Pataryas HA, Stamatoyannopoulos G. Hemoglobins in human fetuses: evidence for adult hemoglobin production after the 11th gestational week. Blood. 1972;39:688.
18. Scammon RE, Calkins LA. The relation of the body weight and age of the human fetus. Pro Soc Exp Biol Med. 1924;22:175.
19. Stockman JA III, deAlarcon PA. Hematopoiesis and granulopoiesis. In: Polin RA, Fox WW (eds). Fetal and Neonatal Physiology. Philadelphia, Saunders. 1992.p.1327.
20. Streeter GL. Weight, sitting height, head size, foot length and menstrual age of human embryo. Contributions Embryol. Carnegie Inst. 1920;11:143.
21. Tavian M, Péault B. Embryonic development of the human hematopoietic system. Int J Dev Biol. 2005;49:243.
22. Thorpe-Beeston JG, Nicolaides KH, Felton CV, et al. Maturation of the secretion of thyroid hormone and thyroid-stimulating hormone in the fetus. N Engl J Med. 1991;324:532.
23. Walker J, Turnbull EPN. Haemoglobin and red cells in the human foetus and their relation to the oxygen content of the blood in the vessels of the umbilical cord. Lancet. 1953; 2:312.
24. Watkins JB. Physiology of the gastrointestinal tract in the fetus and neonate. In: Polin RA, Fox WW (eds). Fetal and Neonatal Physiology. Philadelphia, Saunders, 1992.p.1015.
25. Whitsett JA. Composition of pulmonary surfactant lipids and proteins. In: Polin RA, Fox WW (eds). Fetal and Neonatal Physiology. Philadelphia, Saunders, 1992. p. 941.
26 Wladimiroff JW, Campbell S. Fetal urine-production rates in normal and complicated pregnancy. Lancet. 1974;1:151.

LONG QUESTIONS

1. Discuss the fetal circulation and its adaptations at birth.
2. What are the key milestones of growth in the fetus? What factors affect fetal growth?
3. What is pulmonary surfactant? Discuss its production, importance and role in neonatal life.

SHORT QUESTIONS

1. How is regular breathing established in newborn?
2. List the changes that occur in the circulatory system of the infant immediately after birth.
3. How does fetal circulation differ from adult circulation?
4. Write brief about fetal nutrition.
5. Write a short note on Chemerism
6. What are the components of Meconium
7. What are the chief characteristics of fetal hemoglobin?

MULTIPLE CHOICE QUESTIONS

1. Which day after ovulation primitive fetal circulation established?
   a. 10   b. 12
   c. 21   d. 28
2. In which of the following does fetal hemopoiesis first occur?
   a. Fetal liver   b. Fetal bone marrow
   c. Fetal spleen   d. Yolk sac
3. When do fetal breathing movements commence?
   a. 8 weeks   b. 11 weeks
   c. 16 weeks   d. 24 weeks
4. Type of Hb which has least affinity for 2, 3-Diphosphoglycerate (2, 3-DPG) or (2, 3-BPG):
   a. Hb A   b. Hb F
   c. HbB   d. Hb A2
5. All of the following are derivatives of neural crest, except:
   a. Melanocyte   b. Adrenal medulla
   c. Sympathetic ganglia   d. Cauda equina
6. Surfactant production in lungs starts at:
   a. 28 weeks   b. 32 weeks
   c. 34 weeks   d. 36 weeks
7. Surfactant is produced by:
   a. Type II Pneumocytes   b. Type I Pneumocyte
   c. Macrophages   d. Endothelial cell
8. Surfactant is made up of:
   a. Fibrin   b. Mucoprotein
   c. Phospholipids   d. Fibrinogen
9. Which of the following vessels do not carry deoxygenated blood in fetal circulation?
   a. Pulmonary artery   b. Umbilical artery
   c. Umbilical vein   d. Pulmonary vein
10. Fetal period starts at:
    a. 9 weeks   b. 3 weeks
    c. 6 weeks   d. 12 weeks
11. The fetal circulation is first intact and functional, separated from maternal circulation at the age of:
    a. 8 days   b. 17 days
    c. 21 days   d. 25 days

Answers

1. c   2. d   3. b   4. b   5. d   6. a
7. a   8. c   9. c   10. a   11. d

2.3 CLINICALLY RELEVANT EMBRYOLOGY FOR OBSTETRICIANS

Madhuri Arvind Patel, Hemraj R Narkhede, Navin Srinivasan

INTRODUCTION

The process of progressing from single cell through the period of establishing organ primordia (first 8 weeks of development) is called embryogenesis. To improve better understanding of deviation from normal development, it is imperative to describe the different "phases" of fetal development and growth.[1]

In embryology, fertilization is taken as reference point for describing the development which is also called ovular age of the embryo. But in clinical practices we use menstrual age as reference point hence, while applying embryology knowledge in clinical practice, we should add roughly 2 weeks to embryonic age **(Fig. 1)**.[2]

Ovular phase: First 4 weeks after fertilization, in this phase a series of rapid mitotic divisions occur to form blastula. The organ anlagen are relatively positioned by the process of gastrulation.[2]

Embryonic phase: It starts from 3rd week until the end of 8th week; organogenesis occurs in this period and during this period three germ layers: (1) ectoderm, (2) mesoderm, and (3) endoderm give rise to number of specific tissues and organs.[2]

Fetal phase: It is interval from completion of organogenesis until delivery **(Table 1)**.

Natural events or insult that affects the development of individual life may occur at any phase. Also, time of occurrence of such event will determine the extent of damage. For example, monozygotic twinning where timing of insult has dramatic and profound effects upon subsequent development.[1]

In about 25–30% of monozygotic twins, the zygotic division occurs within 72 hours of fertilization, i.e., before morula stage which will give rise to dichorionic diamniotic twins similar to dizygotic twins. In approximately 65% of monozygotic twins, division occurs after 4–8 days of fertilization resulting into monochorionic diamniotic twins. In about 5% of monozygotic twins, division occurs after 8 days of fertilization giving rise to monochorionic monoaminotic twins. Very rarely in 1/50,000 live birth incomplete division will result after 13 days of fertilization giving rise to conjoined twins.[1]

A *mutagen* is a chemical or physical agent that induces genetic mutation.[3]

A *teratogen* is an agent or factor that causes the production of physical defects in developing embryo.

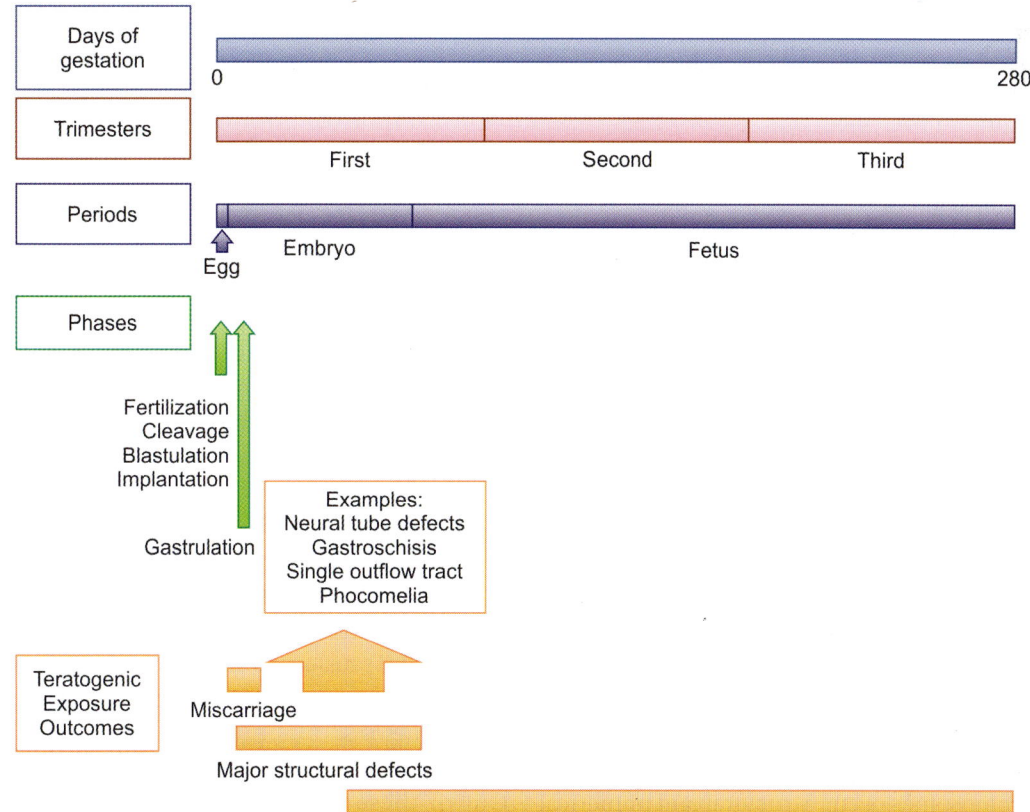

Fig. 1: Timeline of embryogenesis and effect of teratogen exposure.

TABLE 1: Congenital malformation in fetus/infant of diabetic mother.[3]		
System	**Malformation**	**Age of gestation (weeks)**
Nervous	Anencephaly, holoprosencephaly, microcephaly	4
Skeletal	Sacral agenesis, caudal agenesis	3
Cardiovascular	Ventricular septal defect (VSD), transposition of great vessels, patent ductus arteriosus (PDA), pulmonary stenosis	5–6
Renal	Duplication of ureter, renal agenesis	5
Other	Hypospadias	4

Wilson's criteria for identification of teratogens:[3]
1. An abrupt increase in the incidences of particular defect or association of defects (syndrome)
2. Coincidence of this increases with a known environmental change (e.g., new drug)
3. Known exposure to the environmental change early in pregnancy causing characteristically defective infants
4. Absence of other factors common to all pregnancies yielding infants with the characteristic defect or defects.

TYPES OF BIRTH DEFECTS[3]

Anomaly is a structural feature that departs from the normal.

Association is a grouping of anomalies that frequently occur together but are not actual syndromes.

Deformation is an abnormal form, shape, or position caused by mechanical forces.

Disruption is morphologic defect resulting from extrinsic breakdown or interference with normal development.

Malformation is a morphologic defect resulting from abnormal development.

Sequence is a pattern of defects that results from single event early in pregnancy.

Syndrome is a recognizable pattern of structural defects often with a predictable natural history that can be identified on several patients, thus allowing diagnosis and classification.

CHROMOSOMAL THEORY OF INHERITANCE[1]

Primary oocytes and primary spermatocytes both undergo meiosis I and meiosis II giving rise to gametes. Meiosis is reduction division unique for maintenance of 46 chromosomes (diploid). Crossovers are critical event in meiosis I in which interchange of chromatid segments between paired homologous chromosomes occur. Structural and numerical abnormalities of chromosomes are responsible for majority of birth defects and spontaneous abortions **(Figs. 2 and 3)**.[1]

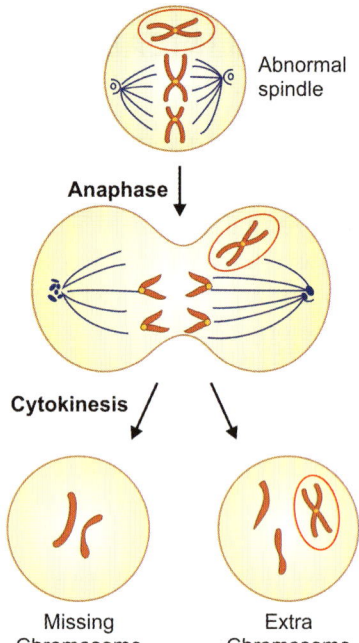

Fig. 2: Mitosis (nondisjunction).

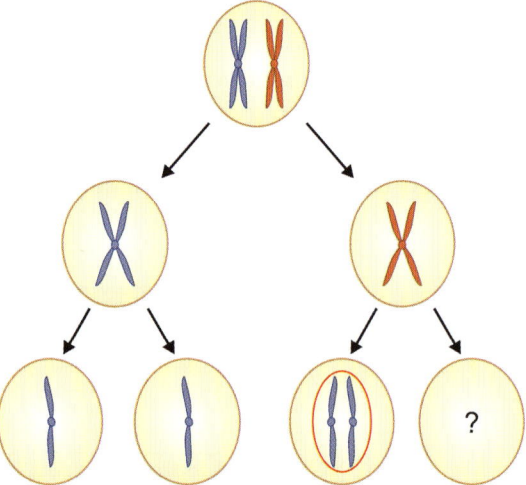

Fig. 3: Meiosis (nondisjunction).

As maternal age advances, i.e., after 35 years, a chance of nondisjunction increases. Rarely, during mitosis, nondisjunction occurs in embryonic cells, which result into *mosaicism*.[1] Other mechanisms like translocation in which chromosome breaks and piece of one chromosome gets attached to another. Such translocation may be balanced or unbalanced. In balanced, breakage and reunion occurs between two chromosomes, but no critical material is lost and individuals are normal. In unbalanced, translocation part of one chromosome is lost and altered phenotype is produced. Translocations are particularly common between chromosomes 13, 14, 15, 21, and 22 because they cluster during meiosis.[1]

Out of all conceptions, 50% get aborted spontaneously. Out of these abortions, 50% have major chromosomal abnormality. Thus, out of all conceptions, 25% have major chromosomal defect.[2]

Recurrent pregnancy losses due to chromosomal abnormalities:[1]
- Numerical abnormalities (50%)
- Structural abnormalities
  - Most common numerical abnormality—aneuploidy
  - Most common aneuploidy—trisomy (trisomy 16, 18, 13, and 21)
  - Most common mechanism for aneuploidy—nondisjunction > translocations
  - Translocations are common between chromosomes: 13, 14, 15, 21, and 22 as they cluster during meiosis.

Numerical Abnormalities

Trisomy 21 (Down Syndrome) (Fig. 4)[1]

Mechanism: Meiotic nondisjunction at oogenesis.

Features: Growth retardation, craniofacial abnormalities, upward slanting eyes, epicanthal folds, flat facies, low-set ears, cardiac defects, hypotonia, increased chance of leukemia, infections, thyroid dysfunction, premature aging, and early-onset Alzheimer's disease.

Incidence increases with increase in maternal age.

Prediction of Down syndrome:
- *Double marker test:* Done between 11^{+5} and 13^{+5} weeks.[2]
- *Triple/quadruple marker test:* 16–18 weeks **(Table 2)**.[2]

- Nuchal translucency-nasal bone (NT-NB) scan: Done between 11^{+5} and 13^{+5} weeks, NT > 3 mm and nuchal fold thickness > 6 mm are considered an increased risk for fetal aneuploidy and various structural anomalies like heart defects. NT implies the maximum thickness of the subcutaneous translucent area between the skin and soft tissue overlying the fetal spine at the back of the neck.[2]

Trisomy 18 (Edwards Syndrome)

Features: Growth retardation, intellectual deficit, micrognathia, flexed fingers and hands, cardiac, renal defects, etc.[1]

Trisomy 13 (Patau Syndrome)

Incidence: 1/20,000 births.

Features: Holoprosencephaly, cardiac defects, deafness, and eye defects—microphthalmia, anophthalmia, colobomas.[1]

Klinefelter Syndrome

Male babies with an extra X chromosome (47,XXY), caused by meiotic nondisjunction of XX chromosomes (1/500 newborns), characterized by infertility (seminiferous tubule hyalinization), gynecomastia. Karyotype is diagnostic, demonstration of Barr body in a male buccal smear.[4]

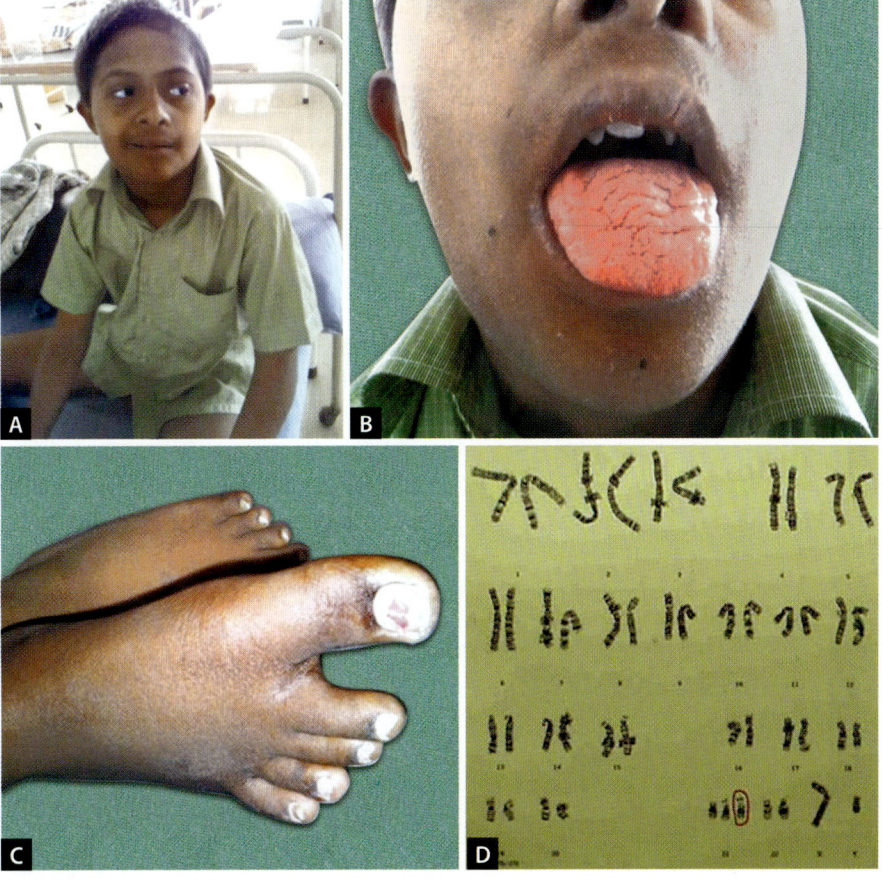

Figs. 4A to D: Phenotype features of Down syndrome. (A) Note the striking facial features; (B) Scrotal tongue; (C) Sandle big toe; (D) Chromosomal pattern showing trisomy 21.

Turner Syndrome (Fig. 5)[4]

Genotype: Female babies with 45,XO—only monosomy that is compatible with life.

Mechanism: 80%—nondisjunction of male gamete.

Features: Short stature, webbed neck, low-set ears and hairline, widely spaced nipples (shield chest), short fourth metacarpals, wide elbow carrying angle (cubitus valgus), poor sexual development—streak ovaries.

Diagnosis done by characteristic phenotype, findings of hypergonadotropic hypogonadism.

Karyotype—One sex chromosome; few may show presence of Y chromosome. Barr body negative females.

TABLE 2: Variations in triple markers in various anomalies.[2]

	Alpha-fetoprotein (AFP)	Estriol	Human chorionic gonadotropin (hCG)
Down syndrome	Low	Low	High
Trisomy 13	Normal	No data	Low
Trisomy 18	Low	Low	Low
Open neural tube defects	High	Normal	Normal

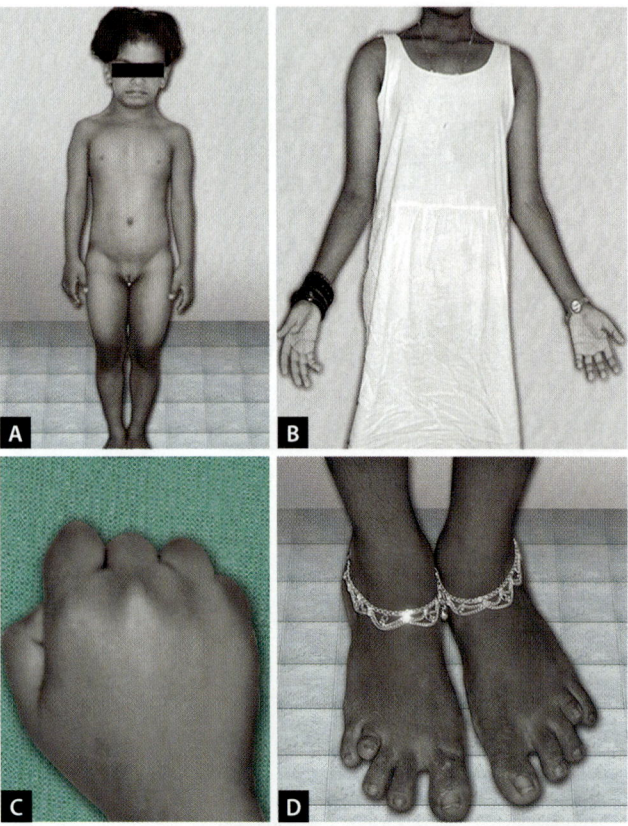

Figs. 5A to D: Phenotype features of Turner syndrome. (A) Note the short stature, typical facies, webbing of neck, shield chest; (B) Increased carrying angle: Cubitus valgus; (C) Knuckle sign—Brachymetacarpal; (D) Brachymetatarsal

Medical problems in Turner syndrome:[4]
- *Cardiovascular anomalies:* Bicuspid aortic valve, coarctation of the aorta, mitral valve prolapse, and aortic aneurysm.
- *Renal anomalies:* Horseshoe kidney, unilateral renal agenesis, pelvic kidney, rotational abnormalities, and partial or complete collecting system duplication.
- *Autoimmune disorders:* Autoimmune thyroiditis, type I diabetes, hepatitis, thrombocytopenia, and celiac disease.
- Sensorineural hearing loss.

Cataracts and Nystagmus

Attention-deficit/hyperactivity disorder (ADHD): Overall mortality is increased threefold because of circulatory disease, diabetes, and liver and renal problems.

Additional and periodic medical evaluation should include—echocardiography, renal ultrasonography (USG), thyroid-stimulating hormone (TSH) and free T4, complete blood count, fasting glucose, lipid profile, renal function tests, and liver enzymes, antiendomysial antibodies, and audiometry.

Structural Abnormalities

One or more chromosomes may undergo breakage (due to environmental factors like viruses, radiation, drugs). The broken piece of chromosome may be lost resulting in partial deletion of genes.[5]

Cri du Chat Syndrome

Partial deletion of 5p, characterized by cat-like cry, microcephaly, congenital heart defects.

Microdeletions[5]

Angelman syndrome: Maternal 15q11-13 microdeletion, characterized by intellectual disability, poor motor development, prone to unprovoked and prolonged period of laughter.[5]

Prader–Willi syndrome: Paternal 15q11-13 microdeletion, characterized by hypotonia, obesity, hypogonadism, undescended testis.[5]

Y chromosomal microdeletion: Azoospermic factor c (AZFc) deletion causes azoospermia.[5]

Miller–Dieker syndrome: Deletion 17q13 causing lissencephaly, developmental delay, seizures, cardiac and facial abnormalities.

Fragile sites and trinucleotide repeat sequence—fragile X syndrome: CGG repeats, FMR1 locus on Xq27, normal (5–200), > 99 (FMR1 premutation), > 200 (FXTAS—fragile X syndrome, ataxia telangiectasia)—large ears and jaws, large testis, and premature ovarian failure.[4]

Abnormal Gametes

- *Teratospermia:* Morphologically abnormal sperms
- Multinucleated/Parthenogenetic oocytes
- *Abnormal pronuclei:* Asymmetrical/single bull's eye
- *Abnormal polar bodies:* Unequal number of nuclear precursor bodies (NPBs), different positions.

OVULAR PHASE

First Week

When zygote divides in two cells stage, it undergoes series of mitotic divisions, which increases in number of cells **(Fig. 6)**. The cells are called blastomeres. After 8 cells stage, cells become compacted and increase their contact with each other and is called morula. Morula is further divided into inner cell mass and surrounding cells are called outer cell mass. Inner cell mass gives rise to embryo proper and outer cell mass forms the trophoblast (placenta).[1]

As morula enters uterine cavity, fluid seeps in and solid morula is converted into cyst called blastocyst **(Fig. 7)**. On 6th day, zona pellucida disappears and trophoblast over inner cell mass (embryoblast) begins to penetrate into endometrium. L-selectin on trophoblast and its carbohydrate receptors on endometrium mediate initial attachment of blastocyst to uterus.

Thus, during 1st week of development, the zygote has crossed morula and blastocyst stage and has begun to invade endometrium.[1]

- Trophoblastic L-selectins and carbohydrate receptors on the uterine epithelium mediate implantation.[1]
- After capture of blastocyst, there occurs invasion of trophoblast into endometrium, mediated by integrin, laminin, and fibronectin.[1]
- Integrin receptor for laminin promotes attachment.[5]
- Integrin receptor for fibronectin promotes migration.[5]

Embryonic stem cells (ESCs):[2] They are derived from inner cell mass/embryoblast. ESC is pluripotent, can form any cell type. They are widely used for treatment of diseases: diabetes, Alzheimer's disease, parkinsonism, anemia, and spinal cord injuries.

They are obtained in vitro fertilization (IVF) embryos by *reproductive cloning.*[2]

Newer technique—therapeutic cloning/somatic nuclear transfer: Devised to extract nuclei from adult cells (e.g., skin) and introduce into enucleated oocytes, which are harvested. This process has lesser risk of immune rejection.[2]

Abnormal zygotes: Usually, they are lost within 2–3 weeks post fertilization.

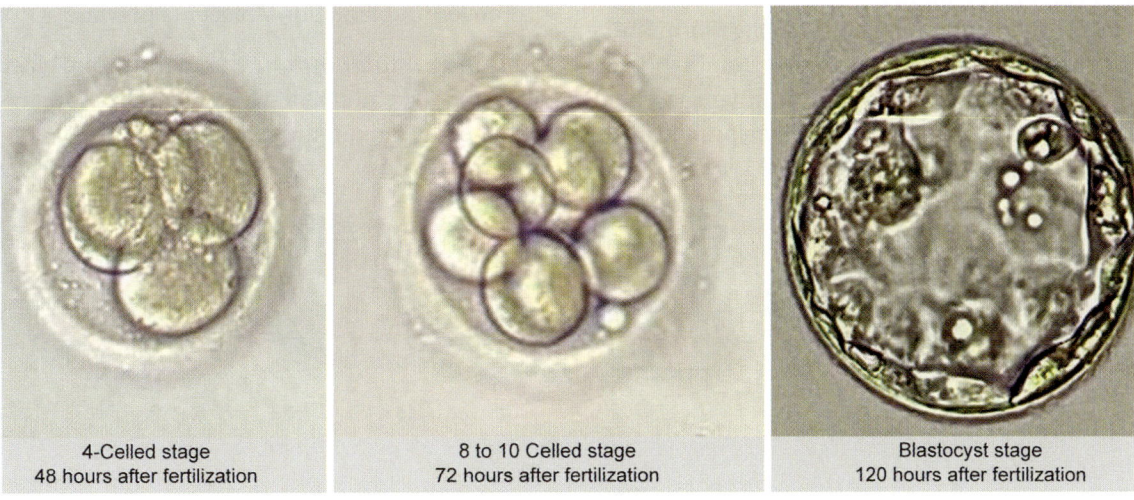

Fig. 6: Morulation and blastulation in the laboratory.

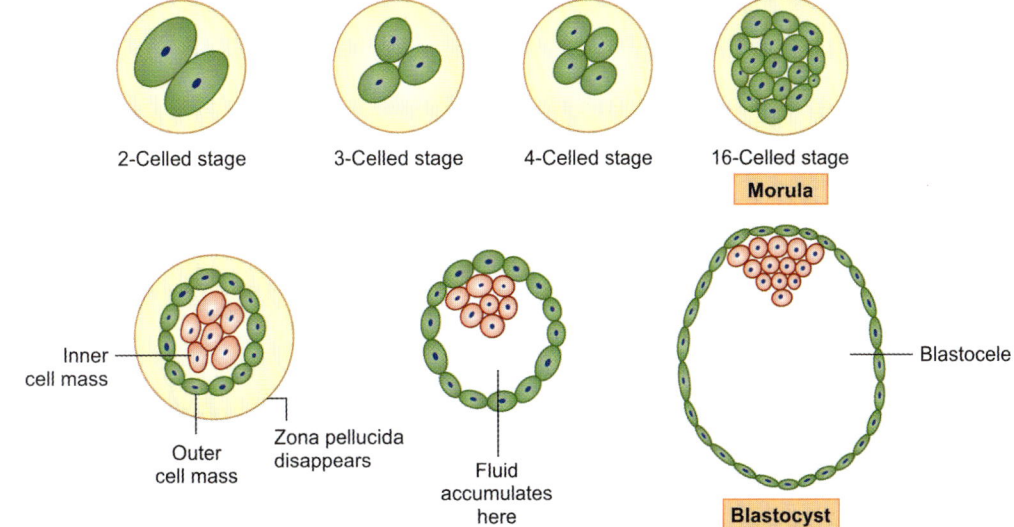

Fig. 7: Morulation and blastulation.

Unequal blastomeres: Fragmentation defects, expanded blastocyst, zona thinning.

Second Week

At start of 2nd week, blastocyst is partially embedded in endometrial stroma. The trophoblast divides into inner cytotrophoblast and outer syncytiotrophoblast, which erodes into maternal tissues. Cavities are formed into syncytiotrophoblast and after maternal sinusoid are eroded, maternal blood fills the lacunae. At the 2nd week, primitive uteroplacental circulation gets established and cytotrophoblast forms primary villi.[1]

Syncytiotrophoblast secrets human chorionic gonadotropin (hCG) by the end of 2nd week and by this stage quantity of this hormone is sufficient to be detected by radioimmunoassay for diagnosis of pregnancy.[1]

Inner cell mass (embryoblast) gives rise to bilaminar disk **(Fig. 8)**. A layer adjacent to blastocyst forms hypoblast and other layer epiblast. Cavity which forms in epiblast is called amniotic cavity. At anembryonic pole, cells originating from hypoblast form the thin membrane that lines the inner surface of trophoblast. This membrane and hypoblast form lining of primitive yolk sac. The cells originated from hypoblast proliferate and form new cavity in primitive sac called secondary yolk sac which is much smaller than primitive sac.[1]

Secondary yolk sac is the first element seen in gestational sac on USG and denotes true gestational sac.[1]

At 13th day of development, the surface defect in the endometrium usually gets sealed off; however, bleeding may occur at implantation site due to increased blood flow into lacunar spaces. This bleeding occurs at 28th day of menstrual cycle which is mistaken as menstrual period causing errors in dating of pregnancy.[1]

The new cells are formed between inner surface of cytotrophoblast and outer surface of primitive yolk sac. These cells form loose connective tissue, the extraembryonic mesoderm. Soon large cavities form in extraembryonic mesoderm coalesces to form chorionic cavity. The extraembryonic mesoderm lining the cytotrophoblast and amnion is called extraembryonic somatopleuric mesoderm. The lining covering the yolk sac is called extraembryonic splanchnopleuric mesoderm **(Fig. 9)**.

Abnormal site of implantation—ectopic pregnancy:
- Most common location of ectopic pregnancy—fallopian tube (ampulla)
- Too low implantation—placenta previa.

Abnormal implantation: Syncytiotrophoblast secretes beta-hCG. By end of 2nd week of fertilization, levels can be estimated by radioimmunoassay.

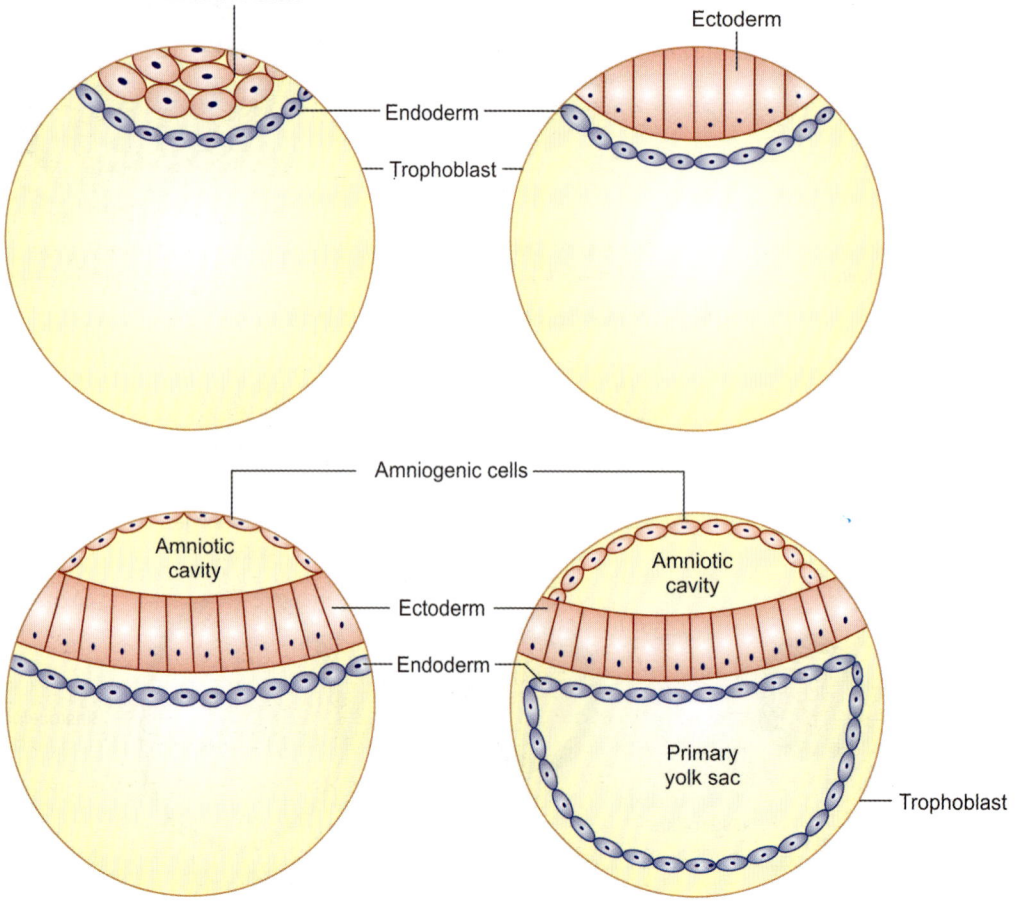

Fig. 8: Formation of bilaminar germ disk.

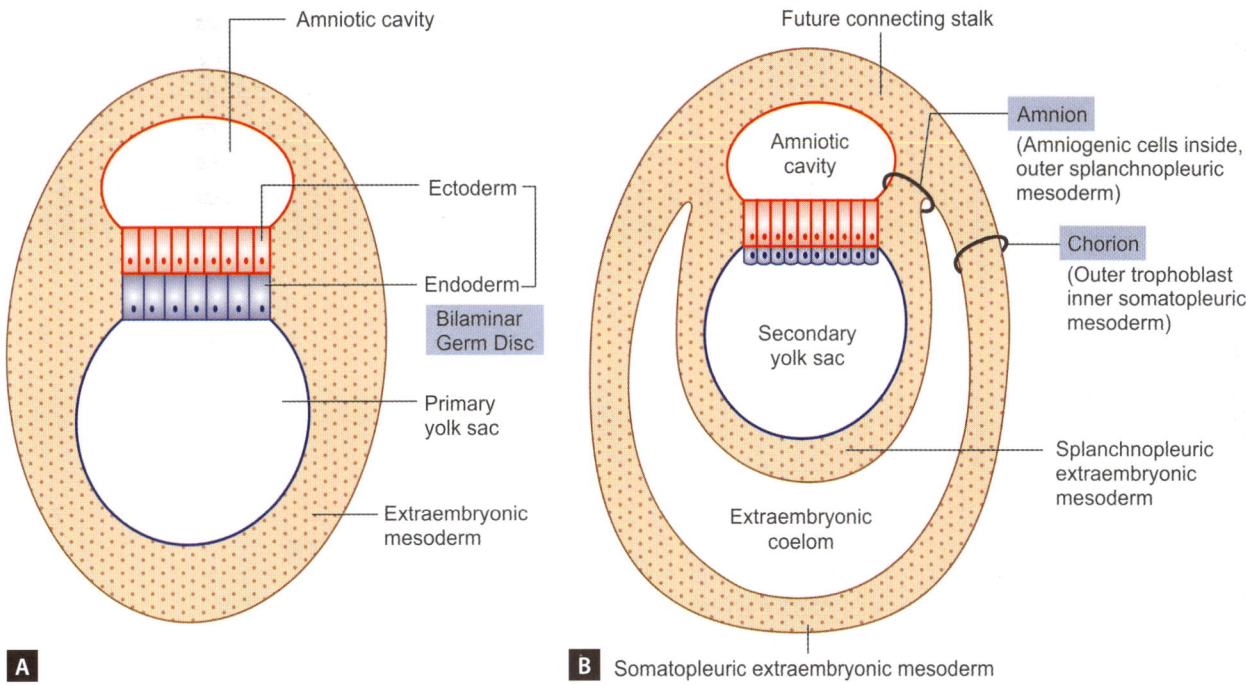

Figs. 9A and B: Formation of extraembryonic mesoderm.

Hartmann's sign: A small blood clot forms at the implantation site, *the Schlusskoagulum*, whose presence may be detected clinically by *spotting (Hartmann's sign)* and may lead to misinterpretation of the length of gestation.[5]

Protection against rejection:[5]
- Trophoblast lacks major histocompatibility complex class 1 (MHC-1), instead has human leukocyte antigen (HLA)—G, E, and C.
- Th2 > Th1, cell-mediated immunity to humoral immunity shift. Diseases that are mediated by cell-mediated immunity resolve (rheumatoid arthritis, multiple sclerosis) and humoral immunity mediated diseases flare up [systemic lupus erythematosus (SLE)] in pregnancy.

Third Week: Gastrulation

In 3rd week, all three germ layers are established **(Fig. 10)**. Gastrulation is process of formation of ectoderm, mesoderm, and endoderm in embryo. It begins with the formation of primitive streak on the surface epiblast. Cephalic end of primitive streak called primitive node which is slightly elevated area surrounding small pit, primitive pit. Cells of epiblast proliferate and arrive in the region of streak. These cells go below epiblast called invagination. These cells displace hypoblast and thus the endoderm is formed. Other cells come to lie in between epiblast and endoderm to form mesoderm. The remaining epiblast is called ectoderm. Notochord is formed from notochord plate between ectoderm and endoderm at center cranially to primitive node.[1]

At initiation of gastrulation, beginning of 3rd week after fertilization, cell populations are designed for various organ systems; therefore, this period becomes very crucial for the development of organs **(Fig. 11)**. Teratogens if present at this time will result in severe malformations.[1]

Gastrulation and Teratogenesis

Beginning of 3rd week of development is a highly sensitive stage for teratogenic insult. As described in **Tables 3 and 4**, the fetal development can be affected by infections and drugs.

Holoprosencephaly[2]

In early normal brain development, the prosencephalon or forebrain divides into the telencephalon and diencephalon. With holoprosencephaly, the prosencephalon fails to divide completely into two separate cerebral hemispheres and into underlying diencephalic structures.[2]

Cause: High alcohol doses taken 2 weeks post fertilization/4 weeks post last menstrual period (LMP)—damage cells on the midline of germ disk, causing defect in central craniofacial structures. It can be due to an obstructive process (aqueductal stenosis), or secondary to a destructive process (porencephaly or an intracranial teratoma).[6]

Features: Small forebrain, two lateral ventricles merge into single ventricle and eyes are placed closer (hypotelorism), cyclopia, or microphthalmia; lips—median cleft; or nose—ethmocephaly, cebocephaly, or arhinia with proboscis.[6]

Main forms of holoprosencephaly: Alobar, semilobar, and lobar types.

The alobar form accounts for 40–75% of cases, and approximately 30–40% have a numerical chromosomal abnormality, particularly trisomy 13.[2]

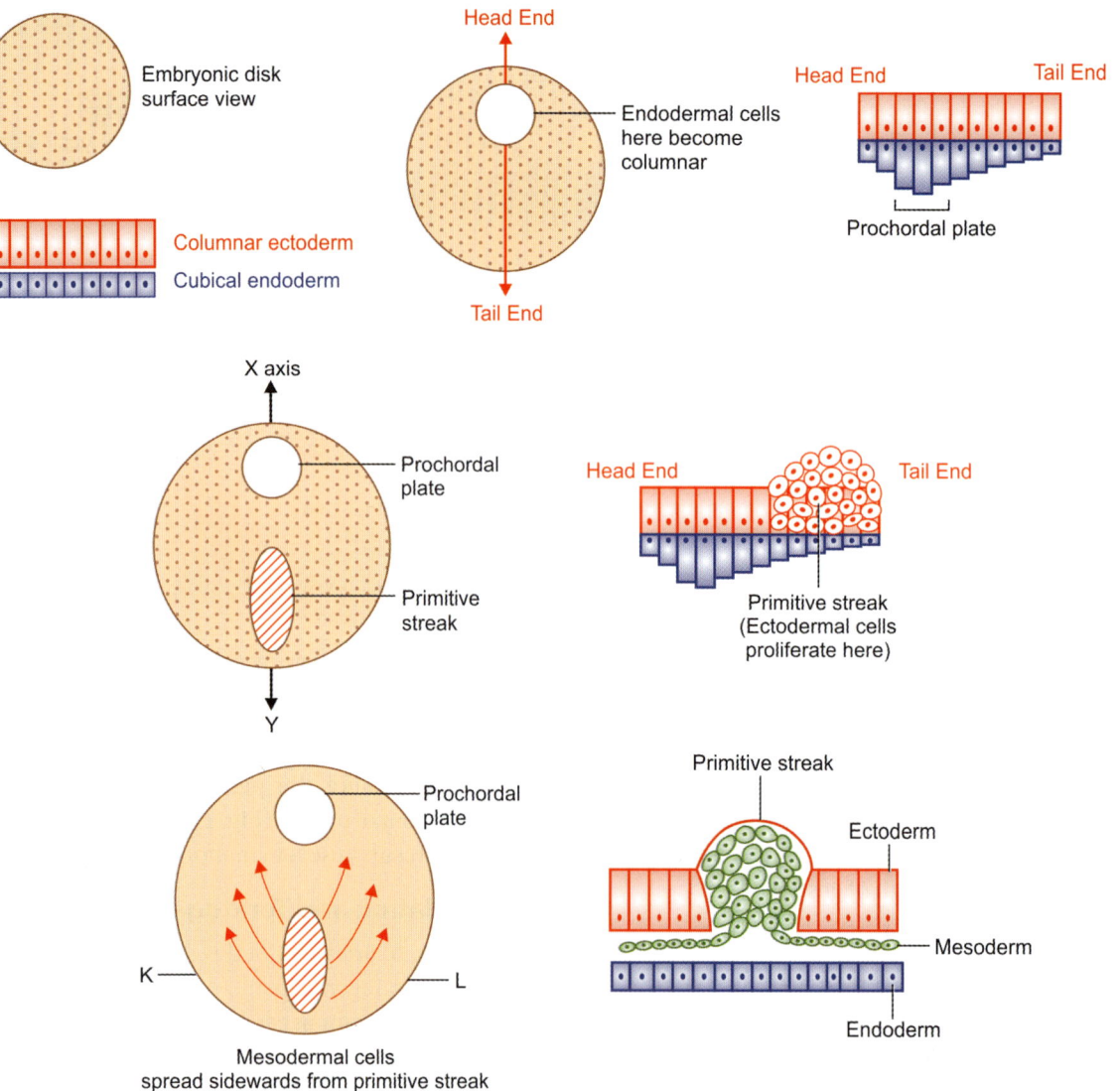

Fig. 10: Formation of intraembryonic mesoderm.

Initial evaluation includes a specialized examination of fetal anatomy, fetal karyotyping, and testing for congenital infections such as cytomegalovirus and toxoplasmosis.[2]

Caudal Dysgenesis/Sirenomelia[6]

Cause: Insufficient mesoderm formation in caudal-most region of the embryo, causing abnormalities of lower limbs, urogenital system (intermediate mesoderm) and lumbosacral vertebrae, associated with maternal overt diabetes.[6]

Features: Hypoplasia, fusion of lower limbs, vertebral anomalies, imperforate anus, urogenital abnormalities.[6]

Caudal Regression Sequence: Sacral Agenesis[2]

It is 25 times more common in pregnancies with pregestational diabetes.

Sonographic findings include a spine that appears abnormally short, lacks the normal lumbosacral curvature, and terminates abruptly above the level of the iliac wings. Shield-like pelvic bones with no sacrum in between.

Situs Inversus[1]

Cause: Disruption of 5-hydroxytryptamine (5-HT) in mothers taking antidepressants/selective serotonin reuptake inhibitors (SSRIs). (5-HT/serotonin plays an important role in laterality of the visceral placement).[1]

Features: Transposition of thoracic and abdominal viscera.[1]

Sacrococcygeal Teratoma[2]

Cause: Mature, immature or malignant tumor of infancy, which arises from the totipotent cells along with Hansen's node, anterior to the coccyx.[2]

The American Academy of Pediatrics classification of sacrococcygeal teratoma (SCT) includes four types:[6]
- *Type 1:* External tumor with a minimal presacral element
- *Type 2:* Mainly external but with a significant intrapelvic element
- *Type 3:* Mainly internal with abdominal extension
- *Type 4:* Purely internal with no external component.

SECTION 2: Normal Pregnancy

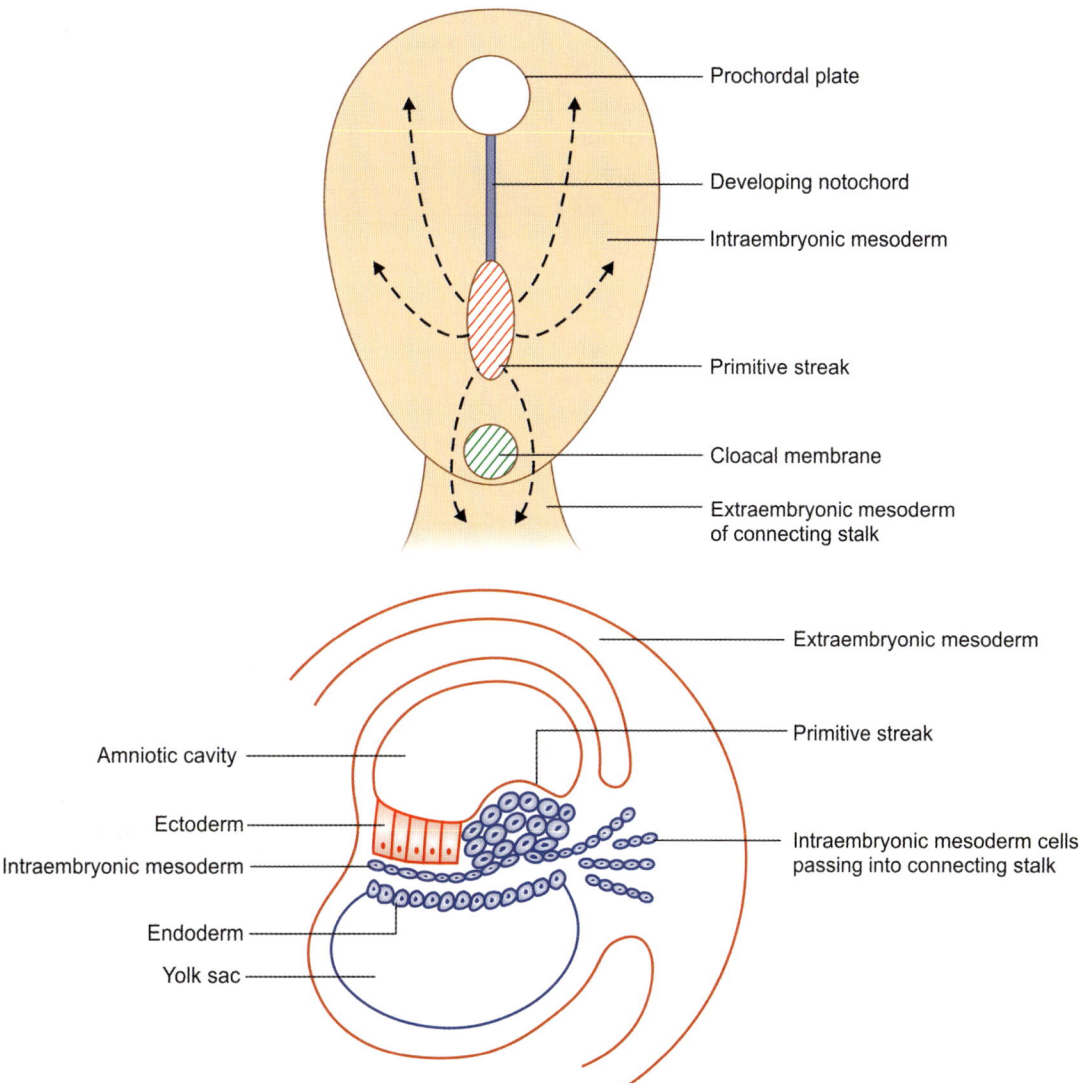

Fig. 11: Migration of intraembryonic mesoderm.

TABLE 3: Perinatal infection and fetal defects.[7]

Maternal viral disease	Fetal effects
Herpes	Microcephaly with intracranial calcification, retinal dysplasia, microphthalmos
Mumps	Fetal death, various malformation, endocardial fibroelastosis
Rubella	Blueberry muffin babies, microcephaly, cataract, chorioretinitis, heart defects

TABLE 4: Teratogenic drug defects.[8]

Maternal exposure	Fetal or neonatal defects
Alcohol	Short palpebral fissure, short upturned nose with hypoplastic philtrum, hypoplastic maxilla, thinned upper vermilion, micrognathia
Chloroquine	Deafness
Nitrofurantoin	Megaloblastic anemia
Vitamin A	Craniofacial defects
Vitamin D	Supravalvular aortic stenosis, elfin facies
Diethylstilbestrol	Vaginal adenosis, uterine, cervical and vaginal malformation
Oral contraceptive	Anomalies of genitalia, limbs reduction defects
Warfarin	Chondrodysplasia punctata
Phenytoin	Cleft lip, cleft palate, microcephaly, limb defects
Valproic acid	Cleft lip, cleft palate, neural plate defects
Thalidomide	Phocomelia

On USG, SCT appears as a solid and/or cystic mass which arises from the anterior sacrum and extends inferiorly and externally as it grows. Hydramnios is frequent, and hydrops may develop from high-output cardiac failure.[2]

Fetuses with tumors > 5 cm need cesarean delivery.

■ EMBRYONIC PHASE/ORGANOGENESIS

In this period (3rd–8th week), three basic germ layers give rise to specific tissues and organs.

Ectoderm

At the beginning of 3rd week, ectoderm has shape of disk which is broader at cranial end and narrow at caudal end. Fibroblast growth factor (FGF) suppresses the activity of bone morphogenetic protein-4 (BMP-4) and transforming growth factor-beta (TGF-β) causes induction of neural plate. FGF also upregulates expression of *chordin and noggin* which inhibits BMP-4 activity.[1]

Bone morphogenetic protein-4 causes ectoderm to form epidermis and mesoderm to form intermediate and lateral plate mesoderm. If BMP-4 is absent, inactivated ectoderm develops into neural tissues. Follistatin, *chordin*, and *noggin* inactivate BMP-4 which is present in primitive node, notochord, and prechordal mesoderm. These three factors are responsible for the development of forebrain and midbrain. In caudal plate (hindbrain and spinal cord), development will depend on secretion of two proteins, WNT-3A and FGF.[1]

Ectodermal Derivatives (Fig. 12)[1]

It gives rise to organs and structures that maintain contact with outside world.

- Central nervous system—neurulation (regulated by FGF, BMP-4, TGF-β, noggin, chordin, follistatin, WNT-3A, retinoic acid)
- Peripheral nervous system
- Sensory epithelium of ear, nose, and eye
- Epidermis—subcutaneous glands and nails
- Mammary gland
- Pituitary gland
- Enamel of teeth.

Neurulation is process of formation of neural tube from neural plate. At the end of 3rd week, lateral edge of neural plate becomes elevated to form neural fold and depressed mid region is called neural groove. Gradually the neural fold approaches each other in midline and fuses to form tube. Fusion begins in the cervical region (5th somite level) and proceeds cranially and caudally. Before fusion is completed, cephalic and caudal ends communicate with amniotic cavity through anterior (cranial) and posterior (caudal) neuropores.[6]

Closure of the cranial neuropore occurs at day 25 (18–20 somite stage) and caudal at day 28 (25 somite stage) **(Table 5)**. Neurulation is then complete and the central nervous system is represented by a closed tubular structure with narrow caudal portion, spinal cord, and broad cephalic portion called brain vesicles.[6]

Neural crest cells are the cells dissociated from neural fold (crest) after fusion to form neural tube. These cells migrate and displace to enter the underlying mesoderm.[1]

Neural crest cells at trunk region leave the neuroectoderm after formation of neural tube along the dorsal and ventral pathway. Dorsal pathway cells give rise to melanocyte in skin and hair follicle. Ventral pathway cells become sensory ganglia, sympathetic and enteric neurons, Schwann cells and cells of adrenal medulla.[1]

Neural crest cells at cranial region migrate before closure and contribute to craniofacial skeleton, neurons of cranial ganglia, glial cells, and melanocytes.[1]

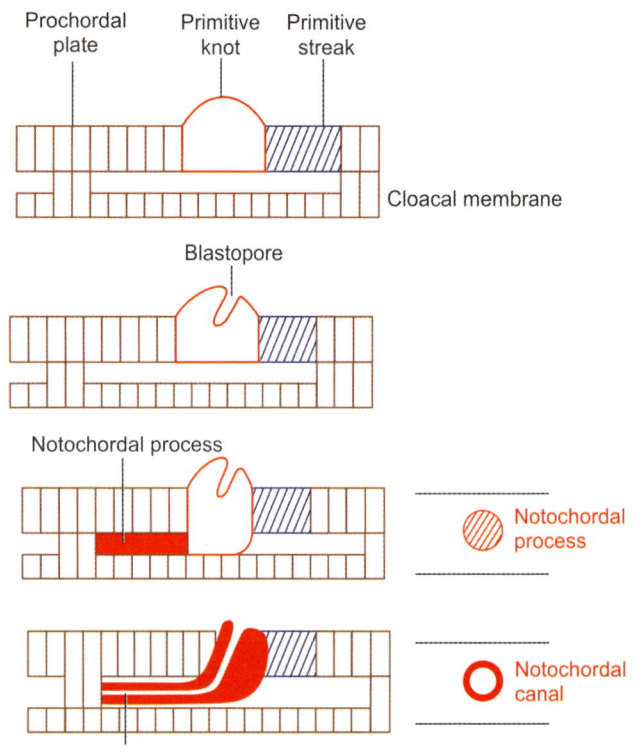

Fig. 12: Ectoderm development—notochord.

TABLE 5: Embryo age by somites.

Age in days	Number of somites
20	1–4
21	4–7
22	7–10
23	10–13
24	13–17
25	17–20
26	20–23
27	23–26
28	26–29
30	34–35

Neural Tube Defects[2]

Neural tube defects (NTDs) constitute the second most common class of fetal malformations.

Periconceptional folic acid supplementation reduces recurrence of NTDs (recurrence risk of NTDs without periconceptional folic acid supplementation: 3–5%).

Anencephaly: Absence of cranium and telencephalic structures, the skull base and orbits are covered only by angiomatous stroma. On USG, Mickey Mouse ear sign or frog eye sign is seen.[2]

Acrania: Absence of the cranium, with protrusion of disorganized brain tissue, gives a shower cap appearance on USG.[2]

Cephalocele: Herniation of meninges through a cranial defect, typically located in the midline occipital region. It is an important feature of the autosomal recessive Meckel–Gruber syndrome, which includes cystic renal dysplasia and polydactyly.[2]

Encephalocele: Brain tissue herniating through the skull defect.

Spina bifida:[2] It is a defect in the vertebrae, especially the dorsal arch, with exposure of the meninges and spinal cord. Most cases are open spina bifida—the defect includes the skin and soft tissues.

- Herniation of a meningeal sac containing neural elements is termed a *myelomeningocele.*
- When only a meningeal sac is present, the defect is a *meningocele.*
- Spina bifida (*Chiari II malformation/Arnold-Chiari malformation*) on second-trimester sonography shows scalloping of the frontal bones—*the lemon sign*, and anterior curvature of the cerebellum with effacement of the cisterna magna—*the banana sign.* These findings occur because of downward displacement of the spinal cord that pulls a portion of the cerebellum through the foramen magnum and into the upper cervical canal.

Ventriculomegaly:[2] Distended cerebral ventricles by cerebrospinal fluid (CSF) are a nonspecific marker of abnormal brain development.

- Normal ventricular atrium measures between 5 and 10 mm from 15 weeks until term.
- Mild ventriculomegaly: 10–15 mm.
- Overt or severe ventriculomegaly: >15 mm.

Cerebrospinal fluid is produced by the choroid plexus, which is an epithelium-lined capillary sinus and loose connective tissue found in the ventricles. A *dangling choroid plexus* is found in USG of severe ventriculomegaly.

Agenesis of the corpus callosum:[2] The corpus callosum is the major fiber bundle connecting the two cerebral hemispheres.

With complete agenesis of the corpus callosum, a normal cavum septum pellucidum cannot be seen sonographically, and the frontal horns are displaced laterally. There is mild enlargement of the atria posteriorly—such that the ventricle has a characteristic "teardrop" appearance.

Dandy-Walker malformation—vermian agenesis:[2] Posterior fossa abnormality—agenesis of the cerebellar vermis, posterior fossa enlargement, tentorial elevation. Sonographically, fluid in the enlarged cisterna magna visibly communicates with the fourth ventricle through the cerebellar vermis defect, with visible separation of the cerebellar hemispheres.

Mesoderm

At 17th day, cells close to midline proliferate to form thickened plate of tissue known as paraxial mesoderm and more laterally mesoderm layer remains thin called lateral plate mesoderm **(Fig. 13)**. Lateral plate mesoderm shows small cavities, which coalesce to form two layers of mesoderm, somatic/parietal and splanchnic/visceral mesoderm. Intermediate mesoderm connects to paraxial and lateral plate mesoderm.[1]

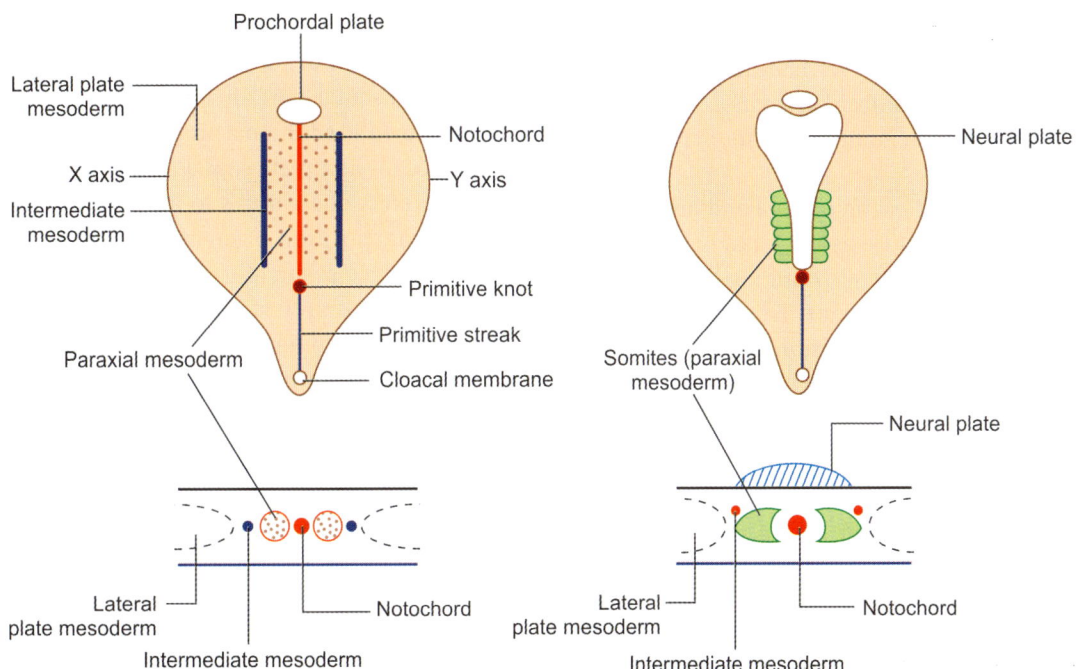

Fig. 13: Mesodermal development.

Paraxial Mesoderm

Paraxial mesoderm is organized into segments known as somitomeres, start at cephalic region proceed caudally. First pair of somites arises in the occipital region of the embryo at approximately 20th day of development. Further caudal development occurs at the rate of 3 per day till 5th week, 42–44 somite pairs are present, 4 occipital, 8 cervical, 12 thoracic, 5 lumbar, 5 sacral, and 8–10 coccygeal pairs. First 5 and last 8–10 coccygeal somites disappear. Medicolegally age of embryo can be accurately determined during early pregnancy by counting the somite.[4]

Somite differentiation: Each somite forms its own sclerotome (tendon, cartilage, and bone component), its own myotome (segmental muscle component), and its own dermatome which form dermis of back. Each myotome and dermatome has its own segmental nerve supply.[1]

Intermediate Mesoderm

It differentiates into urogenital structure. In cervical and upper thoracic region, it forms segmental cluster of cells called nephrotomes and caudally unsegmented mass of tissue known as nephrogenic cord.[1]

Lateral Plate Mesoderm

It splits into parietal (somatic) and visceral (splanchnic) layers. Parietal layer lines the intraembryonic cavity and visceral layer surround the organs.[1]

Parietal layer with overlying ectoderm forms the lateral body wall folds. These two lateral fold contributed by head and tail fold close the ventral body wall. Parietal layer of lateral plate mesoderm with migrated sclerotome and myotome form costal cartilages, limb muscles and most of the body wall muscle. Mesodermal cells of parietal layer form the mesothelial lining of peritoneum, pleural and pericardial cavities.[1]

Visceral layer along with embryonic endoderm form the wall of gut tube.

Blood arise from blood island or pool and angiogenesis which entail sprouting from existing vessels. First blood pool is seen in the mesoderm surrounding the wall of the yolk sac at 3 weeks of development. This mesoderm cells form hemangioblast which is common precursor to blood cells and vessels. This yolk sac island is transitory. Definitive hematopoietic stem cells are derived from mesoderm surrounding the aorta, in the area near developing mesonephric kidney known as aorta-gonad-mesonephros (AGM) region.[1]

Cells of AGM colonize liver which becomes major hematopoietic organ of embryo and fetus from 2nd to 7th month of development. Stem cells from liver colonize the bone marrow in the 7th month and liver loses its hematopoietic function.[1]

Capillary Hemangiomas[1]

Abnormally dense collection of capillary blood vessels.

Most common tumors of infancy (10% of births) are associated with craniofacial structures.

Facial lesions may be focal or diffuse, diffuse ones cause more complications like ulcerations, scarring, airway obstruction (mandibular hemangiomas).

Insulin-like growth factor-2 (IGF-2)—responsible for formation of hemangiomas.

Development of Cardiovascular System[1]

The entire cardiovascular structure is derived from mesodermal germ layer. It includes heart, blood vessels, and blood cells. Heart is developed from cardiogenic area which is initially anterior to oropharyngeal membrane and neural tube. But as brain forms, it grows cephalad and extends over the cardiogenic area. After the cephalic, lateral folding develops heart and comes to lie in thoracic region. Heart tube is lined by endothelium from inside and myocardial cells from outside. This tube continues to elongate and undergoes folding which is completed by 28th day. Tube is divided into cranial to caudal, atrioventricular canal, aortic root, bulbus cordis, conus cordis, truncus arteriosus, ventricle, atrium, sinus venosus, respectively. Bulbus cordis forms right ventricle, conus cordis forms outflow tract of both ventricles, truncus arteriosus will form roots and proximal portion of the aorta and pulmonary trunk.

Heart septum is formed between 27th and 37th day of development [crown-rump length (CRL) 5–17 mm]. Septum is formed by two active growth of tissue approaching each other or overgrowth of one active tissue from one margin to another. Such active tissue is called endocardial cushion. It helps in formation of membranous part of atrial and ventricular septa. Muscular portion of septa is derived from growing cardiac muscles. Muscular part always fails to reach membranous part on its own so additional proliferation by nearby structures is required for complete septal formation.[7,9] An endocardial cushion defect contributes to atrial and ventricular septal defects, transposition of great vessels, tetralogy of Fallot. Due to the same origin of endocardial cushion, conotruncal cushion, and neural crest cells, heart and craniofacial defects occur by the same teratogenic insult. Heart and vascular abnormality are common accounting to 1% of total birth defects in live born.[7] About 8% of heart defects are due to genetic causes and 2% are due to teratogens and genetic factor interplay.[7] Diabetes, rubella, thalidomide, alcohol, vitamin A are classic examples for cardiac anomalies. Heart malformations are associated with 6–10% of newborns resulting due to unbalanced translocation. About 33% of children with chromosomal abnormalities have heart defects, nearly 100% in trisomy 18.[7] Atrial septal defect has incidence of 6.4/10,000 births which is more common in females.

Mostly it is ostium secundum defect due to reabsorption of septum primum or short development of septum secundum.

Ventricular septal defect may involve membranous or muscular part and is most common congenital heart defect (12/10,000). In 80% of cases, it involves muscular portion and closes as child grows.[1]

Endoderm

Endodermal Derivatives[1]

- Epithelial lining of primitive gut
- Respiratory tract epithelium
- Parenchyma of thyroid/parathyroid/liver/pancreas
- Reticular stroma of tonsil, thymus
- Epithelium of urinary bladder and urethra
- Epithelium of tympanic cavity and auditory tube.

This layer gives rise to gastrointestinal tract. Head tail and lateral fold of endoderm is incorporated inside the body of embryo to form tube called gut tube **(Fig. 14)**. This tube is divided into foregut, midgut, and hindgut. Midgut communicates with the yolk sac by the way of broad stalk called vitelline duct. This vitelline duct elongates and thins to give rise to umbilical cord. At cephalic end of foregut oropharyngeal membrane separates stomodeum (primitive oral cavity) from pharynx.[1]

At the caudal end of hindgut, cloacal membrane which is lined by endoderm inside and ectoderm outside breaks down in the 7th week to create opening for anus. Another result of folding of body walls is partial incorporation of allantois into the body of embryo where it forms the cloaca.[1]

Endoderm in further development gives rise to epithelial lining of respiratory tract, urinary bladder, urethra, tympanic cavity, auditory tube, parenchyma of thyroid gland, parathyroids, liver, and pancreas.

Formation of Body Cavity

At end of 3rd week, somatopleuric and splanchnopleuric mesoderms constitute the primitive body cavity and by 4th week, lateral body folds fuse to close the ventral body wall. Parietal layer of serous membranes line peritoneal, pleural, and pericardial cavities. Visceral layer of serous membranes surround abdominothoracic organs. Visceral and parietal layers are continuous over each other as *dorsal mesentery* that suspends gut tube from posterior body wall into the peritoneal cavity. Mesentery provides pathway for blood vessels, nerves, and lymphatics.[1]

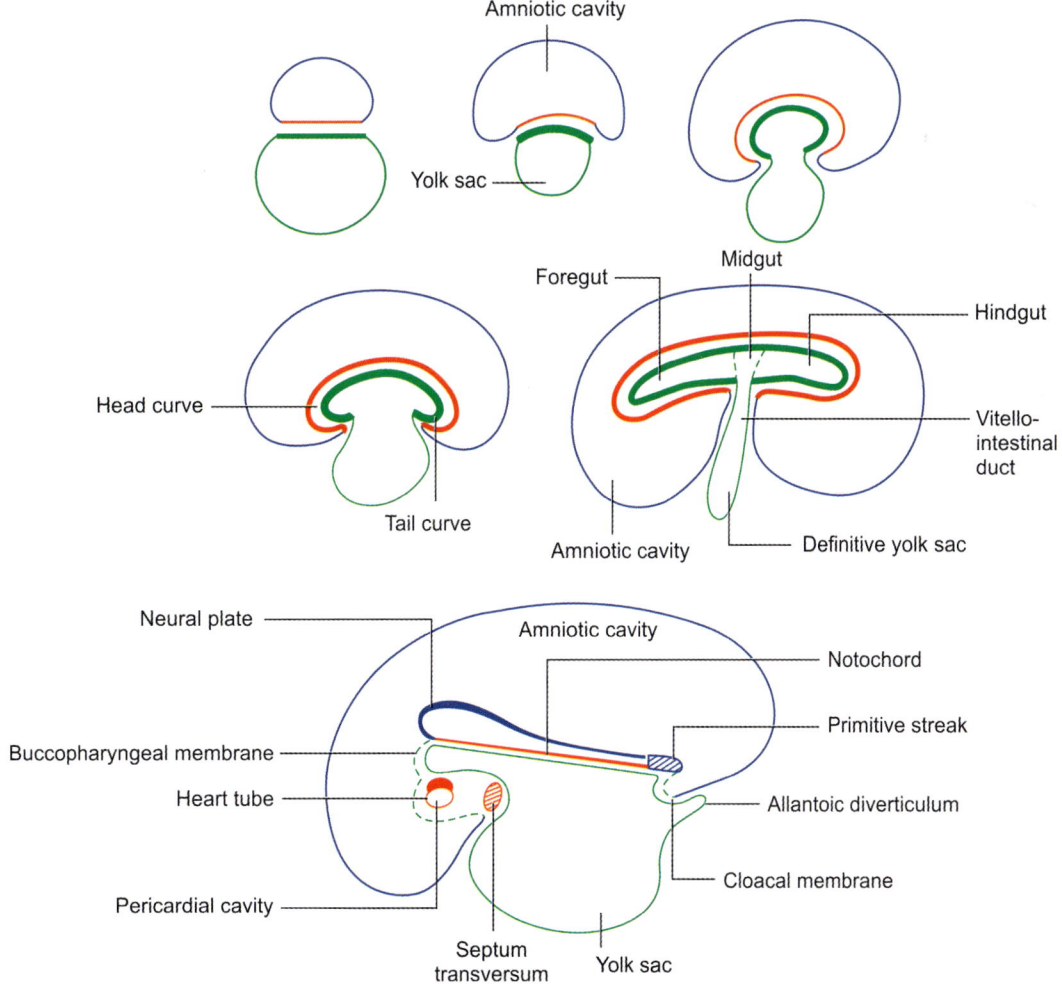

Fig. 14: Endodermal development—gut tube formation.

Ventral Body Wall Defects

Ventral body wall defects occur in thorax, abdomen, and pelvis. These defects may involve heart, abdominal viscera, and/or urogenital organs.

Ectopia Cordis[1]

Cause: Lateral body wall folds fail to close in midline in thoracic cavity placing heart outside thoracic cavity.

Associations: Sternal and upper abdominal wall abnormalities (pentalogy of Cantrell)[1] including ectopia cordis, anterior diaphragmatic defects, sternal defects, omphalocele, gastroschisis.

Gastroschisis[1]

Cause: Lateral body wall folds fail to close in midline in abdominal area placing intestinal loops outside abdominal cavity, which now lie freely in the amniotic cavity.

The defect lies just *right to the umbilicus*.[1]

Incidence: 3–4/10,000 live births.[1]

Diagnosis: USG.

Affected bowel loops may undergo volvulus or corrosive effect due to exposure to amniotic fluid.[1]

Bladder Exstrophy/Cloacal Exstrophy

Cause: Body wall closure defect in the pelvic area, placing bladder (bladder exstrophy) or bladder and rectum outside pelvic cavity (cloacal exstrophy).

Omphalocele

Cause: The primary reason is not due to inhibition of ventral body wall closure. This occurs when a *portion of gut tube fails to return back into abdominal cavity following its physiological herniation (6–10 weeks) into umbilical cord*.[1]

Features: Bowel loops and other viscera may herniate through the defect. But, since the umbilical cord is *covered by a reflection of the amnion*, defect is also covered by this epithelial layer (in gastroschisis, there is no such covering).

Incidence: 2.5/10,000 live births.[1]

Diaphragm and Thoracic Cavity

The septum transversum appears as a thick plate of mesodermal tissue that occupies the space between thoracic cavity and yolk sac stalk. This septum is derived from visceral/splanchnopleuric mesoderm surrounding heart and is placed between the primitive abdominal and thoracic cavities. This septum has large openings known as *pericardioperitoneal canals* on each side of foregut.[1] When lung buds begin to grow they expand caudolaterally into these canals. Mesoderm of body wall splits into components: definitive wall of thorax and pleuropericardial membranes that contain common cardinal veins and phrenic nerves. With descent of heart, the pleuropericardial membranes are drawn out like a mesentery, they divide pleuropericardium into a *definitive pericardial cavity* and *two pleural cavities*. During further development, pleuroperitoneal openings are closed by crescent-shaped folds known as *pleuroperitoneal folds*.[1] By 7th week, they fuse with mesentery of esophagus forming the septum transversum. Later myoblasts originating from 3rd–5th cervical somites penetrate to form musculature of the diaphragm.

Diaphragm is derived from:
- Septum transversum—central tendon of diaphragm
- Two pleuroperitoneal membranes
- Muscular components from 3–5 cervical somites, which are supplied by phrenic nerves
- Mesentery of esophagus—crura of the diaphragm.

Diaphragm develops in cervical somite area and later descends to thoracic region because of differential growth of dorsal and ventral aspects of embryo.

Diaphragmatic Hernia[2]

Pleural and peritoneal cavities are continuous with one another along posterior body wall.

Abdominal viscera herniate into pleural cavity. It is more commonly on left side (80–90% cases intestinal loops, stomach, spleen, and part of liver enter thoracic cavity). Abdominal viscera in chest push the heart anteriorly and compress lungs, which become hypoplastic.

Mortality rate—75% (due to pulmonary hypoplasia).[5]

On USG, the most common finding in a left-sided congenital diaphragmatic hernia (CDH)—repositioning of the heart to the mid or right hemithorax. Additional findings include the stomach bubble or intestinal peristalsis in the chest and a wedge-shaped mass (liver) in the left hemithorax. Liver herniation is the strongest predictor of outcome in fetuses with isolated CDH. It complicates at least 50% of cases and is associated with a 30% reduction in the survival rate.[2]

Predictors of survival—sonographic lung-to-head ratio (LHR), magnetic resonance imaging (MRI) measurements of lung volume, and the degree of liver herniation.[1]

Lung-to-head ratio—measurement of the right lung area, taken at the level of the four-chamber view of the heart, divided by head circumference.[1]

Liver volume might be a more reliable predictor because lungs are inherently more compressible than liver.

Treatment—*tracheal occlusion/fetoscopic endotracheal occlusion (FETO)*: Fetal lungs normally produce fluid and fetuses with upper airway obstruction develop hyperplastic lungs, that push bowel loops back into the abdomen is the rationale for tracheal occlusion in CDH. EXIT Procedure.[2]

External Appearance

At the end of 4th week (at 28 somite stage) after fertilization, main external features are of the somites and pharyngeal arches.[2] During 2nd month, external appearance changes by increase in head size, formation of limbs, face, ear, nose, and eye. By the beginning of 5th week, forelimbs and hindlimbs appear as paddle-shaped buds.

■ CONCLUSION

Exact knowledge is very important in management of pregnancy exposed to teratogen or history of anomalies in past pregnancy. Detailed knowledge can help in performing and interpreting USG report in early months of pregnancy. Organogenesis period is very crucial in development of organ systems. Women may have exposure to infections and teratogens in this near date period and may not be aware of the pregnancy hence, require careful evaluation.

■ REFERENCES

1. Sadler TW. Langman's Medical Embryology, 11th edition. Philadelphia: Wolters Kluwer Health/Lippincott Williams and Wilkins; 2010.
2. Cunningham FG, Leveno KJ, Bloom SL, Dashe JS, Hoffman BL, Casey BM, Spong CY. Williams Obstetrics, 25th edition. New York: McGraw-Hill Education; 2018.
3. Moore KL, Persaud TV, Torchia MG. The Developing Human: Clinically Oriented Embryology, 10th edition. Philadelphia: Saunders; 2015.
4. Fritz MA, Speroff L. Clinical Gynecologic Endocrinology and Infertility, 8th edition. Philadelphia: Wolters Kluwer Health/Lippincott Williams and Wilkins; 2011.
5. Creasy RR, Resnik R, Iams JD. Maternal-Fetal Medicine: Principles and Practice. Philadelphia: WB Saunders; 2004.
6. Moore KL, Persaud TV, Torchia MG. Before We Are Born: Essentials of Embryology and Birth Defects, 9th edition. Philadelphia: Saunders; 2015.
7. Schoenwolf GC, Bleyl SB, Brauer PR, Francis-West PH. Larsen's Human Embryology, 5th edition. New York; Edinburgh: Churchill Livingstone; 2015.
8. Moore KL, Persaud TV, Torchia MG. Before We Are Born: Essentials of Embryology and Birth Defects, 7th edition. Philadelphia, PA: Saunders; 2008.
9. Gilbert SF. Developmental Biology, 6th edition. Sunderland, MA: Sinauer Associates; 2000.

■ LONG QUESTIONS

1. Discuss the stage of gastrulation and the impact of teratogens on the fetus at this stage.
2. Discuss the formation of the notochord and pathogenesis of neural tube defects.

■ SHORT QUESTIONS

1. What are Wilson's criteria for identification of teratogens?
2. What is the importance of the formation of the bilaminar germ disc?
3. Name the important ectodermal derivatives.
4. What are the important ventral body defects seen in the fetus?

■ MULTIPLE CHOICE QUESTIONS

1. The following is a criterion for identifying a teratogen:
    a. A gradual increase in incidence of a defect
    b. Coincidence of increase in defects with a known environmental change
    c. High usage of a drug in a population
    d. Confounding or multiple factors that could cause defect
2. The following is true about holoprosencephaly:
    a. Associated with high maternal alcohol intake
    b. Prosencephalon divides completely into two separate cerebral hemispheres
    c. Large forebrain formation
    d. All fetuses have Karyotype abnormalities
3. The greatest association of caudal regression syndrome is with the following maternal condition:
    a. Alcohol abuse   b. Opioid abuse
    c. SSRI treatment   d. Maternal diabetes
4. Heart septum is formed between:
    a. 7th and 17th day of development
    b. 17th and 27th day of development
    c. 27th and 37th day of development
    d. 37th and 47th day of development
5. The predictors of neonatal survival with isolated diaphragmatic hernia are all, except:
    a. Fetal gender
    b. Lung to head ratio
    c. Liver herniation
    d. MR measured lung volume

Answers

1. b   2. a   3. d   4. c   5. a

2.4 MATERNAL ADAPTATIONS IN NORMAL PREGNANCY

Sadhana Gupta, Hema J Shobhane

PHYSIOLOGICAL ADAPTATION DURING PREGNANCY: OVERVIEW

Physiological adaptation occurs in pregnancy to support by nurture the developing fetus and prepare the mother for optimum parturition. Many of these changes influence normal biochemical values while others may mimic symptoms of medical disorders. It is significant to differentiate between normal physiological adaptation and disease pathology. Plasma volume increases progressively during normal pregnancy. Maximum of this 50% increase occurs by 34 weeks' gestation and is proportional to the growth and birth weight of the baby. Because the expansion in plasma volume is greater than the increase in red blood cell mass, there is a down fall in hemoglobin concentration, hematocrit, and red blood cell count. Despite of this hemodilution due to physiological anemia, there is usually no change in mean corpuscular volume (MCV) or mean corpuscular hemoglobin concentration (MCHC). Changes in the cardiovascular system in pregnancy are remarkable and begin very early in pregnancy, such that by 8 weeks' gestation, the cardiac output has already increased by 20%. As a consequence of renal vasodilatation, renal plasma flow and glomerular filtration rate (GFR) both increases, compared to non-pregnant woman's level, by 40–65 and 50–85%, respectively. There is a significant increase in oxygen requirement during normal pregnancy. This is due to a 15% increase in the metabolic rate and a 20% increased consumption of oxygen. There is a 40–50% increase in minute ventilation, due to an increase in tidal volume, rather than in the respiratory rate. Nausea and vomiting are common complaints in early pregnancy, affecting 50–90% of pregnancies. This can be a protective and an adaptive mechanism of pregnancy, aiming at preventing pregnant women from consuming potentially teratogenic and harmful substances. Pregnant women require an increased intake of nutritive substances like protein during pregnancy. Amino acids are actively transported across the placenta to fulfill the needs of the development of fetus. Energy requirement during pregnancy, protein catabolism is decreased as fat stores are used to provide for energy metabolism. Serum concentrations of thyroid-stimulating hormone (TSH) are decreased slightly in the first trimester in response to the thyrotropic simulative effects of increased levels of human chorionic gonadotropin. During pregnancy, levels of TSH increase again at the end of the first trimester, and the upper limit in pregnancy is raised to 5.5 μmol/L compared with the level of 4.0 μmol/L in the non-pregnant women. Central nervous system changes are relatively few and usually subtle. Woman often reports problems with attention, concentration, and memory during pregnancy and in puerperium.

REPRODUCTIVE SYSTEM

Uterus

Uterus increases in weight from 60 to 1100 g at term and is transformed from almost solid structure to a relatively soft, thin walled muscular, indentable organ with capacity of 5–20 L to accommodate the fetus, placenta, and amniotic fluid with in the uterine cavity. Early uterine hypertrophy is due to effects of estrogen and progesterone but after 12 weeks, uterine hypertrophy is due to mechanical distension due to growth of products of conception in the uterine cavity. The uterine enlargement is normally symmetrical and more marked in fundus, and leads change of pear shape organ to globular form and later on ovoid shape. During pregnancy, as the uterus continues to enlarge, it contacts the anterior abdominal wall, displaces the intestine laterally and superiorly, and continues to rise, ultimately reaching almost to the liver **(Figs. 1A to D)**. After conception uterus undergoes irregular contraction from

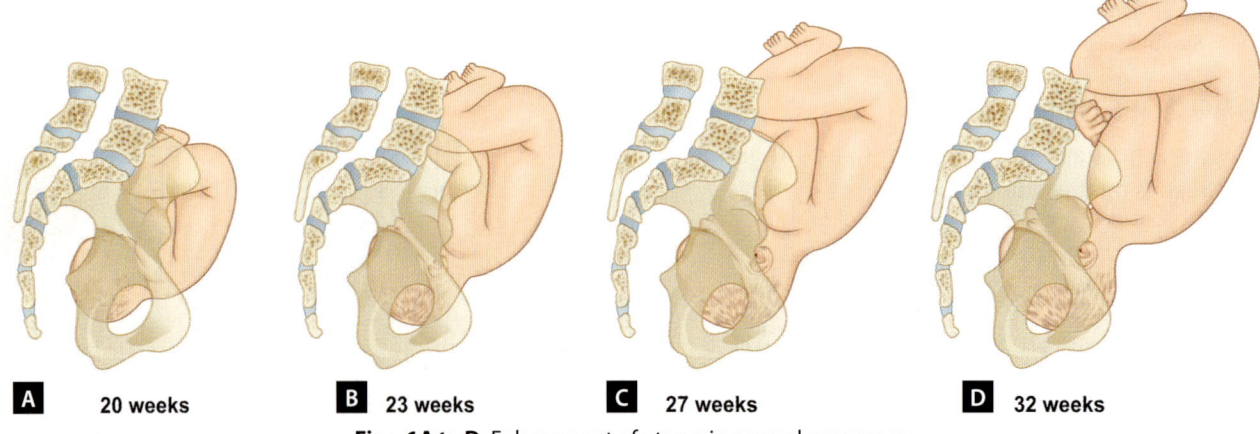

A 20 weeks **B** 23 weeks **C** 27 weeks **D** 32 weeks

Figs. 1A to D: Enlargement of uterus in normal pregnancy.

the first trimester around, which is normally painless. Mostly such contractions appear unpredictable, sporadically and usually nonrhythmic (Braxton Hicks contractions). During the last weeks of gestation, the contractions may be more frequent and regular and uncomfortable, accounting for so called false labor.

Uteroplacental blood flow is essential during pregnancy for growth and metabolism of the fetus and placenta, as well as removal of most metabolic wastes of fetus. Uteroplacental blood flow is ranging from 450 to 650 mL/min, and dependent on adequate perfusion of the intervillous space which is regulated by vasodilatation and continuing growth of placental vessels in influences of mainly estrogen stimulation, progesterone, and nitric oxide.

Cervix

During pregnancy, cervix is more edematous, vascular, soft and cyanosed due to hypertrophy and hyperplasia of cervical glands and rearrangement of collagen tissues and smooth muscles to permit maintenance of a pregnancy, dilatation of cervix to aid labor and further regain almost near to prepregnant status. Soon after conception cervical canal is filled with mucoid plug and this mucoid plug is expelled at onset of labor, resulting in a blood stained discharge of mucus plug, and is called bloody show. Dried cervical mucus examined microscopically has characteristic patterns such as crystallization, or beading, as a result of progesterone, and on the other hand fern-like pattern is observed as a result of rich sodium chloride due to effects of estrogen or amniotic fluid leakage **(Fig. 2)**.

Ovaries

There is persistence and growth of the corpus luteum which reaches its maximum at 8 weeks of gestation, and secretes progesterone and estrogen before placenta assumes its own functions. The function of hormones, not only controls the formation and maintenance of decidua of pregnancy, but also inhibits ripening of the follicles in the ovaries. Thus, not only the ovarian but uterine cycle of the normal menstruation also remain suspended.

Pregnancy luteoma and theca lutein cysts are two physiological, nonmalignant conditions need observations and expectant treatment or no treatment is required for these cysts. The abnormal luteal tissues disappears spontaneously when the pregnancy is terminated or after delivery.

Breasts

The breasts will have tenderness due to progressive development of more ducts, formation of more number of alveoli and deposition of fat. Nipples become larger, more deeply pigmented, and more erectile with expression of thick, yellowish fluid known as colostrum. The areolae become broader, darker and more pigmented. Many numbers of small elevations of sebaceous glands scattered through the areolae known as glands of Montgomery **(Fig. 3)**.

■ SKIN

Like other organ systems, the skin also undergoes significant changes during pregnancy. Multiple reddish, slightly depressed streaks commonly develop in the abdominal skin, and are called striae gravidarum. Hyperpigmentation develops in 90% of women and more with darker complexion in comparison to lighter complexion. The midline of abdominal skin, linea alba becomes more brownish black color to form linea nigra. Sometimes irregular brownish patches of varying size appear on the maxillary areas of face and neck, giving rise to chloasma or melasma gravidarum, mask or sign of pregnancy. Most physiologic skin conditions related to gestation resolve after childbirth. However, they may cause significant concern or cosmetic distress or mistaken for one of the specific dermal disorders of pregnancy[1] **(Fig. 4)**.

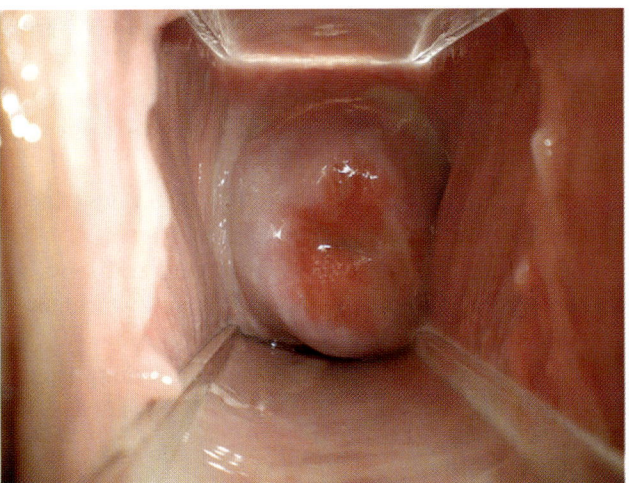

Fig. 2: An extension of proliferated columnar endocervical glands during pregnancy.

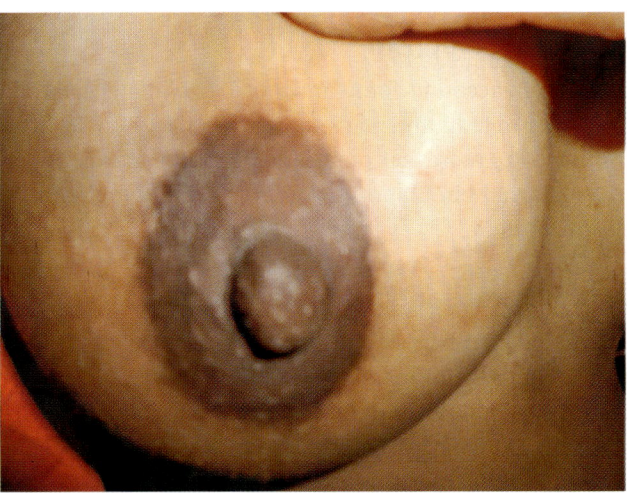

Fig. 3: The areola becomes broader and more deeply pigmented, glands of Montgomery scattered through the areolae.

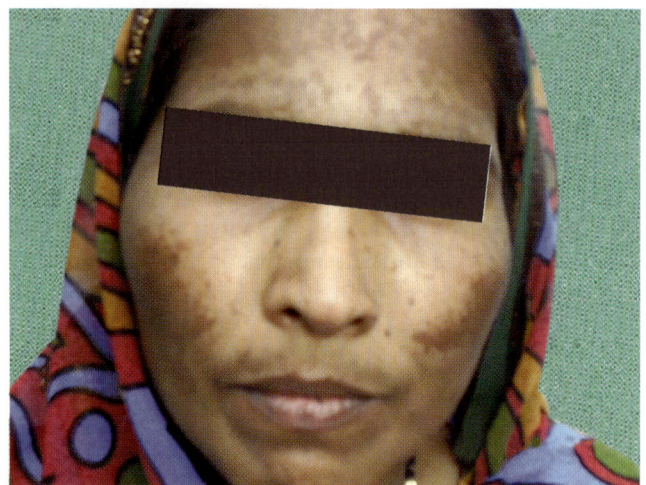

Fig. 4: Irregular brownish patches of varying size on face occur during pregnancy.

TABLE 1: The contributions of different organs in weight gain.	
Tissues/Fluid	**Gain (g)**
Fetus	3,400
Placenta	650
Amniotic fluid	800
Uterus	970
Mammary glands	400
Blood extracellular	1,250
Extravascular fluid	1,700
Fat	3,500

■ METABOLIC CHANGES

Many maternal metabolism changes substantially during the pregnancy. Early pregnancy can be viewed as an anabolic state and in contrast, late pregnancy is better characterized as a catabolic state.

Weight Gain

Maternal weight gain is 0.35 kg/week, 0.45 kg/week and 0.35 kg/week respectively in early, mid and in later part of pregnancy. The average total weight gain is 12.5 kg. The contribution to this weight gain from identified sources is given in **Table 1**.

Water Metabolism

Increased water retention near about 6.5 L is a normal maternal adaptation during pregnancy. At term water content of fetus, placenta and amniotic fluid constitutes about 3.5 L and another 3 L of water is added by increase in maternal blood volume, uterus and both breast.

Protein Metabolism

The protein accounts for near about 1 kg of maternal weight gain. At term fetus and placenta contain 500 g of protein and another 500 g more of protein is added to the uterus, breasts, and maternal circulation in the form of hemoglobin and plasma protein.

Carbohydrate and Fat Metabolism

Early gestation can be viewed as an anabolic state in the mother with an increase in maternal fat stores and slight increases in insulin sensitivity. Hence, nutrients are stored in early pregnancy to meet the fetoplacental and maternal demands of late gestation, parturition and lactation. In contrast, late pregnancy is better characterized as a catabolic state with decreased insulin sensitivity (increased insulin resistance).[2,3] An increase in insulin resistance results in increase in maternal glucose and free fatty acid concentrations, allowing for greater substrate available for fetal growth.[4,5]

Acid–Base Equilibrium

The pregnant woman hyperventilates and leads to respiratory alkalosis by lowering the PCO_2 of blood. There is a moderate reduction in plasma bicarbonate thus there is only a minimal increase in blood PH.

Mineral Metabolism

The requirements of iron during pregnancy are considerable and often exceed the amount available. Serum concentration of Na, K decreases due to expanded plasma volume in pregnancy. Calcium and magnesium levels also decrease for compensation of increase fetal demand. But there is no change of serum phosphorus level during pregnancy.

■ HEMATOLOGICAL CHANGES

Blood Volume

Plasma volume increases by over 40% but red cell volume only to half that extent during pregnancy. This disproportionate increase in plasma volume leads to hemodilution in pregnant woman. The maternal blood volume increases markedly during pregnancy by 40–45% after 32–34 weeks of pregnancy to fulfill the important functions.

- Deliver the demands of the enlarged uterus with its greatly hypertrophied vascular system.
- To protect the mother and growing fetus against the deleterious effects of impaired venous return in the supine and erect posture.
- To safeguard the mother against the deleterious effects of blood loss associated with parturition.
- To provide an abundance of oxygen, nutrients and elements to support the rapidly growing placenta and fetus.

Changes in cellular composition of blood during pregnancy are listed in **Table 2**.

Iron Metabolism

Total iron content of normal adult woman ranges from 2 to 2.5 g and total iron requirement of normal pregnancy is about

TABLE 2: Changes in cellular composition of blood.

Component	Changes
• Total white blood cell count	• Increase
• Neutrophil	• Increase
• Lymphocyte	• No change
• Eosinophil	• Fall sharply during labor and delivery
• Platelet	• Decrease
• Red cell count	• Decrease
• Hematocrit (packed cell volume)	• Decrease
• Hemoglobin concentration	• Decrease (acceptable minimum 11 g/dL)
• Mean cell hemoglobin concentration	• No change
• Mean cell volume	• Small increase
• Red cell fragility	• Increase
• ESR	• Increase

(ESR: erythrocyte sedimentation rate)

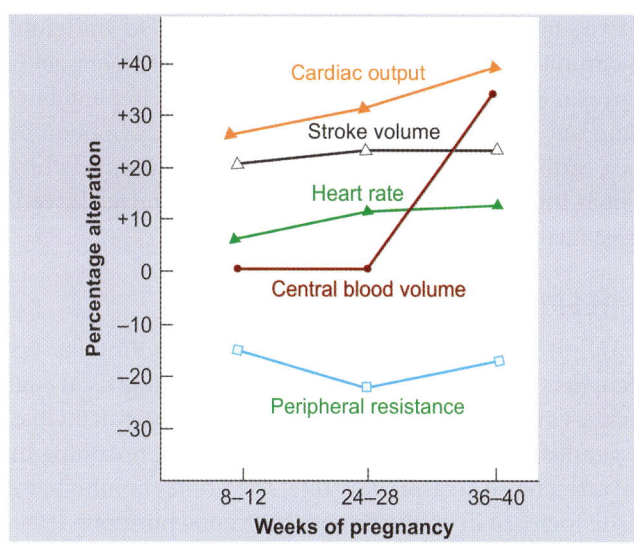

Fig. 5: Cardiovascular changes in pregnancy (% alteration over nonpregnant level occurring in pregnancy).

1,000 mg, in this 300 mg to the fetus and placenta, 500 mg to RBCs and 200 mg is excreted by various routes in pregnancy. So the daily iron requirement is 6–7 mg/dL in pregnant woman. The amount of iron absorbed from diet together with that mobilized from stores is usually not sufficient to meet the demands imposed by pregnancy.

■ IMMUNOLOGICAL FUNCTION

Pregnancy is considered immunosuppressive state with somewhere suppression of both humoral and cell mediated immunological functions to accommodate the semiallogeneic fetal graft in uterus. Pregnant woman is more likely susceptible to the infectious disease due to immune suppression.[6]

Leukocytes

The total blood white blood cells count increases during normal pregnancy from prepregnancy level from 5,000 to 1,2000/uL. Reduced polymorphonuclear leukocyte adherence has been reported mainly in the third trimester. These physiological changes may predispose pregnant woman to infection.

Inflammatory Markers

Many markers, such as leukocyte alkaline phosphatase, C-reactive protein, erythrocyte sedimentation rate and complement factors C3 and C4, are elevated in response to inflammation but no one is specific and reliable during pregnancy.

■ COAGULATION AND FIBRINOLYSIS

During normal pregnancy, both coagulation and fibrinolysis are augmented then normal adult woman but remain balanced to maintain hemostasis. Circulatory levels of several coagulation factors elevated in pregnancy. Fibrinogen factor I and factor VIII level increases markedly whereas factors VII, IX, X and XII increases to a lesser extent in blood. Plasma fibrinogen concentration begins to increase from non-pregnant level (1.5–4.5 g/L) during the third month of pregnancy and progressively rise by nearly double by late pregnancy (4–6.5 g/L).

Plasma levels of factor VI, VIII, IX and XII together with fibrin degradation products are increases during pregnancy. Factor IX and antithrombin III level decreases in pregnancy. Fibrinolytic activity is more depressed during pregnancy. Understanding the physiological alteration of coagulation and fibrinolytic system in pregnancy is important for management of hemorrhage and thromboembolic disorders.

■ CARDIOVASCULAR SYSTEM

Physiological adaptation to pregnancy involves enormous changes in maternal cardiovascular system. In pregnant woman, cardiac output increases in early pregnancy as early as 5th week of gestation due to increased heart rate, soon followed by an increased stroke volume. Cardiac output then rises from 7 L/min at 8–11 weeks to 9 L/min at 36–39 weeks in pregnant woman. Cardiac output continues to increase until middle of pregnancy, and remains stable afterward with small decline in last weeks of pregnancy and opposite to this blood pressure decreases in early pregnancy, minimum in mid-pregnancy and then returning to baseline at term during pregnancy. Peripheral vascular resistance is decreased throughout pregnancy **(Fig. 5)**. Myocardial contractility is increased during all trimesters of pregnancy, thus it leads mild ventricular hypertrophy in heart. The increase in preload, which develops in concert with the increment in blood volume, leads to an increase in left atrial diameter of heart. During labor, both cardiac output and blood pressure increase.[7] This causes a hemodynamic burden on patients with underlying heart disease, and is associated with significant morbidity and mortality during pregnancy.[8,9]

The maternal uterine vasculature may also vulnerable to chronic binge like alcohol due to its negative impact on estrogen actions on the uterine vasculature[10] in pregnancy. Maternal smoking during pregnancy not only impede her own cardiovascular adaptations but also causes low birth weight, intrauterine fetal growth retardation and fetal arterial resistance adaptations during childhood.[11]

■ RESPIRATORY TRACT

During pregnancy, the diaphragm rises by 4 cm, the transverse diameters of the chest increased by 2 cm and subcostal angle increases from 68 to 103 degrees. Overall there is an increase in ventilation attributed to a greater depth of breathing but not an increase in respiratory rate. The prime stimulus to this is the increase in circulating progesterone hormone levels. Many evidence suggests presently, neither pregnancy nor advancing gestation are associated with reduced aerobic working capacity or increased breathlessness at any given work rate or ventilation during exhaustive weight-supportive exercise.[12]

Oxygen consumption increases during pregnancy from 250 to 300 mL/min due to increased demand pregnant woman and her growing fetus. Because this 20% increase is less than 50% for alveolar ventilation, there is an effective hyperventilation. Both alveolar and arteriolar PCO_2 are reduced (35–40 mm Hg in nonpregnant, 30 mm Hg in pregnancy). Hyperventilation and attendant hypocapnia/alkalosis of human pregnancy results from a complex interaction of pregnancy induced changes in alertness, wakefulness and central chemoreflex drives to breath, acid–base balance, metabolic rate, and cerebral blood flow.[13]

■ RENAL SYSTEM

In pregnant woman, the length of kidney increases by 1–1.5 cm. The renal and pelvis also dilated in pregnancy and entire dilated collecting system may contain up to 200 mL of urine, which predispose to ascending urinary infection in pregnancy. In pregnancy, glomerular filtration rate (GFR) and effective renal plasma flow (ERPF) increases approximately 50–80% above nonpregnant levels for adequate renal perfusion. The increments occur shortly after conception and persist throughout the second trimester, with some reduction in third trimester in pregnancy.[14,15] The interpretation of tests for renal function also varies due to physiological changes during pregnancy. Serum creatinine levels decrease during normal pregnancy from a mean of 0.7 to 0.5 mg/dL and value less than 0.9 mg/dL suggest underlying renal disease and should prompt further evaluation to rule out renal cause. Creatinine clearance in pregnancy averages about 30% higher than the 100–150 mL/min in nonpregnant woman. Creatinine clearance is a useful test to estimate renal function provided that complete urine collection is made during an accurately timed period. If either is done incorrectly, results are misleading.

■ GASTROINTESTINAL TRACT

Various physiological changes occur in the gastrointestinal system in pregnant woman. The gum may become hyperemic due to increased vascularity, which causes pregnancy does not predispose to tooth decay or infection. Reduced competence of esophageal sphincter due to progesterone hormone may lead to reflex esophagitis. Pregnant woman is associated with greater production of gastrin which increases stomach volume and acidity of gastric secretion. Gastrointestinal tract tone and motility are also reduced, especially during labor, and the emptying time increased from 50 to 100 minutes. In pregnancy up to 90% of women will suffer from nausea and vomiting of pregnancy, which lead significant physical and psychological morbidity.[16] Small and large intestines have reduced motility due to mechanical pressure from gravid uterus and progesterone hormone effects. Knowledge of the underlying physiologic alterations in gastrointestinal motility during pregnancy and safe treatment options is essential to the care of pregnant patient[17] for gastrointestinal problems. Gallbladder motility and emptying rate is reduced and leads bile stasis and formation of gallstone in pregnancy. Liver has shown no distinct morphology. Albumin concentration may be near 3.0 g/dL compared with 4.3 g/dL in nonpregnant state. Total albumin is increased, however, because of a greater volume of distribution from plasma volume increase in pregnancy.

■ ENDOCRINE SYSTEM

Pituitary Gland

During normal pregnancy, the pituitary gland enlarges by approximately 135%. Although it has been suggested that the increase may be sufficient to compress the optic chiasma and reduce visual fields, impaired vision due to physiological pituitary enlargement during normal pregnancy is rare. Placental growth hormone is a major determinant of maternal insulin resistance after mid-pregnancy. Mid-trimester maternal insulin resistance is associated with subsequent preeclampsia.[18]

Thyroid Gland

Physiological changes of pregnancy cause the thyroid gland to increase production of thyroid hormones by 40–100% to meet maternal and fetal needs. Two pregnancy related hormones—human chorionic gonadotropin (hCG) and estrogen cause increased thyroid hormone levels in the blood. Made by placenta, hCG is similar to TSH and mildly stimulates the thyroid to produce more thyroid hormone. Increased estrogen produces higher levels of thyroid binding globulin, a protein that transports thyroid hormone in blood. These normal hormonal changes can sometimes make thyroid function tests during pregnancy difficult to interpret. Thyroid hormone is critical to normal development of the baby's brain and nervous system. During the first trimester, the fetus depends on the mother's supply of thyroid hormone, which it gets through placenta. At 10-12 weeks, the baby's thyroid begins to function on its own. The baby gets its supply of iodine, which the thyroid gland uses to make thyroid hormone, through the mother's diet. Women need more iodine when they are pregnant—about 250 µm/day. The thyroid gland enlarges slightly in healthy women during pregnancy, but not enough to be detected by the physical examination. A noticeably enlarged gland can be a sign of thyroid disease and should be evaluated. Higher levels of thyroid hormone in the blood, increased thyroid size, and other symptoms common to both pregnancy and thyroid disorders such as fatigue can make thyroid problems hard to diagnose in pregnancy. Physiologic changes in pregnancy serum thyroid stimulating hormone and free T4 are two specific tools to diagnose thyroid functions. Free T4 is more specific because it is either not altered or slightly altered during pregnancy and any alteration indicates thyroid dysfunction[19] (**Fig. 6**).

Parathyroid Glands

During pregnancy and lactation, mothers require an adequate amounts of calcium to pass on to the developing fetus and neonate, infant on breast feeding, respectively.[20] The regulation of calcium concentration is closely interlinked to magnesium, phosphate, parathyroid hormone, vitamin D, and calcitonin physiology. Physiological hyperparathyroidism occurs during pregnancy to deliver the fetus with adequate

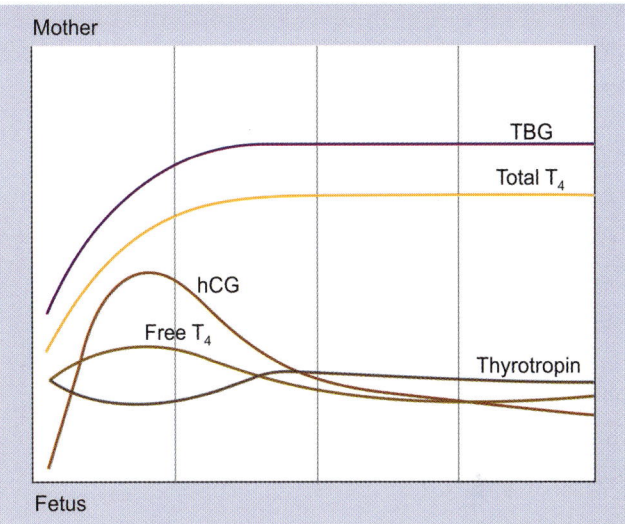

Fig. 6: Changes in maternal thyroid function during pregnancy, showing rise in thyroid binding globulin (TBG), total T4 due to rise in human chorionic gonadotropin (hCG), which has thyrotropin like activity.

TABLE 3: Physiological adaptation in pregnancy with its clinical significance.		
Systems summary	**Changes in pregnancy**	**Impact**
Reproductive system		
Vaginal pH	Decreased	Increased risk for chorioamnionitis
Cervix vascularity	Increased	Softening of cervix
Cervical mucus glands	Increased secretion	Mucus plug acts as seal for prevention of infection
Uterus weight	Increased	50 mg uterus turns in to 1000 mg
Uterus height and vascularity	Increased	Adopted to give space and nutrition for adequate growth of fetus
Ovary corpus luteum	Estrogen and progesterone increased secretion	Maintain environment of growing ovum
Cardiovascular system		
Plasma volume and RBC expansion	Increased by 40–50%, RBC expansion by 20%	Hypervolemia fulfills metabolic demands, nutrition, decreased VR, parturition blood loss Greater reduction of oxygen supply to tissues
Peripheral vascular resistance	Decreased	Masking of initial signs of sepsis
Heart rate at rest	Increased by 10–20 bpm	For compensation of increased metabolic state of pregnancy
Cardiac output	Increased by 40% Significantly reduced by pressure of gravid uterus on IVC	Increased CPR circulation demands
Uterine blood flow	10% of cardiac output at term	Potential for rapid massive hemorrhage
Systemic vascular resistance	Decreased	Sequesters blood during CPR
Arterial blood pressure	Decreased by 10–15 mm Hg	Decreased reserve

Contd...

Contd...

Systems summary	Changes in pregnancy	Impact
Venous return	Decreased by pressure of gravid uterus on IVC	Increased CPR circulation demands. Decreased reserve
Respiratory system		
Tidal volume	Increased	To compensate increase oxygen requirement
Residual volume	Decreased	Decrease buffering capacity. Acidosis more likely
Arterial PCO_2	Lower	Facilitate transfer of carbon dioxide from fetus to mother
Laryngeal edema	Increased	Decreased endotracheal diameter
Oxygen	Increased by 30%	Prone for hypoxia, hyperventilation, dyspnea
PaO_2	Increased	To facilitate the transfer of oxygen from mother to fetus
Gastrointestinal system		
Lower esophagus sphincter tone	Decreased	Pyrosis (heart burn)
Stomach emptying time	Delayed	Regurgitation and aspiration
Endocrine system		
Pituitary gland size	Increased by 135%	Compress the optic chiasma to reduce visual fields
Thyroid gland	Boosts production of thyroid hormones by 40–100%	To meets maternal and fetal needs
Renal system		
Ureteral pressure	Decreased due to dilatation, relaxation of smooth muscles	Favorable to pyelonephritis
Intravesical pressure	Increased	Some degree of urinary incontinence.
Renal plasma flow and GFR	Increased	Decreased urea and creatinine average value
Coagulation system		
Factors VII, VIII, IX, XII, von Willebrand, fibrinogen	Increased	Increased risk of thrombotic events
Protein S, fibrinolytic activity	Decreased	Increased risk of DIC
Metabolic changes		
Protein	Increased by 1,000 mg	Growth of fetus, placenta, contractile protein of uterus, mammary glands, hemoglobin, and plasma proteins
Carbohydrates	Mild fasting hypoglycemia, postprandial hyperglycemia, hyperinsulinemia	Reduced Insulin sensitivity. Ketonemia in prolonged fasting
Musculoskeletal system		
Lordosis	Progressive	Compensating for the anterior position of the uterus
Pubic symphysis, sacroiliac, sacrococcygeal joints	Relaxed	Helps in contribution of altered maternal posture and facilitate labor
Central nervous system		
Middle and posterior cerebral arteries blood flow	Decreased	Transient decline in memory
Sleep apnea	Increased	Postpartum depression, postpartum blues
Vitrous humur outflow	Increased	Intraocular pressure drops
Corneal thickness	Increased	Difficulty in previously comfortable contact lenses

calcium. In the pregnant woman there are physiological mechanisms that support the necessary calcium fluxes across the placenta and mammary glands and that are unresponsive to increase in calcium intake. In contrast, there is unlikely to be an additional requirement for vitamin D during pregnancy and lactation. Many women have poor vitamin D status. This places them at risk of bones without adequate calcium such as osteomalacia and their infants at risk of rickets, compromised skeletal growth and other outcomes.[21]

■ MUSCULOSKELETAL SYSTEM

Progressive lordosis is a typical feature of normal pregnancy. Compensating for the anterior position of the enlarging uterus, the lordosis shifts the center of gravity back over the lower extremities of the body. The sacroiliac, sacrococcygeal, and public joints have increased mobility, laxity during pregnancy.

■ CENTRAL NERVOUS SYSTEM

Women often report problems such as attention, concentration, and memory during pregnancy, specifically in third trimester, but it is transient and quickly resolved after delivery. Women have difficulty going to sound sleep, frequent awakening, fewer hours of night sleep, and reduced sleep efficiency which begin as early as about 12 weeks and extending through the first 2 months after delivery. The greatest disruption of sleep is encountered postpartum and may contribute to postpartum blues or to Frank depression due to this American College of Obstetricians and Gynecologists (2002) suggested education and counseling during pregnancy, especially in third trimester to all pregnant women.

■ CONCLUSION

There are numerous and profound changes that occur in the mother's body during pregnancy. A summary of these changes is presented in **Table 3**. It is important for the clinician to understand these changes to appreciate the differences between normal physiology and evolving pathological adaptations.

■ REFERENCES

1. Geraghty LN, Pomeranz MK. Physiologic changes and dermatoses of pregnancy. Int J Dermatol. 2011:50(7)771-82.
2. Lain KY, Catalano PM. Metabolic changes in pregnancy. Clin Obstet Gynecol. 2007:50(4):939-48.
3. Butte NF. Carbohydrate and lipid metabolism in pregnancy: normal compared with gestational diabetes mellitus. Am J Clin Nutr. 2000;71(5 Suppl):1256S-61S.
4. Catalano PM, Huston L, Amini SB, Kalhan SC. Longitudinal changes in glucose metabolism during pregnancy in obese women with normal glucose tolerance and gestational diabetes mellitus. Am J Obstet Gynecol. 1999;180(4):903-16.
5. Borden G. Fuel metabolism in pregnancy and in gestational diabetes mellitus. Obstet Gynecol Clin North Am. 1996;23(1):1-10.
6. Mor G, Cardenas I. The Immune system in pregnancy: a unique complexity. Am J Reprod Immunol. 2010;63(6):425-33.
7. Duvekott JJ, Peeters LL. Maternal cardiovascular hemodynamic adaptation to pregnancy. Obstet Gynecol Surv. 1994;49(12 Suppl):S1-14.
8. Abbas AE, Lester SJ, Connolly H. Pregnancy and cardiovascular system. Int J Cardiol. 2005;98(2):179-89.
9. Moll W. Physiological cardiovascular adaptation in pregnancy—its significance for cardiac diseases. Z Kardiol. 2001;90(Suppl 4):2-9.
10. Ramadoss J, Jobe SO, Magness RR. Alcohal and maternal uterine vascular adaptations during pregnancy-part I: effects of chronic in vitro binge-like alcohol on uterine endothelial nitric oxide system and function. Alcohol Clin Exp Res. 2011;35(9):1686-93.
11. Geelhoed JJ, EL Marroun H, Verburg BO, van Osch-Gevers, Hofman A, Huizink AC, et al. Maternal smoking during pregnancy, fetal arterial resistance adaptations and cardiovascular function in childhood. BJOG. 2011;118(6)755-62.
12. Jensen D, Webb KA, O'Donnell DE. Chemical and mechanical adaptations of the respiratory system at rest and during exercise in human pregnancy. Appl Physiol Nutr Metab. 2007;32(6):1239-50.
13. Jensen D, Duffin J, Lam YM, Webb KA, Simpson JA, Davies GA, et al. Physiological mechanism of hyperventilation during human pregnancy. Respir Physiol Neurobiol. 2008;161(1):76-86.
14. Davison JM. Kidney function in pregnant women. Am J Kidney Dis. 1987;9(4):248-52.
15. Jeyabalan A, Latin KY. Anatomic and functional changes of the upper urinary tract during pregnancy. Urol Clin North AM. 2007;34(1):1-6.
16. Hauth JC, Clifton RG, Roberts JM, Myatt L, Sponge CY, Leveno KJ, et al. Maternal insulin resistance and preeclampsia. Am J Obstet Gynecol. 2011;204(4):327.e1-6.
17. Ebrahimi N, Maltepe C, EinarsonA. Optimal management of nausea and vomiting of pregnancy. Int J Womens Health. 2010;2:241-8.
18. Baron TH, Ramirez B, Richter JE. Gastrointestinal motility disorders during pregnancy. Ann Intern Med. 1993;118(5):366-75.
19. Casy BM, Leveno KJ. Thyroid disease in pregnancy. Obstet Gynecol. 2006;108:1283-92.
20. Kovacs CS. Vitamin D in pregnancy and lactation: maternal, fetal, and neonatal outcomes from human and animal studies. Am J Clin Nutr. 2008;88(2):520S-528S.
21. Prentice A. Milk intake, calcium and vitamin D in pregnancy and lactation: effects on maternal, fetal and infant bone in low- and high-income countries. Nestle Nutr Workshop Ser Pediatr Program. 2011:67:1-15.

■ LONG QUESTIONS

1. Describe the cardiovascular adaptations during pregnancy.
2. Write on metabolic changes during pregnancy.

SHORT QUESTIONS

1. What are the normal physiological changes in genital tract?
2. Write short note on hematological changes during pregnancy.
3. Justify, pregnancy is a physiological hyperthyroid state.
4. Give brief description of coagulation and fibrinolysis during pregnancy.

MULTIPLE CHOICE QUESTIONS

1. The uterine flow at term is:
   a. 150 mL/min
   b. 200 mL/min
   c. 650 mL/min
   d. 1000 mL/min
2. Increased calories required during pregnancy:
   a. 300
   b. 550
   c. 800
   d. 400
3. Which of the following is truly physiological in pregnancy:
   a. Albuminuria
   b. Increased BP
   c. Mild pedal edema
   d. Increased GFR
4. In early pregnancy:
   a. Decreased stroke volume
   b. Increased peripheral vascular resistance
   c. Decreased renal blood flow
   d. Increased renal blood flow
5. True about various changes in pregnancy is:
   a. Fibrinogen levels are increased
   b. Uric acid levels are increased
   c. Serum sodium is increased
   d. Serum K is increased
6. Which of the following is not increased in pregnancy:
   a. Globulin
   b. Fibrinogen
   c. Uric acid
   d. Leukocyte
7. Physiological changes of pregnancy include:
   a. Insulin level increase
   b. Increased BMR
   c. Hypothyroidism
   d. GH decreases
8. What are maternal physiological changes in pregnancy:
   a. Increased cardiac output
   b. Increased tidal volume
   c. Increased vital capacity
   d. Decreased plasma protein concentration.
9. Serum creatinine level during normal pregnancy:
   a. 0.7 to 0.5 mg/dL
   b. 1.5 mg/dL
   c. 0.9 mg/dL
   d. 1 mg/dL
10. Cervical mucus is showing beading or crystallization during pregnancy:
    a. Progesterone effect
    b. Estrogen effect
    c. Due to presence of sodium chloride
    d. None

Answers
1. c 2. a 3. c, d 4. d 5. a 6. c
7. a, b 8. a, b, d 9. a 10. a

2.5 PRECONCEPTION AND ROUTINE ANTENATAL CARE

Vanita Suri, Bharti Sharma

OVERVIEW

Preconception and antenatal care is the integral part of continuum of care not only to prevent maternal and perinatal mortality and morbidity but are also crucial for women's health throughout the life span.[1-3] It is an excellent example of preventive medicine. Over years there has been marked improvement in healthcare facilities, still the pregnancy-related preventable perinatal morbidity and mortality remains unacceptably high. In 2015, an estimated 303,000 women died from pregnancy-related causes and 2.6 million babies were stillborn worldwide. Many of these adverse outcomes can be prevented by providing quality preconceptional and antenatal care.

PRECONCEPTION CARE

Definition

Preconception care is the provision of biomedical, behavioral, and social health interventions to women and couples before conception occurs.[4]

Aim of Preconception Care

- Optimize the maternal health
- Address the modifiable factors
- Educate about health pregnancy.

Preconception Counseling and Intervention

The following points serve as the basis for preconception counseling:

1. *Timing of preconception counseling*: Any encounter with a reproductive aged woman is an opportunity to counsel her about the healthy habits which may improve her reproductive outcome.
2. *Family planning and spacing*: Family planning is foundational aspect of preconception counseling to avoid unplanned pregnancies.
3. *Review of medical and surgical histories in detail*: Chronic medical diseases like diabetes, hypertension, autoimmune disorders, thyroid disorders, epilepsy, etc. have implications on pregnancy outcome and should be optimized before planning pregnancy.

4. *Review of current medications*: The potential effect of medicine and potential teratogenicity should be reviewed and discussed.
5. *Review the family and genetic history*: Inquire about the history of any genetic disorder, mental disorder, birth defects, etc. in the family.
6. *Prepregnancy immunization*: Review the immunization status and ideally it is best to administer vaccine before pregnancy to avoid exposure to the fetus. Women who receive live virus vaccine should avoid conception at least 1 month after immunization. Rubella and hepatitis B should be given to nonimmune women.
7. *Infectious disease screening*: Sexually transmitted infections which include syphilis, human immunodeficiency virus (HIV), hepatitis B and C should be screened and treated before conception.
8. *Substance abuse assessment*: Inquire regarding smoking, alcohol consumption, or any other substance abuse and suggest stopping before planning pregnancy.
9. *Intimate partner violence*—should also be taken care.
10. *Nutritional conditions*:
    i. Assess the nutritional status and encourage achieving the healthy body weight.
    ii. Screening for anemia—supplementing iron and folic acid
    iii. Preconception folic acid supplementation
    iv. Iodized salts
    v. Optimization of body mass index (BMI) and weight gain.
11. *Assessing risks* of Rh alloimmunization, history of recurrent stillbirths, and patients at high risks for having fetuses with aneuploidy are evaluated.

ANTENATAL CARE

Antenatal care is the provision of quality health care by implementing timely and appropriate evidence-based practices during pregnancy and childbirth.[2] It is important in establishing an individualized plan according to the needs of the woman and her family. It provides an opportunity for health promotion, screening, diagnosis, and prevention of disease. The concept of antenatal care is almost 100 years old (United Kingdom in 1929) and the main objective was to achieve safe motherhood. Now the safe motherhood is not just the prevention of morbidity or mortality, it also encompasses respect for women's basic human rights, to provide respectful maternity care to every pregnant woman.[3,5]

Antenatal care comprises the following:
- Provision of services:
  - Readily available and provide regular antenatal care from early pregnancy to postpartum period
  - Access to emergency services on a 24-hour basis
  - Proper documentation and maintenance of antenatal records
- Management of modifiable risk factors and complications during pregnancy
- Timely referral to higher center.

Objectives of Antenatal Care
- To reduce maternal mortality and morbidity (maternal near-misses)
- To reduce preterm births, intrauterine growth retardation, congenital anomalies, and failure to thrive
- To promote health supervision, and healthy fetal growth and development
- To prepare the mother physically and mentally for normal vaginal delivery.

Antenatal Care Model
In 1990, World Health Organization (WHO) introduced the concept of focused antenatal care model (FANC), a goal-oriented approach to deliver evidence-based intervention in four antenatal visits. With this approach, there was marked rise in antenatal care utilizations, especially in low- and middle-income countries (LMICs) but the perinatal mortality still remains high. In 2016, WHO came up with the "new WHO antenatal care model" which recommends minimum of *eight contacts* between pregnant woman and the healthcare providers.[3,5] The new WHO model emphasizes on:
1. Patient-centered health care
2. Human right-based approach—respectful maternity care
3. Ensure "positive pregnancy experience"*[3]

Antenatal Care Contacts Schedule
Women who receive early and regular antenatal care are likely to have healthy babies. The frequency of antenatal visit should be individualized; a woman with an uncomplicated first pregnancy is examined every 4 weeks for the first 28 weeks of gestation, every 2 weeks until 36 weeks of gestation and weekly thereafter. As per "WHO new antenatal care model", every pregnant woman should have eight contacts during her pregnancy, elaborated in **Table 1**.[5]

First Antenatal Visit
First antennal visit is the single most important visit for risk assessment and patient education, especially in LMICs where most of the pregnancies are unplanned or without any preconception visit. At first visit, following information should be discussed with each woman:
- Scope of care and facilities available in that particular facility

---

*Positive pregnancy experience is defined as maintaining physical and sociocultural normality, maintaining a healthy pregnancy for mother and baby (including preventing and treating risk, illness and death), having an effective transition to positive labor and birth, and achieving positive motherhood (including maternal self-esteem, competence, and autonomy).

TABLE 1: Summary of antenatal care contacts.

Contacts	Examination	Investigations	Treatment
Contact 1: up to 12 weeks	Detailed history General physical examination	Hemogram Urine routine microscopy and culture sensitivity Oral glucose tolerance test (OGTT) with 75-g glucose ABO Rh grouping—wife Husband (if wife's blood group is negative) Indirect Coombs test (ICT) if Rh negative The venereal disease research laboratory (VDRL) (both husband and wife) Hepatitis B surface antigen (HBsAg) Human immunodeficiency virus (HIV) Hepatitis C virus (HCV) Thyroid function test Ultrasound [11–13 weeks, nuchal translucency (NT), nasal bone (NB) scan]	Folic acid 400 μg once daily
Contact 2: 20 weeks*	History Examination Blood pressure	Anomaly scan (18–20 weeks)[6] Urine for albumin and sugar	Iron and folic acid supplementation: 60 mg elemental iron and 400 μg folic acid The equivalent of 60 mg of elemental iron is 300 mg of ferrous sulfate, 180 mg of ferrous fumarate or 500 mg of ferrous gluconate Calcium supplementation 1 g/day Tetanus toxoid injection
Contact 3: 26 weeks	History Examination Blood pressure Inquire about fetal movements	Repeat ICT in Rh negative OGTT with 75-g glucose	Continue iron and calcium
Contact 4: 30 weeks Contact 5: 34 weeks Contact 6: 36 weeks Contact 7: 38 weeks Contact 8: 40 weeks	History Examination Blood pressure Inquire about fetal movements	Ultrasound for fetal growth if indicated Hemoglobin (Hb) Urine for protein	Continue iron and calcium

*Antenatal contact should preferably be at 16–18 weeks, so that report of anomaly scan and aneuploidy screen can be collected and managed before 20 weeks. As per the Medical Termination of Pregnancy (MTP) law, MTP can be performed till 20 weeks so it is preferable to have antenatal contact before 18 weeks.

- Determination of gestational age by clinical dating and ultrasound dating
- Investigations required and their indications
- Expected course of pregnancy and anticipated antenatal contacts (visits)
- Patient education on nutrition, exercise, nausea, vomiting, vitamin, teratogens, dental care, working, and air travel
- Sensitize regarding the warning signs and symptoms to be reported to healthcare facility
- To discuss about the place, time, and mode of delivery
- Cost to the patient of antenatal care, delivery, and neonatal care first visit
- Risk counseling, including substance use and abuse
- Psychosocial support in pregnancy and postpartum period.

Subsequent Routine Visits

- During each visit; healthcare worker should inquire about fetal movements (after quickening), pain abdomen/contractions, and leakage of fluid or vaginal bleeding.
- Should evaluate woman's blood pressure (BP), weight, uterine size for progressive growth and consistency with estimated period of gestation and fetal heart activity.
- Routine investigations include hemogram, urine albumin, and sugar and blood group testing. Special individualized investigations should also be done.
- Patient and her attendant should be educated about childbirth, anticipating labor or preterm labor, breastfeeding, newborn care, and postpartum contraception. Options about labor analgesia and cord

blood banking should also be given depending upon availability of facilities.

History Taking

The detailed history should be taken and all the relevant information should be recorded in the antenatal card. Every healthcare facility should provide the antenatal case record and ensure that each pregnant woman carries her case records during each antenatal visit to improve the continuity, quality, and her pregnancy experience.

General Information of Pregnant Woman

Name, age, date of first examination, religion, education, occupation, husband's name and address, and occupation with monthly income should be recorded.

Duration of marriage: It is important to note the fecundity and fertility.

Menstrual history: Ask about the length of menstrual cycle as previous prolonged and irregular cycle (>28 days) may change the expected date of of delivery (EDD).

Calculation of Period of Gestation

The first date of the last menstrual period (LMP) when known should be recorded and the reliability of the LMP should be ensured. The factors like mother's uncertainty (mention sure of dates or not), use of oral contraceptive pills within the past 6 months, irregular cycles or lactation should be noted. Ask about the period of amenorrhea and when was the urine pregnancy test done to confirm the pregnancy.

How to Calculate the Expected Date of Delivery?

- The average duration of pregnancy is 266 days from conception and 28 days from the date of LMP in women with 28 days cycle. Traditionally EDD is calculated from Naegele's rule: add 7 days to the first day of LMP and count back 3 months. For example of first day of LMP be March 22, the EDD will be December 29.
- Previous 1st trimester ultrasonography (USG) if available: crown-rump length (CRL) measurement in 1st trimester of pregnancy is most accurate to determine gestational age. CRL predicts menstrual age with a variation of ±3 days when it is obtained between 7 and 10 weeks and is most accurate for dating.
- From the date of quickening—22 weeks should be added to the date of quickening to calculate the probable date of delivery.

Presenting Complaints

Any complaint should be noted with onset, progression, and duration. If there is no complaint, then inquire about the appetite, urinary, and bowel habits.

History of Present Pregnancy

Trimester-wise history to be asked and documented as:
- *First trimester*: Ask about excessive nausea, vomiting, bleeding per vaginum, fever with rash, folic acid intake, other drug intake, and exposure to teratogen or irradiation exposure.
- *Second trimester*: Ask for quickening, any history of urinary tract infection, tetanus immunization, and intake of iron and calcium tablets.
- *Third trimester*: History of headache, blurring of vision, epigastric pain or any high BP record, fever, bleeding per vaginam, and decreased fetal movements should be asked. Any history of medical or surgical intervention during pregnancy should be noted.

Obstetrics History

The past obstetrics history is relevant in multipara and should be recorded in chronological order detail as given in **Tables 2 and 3**.

Past history: It constitutes relevant history of past medical and surgical illness. Previous history of blood transfusion, corticosteroid therapy, etc. should be elicited.

Family history: Family history of hypertension, diabetes, tuberculosis (TB), hereditary disease or multiple pregnancy in family should also be inquired.

Personal history: Sleep, appetite, bowel and bladder habits. Smoking, alcohol or any substance abuse should be inquired.

Clinical Examination

Clinical examination includes general examination, height, maternal weight, and BMI: prepregnancy weight in kg/height in m^2.

Ideally prepregnancy BMI should be taken into account and usually gestational weight gain occurs after 20 weeks of gestation. The range of weight gain varies according to prepregnancy BMI **(Table 4)**.

- *Build* (obese, average, or thin), *nutrition* (good/average/poor)
- *Pallor*—examine the nails, conjunctiva
- *Jaundice*—examine sclera for jaundice
- *Oral cavity*—look for oral hygiene, gingivitis or dental caries
- *Neck*—examine the neck for enlarged thyroid, Jugular venous pressure and lymphadenopathy
- *Edema of legs and feet*
- *Pulse*—rate, rhythm, and volume of pulse. Look for radioradial, radiofemoral delay, and palpate all peripheral pulses.
- *Blood pressure*:
   How to measure the BP in pregnancy?
   - Remove tight clothing, ensure arm is relaxed and supported at heart level

TABLE 2: Format for documentation of obstetric history.

Obstetrics formula: Gravida................. Parity................. Abortion................. Living .... Issues.........

S. No.	Parity	Date/month/year of delivery	Pregnancy detail	Delivery details	Baby details
			Trimester-wise Whether it was spontaneous onset of labor or induction Indication of induction Method of induction	Mention the mode of delivery Any intrapartum complication Cesarean delivery: indication Mention the day of suture removal History of puerperal sepsis, secondary postpartum hemorrhage (PPH), deep vein thrombosis, surgical site infection, etc. Duration of hospital stay	Weight, sex, APGAR Need for the neonatal intensive care unit (NICU) admission Immunization status Current health status
			Abortion Spontaneous or induced Early ultrasound findings	Medical method or surgical (D and C) Details of postabortal complications	Results of investigations, e.g., histopathology report of products of conception or karyotype report, etc.

TABLE 3: Terminology for obstetric formula.

Terminology:
- Gravidity—refers to the number of times a woman has been pregnant
- Parity—refers to number of potentially viable children she has delivered
- Nulligravida—is one who is not now and never has been pregnant
- Primigravida—is one who is pregnant for the first time
- Multipara—is one who has delivered two or more children
- Parturient—is a woman in labor
- Puerpera—is a woman who has recently given birth (up to 6 weeks)

TABLE 4: The range of weight gain during pregnancy.

Body mass index	Weight gain in pregnancy
<18.5 kg/m² —underweight	12.5–18 kg
18.5–24.9 kg/m² —normal weight	11.5–16 kg
25–29.9 kg/m² —overweight	7–11.5 kg
>30 kg/m² —obese	5–9 kg

- Use cuff of appropriate size
- Inflate the cuff to 20–30 mm Hg above palpated systolic BP
- Lower column slowly, by 2 mm Hg per second or per beat
- Read BP to the nearest 2 mm Hg
- Measure diastolic BP as disappearance of sounds (phase V).
■ *Breast*: Examination of breast is desirable to note the inverted or cracked nipple which can be corrected for breastfeeding after delivery.

■ *Cardiovascular system*: Auscultation of all four areas (mitral, tricuspid, aortic, and pulmonary) should be done to rule out heart disease.
■ *Respiratory system*: Count the respiratory rate and look for type of breathing. Auscultation should be done for breath sound and any adventitious sounds (rhonchi, crepitations, and pleural rub).
■ *Abdominal examination and obstetrics examination*: Inspect the abdomen and look for any other abnormality other than gravid uterus. On palpation, the fundal height, presentation, and position of the fetus should be looked for and fetal heart rate using stethoscope or Doppler. The symphysis fundal height (SFH) should be measured for fetal growth assessment **(Fig. 1)**.
In 3rd trimester, Leopold's maneuvers are performed to ascertain the presentation of the fetus (first Leopold—fundal grip), position of the back, limbs, anterior shoulder (second Leopold—lateral grip), precise presenting area, attitude, and engagement (third and fourth Leopold) **(Fig. 2)**. Estimation of fetal weight (EFW) assessed clinically by Johnson's formula. (SFH in centimeter minus 12 if head unengaged and minus 11 if head engaged multiplied by 155 gives EFW in grams). USG is used to calculate EFW by Hadlock's formula. Subjective assessment of liquor should also be done.
■ *Vaginal examination*: Vaginal examination is routinely not recommended in early pregnancy unless indicated (pelvic pathology, ectopic pregnancy, etc.) as ultrasound is usually available to diagnose the early pregnancy nowadays. Routine pelvis assessment to predict the cephalopelvic disproportion or preterm labor is also not recommended.

ANTENATAL CARE PACKAGE

Antenatal care package is comprises of mainly five components or interventions highlighted in **Table 5**.

SECTION 2: Normal Pregnancy

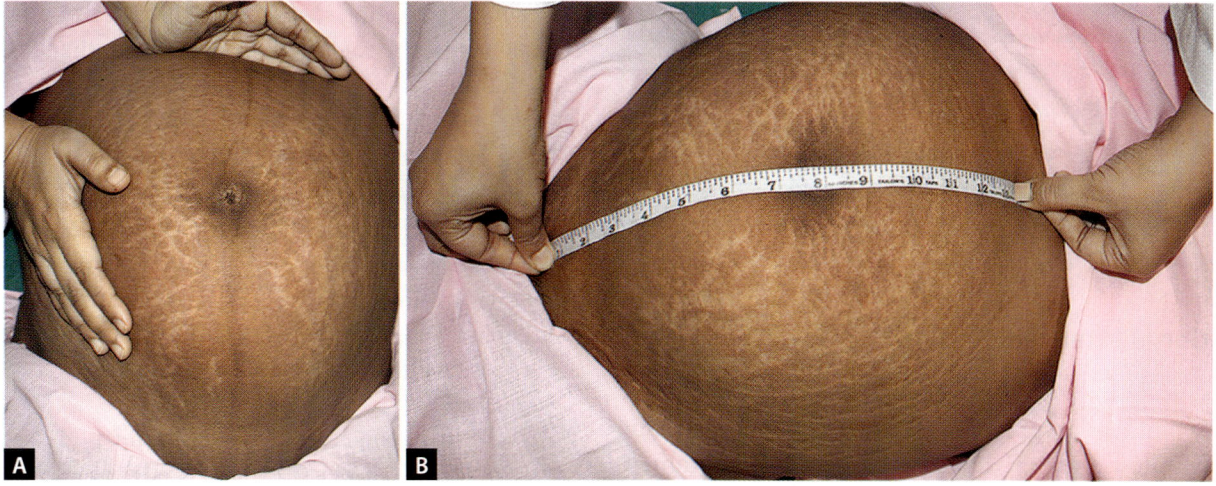

Figs. 1A and B: Measurement of symphysis-fundal height. (A) Marking the fundal height and correction of dextrorotation; (B) Measurement of distance between the fundus and the pubic symphysis.

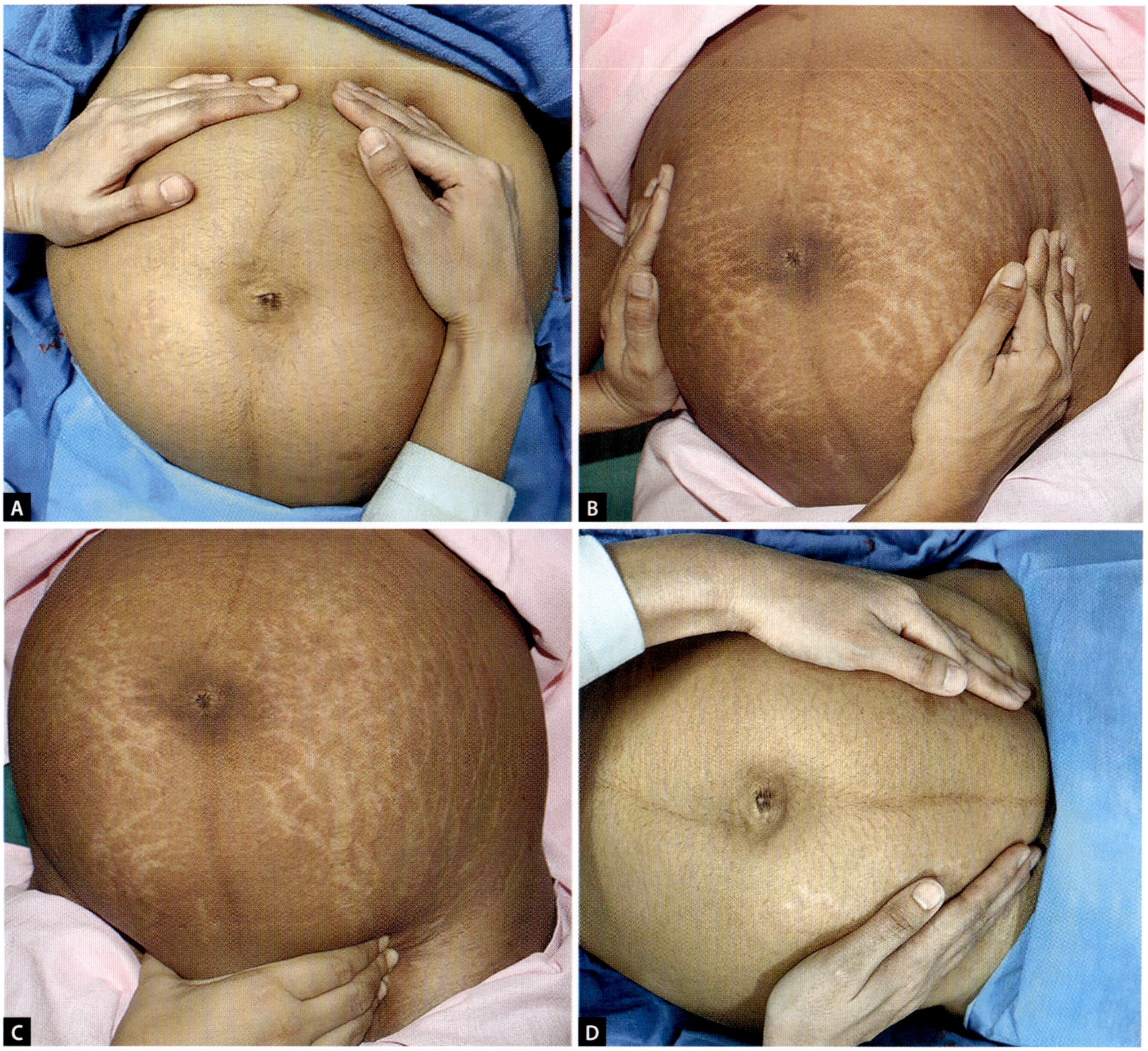

Figs. 2A to D: Leopald's maneuver. (A) First; (B) Second; (C) Third; (D) Fourth.

TABLE 5: Components of antenatal care.

1. Nutritional interventions
2. Maternal and fetal assessment
3. Preventive measures
4. Interventions for common physiological symptoms
5. Health system interventions to improve the utilization and quality of antenatal care

Nutritional Interventions

Diet

Healthy diet during pregnancy should contain adequate carbohydrates, protein, vitamins, and minerals, obtained through consumption of variety of food like green vegetables, meat, fish, beans, nuts, whole grains, and fruits.

The average pregnant woman requires about 2,400 calories/day (300 calories/day extra).

Iron and Folic Acid Supplementation

- Daily oral iron and folic acid supplementation with 30–60 mg of elemental iron and 400 μg of folic acid is recommended to prevent maternal anemia, puerperal sepsis, low birth weight, and preterm birth.
- If daily iron is acceptable due to side effects, intermittent oral iron and folic acid supplementation with 120 mg elemental iron and 2,800 μg of folic acid once weekly is recommended.

Calcium Supplements

Daily supplementation of 1.5–2.0 g oral elemental calcium is recommended to reduce the risk of preeclampsia.

Vitamin A Supplements

- Only in area where vitamin A is a severe public health problem (>5% of women in a population have a history of night blindness in their most recent pregnancy in the previous 3–5 years that ended in a live birth or if >20% of pregnant women have serum retinol level <0.70 μmol/L).
- Supplementation of zinc, micronutrients, vitamin B_6, vitamin E, D, and C are not recommended to improve the maternal and perinatal outcomes.

Maternal and Fetal Assessment

Maternal Assessment

Screening for infections:
- *Asymptomatic bacteriuria:* Women should be offered routine screening by midstream urine culture early in pregnancy to reduce the risk of pyelonephritis.
- Hepatitis B virus.
- HIV—should be offered at early pregnancy as appropriate intervention can reduce mother to child transmission of HIV infection.
- *Syphilis:* Screening should be done in early pregnancy as timely treatment is beneficial to the mother and baby.
- Hepatitis C virus, rubella, bacterial vaginosis, group B streptococcus (GBS), toxoplasmosis, and cytomegalovirus (CMV) screening is not recommended routinely.

Screening for clinical condition:
- Gestational diabetes mellitus (GDM): GDM should be diagnosed at any time in pregnancy if one or more of the following criteria are met (WHO) or by the Diabetes in Pregnancy Study Group of India (DIPSI).[7]
  - Fasting plasma glucose 5.1–6.9 mmol/L (92–125 mg/dL)
  - 1-hour plasma glucose 10.0 mmol/L (180 mg/dL) following 75-g glucose load
  - 2-hour plasma glucose 8.5–11.0 mmol/L (153–199 mg/dL) following 75-g glucose load.

"*DIPSI:* A modified version of WHO criteria is a one-step procedure with a single glycemic value". The pregnant woman is given a 75-g oral glucose load, irrespective of whether she is in the fasting or nonfasting state and without regard to the time of the last meal. A venous blood sample is collected at 2 hours for estimating plasma glucose. GDM is diagnosed if 2-hour plasma glucose is ≥140 mg/dL.

- *Preeclampsia:* Blood pressure measurement and urinalysis for protein should be carried out at each antenatal visit to screen for preeclampsia. More frequent BP monitoring should be done in women with following risk factors:
  - Age 40 years or older
  - Nulliparity
  - Interpregnancy interval of >10 years
  - Family history of preeclampsia
  - Previous history of preeclampsia
  - Body mass index 30 kg/m² or above
  - Preexisting vascular disease such as hypertension
  - Preexisting renal disease
  - Multiple pregnancy.
- *Preterm birth:* No screening recommended.
- *Placenta previa:* Because most low-lying placentas detected at the routine anomaly scan will have resolved by the time the baby is born, only a woman whose placenta extends over the internal cervical os should be offered another transabdominal scan at 32 weeks.
- *Tuberculosis:* In settings where the TB prevalence in the general population is 100/100,000 population or higher, systemic screening for active TB should be considered as a part of antenatal care.

Fetal Assessment

- *Symphysis fundal height*: Along with abdominal palpation, SFH should be recorded and documented at each visit to assess the fetal growth.
- *Ultrasound*: One ultrasound scan before 20 weeks (18–19 weeks) of gestation is recommended to estimate gestational

age, detect fetal anomaly and multiple pregnancies, reduce induction of labor for post-term pregnancy, and improve a woman's pregnancy outcome.[7] The common conditions during pregnancy are elaborated trimester wise in **Table 6** when an ultrasound is needed in routine care. Routine USG after 20 weeks is not recommended except for the confirmation of suspected fetal malpresentation and placental localization in cases of placenta previa (covering os).

- *Daily fetal movement count* is only recommended in the context of rigorous research.
- *Routine Doppler ultrasound* is not recommended to improve the maternal-perinatal outcome.
- Ultrasound biometry and EFW for fetal growth and modified biophysical profile (BPP) to assess fetal well-being in 3rd trimester are recommended in indicated cases.
- *Routine antenatal cardiotocography* is not recommended in uncomplicated pregnancies.

Antenatal screening:

For hemoglobinopathy:
- Screening for sickle cell diseases and thalassemias should be offered to all women as early as possible in pregnancy (10 weeks).
- If the woman is identified as a carrier, then husband should be offered counseling and screening.

Aneuploidy screening:
- All pregnant women should be offered screening for Down's syndrome with proper counseling and need for diagnostic test further.
- Ultrasound screening for fetal anomalies (level II) should be routinely offered between 18 and 20 weeks of gestation.
- Fetal echocardiography involving the four-chamber view of the fetal heart and outflow tracts is recommended as part of the routine anomaly scan.
- The "combined test" (nuchal translucency, beta-human chorionic gonadotropin, pregnancy-associated plasma protein-A) should be offered to screen for Down's syndrome between 11 weeks 0 days and 13 weeks 6 days. In 2nd trimester, quadruple test should be offered between 15 weeks 0 days and 20 weeks 0 days.

Preventive Measures

- *Asymptomatic bacteriuria*: A 7-day antibiotic regimen is recommended to prevent persistent bacteriuria, preterm birth, and low birth weight.
- *Recurrent urinary tract infection*: Antibiotic prophylaxis should be given.
- *Antenatal anti-D immunoglobulin* administration in nonsensitized Rh-negative pregnant women at 28 and 34 weeks of gestation.
- *Preventive anthelmintic treatment and malaria prevention intermittent preventive treatment in pregnancy*—recommended in endemic areas after 1st trimester.
- *Immunization in pregnancy*:
  - Tetanus toxoid (TT)—vaccination recommended for all. Two doses, minimum 1 month apart. If a woman has not previously been vaccinated or immunization status is unknown, two doses of TT/Td, one month apart is recommended. If any woman has had 1–4 doses of TT/Td in the past, give one booster dose in 3rd trimester.

As per the recommendations of National Technical Advisory Group on Immunization and Ministry of Health and Family Welfare, TT has been replaced by Td—Tetanus and adult diphtheria in India's immunization program for all age groups, including pregnant women.[8]

  - Influenza vaccine—recommended, can be given in any trimester.
  - Tdap—recommended 27–36 weeks of gestation.
  - Hepatitis A, hepatitis B, and pneumococcal vaccine can be given in any trimester if indicated.

Interventions for Common Physiological Symptoms

Common physiological symptoms of pregnancy and their management are given in **Table 7**.

TABLE 6: Indications for fetal ultrasonography during pregnancy.

1st trimester	2nd and 3rd trimester
• To confirm the presence of an intrauterine pregnancy and confirmation of cardiac activity • To diagnose a suspected ectopic pregnancy • To evaluate vaginal bleeding • To estimate gestational age • To diagnose multiple gestation • To screen for fetal aneuploidy (NT/NB scan) and certain fetal anomalies • To evaluate maternal pelvic or adnexal masses or uterine abnormalities • As adjunct for procedures like chorionic villus sampling, embryo transfer, etc.	• Fetal number • Cardiac activity • Placental position • Detailed targeted anatomic examination in cases of suspected anomaly • Fetal biometry • Evaluation of fetal presentation • Amniotic fluid volume • Biophysical profile (BPP) and modified BPP • If indicated Doppler assessment in case of suspected fetal growth restriction (FGR)

TABLE 7: Management of common physiological symptoms of pregnancy.

Symptoms	Management
Nausea and vomiting	• Ensure the woman that it gets resolved within 16–20 weeks of gestation • Nonpharmacological: ginger, chamomile, acupuncture • Pharmacological: antihistamines
Heartburn	• Lifestyle and diet modification • Antacids may be offered to women whose heartburn remains troublesome despite lifestyle and diet modification
Leg cramps	• Magnesium, calcium supplements • Hot fomentation
Low back and pelvic pain	Regular exercise, massage therapy, physiotherapy, acupuncture
Constipation	Diet modification, such as bran or wheat fiber supplementation
Varicose veins and edema	Compression stockings, leg elevation, and water immersion
Vaginal discharge	• Women should be informed that an increase in vaginal discharge is a common physiological change that occurs during pregnancy • If it is associated with itch, soreness, offensive smell or pain on passing urine, there may be an infective cause and investigation should be considered • One-week course of a topical imidazole is an effective treatment and should be considered for vaginal candidiasis infections in pregnant women

Health System Interventions to Improve the Quality and Utilization of Antenatal Care

Various interventions and innovations are being planned and recommended by WHO and various healthcare organization of different countries, to improve the antenatal care utilization, care seeking behavior, and quality of care. These are:
- *Group antenatal care:* Healthcare provider provides antenatal care and information to group of pregnant women (8–12 in number) in place of individualized care and it has been found to have better perinatal outcome
- Midwife-led continuity of care model
- Community-based interventions to improve the communication and support
- Birth preparedness and complication readiness
- Recruitment and retention of staff in rural and remote areas.

Birth Preparedness and Complication Readiness

Birth preparedness and complication readiness is one of the most essential components of antenatal care package to ensure quality care during pregnancy, childbirth, and after birth.[9] Ideally the women and their husbands and family members should be sensitized by healthcare provider and prepared for childbirth and how to respond to any complications.

Birth preparedness consists of following elements:
- The desired place of birth
- Identification of skilled birth attendant or ASHA who would accompany her to healthcare facility
- Preparedness for birth and possible complications
- Aware of signs of onset of labor and danger signs during pregnancy and after birth
- Woman and her family should be aware of facility available at desired place of birth and referral center
- Woman's rights during childbirth
- Birth companion identification
- Things to bring to the healthcare facility (baby's clothes, etc.)
- Identified support (relative or neighbor) to look after other children at home
- Transport facility
- Facility of blood bank and compatible blood donor.

LIFESTYLE CONSIDERATIONS AND ANTENATAL ADVICE

- *Working during pregnancy*:
  - Women should be reassured that it is safe to continue working during pregnancy and can perform usual activities throughout pregnancy.
  - A woman's occupation during pregnancy should be ascertained to identify those who are at increased risk through occupational exposure.
  - Advised to rest for at least 2 hours in the afternoon and 8 hours at night.
- *Medication during pregnancy*:
  - Prescription medicines should be used as little as possible during pregnancy and should be limited to circumstances in which the benefit outweighs the risk.
  - Over-the-counter medicines should be used as little as possible during pregnancy.
- *Exercise in pregnancy*:
  - Beginning or continuing a moderate course of exercise during pregnancy is not associated with any adverse outcomes.
  - Activities like contact sports, high-impact sports, and vigorous racquet sports that may involve the risk of abdominal trauma, falls or excessive joint stress, and scuba diving, which may result in fetal decompression disease, should be avoided during pregnancy.
- *Sexual intercourse in pregnancy*:
  - Pregnant woman should be informed that sexual intercourse in pregnancy is not known to be associated with any adverse outcomes. It should be avoided if there is risk of abortion or preterm labor.
- *Air travel during pregnancy*:
  - Women should be informed that long-haul air travel is associated with an increased risk of venous thrombosis,

although whether or not there is additional risk during pregnancy is unclear.
- In the general population, wearing correctly fitted compression stockings is effective at reducing the risk.
- *Car travel during pregnancy*:
  - Pregnant women should be informed about the correct use of seat belts (that is, three-point seat belts "above and below the bump, not over it").
- *Smoking and alcohol*:
  - Both smoking and alcohol are harmful to maternal and fetal health and should be avoided and stopped.
- *General advice*:
  - All pregnant women should be advised to attend antenatal clinic on scheduled date of visits and should have minimum of eight contacts during pregnancy to reduce perinatal mortality and improve experience of care.

Preconception and antenatal care are the pillars for the foundation of safe motherhood and optimal perinatal outcome.

ANTENATAL CARE DURING COVID-19 PANDEMIC

All the pregnant women should be advised to use the mask and maintain social distancing to reduce the risk of infection and practice hand hygiene. They should be advised to attend routine antenatal care, tailored to minimum, at the discretion of the healthcare provider at 12, 20, 28, and 36 weeks of gestation, unless they meet current self-isolation criteria.[10] Teleconsultation can be provided wherever feasible and any woman who has a routine appointment delayed for >3 weeks should be contacted.

For women who have had symptoms, appointments can be deferred until 7 days after the start of symptoms, unless symptoms become severe. Daily fetal movement count to be maintained.

For women who are self-quarantined because someone in their household has possible symptoms of coronavirus disease 2019 (COVID-19), appointments should be deferred for 14 days.

REFERENCES

1. Kilpatrick SJ, Papile LA, Macones GA, Watterberg KL. Guidelines for Perinatal Care, 8th edition. Elk Grove Village, IL: American Academy of Pediatrics; 2017.
2. National Institute for Health and Care Excellence. Antenatal care for uncomplicated pregnancies. NICE; 2008. [online] Available from: https://www.nice.org.uk/guidance/cg62 [Last accessed October, 2021].
3. World Health Organization. WHO recommendations on antenatal care for a positive pregnancy experience. WHO; 2016. [online] Available from: https://www.who.int/publications/i/item/9789241549912 [Last accessed October, 2021].
4. American Society for Reproductive Medicine, American College of Obstetricians and Gynecologists' Committee on Gynecologic Practice. Prepregnancy counseling: Committee Opinion No. 762. Fertil Steril. 2019;111(1):32-42.
5. Tunçalp Ö, Pena-Rosas JP, Lawrie T, Bucagu M, Oladapo OT, Portela A, et al. WHO recommendations on antenatal care for a positive pregnancy experience—going beyond survival. BJOG. 2017;124(6):860-2.
6. Guidelines on use of ultrasonography during pregnancy. (2011). Ministry of Health and Family Welfare, Government of India. [online] Available from: http://www.nrhmhp.gov.in/sites/default/files/files/Approved-%20Guidelines%20on%20use%20of%20Ultrasonography.pdf [Last accessed October, 2021].
7. Seshiah V, Das AK, Balaji V, Joshi SR, Parikh MN, Gupta S, et al. Gestational diabetes mellitus—guidelines. J Assoc Physicians India. 2006;54:622-8.
8. Tetanus and adult diphtheria (Td): operational guidelines. (2017). Ministry of Health and Family Welfare, Government of India. [online] Available from: https://nhm.gov.in/New_Updates_2018/NHM_Components/Immunization/Guildelines_for_immunization/Td_vaccine_operational_guidelines.pdf [Last accessed October, 2021].
9. WHO recommendation on birth preparedness and complication readiness interventions. Geneva: World Health Organization; 2015.
10. Guidance for management of pregnant women in COVID-19 pandemic. [online] Available from: https://www.icmr.gov.in/pdf/covid/techdoc/Guidance_for_Management_of_Pregnant_Women_in_COVID19_Pandemic_12042020.pdf [Last accessed October, 2021].

LONG QUESTIONS

1. What is new WHO antenatal care model? How does it differ from focused antenatal care model?
2. Define antenatal care. What are the components of antenatal care?

SHORT QUESTIONS

1. Preconception care and counseling.
2. Birth preparedness and complication readiness.
3. Antenatal immunization.
4. Role of obstetric ultrasound in uncomplicated pregnancy.
5. How to calculate the expected date of delivery?

MULTIPLE CHOICE QUESTIONS

1. Preconception counseling includes all, except:
   a. Folic acid supplementation
   b. Infection screening
   c. Calcium supplementation
   d. Screening for anemia
2. According to WHO antenatal care model, minimum number of "contacts" should be:
   a. 4   b. 6
   c. 8   d. 10
3. Expected date of delivery is calculated by all, except:
   a. 9 calendar months plus 7 days
   b. 10 lunar months
   c. 280 days or 40 weeks
   d. 266 days or 38 weeks

4. The recommended dose of daily oral iron to prevent maternal anemia is:
   a. 300 mg of ferrous sulfate
   b. 600 mg of ferrous sulfate
   c. 120 mg of elemental iron
   d. None of the above
5. True or false:
   a. Routine Doppler ultrasound examination is recommended for uncomplicated cases to improve the perinatal outcome.
   b. Antibiotic prophylaxis should be prescribed for asymptomatic bacteriuria.
   c. Only undernourished pregnant women should be counseled for healthy eating.
   d. Midstream urine culture should be done for all pregnant women.
   e. Routine antenatal cardiotocography is not recommended to improve the perinatal outcome.
6. All of the following interventions are recommended to improve the quality of antenatal care, except:
   a. Group antenatal care
   b. Birth preparedness
   c. To maintain antenatal record notes/sheet at health care facility
   d. Ask every woman to carry case records along for each antenatal visit
7. All of the following vaccines can be given in antenatal period, except:
   a. Combined tetanus, diphtheria, and acellular pertussis (Tdap)
   b. Tetanus toxoid
   c. Influenza
   d. Human papillomavirus (HPV)
8. Naegele's rule is used to calculated the:
   a. Fundal height
   b. Period of gestation
   c. Expected date of delivery
   d. None of the above
9. All of the following are physiological symptoms of pregnancy, except:
   a. Heartburn   b. Leg cramps
   c. Constipation   d. Spotting per vaginum
10. The common indications for obstetric ultrasound in pregnancy are all, except:
    a. Bleeding per vaginum
    b. To detect anomaly
    c. Assessment of fetal growth
    d. Placental grading

Answers

1. c   2. c   3. d   4. a
5. a—F, b—T, c—F, d—T, e—T,   6. c,   7. d
8. c   9. d   10. d

2.6 MINOR AILMENTS IN PREGNANCY AND CARE

Aswath Kumar

OVERVIEW

The female body undergoes physiological adaptation during pregnancy. Some of these changes or their effects can lead to minor ailments which can cause discomfort to the pregnant female. Most of these complaints can be dealt with minor adjustments in the lifestyle and medication. This chapter addresses on aspects to consider when a physician comes across patients having such pregnancy related discomforts.

Pregnant women should avoid medications wherever possible, and non-pharmacological and emotional support to the woman is beneficial to alleviate most of the minor ailments in majority of the occasions.

NAUSEA AND VOMITING

It is the most common complaint that affects 80–90% patients especially during the first half of pregnancy. It usually commences by 4–8 weeks of gestation and subsides by 16–20 weeks in most of the patients. It significantly affects the patient's quality of life. Though the symptoms continue throughout the day, termed as "morning sickness" as it tends to worse in the morning.

Multifactorial: Predominantly attributed to the emetic stimuli caused by the rising hormone levels in early pregnancy especially human chorionic gonadotropin (hCG), estrogen, progesterone, leptin, placental growth hormone, thyroxin, prolactin, ACTH, etc.

Molar pregnancies and multifetal gestations can lead to excess vomiting due to exposure to increased levels of these pregnancies related hormones in blood.

Hyperemesis gravidarum (HG): Severe intractable vomiting associated with a triad of >5% weight loss, dehydration and electrolyte imbalance requiring hospital admission. It is a diagnosis of exclusion.

Complications

- Acute renal failure
- Mallory Weiss tear due to retching

- Pneumothorax, pneumomediastinum, diaphragmatic rupture
- Wernicke's encephalopathy due to thiamine deficiency
- Vitamin K deficiency
- Gastroesophageal rupture (Boerhaave syndrome).

History
- Previous history of nausea and vomiting in pregnancy (NVP)/HG
- Inability to tolerate food and fluids, effect on quality of life
- *History to exclude other causes:*
  - Abdominal pain
  - Urinary symptoms
  - Infection
  - Drug history
  - Chronic *Helicobacter pylori* infection.

Examination
- Temperature
- Pulse, BP
- Oxygen saturation
- Respiratory rate
- Abdominal examination
- Weight
- Signs of dehydration
- Signs of muscle wasting.

Investigations
- *Urine dipstick:* Quantifies ketonuria as 1+ ketones or more
- *Urea and electrolytes:* To rule out
  - Hypokalemia/hyperkalemia
  - Hyponatremia
  - Dehydration
  - Renal disease
- *Full blood count:* To rule out
  - Infection
  - Anemia
  - Hematocrit
  - *Blood glucose monitoring:* Exclude diabetic ketoacidosis if diabetic
- *Ultrasound scan:*
  - Confirm viable intrauterine pregnancy
  - Exclude multiple pregnancy and trophoblastic disease
- In refractory cases or history of previous admissions, check:
  - *Thyroid function tests (TFTs):* Hypothyroid/hyperthyroid
  - *Liver function tests (LFTs):* Exclude other liver disease such as hepatitis or gallstones, monitor malnutrition
  - Calcium and phosphate

- *Amylase:* Exclude pancreatitis
- *ABG:* Exclude metabolic disturbances to monitor severity.

Treatment

Nonpharmacological Measures for Mild Disease
- Emotional support
- Small but frequent meals
- Rest, avoid large drinks
- Ginger[1,2]
- Acupressure[3] (at PC6 which is located about 2.5 finger breadths up from the wrist crease on the inside of the forearm, between the tendons of palmaris longus and flexor carpi radialis).

Pharmacological Therapy for Mild to Moderate Disease
There are abundant data on the safety of antihistamines, phenothiazines, and metoclopramide in early pregnancy and treatment should therefore not be withheld on the basis of teratogenicity concerns.
- Vitamin B6 with Doxylamine, Vitamin B12
- Antihistamines such as promethazine and cyclizine
- Antiemetics such as metoclopramide and prochlorperazine, serotonin antagonists like ondansetron.[4]

Management of Severe Disease
- Hospitalization and correction of dehydration with intravenous crystalloids **(Table 1)**
- Correction of ketonemia and hypokalemia
- Parenteral metoclopramide, promethazine or ondansetron
- Thiamine 100 mg intravenously added to IV fluids
- Corticosteroids for intractable vomiting (100 mg IV twice daily followed by oral prednisolone slowly tapered)—not routinely recommended due to teratogenic effects
- Enteral or parenteral nutrition if not better.

The Pregnancy Unique Quantification of Emesis (PUQE) aimed primarily at helping clinicians to evaluate the clinical status of NVP **(Table 2)**. It is a validated NVP severity index and covers symptoms in the previous 12 hours.

Differential Diagnosis
- Acute gastroenteritis
- Pancreatitis
- Cholecystitis
- Hepatitis
- Peptic ulcer disease
- Pyelonephritis
- Severe preeclampsia
- Acute fatty liver of pregnancy.

TABLE 1: Fluid management.[5]

Type of fluid	Quantity/rate	Comments
0.9% sodium chloride	1–2 L. Initial rate 1L/h	Further IV fluids should be given at a rate of 1L/1–2 h or slower to correct dehydration and electrolytes (see below)
4% dextrose and 0.18% sodium chloride or 5% dextrose	1L. Initial rate 1L/2h	Consider as an option if minimal oral intake, starvation or uncontrolled nausea and only after correction of thiamine deficiency and exclusion of hyponatremia
Add electrolytes as required Potassium chloride	30–40 mmol/L Maximum infusion rate 10 mmol over 1 h	Administer with caution as per local protocol. Preferred product is premixed 30 mmol potassium chloride in 1 L bags of 0.9 sodium chloride. Use large peripheral vein or central venous access only
Magnesium sulfate	10–20 mmol/day over 20–40 min	Dilute with 100 mL 0.9% sodium chloride. Use large peripheral vein or central venous access only

TABLE 2: The Pregnancy Unique Quantification of Emesis (PUQE).[6]

Circle the answer that suit the best your situation for the last 12 hours

1. In the last 12 hours, for how long have you felt nauseated or sick to your stomach?

Not at all	≤1 hour	2–3 hour	4–6 hour	>6 hour
(1)	(2)	(3)	(4)	(5)

2. In the last 12 hours, have you vomited or thrown up?

≤7 times	5–6 times	3–4 times	1–2 times	I did not throw up
(5)	(4)	(3)	(2)	(1)

3. In the last 12 hours, how many times have you had retching or dry heaves without bringing anything up?

None	1–2 times	3–4 times	5–6 times	≥7 times
(1)	(2)	(3)	(4)	(5)

Total score (sum of replies to 1,2, and 3): mid NVP, ≤6, moderate NVP, 7–12; severe NVP, ≥13. (From Koren G, Boskovic R, Hard M, Maltepe C, Navioz Y, Einarson A. Motherisk-PUQE) (Pregnancy-unique quantification of emesis and nausea) scoring system for nausea and vomiting of pregnancy. Am J Obstet Gynecol 2002;186:S228-31. With permission.) Lacasse. Validity of the modified-PUQE. Am J Obstet Gynecol 2008.

GASTROESOPHAGEAL REFLUX AND HEARTBURN

Incidence

It affects 60–70% patients in the later months of pregnancy.

Etiology

These occur due to the increased levels of progesterone combined with upward displacement and compression of the stomach by uterus and the decreased tone of the lower esophageal sphincter.

Treatment

Nonpharmacological Measures

- Eating small meals at frequent intervals
- Reducing intake of caffeine and spices
- Avoiding sleeping immediately post meal
- Sleeping in a propped-up position
- Avoid bending over or lying flat.

Pharmacological Measures

- Antacids such as calcium carbonate, aluminum hydroxide and magnesium trisilicate or magnesium hydroxide are the first-line of treatment.
- H2-antagonists such as ranitidine and proton pump inhibitors like omeprazole can be administered safely without any fear of teratogenic effects.[7]

CONSTIPATION

Etiology

- Due to increased levels of progesterone causes reduced gastrointestinal motility.
- Iron supplementation given to most women during pregnancy is also an additive factor to be considered.

Treatment

- Increasing dietary fibers.
- Maintaining adequate hydration.

- Dry husk or ispaghula sachets.
- Anthraquinone derivatives and lactulose are not reported to have any fetotoxic effects.
- Phosphate and sodium enemas and macrogols can also stimulate uterine contractions apart from causing fluid and electrolyte imbalances. Hence, it is best to **avoid** them near term.
- Liquid paraffin is also **not** recommended in most cases as it reduces the absorption of the fat-soluble vitamins that indirectly interferes with fetal growth.

PAIN

Types
Musculoskeletal, backache and headache.

Etiology
- Due to the excess strain on the ligaments of the spine due to the increasing weight of the fetus
- Relaxation induced by pregnancy among the pelvic ligaments.

Treatment
- Rest
- Application of heat or cold
- Paracetamol is the treatment of choice for all types of pain in pregnancy and shown to be free of teratogenic effects[8]
- Nonsteroidal anti-inflammatory drugs (NSAIDs) though effective are best avoided after 28 weeks gestation due to increased incidence of premature closure of the ductus arteriosus.

VAGINAL CANDIDIASIS

Incidence
The most common fungal infection occurring in pregnancy.

Etiology
It is due to increased glycogen content in the vagina.

Treatment
- Local clotrimazole and miconazole are the recommended drugs and have no known or reported fetotoxic effects.[9]
- Oral fluconazole therapy though used has to be advised with caution as cases of Antley-Bixler syndrome (multiple congenital abnormalities) have been reported with doses of fluconazole exceeding 400 mg/day.[10]

FREQUENT MICTURITION AND RETENTION OF URINE

It is one of the earliest signs of pregnancy.

Etiology
It is due to the enlarging uterus pressing over the bladder. During the late stages of pregnancy, it is predominantly due to the fetal head that presses on to the bladder.

Treatment
- Reassurance
- Drinking plenty of water throughout the day to maintain adequate hydration
- If associated with hematuria or with suprapubic pain, it is recommended to evaluate the patient (urine microscopy and urine culture and sensitivity to be done)
- If urinary tract infections (UTIs) detected, start antibiotics usually nitrofurantoin.

HEMORRHOIDS (FIG. 1)

Etiology
- Increased pressure on the pelvic veins
- Relaxation of the blood vessel walls due to the effect of progesterone
- Additive constipation.

Symptoms
- Itching
- Tenderness or even mild bleeding.

Treatment
- Reassurance as they resolve after pregnancy
- Maintain good perianal hygiene
- If complaints of soreness and pruritus, emollient lotions and creams can be applied
- Large asymptomatic hemorrhoids can either be given an ice massage or can simply be reposted gently following aseptic precautions

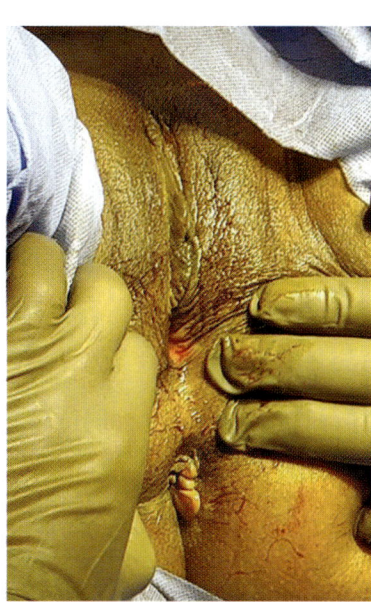

Fig. 1: Hemorrhoids.

- Surgery for hemorrhoids is usually not recommended during pregnancy as most of them resolve once the pregnancy ends.

VARICOSE VEINS

Etiology

- Increased pressure on the veins
- Increased fluid retention
- Acquire with increasing maternal age
- Advance with gestational age
- Cosmetic discomfort in the patients.

Treatment

- Lifestyle modifications such as avoiding prolonged standing at work
- Wearing stockings to aid in venous return from the legs
- Avoid gaining excess weight during pregnancy
- Sleeping with legs raised can all reduce the varicosities
- Stretch panties are available in cases of vulvar varicosities, though benign are associated with an increased risk of severe bleeding while giving episiotomies to aid delivery.

PEDAL AND PALMAR EDEMA (FIG. 2)

These are seen in a lot of uncomplicated pregnancies, as there is excess water storage in the body as a part of the physiological adaptation. It is usually relieved completely by rest and lying down supine. Pathological edema that does not respond to rest or foot end elevation has to be evaluated for associated blood pressure changes.

PRURITUS

Pruritus in pregnancy is caused due to increased blood supply to the skin, which increases skin secretions, as well as due to stretching induced by the 3rd trimester of pregnancy. This uncomplicated pruritus needs emollients and skin soothers as pruritus disappears after pregnancy. However, obstetric cholestasis of pregnancy is to be excluded by doing the liver function tests and if detected warrants monitoring and medication to reduce the bilirubin levels and an early termination of pregnancy.

SKIN CHANGES (FIG. 3)

These include linea nigra, striae gravidarum and chloasma of pregnancy. Patient counseling and reassurance is important as these can be of significant cosmetic concern. Usually, the chloasma of pregnancy and the striae gravidarum fade away following pregnancy, not completely however. The role of emollients and lotions in reducing the incidence and recovery is debatable but can be prescribed when needed.

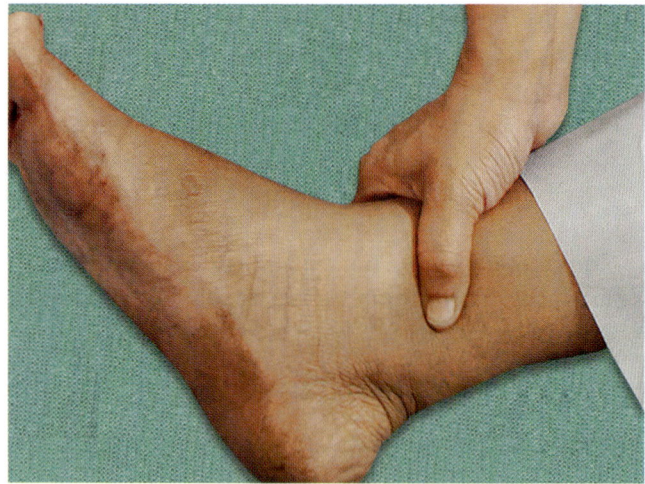

Fig. 2: Demonstration of pedal edema.

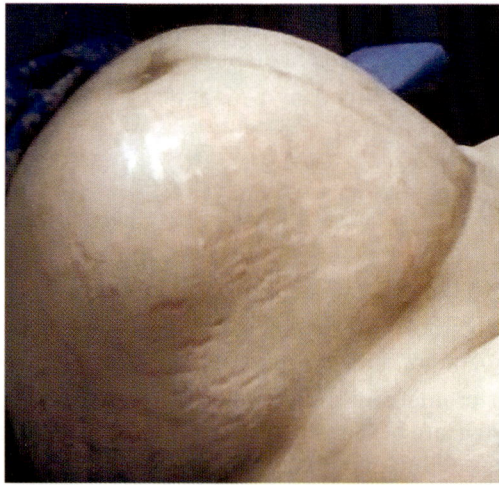

Fig. 3: Striae gravidarum and linea nigra.

ORAL HYGIENE

It has to be adequately maintained during pregnancy as the chances of bleeding and swelling of gums increases during pregnancy as well as periodontal infections are postulated to have an increased risk with preterm labor.

CARPEL TUNNEL SYNDROME

Carpel tunnel syndrome (CTS) is due to compression of the median nerve in pregnancy is due to fluid retention within the carpal tunnel space. The true cause of pregnancy-related CTS is unknown. It is thought to be multifactorial, with median nerve compression, as a consequence of normal physiologic changes of pregnancy.

A thorough history and physical examination are warranted. The history should elucidate the duration, quality, and consistency of symptoms and also inquire about gestational age, weight gain, nulliparity, excessive edema, previous pregnancy related CTS, and any current complications.

Clinical Presentation

Numbness and pain in the palmar thumb, index finger, long finger, and radial half of the ring finger or aching in the thenar eminence, weakness in thumb opposition, and thenar atrophy. Imaging modalities such as ultrasonography or magnetic resonance can be effective in determining median nerve compression at the wrist. Nerve conduction studies and electromyography are used to evaluate the health of an axon, the associated myelin, and the innervation of specific muscles.

Conservative treatment is the initial route with nighttime neutral wrist splints and local corticosteroid injections into the carpal tunnel. Unlike nonpregnant patients, up to 85% of cases of pregnancy-related CTS resolve within 2–4 weeks of delivery, therefore the goal is to keep patients comfortable as they progress through pregnancy.

CONCLUSION

- Majority of the minor ailments need minimal medical intervention but can cause significant discomfort.
- Vomiting being the most common ailment responds to lifestyle changes; though medical interventions are frequently needed, are found to be safe.
- Paracetamol is the drug of choice for any type of pain in pregnancy.
- Antacids can be safely prescribed in pregnancy for GI symptoms.
- Nitrofurantoin is the drug of choice for symptomatic UTIs.
- Hemorrhoids and varicose veins are caused due to the pressure symptoms and typically resolve spontaneously after pregnancy on most occasions.
- While considering pruritus, liver abnormality has to be ruled out.
- Skin changes though typically disappear after pregnancy but can be a cause of significant cosmetic discomfort.

REFERENCES

1. Borrelli F, Capasso R, Aviello G, Pittler MH, Izzo AA. Effectiveness and safety of ginger in the treatment of pregnancy-induced nausea and vomiting. Obstet Gynecol. 2005;105(4):849-56.
2. Sonkusare S. The clinical management of hyperemesis gravidarum. Arch Gynecol Obstet. 2011;283(6):1183-92.
3. Norheim AJ, Pedersen EJ, Fønnebø V, Berge L. Acupressure treatment of morning sickness in pregnancy. A randomised, double-blind, placebo-controlled study. Scand J Prim Health Care. 2001 Mar;19(1):43-7.
4. Berkovitch M, Mazzota P, Greenberg R, Elbirt D, Addis A, Schuler-Faccini L, et al. Metoclopramide for nausea and vomiting of pregnancy: a prospective multicenter international study. Am J Perinatol. 2002;19(6):311-6.
5. Lowe SA, Armstrong G, Beech A, Bowyer L, Grzeskowiak L, Marnoch CA, et al. SOMANZ position paper on the management of nausea and vomiting in pregnancy and hyperemesis gravidarum. Aust N Z J Obstet Gynaecol. 2020;60(1):34-43.
6. Lacasse A, Rey E, Ferreira E, Morin C, Bérard A. Validity of a modified Pregnancy-Unique Quantification of Emesis and Nausea (PUQE) scoring index to assess severity of nausea and vomiting of pregnancy. Am J Obstet Gynecol. 2008;198(1):71.e1-7.
7. Diav-Citrin O, Arnon J, Shechtman S, Schaefer C, van Tonningen MR, Clementi M, et al. The safety of proton pump inhibitors in pregnancy: a multicentre prospective controlled study. Aliment Pharmacol Ther. 2005;21(3):269-75.
8. Shaheen SO, Newson RB, Smith GD, Henderson AJ. Prenatal paracetamol exposure and asthma: further evidence against confounding. Int J Epidemiol. 2010;39(3):790-4.
9. Czeizel AE, Kazy Z, Puhó E. Population-based case-control teratologic study of topical miconazole. Congenit Anom. 2004;44(1):41-5.
10. Unbound Medicine. Maternal use of fluconazole and risk of congenital malformations: a Danish population-based cohort study. [online] Available from: https://www.unboundmedicine.com/medline/citation/18400803/Maternal_use_of_fluconazole_and_risk_of_congenital_malformations:_a_Danish_population_based_cohort_study_.[Last Accessed October, 2021].

LONG QUESTION

1. Discuss the management of hyperemesis gravidarum.

SHORT QUESTIONS

1. Explain the evaluation of a patient with pruritus.
2. Which are the minor ailments caused due to pressure of the gravid uterus?
3. What are the non-pharmacological and pharmacological management of heartburn in pregnancy?

MULTIPLE CHOICE QUESTIONS

1. What is the drug of choice for backache in pregnancy?
   a. Ibuprofen
   b. Nimesulide
   c. Paracetamol
   d. Indomethacin
2. What is the treatment of choice for managing asymptomatic hemorrhoids in pregnancy?
   a. Simple repositioning
   b. Stool softeners
   c. Reassurance
   d. Surgical management
3. Which comorbidity predisposes to genital candidiasis in pregnancy?
   a. Preeclampsia
   b. GDM
   c. Preterm labor
   d. PPROM

Answers
1. c   2. c   3. b

2.7 NORMAL LABORATORY VALUES IN PREGNANCY

Sumitra Yadav, Shraddha Paliwal

■ INTRODUCTION

There are many physiological changes occurring during normal pregnancy which can result in significant alterations in laboratory values that are considered abnormal in a nonpregnant woman. This is principally a phenomenon of maternal adaptation to increasing demands of the growing fetus. For the benefit of the practicing gynecologist and postgraduate students, we are providing a ready reckoner table values of laboratory investigations.

■ HEMATOLOGICAL CHANGES

Blood Volume

There is increased vascularity of enlarging uterus due to change in uteroplacental circulation in the pregnancy. The blood volume increases from about 6th week, expands rapidly thereafter to maximum 40–50% above the nonpregnant level at 30–34 weeks. All the blood parameters are affected due to increased blood volume.

Plasma Volume

It starts to increase by 6 weeks and reaches a maximum at 30 weeks of gestation. The rate of increase is almost similar to that of blood volume but the maximum is reached to the extent of 50%.[1]

RBC and Hemoglobin

The RBC volume is increased to the extent of 20–30%. RBC mass begins to increase at about 10 weeks and continues till term. Reticulocyte count increases by about 2% due to increased level of erythropoietin.[1]

The disproportionate increase in plasma and RBC volume produces a state of hemodilution (fall in hematocrit) during pregnancy **(Tables 1 and 2)**. The advantage of relative hemodilution results in diminished blood viscosity, helps in optimum gaseous exchange between the maternal and fetal circulation.[1]

■ LEUKOCYTES AND IMMUNE SYSTEM

Neutrophilic leukocytosis occurs to extent of 8,000/mm³ and even to 20,000/mm³ in labor. The major change in the immune system is toward humoral and innate immune responses from cell mediated cytotoxic immune response.[2]

TABLE 1: Principal blood changes during pregnancy.

Parameters	Nonpregnant	Pregnancy near term	Total increment	Change
Blood volume (mL)	4,000	5,500	1,500	+30–40%
Plasma volume (mL)	2,500	3,750	1,250	+40–50%
Red cell volume (mL)	1,400	1,750	350	+20–30%
Total hemoglobin (g)	475	560	85	+18–20%
Hematocrit (whole body)	38%	32%		Diminished

TABLE 2: Hematological indices.

Indices	Nonpregnant	1st trimester	2nd trimester	3rd trimester
Hemoglobin (g/dL)	12–15.8	11.6–13.9	9.7–14.8	9.5–15
Hematocrit (%)	35.4–44.4	31.0–41.0	30.0–39	28–40
MCH (pg/cell)	27–32	30–32	30–33	29–32
MCV (xm³)	79–93	81–96	82–97	81–99
MCHC	32–36%	32–35%	31–35%	30–35%
Platelet (×10⁹/L)	165–415	174–391	155–409	146–429
RBC (×10⁶ mm³)	4.0–5.2	3.42–4.55	2.81–4.49	2.71–4.43
RDW (%)	<14.5	12.5–14.1	13.4–13.6	12.7–15.3
WBC (×10³/mm³)	3.5–9.1	5.7–13.6	5.6–14.8	5.9–16.9

(MCHC: mean corpuscular hemoglobin concentration; MCV: mean corpuscular volume; RDW: red cell distribution width)

CARDIAC MARKERS IN PREGNANCY

There is morphological and functional changes such as increased LV mass, increased LA volume and reduced early to late diastolic transmitral flow velocity ratio by the onset of labor due to increase in blood volume by 40%. Because of auto transfusion of 300–500 mL of blood from uterus into systemic circulation occurs after each uterine contraction, there is further increase in cardiac output. These changes results in the transit rise in N terminal proB type natriuretic peptide (NT-proBNP) on postpartum day 3 and therefore, heart failure is commonly to occur within 1 week after delivery among women with structural heart diseases. Therefore, it is beneficial to screen pregnant women at higher risk of heart failure using biomarkers such as brain natriuretic peptide (BNP)/NT-proBNP and troponin I. In patients with heart failure caused by peripartum cardiomyopathy, raised levels of both troponin I and NT proBNP are seen while high sensitivity troponin T has prognostic value in patients with chronic heart failure.[3]

BLOOD COAGULATION FACTORS

Pregnancy is a hypercoaguable state with increase in levels of factors VII, VIII and X, and marked increase in level of plasma fibrinogen. Accelerated erythrocyte sedimentation rate (ESR) seen during pregnancy is because of elevated fibrinogen level **(Table 3)**. The effect of pregnancy on the coagulation factors seen from 12 weeks of pregnancy, and the amount of fibrinogen in late pregnancy is twice that of fibrinogen level in nonpregnant state **(Table 4)**. The placenta is rich in tissue factor (thromboplastin), which will produce fibrin formation within 12 seconds. Gestational thrombocytopenia may be due to hemodilution and increased platelet consumption. Level of coagulation factors normalize within 2 weeks postpartum.[4]

TOTAL PROTEIN

Total plasma protein increases from the normal 180 g to 230 g at term. Plasma protein concentration falls from 7 to 6 g% due to hemodilution, resulting in decreased colloid osmotic pressure leading to better absorption and assimilation of substances **(Table 5)**. The normal albumin:globulin ratio of 1.7:1 is decreased to 1:1.[5]

CARBOHYDRATE METABOLISM

Pregnancy is characterized by maternal hyperinsulinemia and insulin resistance which becomes most marked in third trimester. Human placental lactogen (HPL) is the hormone mainly responsible for insulin resistance and lipolysis.[6]

Therefore, gestational diabetes mellitus (GDM) is diagnosed by screening test (diagnostic test for sugar intolerance by either one or two step test) **(Table 6)**.

1. *50 g oral glucose challenge test (GCT)—two step test*: In India, ideally all pregnant women must be screened for gestational diabetes, as we belong to moderate risk group, with a 50 g oral glucose load at any prandial status between 24 and 28 weeks of gestation. Blood glucose estimation done 1-hour later if the blood sugar is more than 140 mg% the test is considered positive and glucose tolerance test (GTT) is recommended.[6]

2. *One step screening and diagnostic test (DIPSI):* This is simple one step test. In this, 2 hr postprandial blood sugar is measured after ingestion of 75 g of oral glucose at any prandial state, value more than 140 is diagnostic of GDM.[6]

3. *100 g oral glucose tolerance test (OGTT):* After an overnight fast of at least 8-hour FBS value is obtained.
   The patient is next asked to drink a solution containing 100 g of glucose in 200–400 mL of water over a period of about 5 min. Blood sugar values are obtained at 1, 2 and 3 hour interval.[6]

TABLE 3: Changes in coagulation during pregnancy.

Increased	Unchanged	Decreased
Fibrinogen	II	XI
VII	V	XIII
VWF: C (function)	IX	Platelets
VWF: Ag (antigen)	Protein C	Protein S
VWF: Roc (ristocetin cofactor activity)	TFPI	
X	Antithrombin III	
XII	Plasminogen	
Fibrinopeptide A	Prekallikrein	
PAI–I		
PAI–II		
α2-macroglobulin		

TABLE 4: Changes in blood coagulation factors.

Parameters	Nonpregnant	Pregnancy near term	Change
Platelets (mm³)	160,000–200,000	Conflicting observation	Static or 15% reduction of the count
Fibrinogen (mg%)	200–400	300–600	+50%
Fibrinolytic activity	–	Depressed	–
Clotting time	–	Unaffected	–
ESR	10 mm/h	40 mm/h	Marked increase (4 times)

TABLE 5: Plasma protein changes during pregnancy.

Parameters	Nonpregnant	Pregnancy near term	Change
Total protein (g)	180	230	Increased
Plasma protein concentration (g/100 mL)	7	6	Decreased
Albumin (g/100 mL)	4.3	3	Decreased (30%)
Globulin (g/100 mL)	2.7	3	Slightly increased
Albumin: Globulin	1.7:1	1:1	Decreased

TABLE 6: Screening tests for GDM.

Criteria*	Fasting	1-hour	2-hour	3-hour
National Diabetes Data Group (NDDG) (O'Sullivan)	105	190	165	145
Carpenter and Coustan	95	180	155	140

*All value in mg/dL

TABLE 7: Interpretation of 75 g WHO OGTT.

Interpretation	Fasting	2-hour
Impaired	110–125	140–199
GDM	>126	>200

TABLE 8: Changes in lipid metabolism.

Parameters	Nonpregnant	Pregnancy near term	Change
Total lipid (mg/100 mL)	650	1,000	+50%
LDL and cholesterol (mg/100 mL)	180	260	+40%
HDL (mg/100 mL)	60	70	+15%
Triglycerides (mg/100 mL)	80	160	+50%

Glucose tolerance test is considered abnormal if:
- Fasting is abnormal
- Any two or more values are abnormal
- Any value >200 mg/dL is abnormal
- If any value is abnormal (not fasting) the test is considered normal
- If all values are at borderline, test should be repeated.

4. *Fasting and postprandial blood sugar:* FBS of less than 92 mg/dL or 2-h post lunch blood sugar (PLBS) <140 mg/dL, both values are in normal range. If anyone value is abnormal, a full GTT is recommended.[6]
5. *Modified World Health Organization (WHO) GTT Criteria:* In this, women is given 75 g of oral glucose instead of 100 g, after overnight fasting and blood is drawn at fasting and 2 hour **(Table 7)**.

LIPID METABOLISM

Hyperlipidemia of normal pregnancy is not atherogenic in nature. HDL level increased, LDL is utilized for placental steroid synthesis **(Table 8)**. Leptin, a peptide hormone, is secreted by adipose tissue and placenta. It regulates the body fat metabolism.[7]

LIVER FUNCTION TEST IN NORMAL PREGNANCY

The liver in pregnancy does undergo some physiological changes, which are due to redistribution of blood into the splanchnic circulation and great veins **(Table 9)**. The proportion of cardiac output perfusing the liver falls from 35 to 25% but the total blood flow to liver is unchanged.

There is rise in levels of serum alkaline phosphatase which mostly is due to placental production. Aspartate transaminase, alanine transaminase, gamma-glutamyltransferase, and total bilirubin each fall during pregnancy, the upper limit of normal being about 25% lower than the nonpregnant women, mainly due to hemodilution.[8]

THYROID PHYSIOLOGY IN PREGNANCY

Thyroid binding globulin increases in first 2 weeks of pregnancy till 20 weeks and remains elevated till delivery because of estrogenic stimulation. It leads to elevation in serum total T4 and total T3 concentration but reduction of free thyroid hormones.

First trimester elevation of hCG level (cross reactivity of a subunit of TSH) resulting in partial inhibition of pituitary glands, therefore there is transient decrease in TSH level between 8 and 14 weeks of pregnancy.

Plasma iodide level decreases in pregnancy because of following reasons:
1. Increase of type III 5-deiodinase due to increased placental tissue
2. Increase in GFR resulting in increased renal clearance of iodide
3. Increase in thyroid gland in 15% women
4. Increased fetal use of iodide.

The test results change significantly in pregnancy influenced by serum thyroxin-binding globulin (TBG) concentration. Therefore, accurate assessment can only be obtained by free thyroid hormones and TSH **(Tables 10 and 11)**.[9]

TABLE 9: Liver function tests in normal pregnancy.

	Nonpregnant	First trimester	Second trimester	Third trimester
AST µ/L	7–40	10–28	11–29	11–30
ALT µ/L	0–40	6–32	6–32	6–32
Bilirubin µmol/L	0–17	4–16	3–13	3–14
GGT µ/L	11–50	5–37	5–43	5–41
Alkaline phosphatase µ/L	30–130	32–100	43–135	130–418

(ALT: alanine aminotransferase; AST: aspartate aminotransferase; GGT: gamma-glutamyl transferase)

TABLE 10: Thyroid physiology in pregnancy.

Parameter	Nonpregnant	First trimester	Second trimester	Third trimester
T4 (µg/dL)	5–11	35% increase	65% increase	65% increase
Free T4 (ng/dL)	0.7–2.2	No change	No change	No change
TSH (mIU/L)	0.3–5.0	0.1–2.5	0.2–3	0.3–3
T3 (ng/mL)	70–200	30% increase	50–70% increase	50–70%
Free T3 (pg/mL)	200–500	No change	No change	No change

TABLE 11: Levels of thyroid function tests in pregnancy.

Maternal status	TSH	FT4	Free thyroxin index	Total T4	Total T3	Resin T3 uptake
Pregnancy	No change	No change	No change	Increase	Increase	Decrease
Hyperthyroidism	Decrease	Increase	Increase	Increase	Increase or no change	Increase
Hypothyroidism	Increase	Decrease	Decrease	Decrease	Decrease or no change	Decrease

ACID–BASE BALANCE

Hyperventilation in pregnancy resulting into changes in acid-base balance. The arterial $PaCO_2$ decreased from 38 to 32 mm Hg and PaO_2 increased from 95 to 105 mm Hg **(Table 12)**. These help in transfer of O_2 from mother to fetus and CO_2 from fetus to mother. The pH increases by 0.02 unit, thus pregnancy is a state of respiratory alkalosis.[10]

RENAL FUNCTION TEST

Renal plasma flow increased by 50–75%, maximum at 16 weeks and maintained till 34 weeks, then decreased by 25% **(Table 13)**. Glomerular filtration rate is raised by 50% in pregnancy, resulting in decrease in maternal plasma level of creatinine, uric acid and blood-urea-nitrogen (BUN).[11]

SERUM LACTATE LEVELS

Venous lactic acid levels is a screening test in both pregnant and nonpregnant woman except during labor, level is increased due to maximal skeletal muscle contraction.

Lactic acid level is currently actively researched for its role in pregnancy associated sepsis (PAS). Lactic acid level ≥4 mmol/L is associated with severity and culture positivity in PAS. A serum lactic acid level ≥3 mmol/L is seen in organ failure. Therefore, if lactic acid levels are raised, culture and identification of microorganism and appropriate antibiotic administration should be considered.[12]

CALCIUM METABOLISM AND SKELETAL SYSTEM[13]

The demand of calcium increases in pregnancy by growing fetus to the extent of 28 g. 80% of which is required in the last trimester for fetal bone mineralization **(Table 14)**. Daily requirement of calcium during pregnancy and lactation is 1–1.5 g. Maternal total calcium level falls but serum ionized calcium level is unchanged. Calcium absorption from intestine and kidney are doubled due to increase in 1,25-dihydroxy vitamin D3. The increase in Calcitonin levels is by 20%. Serum phosphate level remains unchanged.

URINE ANALYSIS

It gives valuable information to the treating obstetrician **(Tables 15 to 18)**.[14]

TABLE 12: Acid–base changes.

Parameters	Nonpregnant	Pregnancy near term	Change
Arterial PO$_2$	95 mm Hg	106 mm Hg	Increased
Arterial PCO$_2$	38 mm Hg	32 mm Hg	Diminished
pH	7.40	7.42	Slightly increased
Plasma HCO$_3$	26 mmol/L	22 mmol/L	Decreased

TABLE 13: Renal function parameters.

Parameters	Nonpregnant	First trimester	Second trimester	Third trimester
Renal plasma flow (mL/min)	492–696	696–985	612–1170	595–945
GFR (mL/min)	106–132	131–166	135–170	117–182
Urine osmolarity (mOsm/kg)	500–800	326–975	278–1066	238–1034
24-h creatinine excretion	8.8–14	10.6–11.6	10.3–11.5	10.2–11.4

TABLE 14: Pregnancy-induced changes in calcium metabolism.

Parameters	Non-pregnant	First trimester	Second trimester	Third trimester
1,25-dihydroxy vitamin D (pg/mL)	51	94	118	117
25-hydroxy vitamin D (ng/mL)	14	16	18	16
Intact parathyroid hormone (ng/mL)	25	13	16	14
Ionized calcium (mg/dL)	5.2	4.9	5.1	5.3
Total calcium (mg/dL)	10.3	9.2	9.3	9.6

TABLE 15: Types of urine samples.

Sample type	Sampling	Purpose
Random specimen	No specific time, most common	Routine screening, chemical and microscopic
Morning sample	First urine in morning, most concentrated	Pregnancy test, microscopic
Clean catch	Discard first few mL, collect the rest in sterile container	Culture and sensitivity
24 hours	All urine passed during day and night and next day first sample is collected	Used for quantitative and qualitative analysis of substance
Postprandial	2 hours after meal	Determine glucose in diabetes monitoring
Suprapubic aspired	Needle aspiration	Obtaining sterile urine

TABLE 16: Physical examination of a urine sample.

Components	Normal	Abnormal
Volume	600–2,000 mL/24 hours	<100 mL—anuria, <400 mL—oliguria, >2,500 mL—polyuria
Odor	Uriniferous	Fruity–acetone in DKA, ammonical—UTI
Color	Pale yellow or amber yellow (urobilinogen)	*Colorless:* CRF, DI *Orange:* Drug rifampicin, carotenoids *Yellowish brown:* Jaundice *Red:* Blood *Black:* Methemoglobin, malignant malaria *Smoky urine:* Due to RBC in acute glomerulonephritis *White:* Chyluria *Portwine:* Porphyria
Deposits	Absent	Crystals, salt and cells

Composition of proteinuria:
One-third albumin + two-thirds globulin (Tamm–Horsfall mucoprotein 25%)

- Measurement done by *Urine dipstick*
- *Principle:* It analyzes the albumin concentration via calorimetric reaction between albumin and tetrabromophenol blue producing different shades of green.
- *Negative:* Normal
- *Trace:* 15–30 mg/dL
- + – 30–100 mg/dL
- 2+ – 100–300 mg/dL
- 3+ – 300–1,000 mg/dL
- 4+ – >1,000 mg/dL.

SECTION 2: Normal Pregnancy

TABLE 17: Chemical examination of a urine sample.

Components	Normal	Abnormal and clinical significance
pH	4.6–8	Acidic in metabolic and respiratory acidosis, large intake of fruits Alkaline—vegetarian, metabolic and respiratory alkalosis, UTI with urea splitting bacteria
Specific gravity	1.015–1.025	Increased in dehydration, DM, ARF Decreased in diabetes insipidus
Blood	Absent	Presence indicates renal disease
Ketones	Absent	Diabetes and starvation ketoacidosis
Bilirubin	Absent	Liver disease
Urobilinogen	Absent	Hemolytic anemia and liver disease
Nitrite	Absent	UTI
Leukocyte esterase	Absent	UTI
Protein	Absent	Proteinuria prerenal, renal and postrenal
Glucose	Absent	Glycosuria: GDM, uncontrolled DM

TABLE 18: Microscopic examination (40X Objective) of a urine sample.

Components	Normal	Abnormal and clinical significance
RBCs	2–5 cell/HPF	Renal disease Urinary system bleeding
Pus cells	2–4 cells/HPF	UTI and genital tract infection
Mucus	Few	More in UTI, ulcerative colitis and kidney stones
Epithelial cells	1–5 cells/HPF	Renal disease, UTI, liver disease
Crystals	Absent	Acidic urine-calcium oxalate and urate alkaline urine-triple phosphate
Bacteria	Absent	UTI
Yeast	Absent	Fungal infection
Parasites	Absent	*Schistosomiasis haematobium*, *Trichomonas vaginalis*

Urinary Protein/Creatinine Ratio in Hypertensive Pregnant Women (Spot Protein Creatinine Ratio)

The protein/creatinine ratio measured in a single random urine sample taken from hypertensive pregnant women has good sensitivity and specificity for diagnosis of 24 h proteinuria ≥300 mg. 24 h urine collection is inconvenient and time consuming process resulting in delayed management of patient. The protein/creatinine ratio could not replace 24 h urine protein measurements for diagnostic test. It could be used as a rapid alternative test to prevent any delay in the management of patients with poor clinical status.[15]

TABLE 19: Serum human chorionic gonadotropin (hCG) level.

3 weeks LMP	5–50 mIU/mL
4 weeks LMP	5–426 mIU/mL
5 weeks LMP	18–7340 mIU/mL
6 weeks LMP	1,080–56,500 mIU/mL
7–8 weeks LMP	7,650–229,000 mIU/mL
9–12 weeks LMP	25,700–288,000 mIU/mL
13–16 weeks LMP	13,300–254,000 mIU/mL
17–24 weeks LMP	4,060–165,400 mIU/mL
25–40 weeks LMP	3,640–111,000 mIU/mL
Nonpregnant	55–200 ng/mL

(LMP: last menstrual period)

Urinary Albumin/Creatinine Ratio for the Detection of Significant Proteinuria in Preeclampsia

The albumin/creatinine ratio (ACR) is used to detect abnormal amount of albumin in the urine outside pregnancy but there is little evidence on its significance in pregnancy. Microalbuminuria is defined as urine albumin excretion higher than 30 mg/24 h which corresponds to an albumin/creatinine ratio of 2.9.[15]

HORMONAL CHANGES IN PREGNANCY

In pregnancy, placenta produces variety of hormones of which protein and steroidal hormones are significantly important.

Human Chorionic Gonadotropin

Human chorionic gonadotropin is a glycoprotein. Its molecular weight is 40,000 Dalton. It consists of a hormone nonspecific alpha (92 amino acids) and hormone specific beta (145 amino acids) subunits. hCG is a chemically and functionally similar to pituitary luteinizing hormone **(Table 19 and Fig. 1)**.

It acts as stimulus for the secretion of progesterone by corpus luteum of pregnancy till 6 weeks. hCG also stimulates Leydig cells of male fetus to produce testosterone thus indirectly involved in development of male external genital. It also stimulates secretion of relaxin from the corpus luteum.

Human chorionic gonadotropin is produced by syncytiotrophoblast of the placenta and secreted into blood of both mother and fetus. The plasma life span of hCG is about 24–36 hour. During pregnancy in early the doubling time of hCG is 24–72 hour maximum level ranges from 100 to 200 IU/mL between 60 and 70 days. The concentration falls slowly reaching a low level of 10–20 IU/mL after 2 weeks of pregnancy.[16]

Human chorionic gonadotropin tested by many different ways:

Urine test sensitivity upto 10–20 IU/mL (most commonly available) but sensitivity is low. Qualitative methods are ELISA,

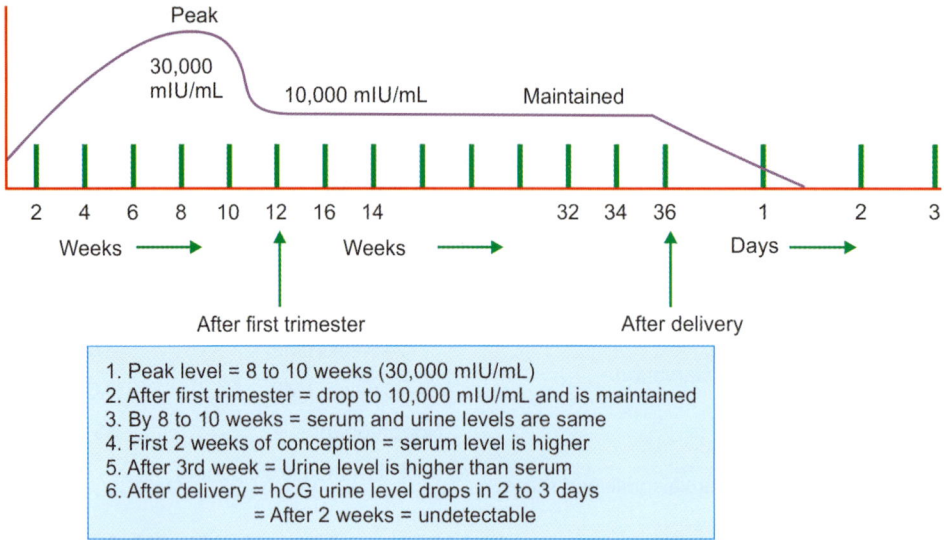

Fig. 1: Human chorionic gonadotropin (hCG) level during pregnancy.

radioimmunoassay (RIA), immunoradiometric assay (IMRA), most sensitive is IMRA up to 0.05IU/mL can be detected.

There are multiple reasons hCG levels can be raised (cause serum false positive).

- Ectopic production of hCG (hydatidiform mole, choriocarcinoma, and germ cell tumors, multiple myeloma, stomach, liver, lung, bladder, pancreatic, breast, colon, cervical, and endometrial cancer)
- Heterophile antibodies
- Rheumatoid factors
- Chronic renal failure or on hemodialysis.

Serum false negatives:
- Just after conception
- *Hook effect:* When hCG levels are about 500,000 mIU/mL, there are so many hCG molecules that they saturate both the tracer and the antibodies separately, which does not allow for the sandwiching of the tracer-hCG-antibody required for the measurement. All of the complexes are washed away, resulting in a false-negative result.

Human Placental Lactogen

It is also known as human chorionic somatomammotropin, synthesized by syncytiotrophoblast of placenta. It is a polypeptide hormone. hPL is first detected during 3rd week of gestation. The level progressively increases from 5 to 25 µg/mL. It decreases maternal insulin sensitivity leads to increase in maternal glucose levels. It decreases maternal glucose utilization which gives adequate fetal nutrition.

Act as potent angiogenic hormone helps to develop fetal vasculature. It promotes mammogenesis. HPL values increase with multiple pregnancies, molar pregnancy, diabetes, Rh incompatibility. And found decrease in toxemia, choriocarcinoma, placental insufficiency.[17]

Pregnancy Specific Beta-1 Glycoprotein

It is produced by trophoblast cells. It can be detected after 18–20 days after ovulation in maternal serum. Human pregnancy specific beta-1-glycoproteins (PSGs) has immunomodulatory roles during pregnancy; PSGs induce transforming growth factor beta 1 (TGFβ-1), which inhibits T-cell function and has proangiogenic properties. It is inducer of proangiogenic growth factors resulting in establishment of the vasculature at the maternal-fetal interface. PSG-1 stimulates upregulation of TGFβ1 and VEGFA in human monocytes, macrophages, and two human extravillous trophoblast cell lines.

STEROID HORMONE PRODUCTION AND USES

Progesterone

Progesterone is produced by the corpus luteum till 10 weeks of pregnancy. At term pregnancy, progesterone levels range from 100 to 200 ng/mL and the placenta produces about 250 mg/day. Half-life of progesterone is 24–48 h. Progesterone act as precursor for many steroidal hormones.

The maternal levels of 17 α-hydroxyprogesterone rises in early pregnancy due to activity of the corpus luteum. Its value decreased to baseline levels by 10th week of pregnancy indicating that the placenta has little 17α-hydroxylase activity. However, during 32nd week there is a secondary rise in 17α-hydroxyprogesterone due to placental utilization of fetal precursors for prevention of preterm labor. Progesterone has role in suppressing the maternal immunologic response to fetal antigens, which prevents maternal rejection of the trophoblast. Progesterone maintains uterine quiescence by stabilizing lysosomal membrane and inhibiting prostaglandin synthesis.[18]

Estrogen

Estriol is the important and specific pregnancy estrogen. Main site of its production is syncytiotrophoblast. It is detected in first 9 week (0.05 ng/mL) gradually increases to 30 ng/mL at term. It half-life is 36 hour. It causes development of uterus, mammogenesis, and increases HDL cholesterol.[18]

■ CONCLUSION

It is important to understand that normal laboratory values of clinical importance change during pregnancy due to physiological changes. Hence, labeling a value as abnormal during pregnancy, one must be familiar with the normal altered values of the investigative parameters.

■ REFERENCES

1. RodgerM, Sheppard D, Gandara E, Tinmouth A. Haematological problems in obstetrics. Best Prac Res Clin Obstet Gynaecol. 2015;29(5):671-84.
2. Ramsay M. The Obstetric Hematology Manual. In: Pavord S, Hsunt B (Eds). Normal Hematological Changes during Pregnancy and the Puerperium. Cambridge: Cambridge University Press; 2010. pp. 3-12.
3. Elkayam U. Clinical characteristics of peripartum cardiomyopathy in the United States: diagnosis, prognosis and management. J Coll Cardiol. 2011;58:659-70.
4. Norris LA. Blood coagulation. Best Pract Res Clin Obstet Gynaecol. 2003;17:369-83.
5. Romero R, Erez O, Maymon E, Chaemsaithong P, Xu Z, Pacora P, et al. The maternal plasma proteome changes as a function of gestational age in normal pregnancy: a longitudinal study. Am J Obstet Gynecol. 2017;217(1):67.E1-67.
6. Angueira AR, Ludvik AE, Reddy TE, Wicksteed B. New insights into gestational glucose metabolism: lessons learned from 21st century approaches. Diabetes. 2015;64:327-34.
7. Butte NF. Carbohydrate and lipid metabolisms in pregnancy; normal compared with gestational diabetes mellitus. Am J Clin Nutr. 2000;71;1255.
8. Al-Jameil N, Hajira HT, Al-Mayouf H, Al-Otay L, Khan FA. Liver function test as probable markers of preeclampsia: a Prospective study conducted in Riyadh. J Clin Anal Med. 2015;6:461-4.
9. El Baba KA, Azal ST Thyroid dysfunction in pregnancy. Int J Gen Med. 2012;5:227-30
10. Gaberscek S, Zaletel K. Thyroid Physiology and autoimmunity in pregnancy and after delivery. Exp Rev Clin Immunol. 2011;7(5):697-706.
11. Hagewald MJ, Crapo RO. Respiratory physiology in pregnancy. Clin Chest Med. 2011;32:1-13.
12. CheungKL, Lafayette RA. Renal Physiology of pregnancy. Adv Chronic Kidney Dis. 2013;20(3):209-14.
13. Bauer Me, Balisteri M, MacEachern M, Cassidy R Schoenfeid R, Sankar K, et al. Normal Range for Maternal LACTIC Acid during Pregnancy and Labor: a Systematic Review and Meta-Analysis of observational Studies. Am J Perinatol. 2019;36(9);898-906.
14. Woodrow JP, Sharpe CJ, Fudge NJ, Hoff AO, Gagel RF, Kovas CS. Calcitonin plays a critical role in regulating skeletal mineral metabolism during pregnancy. Endocrinology. 2006;147(9): 4010-21.
15. Simerville JA, Maxted WC, Pahira JJ. Urinalysis: a comprehensive review. Am Fam Physician. 2005;71(6):1153-62.
16. Hoberman A, Wald ER, Penchansky L, Reynolds EA, Young S. Enhanced urinalysis as a screening test for urinary tract infection. Pediatrics. 1993;91(6):1196-9.
17. Morris RK, Riley RD, Doug M, Deeks JJ, Kilby MD. Diagnostic accuracy of spot urinary protein and albumin to creatinine ratios for detection of significant proteinuria or adverse pregnancy outcome in patients with suspected preeclampsia: systematic review and meta-analysis. BMJ. 2012;345:E4342.
18. HCG-Cole LA. Biological functions of hCG and hCG related molecules. Rep Biol Endocrinol. 2010;8:102.
19. Newbern D, Freemark M. Placental hormones and the control of maternal metabolism and fetal growth. Curr Opin Endocrinol Diabetes Obes. 2011;18:409-16.
20. Arikn I, BarutA, Harma M, Harma IM. Effect of progesterone as a tocolytic and in maintainance theraphy during preterm labor. Gynecol Obstet Invest. 2011;72:269-73.
21. Tonguc E, Var T, Ozyer S, Citil A, Dogan N. Estradiol supplementation during the luteal phase of in vitro fertilization cycle: a prospective randomised study. Eur J Obstet Gynecol Reprod Biol. 2011;154:172-6.

■ LONG QUESTIONS

1. Discuss the changes to the hematological laboratory parameters in pregnancy.
2. Why is pregnancy a hypercoagulable state? Explain on the basis of the changes in coagulation laboratory parameters.

■ SHORT QUESTIONS

1. What is hemodilution? How does it impact the parameters of complete blood count?
2. What is the effect of pregnancy on renal function tests?
3. What is physiological glycosuria in pregnancy? What laboratory parameters are affected by it?
4. When does beta-hCG become detectable in a normal pregnancy and when does it peak?

■ MULTIPLE CHOICE QUESTIONS

1. The following changes occur in lipid metabolism, except:
    a. Increased HDL level
    b. LDL is utilized for placental steroid synthesis
    c. Triglycerides level is increased by 50% as compare to non-pregnant state
    d. Hyperlipidemia in pregnancy is atherogenic in nature
2. Which of the following is not a physiological change occurred in pregnancy?
    a. Rise in serum alkaline phosphatase
    b. Cardiac output perfusing the liver falls from 35% to 25%
    c. Plasma iodide level is increased
    d. Pregnancy is a state of respiratory alkalosis

3. Daily requirement of calcium during pregnancy and lactation is:
   a. 1–1.5 g
   b. 2–2.5 g
   c. 0.5–0.8 g
   d. Less than 0.5 g
4. Composition of proteinuria in pregnancy:
   a. 1/2 albumin + 1/2 globulin
   b. 1/3 albumin + 2/3 globulin
   c. 2/3 albumin + 1/3 globulin
   d. Only albumin
5. Ideal type of urine sample for pregnancy test is:
   a. Random sample
   b. Morning sample
   c. Clean catch sample
   d. 24 hr collected urine
6. All of the following can be a reason for false positive serum hCG level, except:
   a. Heterophile antibodies
   b. Ectopic production of hCG
   c. Chronic renal failure
   d. Hook effect
7. The clotting factor which is not increased in pregnancy:
   a. Factor 2
   b. Factor 7
   c. Factor 10
   d. Factor 11
8. The following changes occur urinary system in pregnancy, except:
   a. Increased GFR
   b. Increased RBF
   c. Hypertrophy of bladder musculature
   d. Increased activity of uterus
9. Which of the following is least likely physiological change in pregnancy?
   a. Increase in intravascular volume
   b. Increase in cardiac output
   c. Increase in stroke volume
   d. Increase in peripheral vascular resistance
10. Which of the following statement for changes in pregnancy is false?
    a. Fibrinogen levels are increased
    b. Uric acid level are increased
    c. Serum potassium is decreased
    d. Sodium retention

Answers

1. d   2. c   3. a   4. c   5. b   6. d
7. d   8. d   9. d   10. b

SECTION 3

Fetal Evaluation

3.1 GENETICS AND GENOMICS FOR THE OBSTETRICIAN

Pragya Mishra Choudhary, Manisha Madhai Beck

INTRODUCTION

Genetics is the study of heredity and variation of inherited characteristics. Genomics, on the other hand, studies the interaction of individual genes with each other and with the environment in order to identify their combined influence on the growth and development of the organism. Genetic literacy among the obstetricians is the need of the hour since there is an increase in the diagnosis of fetal congenital malformations with better ultrasonography (USG) facilities available, increased availability of genetic tests that can be offered for various conditions and increased awareness in the society towards these, which lead to people with underlying genetic conditions in family, coming up for preconception counseling.

BASIC CONCEPTS

- *Genome*: Each nucleated cell has 23 chromosomes. *Genome refers to the genetic information encoded by a full set of haploid chromosomes. The Human Genome Project* (world's largest collaborative biological project), which was completed in 2003, identified >25,000 genes and allows mapping of the entire human deoxyribonucleic acid (DNA). Human genome has 3 billion (3×10^9) base pairs.
- *Chromosomes* **(Fig. 1)**: Genetic information of the genome is packaged into chromosomes. Somatic cells are diploid (have 46 chromosomes, one set each from father and mother). Germ cells like sperm or ova, on the other hand, are haploid (contain only one set of 23 chromosomes). *Chromosomes are arranged in decreasing order of their length.*
- *Genes*: This is the basic functional unit of the genome. It occupies specific site on chromosome called *locus* and is made of *nucleotides* (DNA sequences), which encode for proteins. Each gene has two types of regions, *exons* and *introns*. Exons are the part of gene, which contain DNA sequences that code for proteins whereas introns do not

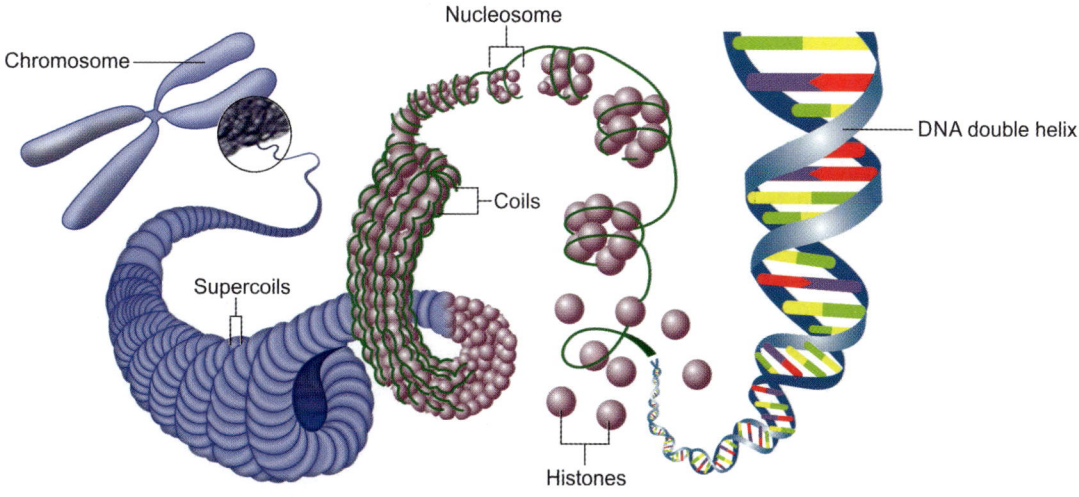

Fig. 1: Structure and packaging of human chromosome. (DNA: deoxyribonucleic acid)
(*Source:* https://pmgbiology.com/2015/10/13/chromosomes-a-understanding-for-igcse-biology/)

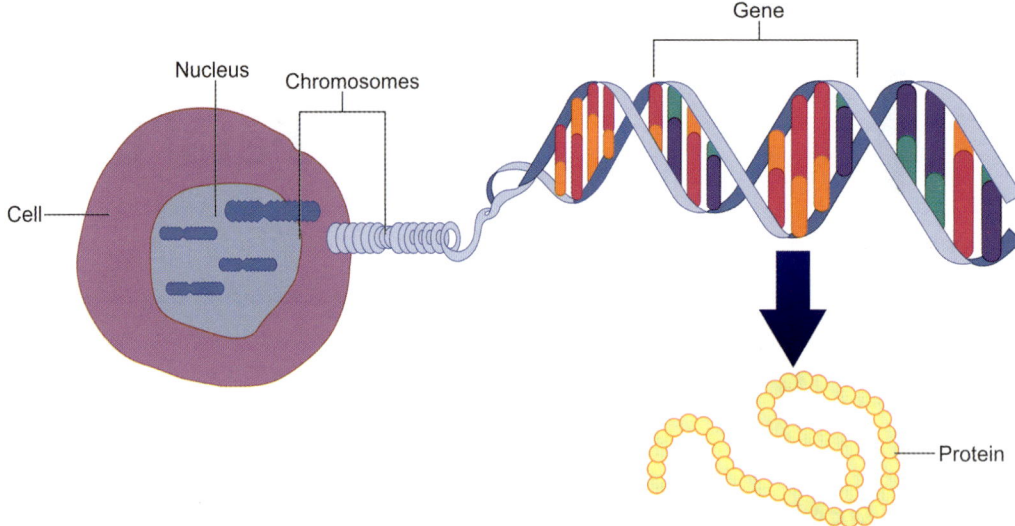

Fig. 2: Structure showing relationship between deoxyribonucleic acid (DNA), genes, and chromosomes.
(*Source:* socratic.org)

code for proteins. Genes are responsible for inheritance of specific traits.
- *Alleles*: An allele is a variant form of gene. Each gene resides at a specific locus of chromosome in two copies, one derived from each parent. The two copies of genes may not be similar. When the two copies of genes differ from each other, they are called alleles. According to American College of Medical Genetics and Genomics, variants may be classified as benign, likely benign, pathogenic, likely pathogenic, and uncertain significance.
- *Exome*: Part of the genome, which is made up of exons that code for proteins.
- *DNA* **(Fig. 2)**: Basic genetic material, which serves as building blocks for genes and chromosomes. The human DNA is 2 meters long and is made up of 25,000–30,000 genes. It is a double helical structure made up of nucleotides. DNA wraps around histone proteins to form nucleosomes. Chromatin is formed when nucleosomes loop around nonhistone proteins scaffold. As the chromatin enters into cell cycle, it condenses to form chromosomes, typically seen during metaphase.
- *Genotype*: Genes at a single locus on homologous chromosomes.
- *Phenotype*: Observable characteristics (morphological/cellular/biochemical/clinical) of an organism due to expression of the genotype and its interaction with environment.
- *Penetrance*: Percentage of people with predisposing genotype who are actually affected.
- *Proband*: Index case affected with genetic disorders.
- *Consultand*: Person requesting genetic counseling.

TYPES OF GENETIC DISORDERS

There are different types of genetic disorders which are presented in **Flowchart 1**.

Chromosomal Disorders

These are either numerical or structural. There are two types of numerical aberrations: aneuploidy and polyploidy.
- *Polyploidy*: The cell contains chromosomes in multiples of 23. For example, in triploidy, there are 69 chromosomes and in tetraploidy there are 92 chromosomes.
- *Aneuploidy*: Number of chromosomes in a cell is not a multiple of 23. In monosomy, instead of two copies of a chromosome, there is only one copy. For example, Turner syndrome is due to monosomy X or XO, only one copy of X chromosome present instead of two copies. In trisomy, one extra copy of specific chromosome present in an otherwise diploid cell. For example, Edwards' syndrome is due to trisomy 18 wherein an extra copy of chromosome 18 is present and trisomy 21 (Down syndrome) has an extra copy of chromosome 2.
- *Structural abnormalities* are of two types: balanced and unbalanced rearrangements. *In balanced rearrangements, there is no loss or gain of chromosomal segments.* In unbalanced rearrangements, there is either loss or gain of genetic material.
- *Deletion*: Loss of part or segment of chromosome. For example, deletion of terminal part of short arm of chromosome 5(5p-) leads to cri du chat syndrome. Deletion syndromes cause more serious phenotypic and functional abnormalities than duplication syndromes.
- *Duplication*: Extra copy of chromosomal segment or part leading to partial trisomy.
- *Inversion*: A segment of chromosome is broken at two places and rejoined in reverse orientation. *Pericentric inversions* **(Fig. 3)** involve breakage on either side of centromere. In *paracentric inversions* **(Fig. 4)**, the break points are on one side of the centromere.
- *Translocation*: Transfer of a segment of chromosome to another chromosome. The rearranged chromosome

SECTION 3: Fetal Evaluation | 115

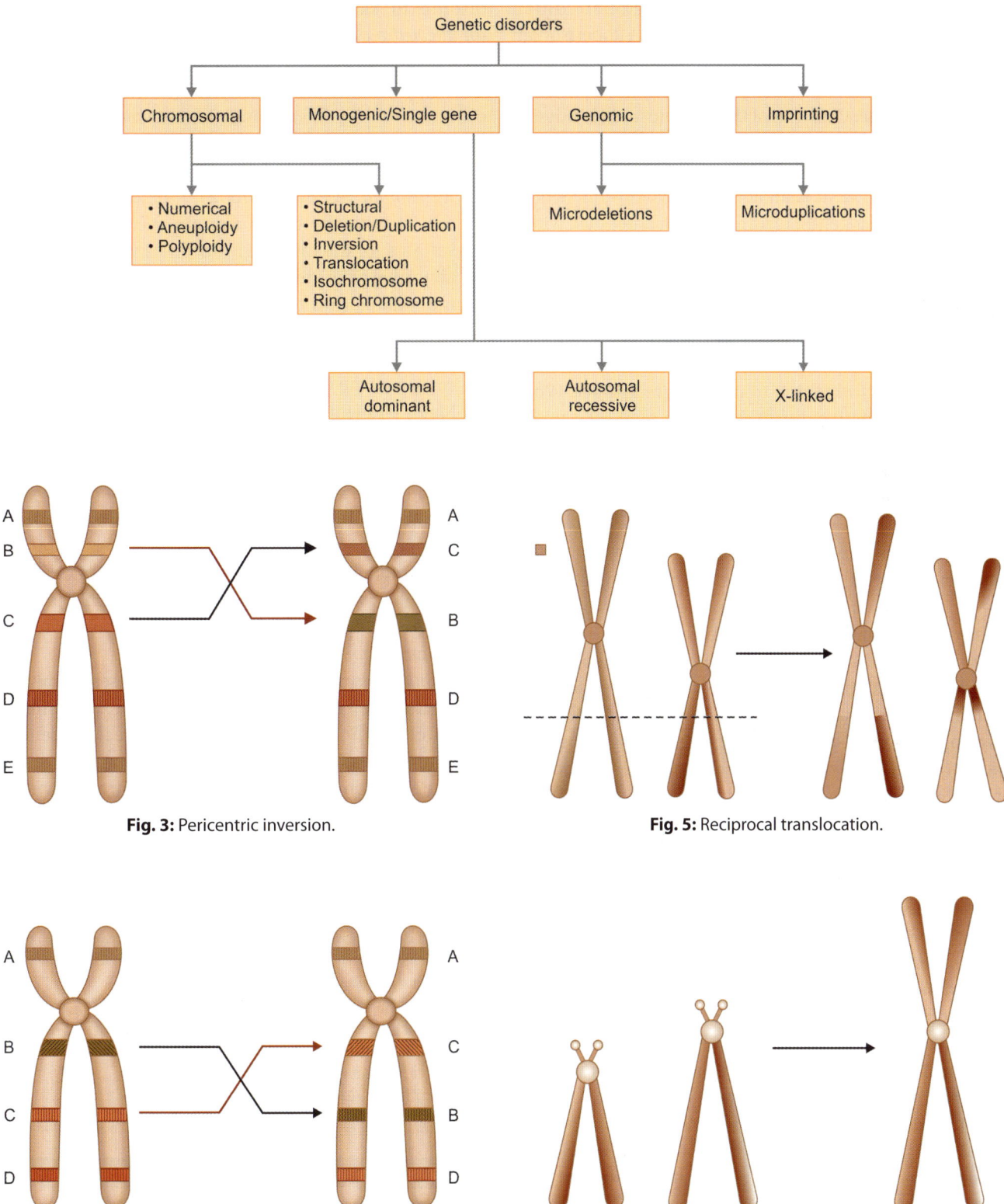

Flowchart 1: Types of genetic disorders.

Fig. 3: Pericentric inversion.

Fig. 4: Paracentric inversion.

Fig. 5: Reciprocal translocation.

Fig. 6: Robertsonian translocation.

is called a derivative (der) chromosome. *Reciprocal translocations* **(Fig. 5)** are due to mutual exchange of genetic material between two chromosomes. In *Robertsonian translocation* **(Fig. 6)**, two long arms of acrocentric chromosomes join together to form metacentric chromosome. This is nonreciprocal. For example, Robertsonian translocation between chromosomes 14 and 21 can lead to trisomy 21 (Down syndrome) and between chromosomes 13 and 14 der (13;14)(q10;q10), the most common Robertsonian translocation, can lead to Patau syndrome. A Robertsonian translocation carrier has only 45 chromosomes in numbers but the genetic material is balanced.

- *Isochromosome*: One arm of the chromosome is missing and the other arm of same chromosome is duplicated in a mirror image fashion.
- *Ring chromosome*: It is an aberrant chromosome whose ends are fused together to form a ring. It is denoted with r.

Chromosomal Mosaicism

When two or more cytogenetically distinct cell lines arise from a single zygote, it is called chromosomal mosaicism, which can be true or pseudo.

Pseudomosaicism is due to cell culture artifact. When several amniotic fluid cultures show abnormal cells, which represent the true fetal chromosomal complement, it is called *true mosaicism*.

Confined placental mosaicism is present in 2% of placentas and generally has a good outcome. However, if there is mosaicism for chromosomes 6, 7, 11, 14, or 15, it is important to test for *uniparental disomy* as it can have adverse fetal outcome. Confined placental mosaicism for trisomy 16 essentially has a bad prognosis.

Some autosomal disorders such as osteogenesis imperfecta, achondroplasia, and X-linked disorders like Duchenne muscular dystrophy can arise de novo in the offspring of normal parents, which can be as a result of *gonadal mosaicism*. Gonadal mosaicism also accounts for 6% disease recurrence after birth of a child with "new" mutation.

Single Gene/Monogenic Disorders

Diseases caused by abnormalities in a single gene are called monogenic or single gene disorders, e.g., thalassemia and spinal muscular atrophy. They exhibit Mendelian patterns of inheritance, e.g., autosomal dominant (AD), autosomal recessive (AR), or X linked.

- *Autosomal dominant* (**Box 1**): All autosomal genes are found in pairs, one copy each on one of the homologous chromosomes. A disease or trait is said to be AD if the mutant gene causing it as dominant, that is, it determines the phenotype of the individual in preference to its counterpart normal gene. This means one mutant gene is enough to cause the disease or the trait.

  Penetrance, expressivity, presence of codominant genes are the determining factors for the phenotype of an AD condition.

  These diseases can be inherited by either sexes and there is male-to-male transmission as opposed to X-linked inheritance where there is no male-to-male transmission. Phenotype appears in every generation, provided there is complete penetrance. Incomplete *penetrance* may allow disorder to "skip" generations. *Each affected individual has an affected parent. There is a 50% chance of recurrence with each pregnancy.*

  Expressivity is the extent or degree to which the gene expresses itself in different individuals which can be variable and range from mild to severe expression, neurofibromatosis being a good example.

- *Autosomal recessive* (**Box 2**): Phenotype is expressed only if both the genes contain the same pathogenic variants for the disease. Individuals who have only one abnormal gene are called heterozygotes and are carriers. Individuals with both genes affected are homozygotes and have the disease. Phenotype is seen in siblings and offspring (homozygotes) and not in parents who are carriers of the disease (heterozygotes).

  Males and females are equally affected and there is 25% recurrence risk in each pregnancy. *If one parent is a carrier of the disease none of the offspring will be affected. If both parents are carriers of the disease, then 25% of the offspring will be normal, 50% will be heterozygous carriers and 25% will be affected.*

  If an individual contains two different mutant alleles/pathogenic variants for cystic fibrosis, they will have cystic fibrosis, even though both mutant alleles are not similar. This is called *compound heterozygosity*.

- *X-linked recessive* (**Box 3**): These diseases mainly affect men as they have only one copy of the X chromosome. Women who carry the X-linked recessive genes are usually unaffected. These are never transmitted from father to son as sons inherit only Y chromosome from their fathers. Mutant gene is transmitted from the affected man through his daughters.

  A woman carrying X-linked recessive gene has 50% chance of passing it on in each pregnancy. Her sons have

---

BOX 1: Common autosomal dominant disorders.

Autosomal dominant disorders:
- Adult onset polycystic kidney disease
- Familial hypercholesterolemia
- Huntington disease
- Achondroplasia
- Neurofibromatosis
- Myotonic dystrophy

BOX 2: Common autosomal recessive disorders.

Autosomal recessive disorders:
- Thalassemia
- Cystic fibrosis
- Hemochromatosis
- Xeroderma pigmentosum
- Infantile polycystic kidney disease
- Spinal muscular atrophy
- Inborn errors of metabolism, e.g., Tay–Sachs and phenylketonuria

> **BOX 3:** Common X-linked recessive disorders.
>
> *X-linked recessive disorders:*
> - Color blindness
> - Hemophilia A
> - Duchenne muscular dystrophy
> - Hunter syndrome
> - Fragile X

> **BOX 4:** Common X-linked dominant disorders.
>
> *X-linked dominant:*
> - Hypophosphatemic rickets
> - Rett syndrome
> - Incontinentia pigmenti type I
> - X-linked lissencephaly

50% chance of inheriting the disease while 50% daughters will be carriers.

- *X-linked dominant* (**Box 4**): Predominantly affects females, as they tend to be lethal in male offspring. *Pattern of inheritance through affected females are similar to AD: 50% offspring are affected irrespective of the sex.*
- *Codominant*: If the genes in a pair are different from each other yet both express themselves in an individual, they are said to be codominant. For example, genes that determine the blood type are codominant because the individual expresses both A and B antigen simultaneously. Genes for hemoglobinopathies are known to be codominant. For example, individual who has gene which directs production of HbS and gene which directs production of HbC will have both HbS and HbC.

Genomic Disorders

These disorders are caused by small, submicroscopic deletions, or duplications in part of the genome. These are known as *microdeletions* or *microduplications*. Microdeletion involves deletion of genes located together in a chromosome. These cannot be picked up by conventional cytogenetic techniques and need molecular cytogenetic techniques such as fluorescence in situ hybridization (FISH) and chromosomal microarray (CMA). The most common example of microdeletion syndrome is *DiGeorge syndrome*, caused by deletion of long arm of chromosome 22 (del 22q11.2) characterized by conotruncal anomalies, thymic hypoplasia, abnormal facies, micrognathia, and ear abnormalities.

Imprinting Disorders

The function of genes varies based on the sex of parent from whom they are inherited because of a process called imprinting. It is a mechanism for *epigenetic* control of gene expression. The typical example of imprinting disorder is *deletion of chromosome 15q11-13*. If the segment of maternally derived chromosome 15 is deleted, the result is *Angelman syndrome*. If paternally derived chromosome 15 segment is deleted, it results in *Prader–Willi syndrome*. Both of these phenotypes are totally different.

Deletion need not always be the cause for different phenotypes. For example, if the fetus inherits two normal, intact chromosomes 15 from the father and none from the mother, it will develop features of Angelman syndrome since maternal contribution is missing. Similarly, if the fetus inherits both chromosomes 15 from mother and none from father, it will manifest features of Prader–Willi syndrome. This phenomenon is known as *uniparental disomy*.

Polygenic and Multifactorial Disorders

Polygenic disorders occur due to combined effect of many genes. Multifactorial disorders, on the other hand, are caused by interaction between genetic and environmental factors. Familial clustering and occurrence in identical twins provide evidence for genetic contribution. However, these do not show typical inheritance patterns similar to single gene disorders due to interaction with environmental factors. *Neural tube defects, congenital heart defects, cleft palate, gestational diabetes mellitus (GDM), and preeclampsia syndrome* are some examples of multifactorial disorders.

OBSTETRIC CONDITIONS WITH GENETIC ETIOLOGY

It is important for obstetricians to be familiar with common obstetric conditions with genetic etiology. Having an awareness of these conditions will help the clinicians in providing counseling. This will, in turn, help the parents in deciding for or against a genetic test via invasive diagnostic methods such as chorionic villus sampling, amniocentesis, cord blood sampling of fetus, or peripheral blood sampling of parents. Also having the knowledge of the recurrence risk for a particular condition would help in counseling for subsequent pregnancies.

Spontaneous Miscarriage

One-fifth (15–20%) of clinically recognized pregnancies end up in miscarriage, with 80% losses in the first trimester. These are mostly sporadic with aneuploidy such as trisomy 13, 16, and 21, monosomy X, and triploidy being the cause in 50–70%. The most common chromosomal abnormalities in early pregnancy losses are monosomy X (20%) and triploidy (15%).

In these cases, where the conceptus or abortus is aneuploid the chances of recurrence is much less (15%) compared to when it is euploid and thus helps in patient counseling and giving prognostic information regarding future obstetric outcome. Parental karyotyping is not required in these cases as a vast majority of them are normal.

Recurrent Pregnancy Loss

Recurrent pregnancy loss (RPL) is defined as three or more consecutive first trimester losses. The incidence of genetic etiology in RPL has been well established with causes being fetal chromosomal abnormalities, parental balanced translocation, and single gene disorders such as inherited thrombophilia, alpha thalassemia major, and X-linked lethal conditions.

Presence of balanced translocations has been found in 3.5–5% couples being evaluated for RPL. If either parent is a carrier of balanced translocation, the fetus can have unbalanced translocation resulting in abnormal live born, mental retardation, or recurrent miscarriage. There is 10–30% chance of unbalanced translocation in the fetus if parents are carriers of reciprocal and Robertsonian translocations.

Chromosomal microarray of the products of conception is preferred over conventional karyotype since it does not require actively dividing cells for detection of chromosomal aberration. If products of conception are not available, peripheral blood of both parents can be used to look for balanced translocations.

Molar Pregnancy

A partial hydatidiform mole occurs as a result of triploidy which occurs when either one egg is fertilized by two sperms or when there is a failure in one of the meiotic divisions leading to a diploid set of chromosomes in either the egg or more commonly the sperm.

If the extra set of chromosomes is from the father (diandric), it results in a partial hydatidiform mole with abundant placental tissues and abnormal fetal structures. If it is, on the other hand, derived from the mother (digynic) it results in a triploidy with a small placenta and a growth restricted fetus. Triploidy frequently results in fetuses with dysmorphic features and has a recurrence risk of 1–1.5% if the fetus survives the first trimester and hence prenatal diagnosis is important in subsequent pregnancies.

A complete hydatidiform mole is an example of imprinting important to obstetricians. If the diploid set of chromosomal complement is of paternal origin there is abundant growth of placental tissues and no fetal structures whereas if the diploid set of chromosomal complement is maternal in origin it results only in development of fetal structures as seen in partial mole.

Nonimmune Fetal Hydrops

Nonimmune hydrops is defined as presence of fetal hydrops in the absence of rhesus or ABO incompatibility. It is characterized by presence of fetal subcutaneous edema and presence of fluid in at least two visceral cavities such as presence of pleural or pericardial effusion or ascites. Fetal chromosomal disorders, cardiac defects, and genetic syndromes constitute important cause of nonimmune hydrops fetalis in 8–9% cases.

Chromosomal disorders which can lead to nonimmune hydrops are monosomy X, trisomy 21, 13, 15, 16, and 18, partial duplication of chromosomes 11, 15, 17, and 18, and cri du chat syndrome which is due to deletion of 5p. Genetic syndromes, which can cause nonimmune hydrops, are Opitz–Frias syndrome, myotonic dystrophy, Cornelia de Lange syndrome, and Noonan syndrome. Hence, fetal karyotyping and DNA analysis form an important part in the diagnostic work up of nonimmune hydrops. It is also important to do a detailed anomaly scan to rule out fetal cardiac defects and skeletal dysplasia.

Fetal Growth Restriction

Chromosomal aneuploidies, especially autosomal trisomies, can lead to fetal growth restriction (FGR) as these have placentae with reduced number of small muscular arteries in the tertiary stem villi. These usually manifest as early onset FGR, often diagnosed at the time of morphology scan. Early-onset FGR is most marked in cases of trisomy 18.

Growth restriction in cases of trisomy 13 and 21 is not as severe as compared to trisomy 18. Turner syndrome (45, X) and Klinefelter syndrome (47 XXX) do not have significant FGR. Confined placental mosaicism with patches of trisomy 16 or others can be a cause for unexplained FGR which probably results from impaired function of the placenta due to aneuploidy.

Late Intrauterine Deaths and Stillbirths

Chromosomal abnormalities are implicated as a cause of stillbirths in 8% cases. In the absence of dysmorphic features, up to 5% of stillbirths are due to chromosomal abnormalities. Risk of stillbirth is higher in fetuses with confined placental mosaicism. Earlier, karyotyping was used in the laboratory evaluation of stillborn fetuses but in only one-third of cases culture could be carried out successfully in macerated tissue.

Recently, molecular cytogenetic technique, CMA, is increasingly being used in investigating the cause of stillbirth. Unlike conventional cytogenetics, CMA does not require dividing cells and can pick up submicroscopic duplications and deletions such as 22q11.2 microdeletion syndrome also known as DiGeorge syndrome which can be a cause of stillbirth. Tissues, which can be used for CMA could be fetal, placental, or amniotic fluid.

Intrahepatic Cholestasis of Pregnancy

This is a reversible form of cholestasis, seen in third trimester of pregnancy, characterized by pruritus, jaundice, increased bile salts, and abnormal liver enzymes which resolve postdelivery. The recurrence risk in subsequent pregnancies is 45–70%.

Heterozygous mutation in *ATP8B1* gene on chromosome 18q21 has been implicated in cholestasis of pregnancy. Children who were diagnosed to have progressive familial intrahepatic cholestasis (PFIC) had mothers whose pregnancies were affected with intrahepatic cholestasis. One of the genes mutated in PFIC is ATP8B1.

Gestational Diabetes Mellitus

Gestational diabetes mellitus is the result of interaction between genetic and environmental factors, hence is multifactorial in origin. Insulin resistance in pregnancy leads to GDM in only few women. Also, familial clustering of GDM supports genetic basis.

Genes related to beta-cell function have been implicated in the pathogenesis of GDM. Polymorphisms of genes such as TCF7L2 on chromosome 10; FTO on chromosome 16 and GCK (glucokinase) on chromosome 7 are some of those described in literature. These have also been associated with maturity-onset diabetes of the young (MODY).

Preeclampsia Syndrome

It has been well-established that preeclampsia is a disease of multifactorial and polygenic inheritance. Environmental and genetic factors interact with each other in the development of preeclampsia. Incidence in daughters and sisters of mothers with preeclampsia is 20–40% and 11–37%, respectively and incidence in twins is even higher of about 22–47%. Interaction between hundreds of genes inherited from both parents have been ascribed in the development of preeclampsia, some of them being MTHFR (C6771), F5 (Leiden), AGT (M235T), HLA (Various) and NOS3 (Glu298Asp). Even fetal genes on chromosome 18 have been linked to a hereditary predisposition for preeclampsia.

Prenatal Diagnosis in Presence of Fetal Malformations

Fetal malformations are intrinsic defects in the formation of a fetal structure/s. Most of these are likely to have genetic etiology. These may be isolated or associated with other malformations and/or underlying growth problems, which indicate presence of underlying genetic syndrome. For example, presence of fetal exomphalos or omphalocele is associated with trisomy 21 in 30% cases.

A specific spectrum of abnormalities may point to a specific genetic condition. For example, Meckel-Gruber syndrome is classically associated with occipital encephalocele, polydactyly and bilateral multicystic dysplastic kidneys. Presence of multiple abnormalities is usually associated with a genetic condition whereas an isolated abnormality may or may not be associated.

Preimplantation genetic diagnosis (PGD) is a method to diagnose defects in an embryo, prior to implantation in in vitro fertilization (IVF) procedures. After IVF, one or two cells are removed from eight-cell embryo-blastocyst. DNA is amplified using polymerase chain reaction (PCR) and analyzed by various techniques. The most common test done is FISH leading to diagnosis of chromosomal and genetic defects.

TYPES OF GENETIC TESTS

A basic knowledge of what genetic tests to do, and when, is a must for any obstetrician. The most common application in obstetrics is for prenatal diagnosis of chromosomal disorders or genetic syndromes.

Most common samples used for prenatal diagnosis include amniotic fluid and chorionic villi, along with fetal cord blood, which is less commonly used. Of late, maternal blood is being used to extract cell free fetal DNA and used for aneuploidy detection in the fetus.

Chromosomal abnormalities are detected using either conventional cytogenetics (karyotyping) or molecular cytogenetic techniques such as FISH, quantitative fluorescent polymerase chain reaction (QF-PCR), and multiplex ligation-dependent probe amplification (MLPA).

Indications for fetal cytogenetic evaluation include: (1) Presence of fetal malformations on USG, (2) Abnormal first or second trimester aneuploidy screen, (3) Abnormal noninvasive prenatal test (NIPT), (4) One of the parents is a carrier of chromosomal structural rearrangement, (5) History of previous offspring with chromosomal disorder, e.g., Down syndrome, and (6) advanced maternal age ≥35 years at the time of delivery (this indication is rarely used now).

Genomic disorders are picked up using CMA, clinical exome sequencing (CES), whole exome sequencing (WES), and whole genome sequencing (WGS). Each of these tests has a specific indication for doing them.

Conventional Cytogenetics (Karyotyping)

Karyotyping is done on dividing cells or cells which can be stimulated to divide. It is almost 99% accurate and can detect aneuploidy, mosaicism, and structural rearrangements such as translocation, deletion, and duplication of 5–10 megabases (Mb) in size.

In order to obtain dividing cells, the amniotic fluid or chorionic villi sample needs to be cultured. Cell culture takes a minimum of 10–14 days. Fetal cord blood, however, takes 36–48 hours for culture but is not commonly used. The rapidly dividing cells are arrested in metaphase and banding is done using the Giemsa stain. Each haploid set of chromosome yields 450–550 G-bands in metaphase.

The *advantages* of conventional karyotyping are that it can detect balanced chromosomal rearrangements and hence is the first-line test in the investigation of couples with RPL. It is considered as gold standard for detection of autosomal trisomies and sex chromosome aneuploidies. Hence, it is quite useful in prenatal diagnosis.

The *disadvantages* of conventional karyotyping are long duration of cell culture and cell culture failure, this leads to delayed and sometimes, even, inconclusive results. It cannot pick up structural arrangements which are <5 Mb, for which CMA is preferred.

Fluorescence in Situ Hybridization

Fluorescence in situ hybridization is used in the detection of specific chromosomal abnormalities such as those of chromosomes 13, 18, 21, X, and Y and also in cases of suspected microdeletion or duplication syndromes. It is usually performed on uncultured interphase cells with fluorescent-labeled probes designed specifically for the target chromosomes. The number of copies of targeted chromosome is determined by the number of fluorescent signals obtained.

The main *advantage* of FISH is that it is a rapid test for aneuploidy detection and takes just 1–2 days. However, the *disadvantage* is that it does not analyze the full chromosome complement, and cannot detect structural alterations in the chromosomes.

Fluorescence in situ hybridization cannot be used as a stand-alone test to guide obstetric decisions. The findings on FISH need to be backed up by a confirmatory test such as karyotyping or CMA. It is also a nonautomated technique and requires a skilled technician.

Quantitative Fluorescent Polymerase Chain Reaction

This assay has been widely used for the past 20 years for rapid aneuploidy detection, especially in the context of prenatal diagnosis. Fluorescent labeled primers are used to amplify specific DNA markers of chromosomes 13, 18, 21, X, and Y using PCR. The amplified products are then separated using electrophoresis. The copy number of a specific sequence of each chromosome is determined by intensity of fluorescent signal. The sensitivity and specificity of the assay is in the range of 95–100%.

Multiplex Ligation-dependent Probe Amplification

This is also a PCR-based method, which is less labor intensive and relatively cheaper than FISH. It is also been validated for rapid aneuploidy detection in prenatal diagnosis. It has 100% sensitivity and specificity for detection of nonmosaic aneuploidies. One of the *major drawbacks* of this method is its failure to detect triploidy in a female fetus.

Chromosomal Microarray

The technique of CMA uses chips with reference DNA fragments or oligonucleotides of known sequence to which the test fetal DNA (extracted from amniotic fluid or chorionic villi) is hybridized and compared. Copy number variants in fetal DNA are detected in reference to standard chip DNA. It can be done on the comparative genomic hybridization (CGH) platform or single nucleotide polymorphism (SNP) platform or both.

The *advantages* of CMA are that it studies chromosomes at a very high resolution, unlike conventional karyotype, and can detect gains or losses as small as 50–100 kilobases (Kb). FISH and MLPA also provide higher resolution than conventional method but these studies only targeted regions in the genome. On the other hand, CMA provides whole genome coverage at a high resolution.

Chromosomal microarray can detect additional chromosomal abnormalities, over conventional karyotype, in 6–7% fetuses with congenital malformations on USG. Hence, it is rapidly gaining popularity as first-line investigation in such cases.

Also it can be done directly on DNA extracted from amniotic fluid or chorionic villi and does not require cell culture. Hence, it can be used for genetic evaluation of nonviable tissues such as products of conception in cases of RPL or tissues from a stillborn fetus.

It has a rapid turnover as the results take only 3–5 days. The SNP platform has added advantages of diagnosing uniparental disomy and consanguinity as it can detect *absence of heterozygosity*. The SNP array can also detect triploidy.

The main *disadvantage* of CMA is that it cannot detect balanced chromosomal structural rearrangements. Variants of unknown significance seen in 1–2% cases pose a challenge to genetic counseling. Another limiting factor to its use is cost factor.

Whole Genome Sequencing and Whole Exome Sequencing

The next-generation sequencing techniques are mainly useful in the diagnosis of suspected fetal genetic disorders where CMA has failed to give a diagnosis. The American College of Obstetricians and Gynecologists recommends that WGS and WES should only be used in cases of recurrent or lethal anomalies where other tests have been noninformative.

Whole genome sequencing is used for sequencing the entire genome, including the noncoding (introns) and coding regions (exons). This is not routinely performed in clinical practice. WES, on the other hand, sequences only the protein coding regions of genome called exons. This has greater clinical relevance as most of the understanding of Mendelian inherited disorders is derived from research on variants in the exome.

Whole exome sequencing cannot detect trinucleotide repeats; aneuploidy; microdeletions and duplications and structural chromosomal abnormalities such as translocation;

inversion, etc. Moreover, the amount of information generated by these tests is so extensive that it makes analysis time consuming and counseling difficult due to presence of large number of variants of unknown significance. To curtail this problem, *trio sequencing* is used where DNA of both parents and fetus are sequenced together to filter out the irrelevant variants.

CONCLUSION

Knowledge of genetics and genomics is very important for today's obstetricians. With the widespread use of antenatal scans, detection rate of fetal malformations is on the rise. Also there is increasing awareness among people, of genetic conditions existing in their region or family. This leads to more couples seeking prenatal diagnosis. Since the obstetrician is the primary care giver, such knowledge will help in providing appropriate counseling.

FURTHER READING

1. ACOG Technology Assessment paper No. 14: Modern Genetics in Obstetrics and Gynaecology. Obstet Gynecol. 2018;132:e143-68.
2. Armengol L, Nevado J, Serra-Juhe C, Plaja A, Mediano C, García-Santiago FA, et al. Clinical utility of chromosomal microarray analysis in invasive prenatal diagnosis. Hum Genet. 2012;131(3):513-23.
3. Cirigliano V, Voglino G, Ordonez E, Marongiu A. Rapid prenatal diagnosis of common chromosome aneuploidies by QF-PCR, results of 9 years of clinical experience. Prenat Diagn. 2009;29(1):40-9.
4. Committee on Genetics and the Society for Maternal-Fetal Medicine. Committee Opinion No. 682: Microarrays and next-generation sequencing technology: the use of advanced genetic diagnostic tools in obstetrics and gynecology. Obstet Gynecol. 2016;128:e262-8.
5. Cunningham GF, Leveno KJ, Bloom SL, Spong CY. Williams Obstetrics, 25th edition. New York: McGraw Hill Medical; 2018.
6. Deka D, Malhotra N. An Introduction to Genetics and Fetal Medicine, 2nd edition. New Delhi: Jaypee Brothers Medical Publishers (P) Ltd.; 2010.
7. Delhanty JD. Molecular cytogenetics in obstetric practice. Obstet Gynaecol. 2006;8:171-6.
8. de Wit MC, Srebniak MI, Govaerts LC, Van Opstal D, Galjaard RJ, Go AT. Additional value of prenatal genomic array testing in fetuses with isolated structural ultrasound abnormalities and a normal karyotype: a systematic review of the literature. Ultrasound Obstet Gynecol. 2014;43(2):139-46.
9. Drury S, Williams H, Trump N, Boustred C, GOSGene, Lench N, et al. Exome sequencing for prenatal diagnosis of fetuses with sonographic abnormalities. Prenat Diagn. 2015;35(10):1010-7.
10. Hillman S, Mc Mullar DJ, Maher ER, Kilby MD. The use of chromosomal microarray in prenatal diagnosis. Obstet Gynaecol. 2013;15:80-4.
11. Horgan RP, Kenny LC. 'Omic' Technologies: genomics, transcriptomics, proteomics and metabolomics. Obstet Gynaecol. 2011;13:189-95.
12. Lander ES, Linton LM, Birren B, Nusbaum C, Zody MC, Baldwin J, et al. Initial sequencing and analysis of the human genome. Nature. 2001;409:860-921.
13. Manning M, Hudgins L. Professional Practice and Guidelines Committee. Array-based technology and recommendations for utilization in medical genetics practice for detection of chromosomal abnormalities. Genet Med. 2010;12(11):742-5.
14. Mann K, Donaghue C, Fox SP, Docherty Z, Ogilvie CM. Strategies for the rapid prenatal diagnosis of chromosome aneuploidy. Eur J Hum Genet. 2004;12:907-15.
15. Online Mendelian Inheritance in Man. Cholestasis, Intrahepatic of pregnancy-1; ICP1. [online] Available from / www.omim.org/entry/147480. [Last accessed October, 2021].
16. Pop M, Salzberg SL. Bioinformatics challenges of new sequencing technology. Trends Genet. 2008;24(3):142-9.
17. Reddy UM, Page GP, Saade GR, Silver RM. Karyotype versus microarray testing for genetic abnormalities after stillbirth. N Engl J Med. 2012;367:2185-93.
18. Rosik J, Szostak B, Machaj F, Pawlik A. The role of genetics and epigenetics in the pathogenesis of gestational diabetes mellitus. Ann Hum Genet. 2020;84:114-24.
19. Royal College of Obstetricians and Gynaecologists. Recurrent Miscarriage, Investigation and Treatment of Couples (Green-top Guideline No. 17). London: Royal College of Obstetricians and Gynaecologists; 2011.
20. Tobias ES, Connor JM. Medical Genetics for the MRCOG and Beyo**nd,** 2nd edition. Cambridge: Cambridge University Press; 2014.
21. van Opstal D, Boter M, de Jong D, van den Berg C, Brüggenwirth HT, Wildschut HIJ, et al. Rapid aneuploidy detection with multiplex ligation-dependent probe amplification: a prospective study of 4000 amniotic fluid samples. Eur J Hum Genet. 2009;17(1):112-21.
22. World Health Organization. WHA 57.13: Genomics and World Health, Fifty Seventh World Health Assembly Resolution. Geneva: World Health Organization; 2004.

LONG QUESTIONS

1. What are the various types of genetic and chromosomal tests available for obstetric diagnosis?
2. Evaluate the role of genetic etiology in pregnancies with adverse obstetric outcome.

SHORT QUESTIONS

1. What is a Robertsonian translocation?
2. What is chromosomal mosaicism?
3. Describe the inheritance pattern in autosomal recessive disorders.
4. What are imprinting disorders?

MULTIPLE CHOICE QUESTIONS

1. All are examples of single gene disorders, except:
   a. Thalassemia
   b. Phenylketonuria
   c. Fragile X syndrome
   d. Neural tube defects
   e. Duchenne muscular dystrophy

2. All of the following regarding modes of inheritance are true, except:
   a. Autosomal dominant disorder: If one parent is affected then 50% of offspring will be affected
   b. Autosomal recessive disorder: If one parent is a carrier then 25% of the offspring will be affected
   c. X-linked recessive disorder: If mother is a carrier then 50% of male offspring will be affected and 50% of female offspring will be carriers
   d. X-linked dominant disorder: 50% of offspring will be affected irrespective of sex
3. All for the following statements are true, except:
   a. The incidence of chromosomal anomalies in the POC in spontaneous miscarriage is 50–70%
   b. Chromosomal anomalies account for 3.5–5% of recurrent pregnancy loss (RPL)
   c. In RPL about 25–32% of POC have abnormal karyotype
   d. In RPL where one partner is a carrier of balanced translocation the likelihood of normal pregnancy is 30%
   e. Approximately 85% of patients with an aneuploid abortion have a good prognosis
4. If one of the parents has balanced translocation of chromosome 21 then the following can happen:
   a. Unbalanced translocation in the offspring
   b. Recurrent pregnancy loss
   c. Mental retardation
   d. Stillbirth
   e. 100% will be abnormal live born
5. None of these can detect balanced chromosomal translocation, except:
   a. Karyotyping
   b. FISH
   c. QF-PCR
   d. CMA
6. The following may be involved in the survival of aneuploid fetuses at times, except:
   a. Confined placental mosaicism
   b. Trisomic correction
   c. Uniparental disomy
   d. Robertsonian translocation

Answers
1. d 2. b 3. d 4. e 5. a 6. d

3.2 FETAL ABNORMALITIES: DEFINITIONS, ETIOLOGY, AND PATHOPHYSIOLOGY

Mandakini Pradhan

INTRODUCTION

Fetus is formed as a result of fusion of two gametes, i.e., fusion of two haploid cells results in formation of one diploid cell which subsequently grows into an embryo and a fetus. During this period of well-coordinated process many chemicals, biochemical, and signaling pathways get activated and inactivated. Many developmental genes play a role by switching on and off. Thereby proteins which are active in one phase of development become inactive during development or after birth. The simplest example is gamma genes of hemoglobin (Hb) which is active in fetal life making HbF ($\alpha 2\gamma 2$) and absent in adult life, i.e., HbA ($\alpha 2\beta 2$).

Normal process of fetal development may be interrupted by inherited abnormalities or acquired abnormalities. Many of such embryo gets aborted before reaching the fetal stage and goes unnoticed or uninvestigated. Hence, abnormality detected in newborn or in infant is much less than what occurs at conception.

DEFINITION

Fetal abnormalities are the birth defects detected in utero or after birth. The abnormalities may be structural defect or functional defect of the organ which may or may not lead to life-threatening abnormality of the newborn.

Terminology that are useful for understanding fetal malformations are:
- A *malformation* signifies that fetal growth and development did not proceed normally due to underlying genetic, epigenetic, or environmental factors that altered the development of a structure.
- A *deformation* is caused by an abnormal external force on the fetus during in utero development that resulted in abnormal growth or formation of the fetal structure. For example, in oligohydramnios causing Potter sequence.
- *Disruption* is arrest of growth of a normally formed structure as seen in amniotic band which results in abnormalities of the structure involved including limb or face abnormalities.
- *Major fetal abnormalities* are those which involve a major organ like heart or brain and may lead to life-threatening consequences. It is an abnormality and not a variation of spectrum of normal structure.
- *Minor anomalies* are variation of normal spectrum or involves minor organ like extra fingers or ear abnormality. It may be seen in normal population.

- A *syndrome* is defined as presence of a group of major or minor anomalies that occur together in a predictable fashion and usually due to a single underlying cause.
- An *association* is a group of anomalies that occur together more frequently than would be expected by chance alone but that do not have a predictable pattern of recognition and/or a suspected unified underlying etiology.
- A *sequence* is a group of related anomalies that generally stem from a single initial major anomaly that alters the development of other surrounding or related tissues or structures. For example, renal abnormalities leading to oligohydramnios leading to flat face and pulmonary hypoplasia.
- A *field defect* is used to describe malformation of a particular region or developmental origin. Neural tube defect resulting in club foot and bowel and bladder dysfunction is an example of sequence or field defect.
- *Dysplasia* is due to intrinsic cellular defect of a tissue which is not normally maintained throughout growth and development. Example of such defect is skeletal dysplasia leading to short stature due to dysplasia in the developing bone.

ETIOLOGY

Fetal abnormalities may be due to maternal infection being transmitted to fetus, chromosomal abnormality or single gene disorder in the fetus, nutritional deficiency in the mother, or maternal drug intake during organogenesis period or may not have any definite cause.

Maternal Infection

Maternal infections such as varicella or chicken pox, rubella, cytomegalovirus, toxoplasmosis, parvovirus B19, *Treponema,* or more recently Zika have been associated with fetal infection and affection. All these maternal infections can get transmitted to fetus in first trimester of pregnancy. It can cause fetal death as in *Treponema* infection, microcephaly as in Zika, fetal anemia as in parvovirus B19 infection, limb reduction defect in varicella infection **(Fig. 1)**, chorioretinitis and cardiac defect in rubella, and hepatosplenomegaly and thrombocytopenia **(Fig. 2)** in cytomegalovirus infection.

Environmental Factors

Exposure of fetus to alcohol, tobacco, radiation, and drugs during organogenesis period of pregnancy may increase the risk of having a fetus being affected with malformation. Maternal smoking during pregnancy may lead to fetal growth restriction, miscarriage and stillbirth, and cleft lip and palate. Excessive maternal alcohol ingestion may lead to fetal alcohol syndrome having abnormal facial features and mental retardation.[1,2] Maternal exposure to thalidomide leading to phocomelia is the best example of drugs causing teratogenicity. Exposure to valproic acid may cause neural tube defect; angiotensin-converting enzyme inhibitor can cause renal abnormality. Hence, the need for switching onto safer drugs in periconceptional period is necessary.

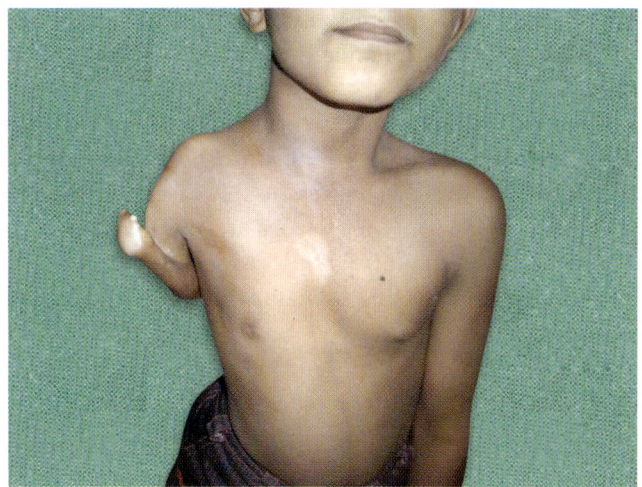

Fig. 1: Limb reduction defect and cicatrization on skin due to maternal varicella infection.

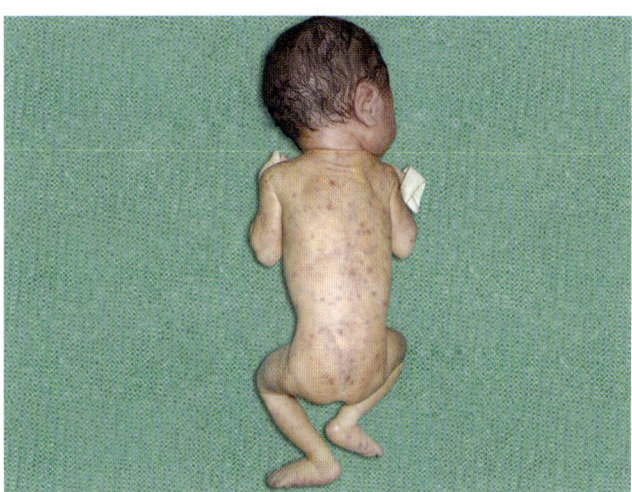

Fig. 2: Petechiae due to maternal CMV infection.

Maternal Nutritional Deficiency

Deficiency of folic acid in periconceptional period leading to neural tube defect is very well known. Deficiencies like micronutrients causing fetal abnormalities are reported off and on.

Chromosomal Abnormalities

Both numerical and structural chromosomal abnormality may be the cause of fetal abnormality. Example of numerical chromosomal abnormalities are triploidy (69 chromosome), trisomies of 21, 13, and 18 (47 chromosome in cell), abnormality of sex chromosome as in Turner syndrome with having one X chromosome, and Klinefelter syndrome having three sex chromosomes. These are usually due to nondisjunction during gametogenesis and are rarely due to translocation carrier status of the parents, whereas structural chromosomal abnormalities resulting in fetal malformation are mostly due to a balanced carrier state in one of the parents.

Children with behavioral abnormality and developmental delay are found to have chromosomal microarray abnormality (CMA) in as high as 10–15% cases. With normal chromosomal pattern, 3–6% fetuses are found to have CMA with and without malformations, respectively. Hence, the need for providing testing prenatally in such a situation is necessary.[3,4]

Single Gene Disease

Chromosomal disorder is due to nondisjunction and may be de novo, i.e., first time seen in the family unless one of the parent is a balanced carrier of the abnormality. Unlike that, single gene diseases follow a specific pattern of inheritance. For example, beta-thalassemia which is an autosomal recessive condition with both parents being carrier of the gene defect and clinically normal. Many of the conditions are more common in some ethnic group. Rare autosomal disorder is seen in consanguineous couple, i.e., when the couple is blood relative. Autosomal dominant condition like achondroplasia or osteogenesis imperfecta is usually due to a new mutation in the fetus and has less recurrence risk.

The cause of the congenital abnormalities could be genetic, environmental, or multifactorial. The proportion of genetic causes is gradually increasing with the advent of sequencing of human genes.

■ PREVENTION

Various health measures enforced or practiced may decrease the occurrence of congenital anomalies and it is specific to the cause of the defect.

Preventive steps includes:
- Women in reproductive age group to have healthy diet and appropriate weight.
- Women planning pregnancy should have folic acid before becoming pregnant.
- Women should avoid smoking and stop alcohol intake.
- Reduce or eliminate exposure to environmental hazardous substances (such as heavy metals and pesticides), medical radiation, etc.
- Vaccination of women before pregnancy such as vaccination for rubella and hepatitis B infection.
- Control or treatment of the chronic diseases such as diabetes, hypertension, and heart diseases.
- Switching onto safer drugs for chronic disease like antiepileptics, especially valproic acid and antihypertensive like ACE inhibitors.
- Emphasizing to continue with drugs for chronic disease like systemic lupus erythematosus (SLE) or idiopathic thrombocytopenic purpura (ITP) after becoming pregnant and need for switch over of drugs like oral anticoagulant after pregnancy.
- Screening for infection and treating that such as syphilis, human immunodeficiency virus (HIV), and tuberculosis.

Screening

Couple at higher risk of congenital malformation or fetal and neonatal abnormalities may be screened in preconception period and hence the need of a *preconception clinic*. Screening may be conducted at various periods such as premarital, preconception, and if not done yet then in early pregnancy or after pregnancy.

Screening includes a detailed family history including three-generation pedigree drawing, consanguinity, history of recurrent pregnancy loss, malformation, and mental subnormality in the family.

Premarital Screening

To look for common disorder such as hemoglobinopathies and the disease specific to the family as per history.

Preconception Screening

It should include screening for hemoglobinopathies if not done earlier and advice for stoppage of substance abuse and advice for intake of folic acid.

During Pregnancy

Apart from the disease or steps mentioned above, it must include looking into structural malformation of the fetus by ultrasound examination at 18–20 weeks of pregnancy. In addition, ultrasound examination at 12–13 weeks may be done as per policy and after counseling the couple and to look for risk for fetal chromosomal aneuploidy.

Neonatal Screening

It includes screening for congenital hypothyroidism and other metabolic disorder as per government guideline. Examination to look for malformation is done in delivery room and evaluation of hearing is being done to detect auditory impairment early.

■ TREATMENT

Treatment option of fetal abnormalities depends on the type of defect and cause. Some fetal abnormalities can be corrected or symptomatically treated in utero as in congenital diaphragmatic hernia, posterior urethral valve, unilateral pleural effusion, etc. Most isolated structural abnormalities are corrected in neonatal period after surgery. Few structural malformations may be followed up for various duration to see for progress and need for intervention like unilateral multicystic kidney disease. Detection and treatment are possible for condition like congenital hypothyroidism.

KEY MESSAGES

- More than 3 lakhs newborn die every year, worldwide in first 4 weeks of life, due to congenital malformation.
- Occurrence can be prevented by measures such as intake of folic acid for prevention of neural tube defect and identification of fetal malformation by careful ultrasound examination of all pregnant women at 18–20 weeks of pregnancy.
- Birth of any malformed fetus needs proper evaluation to identify the cause and prevent recurrence in future pregnancy. That may include description of all malformation, X-ray if skeletal defect, chromosomal analysis, and microarray analysis of the cord blood. If both the investigations are normal, then an advice for clinical exome sequencing will detect rare genetic cause of malformation.
- Identification in fetal life warrants similar investigation as above antenatally and consultation with pediatrician and pediatric surgeon may help in better explaining the further course of the disease. That prepares the family for minor or major intervention if required in neonatal period.
- The most common cause of mental subnormality is trisomy 21 and women can be screened early during antenatal period with high accuracy.
- Beta-thalassemia being the most common single gene disorder and can be eradicated by screening of all pregnant women.

REFERENCES

1. Ericson A, Källén B, Westerholm P. Cigarette smoking as an etiologic factor in cleft lip and palate. Am J Obstet Gynecol. 1979;135:348-51.
2. Knight AH, Rhind EG. Epilepsy and pregnancy: a study of 153 pregnancies in 59 patients. Epilepsia. 1979;16:99-110.
3. Lee JS, Hwang H, Kim SY, Kim KJ, Choi JS, Woo MJ, et al, Chromosomal microarray with clinical diagnostic utility in children with developmental delay or intellectual disability. Ann Lab Med. 2018;38(5):473-80.
4. Levy B, Wapner R. Prenatal diagnosis by chromosomal microarray analysis. Fertil Steril. 2018;109(2):201-12.

LONG QUESTIONS

1. Describe the causes of fetal malformation.
2. Describe the difference between malformation, disruption and deformation giving example of each.
3. Enumerate the environmental causes in fetal growth abnormality.
4. How can we prevent fetal malformation?
5. Explain the term sequence and association and give example of each.

SHORT QUESTIONS

1. Major fetal malformation and its implication.
2. Autosomal recessive disorder with example.
3. Role of pre-conceptional counseling.
4. Folic acid and fetal malformation.
5. Fetal syndromes.

MULTIPLE CHOICE QUESTIONS

1. All regarding fetal malformation are true, except:
   a. Maternal uncontrolled diabetes can cause fetal neural tube defect
   b. Fetal deformation is due to severe oligohydramnios
   c. Fetal disruption is due to short umbilical cord
   d. Detection of fetal malformation requires termination of pregnancy
2. All are true about fetal defect, except:
   a. All fetal malformations are inherited
   b. Defects in few genes is the usual cause of one fetal syndrome
   c. Neural tube defect causing club foot is an example of field defect
   d. Group of fetal anomalies arising following a single major anomaly is called sequence
3. Maternal infection during pregnancy can cause all, except:
   a. Zika infection can cause microcephaly
   b. Treponema infection can cause fetal death
   c. Rubella can cause neonatal rash
   d. Varicella can cause limb reduction defect
4. True regarding chromosomal abnormalities, except:
   a. Down syndrome is an example of numerical chromosomal abnormality
   b. Couple with recurrent spontaneous abortion due to balanced translocation carrier should have a chromosomal microarray analysis
   c. Klinefelter syndrome is an example of sex chromosome abnormality
   d. Live cells are required for chromosomal analysis
5. Regarding screening for fetal abnormalities:
   a. All neonates should be screen for all metabolic disorder
   b. Only women with prior history of neural tube defect fetal affection are to be prescribed folic acid before pregnancy
   c. Steroid for SLE is to be tapered before planning pregnancy
   d. Thalassemia can be prevented by screening of couple

Answers									
1.	d	2.	b	3.	c	4.	b	5.	d

3.3 ULTRASOUND IN FIRST TRIMESTER: MILESTONES AND PATHOLOGY

PK Shah, Pooja Lodha

INTRODUCTION

Care during "pregnancy" has extended beyond care of the pregnant woman. Fetal surveillance and care is now an integral part of antenatal care. Ultrasonography (USG) is instrumental in the care of the fetus. In the last three to four decades, routine ultrasound examination of the embryo/fetus has become an extended armamentarium in the standard pregnancy care. The accurate information, which is provided by the ultrasound, facilitates delivery of optimized antenatal care with best outcomes for the mother and baby both. This chapter aims to systematically elaborate various normal and abnormal aspects of USG in pregnancy in the first trimester.

SONOEMBRYOLOGY

The ultrasound examination of early pregnancy is known as sonoembryology. The routine use of ultrasound in pregnancy has led to remarkable progress in the visualization of early embryos and fetuses and in the development of sonoembryology. New technology moved embryology from postmortem studies to the in vivo environment. The embryonic development, its anatomy and physiology, is a field where medicine exerts its greatest impact on early pregnancy at present time, and it opens fascinating aspects of embryonic differentiation.

A transvaginal sonography and quantitative testing of serum levels of the beta-human chorionic gonadotropin (beta-hCG) are the standard means of establishing the presence of viable intrauterine pregnancy (IUP)—single and multifetal gestation, failed IUP, ectopic pregnancy and rarely, heterotrophic pregnancy. **Figures 1A to G** demonstrate various findings of an early pregnancy ultrasound. Early USG also helps diagnose bleeding near the embryo and uterine/adnexal pathologies such as uterine Müllerian anomalies, fibroids, and ovarian masses.[1] In absence of any warning

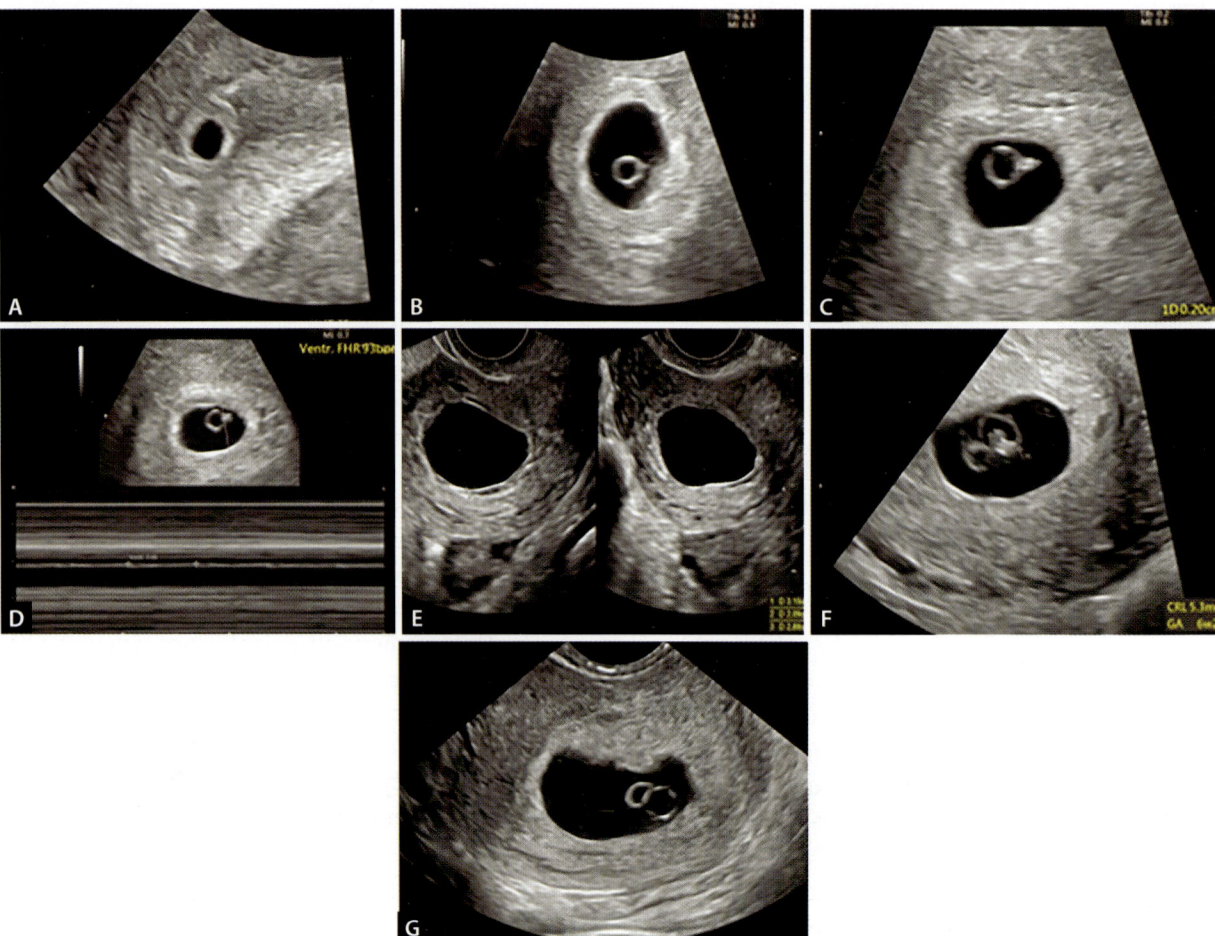

Figs. 1A to G: An atlas of first trimester ultrasound findings. (A) Early pregnancy; small intrauterine gestational sac; (B) Yolk sac—regular and anechoic; (C) Fetal pole; (D) Fetal cardiac activity; (E) Blighted ovum; (F) Missed miscarriage, absent fetal cardiac activity; (G) Double yolk sac, no embryo visualized; (A-D) Normal; (E-G) Pathological.

symptoms (pain/bleeding/known high-risk pregnancies), few guidelines advice against a routine early pregnancy USG. Yet, early USG in pregnancy is almost a norm if not a rule, as it is helpful in the ways mentioned in the section above. Also, it alleviates patient's anxiety.

The timeline of normal early pregnancy development is listed in the **Table 1**.

Tables 2 and 3 enlist USG features which raise suspicion/confirm pregnancy failure.

Diagnostic and management guidelines[1] related to the possibility of a viable intrauterine or pregnancy in a woman with a pregnancy of unknown location is mentioned in **Table 4**.

11–13[+6] WEEKS: A WINDOW OF FETOMATERNAL WINDOW OF OPPORTUNITY

Over generations, pregnancy care typically included management of problems only after they developed. But over the last decade, this pyramid of antenatal care has inverted[2] and has seen a sea change as demonstrated by the illustrations **(Fig. 2)**.

Although the first trimester technically closes at 12 weeks gestation, the 11–13[+6] weeks USG is included in the study of first trimester scan for all practical purposes.

This scan is known as "nuchal translucency (NT) scan", level I USG or 12 weeks scan. Considering the vast advantages it offers, the role of this scan includes measurement of NT, but is not limited to it. The 11–13[+6]-week scan provides the opportunities as mentioned below.
- Accurate dating
- Assessment of early anatomy
- Screening for chromosomal abnormalities by itself or with serum screening

TABLE 1: Development milestones.

Time period	Developmental milestone
Week 0	Last menstrual period
Week 2	Conception
Week 4.5–5	Gestational sac appears
Week 5–5.5	Yolk sac appears
Week 6	Embryo appears, fetal cardiac pulsations begin—physiological bradycardia (up to 100 bpm) Umbilical cord and vitelline duct seen Embryo appearance on transvaginal ultrasonography (USG): Rounded bulky head and thin body
Week 6.5–7	Amniotic membrane appears, fetal cardiac pulsations (up to 120 bpm)
Week 7–8	Spine develops
Week 8	Head curvature separates from body and limb buds appear
Week 8–8.5	Intrinsic motion of embryo begins
Week 8–10	Rhombencephalon develops

TABLE 2: Findings related to pregnancy failure.

Findings diagnostic of pregnancy failure*	Findings suspicious for pregnancy failure[†]
Crown-rump length ≥ 7 mm and no cardiac activity	Crown-rump length < 7 mm and no cardiac activity
Mean gestational sac diameter ≥ 25 mm and no embryo	Mean sac diameter of 16–24 mm and no embryo
Absence of embryo with cardiac activity ≥ 2 weeks after ultrasonography (USG) that showed gestational sac only (without yolk sac)	Absence of embryo with heartbeat 7–13 days after a scan that showed a gestational sac without a yolk sac
Absence of embryo with cardiac activity ≥ 11 days after USG that showed gestational sac with yolk sac	Absence of embryo with heartbeat 7–10 days after a scan that showed a gestational sac with a yolk sac
	Absence of embryo ≥6 week after last menstrual period
	Empty amnion (amnion seen adjacent to yolk sac, with no visible embryo)
	Enlarged yolk sac (>7 mm)
	Small gestational sac in relation to the size of the embryo (<5 mm difference between mean sac diameter and crown-rump length)
Findings diagnostic of pregnancy failure	Findings suspicious for pregnancy failure
Crown-rump length ≥ 7 mm and no cardiac activity	Crown-rump length < 7 mm and no cardiac activity
Mean gestational sac diameter ≥ 25 mm and no embryo	Mean sac diameter of 16–24 mm and no embryo
Absence of embryo with cardiac activity ≥ 2 weeks after USG that showed gestational sac only (without yolk sac)	Absence of embryo with heartbeat 7–13 days after a scan that showed a gestational sac without a yolk sac

*Criteria are from the Society of Radiologists in Ultrasound Multispecialty Consensus Conference on Early First Trimester Diagnosis of Miscarriage and Exclusion of a Viable Intrauterine Pregnancy, October 2012.
†When there are findings suspicious for pregnancy failure, follow-up USG at 7–10 days to assess the pregnancy for viability is generally appropriate.

- Screening for preeclampsia, fetal growth restriction, and preterm birth
- Determination of chorionicity in multiple pregnancy.

SCREENING FOR ANEUPLOIDIES (CHROMOSOMAL ABNORMALITIES)

For whom to perform aneuploidy screening?

Every woman, irrespective of age, has a risk that her fetus may have aneuploidy. Although the risk for aneuploidies increases with age, there are more number of women who deliver in the age group <35 years therefore more number of Down syndrome babies are born to young women.

TABLE 3: Poor prognostic indicators in the first trimester.

Ultrasonography (USG) indicators of poor prognosis in a viable intrauterine pregnancy

Element/feature	USG appearance
Gestational sac	Disproportionate to embryo, irregular, and low lying
Yolk sac	Calcified and enlarged > 7 mm
Amnion	Empty, enlarged, or expanded
Embryo	Abnormal shape
Cardiac activity	Bradycardia < 85 bpm
Chorionic villi	Hydropic/jelly like
Subchorionic hemorrhage	Large, more than two-thirds of gestational sac, sac separation

TABLE 4: Diagnostic and management guidelines related to the possibility of a viable intrauterine pregnancy in a woman with a pregnancy of unknown location.*

Finding	Interpretation
No intrauterine fluid collection and normal adnexa on USG	A single measurement of hCG does not reliably distinguish between ectopic and intrauterine pregnancy (viable or nonviable) If a single hCG measurement is <3,000 mIU/mL, presumptive treatment for ectopic pregnancy with the use of methotrexate or other pharmacologic or surgical means should not be undertaken, in order to avoid the risk of interrupting a viable intrauterine pregnancy If a single hCG measurement is ≥3,000 mIU/mL, a viable intrauterine pregnancy is possible but unlikely. However, the most likely diagnosis is a nonviable intrauterine pregnancy, so it is generally appropriate to obtain at least one follow-up hCG measurement and follow-up USG before undertaking treatment for ectopic pregnancy
USG not yet performed	The hCG levels in women with ectopic pregnancies are highly variable, often <1,000 mIU/mL and the hCG level does not predict the likelihood of ectopic pregnancy rupture Thus, when the clinical findings are suspicious for ectopic pregnancy, transvaginal ultrasonography is indicated even when the hCG level is low

(hCG: human chorionic gonadotropin; USG: ultrasonography)
*Criteria are from the Society of Radiologists in Ultrasound Multispecialty Consensus Conference on Early Trimester Diagnosis of Miscarriage and Exclusion of a Viable Intrauterine Pregnancy, October 2012.

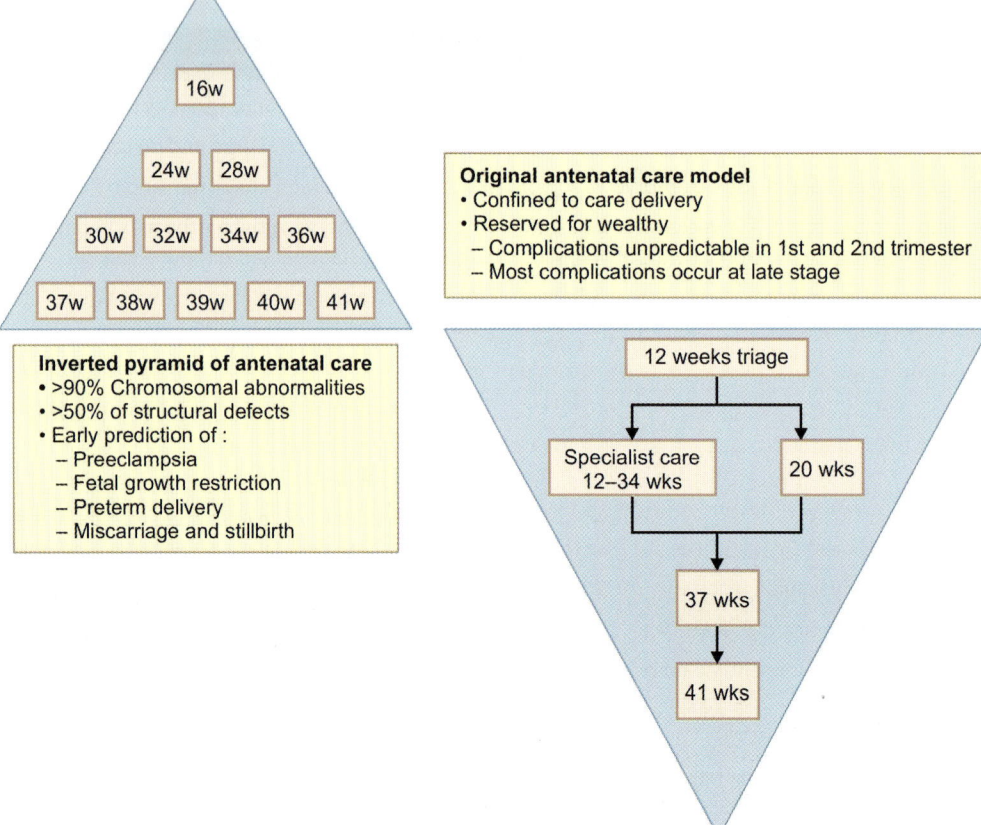

Fig. 2: Antenatal care pyramids. (w: weeks; wks: weeks)

Aneuploidy screening is recommended for all as a standard of care; irrespective of the age.[3]

What is the best mode of aneuploidy screening for all?
A double marker blood test combined with USG markers at 11–13^{+6} weeks is a near ideal method of aneuploidy screening for all. This is known as *"combined first trimester screening for aneuploidies"*.

Which chromosomal abnormalities are commonly screened for?
Down syndrome (trisomy 21), *Edward syndrome* (trisomy 18), and *Patau syndrome* (trisomy 13) are the commonly screened chromosomal abnormalities.[3] Edward and Patau fetuses show gross abnormalities and are less likely to be missed on USG. High proportion of these fetuses have an intrauterine demise, and those which survive till birth, eventually die early in life. Down syndrome fetuses may show relatively subtle findings, making their diagnosis more challenging than the others.

When is the ultrasonography for aneuploidy screening recommended?
The USG for aneuploidy screening is recommended between 11 and 13 weeks +6 days gestational age (GA); more precisely, it should be done when the fetal crown-rump length (CRL) is between 45 and 84 mm.[3]

What are the aneuploidy markers at 11–13^{+6} weeks?
The aneuploidy markers at the first trimester scan are NT, nasal bone (NB), tricuspid regurgitation (TR), and ductus venosus (DV). While NT and NB are vital as chromosomal markers, TR and DV are relatively new, and can be considered optional depending upon the standard care of locality.

What is the single most important marker for chromosomal abnormality and how is it measured?
Nuchal translucency is the most important marker for chromosomal abnormality. The correct midsagittal section is extremely vital for measurement of NT **(Fig. 3)**. The Fetal Medicine Foundation has given criteria for measurement of NT at 11–13^{+6} weeks GA.[3] They are mentioned in **Table 5**.

Higher the NT, more the risk of underlying chromosomal abnormality. High NT is associated with not only chromosomal abnormalities, but also with genetic syndromes, structural defects, fetal infections, and eventually long-term neurodevelopmental outcomes. NT is a function of CRL, and the value >95th centile for CRL is considered pathological. NT of >3 mm demands detailed further workup (invasive testing for karyotype, structural survey, and infection screen, etc.).

There could be varied causes for high NT. Various causes for increased NT are mentioned in **Figure 4**.

As seen in the exhaustive list; apart from aneuploidies, increased NT could be due to underlying structural defects (cardiac and extracardiac), musculoskeletal dysplasia, metabolic disorders, infections, and genetic syndromes.

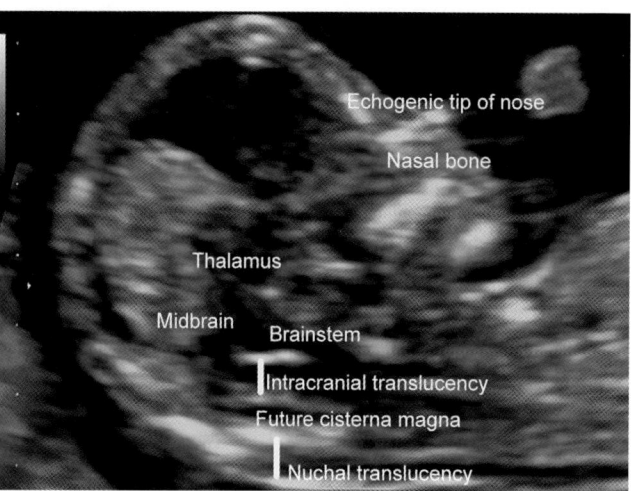

Fig. 3: Correct midsagittal section.

TABLE 5: The Fetal Medicine Foundation (FMF) criteria for measuring nuchal translucency (NT).

Nuchal Translucency: FMF Criteria	
Criteria	**Details**
Image magnification	Fetal head and thorax should occupy the whole screen
When to measure	When CRL is between 45–84 mm
Fetal position	Midline sagittal section
Fetal skin and amnion	Differentiate skin and amnion (Do not include amnion in measurement of NT)
Fetal attitude	Neutral – nor flexed/extended
When to measure NT	Widest part available
How to measure NT	Caliper not visible Machine setting – Gain down

(CRL: crown-rump length)

Due to the varied causes of high NT, and the spectrum of implications, it can be a difficult task to counsel the couple. The algorithm **(Fig. 5)** states the approach towards a fetus with increased NT.

It is important to note that not all fetuses with increased NT are abnormal. But a thorough workup is essential to help prognostication and aid decision making. One of the commonly used statistical charts which aids counseling and decision making in a case with high fetal NT has been provided by the Fetal Medicine Foundation **(Fig. 6)**.

Which fetal parts/markers can be visualized/measured in a standard midsagittal section at 11–13^{+6} weeks gestational age?
The midsagittal section is the single most important section during this scan.

Following can be visualized on that section:
- NT measurement
- *NB visualization*: Present/absent/hypoplastic

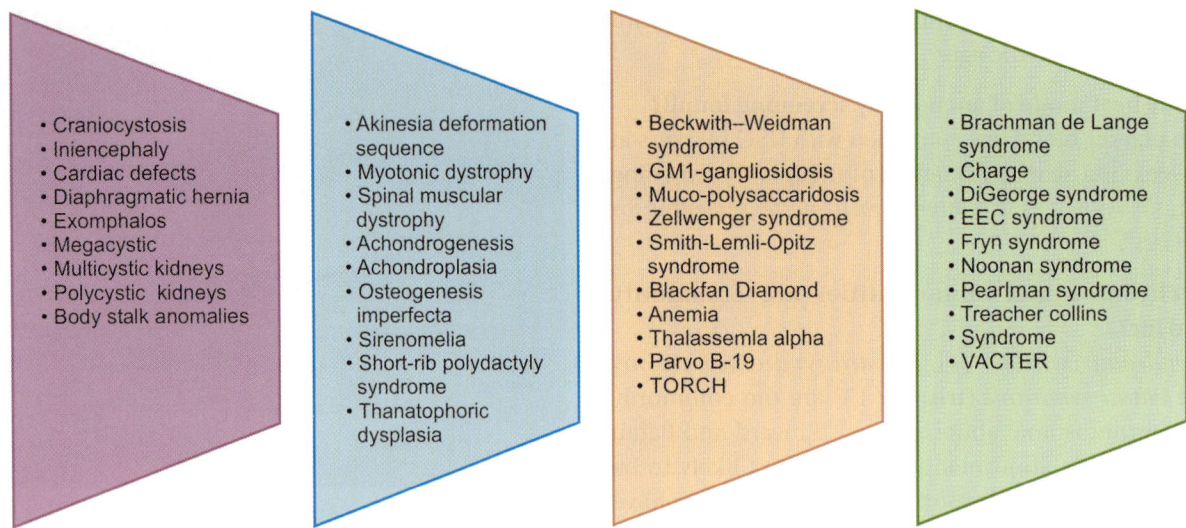

Fig. 4: Fetal abnormalities (other than aneuploidies) associated with high nuchal translucency.

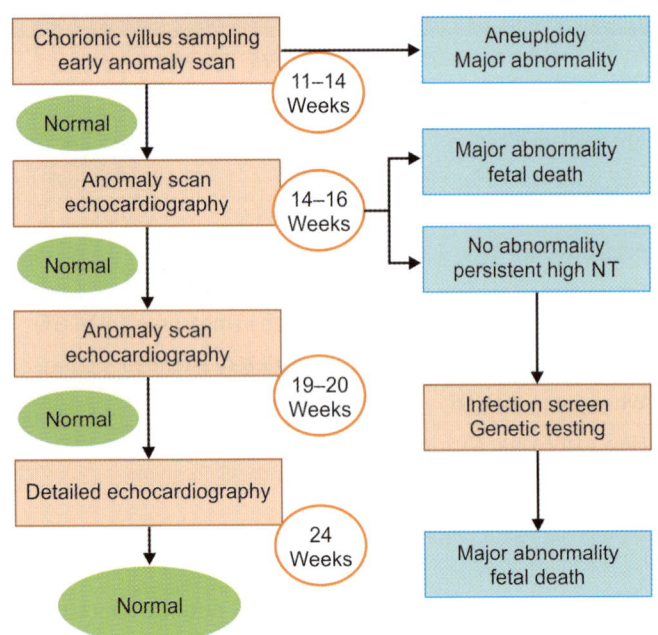

Fig. 5: Algorithm to assess high nuchal translucency (NT).

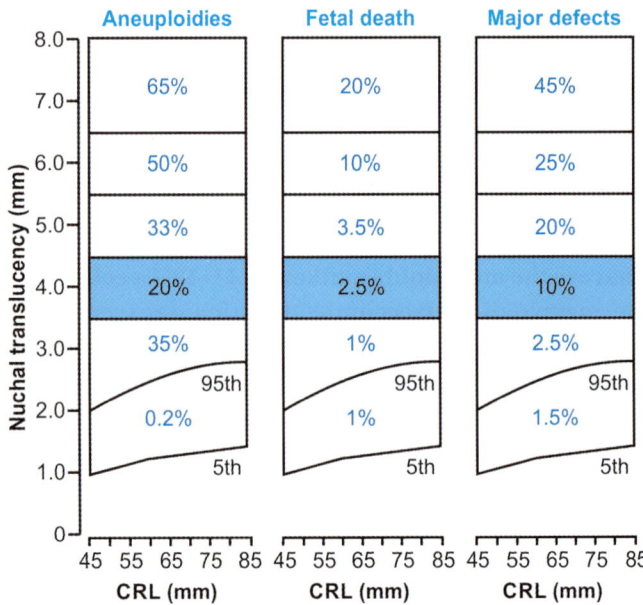

Fig. 6: Probability of abnormal fetal outcomes with increased nuchal translucency. (CRL: crown-rump length)

- *CRL measurement*: 10–14 weeks is an optimal time to assign revised date of delivery if there is a discrepancy of >1 week between CRL and GA by last menstrual period
- *Intracranial translucency (ICT)*: Collapsed/absent intracranial translucency is a surrogate marker for *open neural tube defects* and prompts a detailed spine examination.[4]

SCREENING FOR STRUCTURAL DEFECTS

In the last decade, early diagnosis of structural defects in fetus is an added attraction of a detailed 11–13^{+6} weeks GA scan. Without much addition of expertise/technology (machine), >50% of fetal structural abnormalities can be detected on this first trimester scan. Earlier detection enables early decision making, further testing, and safer and more private termination if opted for.

The basic views which can be visualized at the 11–13^{+6} weeks window are illustrated in the **Figures 7A to I**. Apart from these views, the facial profile and its details are already visualized on the midsagittal section, and the fetal heart is assessed while checking for tricuspid flow.

If the above mentioned fetal views are systematically obtained at the 11–13^{+6} weeks scan; over 60% of fetal structural defects can be identified.[5] **Table 6** depicts some of the anomalies that can be detected at this scan.

The 11–13^{+6} weeks GA window of opportunity also aids prediction of preeclampsia and fetal growth restriction,

SECTION 3: Fetal Evaluation | 131

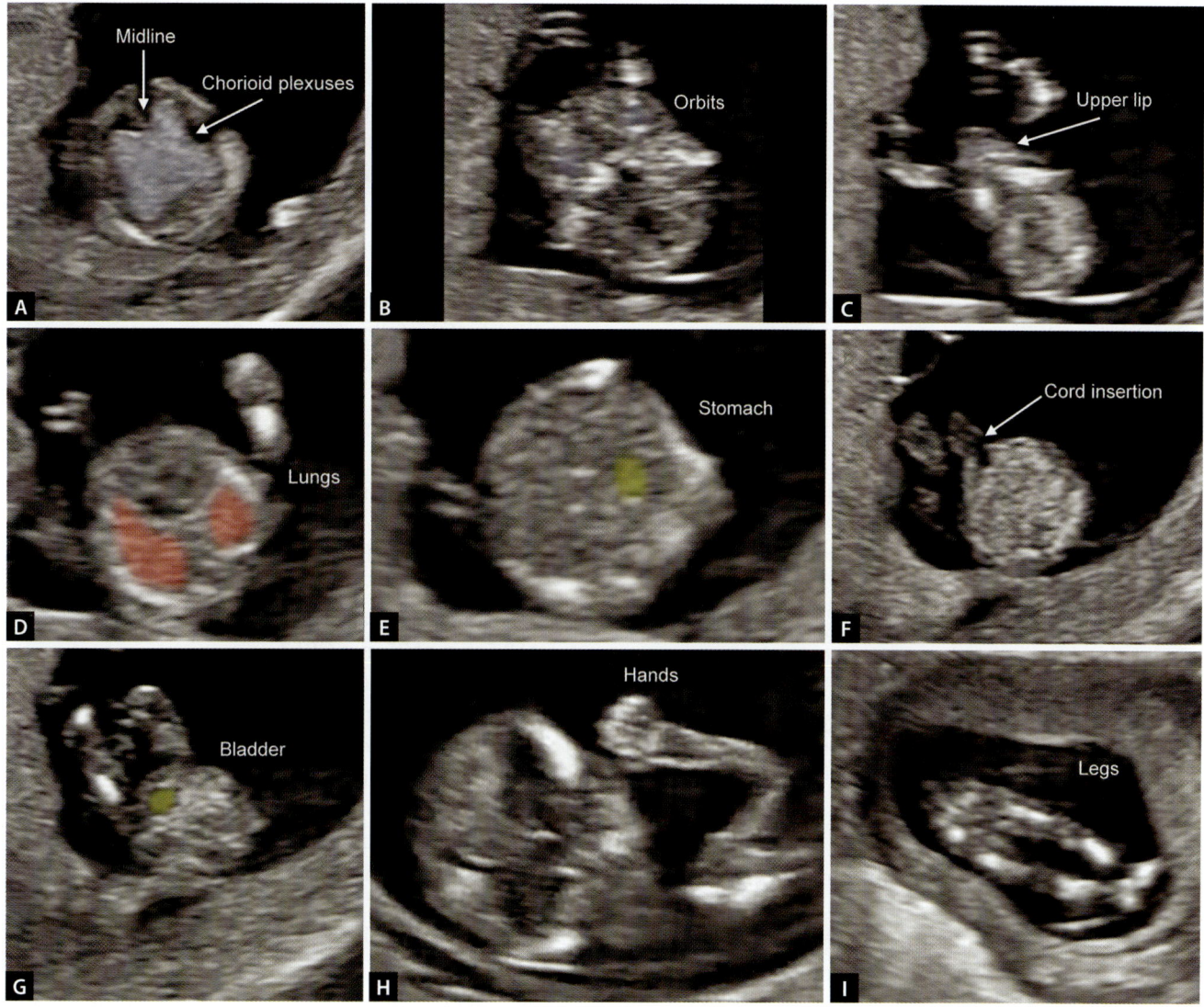

Figs. 7A to I: Early anatomy on the 11–13^{+6} weeks scan. (A) Choroid plexus, skull, and flax; (B) Orbits; (C) Upper lip; (D) Lungs; (E) Stomach; (F) Umbilical cord insertion; (G) Bladder; (H) Hands; (I) Legs.

TABLE 6: Anomalies detected at 11–13^{+6} weeks gestational age scan.

Always detectable anomalies	Potentially detectable anomalies	Undetectable anomalies
Body stalk anomaly	Lethal skeletal dysplasias	Microcephaly
Anencephaly	Diaphragmatic hernia	Cerebellar hypoplasia
Alobar holoprosencephaly	Major cardiac defects	Agenesis of corpus callosum
Exomphalos	Open spina bifida	Achondroplasia
Gastroschisis		Echogenic lung abnormalities
Megacystis		Renal abnormalities
		Bowel obstruction

preterm birth screening, and determining chorionicity. The details of these topics are beyond the scope of this chapter and have been covered in other chapters of this textbook.

The benefits of a thorough screening at 11–13^{+6} weeks window of opportunity is undebatable. It helps in predicting complications of late pregnancy, which were earlier only diagnosed after their onset in the late third trimester. This model of antenatal care facilitates patient specific approach towards monitoring the antenatal care and surveillance.

■ KEY MESSAGES

- 11–13^{+6} weeks GA is a window of opportunity for aneuploidy screening, structural check, preeclampsia and fetal growth restriction screening, preterm birth screening, and determination of chronicity.
- Inverted pyramid of antenatal care is a better model as it predicts adverse events later in pregnancy, at as early at 11 weeks.

- NT is the most important marker for chromosomal abnormalities.
- In fetuses with high NT and a normal karyotype, structural abnormalities and genetic syndromes should be thoroughly screened for.
- More than 60% of all structural abnormalities in the fetus can be detected at 11–13^{+6} weeks if a systematic approach for structural check is followed.

REFERENCES

1. Rodgers SK, Chang C, DeBardeleben JT, Horrow MM. Normal and Abnormal US Findings in Early First-Trimester Pregnancy: Review of the Society of Radiologists in Ultrasound 2012 Consensus Panel Recommendations. Radiographics. 2015;35(7):2135-48.
2. Sonek JD, Kagan KO, Nicolaides KH. Inverted Pyramid of Care. Clin Lab Med. 2016;36:305-17.
3. Nicolaides K. Fetal Medicine Foundation, London, 2004. Available at: www.fetalmedicine.org.
4. Chaoui R, Nicolaides KH. From nuchal translucency to intracranial translucency: towards the early detection of spina bifida. Ultrasound Obstet Gynecol. 2010;35:133-8.
5. Lopes LM, Brizot ML, Lopes MAB, Ayello VD, Schultz R, Zugaib M. Detection of fetal structural abnormalities at the 11-14 week ultrasound scan. Ultrasound Obstet Gynecol. 2003;22:470-8.

LONG QUESTIONS

1. Elaborate on the sonoembryology with schematic illustrations.
2. What are the opportunities which 11–13^{+6} weeks window provides? Elaborate in details.
3. Which are the important structures which should be visualized during the 11–13^{+6} weeks scan? Which abnormalities can be detected so early?
4. What is the inverted pyramid of antenatal care? How has the pattern of antenatal care changed over last decade?

SHORT QUESTIONS

1. What are the criteria which hint towards a pathological/failing early pregnancy?
2. What are the Fetal Medicine Foundation criteria for measuring nuchal translucency?
3. Name the aneuploidy markers at 11–13^{+6} weeks ultrasound.
4. Should all fetuses with high nuchal translucency be terminated? Why/why not?

MULTIPLE CHOICE QUESTIONS

1. At what CRL, if fetal cardiac activity is not seen, it is a sign of pregnancy failure?
    a. 5 mm
    b. 6 mm
    c. 7 mm
    d. 8 mm
2. Which of the following are suspicious indicators for blighted ovum?
    a. 5 mm, and no fetal cardiac activity
    b. 10 mm gestational sac and no embryo
    c. 16–24 mm gestational sac and no embryo
    d. >4 weeks after last menstrual period
3. Which is the most important marker for aneuploidy screening?
    a. Tricuspid regurgitation   b. Nasal bone
    c. Nuchal translucency   d. Ductus venosus
4. Which of the following is true?
    a. Structural check is not possible as early as 11–14 weeks
    b. Complete structural check is possible at 11–14 weeks
    c. Up to 25% of structural defects can be diagnosed at 11–14 weeks
    d. Approximately 50–60% of fetal structural defects can be diagnosed at 11–14 weeks GA
5. What is the approach for a fetus with nuchal translucency of 3.5 mm at 75 mm CRL?
    a. Terminate without any workup
    b. Karyotype, structural check, and decide accordingly
    c. 100% neurodevelopmentally abnormal
    d. Normal, continue without further work-up
6. What further work-up is vital for persistent increased nuchal fold thickness beyond 14 weeks?
    a. Fetal infection   b. Cardiac defects
    c. Microarray   d. All of the above
7. Which of the following cannot be diagnosed at 11–14 weeks USG?
    a. Microcephaly   b. Body-stalk anomaly
    c. Holoprosencephaly   d. Exencephaly
8. Which is the most vital USG view at 11–14 weeks USG?
    a. Coronal views   b. Lateral views
    c. Axial views   d. Midsagittal view
9. For whom should combined first trimester screening for aneuploidies be done?
    a. Maternal age >35 years
    b. Maternal age >40 years
    c. Both of the above
    d. Not for anyone
10. Which is the best time to assign revised dates for pregnancy dating?
    a. 6 weeks   b. 7 weeks
    c. 10–14 weeks   d. After 20 weeks
11. Which of the following is not true as a criterion for measuring NT?
    a. It can be measured in a prone position of the fetus as long as FMF criteria are followed
    b. 75–90% magnification
    c. Midsagittal section
    d. Neutral position of the fetal head

12. Which of the following can be performed at the 11–14 weeks window during pregnancy?
    a. Preeclampsia screening   b. Preterm birth screening
    c. Aneuploidy screening   d. All of the above

13. Which is the best time to perform screening for chromosomal abnormalities?
    a. Before 10 weeks
    b. At 20 weeks–during anomaly scan
    c. 11–13^{+6} weeks
    d. None of the above

14. Which is a better model for antenatal care?
    a. Inverted pyramid of care
    b. Old model of frequent visits, confined to the third trimester
    c. Antenatal visits only in the second trimester
    d. None of the above

Answers
1. c   2. c   3. c   4. d   5. b   6. d
7. a   8. d   9. c   10. c   11. a   12. d
13. c   14. a

3.4 BIOCHEMICAL TEST FOR FETAL SCREENING

Vinita Das, Smriti Agrawal

INTRODUCTION

During the past few decades, there has been a tremendous development of new screening/methods in pregnancy to rule out chromosomal or congenital anomalies in fetus. It is usually seen that the incidence of chromosomal anomalies among pregnant women is high. 40–50% of spontaneously aborted fetus[1] and 5–10% of perinatal deaths are contributed by chromosomal anomalies.[2] The prevalence of chromosomal abnormality in live birth is 0.625% (1 in 160).[1] Chromosomal aberration leads to significant psychological, economical, and social burden on parent couple as well as society.

Of the various aneuploidies defined, the most common are autosomal trisomies (+16) and sex chromosome monosomy (45 XO) among abortions and trisomy 21 among live births. The other trisomies seen are trisomy 18, 13, and Klinefelter syndrome (47 XXY). Trisomy 21 is responsible for causing Down syndrome in 90% of cases. This is the most common genetic cause of mental retardation (20–30%) and thus a focus of most of the genetic screening protocols. Advent of sonography and biochemical markers help in detection of >95% of trisomy affected fetus.

HISTORY

In 1960s, maternal age 35 years or more at the time of delivery was considered a risk factor for Down syndrome. Hence, these women were offered genetic counseling and required tests for diagnosis. However, later on it was realized that most of fetal aneuploidies (70–80%) were seen in younger women (<35 years) and hence there was a need to screen the entire population. *Screening* offers risk assessment and identifies a subset of women whose fetus is at risk for aneuploidies. Screening test should ideally be noninvasive, easy to carry out, and with no associated risk to pregnancy. The test should also have high detection rate (DR) and minimal false positive rate (FPR). Various screening tests are developed lately and involve both biochemistry as well as sonography. The diagnostic tests for confirmation of fetal disorder involve obtaining fetal tissue by invasive procedures such as chorionic villus sampling, amniocentesis that are expensive, require expertise, and are associated with slight risk of miscarriage.

Biochemical screening was introduced in 1984 when an association was found between low serum alpha-fetoprotein (AFP) and Down syndrome. In 1990, human chorionic gonadotropin (hCG) and unconjugated estriol were also used with serum AFP to screen Down syndrome and trisomy 18. Nuchal translucency (NT) as a valid tool was initiated as a part of screening test in 1990s. However, now in an effort to have early diagnosis in first trimester, biochemical markers along with sonology features are used and have DR of >90% with low FPR. It is seen that 70–80% of aneuploidy are seen in women with no obvious risk factor and hence screening for fetal aneuploidy should be offered universally.

Biochemical test

First trimester (up to 14 weeks)	Second Trimester (14–20 weeks)
Free beta-human chorionic gonadotropic (βhCG)	Alpha-fetoprotein (AFP)
Pregnancy-associated plasma protein A (PAPP-A)	Human chorionic gonadotropin (hCG)
	Unconjugated estriol (μE3)
	Inhibin A

Ultrasonography

First trimester (up to 14 weeks)	Second trimester (14–20 weeks)
Nuchal thickness	Major structural defects including neural tube defects
Nasal bone prominence	Soft markers such as choroid plexus cyst, renal pyelectasis, and cardiac echogenic focus. These soft markers modify the priori risk of aneuploidy established by age or prior screening
Ductus venosus blood flow	
Tricuspid regurgitation	

■ FIRST TRIMESTER SCREENING

First trimester screening provides early diagnosis of aneuploidy thus allowing couple safe termination, if required. In this effort, serum marker pregnancy-associated plasma protein A (PAPP-A), free beta-human chorionic gonadotropin (βhCG), and NT have emerged as vital screening tools. The maternal serum concentration of free βhCG is increased to 1.98 multiple of median (MoM) in trisomy 21 pregnancies as compared to chromosomally normal pregnancies. Measuring free βhCG alone in first trimester would identify 35% of fetus with trisomy 21. If it is integrated with maternal age, the DR is increased to 45%. The maternal serum free βhCG is decreased in trisomy 13 and 18. The PAPP-A level normally increases with gestation and is lower in pregnancies with trisomy 21 to 0.43 MoM than in chromosomally normal fetus. When used alone in first trimester, the DR is 40% of fetus with trisomy 21. It is increased to 50% when PAPP-A is used with maternal age.[3]

Nuchal translucency, i.e., physiological collection of fluid under the skin behind the fetal neck, at 11–14 weeks is an important tool to diagnose fetal aneuploidies, fetal cardiac defects, and fetal congenital malformations. Measurement of NT needs optimal standardization. The average DR of aneuploidy with NT measurement is 64–70% with a FPR 5%.[4] Risk of trisomy 21 is higher if NT is more and lower if NT is less. NT is also increased in trisomy 18 and monosomy X. NT when combined with free βhCG and PAPP-A in first trimester has increased the DR to 82–87% with 5% FPR. Apart from other first trimester sonography markers, absence or hypoplasia of nasal bone is the most useful marker due to delayed ossification in Down syndrome. This isolated marker has a DR of 70% with FPR of 2–9% (depending on accuracy). Other markers include absent or reverse a wave in ductus venosus Doppler or regurgitated flow across tricuspid regurgitation (velocity of 80 cm/s for at least 50% of systole). However apart from NT and nasal bone, these ultrasound markers are very objective, need a lot of expertise, and hence not incorporated in routine aneuploidy screening.

TABLE 1: Changes in biochemical and sonological marker in trisomy.

S. No	Marker	Trisomy 13	Trisomy 18	Trisomy 21
1.	βhCG	↓	↓	↑ (1.98 MoM)
2.	PAPP-A	↓	↓	↓ (0.43 MoM)
3.	NT	↑	↑	↑

(βhCG: beta-human chorionic gonadotropin; MoM: multiple of median; NT: nuchal translucency; PAPP-A: pregnancy-associated plasma protein A)

TABLE 2: Percentage detection rate of various markers in trisomy 21 (Down syndrome).[5]

S. No.	Marker	% detection	False positive rate
1.	MA	30%	5–15%
2.	βhCG	35%	
3.	PAPP-A	40%	
4.	NT	64–70%	5%
5.	MA + NT	77%	5%
6.	MA + βhCG + PAPP-A	60%	5%
7.	NT + βhCG + PAPP-A	82–87%	5%
8.	MA + NT + βhCG + PAPP-A	90%	5%
9.	MA + NT + NB	90%	5%
10.	MA + NT +NB + βhCG + PAPP-A	97%	5%
11.	MA + βhCG + PAPP-A ± DV, TR or NB	90%	2–5%

(βhCG: beta-human chorionic gonadotropin; DV: ductus venosus; MA: maternal age; NB: nasal bone; NT: nuchal translucency; PAPP-A: pregnancy-associated plasma protein A; TR: tricuspid regurgitation)

Changes in level of markers in trisomy are given in **Table 1** and the percentage DRs are listed in **Table 2**.

■ SECOND TRIMESTER SCREENING

Among the various biochemical markers, AFP, hCGs, and unconjugated estriol have been widely used. In women with Down syndrome, average maternal serum AFP level and μE_3 are reduced as compared to euploid pregnancies. Intact hCG is increased in trisomy 21. The levels of all the three markers are reduced in trisomy 18.[3] These levels are given in **Table 3**.

The tests used in second trimester are:
- *Double test*: Measurement of serum AFP and hCG
- *Triple test*: Measurement of serum AFP, unconjugated estriol, and human chronic gonadotropin
- *Quadruple test*: Measurement of serum AFP, unconjugated estriol, and hCG and inhibin A
- Integrated test includes measurement of serum analytes in first and second trimester with NT measurement in first trimester. The results are reported only after both first and second trimester screening tests are completed.

TABLE 3: Biochemical markers in trisomy in second trimester.

Marker	Level in T21	Levels in T18
AFP	0.7 MoM ↓	0.6 MoM ↓
µE₃	0.7 MoM ↓	0.5 MoM ↓
βhCG	1.9 MoM ↑	0.3 MoM ↓
Inhibin A	1.7 MoM ↑	-

(AFP: α-fetoprotein; βhCG: beta-human chorionic gonadotropic; MoM: multiple of median)

TABLE 4: Percentage detection rates of various markers in trisomy 21 (Down syndrome).

Screening test	Detection rates
Second trimester	
Double screening (AFP + hCG)	65%
Triple screen (AFP + hCG + µE3)	69%
Quadruple screen (AFP + hCG + µE3 + inhibition A)	81%
First plus second trimester	
Serum integrated screen—PAPPA + quad screen (useful where facility of NT is not available)	85–88%
Integrated (NT + PAPPA + quad screen)	94–96%

Integrated biochemical screening can also be performed using only first and second trimester serum markers without incorporating NT measurement. Advantage of using integrated test is superior sensitivity (DR of 90-96% and FPR 2-5%), however disadvantage is that even positive test in first trimester is not considered for diagnostic testing and there is a longer wait time till results are available.

Biochemical markers in second trimester also help in detection of 80% of open spina bifida and 97% of anencephaly. The DRs[3] of these screening tests are listed in **Table 4**.

Cell-free fetal deoxyribonucleic acid (DNA) is a method of analyzing fetal DNA in maternal circulation. This approach is often called "noninvasive prenatal testing", although the above mentioned biochemical tests are also noninvasive. Source of fetal cell-free DNA (cfDNA) is thought to be syncytiotrophoblast cells. Fetal fraction begins to increase as early as 5 weeks of gestation and is usually measured after 10 weeks of gestation. cfDNA is the most sensitive screening option for trisomy 21, 18, and 13. The DRs along with FPRs are as follows:

Trisomy 21—DR 99.5%, FPR 0.05%; trisomy 18—DR 97.7%, FPR 0.04%; trisomy 13—DR 96.1%, FPR 0.06%; and monosomy X—DR 90.3%, FPR 0.23%.

Percentage of fetal fraction plays a pivotal role in the accuracy of test result. Fetal fraction is influenced by maternal weight, gestational age, aneuploidy, and assay platform. This test is expensive and has false positive and false negative too and confirmation of prenatal diagnosis is done by karyotype analysis by amniocentesis or chorionic villus sampling (CVS) depending on gestation.[6] However, cell-free fetal DNA is an expensive test and has limited role as first-line screening test. As per the Society for Maternal-Fetal Medicine (SMFM) (2012) and American College of Obstetricians and Gynecologists (ACOG), Committee Opinion No. 545, this test is recommended in all women >35 years, ultrasonography features of aneuploidy, previous pregnancy with aneuploidy, positive screening test, and parental balanced translocation. This test is not to be used as primary screening test. This is also because sequential screening is a less specific test and uncovers many nontargeted abnormalities. Moreover, cfDNA may not detect trisomy 13 and 18 as there are more chances of test failure.[7]

SCREENING IN MULTIPLE PREGNANCY

Incidence of multiple pregnancies has risen considerably over the last few years due to more widespread use of assisted reproductive technology (ART) methods and older age at conception. Biochemical screening in twin pregnancy may not be feasible as unaffected twin may mask the affected one. In twin pregnancy, preferred method of aneuploidy screening is combined NT and first-trimester serum screening with PAPP-A and βhCG. It has a sensitivity and specificity of 87.4% [95% confidence interval (CI), 52.6-97.7] and 95.4% (95% CI, 94.3-96.3) in monochorionic twins and 86.2% (95% CI, 72.8-93.6) and 95.2% (95% CI, 94.2-96.0) for dichorionic twins.[8] Stepwise sequential test, which also includes second trimester quadruple test may improve DR. Second trimester analyte screening is offered to those women with multiple pregnancy who present late. Although data are limited, cfDNA has an important role in screening of twin pregnancy.

DIAGNOSTIC TEST

Women with a positive screening test should be offered a diagnostic test that confirms if the fetus is affected by aneuploidy. *Diagnostic tests* include:
- Amniocentesis
- CVS
- Cordocentesis
- Fetal tissue biopsy.

These tests are invasive, need expertise, are expensive, and are associated with risk of miscarriage (0.5% in amniocentesis and 1-2% in CVS).[9]

WHEN TO DO SCREENING?

The timing of prenatal genetic screening test is very important. Early detection has its obvious advantages; however, certain issues such as limited view of sonography in early gestation and placental mosaicism in chorionic tissue may impede the final diagnosis in early pregnancy. cfDNA is available from 10 weeks onwards. First trimester screening including biochemical and sonography is available from 11 to 14 weeks of gestation and quadruple screening from 15 to 22 weeks. Anatomy sonogram is done from 18 to 20 weeks of pregnancy. CVS, a diagnostic test, is done after 10 weeks and amniocentesis after 15 weeks. Presence of cfDNA test and serum screening and NT in first trimester now offers women with early alternative to invasive diagnostic testing. The women who present late for prenatal care can be offered quadruple test in second trimester.[10] These tests are also useful in areas where there is limited access to prenatal care and ultrasound information is needed for dating only.

■ HOW TO CHOOSE THE SCREENING METHOD?

In a large array of screening test that are available, choosing a test can be a big dilemma. Interpretation of biochemical markers in first or second trimester takes into account gestational age, maternal age, maternal weight, spontaneous or ART conception, ethnicity, presence of insulin dependent diabetes, or if there is history of neural tube defects in previous pregnancy. The clinician should wisely choose a strategy depending on the test available in the area and the needs of patient. Regardless of which screening test is decided, the patients should be informed about the detection and FPR and advantages and disadvantages of screening test. Risk and benefits of diagnostic procedure should also be told so they can make informed decisions.

The choice of screening test depends on gestational age at first prenatal visit, number of fetus, availability of NT measurement, risk of invasive procedures and desire for early results. The women who are seen for the first time in first trimester undergo integrated screening. Those who are seen for the first time in second trimester can undergo quadruple screening and ultrasound examination.

The woman who undergo first trimester test and second trimester test for Down syndrome independently have higher DR (94–98%); however, the FPRs are also higher leading to more invasive procedure (11–17%). Hence, it is recommended that woman who undergo first trimester test and want a higher DR should have an integrated or sequential screening test as outlined below. The advantage of sequential screening is that the results of first trimester screen are informed and those at highest risk might opt for a diagnostic procedure and those at low risk can go ahead with second trimester screen for higher DR. While in integrated screening, results are disclosed after second trimester screening is complete.

Two strategies have been proposed according to the ACOG guidelines:[3]
1. Sequential screening
2. Contingent screening

Sequential Screening (Flowchart 1)

Women who present in first trimester are offered first trimester screening test, which includes biochemical as well as NT. Those who test positive are offered diagnostic test like CVS in first trimester. Those who test negative can undergo second trimester serum test for assessment. Final risk assessment incorporates both first and second trimester result. The DR of trisomy 21 with sequential method is 91–95%.[10]

Contingent Screening (Flowchart 2)

The women undergo first trimester screening and if tested positive undergo diagnostic test in the form of CVS. If the test is negative no further testing is required. If the risk is intermediate, only then second trimester test are offered. Final risk assessment incorporates first and second trimester result. The DR of trisomy 21 with contingent sequential method is 91–92%.[10]

To conclude, all the women should be offered screening test that have maximum DR and least FPRs. Availability of ultrasonography facility and expertise to evaluate NT should also be kept in mind. If women are seen in first trimester, it is prudent to offer first trimester combined screening. If CVS is available, diagnostic service can be offered in first trimester itself or else amniocentesis offered in second trimester. In such cases, where CVS is unavailable integrated screening would be a better option. If NT is unavailable, serum biochemical integrated screening can be offered in women. In areas where all screening options are available, it is best to choose integrated/sequential screening for women

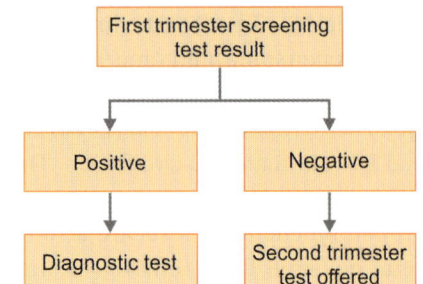

Flowchart 1: Strategy for sequential screening.

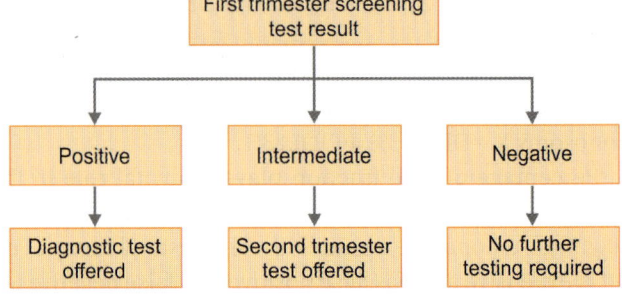

Flowchart 2: Strategy for contingent screening.

who present for prenatal care in first trimester and second trimester screen for women who present later.

Apart from being used to screen aneuploidies, these markers have other research potential as well:
- Low PAPP-A levels at first trimester screening have been found to be associated with higher rates of emergency cesarean section (CS) for fetal distress during labor.[11]
- Various biomarkers such as adiponectin serum and sex hormone-binding globulin (SHBG) at 11–13 weeks of gestation are found to be significant lower for prediction of gestational diabetes mellitus (GDM).[12]
- In a cohort study in a university hospital at Finland, first trimester Down syndrome screening marker (βhCG, PAPP-A, and NT) were correlated and found to be lower with adverse pregnancy outcomes such as preeclampsia, preterm delivery, and small for gestational age pregnancies.[13] There was however no correlation of placental abruption with first trimester biochemical markers.[1]

KEY MESSAGES
- Screening for aneuploidies, especially trisomy 21, should be offered to all pregnant women.
- Choice of screening test depends on the gestational age of patient and the resources available.
- In first trimester, the best option is sequential screening including biochemical and ultrasound markers.
- In second trimester, quadruple test is offered along with sonography.
- cfDNA has excellent DR for trisomy 21, however is expensive. It is not recommended as first-line screening test but helps in reducing the number of invasive tests for diagnosis.
- Diagnostic procedures should be offered to all who are screen positive for aneuploidies.
- Diagnostic procedures include CVS in first trimester and amniocentesis in second trimester.

REFERENCES
1. Valentine GH. Incidence of chromosome disorders. Can Fam Physician. 1979;25:937-9.
2. Alberman ED, Creasy MR. Frequency of chromosomal abnormalities in miscarriages and perinatal deaths. J Med Genetics. 1977;14:313-5.
3. ACOG Committee on Practice Bulletins. ACOG Practice Bulletin No.77: Screening for fetal chromosomal abnormalities. Obstet Gynecol. 2007;109(1):217-7.
4. Nicolaides KH. (2020). The 11–13 weeks scan. [online] Available from: https://fetalmedicine.org/education/the-11-13-weeks-scan. [Last accessed October, 2021].
5. Wright D, Spencer K, Kagan KK, Torring N, Peterson OB, Christou A, et al. First-trimester combined screening for trisomy 21 at 7–14 weeks' gestation. Ultrasound Obstet Gynecol. 2010;36(4):404-11.
6. Harris S, Reed D, Vora NL. Screening for fetal chromosomal and subchromosomal disorders. Semin Fetal Neonatal Med. 2018;23:85-93.
7. American College of Obstetricians and Gynecologists committee on Genetics. Committee Opinion No. 545. Noninvasive prenatal testing for fetal aneuploidy. Obstet Gynecol. 2012;120:1532-4.
8. Bender W, Dugoff L. Screening for aneuploidy in multiple gestations: the challenges and options. Obstet Gynecol Clin N Am. 2018;45:41-53.
9. Brambati B, Lucia T. Chorionic villus sampling and amniocentesis. Curr Opin Obstet Gynecol. 2005;17(2):197-201.
10. Jelin AC, Sagaser KG, MS, Wilkins-Haug L. Prenatal genetic testing options. Pediatr Clin N Am. 2019;66:281-93.
11. Uccela S, Colombo GF, Bulgheroni CM, Serati M, Bogani G, Salvatore S, et al. First-trimester maternal serum screening and the risk for fetal distress during labor. Am J Obstet Gynecol. 2009;201(2):166.e1-6.
12. Nanda S, Savvidou M, Syngelaki A, Akolekar R, Nicolaides KH. Prediction of gestational diabetes mellitus by maternal factors and biomarkers at 11 to 13 weeks. Prenat Diagn. 2011;31(2):135-41.
13. Ranta JK, Raatikainen K, Romppanen J, Pulkki K, Heinonen S. Decreased PAPP-A is associated with preeclampsia, premature delivery and small for gestational age infants but not with placental abruption. Eur J Obstet Gynecol Reprod Biol. 2011; 157(1):48-52.

LONG QUESTIONS
1. What is the ideal method and time to do biochemical screening for fetal aneuploidy in pregnancy?
2. What is the basic difference between integrated screening and sequential and contingent biochemical screening methods?

SHORT QUESTIONS
1. What is the role cfDNA in fetal biochemical screening?
2. What is the appropriate method to do biochemical screening in pregnancy if a woman presents in second trimester for antenatal checkup?
3. What is the method to do fetal biochemical screening in multiple pregnancy and what are the pitfalls?
4. What is integrated screening? Mention its advantages.
5. What are the components of quadruple test? How is it interpreted?

MULTIPLE CHOICE QUESTIONS
1. Low PAPP-A levels at first trimester screening are associated with all, except:
   a. Lower rates of cesarean section for fetal distress in labor
   b. Trisomy 13
   c. Trisomy 18
   d. Trisomy 21
2. All of the following are ultrasonographic markers of fetal aneuploidy, except:
   a. Increased nuchal thickness
   b. Absent nasal bone
   c. Presence of ductus venosus blood flow
   d. Absent tricuspid regurgitation

3. Soft markers of Down syndrome include all, except:
    a. Pyelectasis
    b. Cardiac echogenic focus
    c. Choroid plexus cyst
    d. Renal cyst
4. Components of quadruple test include all, except:
    a. AFP
    b. E$_3$
    c. hCG
    d. Inhibin A
5. As per SMFM (2012) and ACOG cfDNA are recommended in all situations, except:
    a. Age > 35 years
    b. Ultrasonography features of aneuploidy
    c. Positive screening test
    d. Not willing for invasive tests like CVS/amniocentesis
6. What is the best method to screen for aneuploidy in multiple pregnancy in first trimester?
    a. cfDNA
    b. Invasive tests like CVS
    c. Combined NT and biochemical screening
    d. Only biochemical screening
7. cfDNA is available from how many weeks of pregnancy?
    a. 10 weeks
    b. 20 weeks
    c. 30 weeks
    d. At term
8. In sequential screening, negative screening in first trimester should undergo:
    a. Repeat biochemical test in first trimester
    b. Repeat biochemical test in second trimester
    c. No further testing required
    d. Invasive testing
9. In contingent screening, negative screening in first trimester should undergo:
    a. Repeat biochemical test in first trimester
    b. Repeat biochemical test in second trimester
    c. No further testing required
    d. Invasive testing
10. Choice of screening test depends on all of the following, except:
    a. Gestational age at first prenatal visit
    b. Number of fetus
    c. Severity of diabetes
    d. Risk of invasive tests

Answers										
1.	a	2.	d	3.	d	4.	c	5.	d	6. c
7.	a.	8.	b	9.	c	10.	c			

3.5 SECOND-TRIMESTER ANATOMY SCAN

Narendra Malhotra, Neharika Malhotra, Jaideep Malhotra, Rahul Gupta, Nitin Agrawal

INTRODUCTION

Every pregnant woman wonders about the normality of the child that she will bear. One of the most obvious aspects of establishing such normality is the evaluation of the fetal structure. In addition to fetal anatomy, the ultrasound examination will also be informative about the number of fetuses, gestational age, growth, location of the placenta, amniotic fluid volume, soft markers for aneuploidy, and maternal pelvic abnormalities.

There is debate about the gestational age at which the fetal anatomical assessment should be done. Fetal anatomical survey can be carried out at any time of pregnancy. For technical reasons, such as the timing of organogenesis, fetal size, maternal habitus, and legal limits for termination of pregnancy, the mid-trimester period is the ideal time to perform the anatomical survey. A study by Lantz and Chisolm found that the anatomical survey is more likely to be incomplete if done before 18 weeks of gestation in normal sized or overweight women. The timing was not as critical for women who are underweight. The Royal College of Obstetricians and Gynaecologists (RCOG) advises that the ultrasound examination should be done at 22–24 weeks of pregnancy. In our country, till recently, pregnancy termination was legal till 20 weeks only. Therefore, the practice was to offer the scan at 18–19 weeks to strike a balance between maximum diagnostic sensitivity and yet remaining within the 20 weeks period. This practice may change as recent amendments in the medical termination of pregnancy (MTP) act allow termination of pregnancy till 24 weeks for lethal fetal abnormalities.

In terms of public health outcomes, there has been a halving of the infant death rate from congenital abnormalities over the last 2 decades. The second-trimester anatomical survey has contributed significantly to this by allowing an early diagnosis of lethal anomalies allowing the parents to terminate the pregnancy or better preparation for the birth and care of the neonate. It also provides the option of fetal therapy in certain situations.

BASIC COMPONENTS

The main objectives of the second-trimester ultrasound examination are to:
- Establish fetal viability
- Evaluate growth and use the parameters to establish gestational age if an earlier ultrasound has not been done
- Assess fetal anatomy
- Evaluate the placenta, cord, and amniotic fluid

SECTION 3: Fetal Evaluation

- Risk stratification:
  - Soft markers (with or without biochemical screening) for fetal aneuploidy
  - Uterine artery Doppler (with or without biochemical screening) for preeclampsia, growth restriction
  - Cervical length and morphology for preterm labor
- Diagnosis or follow-up of uterine abnormalities or adnexal pathology.

Fetal position is variable and keeps changing in the second-trimester. The lie is described as the relationship of the long axes of the mother and fetus as illustrated in **Figure 1**.

DETERMINING THE FETAL SITUS (TABLE 1)

Normal Fetal Situs

The normal fetal situs can be established by following the steps below:
- Determine fetal lie—vertex, breech or transverse (the back may be anterior or posterior)
- Obtain a transverse cut of the thorax to demonstrate a four-chamber view. The left atrium is nearest the spine and the cardiac axis points to the left **(Fig. 2)**.

WHAT TO LOOK FOR IN FETAL ANATOMY

The fetal anatomical survey can be described to be composed:
- Evaluation of fetal size by standard measurements. At a minimum these should include the biparental diameter, head circumference, abdominal circumference, and femur length.
- Study of the anatomical landmarks and features that establish normalcy and to describe and diagnose deviations from normal.
- Assessment of soft markers for aneuploidy.

Fetal Measurements and Size

It is of critical importance that fetal measurements are taken accurately. Though the pregnancy dates can be established by menstrual dates and earlier ultrasounds, this examination sets a baseline for the growth parameters. Inaccurate measurements can lead to overdiagnosis or missed fetal growth restriction. The measurement planes are

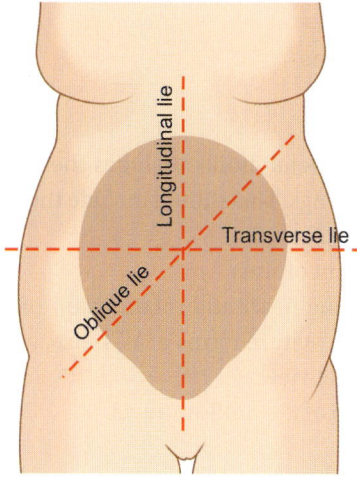

Fig. 1: Schematic diagram showing different lies.
Source: https://radiologykey.com/sonography-of-the-second-and-third-trimesters/

TABLE 1:	Determining fetal situs.	
	Maternal orientation	*Ultrasound transducer*
Fetal left side	Anterior, nearest to maternal abdomen	Nearest to transducer
Fetal left side	Posterior, nearest to posterior uterine wall	Farthest from the transducer
Fetal left side	Right uterine wall, nearest to maternal right	Intermediate depth of transducer relative to the fetal spine
Fetal left side	Left uterine wall, nearest to maternal left	Intermediate depth of transducer relative to the fetal spine

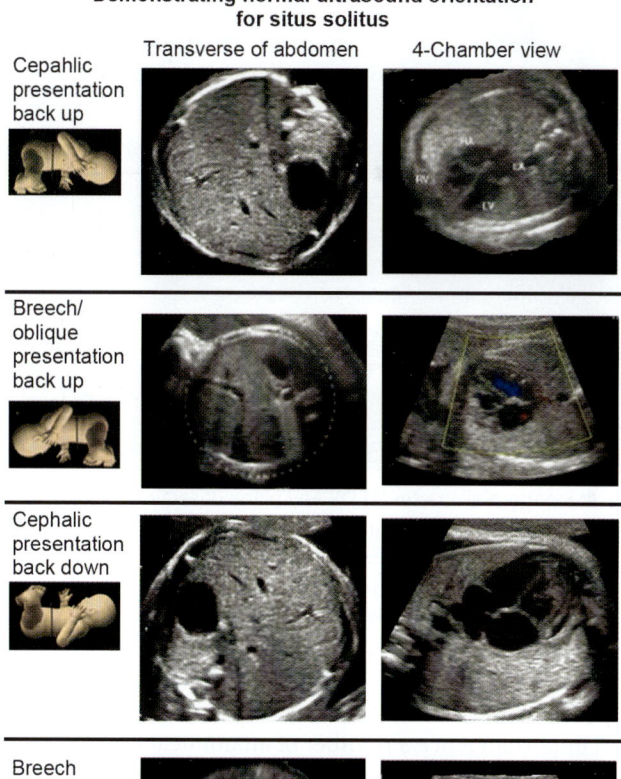

Fig. 2: Different presentations.
Source: https://www.obimages.net/wp-content/uploads/2015/01/1Final.Normalsitus1.png

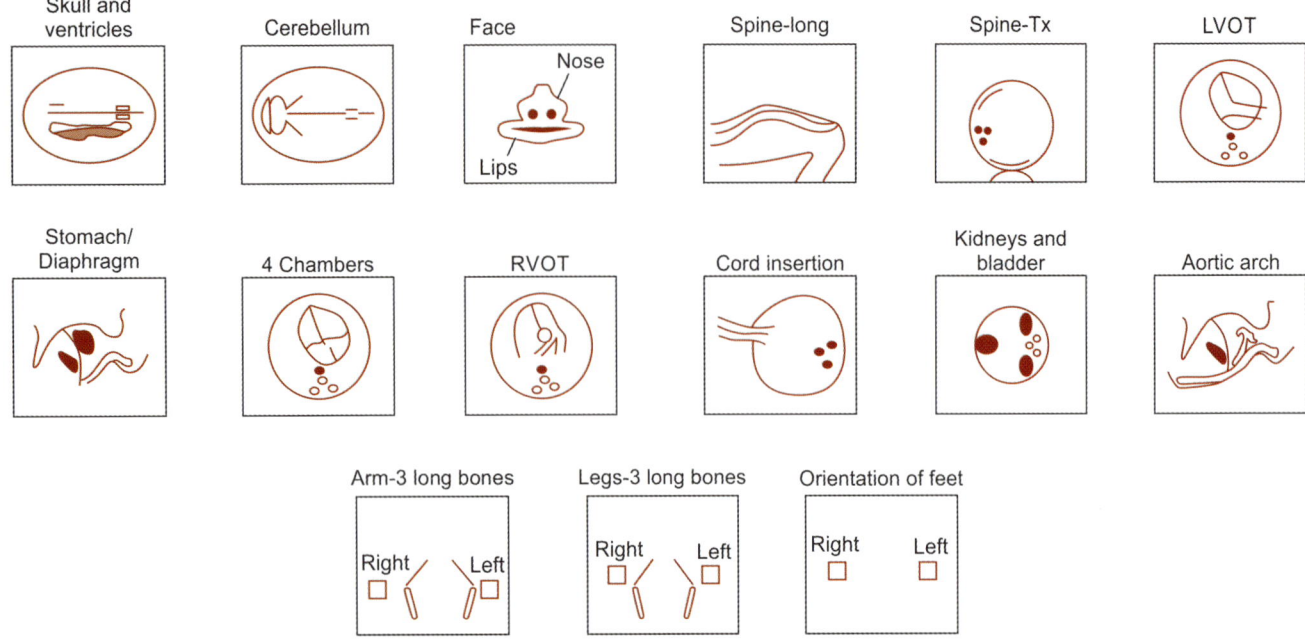

Fig. 3: Shows basic steps of ultrasound.
(LVOT: left ventricular outflow tract; RVOT: right ventricular outflow tract)

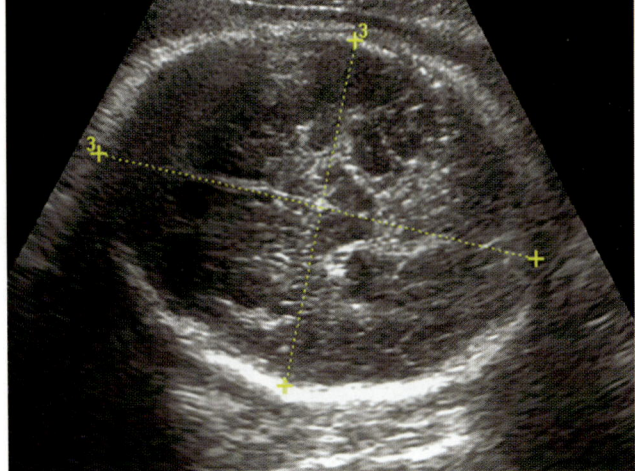

Fig. 4: Biparietal diameter (BPD): Any plane of section that intersects the third ventricle and thalami will allow an accurate measurement of the biparietal diameter. Three criteria should be fulfilled for accurate and standard measurement:
1. The plane of section is taken at the proper craniocaudal plane
2. Transducer is oriented perpendicular to the central axis of the head
3. The plane is properly oriented to the skull base.

also important since a number of anatomical landmarks are described in these planes to establish fetal normalcy.

■ FETAL ANATOMY SURVEY

Fetal brain assessments should include the visualization, description, and documentation of the following basic landmarks **(Figs. 7 to 11)**:
- Shape of fetal skull
- Cavum septi pellucidi
- Midline falx
- Choroid plexus
- Lateral ventricles
- Cerebellum
- Cisterna magna
- Nuchal fold
- Face.

Survey of the fetal thorax includes the evaluation of the fetal heart and lungs. This should include the following at the very least **(Fig. 12)**:
- Establishment of situs
- Position of the heart and relationship of the heart with the thoracic cavity in terms of axis, size, and position
- Four chamber view
- Relationship of the outflow tracts
- Heart rate
- Cardiac wall motion
- Lungs—size/volume and echogenicity.

The fetal abdomen and its contents should be assessed for situs of the stomach and a survey of the bowel, bladder, kidneys, cord insertion and number of cord vessels, and whether a loop of cord is present **(Figs. 13 to 16)**.

The fetal spine should be seen along its entire length from cervical through sacral region in sagittal, coronal, and transverse planes. An effort should be made to visualize the fetal skin line away from the maternal uterine wall **(Figs. 17 and 18)**.

The limbs should be visualized to confirm their presence and that of hands, feet, and digits. The genitalia should be assessed, but there should be no determination or disclosure of fetal gender in our country. Examine the placenta, its position, and appearance. Check for any placental

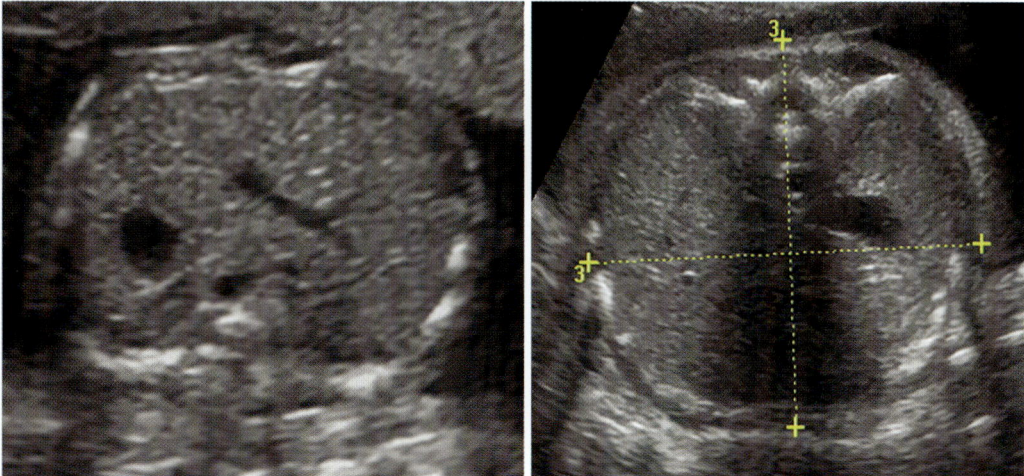

Fig. 5: Abdominal circumference (AC): Measurement should be taken in a plane which meets the following criteria:
- Spherical plane
- Ribs are symmetrical
- Junction of right and left portal vein and body of fetal stomach are visualized. In a plane that is too caudal, GB is visible rather than the stomach. If the plane of section is inclined relative to the body axes, only a long length of the left portal vein is seen instead of the junction of the right and left portal vein.

(GB: gallbladder)

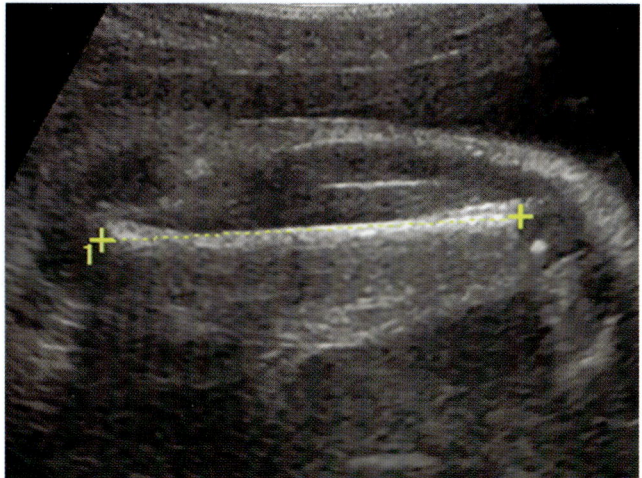

Fig. 6: Femur length (FL) measurement should be taken to include only the ossified portion of the diaphysis and metaphysis. The cartilaginous femoral head, greater trochanter, and distal epiphysis should be excluded to avoid an overestimate. When the distal femoral epiphysis ossifies, it should also be excluded as shown above.

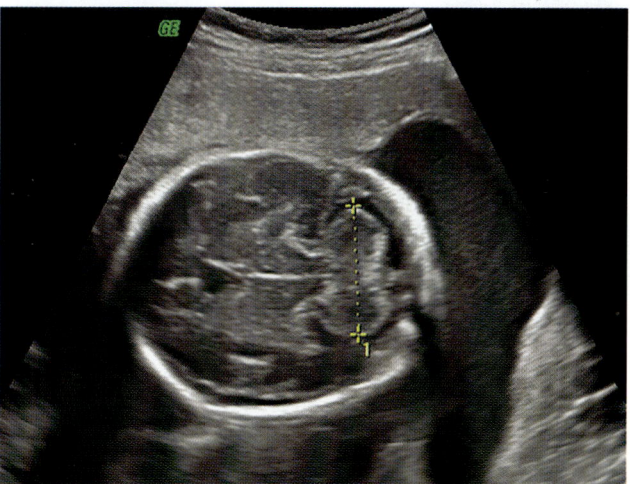

Fig. 7: Transverse section of the fetal skull at the level of cerebellum showing transcerebellar diameter.

abnormalities. The placenta relationship to internal os also to be documented **(Fig. 19)**.

In the mid-trimester, the amniotic fluid is assessed subjectively. It should be reported as normal, increased, decreased, or absent.

Table 2 lists the recommended content of the report.

Besides the correct name, identity and examination date, technical details such as the type of machine, transducer, and routes of scanning should be included. The fetal biometric information, standards, and composite gestational age are important basic information that will help further growth assessments.

If a structure was not seen, this should be reported, along with the reason it was not seen, for example, maternal habitus, fetal position, low-amniotic fluid volume, mistimed examination, etc. If fetal or maternal abnormalities are reported, it should include a description and an interpretation with a differential diagnosis. The obstetrician can be aided with when appropriate, a recommendation for further investigation should be provided. The report should comment on any significant technical difficulty of the examination. Any *significant* fetal or maternal abnormalities need to be reported promptly. The communication should be recorded in the patient's file.

A systematic well-conducted fetal anatomical survey is not an ironclad guarantee against birth defects. There are some limitations and these hold true even in expert hands.

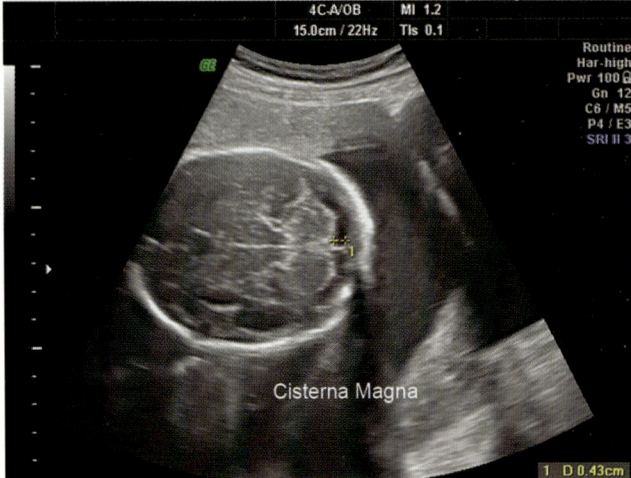

Fig. 8: Cisterna magna.

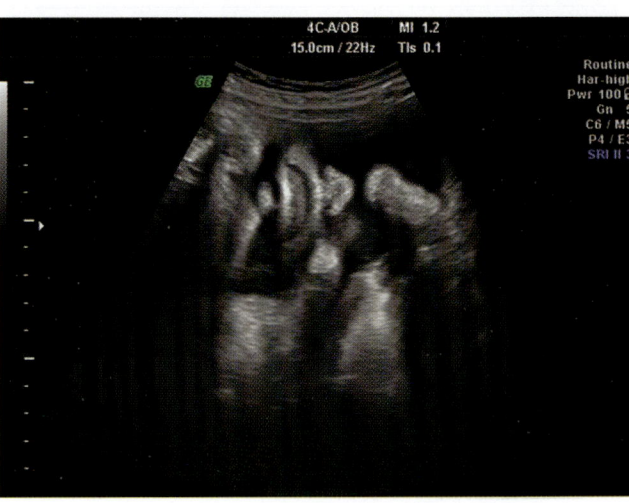

Fig. 11: Fetal face showing the nose and lips.

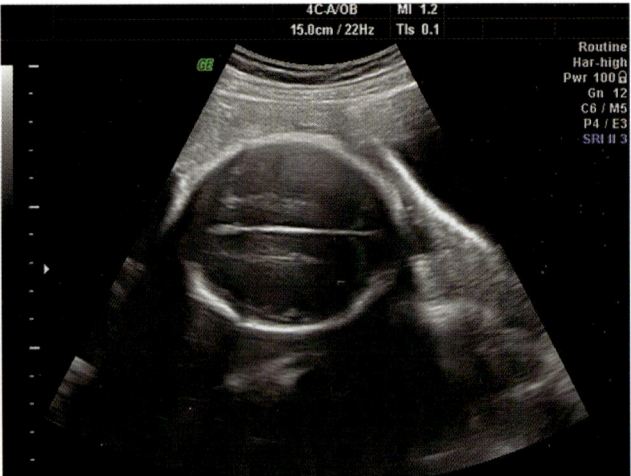

Fig. 9: Transverse section of the fetal skull at the level of lateral ventricles. Falx cerebri is well seen.

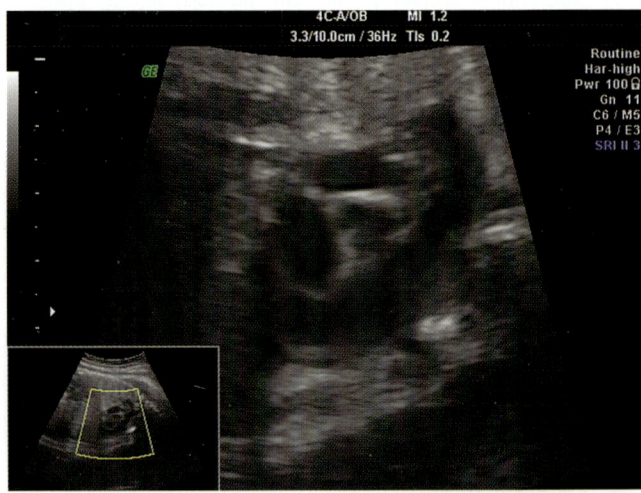

Fig. 12: Fetal heart showing the outflow tracts.

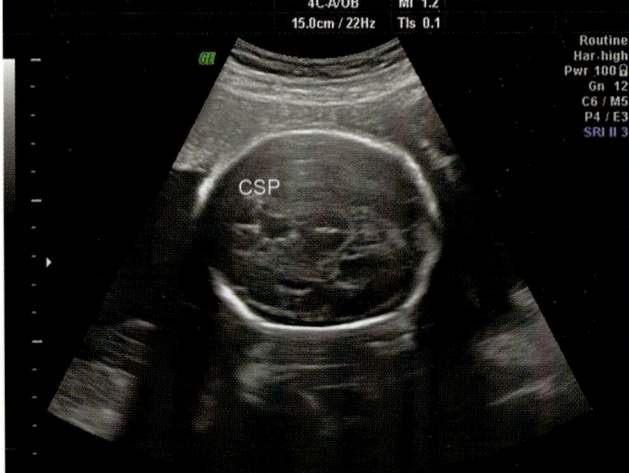

Fig. 10: Box like structure seen anteriorly is the cavum septum pellucidum. (CSP: cavum septum pellucidum)

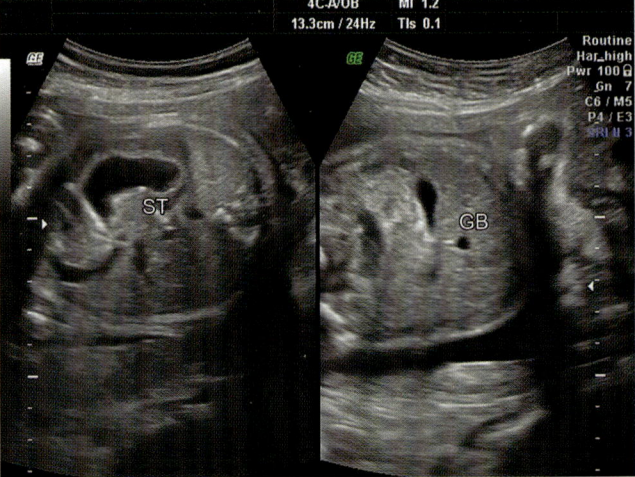

Fig. 13: Fetal abdomen showing the stomach and gallbladder. (GB: gallbladder; ST: stomach)

SECTION 3: Fetal Evaluation

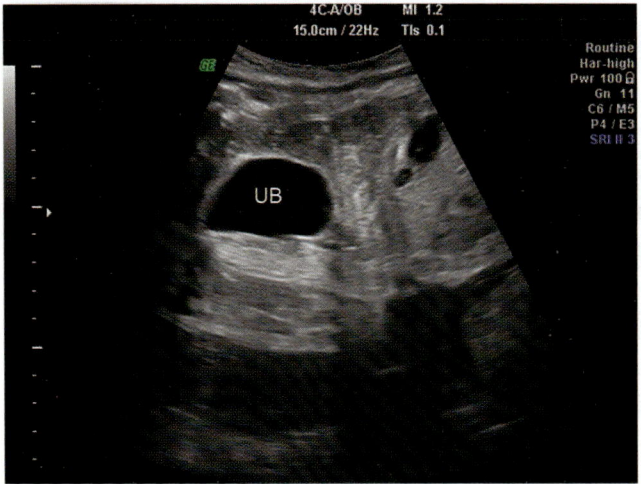

Fig. 14: Fetal pelvis showing the urinary bladder (UB).

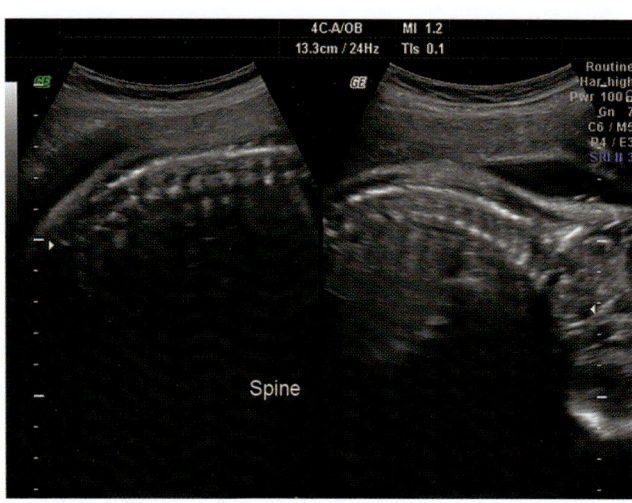

Fig. 17: Fetal spine seen in sagittal section.

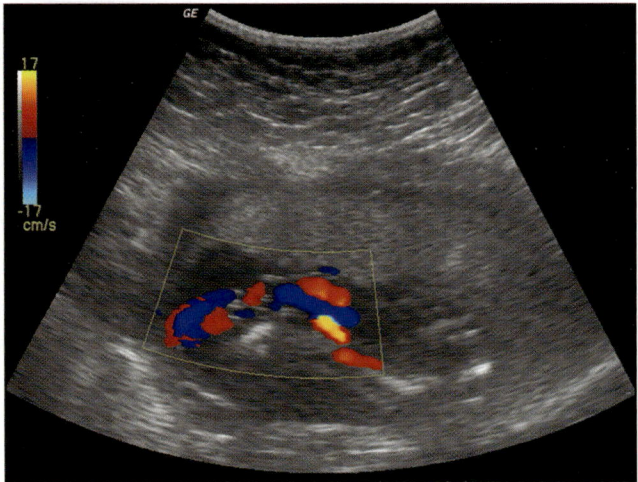

Fig. 15: Normal umbilical cord consists of two arteries and one vein.

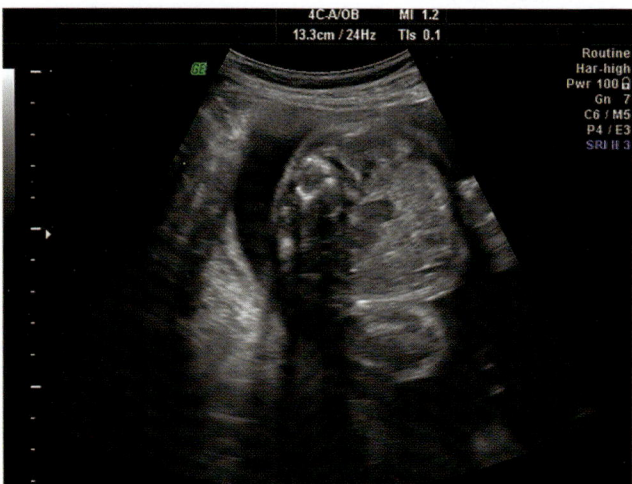

Fig. 18: Fetal spinal vertebra in transverse section.

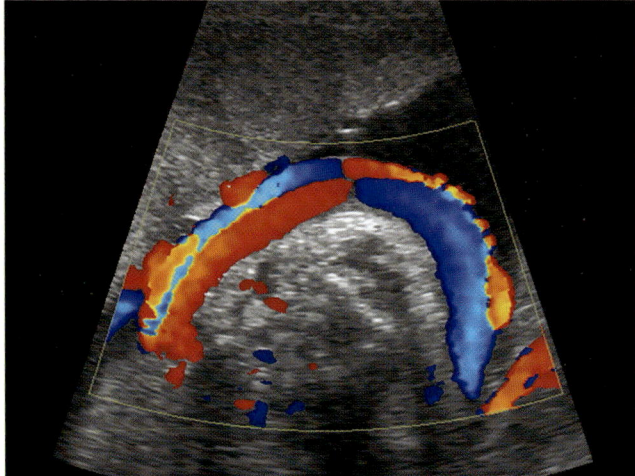

Fig. 16: Nuchal cord. A loop of cord seen around the nape of the neck of fetus.

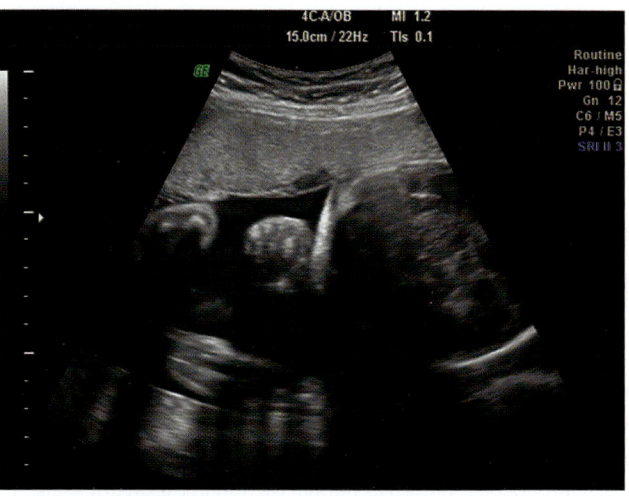

Fig. 19: Placenta seen as homogeneously echogenic structure anteriorly.

PART 1: Obstetrics and Perinatology

TABLE 2: Obstetrical report.

	Content of a complete obstetrical ultrasound report
1	*Patient demographic information:* • Patient name • Indication for consultation • Requesting physician/obstetrician (preferably with contact information) • Starting date of last normal menstrual period (LMP) • Examination date • Date of written report • Name of interpreting sonologist
2	*Number of fetuses and indications of life:* • Presence of cardiac activity for each fetus • If multiple gestation—chorionicity and amnionicity should be reported
3	*Biometry should be reported all in millimeters or in centimeters along with equivalent estimated gestational age for* **(Figs. 1 to 3)**: • Biparietal diameter (*see* **Fig. 4**) • Head circumference • Abdominal circumference (*see* **Fig. 5**) • Femur length (*see* **Fig. 6**) *Should be reported in millimeters if abnormal:* • Nuchal fold • Cisterna magna • Cerebellar diameter • Lateral ventricle width
4	Fetal anatomy should be reported as: normal OR abnormal (with details) OR not seen, with explanation *Should be reported for:* • Cranium • Cerebral ventricles, cavum septi pellucidi, the midline falx, and the choroid plexus • Posterior fossa—cisterna magna, cerebellum • Face—orbits, lips • Spine • Chest • Diaphragm • Lungs • Cardiac four-chamber view • Cardiac outflow tracts • Heart axis • Cardiac situs • Stomach • Bowel • Kidneys • Bladder • Abdominal cord insertion • Number of cord vessels • Upper extremities and presence of hands • Lower extremities and presence of feet
5	*Amniotic fluid amount:* Should be reported as: normal OR increased OR decreased OR absent
6	*Placenta:* Position should be reported as well as relationship to the cervical os
7	*Maternal anatomy uterus, ovaries, cervix, and bladder:* Should be reported as normal OR abnormal OR not seen

It is acknowledged that even in the best of hands and circumstances; the 18–22 weeks scan has limitations and

TABLE 3: Chances of detection of common abnormalities by second-trimester ultrasound (USG).

Fetal anomalies	Chance of being detected by USG
Spina bifida	90%
Anencephaly	99%
Hydrocephalus	60%
Major congenital heart problems	25%
Diaphragmatic hernia	60%
Exomphalos/Gastroschisis	90%
Major kidney problems	85%
Major limb abnormalities	90%
Cerebral palsy	0%
Autism	0%
Down syndrome	40%

cannot detect all fetal and maternal abnormalities. **Table 3** lists the chances of detection of common abnormalities by second-trimester ultrasound. It should be appreciated that though major abnormalities are usually detected, seemingly serious problems such as cardiac defects may have a low detection rate.

SECOND-TRIMESTER SCAN AND ANEUPLOIDY (CHROMOSOMAL MARKERS)

There have been many described approaches to screening for fetal aneuploidy, which affects 0.5–1% of all pregnancies. The second-trimester sonography presents us with one more opportunity to do so. The most common aneuploidy is trisomy 21 and most anatomical features associated with it are included in the standard list of soft markers. Other aneuploidies such as trisomy 18, 13, monosomies, and triploidies also have typical ultrasound features.

Besides major structural defects associated with aneuploidies, the most common soft markers are:
- Nuchal fold
- Limb shortening
- Hyperechoic bowel
- Echogenic cardiac focus
- Pyelectasis
- Choroid plexus cyst.

There is controversy about the significance of soft markers. They may trigger anxiety on the part of parents and unnecessary, invasive and potentially harmful fetal testing. The soft markers should be reviewed in terms of their validity, significance, and numerical risk assessment.

Nuchal Fold Thickness (Fig. 20)

The collection of fluid in the skin behind the neck is useful as a soft marker and is called the nuchal fold thickness. The measurement is done at the transverse plane of the fetal head, measuring from the outer edge of the occipital bone to

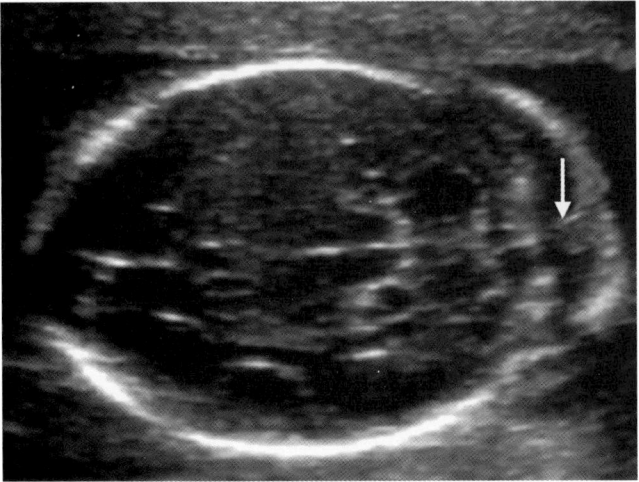

Fig. 20: Nuchal fold thickening.

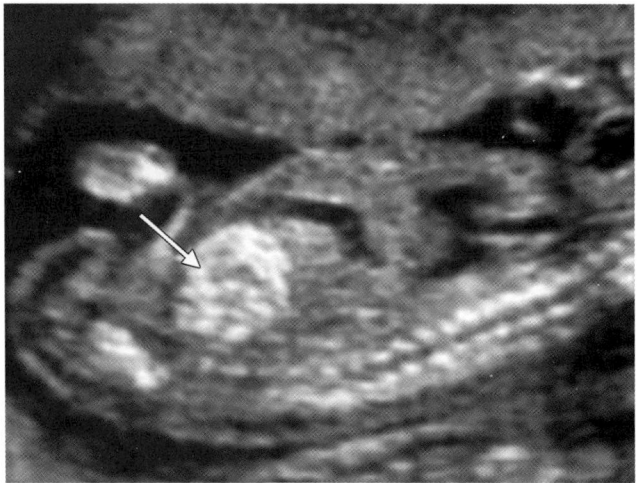

Fig. 21: Echogenic bowel.

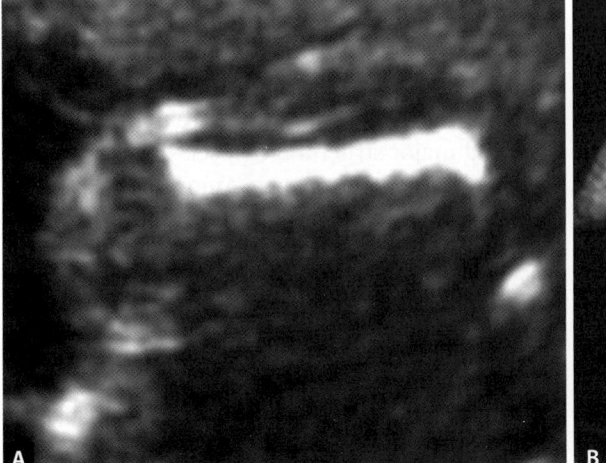
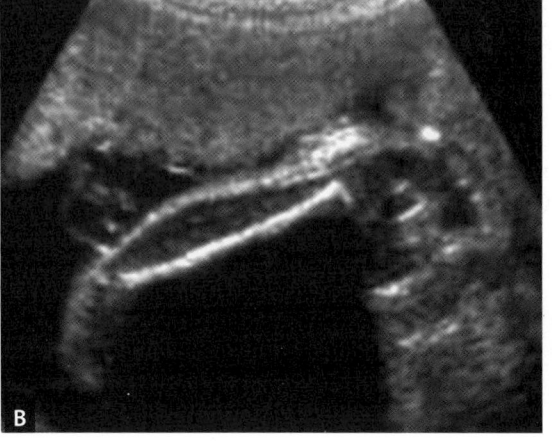

Figs. 22A and B: Measurement of long bones.

the outer edge of the skin. Earlier, the cutoff was 6 mm, but receiver-operator characteristic (ROC) curve analysis suggest the use of a 5 mm cutoff before 20 weeks of pregnancy.

Echogenic Bowel (Fig. 21)

The echogenicity of the bowel wall is compared to that of the adjacent fetal iliac bone. If they are similar in intensity, it is termed as an echogenic bowel. About 1% of fetuses have echogenic bowel. Echogenic bowel is associated with trisomy 21. Besides aneuploidy, it may also be a marker for future growth restriction, fetal TORCH infections, cystic fibrosis or hemoglobinopathies.

Short Long Bones (Figs. 22A and B)

The femur and humerus lengths are predictive of trisomy 21 risk. The measurement of the bones should be standardized and compared to the basic fetal measurement parameter such as biparietal diameter (BPD). The percentile growth for the gestational age should be charted and this will help in identifying the fetus at risk for aneuploidies.

Echogenic Cardiac Foci (Fig. 23)

The papillary muscles in the cardiac ventricles may show a higher echogenicity than the surrounding tissue and may appear similar in echogenicity to the overlying bone. This is termed as an echogenic focus. Artifacts should be eliminated by confirming such a focus from different angles. This warrants a further detailed fetal echocardiographic examination.

In the Asian population, an echogenic focus is seen in 1–5% of the population. However, only 1 in 625 pregnancies with an isolated echogenic focus have aneuploidy (trisomy 21).

Choroid Plexus Cysts (Fig. 24)

The choroid plexus is seen in axial plane of head. Choroid plexus cysts are well circumscribed echo lucent areas. They can be unilateral, bilateral or multiple. About 1–2.5% of fetuses have a choroid plexus cyst and most fetuses will have a single unilateral cyst. These cysts exist for a limited time and usually resolve in fetal life. They do not have any structural or functional significance of their own. Isolated unilateral choroid plexus cysts are also not indicative of a

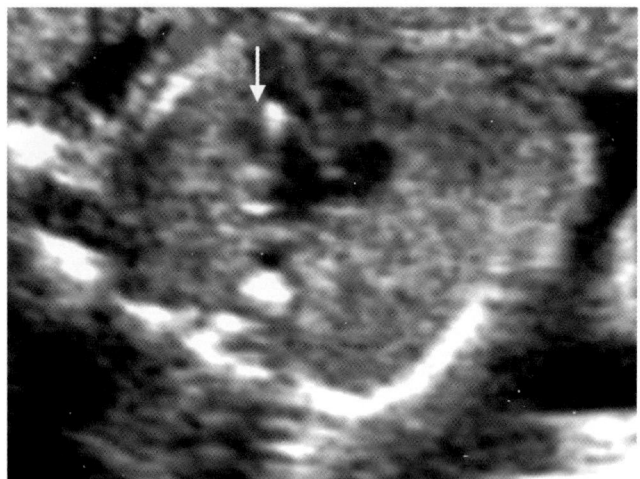

Fig. 23: Intracardiac echogenic focus.

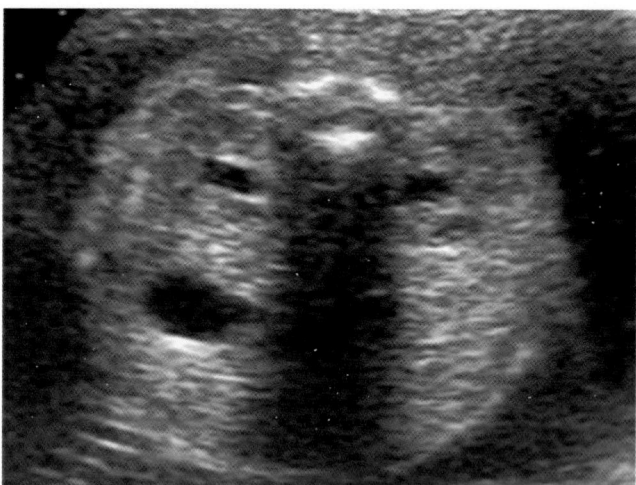

Fig. 25: Mild pyelectasis.

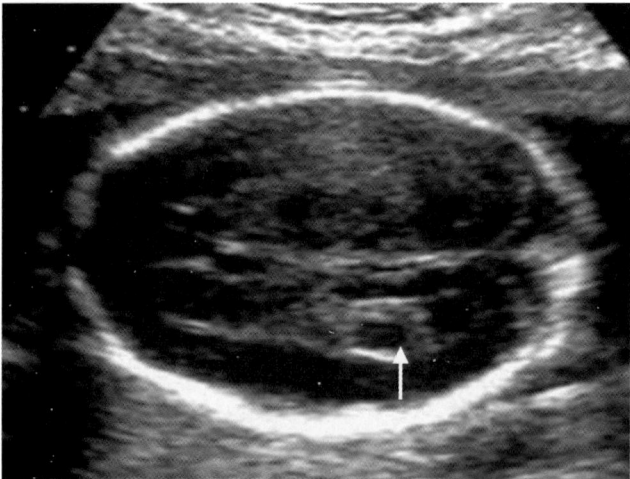

Fig. 24: Choroid plexus cyst.

higher risk of aneuploidy (trisomy 18). However, multiple cysts, bilateral cysts or their findings with other markers should prompt further investigations for aneuploidy.

Mild Pyelectasis (Fig. 25)

Pyelectasis is dilation of fetal renal pelvis and is commonly seen in second-trimester. Mild pyelectasis needs close follow-up. Mild pyelectasis is when renal pelvis is >4 mm and 10 mm.

■ SIGNIFICANCE OF SONOGRAPHIC MARKERS

The assessment of sonographic soft markers in the mid-trimester is also called the genetic sonogram. A well conducted genetic sonogram should describe the presence, absence, and/or appropriate measurements. Modern software give a numerical risk association with the soft markers. The possible results of a genetic sonogram are:

- *Absence of soft markers:* This is of value to reassure the woman that the risk of aneuploidies is low. The numerical risk of aneuploidies can be accurately adjusted. The resultant combined risk will be much lower than that assessed by age and/or biochemistry if normal soft markers are included. This can prevent unnecessary further investigations along the lines of aneuploidy detection.
- *Presence of an isolated soft marker:* The detection of a soft marker is an indication to look and relook at the fetal anatomy to ensure that there are no other soft markers and major structural defects. The isolated soft marker is a matter of controversy. Among the various soft markers, nuchal fold thickness and hyperechoic bowel have a higher predictive value for aneuploidies as compared to the other markers. Usually, the risk of aneuploidy is the same as the baseline age related risk that the woman carries. This risk can be further elucidated by using a quadruple or penta marker test. Today, noninvasive prenatal testing (NIPT) is the most sensitive screening test for aneuploidies and can be offered in such situations. It does have cost implications.

Presence of multiple soft markers: After a detailed structural evaluation, if there are more than one soft markers, an assessment should be made of the risk that this represents in terms of fetal chromosomal status. One of the methods of risk assessment is the index scoring system (ISS) described by Benacerraf et al. A score of 2 is assigned for structural defects and nuchal thickening (≥6 mm) and a score of 1 is assigned for the ultrasound markers echogenic intracardiac focus (EIF), echogenic bowel, pyelectasis, short femur, and short humerus. A score of 2 or more is considered positive. The authors reported a sensitivity of 73% (33 of 45 fetuses) for detecting trisomy 21, with a false-positive rate of only 4% (4 of 106 fetuses). Recent changes in the approach have better mathematical models integrated into the calculation, which has increased the sensitivity to 87% but at a cost of higher false positive rate of 27%. Nyberg et al. use a different approach called the age-adjusted ultrasound risk assessment (AAURA). This applies the likelihood ratios (LRs) from ultrasound markers to the a priori risk based on maternal age. The advantage of this more mathematically complex approach is a patient-specific risk assessment. By using a threshold of 1 in 200, this method has achieved a sensitivity of 74% (105 of 142) in a high-risk population.

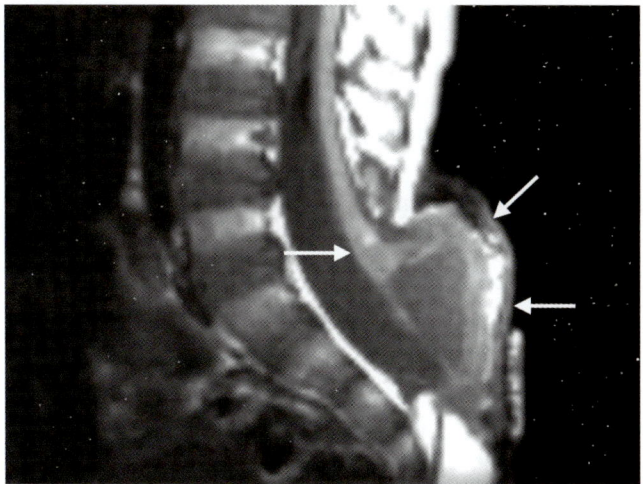

Fig. 26: Meningocele.

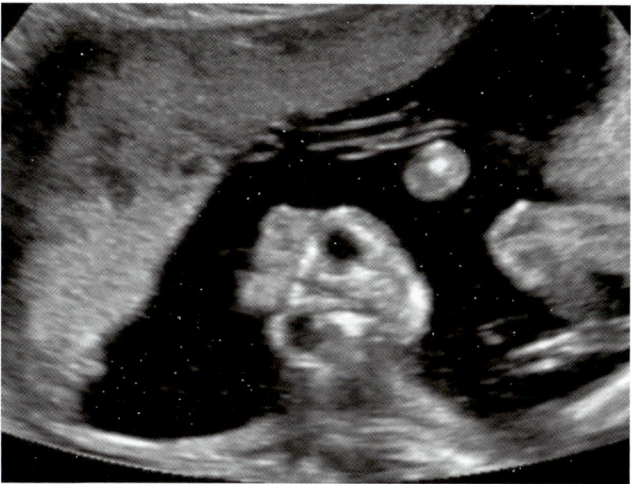

Fig. 27: Anencephaly.

SOME COMMON ANOMALIES

Neural Tube Defects

- Neural tube defects (NTDs) are the types of malformations.
- The most common neural defects are anencephaly, encephalocele/meningocele, and spina bifida **(Figs. 26 to 28)**.
- The incidence ranges from 1 to 5 per 1,000 births.
- Encephalocele and meningocele are defects of the skull.

In the former, brain tissue and meninges protrude through the defect of the skull, while in the latter only the meninges are affected. These defect of the skull can be detected with ultrasound.[17]

Anencephaly is the absence of a major portion of the skull and the brain hemispheres caused by an abnormal closure in the cranial part of the brain. Exencephaly is an early stage of anencephaly, when the brain is still present but is located outside the skull.[18]

Spina bifida is present when the spine does not close properly. There are two types based on what structures are affected:
1. *Occulta*: No protrusion, covered with skin
2. *Cystica:* Protrusion, covered or not covered **(Fig. 26)**
   - *Meningocele*: Contains meninges and cerebrospinal fluid **(Fig. 29)**
   - *Myelomeningocele:* Contains meninges, cerebrospinal fluid, and neural structures.

CONCLUSION

- Ultrasound alone cannot be used to diagnose aneuploidies or exclude aneuploidies.
- Any detection of soft markers on ultrasound need thorough evaluation and further investigations.
- Age of patient, background history, family history, and current ultrasound findings all should be taken into account. Patient should always be offered further testing when in doubt.
- Soft markers are extremely important for high-risk and elderly patients.

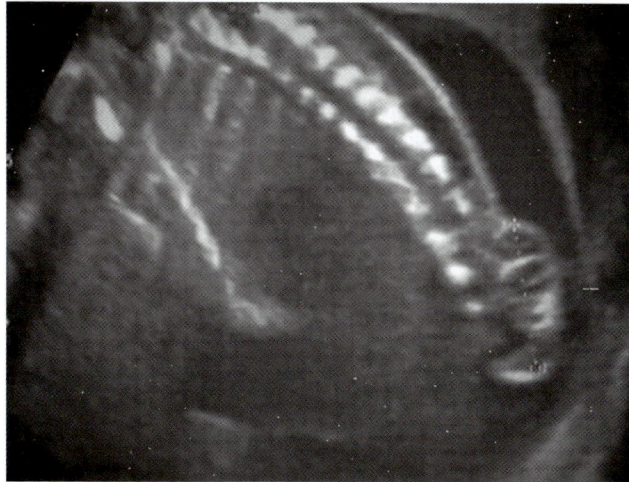

Fig. 28: Spina bifida.

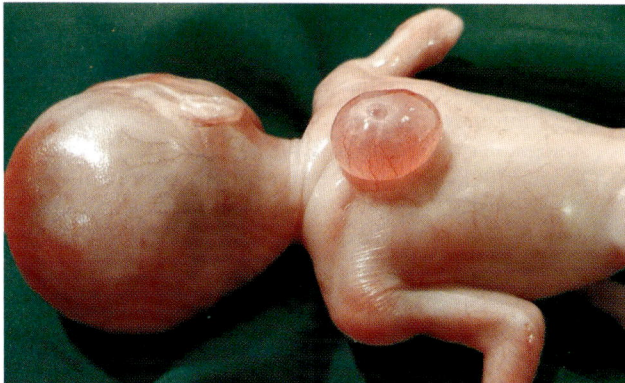

Fig. 29: Meningocele.

- Although there is ongoing debate regarding the clinical use of these markers in low-risk patients, their use in high-risk patients who have normal sonographic findings has been gaining momentum.

REFERENCES

1. ACOG Committee on Practice Bulletins. ACOG Practice Bulletin, No. 58. Ultrasonography in pregnancy. Obstet Gynecol. 2004;104(6):1449-58.

2. Seeds JW. The routine screening obstetrical ultrasound examination. Clin Obstet Gynecol. 1996;39(4):814-30.
3. Liu S, Joseph KS, Wen SW. Trends in fetal and infant deaths caused by congenital anomalies. Semin Perinatol. 2002;26(4):268-76.
4. Souka AP, Pilalis A, Kavalakis I, Antsaklis P, Papantoniou N, Mesogitis S, et al. Screening for major structural abnormalities at the 11- to 14- week ultrasound scan. Am J Obstet Gynecol. 2006;194(2):393-6.
5. Lantz ME, Chisholm CA. The preferred timing of second-trimester sonography based on maternal body mass index. J Ultrasound Med. 2004;23(8):1019-22.
6. Shipp TD, Benacerraf BR. Second trimester ultrasound screening for chromosomal abnormalities. Prenat Diagn. 2002;22(4):296-307.
7. Nyberg DA, Resta RG, Luthy DA, Hickok DE, Mahony BS, Hirsch JH. Prenatal sonographic findings of Down syndrome: review of 94 cases. Obstet Gynecol. 1990;76(3 Pt 1):370-7.
8. Benacerraf BR, Neuberg D, Bromley B, Frigoletto FD Jr. Sonographic scoring index for prenatal detection of chromosomal abnormalities. J Ultrasound Med. 1992;11(9):449-58.
9. Nicolaides K, Shawwa L, Brizot M, Snijders R. Ultrasonographically detectable markers of fetal chromosomal defects. Ultrasound Obstet Gynecol. 1993;3(1):56-9.
10. Nyberg DA, Souter VL, El-Bastawissi A, Young S, Luthhardt F, Luthy DA. Isolated sonographic markers for detection of fetal Down syndrome in the second trimester of pregnancy. J Ultrasound Med. 2001;20(10):1053-63
11. Yeo L, Guzman ER, Day-Salvatore D, Walters C, Chavez D, Vintzileos AM. Prenatal detection of fetal trisomy 18 through abnormal sonographic features. J Ultrasound Med. 2003;22(6):581-90.
12. Benacerraf BR, Frigoletto FD Jr, Laboda LA. Sonographic diagnosis of Down syndrome in the second trimester. Am J Obstet Gynecol. 1985;153(1):49-52.
13. Benacerraf BR, Frigoletto FD Jr. Soft tissue nuchal fold in the second-trimester fetus: standards for normal measurements compared with those in Down syndrome. Am J Obstet Gynecol. 1987;157(5):1146-9
14. Benacerraf BR, Nadel A, Bromley B. Identification of second-trimester fetuses with autosomal trisomy by use of a sonographic scoring index. Radiology. 1994;193(1):135-40.
15. Bromley B, Lieberman E, Benacerraf BR. The incorporation of maternal age into the sonographic scoring index for the detection at 14–20 weeks of fetuses with Down's syndrome. Ultrasound Obstet Gynecol. 1997;10(5):321-4.
16. Nyberg DA, Luthy DA, Williams MA, Winter TC. Genetic sonogram: computerized assessment of risk for Down syndrome based on obstetric US findings during the second trimester. Radiology. 1996;201:160.
17. Tóth Z. A magzat craniospinalis rendellenességei. In: Tóth Z, Papp Z (Eds). Szülészet-Nőgyógyászati Ultrahang-Diagnosztika. Budapest: White Golden Book Kft.; 2006. pp. 175-92.
18. Papp Z. A Szülészet-Nőgyógyászat Tankönyve. Budapest: Semmelweis Kiadó; 2007.

LONG QUESTIONS

1. What is the importance of second-trimester scan? What to look in the second-trimester scan?
2. What are the major and minor markers of aneuploidy?

SHORT QUESTIONS

1. What is "TIFFA"?
2. What do you mean by soft markers of aneuploidy?
3. Difference between nuchal fold thickness and nuchal translucency?
4. What is lemon sign and banana sign?

MULTIPLE CHOICE QUESTIONS

1. Ventriculomegaly is when ventricles are dilated to:
   a. >6 mm
   b. >10 mm
   c. >8 mm
   d. >9 mm
2. Nuchal fold measurement has a cutoff of:
   a. 4 mm
   b. 5 mm
   c. 6 mm
   d. 7 mm
3. Pyelectasis is when the renal pelvis is dilated to:
   a. >1 mm
   b. >2 mm
   c. >5 mm
   d. >10 mm
4. Ideally the second-trimester anomaly scan should be performed at:
   a. 14 weeks
   b. 16 weeks
   c. 20 weeks
   d. 26 weeks
5. The followings are useful in determination of gestational age, except:
   a. Nuchal thickness
   b. Transcerebellar diameter
   c. Biparietal diameter
   d. Interorbital distance
6. A correct section for measuring the abdominal circumference has the following characteristics, except:
   a. Shows fetal stomach
   b. Union of right and left portal vein
   c. Ribs are symmetric
   d. Gallbladder is visible
7. The echogenic bowel is seen in fetuses with the following disorders:
   a. Aneuploidy
   b. Sickle cell anemia
   c. Parvovirus infection
   d. Macrosomia
8. The following statement about choroid plexus cyst is correct:
   a. The fetus has a 2% risk of Down syndrome
   b. Choroid plexus cysts tend to disappear after a few weeks
   c. Neonates are at risk for hydrocephalus
   d. The presence of a choroid plexus cyst is an indication for amniocentesis

Answers
1. b 2. b 3. d 4. c 5. a 6. d
7. a 8. b

3.6 INVASIVE TESTS FOR FETAL DIAGNOSIS

Purnima Satoskar, Shilpa Agrawal

■ INTRODUCTION

Invasive prenatal testing involves obtaining a sample of fluid or tissue from the amniotic sac, placenta, or fetus in order to establish a diagnosis in selected pregnancies in which there is a high risk of fetal abnormality based on history or screening parameters.

■ INDICATIONS

The most common indications for prenatal testing are:
- Increased risk for fetal chromosome abnormalities:
  - Maternal age ≥35 years at estimated date of delivery
  - Positive maternal combined, dual, triple, or quadruple screen
  - Previous child with a chromosome abnormality
  - Chromosome rearrangement in a parent
- Increased risk for a detectable Mendelian disorder:
  - Affected child or family history
  - Positive carrier screen
- Structural fetal anomalies on ultrasound
- Increased risk for polygenic/multifactorial disorder such as neural tube defect:
  - Positive screen [e.g., elevated maternal serum alpha-fetoprotein (MSAFP)]
  - Abnormal ultrasound findings
  - Family history of the condition
- Teratogen exposure (e.g., valproic acid and neural tube defects).

The type of procedure available for diagnosis may depend upon the underlying condition being detected. For example, in cases of increased risk for fetal neural tube defects, chorionic villus sampling (CVS) is not an appropriate test as it cannot obtain amniotic fluid for the AFP and acetylcholinesterase analyses.

■ COUNSELING

Before any invasive tests, nondirective counseling is mandatory. Attitudes and choices of couples are variable and must be considered. Some factors affecting the decisions could be whether pregnancy resulted from the use of assisted reproductive technology after infertility or conceived spontaneously, previous affected children, number of living normal children, religious considerations, and cost of testing.[5]

Options available regarding invasive tests should be explained to the parents.

The discussion should include the risks and benefits of each option available including type of termination of pregnancy in case of abnormal results.

Parents should be made aware of the background risk of spontaneous pregnancy loss of 6–7%.[6]

In twins, particularly in dichorionic twin pregnancies, there is a possibility of discordant karyotypes and options available in that situation should also be discussed.[7]

The counseling should be documented in detail and signed by the patient (preferably couple) and the doctor.

■ PREREQUISITES FOR INVASIVE TESTS

- Detailed counseling and valid indication
- Written informed valid consent
- Maternal blood typing [unsensitized Rh negative patients are given Rh immune globulin (RhIG)]
- Testing for transmittable infections viz. human immunodeficiency virus (HIV), hepatitis B surface antigen, (HbsAg), and hepatitis C virus (HCV)
- Omit tablet aspirin at least 72 hours and low-molecular-weight heparin 24 hours prior to procedure
- Aseptic precautions in a sterile room to be followed
- Maternal abdomen cleaned and prepared with antiseptic solution
- Relative contraindications
- First trimester recent bleeding, abruptio placentae, incompetent cervix, and a history of premature labor.

■ AMNIOCENTESIS

History

Amniocentesis was first used as a blind procedure therapeutically for polyhydramnios and in Rh isoimmunization. It was described as a test of fetal sex determination for X-linked disorders in the 1950s.

In 1966, Steele and Breg successfully cultured fetal cells obtained from amniocentesis, allowing karyotyping of the chromosomes. Bang and Northeved were the first to perform ultrasound-guided amniocentesis in 1972.

Gestational Age

- Early <15 weeks.[1]
- Midtrimester.
- Late or third trimester.
- Genetic amniocentesis is preferably performed later than 15 weeks of gestation, usually between 16 and 18 weeks around 20 mL of amniotic fluid is aspirated.
- *Amniotic fluid composition*: Fetal urine, lung fluid, skin transudate, and water that is filtered across the amniotic membranes, containing electrolytes, proteins, and desquamated fetal cells (amniocytes). It is a source of amniocytes for cytogenetic and molecular analyses.

AFP, acetylcholinesterase, and bilirubin are some of the substances which can be biochemically analyzed.
- Results of fluorescent in situ hybridization (FISH) are usually available in 2 days, whereas results from cell culture take approximately up to 2 weeks.

Tests Done

- Tests on amniotic fluid:
  - Assessing fetal lung maturity—lecithin and sphingomyelin
  - To determine amniotic fluid AFP levels and acetylcholinesterase activity for the diagnosis of fetal open neural tube defects
  - Tests for bilirubin levels in Rh alloimmunization.
- Testing for genetic and chromosomal disorders on fetal cells extracted from amniotic fluid:
  - *Rapid testing*: Results available in 24–48 hours, specifically identifying:
    - Down syndrome (trisomy 21)
    - Edwards syndrome (trisomy 18)
    - Patau syndrome (trisomy 13)
    - Turner syndrome
    - Klinefelter syndrome
    - Other sex chromosome anomalies
    - Specific deletions, e.g., 22q.
  - Chromosome analysis after cell culture (results take about 7–14 days). This will give detailed karyotyping but even this will not identify all chromosomal abnormalities.
  - Other possible tests on fetal cells (appropriate genetic counseling may preclude the need).
  - Direct deoxyribonucleic acid (DNA) analysis techniques (e.g., for cystic fibrosis, thalassemia, Tay–Sachs disease, phenylketonuria, and Duchenne muscular dystrophy).
  - Indirect DNA analysis (e.g., to detect linkage disorders when the exact gene is unknown).
- Intra-amniotic infection to look for pathogenic bacteria.
- *Analysis to detect specific conditions from*: Enzymatic activity in amniocytes (e.g., Tay–Sachs disease) or fluid biochemistry (e.g., 17-OH-progesterone in congenital adrenal hyperplasia).

Procedure of Amniocentesis

- Ultrasound to select the site for needle puncture. Auscultate the fetal heart rate.
- Supine position with empty bladder.
- Abdomen is cleaned with povidone-iodine solution and draped.
- *Needle number*: 20–22 gauge.
- Ultrasound is done to detect number of fetuses, confirm gestational age, check fetal viability, document anatomy, and location of the placenta and cord insertion.
- *Site*: Avoid placenta. If placenta covers entire anterior uterine surface transplacental injection through thinnest part of placenta away from the cord insertion. Stay away from the fetal face and umbilical cord.
- *Antibiotics and tocolysis*: No supporting evidence but may choose to give.
- *Sedation/anesthesia*: Local anesthetic at the insertion site may be given though not mandatory. 1 mL of 1% or 2% lidocaine subcutaneously.
- *Anti D*: If Rh negative.
- *Sample taking*: Discard initial 1–2 mL to avoid maternal contamination.
- *Color of the fluid*: Normally clear.
- *If bloody*: Usual maternal in origin, in transplacental insertion.
- *Brown, dark red, or wine-colored-early intra-amniotic bleeding*: Pregnancy loss eventually occurs in one-third of the pregnancies.
- *Greenish*: Meconium in later gestation.
- Labeled and transported immediately to the genetic laboratory.
- *Post procedure*:
  - Check for the fetal heart rate and show to the mother.
  - Apply dry sterile dressing to the puncture site.
  - The mother should rest for half an hour in left lateral position after the procedure and then resume normal activities.
  - Strenuous exercise and sexual intercourse to be deferred for 48 hours.
  - Patient is asked to report immediately if fever, vaginal bleeding, fluid leakage, and uterine cramping.
  - *Complications*: Higher in the presence of first trimester bleeding or recurrent miscarriage, ultrasonographic demonstration of chorioamniotic separation, discolored amniotic fluid obtained, and/or unexplained elevated MSAFP.
- *Post-procedural loss rates of amniocentesis*: [2]
  - A total of 580 miscarriages occurred following 63,723 amniocentesis procedures. The weighted procedure-related risk of miscarriage following amniocentesis was 0.30%.

Early Amniocentesis

Early amniocentesis is associated with higher procedure-related pregnancy losses, ranging from 2.2–4.8%.

Prior to 15 weeks amniocentesis should be avoided due to higher rates of premature rupture of membranes (PROM), club foot, and amniocyte culture failures (2–5%) than late amniocentesis.

Third Trimester Amniocentesis

- Third trimester amniocentesis is technically easy and associated with less complications. Amniocentesis

later in pregnancy is usually performed for nongenetic indications, such as:
- To confirm fetal lung maturity
- Amnioreduction for severe polyhydramnios
- To confirm a diagnosis of preterm PROM (amniodye test)
- To exclude intra-amniotic infection
- To determine the karyotype with an undertaking from the patient that pregnancy is beyond legal limit of termination of the pregnancy.

Relative contraindications are abruptio placentae, incompetent cervix, placenta previa, and a history of premature labor.

■ CHORIONIC VILLUS SAMPLING

Chorionic villus sampling, also called placental biopsy, is an invasive procedure for prenatal diagnosis with the advantage of early pregnancy, often first trimester, diagnosis.

Gestational Age

Chorionic villus sampling is preferably performed between 10 and 13 weeks of gestation due to an association of CVS performed earlier than 10 weeks with fetal transverse limb abnormalities, micrognathia, and microglossia. Performing CVS after 11 weeks scan can enable screening for aneuploidy as well.

Techniques

Choosing the best approach to the chorion frondosum depends on its localization, the presence of disturbing elements such as fibroids, hyperstimulated ovaries, multiple abdominal scars, frozen pelvis, maternal obesity, and vaginal infections.

The relative filling of the bladder should also be optimized as a tool to significantly adjust the position of the uterus and thus ease of approach to the placenta. Usually an empty bladder is favored for a posterior placenta and a slightly filled bladder for an anterior placenta.

Chorionic villus sampling can be performed either freehand **(Fig. 1)** or with a needle guide. Different techniques used are discussed here.

Transabdominal Technique

The transabdominal approach is performed by inserting a 20-gauge needle (18-gauge after 13 weeks) transabdominally into the placenta under ultrasound guidance. The transabdominal method has the advantage that it can be performed later as well. Placentas especially suitable to the transabdominal approach include those located in the fundus or those located anteriorly in an anteflexed uterus. Transabdominal CVS is also an option in certain circumstances when transcervical sampling is contraindicated (e.g., active herpes or cervical lesions).

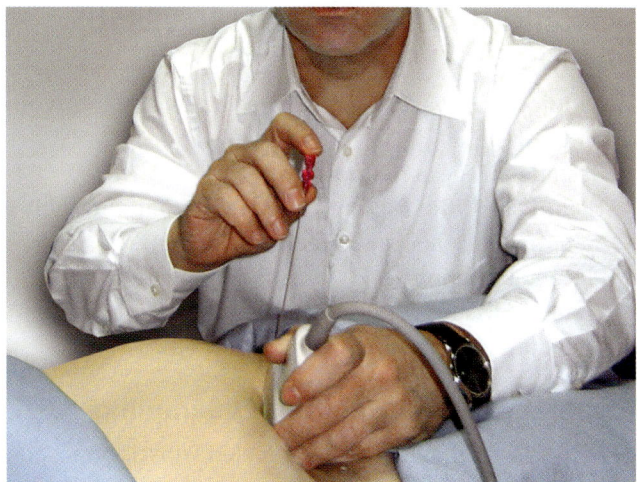

Fig. 1: Single needle and free-hand technique.

Local anesthesia is first given. Visualization of the needle helps to check that the track selected will be in line with the chorion frondosum. Continuous ultrasound guidance is then used to help guide the spinal needle into the chorionic frondosum, remaining parallel to the plate. Vacuum is created. The sample is then obtained by back-and-forth movement of the needle three to four times along the placenta while maintaining negative pressure, taking care to avoid the gestational sac. The needle tip is continuously kept in sight via the ultrasound image.

Transcervical Technique

The transcervical approach is performed most commonly using an aspiration CVS catheter which is inserted through the cervix under ultrasound guidance. The catheter is pliable and can be molded to the same angulation as the uterocervical angle prior to insertion. Alternatively a biopsy forceps appears to be a safe alternative. Absolute contraindications to transcervical CVS include active cervical or vaginal pathology (e.g., infection with herpes, Chlamydia, or gonorrhea). Relative contraindications include cervical canal obstructed by leiomyoma, bleeding from the vagina within 2 weeks of planned CVS, and a markedly retroverted, retroflexed uterus. It may be the favored route for a posterior low-lying placenta.

Transvaginal Chorionic Villus Sampling

Transvaginal CVS is rarely necessary in women having a retroverted retroflexed uterus with a posterior placenta as the only first trimester option.

While increased loss rates associated with the transcervical approach when compared with the transabdominal approach have been reported, the operator should be experienced in both techniques.

Post-procedural Loss Rates

The estimated risk of CVS-associated fetal loss in singletons varies widely (1.3–4.3%).

CHORIONIC VILLUS SAMPLING VERSUS AMNIOCENTESIS[3-5]

The choice of invasive technique for fetal karyotyping depends on:
- Gestational age at referral
- Technical difficulties of the specific patient such as maternal body habitus, scars, and fibroids
- Placental location
- Preferred tissue for the genetic test requested
- Clinicians' experience.

Advantages of Chorionic Villus Sampling

- Affords early diagnosis of an affected fetus as opposed to amniocentesis
- Allows the option for earlier termination of pregnancy
- Lower emotional trauma
- Lower rate of adverse clinical effects
- Early selective feticide in multiple pregnancy
- CVS, in the hands of experienced operators, is at least as safe as second trimester amniocentesis for prenatal diagnosis.[6]

Disadvantages of Chorionic Villus Sampling

- Potential contamination of sample by maternal cells.
- *Confined placental mosaicism*: Chromosomal mosaicism refers to the presence of two or more cell lines with different karyotypes in a single sample. In development, the mosaicism becomes generalized (present in the entire organism) or may be confined to a specific compartment (placenta, fetus, and specific fetal organ system), depending on when the improper chromosome segregation occurs, i.e., in meiosis, early postzygotic mitosis, or late postzygotic mitosis.

If in doubt, a second trimester amniocentesis should be performed.

Advantages of Amniocentesis

- It is technically easier and generally adopted as a safer option in technically challenging patients.
- Confusion due to confined placental mosaicism avoided.

GENETIC TESTS: HOW TO SELECT?[8]

In the most common indication for testing, i.e., an increased risk of aneuploidy based on a positive combined screen or quadruple marker test or noninvasive prenatal testing (NIPT) showing a high risk for aneuploidy, FISH and karyotype are the recommended tests.

Prenatal chromosomal microarray analysis is preferred for a patient with a fetus with one or more major structural abnormalities identified on ultrasonographic examination and who is undergoing invasive prenatal diagnosis. This test can replace the need for fetal karyotype, giving at least 5% increased diagnosis.

In a patient with a structurally normal fetus who is undergoing invasive prenatal diagnostic testing, either fetal karyotyping or a chromosomal microarray analysis can be performed [American College of Obstetricians and Gynecologists (ACOG) and Society for Maternal-Fetal Medicine (SMFM)].

In a previous affected fetus with a known mutation, Sanger sequencing can be done. There is insufficient evidence for clinical and whole exome sequencing for prenatal testing without a definite diagnosis due to the chances of detection variants of uncertain significance leading to difficulties in post-test counseling and subsequent decision making.

In uncertain diagnosis or results, it is a good idea to store DNA for future testing.

CORDOCENTESIS[9]

Cordocentesis [fetal blood sampling (FBS) percutaneous umbilical blood sampling (PUBS), funipuncture] is a procedure for sampling fetal blood from the umbilical cord by a needle that is inserted through the maternal abdominal wall under continuous ultrasonographic monitoring **(Fig. 2)**.

Direct access to the fetal vascular circulation allows improvement of prenatal diagnosis and therapy. Despite its advantages and high acceptance, FBS is relatively invasive and limited to the skilled perinatologist **(Table 1)**.

History

Cordocentesis was first performed by Fernand Daffos in the 1980s. In 1963, Liley was the first to treat fetal anemia by intraperitoneal transfusion of blood. In 1979, Rodeck and Campbell described the ability to perform FBS utilizing a fetoscopic approach, while in 1983, Daffos et al. introduced the technique of ultrasound-guided FBS. Newer, less invasive testing modalities and development of molecular genetic

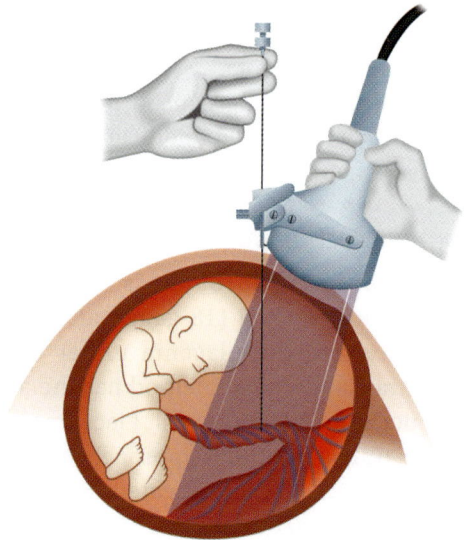

Fig. 2: Transabdominal ultrasound-guided fetal blood sampling in case of posterior placenta.

TABLE 1: Technical aspects of fetal blood sampling.

Prophylactic antibiotics	Insufficient evidence to recommend Centers to individualize
Maternal sedation	Used infrequently
Local anesthesia	Used by some centers
Skin preparation	Preprocedure antibacterial skin preparation and aseptic technique are recommended
Needle guidance	Both needle guide instrument and freehand techniques have been reported and are acceptable; direct needle into target (e.g., umbilical vein) under continuous ultrasound guidance; avoid umbilical arteries
Needle gauge and length	20- or 22-gauge; gauge and length depend on indication Suspicion of thrombocytopenia, gestational age, maternal body habitus, and distance from skin to target
Sampling site	Umbilical vein usually preferred, either at placental cord insertion or fetal cord insertion or free loop Intrahepatic vein Fetal heart (cardiocentesis)
Paralytic agent for transfusion	Pancuronium, atracurium, or vecuronium

(*Source:* Modified and Adapted from Resnik R, Lockwood CJ. Creasy and Resnik's Maternal-Fetal Medicine: Principles and Practice, 8th edition. Amsterdam: Elsevier; 2018.)

techniques have greatly decreased the need for FBS, but still it is an important test for prenatal diagnosis and therapy.

Indications

The most common indication in 1,320 cordocentesis performed between 1989 and 1999 was the fetal risk of thalassemia (61.1%) followed by rapid karyotyping (27.1%).[7]

Indications for cordocentesis may be diagnostic or therapeutic.

Fetal Anemia

Suspected severe fetal anemia is the most common current indication for FBS. Direct measurement of fetal hemoglobin and an accurate diagnosis of fetal anemia can only be made by FBS. Anemia may be suspected due to the presence of maternal alloantibodies, maternal parvovirus exposure or infection, other viral infections, or due to ultrasound findings such as fetal hydrops or abnormal color Doppler. Maternal anti-D alloimmunization is the most common cause of fetal anemia.

Measurement of the peak systolic velocity (PSV) by Doppler velocimetry of the fetal middle cerebral artery (MCA) is a sensitive tool to detect fetal anemia. An MCA-PSV of ≥1.5 multiples of the median is generally considered indicative of moderate or severe fetal anemia and FBS is warranted to directly measure fetal hemoglobin (or hematocrit) levels and determine the need for intrauterine transfusion.[10]

Thrombocytopenia

The diagnosis of fetal thrombocytopenia caused by neonatal alloimmune thrombocytopenia (NAIT) in the current pregnancy can only be made with FBS.

Neonatal alloimmune thrombocytopenia is a disorder in which transplacental passage of maternal antiplatelet antibodies causes fetal (and neonatal) thrombocytopenia. Severe fetal thrombocytopenia as a result of alloimmune thrombocytopenia may lead to cerebral hemorrhage before, during, or after birth and may cause mental handicap or death. Currently, maternal intravenous immunoglobulin, sometimes in conjunction with corticosteroids, is administered to increase the fetal platelet count. FBS can be used to assess the response to maternal therapy provided benefits outweigh the risks of FBS and if vaginal delivery is considered.

Fetal Hydrops

Fetal anemia is one of the most common causes of hydrops. The differential diagnosis of fetal hydrops is extensive but anemia, aneuploidy, and infection are relatively common causes. Initial workup of hydrops involves maternal serum analyses, detailed ultrasound examination, and fetal MCA-PSV. FBS is offered for investigation of nonimmune hydrops, especially if the rest of the workup is negative and the fetal MCA-PSV is elevated.

Chromosomal Abnormalities

White blood cells divide at a rapid rate (48–72 hours) and providing rapid chromosomal diagnosis with good banding. Because of the risks associated with FBS, it is rarely used in current practice and is largely replaced by CVS or amniocentesis with FISH, or by NIPT. If at all used, the indications are possible mosaicism, culture failure after either amniocentesis or placental biopsy, and woman who seeks care late in pregnancy.

Single Gene Defects

It includes mainly diagnosis of hemoglobinopathies, coagulopathies, severe combined immunodeficiency, chronic granulomatous disease, and some metabolic disorders.[6] Usually they are diagnosed earlier in gestation by applying various DNA techniques to chorionic villi or amniocytes. FBS is important for at-risk patients who seek care late in pregnancy and when DNA analysis is not possible.

Inherited Anemias or Hemoglobinopathies

With the advent of modern molecular genetic techniques, fetal diagnosis can reliably be made using DNA obtained via CVS or amniocentesis.[10] Where sophisticated molecular techniques are unavailable and hemoglobinopathies relatively common, FBS continues to be routinely used in the diagnosis of alpha- and beta-thalassemia.

Hypoxia and Acidosis

Suspected fetal hypoxia or acidemia can be confirmed or refuted by fetal blood gas analysis. Fetal acidemia may be excluded by Doppler studies of the fetal vasculature. Increasing evidence shows that chronic fetal acidemia is associated with impaired long-term neurodevelopment, but applications are mainly in a research setting due to its invasive nature.

Fetal Infection

Appropriate fetal blood tests [e.g., infection-specific fetal immunoglobulin M (IgM) or detection of specific genomic material by polymerase chain reaction (PCR)] can determine whether maternal infection has led to fetal infection. Amniotic fluid culture and/or PCR are currently the primary diagnostic modalities. If amniotic fluid is positive, FBS is indicated to assess risk of symptomatic infection in the fetus. Termination of pregnancy can be offered if FBS shows infection. In settings in which PCR is not readily available, FBS has been used for diagnosis, for example in rare cases of fetal varicella with measurement of varicella-zoster virus-specific IgM and viral culture.[12]

Monitoring of Transplacental Therapy

Some fetal diseases are treated by drugs that are given to the mother, cross the placenta, and achieve therapeutic concentrations in the fetus. Examples include antiarrhythmic agents to correct fetal tachyarrhythmias, packed cells to correct anemia, and γ-globulin to improve low fetal platelet counts. An accurate assessment of placental transfer and monitoring of the success of therapy may require FBS.

Fetal Therapy

Access to the fetal circulation offers the possibility of infusing biologic (e.g., blood transfusion) or pharmacologic agents for therapeutic purposes.

There are limited conditions for which a single dose of a medication is useful, and serial or chronic intravascular fetal therapy cannot be done in practice. Fetal hydrops due to supraventricular tachycardia, where transplacental therapy is less effective and a single injection may resolve the arrhythmia. In general, FBS has rarely been used for medical therapy other than transfusions or refractory arrhythmia, and evidence for its benefits is lacking.

Multiple Gestation

In multiple gestations, in which one of the fetuses is abnormal, cordocentesis is also applied for selective termination by potassium chloride injection, which causes cardiac arrest.

Postprocedural Fetal Loss Rates

The procedure-related fetal loss rate of 1.3% is reported. The overall success rate of FBS is high, and blood samples can be obtained in >98% of patients. Counseling for FBS should include discussion about the potential risk of FBS that may include, but may not be limited to: bleeding from puncture site (20–30%); fetal bradycardia (5–10%); pregnancy loss (≥1.3%); and vertical transmission of hepatitis or human immunodeficiency virus. FBS should be performed by experienced operators at centers with expertise in invasive fetal procedures.

Complications of Cordocentesis

- Fetal death
- Bradycardia
- Amnionitis
- Cord hematoma
- Umbilical cord bleeding
- Fetomaternal hemorrhage
- Premature rupture of membranes
- Preterm labor
- Abruptio placentae
- Risk of emergency cesarean section
- Failure to obtain sample.

SPECIAL CONSIDERATIONS IN MULTIPLE PREGNANCY

Chorionic Villus Sampling

Chorionic villus sampling can be tricky in multiple pregnancy with a need to carefully scan the placental locations of each fetus and plan needle entry to minimize error in sampling.

About 2–3% of twin pregnancies having CVS will need resampling because of cross contamination or uncertainty of results.

Measures to reduce cross contamination in multiple pregnancy include:

- Taking the CVS sample near the placental cord insertion for each fetus
- Avoiding the inter twin membrane
- Combined transabdominal and transcervical approach.

Two or more samplings during one procedure have been linked to increased risk of postprocedural miscarriage, implying that the risk may be higher in twin sampling.

In multiple gestation, amniocentesis can be done safely. The rates of pregnancy loss are slightly higher due to the need for two needles insertions. Mapping of twins with respect to position with respect to mother and placental location is very important. Injection of indigo carmine in sampled sac is useful to avoid sampling the same sac twice.

Fetal Bladder Tapping

In fetuses with lower urinary tract obstruction (LUTO), where both kidneys show abnormalities and there is oligohydramnios, placement of vesicoamniotic shunt may help selected fetuses avoid pulmonary hypoplasia resulting from oligohydramnios. The decision to place a shunt depends upon assessment of renal function by urinalysis. Only if renal function is preserved, a shunt may improve prognosis.[11]

The first bladder tap consists of stagnant urine which may not reflect the true levels of urinary components but may be sent for karyotype as it contains fetal cells which can be cultured. The second bladder tap in about 48 hours should be analyzed **(Table 2)**.

Fetal Tissue Biopsy[12]

The concept of ultrasound-guided fetal biopsy as a means for prenatal diagnosis was initially described in the 1970s. This procedure is used to detect hereditary conditions of the fetus that cannot be identified through more conventional methods such as amniocentesis or CVS of the placenta. For example, fetal skin biopsy permits patients who carry an abnormal gene for a severe skin disease to have a pregnancy with the knowledge of whether or not their fetus is similarly affected.

The biopsy is usually performed between 18 and 20 weeks of gestation when skin is well formed. A small amount of intravenous sedation (e.g., diazepam) is used for the mother, if needed. A local anesthetic is used to anesthetize the maternal skin. A sheath (trocar) is inserted into the mother's abdomen and through the gestational sac to reach the fetus under continuous ultrasonic guidance. The trocar permits passage of biopsy forceps that is used to obtain a fetal skin sample from the thorax, back, buttocks, or sometimes the scalp. By sampling fetal liver or muscle other diseases can also be similarly diagnosed. Biopsies of the fetal liver or muscle are performed using a thin needle (typically 16 gauge).

Skin conditions diagnosed by fetal skin biopsy:
- Epidermolysis bullosa
- Ichthyotic disorders
- Oculocutaneous albinism
- Ectodermal dysplasia syndromes.

Results and Risks

Tissue specimens can be analyzed by using light and electron microscopy as well as with a variety of other tests such as enzymes. Fetal tissue biopsies are used to detect skin disorders such as pigment cell disorders, bullous disease, and problems with proper development of epidermal appendages (e.g., ectodermal dysplasias). Over time, fetal tissue biopsies will become less common by using next-generation sequencing (NGS) clinical exome studies to identify mutations by DNA analysis of amniotic fluid, placental tissue, or possibly fetal cells in the maternal circulation. For example, by the discovery of specific gene mutations, the prenatal diagnosis of ornithine transcarbamylase deficiency has recently been made easier. Although this discovery now allows the prenatal diagnosis of this disease by DNA analysis of amniotic fluid or placental tissue, there are still some cases where conventional DNA studies will not be informative for the detected mutation. Fetal liver biopsy could then be used as an alternative diagnostic test.

The main risks associated with fetal tissue biopsies are spontaneous miscarriage, infection, preterm delivery, and possible hemorrhage. In experienced centers, the incidence of fetal loss from skin biopsy has been reported to be <5%.

Fetoscopy

Fetoscopy is a minimally invasive technique for fetal diagnosis and therapy allowing direct visualization of fetus and placenta and membranes **(Fig. 3)**. It requires skills of ultrasonography combined with endoscopy, supportive services including operation theatre, anesthesia, and diagnostic laboratory. Visualization of fetal external body parts **(Fig. 4)**, umbilical cord, placental sinuses, and vessels are quite clear and satisfactory with endoscopes of 2-mm diameter.[13] The applications of endoscopy began with FBS and various fetal biopsies and have now been extended to endoscopic procedures for congenital diaphragmatic hernia and meningomyelocele repair in specialized centers.

TABLE 2: Cut-off values of urinary components of fetal urine on second bladder tap that predict good renal function.

Parameter	Common units	SI Units	Other units
Sodium	<100 mEq/L	<100 mmol/L	<230 mg/dL
Chloride	<90 mEq/L	<90 mmol/L	<319.5 mg/dL
Calcium	<4 mEq/L	<2 mmol/L	<8 mg/dL
Osmolarity	<210 mOsm/L	<210 mOsm/L	–
β2-Microglobulin	<10 mg/L	<0.01 g/L	<1 mg/dL
Total protein	<20 mg/dl	<0.2 g/L	<200 mg/L

(*Source*: Sharma S, Joshi M, Gupta DK, Abraham M, Mathur P, Mahajan JK, et al. Consensus on the management of posterior urethral valves from antenatal period to puberty. J Indian Assoc Pediatr Surg. 2019; 24(1):4-14.)

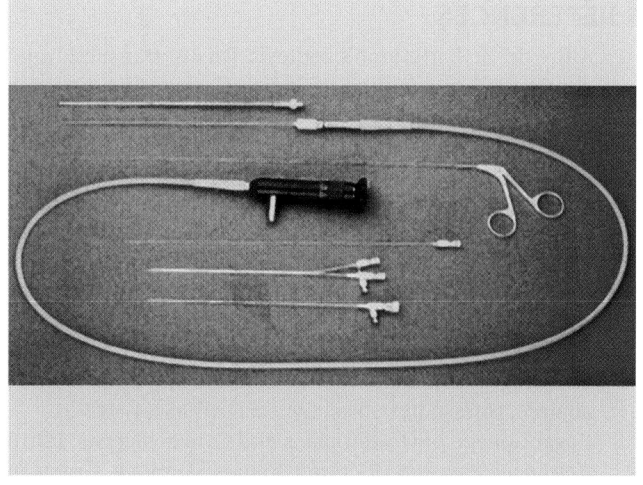

Fig. 3: Fetoscope.

156 **PART 1:** Obstetrics and Perinatology

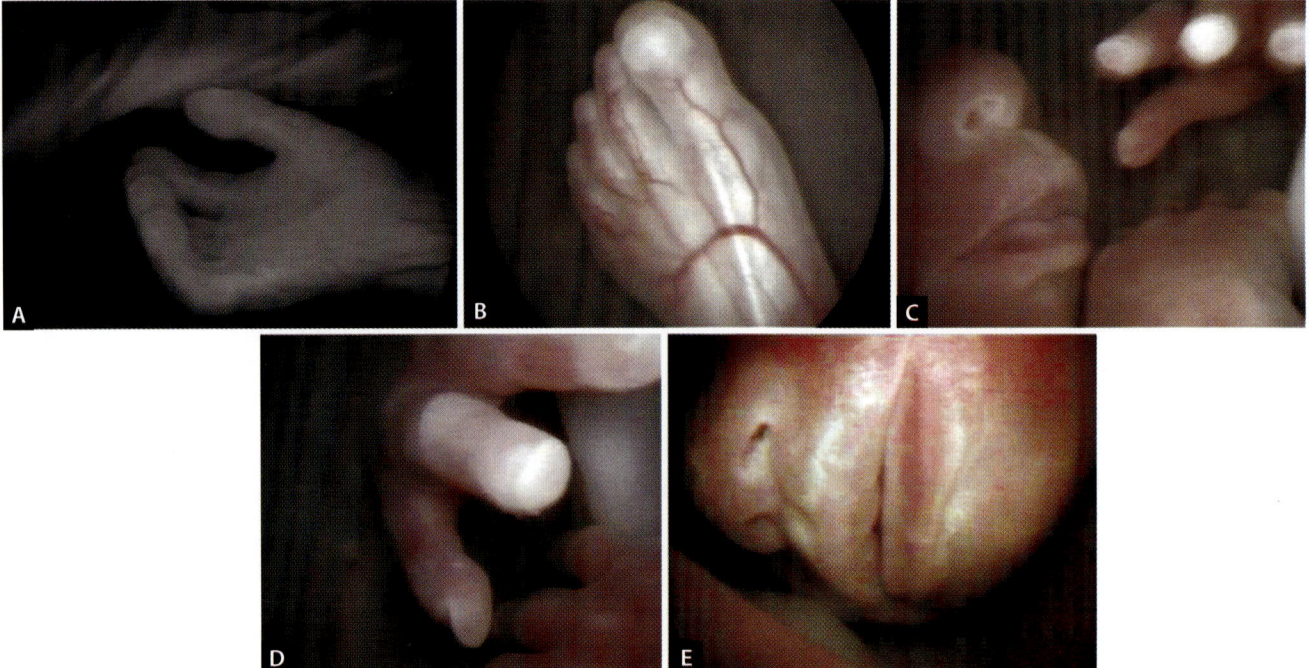

Figs. 4A to E: Fetal imaging through fetoscopy.

Laser ablation of vascular anastomosis in twin-to-twin transfusion has the best fetal salvage rate for the condition.

CONCLUSION

Invasive tests for fetal diagnosis consist of chorionic villus biopsy, amniocentesis, PUBS (cordocentesis), and fetal biopsies.

These tests enable confirmation of a genetic diagnosis or pathological condition in a high risk fetus. Appropriate counseling regarding the indication, options and steps of the procedure, risks and benefits by a fetal medicine specialist, and informed consent is advisable prior to invasive fetal testing. There is a risk of pregnancy loss of 0.5–4% depending upon the procedure. Invasive fetal testing plays a very important role in obtaining a clear diagnosis and guide further decision making in an at-risk fetus.

REFERENCES

1. Alfirevic Z. Early amniocentesis versus transabdominal chorion villus sampling for prenatal diagnosis. Cochrane Database Syst Rev. 2000;(2):CD000077.
2. Antsaklis A, Papantoniou N, Xygakis A, Mesogitis S. Genetic amniocentesis in women 20–34 years old: associated risks. Prenat Diagn. 2000;20:247-50.
3. Alfirevic Z, Mujezinovic F, Sundberg K. Amniocentesis and chorionic villus sampling for prenatal diagnosis. Cochrane Database Syst Rev. 2003;(3):CD003252.
4. Salomon LJ, Sotiriadis A, Wulff CB, Odibo A, Akolekar R. Risk of miscarriage following amniocentesis or chorionic villus sampling: systematic review of literature and updated meta-analysis. Ultrasound Obstet Gynecol. 2019;54(4):442-51.
5. Royal College of Obstetricians and Gynaecologists. (2010). Amniocentesis and Chorionic Villous Sampling. Green-top Guideline No. 8. [online] Available from: https://www.rcog.org.uk/globalassets/documents/guidelines/gtg_8.pdf. [Last accessed October, 2021].
6. Evans MI, Wapner RJ. Invasive prenatal diagnostic procedures 2005. Semin Perinatol. 2005;29(4):215-8.
7. Tongsong T, Wanapirak C, Kunavikatikul C, Sirirchotiyakul S, Piyamongkol W, Chanprapaph P. Cordocentesis at 16–24 weeks of gestation: experience of 1,320 cases. Prenat Diagn. 2000;20(3):224-8.
8. Committee on Genetics and the Society for Maternal-Fetal Medicine. Committee Opinion No.682: Microarrays and next-generation sequencing technology: the use of advanced genetic diagnostic tools in obstetrics and gynecology. Obstet Gynecol. 2016;128:e262-8.
9. Society for Maternal-Fetal Medicine (SMFM); Berry SM, Stone J, Norton ME, Johnson D, Berghella V. Fetal blood sampling. Am J Obstet Gynecol. 2013;209(3):170-80.
10. Mari G, Deter RL, Carpenter RL. Noninvasive diagnosis by Doppler ultrasonography of fetal anemia due to maternal red-cell alloimmunization. N Engl J Med. 2000;342:9-14.
11. Sharma S, Joshi M, Gupta DK, Abraham M, Mathur P, Mahajan JK, et al. Consensus on the management of posterior urethral valves from antenatal period to puberty. J Indian Assoc Pediatr Surg. 2019;24(1):4-14.
12. Cadrin C, Golbus MS. Fetal tissue sampling—indications, techniques, complications, and experience with sampling of fetal skin, liver, and muscle. West J Med. 1993;159(3):269-72.
13. Deka D, Dadhwal V, Gajatheepan SB. The art of fetoscopy: a step toward minimally invasive fetal therapy. J Obstet Gynaecol India. 2012;62(6):655-9.

LONG QUESTIONS

1. Discuss pros and cons of various invasive tests to rule out aneuploidy.
2. Describe various routes and procedure of chorionic villous sampling.

3. Describe complications of invasive testing and discuss how they can be minimized.

SHORT QUESTIONS

1. Write short note on genetic tests on amniotic fluid.
2. Write short note on cordocentesis.
3. Write short note on fetal biopsy.

MULTIPLE CHOICE QUESTIONS

1. Which of the following diagnostic techniques is of no value for the diagnosis of neural tube defects?
    a. Amniocentesis
    b. Chorion villus sampling (CVS)
    c. Maternal serum screening
    d. Ultrasonography
2. Which test is recommended for early diagnosis of Down syndrome if one of the parents is carrying a 14/21 translocation?
    a. CVS at 9 weeks with karyotyping
    b. CVS at 9 weeks with FISH
    c. CVS at 11 weeks with karyotyping
    d. CVS at 11 weeks with FISH
3. The most common approach for intrauterine transfusion is:
    a. Umbilical artery at placental insertion of cord
    b. Umbilical artery at fetal insertion of cord
    c. Umbilical vein at placental insertion of cord
    d. Umbilical vein at fetal insertion of cord
4. The recommendation for genetic testing for structurally anomalous fetus on amniotic fluid is:
    a. FISH and karyotype
    b. Chromosomal microarray
    c. Store DNA
    d. Karyotype is sufficient
5. Which of the following is an unlikely complication of amniocentesis?
    a. Leaking PV
    b. Fetal bradycardia
    c. Chorioamnionitis
    d. Bloody tap
6. A patient undergoes chorionic villous sampling for a positive combined screening for Down syndrome. The report shows normal/trisomy 21 mosaicism. What advice will you give?
    a. Repeat CVS immediately
    b. Final decision after anomaly scan
    c. Amniocentesis and karyotype at 16 weeks
    d. Terminate the pregnancy in view of trisomy 21
7. A G2P1 Rh negative with previous LSCS has an Rh antibody titer of 1:64. Middle cerebral artery peak systolic velocity (MCA PSV) is 2 MoM. How will you proceed?
    a. Repeat MCA PSV in 2 weeks
    b. Repeat MCA PSV in 1 week
    c. Amniocentesis for spectrophotometry
    d. Cordocentesis and transfusion
8. Dual marker test in a primigravida is high risk for trisomy 21 in a pair of diamniotic dichorionic twins at 13 weeks. Placenta is fused and posterior reaching os. How will you proceed?
    a. Repeat the test to rule out erroneous report
    b. Proceed with chorionic villous sampling by combined transabdominal and transvaginal approach
    c. Advise amniocentesis from each sac
    d. Choice of B and C after full counseling about pros and cons
9. A patient with previous beta-thalassemia major child presents at 19 weeks. What test will you advise?
    a. Placental biopsy
    b. Amniocentesis
    c. Cordocentesis
    d. Too late for testing
10. NIPT done in a primigravida shows high risk for Turner syndrome. What will you advise?
    a. Explain features of Turner and offer termination
    b. Explain features of Turner and advise continuation if anomaly scan rules out coarctation of aorta
    c. Confirm with amniocentesis and karyotyping
    d. Can proceed with termination due to very high sensitivity of the test

Answers										
1. b	2. c	3. c	4. b	5. b	6. c					
7. d	8. d	9. c	10. c							

3.7 ANTEPARTUM FETAL SURVEILLANCE TESTS IN THIRD TRIMESTER

Shailesh Kore, Mansi Medhekar

INTRODUCTION

The ultimate aim of antepartum fetal surveillance is prevention of fetal demise and avoidance of unnecessary interventions.

Techniques used for fetal assessment in third trimester are:

- Nonstress test (NST)
- Biophysical profile (BPP)
- Modified BPP
- Contraction stress test (CST), and
- Fetal kick count.

ASSESSMENT OF AMNIOTIC FLUID VOLUME AND DOPPLER VELOCIMETRY ON ULTRASOUND

It is important to understand that when the fetus responds to a slowly progressive (chronic) hypoxemia it undergoes a series of physiological adaptation, which not picked up clinically or via tests like NST or ultrasound at a correct time, it may lead to physiological decompensation and undesirable outcome.[1,2]

Regular fetal antepartum testing usually fails to identify fetuses at risk of death from an acute hypoxemic insult, such as a placental abruption, and therefore it is practically impossible to prevent these fetal deaths.

GOAL

The aim of antepartum fetal assessment is to prevent the adverse outcomes such as intrauterine death or neurologic complications of intrauterine hypoxia by timely noninvasive intervention.

INDICATIONS FOR FETAL SURVEILLANCE

The American College of Obstetricians and Gynecologists (ACOG) recommends antepartum testing for "pregnancies in which the risk of antepartum fetal demise is increased".[3]

Common clinical settings in which antepartum fetal testing is indicated are as follows:
- *Diabetes:* Pregestational diabetes or gestational diabetes treated with oral hypoglycemic drug (OHD) or insulin. Women with gestational diabetes in which glucose levels are normal on nutritional therapy, antepartum fetal testing can be omitted
- *Hypertensive disorders*: Chronic hypertension or pregnancy-associated hypertension
- Fetal growth restriction
- Twin pregnancy
- Post-term pregnancy
- Decreased fetal activity
- Systemic lupus erythematosus
- Antiphospholipid syndrome
- Sickle cell disease
- Alloimmunization
- Oligohydramnios or polyhydramnios
- Prior fetal demise
- *Preterm premature rupture of membranes*: The goal of antenatal testing in this setting is early recognition of intra-amniotic infection necessitating delivery
- Advanced maternal age and obesity
- *Other*: Nonimmune hydrops, maternal cyanotic heart disease, poorly controlled maternal hyperthyroidism, and maternal vascular diseases are associated with an increased risk of fetal demise.

FETAL MOVEMENT COUNTING

Fetal movement kick count is the only antenatal surveillance technique recommended for all pregnant women, even with low risk factors. It is based on maternal awareness of fetal movements.

Decreased placental perfusion and fetal acidemia and acidosis are associated with decreased fetal movements.[4] This is the basis for maternal monitoring of fetal movements or "the fetal movement count test". It requires no technology and is available to all women.

A variety of methods have been described which are as follows:
- The Cardiff method, first reported by Pearson and Weaver suggests a count to 10 movements in a fixed time frame **(Fig. 1)**. The original study required counting for 12 hours. Patient is instructed to start counting movements in morning and note the time when she count 10 movements. If 10 movements are counted in 10–12 hours or less, then fetus is likely in good health. Modified protocols include those of Liston (count to 6 hours)[5] and Moore (count to 2 hours).[6]
- The Sadovsky method suggests a count of movements in a specific time frame (usually 30 minutes to 2 hours).[7]

Though, simple and effective, literature has produced contradictory results about its clinical utility in preventing late fetal deaths.

NONSTRESS TEST

The most commonly used method of antepartum fetal assessment is NST. The NST may be performed with or without sonographic assessment of amniotic fluid volume (AFV). When using AFV assessment, the deepest vertical pocket of fluid, rather than the amniotic fluid index (AFI), may be associated with fewer unnecessary interventions without an increase in adverse perinatal outcomes.[3]

The difference between NST and CST is that the former is primarily a test of fetal condition and the latter is a test of uteroplacental function.

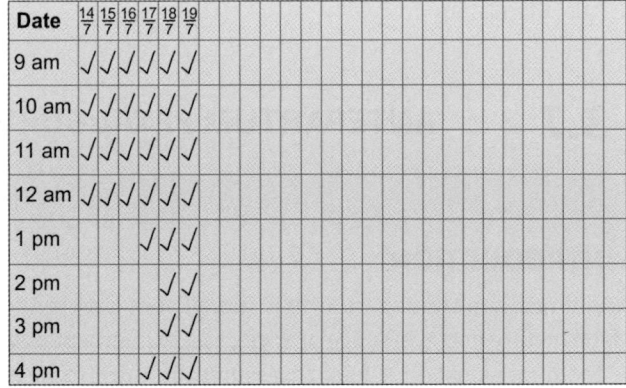

Fig. 1: Cardiff's chart of fetal movement count.

The fetal heart rate (FHR) is normally increased or decreased by autonomic influences mediated by sympathetic or parasympathetic impulses from brainstem center.[8] The NST is based on the hypothesis that the heart rate of a nonhypoxic, nonacidotic fetus will temporarily accelerate in response to fetal movement.

Technique

Nonstress test is performed during the late antenatal period, before the women goes in labor. The uterus is relaxed and the fetus is not exposed to the "stress" of uterine contractions.

The woman should empty her bladder and be positioned on either a bed or a reclining chair in the left lateral recumbent position.[6]

Patient's blood pressure may be taken every 10 or 15 minutes during the procedure because supine hypertension may cause a nonreactive result.

An external transducer is wrapped on the maternal abdomen, over the location of the fetal heart sound (FHS), anterior shoulder being most common, using a coupling jelly. This transducer usually works on principle of Doppler ultrasound.

Another connection to the recording machine is a device for recording fetal movement which is given in patient's hand. Patient is instructed to push the calibration button every time she feels fetal movement.

The FHR tracing is recorded on a standard heat sensitive paper by means of the recording machine. The speed of paper movement should be adjusted to 1 cm/minute. Volume setting of the machine is adjusted such that even patient also can hear fetal heart sounds.

Reactive and Nonreactive Tests

Criteria

The NST is reactive from 32 weeks to term if there are two or more FHR accelerations reaching a peak of at least 15 beats per minute (bpm) above the baseline rate and lasting at least 15 seconds from onset to return to baseline (15 × 15) in a 20-minute period **(Fig. 2)**.[3,9,10]

Before 32 Weeks of Gestation

Before 32 weeks of gestation, a reactive NST may be defined as two accelerations that rise at least 10 bpm above baseline and have a duration of at least 10 seconds (10 × 10).[10]

Due to immaturity of autonomous nervous system in preterm fetuses, acceleratory response to fetal movement is less causing high possibility of false positive result. Hence, these criteria may not be applicable in interpretation of the NST in the premature fetus.

Minimal Duration of Fetal Heart Rate Monitoring

The recommended optimal duration that an NST should be continued is at least for 20 minutes. If the fetal heart acceleratory response does not meet the criteria after 20 minutes of testing, the recording should continue for another 20 minutes.

If there is no acceleration with spontaneous or repeated external stimuli during a 40-minute period, the test is considered *nonreactive* **(Fig. 3)**.

Nonreactivity may be a sign of disruption of fetal oxygenation to the point of metabolic acidosis. Other possible causes of a nonreactive NST include fetal immaturity, fetal sleep, maternal smoking, fetal neurologic or cardiac anomalies, sepsis, or maternal ingestion of drugs with cardiac effects.[11]

Following steps need to be taken if an NST is nonreactive:
- Repeat the test in 30 minutes
- Perform vibroacoustic stimulation to elicit accelerations: The ACOG recommends placing the vibroacoustic stimulation device on the maternal abdomen and applying a stimulus for 1–2 seconds.[3] If no fetal response

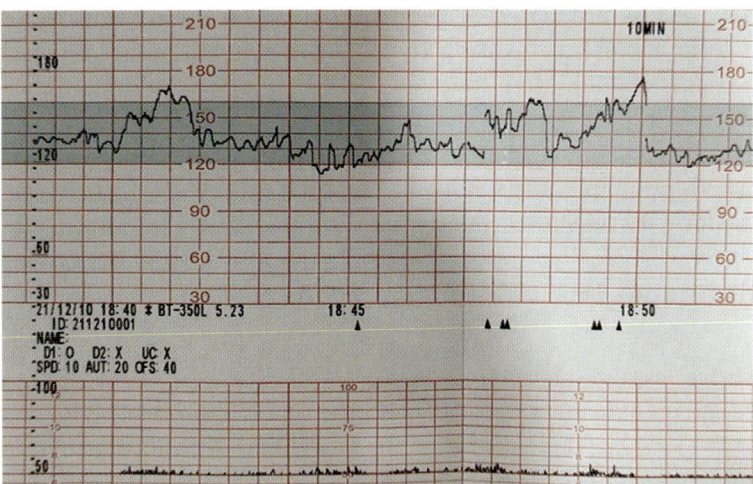

Fig. 2: Reactive nonstress test (NST).

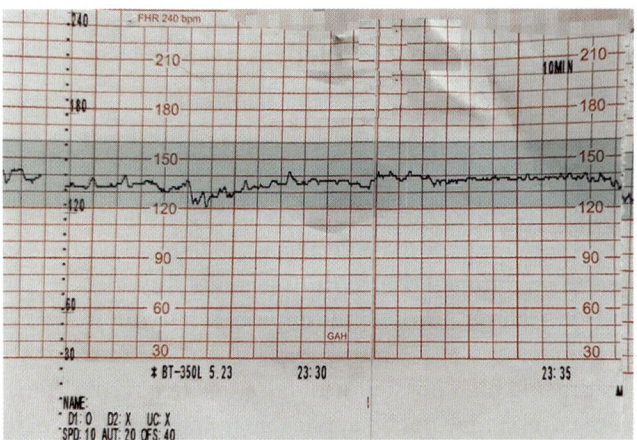

Fig. 3: Nonreactive nonstress test (NST).

occurs, the stimulus may be repeated up to three times for progressively longer durations of up to 3 seconds.
- Perform a back-up test (either CST or complete BPP).
- Before repeating it is prudent to modify factors potentially causing nonreactive results (e.g., smoking).

Reactive Nonstress Tests with Decelerations

The main reason behind FHR decelerations during the NST are variable decelerations, indicating transient episodes of umbilical cord compression. The significance of a reactive NST with FHR decelerations is not very clear.

The ACOG (2007) has concluded that variable decelerations, if nonrepetitive and brief—<30 seconds—do not indicate fetal compromise or the need for any intervention. However, repetitive variable decelerations—at least three in 20 minutes—even if mild or decelerations lasting 1 minute or longer have been shown to have bad prognosis.

Such decelerations may require further evaluation, which might include extended FHR and uterine activity monitoring, ultrasound assessment of fetal growth and anatomy, BPP, AFV, and/or Doppler velocimetry. Management decisions should be guided by the results of the additional evaluation and other details specific to the clinical situation.

In most cases, a normal NST is predictive of good perinatal outcome for at least 1 week (providing the maternal-fetal condition remains stable). More frequent testing is necessary for women with post-term pregnancy, multifetal gestation, type 1 diabetes mellitus, fetal-growth restriction, or gestational hypertension. In these situations, some healthcare providers perform the tests twice-weekly.

Advantages and Disadvantages of Nonstress Tests

- Simple, relatively inexpensive, less time consuming, easy to perform, and can be done on outpatient department (OPD) basis.
- Interpretation of trace requires degree of experience, skill, and training. To be correlated in context of clinical findings.
- High degree of false positive rate and may cause unnecessary intervention, leading to high cesarean rate.
- Fetal sleep pattern or maternal medications can affect result.

Accuracy of Test

The false-negative rate of test is 3.2 per 1,000. Death of fetuses with reactive NST is seen in conditions such as postdatism, diabetes, malformation, and abruption. The false-positive rate is very high, 50% for morbidity and 80% for mortality, indicating that possibility of serious fetal problem is relatively low in nonreactive NST. It also stresses the need of additional testing when test is nonreactive before intervention.

■ CONTRACTION STRESS TEST

The contraction stress test (CST), or oxytocin challenge test, is a test of fetal well-being first described by Ray et al. in 1972.[12] It evaluates the response of the FHR to induced contractions. The aim was to diagnose poor placental perfusion.

The CST should not be used in women in whom vaginal delivery is contraindicated [i.e., women with placenta previa, vasa previa, preterm premature rupture of the membranes (PPROM) or previous classical cesarean section],[13] and when gestation is below 24–28 weeks, at which no intervention is useful for the fetus if test is abnormal.[13]

It is prudent that this test should be performed in centers where emergency cesarean section is available, and the woman should be fully informed of the risks and benefits of the test.

The objective is to induce three contractions, lasting one minute each, within a 10-minute period, and evaluate the fetal heart response to these contractions.

The two commonly used methods to perform the CST are maternal nipple stimulation and an oxytocin infusion. Nipple stimulation is associated with a shorter average testing time than oxytocin infusion with no greater risk of uterine hyperstimulation. If nipple stimulation fails to induce contractions, then oxytocin infusion should be considered.

For oxytocin-induced contractions, the woman is place in semi-recumbent position with an intravenous line in place.[13] An NST is performed prior to the CST. If needed, uterine contractions are induced using exogenous oxytocin, starting at 0.5–1 mU/min, with an increase by 1 mU/min every 15–30 minutes, until optimum contractions are achieved. The tracing is evaluated for baseline rate, baseline variability, and deceleration.[13]

Interpretation

The CST is interpreted as follows:[4]
- *Positive:* A positive (abnormal) test has late decelerations following ≥50% of contractions. The test is positive even if the contraction frequency is less than three in 10 minutes.

- *Negative:* A negative (normal) test has no late decelerations or significant variable decelerations.
- *Equivocal:* An equivocal-suspicious test has intermittent late decelerations or significant variable decelerations, while an equivocal-tachysystolic has decelerations with contractions occurring more frequently than every 2 minutes or lasting longer than 90 seconds.
- *Unsatisfactory:* An unsatisfactory test has fewer than three contractions in 10 minutes (and is not positive as defined above), or is uninterpretable for other reasons.

Advantages and Disadvantages of Contraction Stress Test

The advantage of the CST is that it most closely mimics intrapartum surveillance of the fetus at risk. However, it requires a lengthy observation period and an intravenous (IV) access. It has a high rate of equivocal results. With easy availability of other simpler and reliable tests like BPP and Doppler, role of CST in modern medicine is restricted.

■ BIOPHYSICAL PROFILE (TABLES 1 AND 2)

The fetal BPP is a noninvasive, easily learned and performed antepartum test for evaluating the fetus for signs of compromise. The BPP uses combination of data from two sources (i.e., ultrasonographic imaging and FHR monitoring).

Originally described by manning and colleagues,[14] the BPP has become a standard tool for providing antepartum fetal surveillance.

The BPP integrates five parameters to provide a biophysical profile score (BPS). These parameters include: (1) the NST, (2) ultrasonographic measurement of the AFV, (3) observation of the presence or absence of fetal breathing movements, (4) gross body movements, and (5) fetal tone.

Can the nonstress test be omitted?

The NST does not give any additional benefit when the BPP is 8/8. The predictive value of the four ultrasound biophysical parameters (movement, tone, breathing, and amniotic fluid volume) is equivalent to that of the four ultrasound parameters plus an NST when the four ultrasound parameters are normal (two points for each). An NST should always be performed if any ultrasound-monitored parameter is 0 (i.e., BPP ≤ 6/8).

The Modified Biophysical Profile

The modified BPP was innovated to simplify the examination and reduce the time required to complete testing by focusing

TABLE 1: Determining the BPP score.

Biophysical variable	Normal (score = 2)	Abnormal (score = 0)
Fetal breathing movements	One or more episodes of ≥30 seconds within 30 minutes	Absent or no episode of ≥30 seconds within 30 minutes
Gross body movements	Three or more discrete body/limb movements within 30 minutes	Less than three episodes of body/limb movements in 30 minutes
Fetal tone	One or more episodes of active extension with return to flexion of fetal extremity or opening and closing of hand within 30 minutes	Slow extension with no return or slow return to flexion of a fetal extremity or no fetal movement
NST	Reactive: Two or more episodes of acceleration of ≥15 bpm and of >15 seconds associated with fetal movement within 20 minutes	Nonreactive: Less than two accelerations after 40 minutes
Qualitative AFV	One or more pockets of fluid measuring ≥2 cm in vertical axis	Either no pockets or largest pocket < 2 cm in vertical axis

(AFV: amniotic fluid volume; BPP: biophysical profile; NST: nonstress test)

TABLE 2: Interpretation of biophysical profile (BPP) score.[15,16]

Normal test	10/10, 8/8 (nonstress test omitted), or 8/10 (–2 points for either fetal movement, tone, or breathing but not amniotic fluid)	A BPP score of 8/10 by any combination of parameters is as reliable as a score of 10/10 for the prediction of fetal well-being, as long as no points are deducted for amniotic fluid volume
Equivocal test	6/10 (–4 points for two of fetal movement, tone, breathing, but +2 points for amniotic fluid)	The test is repeated within 24 hours to see if one of the absent acute variables returns to normal or, if the patient is at or near term, delivery is a reasonable option
Abnormal test	6/10 or 8/10 with 0 points for amniotic fluid	The risk of fetal asphyxia within 1 week is 89/1,000 with expectant management
	0 to 4/10: The risk of fetal asphyxia within 1 week is 91–600/1,000 if there is no intervention. Delivery is usually indicated	The risk of fetal asphyxia within 1 week is 91–600/1,000 if there is no intervention. Delivery is usually indicated

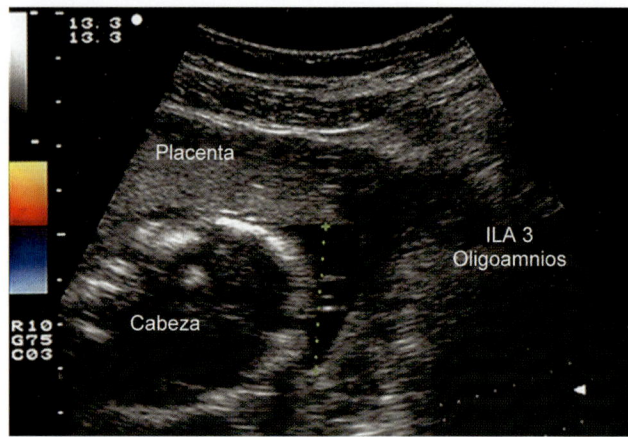

Fig. 4: Oligohydramnios.

on only those components of the BPP that are most predictive of outcome: NST and AFV **(Fig. 4)**. Assessment of only NST and AFV appears to be as reliable a predictor of long-term fetal well-being as the full BPP.[17,18] Since approximately 90% of pregnancies that undergo a modified BPP will have a normal result, only a minority will need to proceed to a full biophysical evaluation, thus saving time and money.[18]

Frequency of Testing

In most high-risk pregnancies weekly testing is recommended, although the standard is twice-weekly testing for pregnancies beyond 40 weeks and for women with insulin-dependent diabetes. Frequency of testing increases in direct proportion to the severity of the maternal or fetal condition.

Reliability of the Biophysical Profile

The BPP is a reliable method of predicting fetal survival. The BPP has a false-negative mortality rate of 0.77 deaths per 1,000 tests. Furthermore, the BPS highly correlates with the antepartum fetal umbilical venous cord pH level.

■ ULTRASONOGRAPHY

Obstetric ultrasound and fetal biometry is mainly useful in monitoring growth of fetus. Lag in biometric measurements, particularly abdominal circumference or estimated fetal weight <10th centile for gestational age in third trimester is considered as diagnosis of fetal growth restriction. Also biometric ratios like head to abdominal ratio or femur to abdominal ratio and plotting of these parameters on customized/population-based growth charts can be useful adjunct to monitor fetal growth and well-being.

Amount of amniotic fluid generally correlates with fetal health. Chronic placental insufficiency is often associated with reduction in amniotic fluid volume. AFI of <5 or single vertical pocket of amniotic fluid <2 is generally associated with fetal hypoxemia and poor fetal outcome.

■ DOPPLER VELOCIMETRY

Measurement of blood flow velocities in the maternal and fetal vessels provides information about uteroplacental blood flow and fetal responses to physiologic changes. Abnormal vascular development of the placenta, such as in preeclampsia, results in progressive hemodynamic changes in the fetoplacental circulation. Doppler indices from the *umbilical artery* increase when 60–70% of the placental vascular tree is compromised;[19] eventually, fetal *middle cerebral artery* impedance falls and fetal *aortic* resistance rises to preferentially direct blood to the fetal brain and heart.[20] Finally, end-diastolic flow in the umbilical artery ceases or reverses and resistance increases in the *fetal venous system* (ductus venosus and inferior vena cava).[20,21] These changes occur over variable periods of time and correlate with fetal acidosis.

As against most other methods of fetal assessment, Doppler-based tests have been rigorously evaluated in randomized trials. Umbilical artery Doppler is the most common Doppler technique used for fetal assessment where fetal hypoxemia is a concern. Fetal middle cerebral artery-peak systolic velocity (MCA-PSV) is the best tool for predicting fetal anemia in at-risk pregnancies.

Umbilical Artery (Figs. 5A to C)

Umbilical artery Doppler assessments are useful for monitoring fetuses with early-onset growth restriction due to uteroplacental insufficiency.[22] The umbilical artery waveform pattern is compatible with a low-resistance system: forward blood flow occurs throughout the cardiac cycle. Umbilical artery flow velocity waveforms of normally growing fetuses have a high-velocity diastolic flow, whereas in growth-restricted fetuses, umbilical artery diastolic flow is diminished, absent, or even reversed in severe cases. In the growth-restricted fetus, absent or reversed end-diastolic flow is associated with fetal hypoxemia and acidemia, and increased perinatal morbidity and mortality.[23]

The ACOG practice guidelines support the use of umbilical artery Doppler assessments in the management of suspected intrauterine growth restriction, but not for normally grown fetuses.[3] Doppler is recommended if the fetus weight on ultrasound is <10th percentile weight for gestational age. When monitoring the growth-restricted fetus, umbilical artery Doppler should be used with standard fetal surveillance (NST and/or BPP score).

There is no strong evidence to support umbilical artery Doppler surveillance in settings other than suspected fetal growth restriction.

Middle Cerebral Artery (Fig. 6)

Doppler assessment of the fetal MCA-PSV is the best tool for monitoring for fetal anemia in at-risk pregnancies, such as those affected by RhD alloimmunization.

SECTION 3: Fetal Evaluation

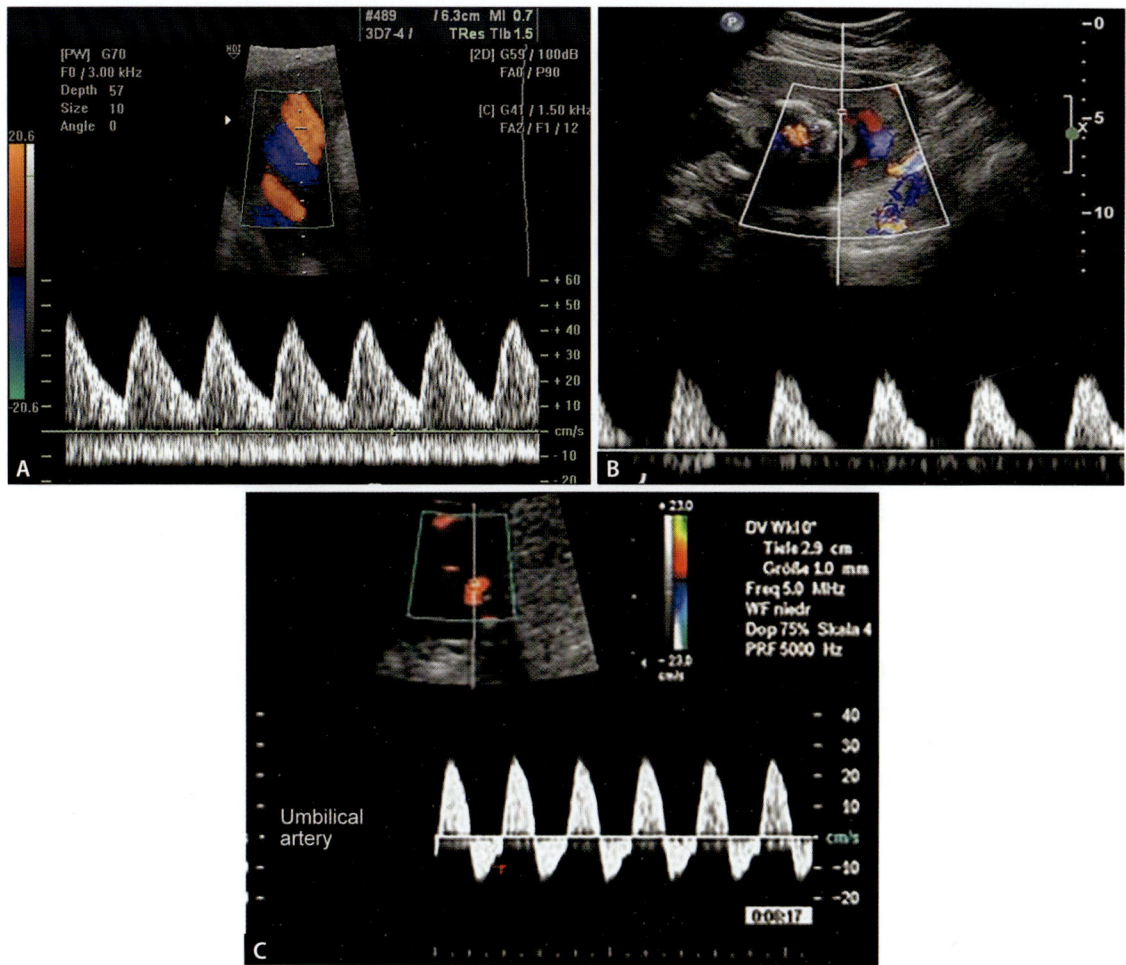

Figs. 5A to C: (A) Normal umbilical artery waveform; (B) Absence of end-diastolic flow velocity (AEDV); (C) Reversal of end-diastolic flow velocity (REDV).

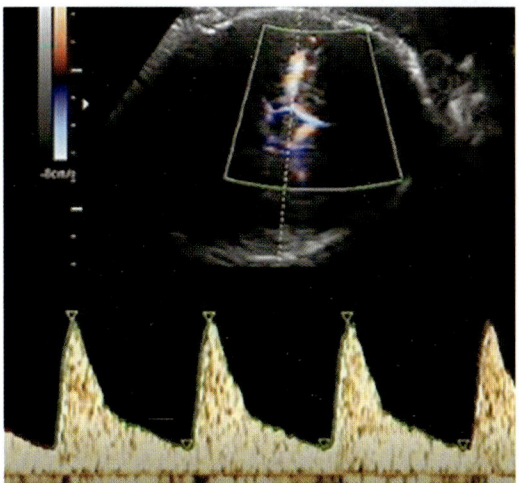

Fig. 6: Flow velocity waveforms in middle cerebral artery (MCA) normal fetus with low diastolic velocity (top) and growth restricted fetus with high diastolic velocity (bottom).

Middle cerebral artery Doppler is an additional tool for surveillance of pregnancies complicated by growth restriction. Its use in this setting is based on the premise that systemic blood flow in these fetuses is redistributed from the periphery to the brain and Doppler measurement of flow velocity in the fetal MCA can detect this brain-sparing effect.[24] Specifically, the cerebroplacental ratio, calculated by dividing the Doppler indices of the MCA by the umbilical artery, is emerging as a potential predictor of adverse outcome for both growth-restricted and appropriately-grown fetuses.

Venous System

The clinical utility of venous Doppler velocimetry is greatest in fetal conditions with cardiac manifestations and/or marked placental insufficiency. These conditions include fetal growth restriction due to placental insufficiency, twin-twin transfusion, fetal hydrops, and fetal arrhythmia.

The fetal precordial veins (ductus venosus and inferior vena cava) and the umbilical vein are the vessels most commonly evaluated in clinical practice. Flow in venous circulation is forward and uniform in normal fetus. Late findings include absent or reversed flow in the ductus venosus (absent or reversed a-wave) or pulsatile umbilical venous flow, occurring approximately 2 weeks after changes are observed in the arterial circulation.[25]

In fetus with absent or reversed end-diastolic arterial flow in the umbilical artery, maternal and fetal medicine experts recommend using this tool to avoid preterm delivery.

In these pregnancies, the absence of abnormal flow patterns in the ductus venosus has been used to support the decision to extend the pregnancy to 32–34 weeks, if the NST and BPP remain reassuring.

Uterine Artery

Investigators have explored the use of uterine artery Doppler for third trimester fetal assessment among women with complicated pregnancies, but its role in these settings has not been clearly defined. Resistance to flow in the uterine arteries normally decreases as pregnancy progresses. Inadequate trophoblast invasion and remodeling of maternal spiral arteries results in a persistent high-pressure uterine circulation and increased impedance to uterine artery blood flow. Elevated resistance indices and/or persistent uterine artery notching at 22–24 weeks of gestation indicate reduced blood flow in the maternal compartment of the placenta and have been associated with development of preeclampsia, fetal growth restriction, and perinatal death.[26]

■ CONCLUSION AND RECOMMENDATIONS

The goal of antepartum fetal surveillance is to prevent fetal death or neurologic injury by identifying the fetus that will benefit from early intervention and to also to prevent unnecessary preterm delivery.

Antepartum testing is based on the premise that the fetus responds to hypoxemia with a detectable sequence of biophysical changes and is indicated in "pregnancies in which the risk of antepartum fetal demise is increased".

The optimal choice of technique(s) for fetal assessment has not been determined and depends on multiple factors, including gestational age, availability, desire for fetal biometry or follow-up of a congenital anomaly, ability to monitor the FHR, and cost. The best evidence supports umbilical artery Doppler assessment for monitoring fetuses with early-onset growth restriction due to uteroplacental insufficiency, given its proven efficacy in reducing perinatal death in this setting when used with standard fetal testing (NST and BPS) and appropriate intervention.

■ REFERENCES

1. Martin CB Jr. Normal fetal physiology and behavior, and adaptive responses with hypoxemia. Semin Perinatol. 2008;32:239-42.
2. Baschat AA, Gembruch U, Harman CR. The sequence of changes in Doppler and biophysical parameters as severe fetal growth restriction worsens. Ultrasound Obstet Gynecol. 2001;18:571-7.
3. Practice bulletin no. 145: antepartum fetal surveillance. Obstet Gynecol. 2014;124:182-92.
4. Bocking AD. Assessment of fetal heart rate and fetal movements in detecting oxygen deprivation in-utero. Eur J Obstet Gynecol Reprod Biol. 2003;110 Suppl 1:S108-12.
5. Baskett TF, Liston RM. Fetal movement monitoring: clinical application. Clin Perinatol. 1989;16(3):613-25.
6. Moore TR, Piacquadio K. A prospective evaluation of fetal movement screening to reduce the incidence of antepartum fetal death. Am J Obstet Gynecol. 1989;160(5 Pt 1):1075-80.
7. Sadovsky E, Weinstein D, Even Y. Antepartum fetal evaluation by assessment of fetal heart rate and fetal movements. Int J Gynaecol Obstet. 1981;19(1):21-6.
8. Matsuura M, Murata Y, Hirano T, Nagatti N, Doi S, Suda K. The effects of developing autonomous nervous system on FHR variabilities determined by the power spectral analysis. Am J Obstet Gynecol. 1996;174:380.
9. Electronic fetal heart rate monitoring: research guidelines for interpretation. National Institute of Child Health and Human Development Research Planning Workshop. Am J Obstet Gynecol. 1997;177:1385-90.
10. Freeman RK, Anderson G, Dorchester W. A prospective multi-institutional study of antepartum fetal heart rate monitoring. II. Contraction stress test versus nonstress test for primary surveillance. Am J Obstet Gynecol. 1982;143:778-81.
11. Oncken C, Kranzler H, O'Malley P, Gendreau P, Campbell WA. The effect of cigarette smoking on fetal heart rate characteristics. Obstet Gynecol. 2002;99:751-5.
12. Ray M, Freeman R, Pine S, Hesselgesser R. Clinical experience with the oxytocin challenge test. Am J Obstet Gynecol. 1972;114(1):1-9.
13. Lagrew DC. The contraction stress test. Clin Obstet Gynecol. 1995;38(1):11-25.
14. Manning FA, Platt LD, Sipos L. Antepartum fetal evaluation: development of a fetal biophysical profile. Am J Obstet Gynecol. 1980;136(6):787-95.
15. Manning FA, Baskett TF, Morrison I, Lange I. Fetal biophysical profile scoring: a prospective study in 1,184 high-risk patients. Am J Obstet Gynecol. 1981;140:289-94.
16. Pillai M, James D. Behavioural states in normal mature human fetuses. Arch Dis Child. 1990;65:39-43.
17. Nageotte MP, Towers CV, Asrat T, Freeman RK. Perinatal outcome with the modified biophysical profile. Am J Obstet Gynecol. 1994;170:1672-6.
18. Miller DA, Rabello YA, Paul RH. The modified biophysical profile: antepartum testing in the 1990s. Am J Obstet Gynecol. 1996;174:812-7.
19. Thompson RS, Trudinger BJ. Doppler waveform pulsatility index and resistance, pressure and flow in the umbilical placental circulation: an investigation using a mathematical model. Ultrasound Med Biol. 1990;16:449-58.
20. Hecher K, Bilardo CM, Stigter RH, Ville Y, Hackelöer BJ, Kok HJ, et al. Monitoring of fetuses with intrauterine growth restriction: a longitudinal study. Ultrasound Obstet Gynecol. 2001;18:564-70.
21. Ferrazzi E, Bozzo M, Rigano S, Bellotti M, Morabito A, Pardi G, et al. Temporal sequence of abnormal Doppler changes in the peripheral and central circulatory systems of the severely growth-restricted fetus. Ultrasound Obstet Gynecol. 2002;19:140-6.
22. Kontopoulos EV, Vintzileos AM. Condition-specific antepartum fetal testing. Am J Obstet Gynecol. 2004;191:1546-51.
23. Karsdorp VH, van Vugt JM, van Geijn HP, et al. Clinical significance of absent or reversed end diastolic velocity waveforms in umbilical artery. Lancet. 1994;344:1664-8.
24. Mari G, Hanif F, Kruger M, Cosmi E, Santolaya-Forgas J, Treadwell MC. Middle cerebral artery peak systolic velocity: a new Doppler parameter in the assessment of growth-restricted fetuses. Ultrasound Obstet Gynecol. 2007;29:310-6.
25. Kiserud T, Eik-Nes SH, Blaas HG, Hellevik LR, Simensen B. Ductus venosus blood velocity and the umbilical circulation in the seriously growth-retarded fetus. Ultrasound Obstet Gynecol. 1994;4:109-14.

26. Papageorghiou AT, Yu CK, Cicero S, Bower S, Nicolaides KH. Second-trimester uterine artery Doppler screening in unselected populations: a review. J Matern Fetal Neonatal Med. 2002;12:78-88.

LONG QUESTIONS

1. Elaborate on various antenatal tests done in third trimester to assess fetal wellbeing.
2. Discuss at length the modality, method, advantages, disadvantages, clinical applications and evidence base for color Doppler as a third trimester fetal wellbeing test.

SHORT QUESTIONS

1. NST.
2. Bio-physical profile.
3. Role of Doppler in third trimester.

MULTIPLE CHOICE QUESTIONS

1. Reactive NST should have following criteria, except:
   a. Tracing of 20 minutes
   b. Minimum three acceleration
   c. Each acceleration of 15 bpm
   d. No spontaneous prolonged deceleration
2. While doing NST, speed of paper should be:
   a. 1 cm/min   b. 2.5 cm/min
   c. 5 cm/min   d. 10 cm/min
3. Minimum period recommended for correct interpretation of NST is:
   a. 5 min   b. 10 min
   c. 20 min   d. 40 min
4. What is recommended frequency of testing (NST) in diabetic woman with 36 weeks POG?
   a. Weekly   b. Daily
   c. Twice weekly   d. Every 15 days
5. Following are components of biophysical profile, except:
   a. Fetal cardiac movement
   b. AFV
   c. Fetal breathing movement
   d. NST
6. Woman undergoing BPP has all parameters normal except AFV of zero, what is interpretation of the test?
   a. Reassuring
   b. Equivocal, requiring repeat testing after 7 days
   c. Abnormal result requiring further testing
   d. Requires immediate intervention/LSCS
7. A 19-year-old nulliparous woman in her 35th week of pregnancy presents with nausea, blurred vision and a weight gain of 4.5 kg per week. Her blood pressure is 160/110 mm Hg. Which of the following tests is the most suitable for the assessment of fetal status?
   a. Amniocentesis for the measurement of the lecithin/sphingomyelin (L/S) ratio
   b. Amniocentesis for the measurement of the creatinine level of the amniotic fluid
   c. Sonographic cephalometry
   d. A non-stress test (NST)
8. Fetal movements count to 10 was devised by:
   a. Mannings   b. Cardiff
   c. Lewis   d. Simson
9. In multi-vessel Doppler flow studies in placental insufficiency, last change suggestive of imminent fetal is:
   a. Brain sparing effect in MCA
   b. Reversal of flow in umbilical artery
   c. Reversal of flow in DV
   d. Pulsatile flow in umbilical vein
10. Cerebroplacental ratio of .... is early sign of hypoxemia in FGR.
    a. <1   b. >1
    c. <1.5   d. <2

Answers
1. b 2. a 3. c 4. c 5. a 6. c
7. d 8. b 9. d 10. a

3.8 COLOR DOPPLER IN OBSTETRICS

Chinmayee Ratha

INTRODUCTION

The use of ultrasound in obstetrics marked a paradigm shift in the pattern of antenatal care in the twentieth century. It became possible to identify fetal conditions as separate clinical entities in pregnancy leading to identification of the fetus as a distinct patient by itself. The next revolutionary advance in fetal assessment was the use of Doppler technology in obstetric scans which opened the gateway to better understanding of fetal hemodynamics and thus define, screen, and diagnose prognosticate stages of fetal health and disease. As things stand today in the clinical settings, a meaningful practice of obstetrics mandates a basic knowledge of interpretation of fetal ultrasound findings including Doppler parameters. This chapter therefore is drafted to introduce the basic concepts of color Doppler to the reader and further elaborate on the rational use of this technology in various obstetric conditions. An attempt has been made to familiarize the reader not only with the theoretical applications of Doppler but also with the recent evidence-based rationale of its use.

BASIC CONCEPTS OF DOPPLER ULTRASOUND

The "Doppler effect"[1] is named after an Austrian physicist Christian Doppler who elucidated this phenomenon in 1842. He observed that there is an *apparent* change in frequency perceived if there is a *relative emotion* between the source of a wave and its receiver. The most common example that all school students have read in their textbooks is that of the change in intensity of the horn of an approaching train while the listener is standing on the railway platform. This "apparent" increase in intensity is due to the change in distance between the source and reception point due to relative motion—there is no actual change in the horn intensity when perceived at the same point with fixed distance from the source.

In ultrasound technology where imaging is based on the science of studying "echoes" from different tissues, the "Doppler effect" helps in studying moving objects within the human body. The most important moving objects are the blood cells in the blood vessels of a live organism and "color Doppler" technology provides an excellent tool to study characteristics of this flow. The use of Doppler as a noninvasive method to assess fetal hemodynamic was first described by Fitzgerald in 1977.[2]

For the sake of preliminary understanding and familiarizing the readers with the entity of "color Doppler" as distinct from a regular ultrasound image, **Figure 1** shows the pictorial representation of a grey scale ultrasound image and comparison with an image of "color Doppler" ultrasound.

COLOR DOPPLER

Therefore, whenever there is active "flow" in a vessel, colored signals can be picked up and this is the basis of color Doppler imaging. The colors are coded by the machine in a manner that the direction of flow determines the color and the intensity of color depends on the velocity. In **Figure 1**, the orange color determines flow towards the probe while the blue color is used for flow in the opposite direction—the color bar on the top left of the image represents the color code for that image. It may be noticed that when there is no flow (i.e., velocity = 0 cm/s), then the color depicted is black. This is why amniotic fluid appears black but blood flowing actively inside vessels appears colored.

It is well known that blood cells "flow" with the blood plasma inside the lumen of blood vessels with a velocity that is determined by the force of cardiac output and the pressure of the lateral walls of the vessels. In technical terms "blood flow" or "perfusion" is the amount of blood passing through mass of tissue in a given unit of time.[3] Adequate tissue perfusion is a prerequisite for optimal functioning of the tissue and any disturbance can adversely affect the same. Objective parameters on color Doppler studies provide a method of studying the parameters determining adequacy of blood flow through a vessel and help in quantifying the degree of compromise based on these findings.

SPECTRAL DOPPLER

While color Doppler can provide qualitative information about blood flow over a large area, quantitative analysis of specific flow parameters in a given region is achieved by complementing color Doppler with spectral flow studies—also known as "pulse wave" Doppler. This spectral flow Doppler involves investigating a small area of a blood vessel by a "gate" and then studying the pattern of flow that emerges to determine if flow is adequate or restricted.

Figure 2 is a depiction of pulse wave Doppler or spectral Doppler.

As is clear by the picture, the spectral Doppler shows a "wave form" of flow in a vessel with the crest of the wave

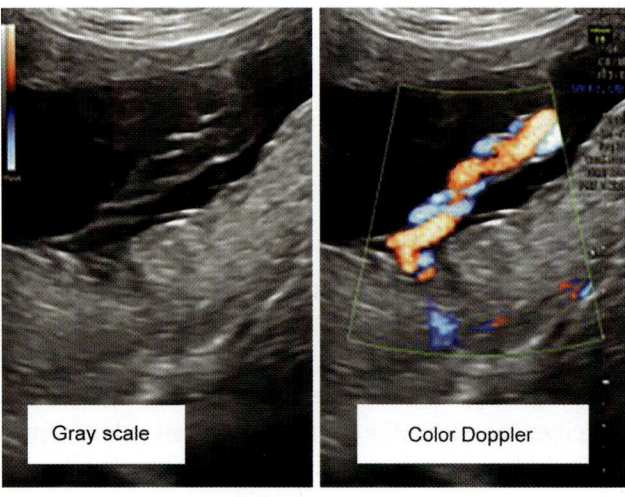

Fig. 1: Image of the placenta and umbilical cord in gray scale and color Doppler.

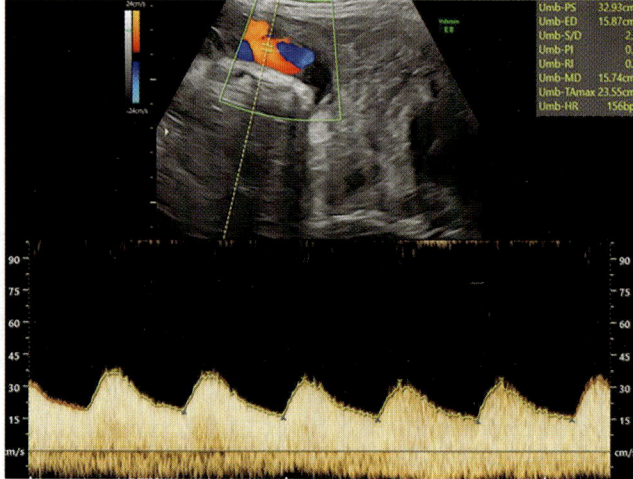

Fig. 2: Spectral flow pattern across umbilical artery.

representing the "peak velocity during cardiac systole" and the trough of the wave representing the "end-diastolic velocity". The flow velocity waveforms in the fetal vessels are largely dependent on the intrinsic hemodynamic factors such as fetal cardiac contractility, blood viscosity, and the compliance of vessel walls which reflect the peripheral resistance.[4] The results of the systolic and diastolic phases of the fetal heart are therefore well represented in the flow patterns and any compromise in the cardiac force or peripheral vessel resistance will lead to alteration of these flow patterns.

DOPPLER FLOW INDICES

It is logical to assume that the quantification of these flow characteristics will provide measurements or "indices" that can be used for clinical correlation to fetal physiology. This is the basis of the premise of using color Doppler technique for representing fetal physiological and pathological states. However, before venturing into the clinical applications of color Doppler technology it is imperative to understand the basics of "flow indices".

Several measurements have been described based on a combination of factors to quantify the Doppler signals accurately and reproducibly. The Doppler flow indices are calculated as ratios between peak systolic velocity (S), end-diastolic peak velocity (D), and the mean or average velocity (A). **Figure 3** shows the formulae for the pulsatility index (PI), resistant index (RI), and the systolic/diastolic (SD) ratios. The most common in clinical practice are PI and RI.[5]

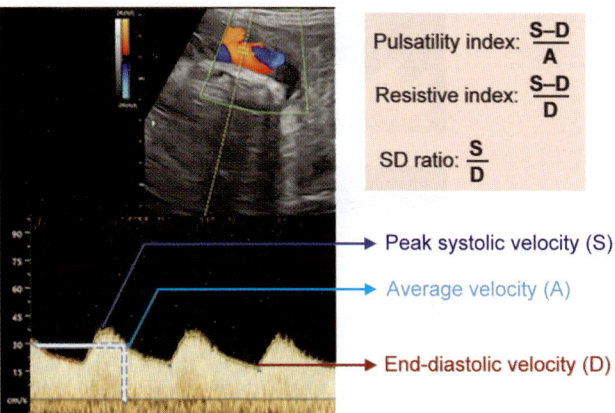

Fig. 3: Doppler flow indices.

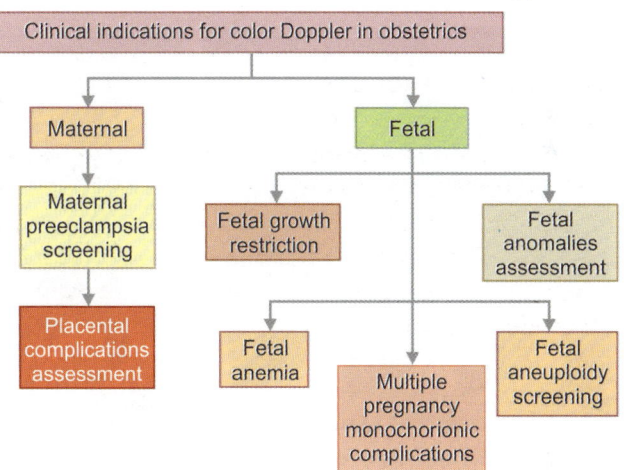

Flowchart 1: Clinical indications for obstetric Doppler.

CLINICAL APPLICATION OF COLOR DOPPLER

After having understood the basics of this brilliant technology, the challenge is to apply its potential into practical and clinical scenarios to optimize the perinatal outcome. The most important uses of color Doppler in clinical obstetrics is in situations affecting either the fetus, the mother or even the placenta. **Flowchart 1** enumerates the major clinical indications for color Doppler in obstetric.

FETAL GROWTH RESTRICTION

Fetal growth restriction (FGR) is a condition where the fetus is unable to attain its own growth potential and may have several causes. Uteroplacental insufficiency is the most common case allocated to FGR which is now classified as either early-onset FGR (starts before 32 weeks) or late-onset FGR (starts after 32 weeks). While "smallness" of the fetus (e.g., weight below the 10th, 5th, or 3rd centiles as the case may be) was considered a prerequisite for FGR, it has now been understood summarily that all small for gestational age (SGA) need not be FGR and all FGR need not be SGA. Fetuses which have growth restriction have a risk of hypoxemia in utero which has potential and adverse long-term neurodevelopmental effects. Therefore in this very context, the role of Doppler becomes very important in diagnosing and prognosticating FGR.

In early-onset FGR, the fetal growth compromise starts with placental dysfunction due to its poor formation. This placenta lacks the adequate number of villi to support fetal growth optimally. Normally the placental bed provides a high compliance and low resistance circulation, but in these cases, the resistance remains high. Fetal umbilical arteries carry blood from the fetus towards the placenta and hence there is increased afterload causing progressive deterioration of umbilical artery (UA) Doppler as shown in **Figure 4**.

As the UA diastolic flow diminishes the risk of fetal hypoxia and acidosis increases. This necessitates the review of the case in context of gestational age to consider the merits of delivery versus in utero continuation.[6] If the gestational age is adequate, delivery may be considered but if the pregnancy has to be prolonged, the other vessel Doppler, e.g., the middle cerebral artery (MCA), the ductus venosus (DV), and the fetal aortic isthmus (AoI) Doppler **(Figs. 5A to C)** will help prognosticate the case further.

The fetal MCA Doppler is considered as a surrogate marker of fetal hypoxia. Normal pattern of flow in fetal MCA

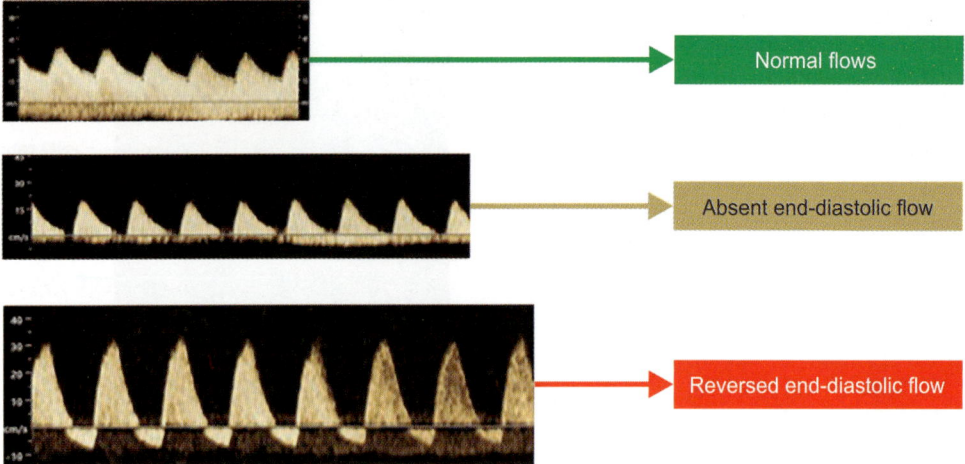

Fig. 4: Serial worsening of umbilical artery Doppler.

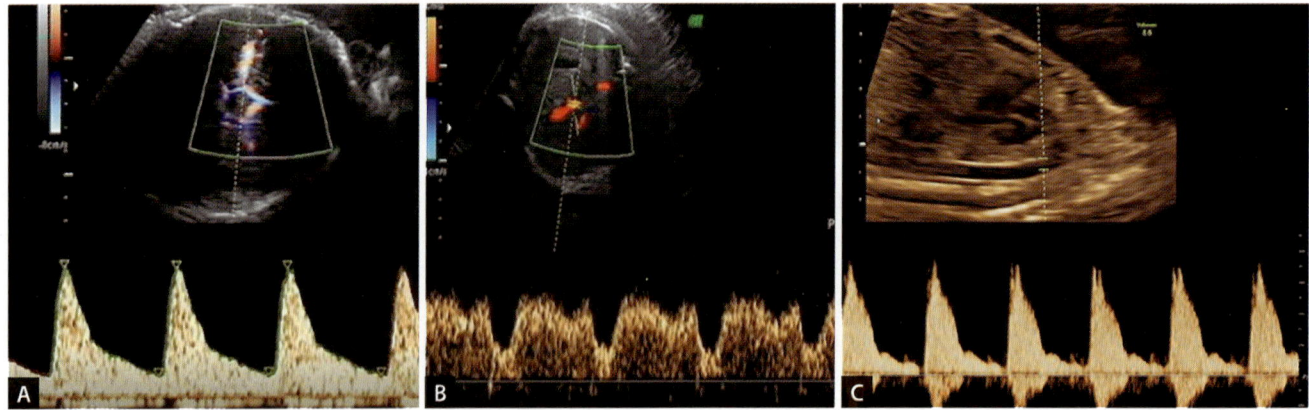

Figs. 5A and C: (A) Fetal middle cerebral artery (MCA); (B) Ductus venosus (DV); (C) Aortic isthmus (AoI) Doppler patterns.

is a high resistance flow but in the presence of hypoxia, the diastolic flow increases leading to a decrease in the MCA PI. Decreased MCA PI and increased UA PI is also known as the "cerebroplacental redistribution" such that it can be used as an index of fetal hemodynamic compromise.[7]

The role of the MCA Doppler is much more crucial in late-onset FGR where the actual "smallness" of the fetus may not be severe but the effect of hypoxemia can be devastating as the fetal reserve is low and the near-term fetus is very sensitive to hypoxia. The cerebroplacental ratio (CPR) is the ratio of the fetal MCA PI to UA PI and it has been shown to be more sensitive to detect circulatory adaptations of the fetus as opposed to only the individual elements of the ratio. A recent systemic review and meta-analysis concluded that calculating the CPR with MCA Doppler can add value to UA Doppler assessment in the prediction of adverse perinatal outcome in women with a singleton pregnancy.[8]

The fetal AoI is a crucial vessel signifying the interface of oxygenated and deoxygenated blood in fetal circulation and the AoI flows help in detecting if the oxygenation of fetal brain is getting compromised at that level.[6] If the AoI Doppler is abnormal, the possibility of residual neurodevelopmental delay increases and hence a decision for delivery may have to be taken depending on the fetal gestational age, availability of neonatal intensive care unit (NICU) facilities, and wishes of the parents.

The fetal DV is the inflow vessel carrying oxygenated blood from the placenta towards the fetal heart. Once the fetal DV flows get compromised there is a serious risk not only of acidosis but of fetal demise in utero. In fact an abnormal fetal DV is a strongest short-term risk factor for intrauterine demise.[6]

■ FETAL ANEMIA

Fetal anemia is an important clinical challenge in obstetrics and there is a potentially successful treatment available for the same in the form of intrauterine blood transfusion. If left unattended, fetal anemia can be lethal due to consequent cardiac failure. Use of the color Doppler technology has revolutionized the noninvasive prenatal diagnosis of fetal anemia. **Figure 6** shows the tall peaks of fetal MCA Doppler in a case of fetal anemia.

The correct technique of obtaining the MCA Doppler for the purpose of screening for fetal anemia is as follows:[9]

- The fetus should be relatively quiet with no major breathing or movements.

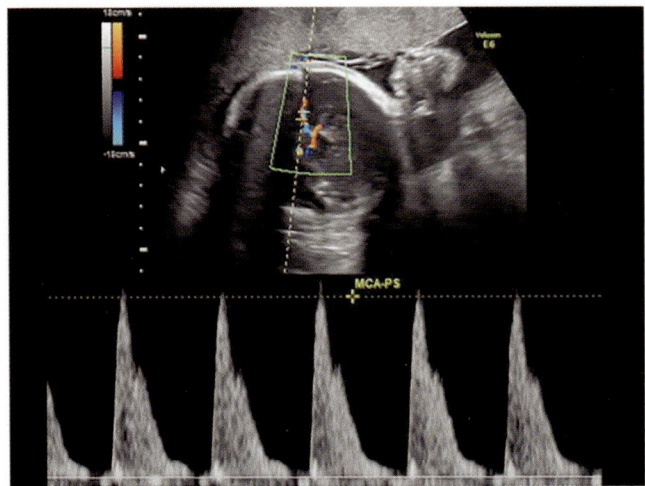

Fig. 6: High fetal middle cerebral artery (MCA) peak systolic velocity (PSV) in fetal anemia.

- Using gray scale imaging the axial section of the fetal head is obtained and the circle of Willis is imaged with color Doppler.
- The picture is zoomed so that the area of the fetal MCA occupies more than half of the screen. The MCA should be visualized for its entire length.
- The sample volume (1-2 mm) is placed soon after the origin of the MCA (at the junction of the proximal one-third and distal two-thirds).
- The direction of blood flow and the ultrasound beam should be parallel to each other.
- The waveforms obtained should be similar to each other and the highest PSV is measured.
- The above steps at least three times to ensure accuracy and reproducibility.

The peak systolic velocity of the fetal MCA is measured in cm/s and converted to "multiples of the median (MoM)"—a statistically easier method of comparison of values. There is a nomogram for the "normal" PSV of the MCA for a particular stage of pregnancy and if the value exceeds beyond 1.5 MoM for that gestation, fetal anemia is diagnosed. The peak systolic velocity of the fetal MCA correlates with fetal anemia closely and over the years it has been proven beyond doubt that this measurement, if done correctly, obviates the need for invasive diagnosis of fetal anemia by fetal blood sampling.[10] Fetal medicine specialists can now diagnose fetal anemia noninvasively and plan for fetal blood transfusion directly. Post-transfusion also this Doppler index helps in monitoring the fetal status and guides the clinician regarding need for repeat procedures.

COLOR DOPPLER IN THE ASSESSMENT OF FETAL ANOMALIES

It is well known that 2–3% of all pregnancies can be affected by fetal structural anomalies. A targeted imaging for fetal anomalies is thus offered to all pregnant women in midtrimester, usually at the 18-20 weeks period.

The practice guidelines for the conduct of the midtrimester anomaly scan do not recommend routine use of color Doppler for the basic scan.[11] However, the expectations from these scans is increasing and in settings where resource crunch is not an issue, there may be a justification of extending the anomaly scan protocol to the use of some added steps in order to improve the detection and delineation of fetal anatomy and its aberrations, if any. While most fetal anomalies can be detected with real time, gray scale ultrasound, color Doppler can help in assisting the diagnosis of some conditions. Few examples of conditions where color Doppler can be a useful adjunct in evaluation of normal anatomy and detection of abnormality include fetal cardiac evaluation[12] (**Fig. 7**), evaluation of kidneys especially when unilateral or bilateral agenesis is suspected or if the kidneys are placed at aberrant locations, e.g., pelvic kidneys (**Fig. 8**), evaluating umbilical cord vasculature (**Fig. 9**), vascular aneurysms, etc.

The use of color flow helps in delineating the anatomical arrangements clearly and reinforces the diagnosis. In conditions like vein of Galen malformations or sacrococcygeal teratomas, the application of color Doppler and the discovery of enhanced blood flows alter the prognosis dramatically. Hence, the role of color Doppler in fetal anatomy evaluation can be considered as a secondary or complimentary adjunct but can be very vital in some cases.

USE OF COLOR DOPPLER IN ASSESSING PLACENTAL ADHERENCE

Morbid adherence of placenta is a clinical nightmare for an obstetrician. There are many reasons in present day obstetrics which have contributed to a phenomenal rise in the incidence of placenta accrete spectrum (PAS) disorders. While a number of gray scale features have been described, color Doppler of the uterine interface with adjoining structures is a very powerful tool to get a preoperative assessment of the degree of invasion. Bridging vessels and conspicuous atypical vasculature is an unequivocally alarming sign for the clinical who can then meticulously plan the surgical procedures at the time of delivery. **Figure 10** shows an example of color flow evaluation of vesicouterine interface in a low lying placenta with suspected morbid adherence.

In a recent systematic review and meta-analysis of prenatal diagnosis of placenta previa and accrete, it was found that loss of clear zone and the presence of bridging vessels, subplacental hypervascularity, and placental lacunae were the most common ultrasound signs of morbid placental adherence.[13]

ROLE OF COLOR DOPPLER IN SCREENING FOR FETAL ANEUPLOIDIES

Screening for fetal aneuploidies is recommended in every pregnancy and the 11-14 weeks scan is an important

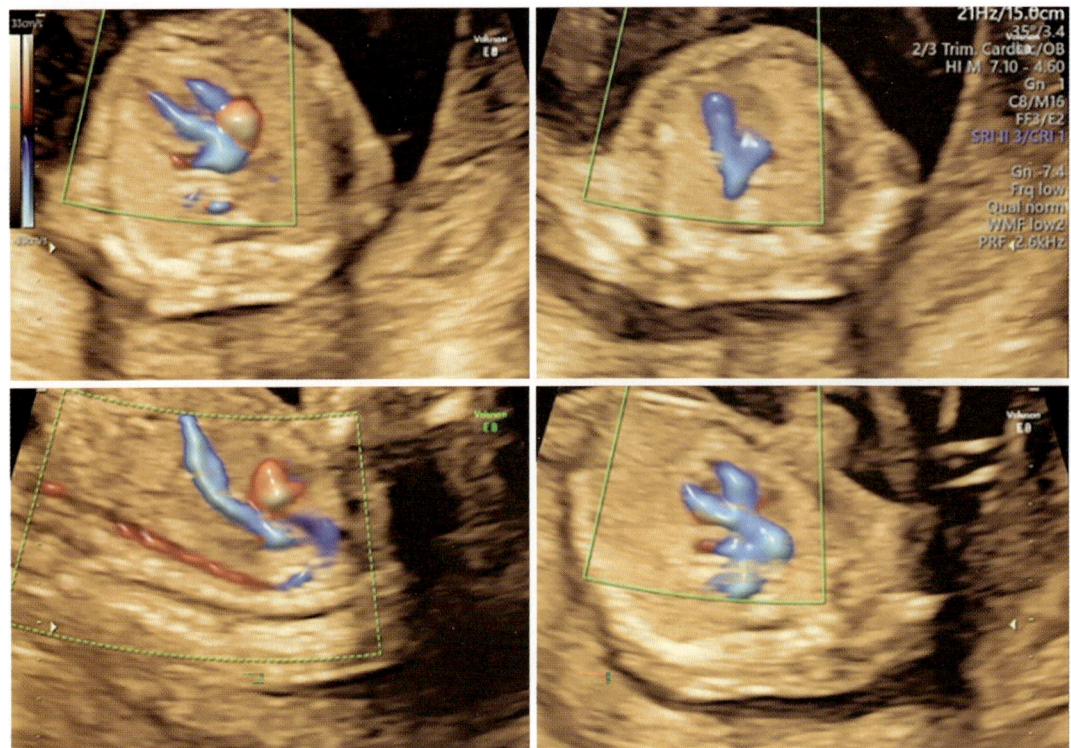

Fig. 7: Color Doppler in assessing the fetal cardiac anatomy.

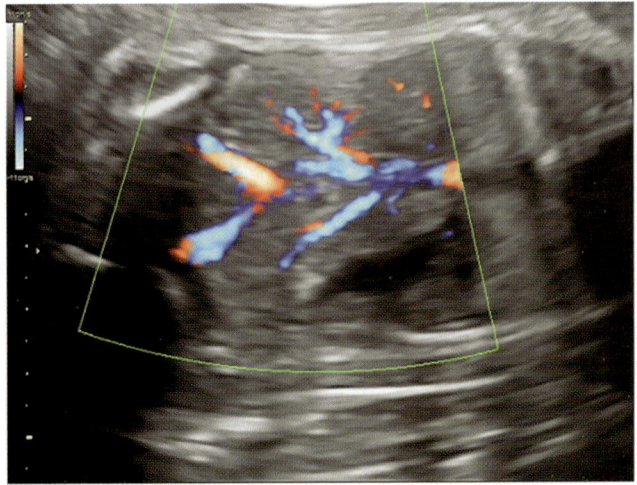

Fig. 8: Renal arteries in pelvic kidneys.

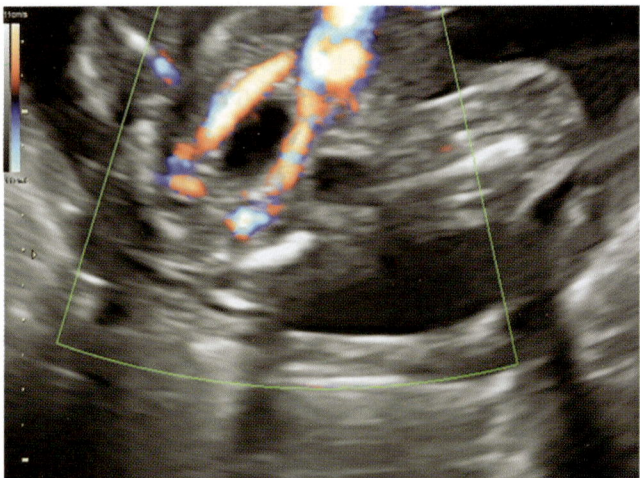

Fig. 9: Two perivesical umbilical arteries.

landmark procedure for the same. The basic protocol for screening at this scan includes primarily the measurement of fetal crown rump length (CRL), heart rate, and nuchal translucency (NT). The extended protocol includes measurement of the fetal DV PI with the use of color flow and spectral Doppler as shown in **Figure 11**.

The inclusion of DV Doppler index increases the sensitivity of aneuploidy screening by providing an independent contribution in the prediction of risk when combined with NT and the maternal serum markers [pregnancy-associated plasma protein A (PAPP-A) and free beta-human chorionic gonadotropin (hCG)]. This increases the detection rate for chromosomal abnormalities to 96% at a false-positive rate of 2.6%. Abnormal DV flow increases the risk of cardiac defects in fetuses with normal or raised NT. In twin pregnancies, abnormal DV flow is associated with chromosomal abnormalities and cardiac defects. In monochorionic (MC) twins, abnormal flow in the DV in at least one of the fetuses increases the risk of developing twin-to-twin transfusion syndrome (TTTS).[14] The DV flows in the first trimester hence form an important prognostic marker in general for fetal wellbeing.

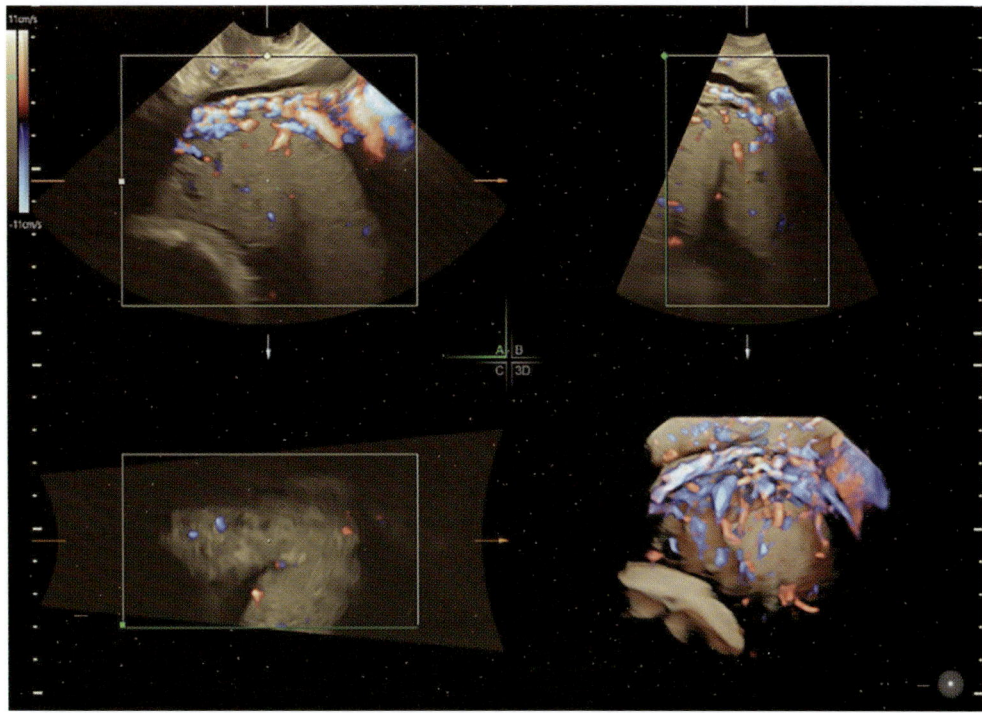

Fig. 10: Uterovesical interface evaluation with color Doppler.

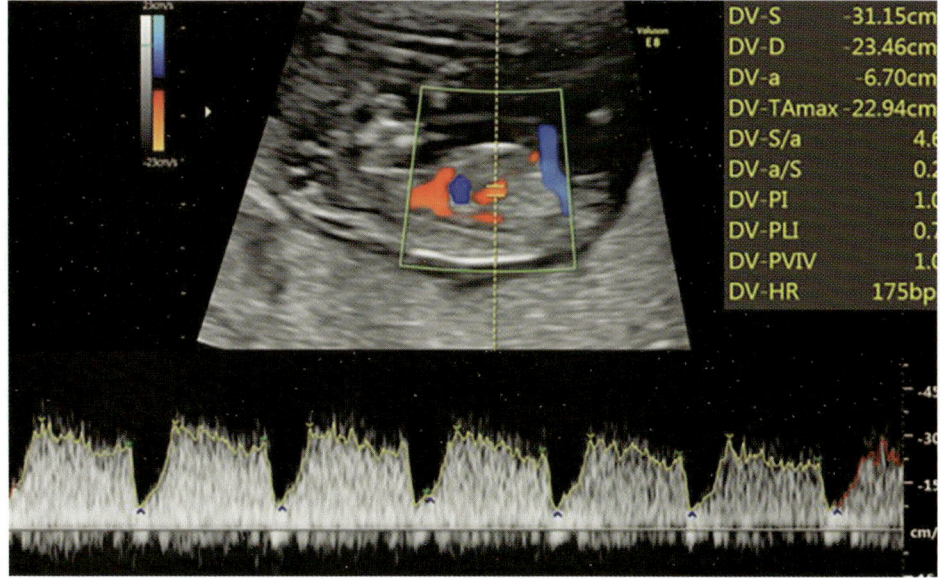

Fig. 11: Color Doppler-assisted ductus venosus (DV) pulsatility index (PI) measurement at the 11–14 weeks scan.

COLOR DOPPLER IN SCREENING FOR MATERNAL PREECLAMPSIA

Preeclampsia remains an important cause of perinatal morbidity and mortality. The most accepted theory of the development of preeclampsia is impaired trophoblastic invasion of the maternal spiral arteries such that the placental bed retains a high resistance to blood flows. Color Doppler of the maternal uterine arteries reflect this physiological process of trophoblastic invasion with the observation that impedance to the flow in uterine arteries decreases with gestation between 6 and 24 weeks and remains constant thereafter.[15]

The uterine artery can be investigated in the first trimester close to the maternal cervix while in the second trimester it is easily seen where it crosses over the external iliac vessels. A spectral flow pattern is obtained and the PI is measured. As there are two uterine arteries—left and right, it is imperative to measure the PI of both the vessels. The final PI considered is a mean of the two values. This mean uterine artery PI again is expressed as an "MoM" for that stage of gestation. If the mean uterine artery PI exceeds 1.5 MoM for that stage of pregnancy, it is reported as high resistance flows and is correlated with an elevated risk of maternal preeclampsia and FGR. **Figure 12** shows the normal pattern of uterine artery blood flow while **Figure 13** shows high resistance flows evident by reduced diastolic component and the presence of an early diastolic notch. While the presence of the "notch" gives a subjective corroboration to the high resistance flow state, its significance in objective risk assessment has diminished and is no longer considered in the risk assessment protocol.

Studies have shown that effective screening for preeclampsia can be achieved by the Doppler measurement of uterine artery PI in first and second trimester by noticing the change in PI which is expected to decrease in normal cases.[15]

The combination of maternal demographic characteristics and uterine artery Doppler and maternal blood pressure measurements is an effective screening tool for the prediction of preeclampsia.[16]

COLOR DOPPLER IN MONOCHORIONIC TWIN COMPLICATIONS

Monochorionic twins have several unique complications which adversely affect the perinatal outcome of both the fetuses. Color Doppler is an important method of diagnosing problems and guiding management in MC twins.[17] It has been mentioned earlier that the fetal DV Doppler study in first trimester can be one of the very early indications of the development of TTTS.

Table 1 enumerates the specific conditions in monochorionic twin pregnancies where color Doppler can be of good clinical use.

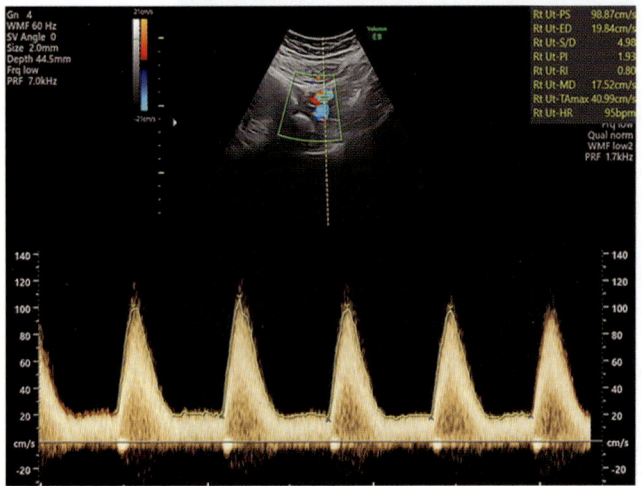

Fig. 12: Normal uterine artery blood flows in pregnancy.

SAFETY CONCERNS WITH COLOR DOPPLER

With the rampant use of ultrasound and Doppler technology in obstetrics, it is logical to have concerns about the safety of the use of color Doppler in obstetrics. There have been some studies relating to possibility of fetal effects (nonright-handedness in boys, growth restriction, etc.) following repeated ultrasound exposure almost 30–40 years back but a Cochrane review in 2010 concluded that no consistent serious adverse effects of obstetric ultrasound have yet been demonstrated. One explanation of the diminishing concerns of fetal safety is that the energy output settings of modern ultrasound machines is very low and highly unlikely to cause fetal effects even in early pregnancy.[18] Nevertheless it is recommended to follow the principle of "as low as reasonably attainable (ALARA)" to ensure minimum exposure to the fetus during color Doppler examination.

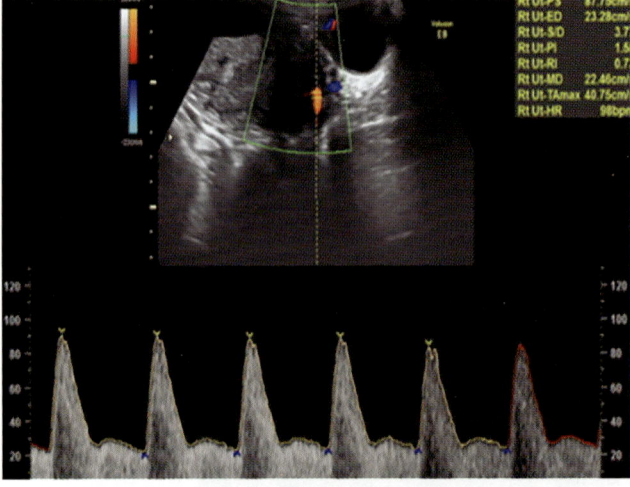

Fig. 13: High resistance flow in uterine artery.

TABLE 1: Use of color Doppler in MC twin pregnancies.			
MC complication	**Clinical challenge**		**Role of color Doppler**
One placenta with two cord insertions	Determine the region of insertion of both cords	Diagnostic	Rule out abnormal insertions like marginal/velamentous
MCMA twins	Possibility of cord entanglement	Diagnostic	Easier to diagnose knots with color Doppler
MCDA–TTTS/sFGR	Hemodynamic risks to both fetuses	Diagnostic	Fetal umbilical Doppler helps in staging the disease
MCDA–TRAP	Vascularity of the TRAP mass determines prognosis	Diagnostic	The blood flow to the TRAP and the consequent hemodynamic changes in the pump twin can help guide treatment decisions
MCDA complications	Needs invasive therapy (LASER/RFA)	Guides therapeutic procedures	Ultrasound-guided therapeutic procedures
(LASER: light amplification by stimulated emission of radiation; MC: monochorionic; MCDA: monochorionic diamniotic; MCMA: monochorionic monoamniotic; RFA: radiofrequency ablation; sFGR: elective fetal growth restriction; TRAP: twin reversed arterial perfusion; TTTS: twin-to-twin transfusion syndrome)			

KEY MESSAGES

- Color Doppler technology is widely used in obstetrics.
- It has both diagnostic and prognostic roles in most cases while it can be used to guide therapy in some situations.
- The common indications for use of color Doppler include extended screening for fetal anomalies, aneuploidies, complications of multiple pregnancy, fetal growth restriction, and fetal anemia.
- Maternal preeclampsia screening and assessment of morbid adherence of placenta can also be helped by color Doppler.
- Safety of color Doppler in pregnancy is established but it is prudent to follow the principle of ALARA.

REFERENCES

1. Giordano N. (2009). College Physics: Reasoning and Relationships. Boston, Massachusetts: Cengage Learning, Inc; 2009. pp. 421-4.
2. Fitzgerald DE, Drumm JE. Non-invasive measurement of the human circulation using ultrasound: a new method. Br Med J. 1977;2:1450-1.
3. Rubin J. Flow quantification. Eur Radiol. 1999;9 Suppl 3:S368-71.
4. Burns PN. Principles of Doppler and color flow. Radiol Med. 1993;85:3-16.
5. Giles WB, Trudinger BJ, Baird PJ. Fetal umbilical artery flow velocity waveforms and placental resistance: pathological correlation. Br J Obstet Gynaecol. 1985;92:31-8.
6. Figueras F, Gratacós E. Update on the diagnosis and classification of fetal growth restriction and proposal of a stage-based management protocol. Fetal Diagn Ther. 2014;36(2):86-98.
7. Dunn L, Sherrell H, Kumar S. Systematic review of the utility of the fetal cerebroplacental ratio measured at term for the prediction of adverse perinatal outcome. Placenta. 2017;54:68-75.
8. Vollgraff Heidweiller-Schreurs CA, De Boer MA, Heymans MW, Schoonmade LJ, Bossuyt PMM, Mol BWJ, et al. Prognostic accuracy of cerebroplacental ratio and middle cerebral artery Doppler for adverse perinatal outcome: systematic review and meta-analysis. Ultrasound Obstet Gynecol. 2018;51(3):313-22.
9. Segata M, Mari G. (2004). Fetal anemia: new technologies. Curr Opin Obstet Gynecol. 2004;16(2):153-8.
10. Mari G. Middle cerebral artery peak systolic velocity for the diagnosis of fetal anemia: the untold story. Ultrasound Obstet Gynecol. 2005;25(4):323-30.
11. Salomon LJ, Alfirevic Z, Berghella V, Bilardo C, Hernandez-Andrade E, Johnsen SL, et al. Practice guidelines for performance of the routine mid-trimester fetal ultrasound scan. Ultrasound Obstet Gynecol. 2011;37(1):116-26.
12. Allan LD, Cook AC, Huggon IC. Fetal Echocardiography: A Practical Guide. Cambridge: Cambridge University Press; 2009.
13. Jauniaux E, Bhide A. Prenatal ultrasound diagnosis and outcome of placenta previa accreta after cesarean delivery: a systematic review and meta-analysis. Am J Obstet Gynecol. 2017;217(1):27-36.
14. Maiz N, Nicolaides KH. Ductus venosus in the first trimester: contribution to screening of chromosomal, cardiac defects and monochorionic twin complications. Fetal Diagn Ther. 2010;28(2):65-71.
15. Plasencia W, Maiz N, Poon L, Yu C, Nicolaides KH. Uterine artery Doppler at 11 + 0 to 13 + 6 weeks and 21 + 0 to 24 + 6 weeks in the prediction of pre-eclampsia. Ultrasound Obstet Gynecol. 2008;32(2):138-46.
16. Kaminopetros P, Higueras MT, Nicolaides KH. Doppler study of uterine artery blood flow: comparison of findings in the first and second trimesters of pregnancy. Fetal Diagn Ther. 1991;6:58-64.
17. Townsend R, Khalil A. Ultrasound surveillance in twin pregnancy: An update for practitioners. Ultrasound. 2018;26(4):193-205.
18. Whitworth M, Bricker L, Neilson JP, Dowswell T. Ultrasound for fetal assessment in early pregnancy. Cochrane Database Syst Rev. 2010;(4):CD007058.

LONG QUESTIONS

1. Describe the progressive changes of fetal Doppler in early-onset fetal growth restriction.
2. How can fetal Doppler be used in fetal anemia?

SHORT QUESTIONS

1. Explain cerebroplacental ratio.
2. Role of color Doppler in screening for fetal aneuploidies.

MULTIPLE CHOICE QUESTIONS

1. Christian Doppler discovered the Doppler effect during study of heavenly bodies. Which of the following is correct about Doppler effect?
    a. There is no apparent motion between source and reception
    b. There is only an apparent change in frequency of the sound
    c. There is a real in frequency of sound at the source
    d. Motion artefacts impede Doppler signals
2. Which of the following is true for spectral Doppler in contrast to plain color Doppler?
    a. It gives little information over a small area
    b. It gives little information over a large area
    c. It gives lot of information over a small area
    d. It gives lot of information over a large area
3. The colors red and blue in a color code for Doppler represent:
    a. Red is oxygenated blood and blue is mixed blood
    b. Red flows towards the probe and blue flows away
    c. Direction of blood flow is same in both
    d. Red is mixed blood blue is deoxygenated
4. Which of the following anomaly detection will not be improved by use of color Doppler?
    a. Thoracic meningomyelocele
    b. Intracranial vein of Galen aneurysm
    c. Muscular VSD
    d. Unilateral pelvic kidney
5. The uterine artery is best localized in second trimester when it:
    a. Branches off the external iliac artery
    b. Crosses over the internal iliac artery

c. Crosses over the external iliac artery
d. Branches from the external iliac artery

6. Raised peak systolic velocity of fetal MCA is when:
   a. The velocity is >50 cm/s
   b. Is >1.5 MoMs for that stage of pregnancy
   c. The cardiac failure has set in
   d. Depends on the maternal blood pressure

7. Which of the following is not a sign of fetal anemia?
   a. Fetal hepatosplenomegaly
   b. Fetal ascites
   c. Raised MCA PI
   d. Fetal tricuspid regurgitation

8. Which of the following is a marker for fetal aneuploidy in first trimester?
   a. Uterine artery mean PI
   b. Ductus venosus PI
   c. Fetal MCA PI
   d. Umbilical artery PI

9. In monochorionic twins, twin-to-twin transfusion can complicate 15% cases. The role of color Doppler in TTTS is most justified as:
   a. Umbilical and ductus venosus Doppler to assess hemodynamics of the fetus
   b. Placental vasculature studies to detect the number and type of AV anastomoses
   c. Evaluation of uterine artery as a risk assessment for IUGR
   d. Cervical evaluation for risk of preterm birth

10. The principle of safety of Doppler ultrasound is based on ALARA. What is ALARA?
    a. As large as regularly attainable
    b. As low as regularly achievable
    c. As large as reasonably achievable
    d. As low as reasonably attainable

Answers
1. b 2. c 3. b 4. a 5. c 6. b
7. c 8. b 9. a 10. d

3.9 FETAL ECHOCARDIOGRAPHY

Jayprakash Shah, Parth Shah

INTRODUCTION

Fetal heart is a not only a complex structure but also always in motion. It is surrounded by bony cage all around, anteriorly by sternum, posteriorly by spine, making is difficult to image by ultrasound. Unless one understands anatomy of heart and its connection in three dimensions, it becomes difficult to have orientation about heart structures. It starts developing from 3rd week and continues to develop till 10th completed week. So, its formation extends right throughout the organogenesis period. That is why it is having association with other malformations. Cardiac malformations occur in 8–13/1,000 live birth,[1] among all pregnancy including still born, the incidence is 30/1,000. Structural cardiac anomalies are most frequently missed fetal malformations.[2,3] It is associated with chromosomal abnormality in approximately 3–18% not 50% of congenital heart defects (CHD) and the incidence is high among the prenatal series compared to neonatal series due to high still birth rate (**Fig. 1**). Prenatal detection can improve the fetal outcome.[4,5] In 274 prenatal confirmed diagnosis of CHD, 109 were found to have aneuploidy in a study published in OB GYN 1993.

ETIOLOGY

Etiology is multifactorial with interplay of chromosomal abnormality and environment factors. Maternal disease, infection, drugs, radiation also play important role in CHD.

INDICATIONS FOR FETAL ECHO

- Routine screening is suggested in all fetuses.
- Parental history of child born with CHD in the same mother
- Familial
  - Family history of CHD
- Predisposing maternal conditions
  - Maternal diabetes
  - Infection during pregnancy
  - Maternal alcoholism
  - Maternal connective tissue disorder
  - Maternal phenylketonuria
- Exposure to teratogens/drug intake
- Abnormal pregnancy progression
  - Polyhydramnios
  - Nonimmune hydrops
  - Dysrhythmias
  - Extracardiac malformations
  - Chromosomal aberrations
  - Symmetrical IUGR.

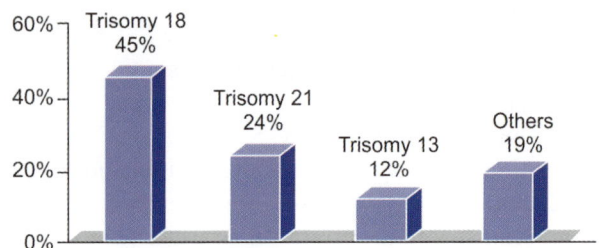

Fig. 1: Chromosomal abnormality in CHD.

FACTORS AFFECTING PRENATAL DETECTION

Prenatal detection rate vary among various study published due to various factors such as examiner's experience, maternal obesity, transducer frequency, abdominal scars, gestational age, amniotic fluid volume, and fetal position.[6,7] Standard technique and a guideline along with the training of the personnel will gradually change the scenario, but still the fact remains that ASD, small VSD and patent ductus are easy to be missed.

FETAL ECHOCARDIOGRAPHY

- **Fetal heart screening**
  - *Basic fetal echocardiography*
    - Detailed 4-chamber view examination
  - *Extended fetal echocardiography*
    - Outflow tracts
      1. Left ventricular outflow tract (LVOT)
      2. Right ventricular outflow tracts (RVOT)
    - Three vessel view
      1. Ductal arch view (3 VV)
      2. Aortic arch view (3 VT view)
- **Advance fetal echocardiography**
  - Color Doppler
  - M mode examination
  - Spectral Doppler
  - 3D/4D ultrasound
    - 3D STIC, Multiplanar, Omniview, TUI with/without color/HD flow
    - 4D STIC Multiplanar, Omniview, TUI with/without color/HD flow

Basic and extended fetal echocardiography guidelines are designed to diagnose and suspect majority of cardiac malformations during 2nd trimester.[8] It will help in improving pick up rate in low risk population screening for cardiac malformations of fetus[9] and if still suspicious, one can refer for advanced fetal echocardiography.

When to do? Timing for Echocardiography

The best time to do echocardiography is 18–22 weeks of pregnancy, to be more accurate it should be done at 22 weeks. This is the time when heart is significantly large, amniotic fluid is relatively more and ribs do not cast a shadow to obscure the imaging of heart. If there is previous history of CHD one can do early echo at 16–18 weeks with reasonable accuracy. Early echo is indicated also in cases where NT was high at 11–13 weeks scan with normal chromosomes, or if the ductus venous flow is abnormal and tricuspid regurgitation is present.

Setting of Machine

It is most important to set the parameters of the machine for optimizing the 2D image, color Doppler settings and 3D-4D settings for fetal echo. It is beyond the capacity of this chapter. Reader is requested to refer relevant chapter from internet or lecture on ISUOG[10] and sonoworld website on this subject by Professor DeVore.

Steps for Fetal Echo

Secret of successful fetal echo is expressed in one word—it is "sequential segmental analysis". CVS is divided in segments:
- Inflow tracts
- Atria
- Ventricles
- Outflow tracts

By sequential it denotes stepwise planes to be seen to establish connection among these segments of the heart.

Making it simple one can say steps of fetal echo are:
1. Define lie and position of fetus
2. Confirm situs of fetal organ
3. Different heart view for fetal heart to define structure of heart and its six connections—3 on right and 3 on left **(Table 1)**. Establish normality.

For this one requires to examine heart in following sections as part of screening. If any suspicious finding is noticed, detailed fetal echo by expert to be done:
- 4 chamber view
- Outflow tracts: LVOT and RVOT
- 3 vessel trachea view and 3 vessel trachea view.

Define Laterality and Abdominal Situs

Determine how the fetus is lying inside the uterus and figure out which is the right and left of the fetus:
- The presentation of the fetus is cephalic, breech or transverse
- The spine is upward toward the transducer, backward or lateral
- Confirm that both the stomach and heart are on the left side.

Obtain the 4-chamber view and maintaining a transverse section of the fetal trunk, angle or slide the transducer downward to the abdomen, in order to image the stomach and situs. Remember "cephalic clockwise". In cephalic presentation of fetus, orientation of fetal organs in abdomen—spine, STOMACH and portal—are in clockwise direction, in that case stomach is on left side. This can be reconfirmed by position of aorta which is anterior to and little to left of fetal spine and IVC is anterior and little to right. Now slide cephalic in transverse section only and confirm to which side heart is tilted. Now if in cephalic presentation, orientation of organs is in anticlockwise directions, stomach

TABLE 1: Six connections of the heart.

Right sided connections	Left sided connections
Inferior vena cava (IVC) and superior vena cava (SVC) connection to right atrium	4 pulmonary connected to left atrium
Right atrium to right ventricle (tricuspid valve)	Left atrium to left ventricle (mitral valve)
Right ventricle to main pulmonary [right ventricle outflow tract (RVOT)]	Left ventricle to ascending aorta [left ventricle outflow tract (LVOT)]

is on right side – wrong side in wrong position. Confirm position of heart in this context and define situs inversus.

Abdominal Situs (Fig. 2)

Simple observation **(Figs. 3 and 4)**
- Fetal cephalic presentation: Abdominal organs are in clockwise rotation such as spine stomach, portal vessel
- Fetal position is breech: Abdominal organs are in anticlock wise rotation such as spine stomach, portal vessel

Importance of Defining Situs (Fig. 5)

Situs solitus: When stomach is on fetal left side and fetal heart is also tilted on the same side, it is termed as situs solitus. In this intracardiac abnormalities are 1%, which is as per prevalent rate of cardiac malformations. Rest of abdominal and cardiac organs are also positioned in their expected position.

Situs inversus: As name suggests, here position of thoracic and abdominal organs are on opposite side – stomach and

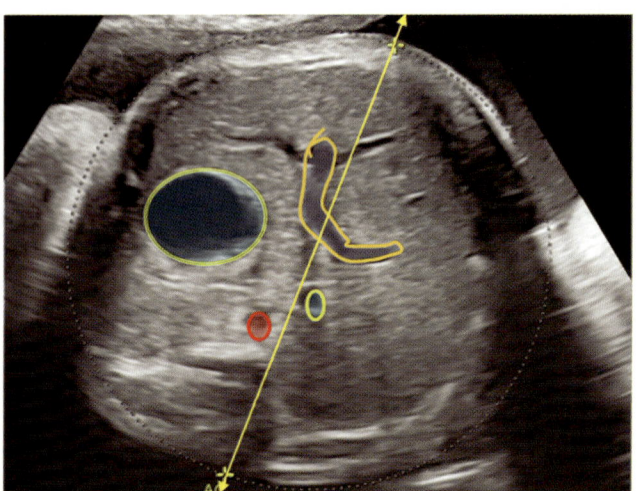

Fig. 2: Abdominal circumference view—cephalic presentation. Central line passing through vertebra. Red circle on aorta to left and anterior of spine. Yellow circle on IVC anterior and to right, big round is stomach on left. Abdominal organs, spine, stomach and portal in clock wise direction

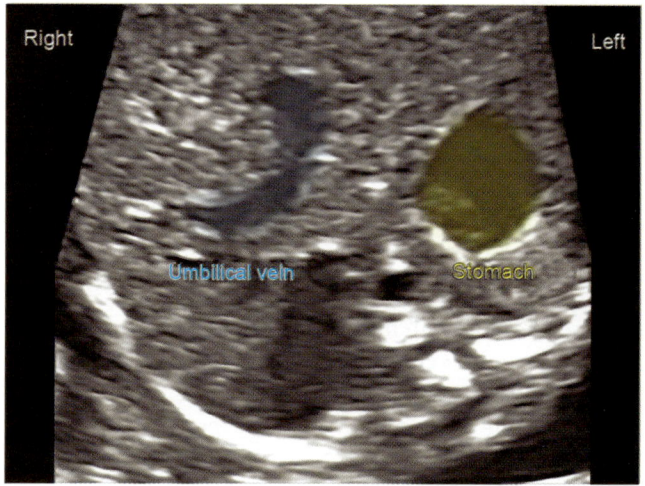

Fig. 3: Breech presentation.

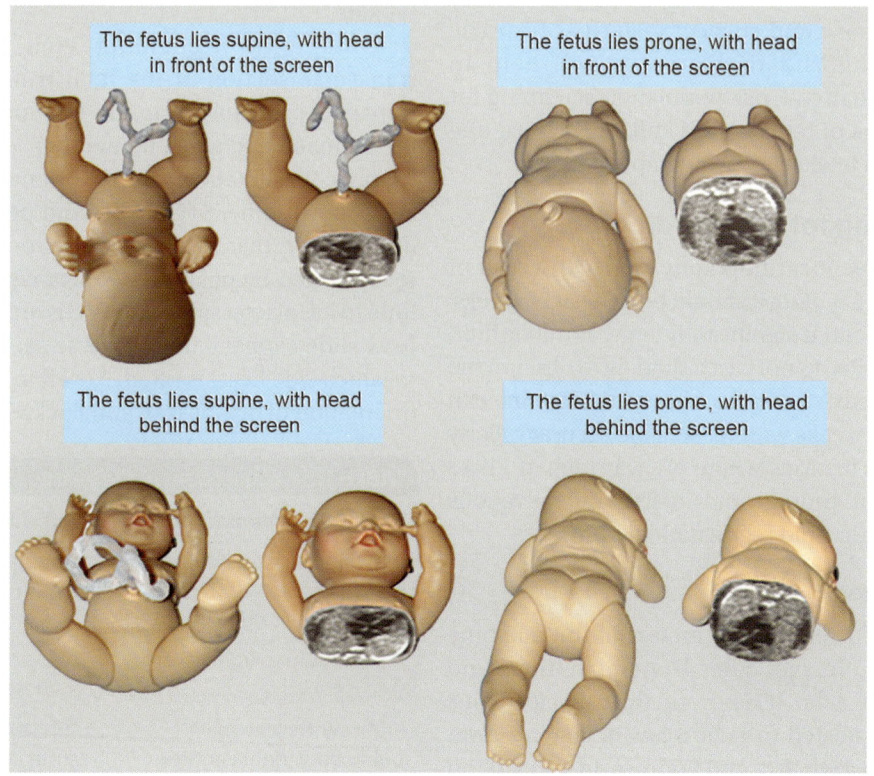

Fig. 4: Fetal cephalic presentation.

SECTION 3: Fetal Evaluation 177

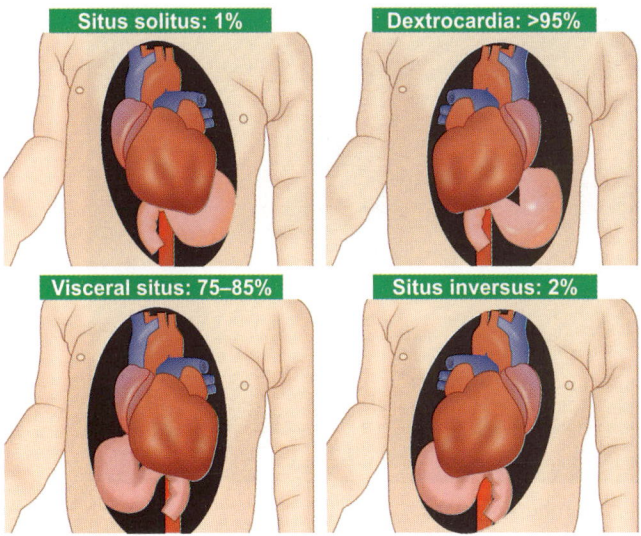

Fig. 5: Understanding situs and its importance in cardiac malformations.

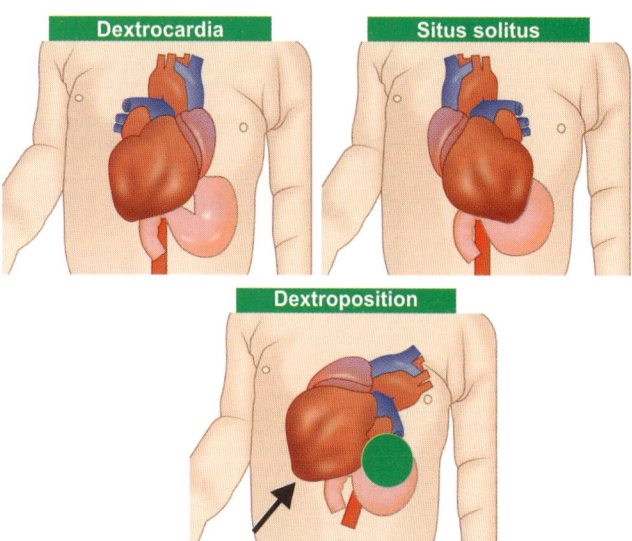

Fig. 6: Understanding different terminology. Dextrocardia where apex is rotated to right is associated with cardiac malformations. Dextroposition is due to pushing of heart with axis towards l left – associated with extracardiac malformations.

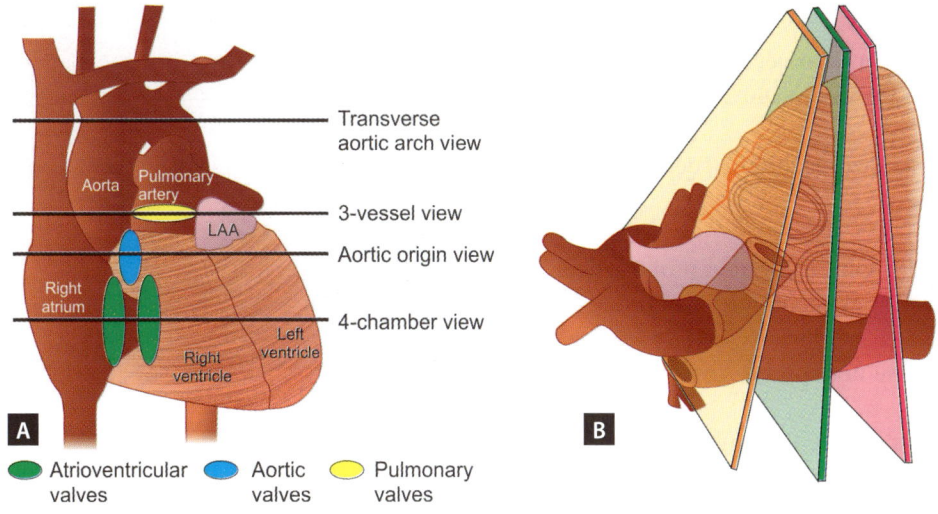

Figs. 7A and B: Normal 4-chamber view.

heart are on right side, liver on left and spleen on right side. In this scenario prevalence of intracardiac malformations are double – 2%.

Visceral situs: In this condition, a single organ like stomach is in the wrong position. With visceral situs prevalence of cardiac malformations is nearly 75–85%

Dextrocardia: When stomach is in normal position – left side but heart with its axis is rotated to right side – it is termed as dextrocardia. Cardiac malformations are highest in dextrocardia – nearly 95%.

Understanding Terminology (Fig. 6)

Dextroposition: In dextroposition, heart is *pushed* to right side with its axis still rotated to left side. This condition is associated with extracardiac malformations so one has to look for thoracic malformations or space occupying lesion on either side.

Dextrocardia: Dextrocardia occurs due to embryonic rotation failure of heart. So heart is rotated to right side in right thorax with axis of heart rotated to right. This is associated with intracardiac malformations.

The basic intracardiac views **(Figs. 7A and B):**
By single sweep from AC upward one can get it.
- The 4-chamber view
- The left ventricular outflow tract (or aortic origin) view (LVOT)
- Right ventricular outflow tract view (RVOT)
- The 3-vessel view (ductal arch view) and 3 vessel trachea view
- The transverse aortic arch view – tracheal view.

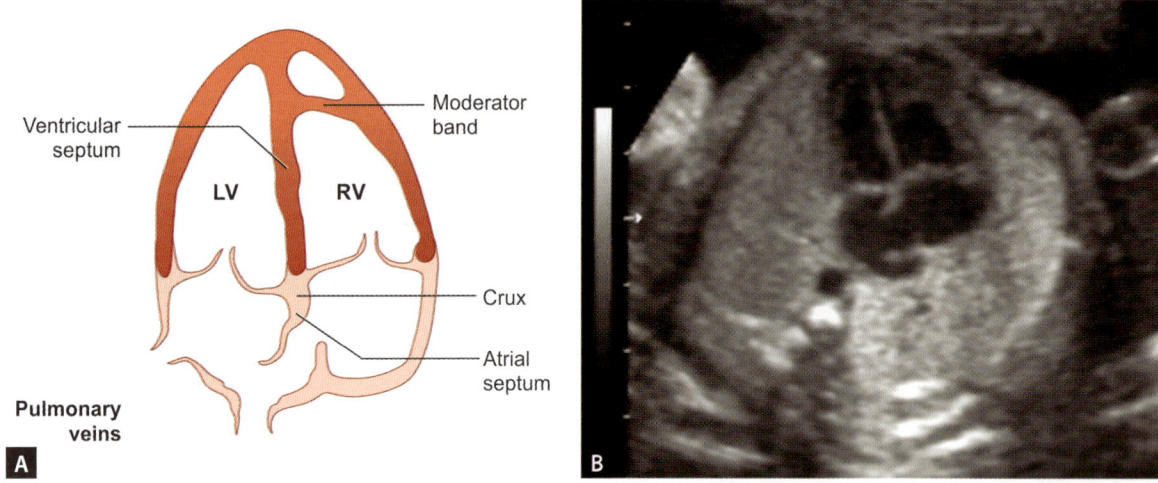

Figs. 8A and B: Demarcation of chambers of heart.

Overview

The 4-chamber view:
- Most important section of the heart and it is essential to evaluate this correctly
- It is much more than 4 chamber count
- It is abnormal in about 60% of major cardiac malformations
- Systematic analysis: Size, position, structure and function of all 4 chambers
- Views
  - Apical view with spine away from probe – ideal
  - Lateral view – apex facing on either side laterally – reasonable
  - Basal view–spine near probe, gives poor imaging of heart
- The rules for analysis of the 4-chamber view are the same no matter which way the fetus is lying.

Defining Chambers (Figs. 8A and B)

- Morphological left atrium
  - Foramen ovale flap in left atrium
  - Pulmonary veins entering in
  - Coronary sinus
- Morphological right ventricle
  - Moderator band
  - Insertion of tricuspid valve lower down
  - Near chest wall anterior most.

Heart Size (Figs. 9A and B)

The heart normally occupies central one-third of the area of the chest.
- Circumference of the heart should be compared to the thoracic circumference (C/T ratio). The normal C/T ratio is around 0.55 (range 0.5–0.6). However, this is not a precise measurement and should only be used as a rough guide.

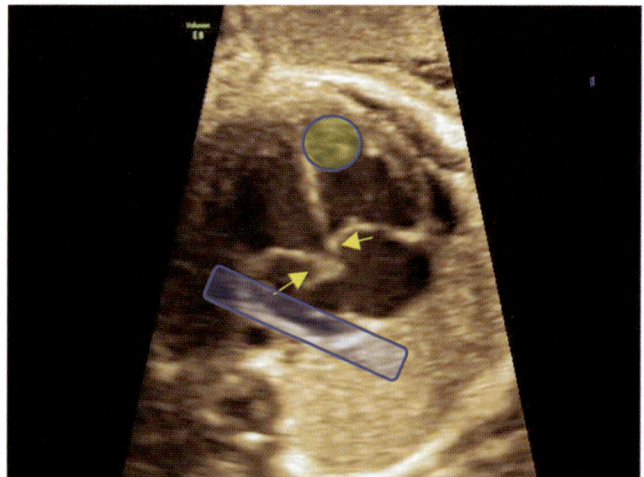

Fig. 9A: Apical 4 chamber view of heart. Note Round circle at moderator band in right ventricle. Both arrows pointing at offset insertion of AV valve. Rectangle on pulmonary veins entering left atrium. Also notice foramen ovale flap in left atrium. This was cephalic presentation with abdominal organ orientation in clockwise direction – Situs solitus.

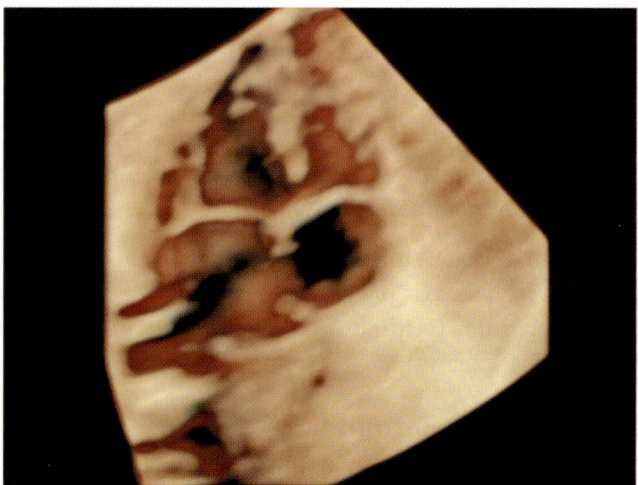

Fig. 9B: Thick slice of STIC showing detail anatomy of 4 chamber with interior of it.

Heart Position

Most of the heart lies in the left chest with tilt of the axis to left at 45° ± 20° to the midline of the thorax with apex pointing to left anterior chest wall **(Figs. 10A and B)**.

- The left atrium (LA) is the most posterior chamber in the normal heart, lying just anterior to the descending aorta, which lies anterior to the spine
- The right ventricle (RV) lies behind the sternum.

Heart Structure (Figs. 11A and B)

There are many structures to note in the 4-chamber view but with experience, this can be achieved within seconds of finding the correct image

- There are two atria of approximately equal size and contract equal and simultaneously
- There are two ventricles of approximately equal size and contract equal and simultaneously
- The crux or center of the heart is formed by the junction of the atrioventricular septum and the septal leaflets of the mitral and tricuspid valves
- There are two atrioventricular valves opening equally, the mitral valve on the left inserted more toward base and the tricuspid valve on the right and inserted more apically and therefore there is "off-setting" of the two valves into the crux
- Remember that valves belong to ventricles, tricuspid valves opens in right ventricle and mitral valve opens in left ventricle
- The apex of the right ventricle is more trabeculated than the left and contains a particularly thick muscle bundle - moderator band
- There is normally a small amount of fluid in the pericardium producing a dark line around the myocardium – measuring less than 2 mm
- The ventricular septum is intact from the apex to the crux

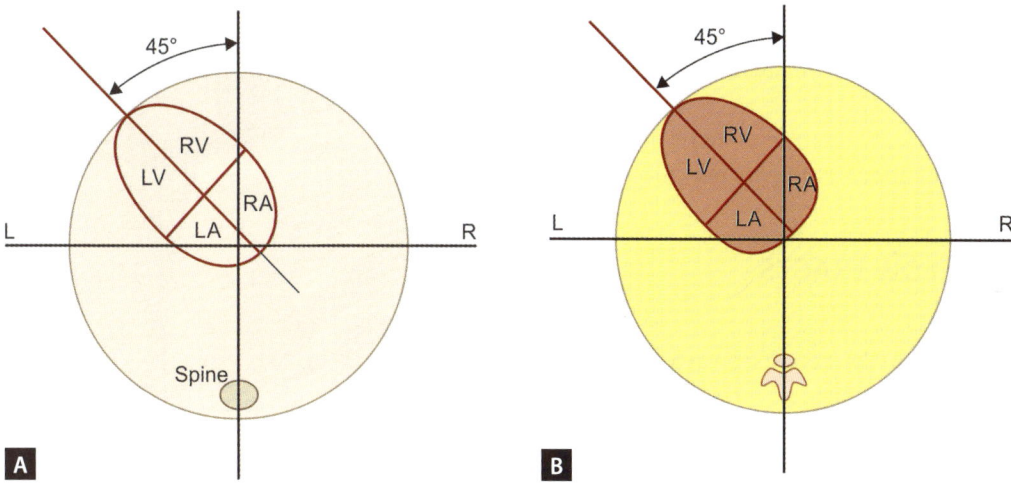

Figs. 10A and B: Cardiac axis and axis deviation.

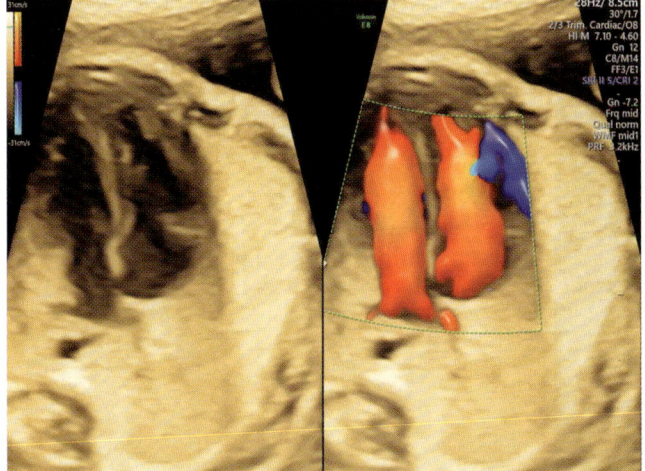

Fig. 11A: Four chamber view with and without color. This image is in ventricular diastole showing blood from left atrium entering in to ventricle with both AV valve open. IVS is intact. Inter-septum is normal and pulmonary veins are seen.

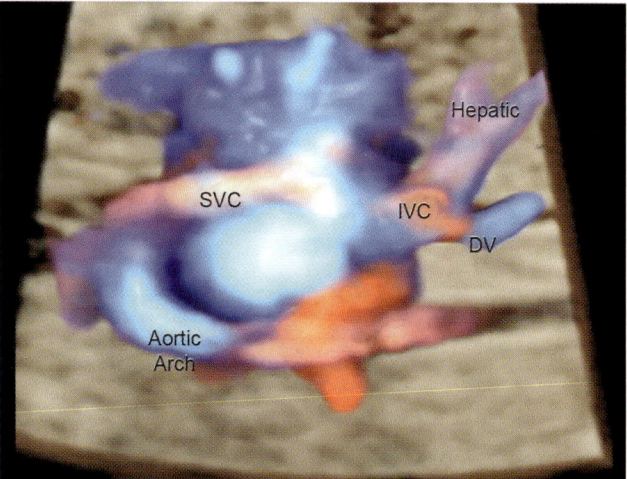

Fig. 11B: Heart in HD flow showing Inflow and outflow tracts.

- The primum atrial septum attaches to the crux. There is a defect in the middle third of the atrial septum (the foramen ovale) which is guarded by the foramen ovale flap in the left atrium
- There is one vessel lying behind the heart (the descending aorta), just to the left of the midline, between the spine and left atrium. Space behind left atrium and spine is less accommodating descending aorta and collapsed esophagus only
- The pulmonary veins attach to the back of the left atrium. Their connection preferably must be confirmed on color flow mapping.

Heart Function

- The two ventricles contract equally and briskly.
- The two atrioventricular (AV) valves open equally and freely. No undue echogenicity or tethering of valves.
- On color flow mapping, there is equal filling of both ventricles and there is no significant AV valve regurgitation
- A small amount of tricuspid regurgitation on color flow mapping is not uncommon with modern sensitive ultrasound machines and is usually of no significance in the 3rd trimester fetus.
- The atria and ventricles contract synchronously and regularly at a rate of about 140 beats per minute with a range of 120–180.

■ NORMAL OUTFLOW TRACTS

Overview

- About 40% of major heart defects are seen in the great artery views. It is therefore important to extend cardiac evaluation from the 4-chamber view to image the outflow tracts
- The great arteries should be analyzed systematically, with reference to size, position, structure and function
- The great artery views include:
  • Left ventricular outflow tract (aortic origin) view
  • Right ventricular outflow tract (RVOT)
  • 3-vessel view
  • 3-VT view.
- If you can recognize an abnormal appearance of any of these views and describe accurately why it is different from normal, you can reach the correct diagnosis
- Establish ventriculoarterial concordance. Additional views or complimentary view
  • Long axis view of the left ventricle
  • Sagittal arch and duct view
  • Long axis view of the duct
  • Long axis view of the arch
  • Short axis view of the left ventricle
  • Tricuspid-aorta view
  • Caval vein view (Hammock view).

Left Ventricular Outflow Tract View (Figs. 12 and 13)

- In the normal heart, the first great artery coming out of heart, seen just above (cranial to) the 4-chamber view, is the aorta

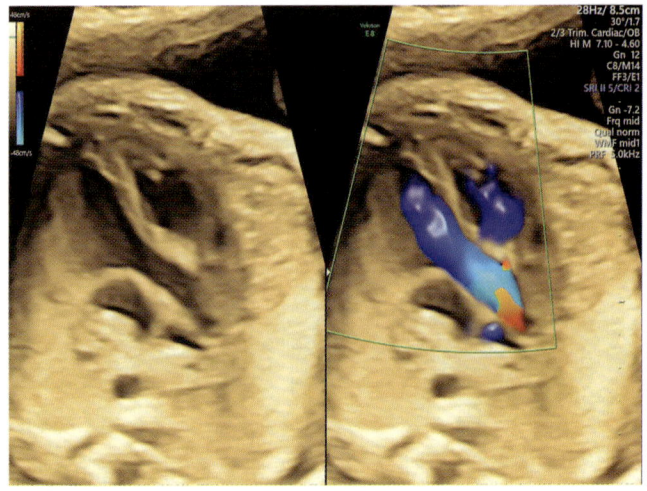

Fig. 12: Left outflow tract. In ventricular systole with open aortic valve and flow from left ventricle to aorta. Note anterior wall of aorta in continuation with IVS and posterior wall of aorta with mitral valve.

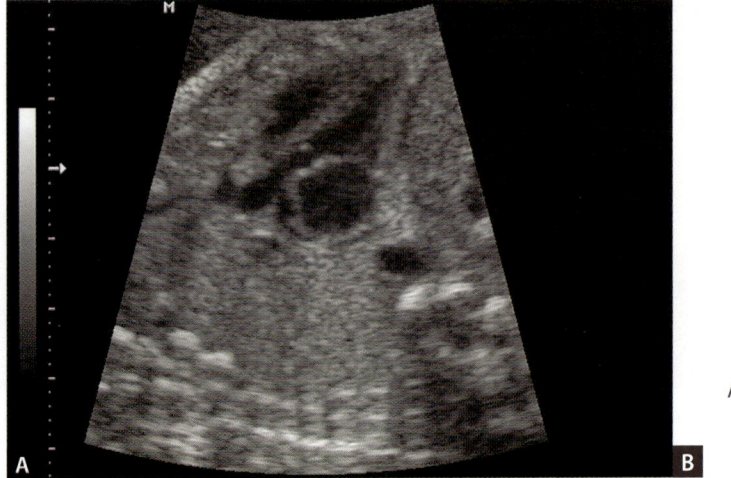
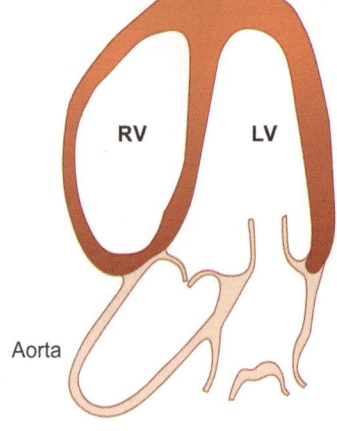

Figs. 13A and B: Left ventricular outflow tract view.

SECTION 3: Fetal Evaluation

- The aorta arises wholly from the left ventricle and initially sweeps out toward the right and then turns back toward descending aorta
- There are no visible branches of the aorta close to the valve (septoaortic concordance)
- The anterior wall of the aorta is continuous with the inter ventricular septum
- The posterior wall of the aorta is continuous with the anterior leaflet of the mitral valve
- The aortic valve opens freely during systole visible as dot in diastole (the valve cusps disappear in systole)
- On color flow mapping there is laminar (non-turbulent) forward flow across the aortic valve and no regurgitation
- No post-aortic valve dilation of vessel.

Right Ventricular Outflow Tract View (Figs. 14A and B)

- Second vessel to come out of heart arising from anterior ventricle (right ventricle) and goes straight to descending aorta, posteriorly is the pulmonary artery
- Divides into two branches immediately after it arise so you will see dilated vessel as its branch. Right pulmonary runs behind ascending aorta and anterior to bronchi toward right lung. Left pulmonary runs downwards and to left lung, before this it gives rise to ductus arteriosus to join descending aorta.

Arterial Crossover (Fig. 15)

- Just above the aortic valve, the pulmonary artery arises from the right ventricle. Note that they arise almost at right angles to each other: The flow is directed cranially and rightward in the aorta and directly posteriorly in the pulmonary artery

- As the probe is moved up toward the head from the view of the aortic origin, the pulmonary artery is seen to crossover the aortic origin
- By moving the ultrasound beam back and forward between the view of the aortic origin and the three-vessel view (which images the pulmonary artery), the relative size and position of the two great arteries can be noted
- On color flow and HD-STI crossover of great vessel can be better appreciated.

The 3-vessel View (Figs. 16 and 17)

Maintaining a transverse section, sweep the probe further up toward the head. Just above the aorta, the pulmonary artery, arising from the right ventricle, crosses over the aortic origin and continues as the arterial duct.

The 3-vessel view is also called line/dot/dot view (Figs. 18 and 19)

- The pulmonary artery is normally slightly bigger than the aorta. (For example, at 20 weeks the pulmonary artery is about 3.5 mm and the aorta is about 3.0 mm). Ratio of PA/Ao is 1 to 2
- The pulmonary valve is anterior and cranial to the aortic valve
- The pulmonary valve opens freely with laminar flow across it
- The pulmonary artery continues as the arterial duct and connects to the descending aorta
- The pulmonary artery branches laterally soon after the valve. The branches of the pulmonary artery are seen just below the level of the arterial duct, therefore just below the 3-vessel view
- In the *video,* the left pulmonary artery is seen better in the black and white image, whereas the right pulmonary artery is more clearly seen by color flow

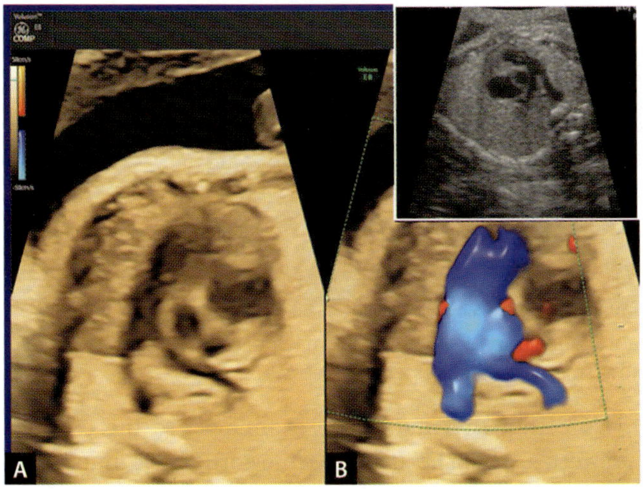

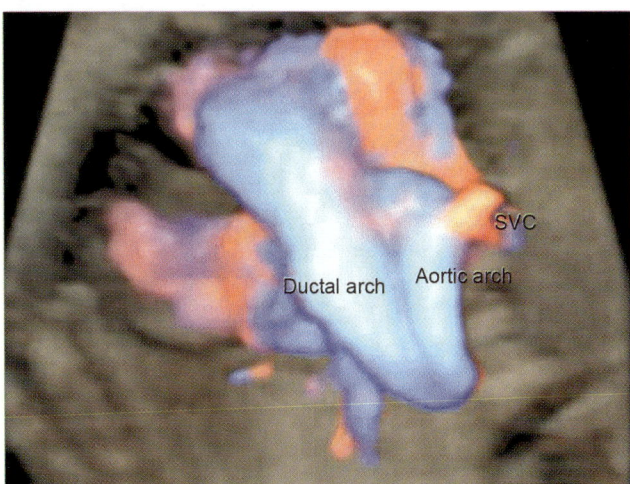

Figs. 14A and B: Right outflow tract. Note vessel connected to right ventricle and immediately divides into two branches. Right pulmonary passes between aorta and bronchi to right lung. Left pulmonary continue as DA to descending aorta.

Fig. 15: HD STIC showing thick slice of 3-vessel trachea view with pulmonary, aorta and SVC. Note aorta and pulmonary crossing at origin and then remain parallel with same color flow.

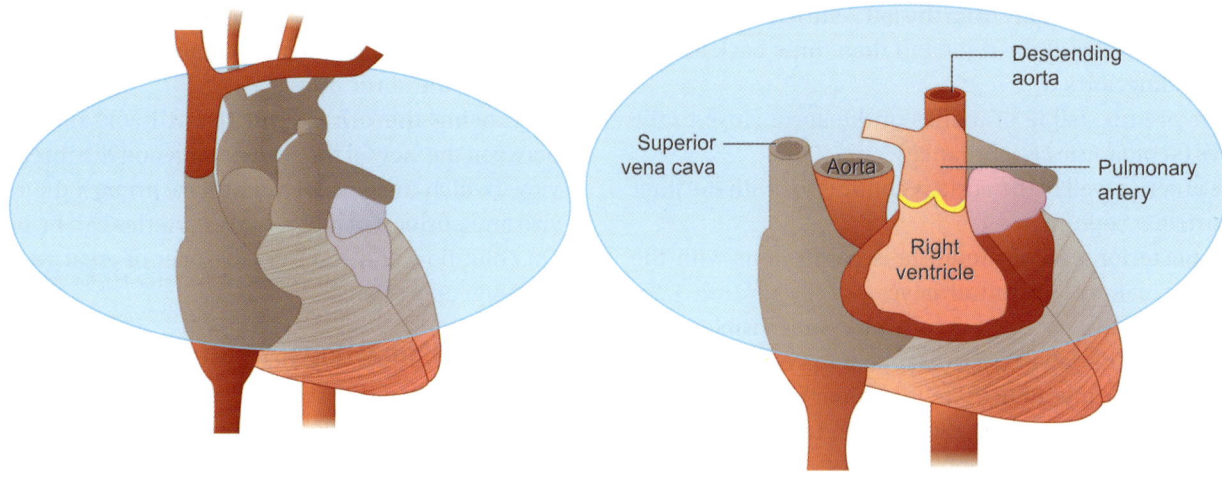

Figs. 16: The 3-vessel view.

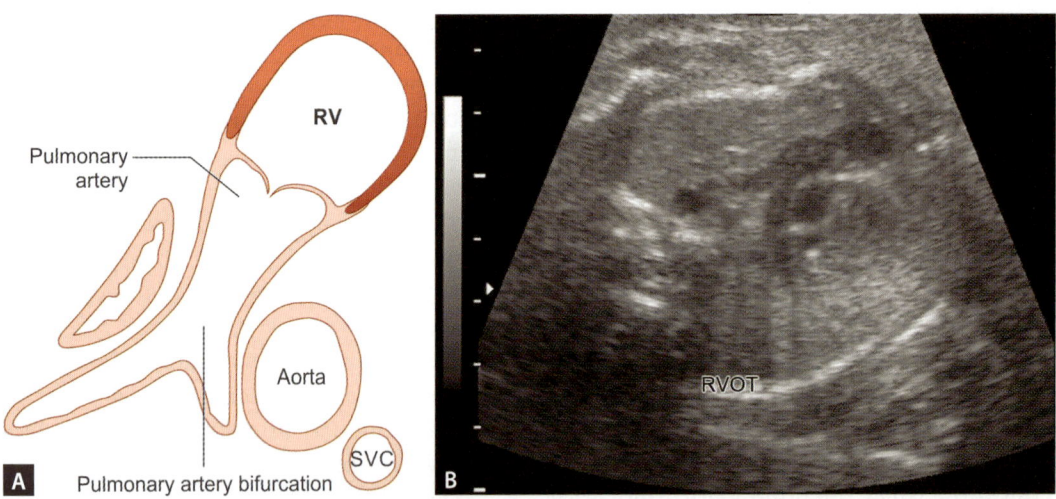

Figs. 17A and B: The 3-vessel view at pulmonary artery bifurcation.

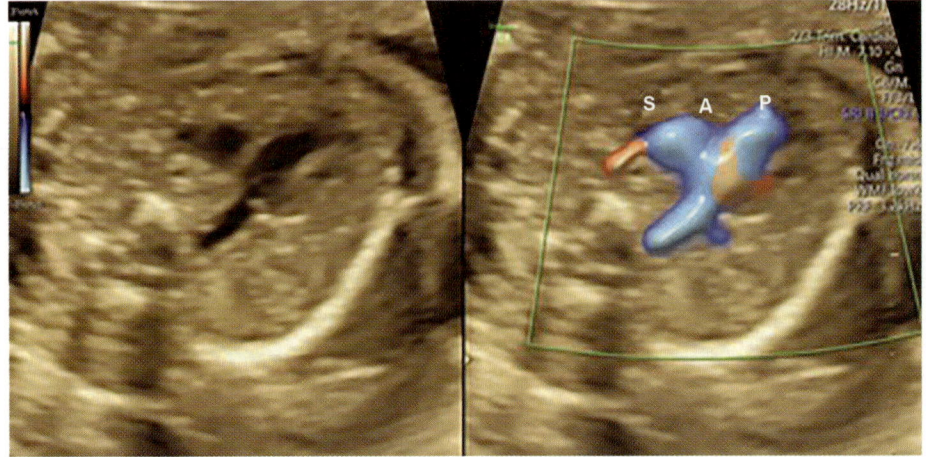

Fig. 18: 3-vessel view showing pulmonary artery, ascending aorta and superior vena cava from left of fetus to right. Both pulmonary and aorta are in same color. Note small red color vessel entering SVC.

- The branching characteristic of the pulmonary artery serves to distinguish this vessel from the aorta, in situations where the great arteries are not normally connected. As the first main branches of the aorta are distal from the valve and are directed superiorly, they are seen in the long-axis views

- Note that the first aortic branches are the coronary arteries, which lie just above the aortic valve, but they are small and they are not normally seen in the fetus.

From left to right pulmonary artery (line), ascending aorta (dot) and superior vena cava (dot) is visible. The aorta is slightly bigger than the superior vena cava.

The transverse aortic arch is seen just above the 3-vessel view. The arch:
- Lies above the arterial duct
- Crosses the midline of the thorax from right to left in front of the trachea
- Has an even caliber along its length
- Demonstrates forward flow on color Doppler.

Transverse Aortic Arch View: 3-VT View (Figs. 20 and 21)

Maintaining a transverse section of the fetal trunk, sweep the beam further up toward the head. Just above the pulmonary artery, the aorta forms the aortic arch.

Arch views: These are additional views which are not in guideline.

Aortic arch view **(Fig. 22):** Aortic arch arises from middle of chest in anteroposterior direction and has a shape of "walking Stick Handle". In both arches it is at cephalic side and from arch three vessels arise – brachiocephalic artery which divides in right common carotid and right subclavian

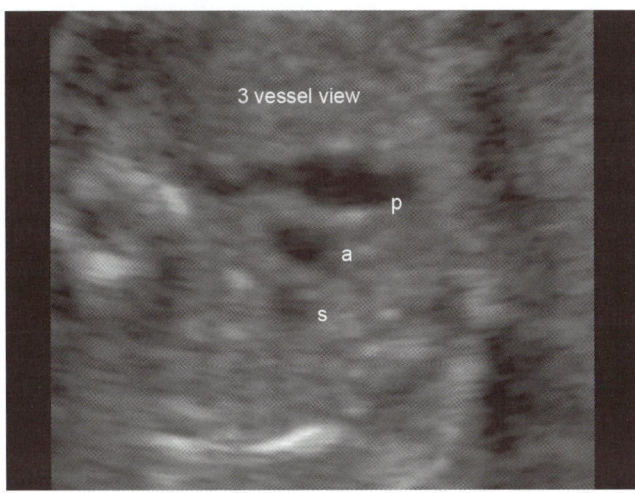

Fig. 19: Transverse aortic arch view.

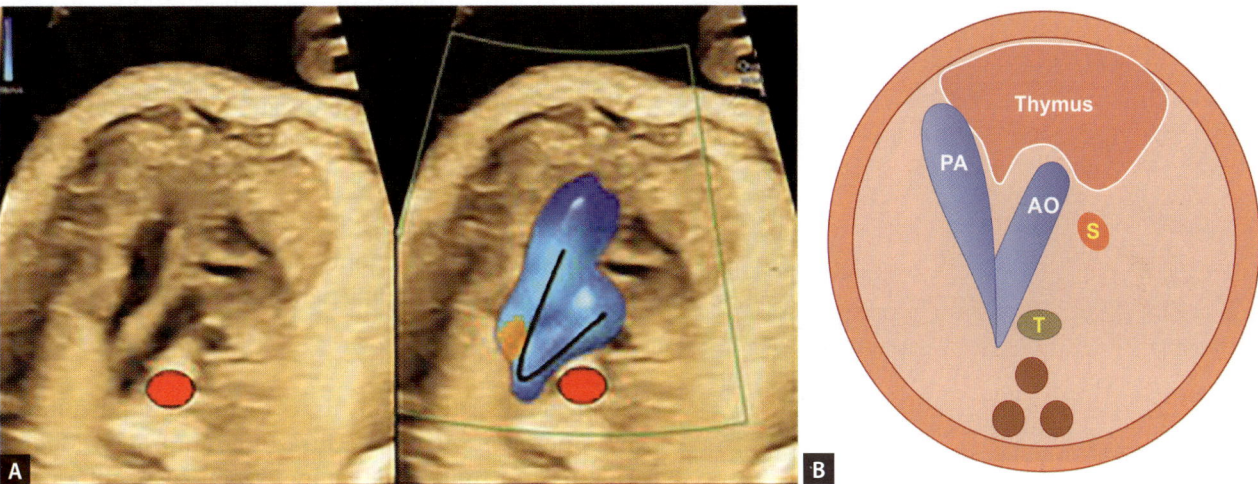

Figs. 20A and B: (A) 3-vessel trachea view showing pulmonary arch (large arm) and aortic arch (small arm) joining to descending aorta forming "V". Note in rec color trachea showing both ductal arch and aortic arch to left of trachea; (B) Same is explained in line diagram.

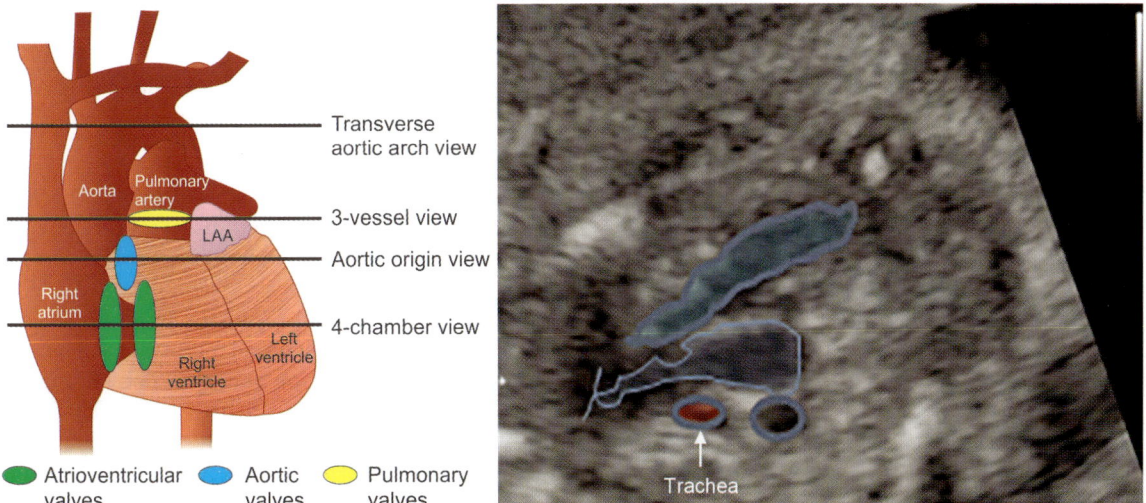

Fig. 21: Position and relations of valves of heart.

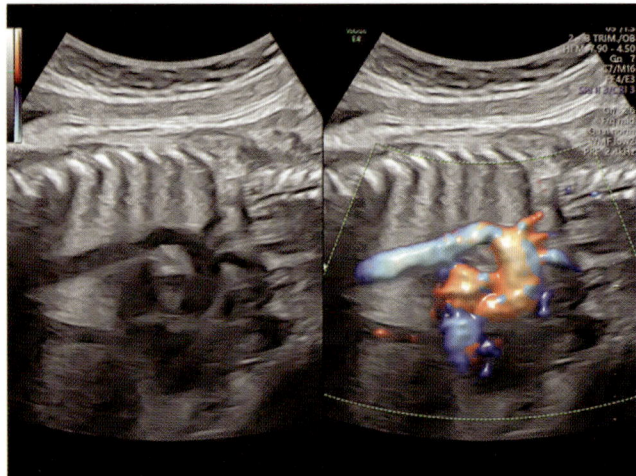

Fig. 22: Aortic arch view showing vessel arising from middle of chest with smooth acute "U" turn and descending down anterior to spine little to left. Note 3 vessel (innominate, left carotid and left subclavian) arising from arch.

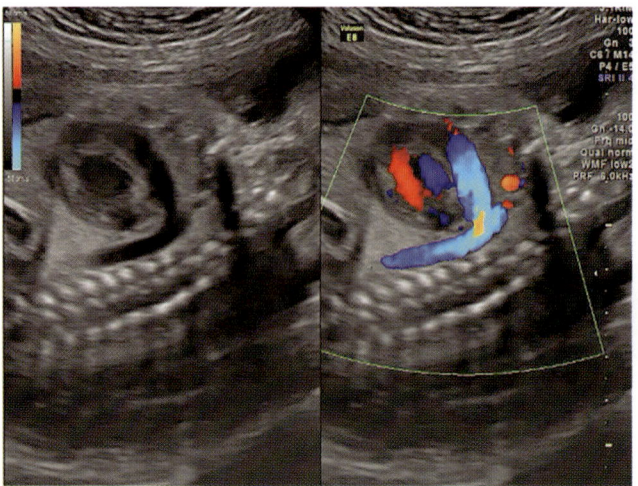

Fig. 23: Ductal arch arising near chest wall and join descending aorta below aortic arch level as ductus arteriosus.

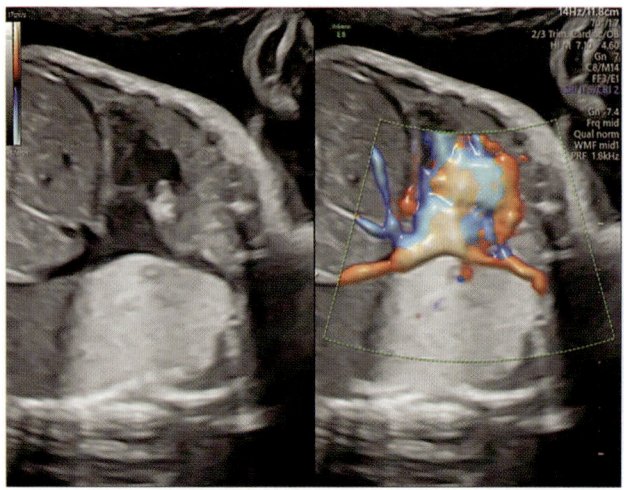

Fig. 24: Hammock view in HD flow showing SVC and IVC entering right atrium.

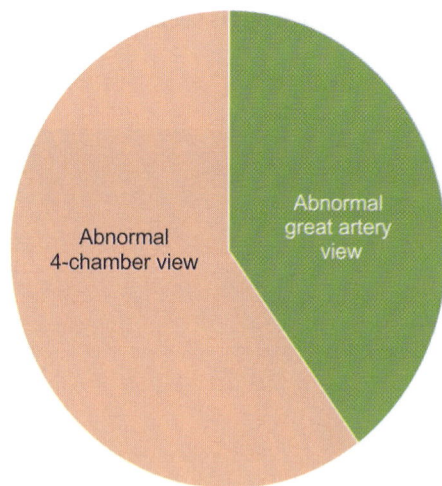

Fig. 25: Advantages of fetal echocardiography.

artery, left common carotid artery and left subclavian artery. This arch runs a little left and anterior to spine.

Ductal arch view **(Fig. 23):** Ductal arch arises from right ventricle and as right ventricle is anterior most, in sagittal view one can notice ductal arch arising from near anterior chest wall and runs backward to spine below the level of aortic arch and joins it after origin of left subclavian artery from the aortic arch. This has a "Hockey stick" appearance just before joining to descending aorta.

Hammock view **(Fig. 24):** This view is in sagittal section little to right of spine where one can see inferior vena cava and superior vena cava joining right atrium.

CONCLUSION

Fetal echocardiography is a recommended guideline by American Society of Ultrasound and Fetal Medicine as a part of routine screening. When suspecting cardiac malformation, advanced fetal echo by trained and experienced person shall be carried out. Association of fetal cardiac malformations with chromosomal abnormality and other malformations leading to adverse perinatal outcome makes it worth to screen the heart by basic and extended fetal heart examination guidelines **(Fig. 25)**.

REFERENCES

1. Ferencz C, Rubin JD, McCarter RJ, Brenner JI, Neill CA, Perry LW, et al. Congenital heart disease: prevalence at livebirth. The Baltimore–Washington infant study. Am J Epidemiol. 1985;121:31-6.
2. Crane JP, LeFevre ML, Winborn RC, Evans JK, Ewigman BG, Bain RP, et al. A randomized trial of prenatal ultrasonographic screening: impact on the detection, management, and outcome of anomalous fetuses. The RADIUS Study Group. Am J Obstet Gynecol. 1994;171:392-9.
3. Abu-Harb M, Hey E, Wren C. Death in infancy from unrecognized congenital heart disease. Arch Dis Child. 1994;71:3-7.

4. Tworetzky W, McElhinney DB, Reddy VM, Brook MM, Hanley FL, Silverman NH. Improved surgical outcome after fetal diagnosis of hypoplastic left heart syndrome. Circulation. 2001;103:1269-73.
5. Bonnet D, Coltri A, Butera G, Fermont L, Le Bidois J, Kachaner J, et al. Detection of transposition of the great arteries in fetuses reduces neonatal morbidity and mortality. Circulation. 1999;99:916-8.
6. DeVore G, Medearis AL, Bear MB, Horenstein J, Platt LD. Fetal echocardiography: factors that influence imaging of the fetal heart during the second trimester of pregnancy. J Ultrasound Med. 1993;12:659-63.
7. Sharland GK, Allan LD. Screening for congenital heart disease prenatally. Results of a 2½-year study in the South East Thames Region. Br J Obstet Gynaecol. 1992;99:220-5.
8. Lee W. American Institute of Ultrasound in Medicine. Performance of the basic fetal cardiac ultrasound examination. J Ultrasound Med. 1998;17:601-7.
9. American Institute of Ultrasound in Medicine. Guidelines for the performance of the antepartum obstetrical ultrasound examination. J Ultrasound Med. 2003;22:1116-25.
10. ISUOG. Cardiac screening examination of the fetus: guidelines for performing the "basic" and "extended basic" cardiac scan. Ultrasound Obstet Gynecol. 2006;27:107-13.

LONG QUESTIONS

1. Discuss the technique of the 4-chamber view in fetal 2D echocardiography.
2. What are the main features of imaging the fetal outflow tracts?

SHORT QUESTIONS

1. What are the indications for fetal 2D echocardiography?
2. What are the technical considerations for timing, machine and limitations of fetal 2D echocardiography?
3. What is the importance of defining situs?
4. Mention the basic intracardiac views on fetal heart imaging.

MULTIPLE CHOICE QUESTIONS

1. Fetal cardiac examination shall be:
   a. Part of fetal screening to all fetus
   b. Not required
   c. Detailed fetal echo is not part of routine screening
   d. It is a job of pediatric cardiologist
2. Why fetal echo is necessary? Which one is not applicable?
   a. It is most common fetal malformation
   b. Fetal cardiac malformations are highly associated with chromosomal abnormalities
   c. Prior information is useful in postnatal management
   d. It is lethal malformation
3. Fetal malformations are having prevalence of:
   a. 1: 2,000 live birth   b. 1: 10,000 Live birth
   c. 1: 80-100 live births   d. Very uncommon
4. As per ISUOG and most Guidelines following is mandatory for screening of fetal heart:
   a. 4 chamber view only
   b. 4 chamber view and 3 VT view
   c. 4 chamber view, Outflow tracts and 3VT view
   d. 4 chamber, out flow g tracts, 3-VT view, sagittal arch views and Hammock view
5. What is optimum time for fetal echo screening?
   a. 16-17 weeks   b. 22-24 weeks
   c. 30 weeks   d. 18-20 week
6. Follow view is not part of fetal echo screening:
   a. 4 chamber view   b. Outflow tracts
   c. Hammock view   d. AC view
7. Order steps for fetal echo in order:
   a. Outflow tracts   b. 4 chamber view
   c. 3 VT view   d. AC View
8. Following statement is true for fetal heart screening:
   a. Only 2 D is sufficient for fetal heart screening
   b. Spectra must for all screening Doppler
   c. 2D and color are needed for fetal heart screening
   d. M Mode is must for fetal heart screening
9. Malaligned VSD is always associated with:
   a. DORV   b. TOF
   c. Truncus arteriosus d. All of above
10. Following CHD can be missed commonly:
    a. TOF   b. AVSD
    c. Malaligned VSD d. ASD
11. Cardiac malformation is more frequent with:
    a. Situs solitus   b. Situs inversus
    c. Ambiguous situs d. Dextrocardia
12. Following is not true to define right ventricle:
    a. Moderator band
    b. Apex is occupied by right ventricle
    c. AV valve is towards apex of heart in right ventricle
    d. Right ventricle is near chest wall
13. In outflow tracts following is not true for aorta:
    a. Aorta comes out of heart as first vessel
    b. Is arises from center of chest
    c. It go anterior and then band backward to descending aorta
    d. It divides in 2 vessels immediately after origin

Answers
1. a 2. d 3. c 4. c 5. b 6. c
7. d→b→a→c 8. c 9. d 10. d 11. d
12. b 13. d

3.10 NONINVASIVE PRENATAL TEST

Hemant Deshpande, Monika Maan Sharma

INTRODUCTION

Prenatal diagnosis of fetal aneuploidy, such as Down syndrome is usually based on a two-stage model: screening tests and invasive diagnostic tests for the high-risk population as determined by the aforesaid screening tests.

Screening tests are directed at the entire population of pregnant women, which are affordable and noninvasive.

They include different combinations of maternal serum biochemical markers and various ultrasound markers; the risk is then computed considering any other risk factors with the women.

Currently, the most commonly employed screening test is the first trimester screening test, which includes maternal age, ultrasound measurement of nuchal translucency in combination with maternal serum levels of pregnancy-associated plasma protein A (PAPP-A), and free beta-human chorionic gonadotropin (beta-hCG) also known as the combined test done at 10–14 weeks of pregnancy.[1,2]

All those cases who fall to be in high-risk group in screening tests or those with family or personal history of chromosomal anomalies or abnormal ultrasound findings are further exposed to the confirmatory invasive diagnostic tests such as chorionic villus sampling (CVS) and amniocentesis where chromosomal analysis of fetal cells is done.

Though diagnostic tests provide definitive results, they are associated with a risk of pregnancy loss.

Chorionic villus sampling can be performed between weeks 10 and 12 and pregnancy, and amniocentesis performed between weeks 15 and 18 of pregnancy. These tests carry up to 1 in 150 or 1 in 100 chance of miscarriage, respectively.

Previously, it was only possible to test for these abnormalities with highly invasive procedures that carried a risk to the pregnancy.

Initial screening with noninvasive prenatal testing (NIPT) which is more reliable and sensitive can help to avoid this potentially unnecessary and invasive testing.

Noninvasive prenatal testing offers such an opportunity. NIPT is a technique that can be used to test a fetus for a range of genetic conditions and variations using a blood sample taken from the pregnant woman. It is referred to as "noninvasive" because it does not involve inserting a needle into the woman's abdomen or cervix, as is the case with invasive testing where cells are taken from the amniotic sac (in amniocentesis) or the placenta (in CVS). There is no risk to mother or baby.

Noninvasive prenatal testing provides the earliest testing available from as early as 9–10 weeks.

- NIPTs usually screen for all of the following seven chromosomal aneuploidies or for a subset of them: Down syndrome (trisomy 21), Edward syndrome (trisomy 18), Patau syndrome (trisomy 13), Turner syndrome (45,X), Klinefelter syndrome (47, XXY), triple X syndrome (47,XXX), and Jacobs syndrome (47,XYY).[3]
- It can provide a definitive diagnosis for some genetic conditions, such as cystic fibrosis, achondroplasia, and Apert syndrome, if they are inherited from the father or arise at conception.
- Since the identification of cell-free fetal deoxyribonucleic acid (cffDNA) in maternal plasma in the late 1990s (Lo et al. 1997), there has been considerable progress in developing safer methods for NIPT based on analysis of fetal DNA circulating in maternal blood. Owing to many advantages, the adoption of NIPT in routine clinical practice was very rapid and global.
- NIPT to detect fetal aneuploidy employs a massive parallel sequencing of cell-free DNA (cfDNA) from maternal blood, is gaining rapid acceptance in obstetrics, given its high sensitivity and specificity for the detection of trisomies 21, 18, and 13, i.e., 99.7%, 97.9%, and 99%, respectively.

Direct analysis of fetal cells from maternal circulation has been difficult given the scarcity of fetal cells in maternal blood (1:10,000–1:1,000,000) and the focus has shifted to the analysis of cffDNA, which is found at a concentration almost 25 times higher than that available from nucleated blood cells extracted from a similar volume of whole maternal blood.

Moreover, the approach using cffDNA provides easier, less labor-intensive, and less time-consuming ways to work with fetal DNA.[4]

WHAT IS CELL-FREE DEOXYRIBONUCLEIC ACID?

- cfDNA is DNA fragments generated from apoptosis of trophoblasts in placenta, which is released into circulation after rapid DNA degradation. The size distribution of these DNA fragments has peaks corresponding to nucleosomes (~143 bp) and chromatosomes (nucleosome + linker histone; ~166 bp).[5] Unlike DNA isolated from circulating fetal cells, cffDNA is actually of placental origin.
- Placental DNA, a surrogate of fetal DNA, enters the maternal bloodstream via apoptosis of trophoblasts in the intervillous space of the placenta, where it mixes with cfDNA of maternal origin.
- During pregnancy, about 10% of cfDNA is of fetal origin (cffDNA) **(Fig. 1)**.[4]

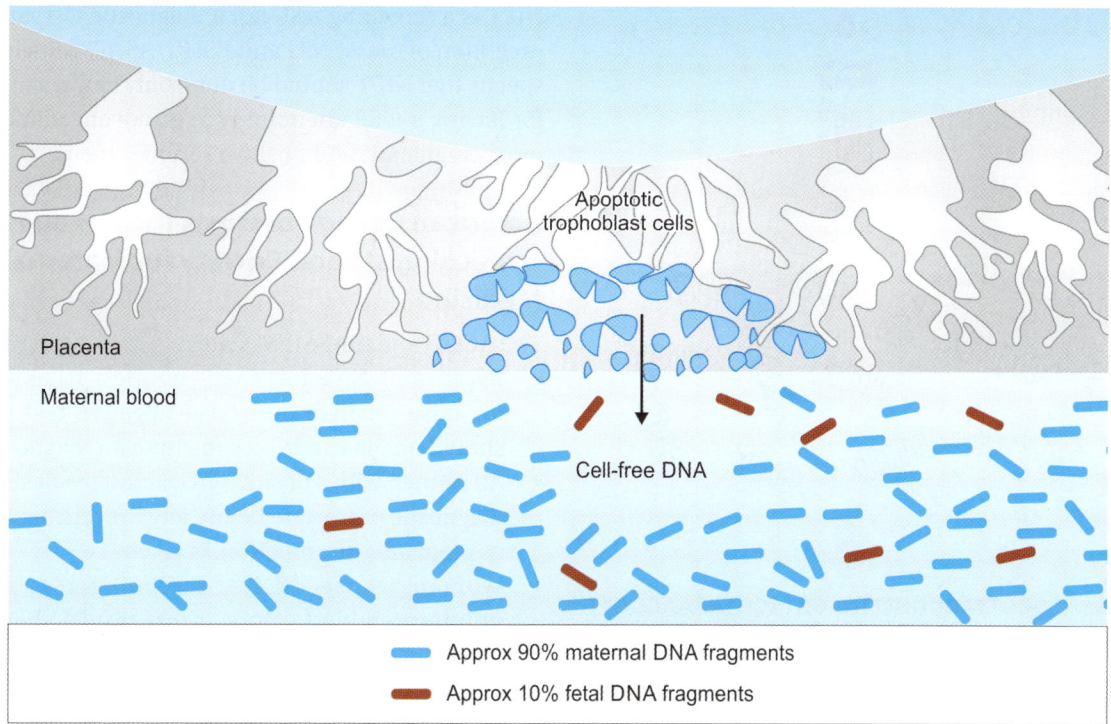

Fig. 1: Maternal and fetal DNA in maternal circulation. (DNA: deoxyribonucleic acid)

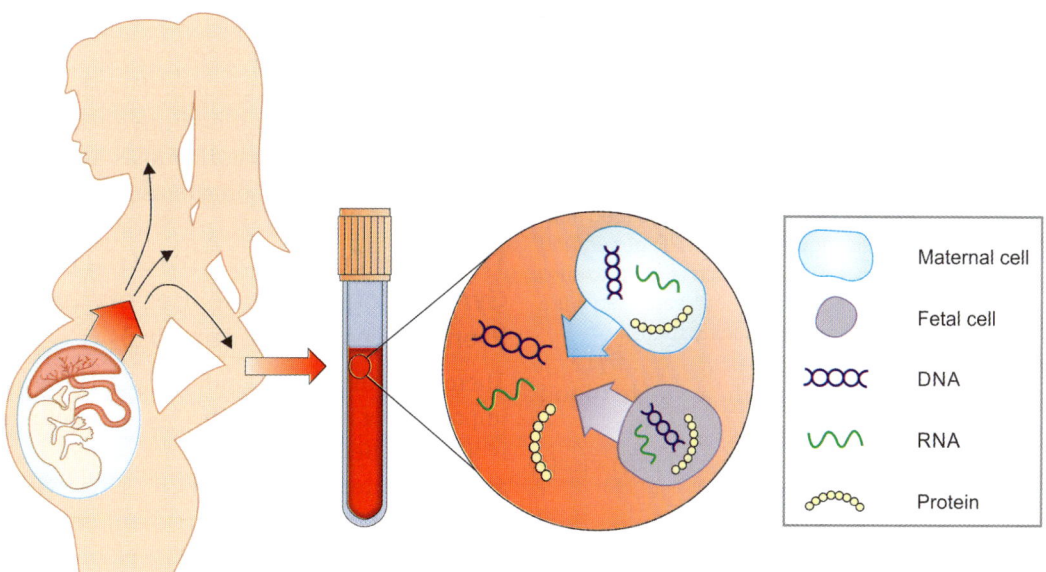

Fig. 2: Principle of noninvasive prenatal testing. Maternal blood consists of maternal and placental cells, which release their DNA content directly into maternal circulation. Therefore, cell-free fetal elements (for example, DNA, RNA, and proteins) are present in the blood of pregnant woman and can be used as biomarkers for prenatal testing and diagnosis.[6] (DNA: deoxyribonucleic acid; RNA: ribonucleic acid)

- Fetal DNA can be detected in as little as 10 μL of maternal plasma and serum.

Noninvasive prenatal testing though a form of advanced screening; positive results require confirmation by a diagnostic test amniocentesis or CVS **(Figs. 2 and 3)**.

There are a number of existing approaches for the determination of fetal deoxyribonucleic acid (DNA) fraction.[8] The principles for these procedures are diagrammatically depicted in **Figure 4**.

WHO GETS NONINVASIVE PRENATAL TESTING DONE?

While all women are offered to undergo NIPT screening, diagnostic tests are typically recommended when the screening tests have shown positive or inconclusive results or women are at an increased risk for genetic disorders, including:

- Advanced maternal age

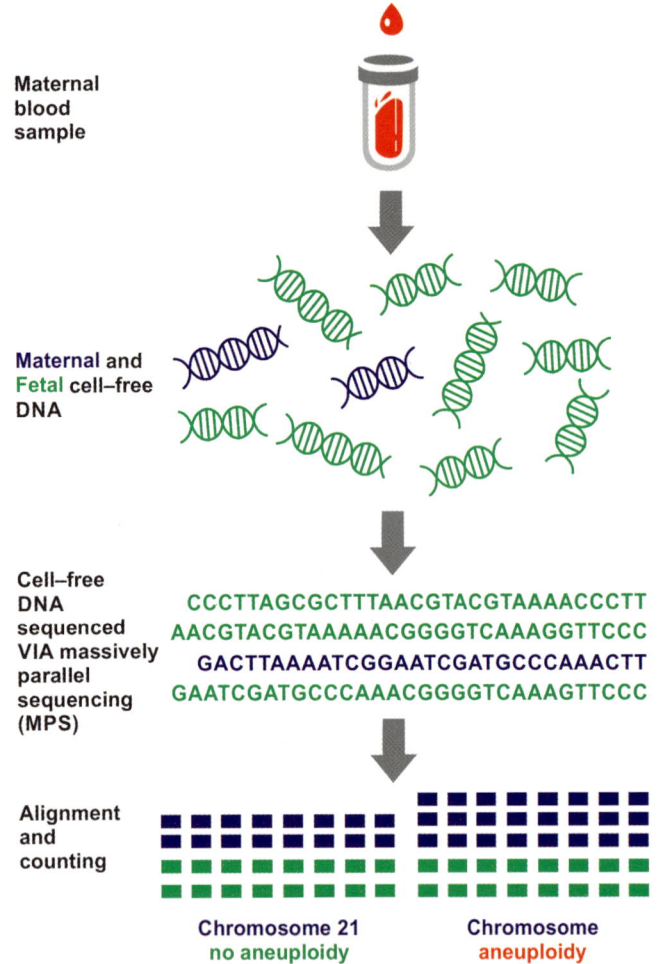

Fig. 3: Massively parallel sequencing and counting for the detection of fetal aneuploidy. Cell-free deoxyribonucleic acid cfDNA is isolated from maternal plasma. The total cfDNA is sequenced by MPS, generating millions of sequence reads. Sequence reads are then aligned to sites from a reference human genome and the aligned reads (tags) are counted for determination of the chromosome ploidy status.[7]

- Chronic maternal conditions, such as high blood pressure, lupus, epilepsy, or diabetes
- History of miscarriages or having a child with birth defects
- Family history of genetic disorders
- Being a carrier of or having a partner who is carrier of a genetic disorder
- Multiple gestation
- Certain ethnicity associated with a higher risk of some genetic disorders.

■ CURRENT GUIDELINES

The Society for Maternal-Fetal Medicine (SMFM), the American College of Obstetricians and Gynecologists (ACOG), the American College of Medical Genetics and Genomics (ACMG), and the European Society of Human Genetics (ESHG) together with the American Society of Human Genetics (ASHG) have issued statements to guide the clinical use of NIPT. These guidelines stress the importance of pre- and post-test genetic counseling; clearly indicate that NIPT is a screening test, not a diagnostic test; and, with the exception of the ACMG and ESHG/ASHG guidelines, clearly specify that NIPT should be done only to women at high risk for having a fetal aneuploidy (e.g., advanced maternal age, prior pregnancy, and positive serum screen).

American College of Obstetricians and Gynecologists and Society for Maternal-Fetal Medicine

The ACOG and the SMFM states:

- Because cfDNA is just a screening test, it has the potential for false-positive and false-negative test results and should not be used as a substitute for diagnostic testing.
- All women with a positive cfDNA test result should have a diagnostic procedure before any irreversible action, such as pregnancy termination, is taken.
- Women whose cfDNA screening test results are uninterpretable (a no call test result) should receive further genetic counseling and be offered comprehensive ultrasound evaluation and diagnostic testing because of an increased risk of aneuploidy.
- The cfDNA screening tests for microdeletions have not been validated clinically and are not recommended at this time.[9]
- Some women who receive a positive test result from traditional screening may prefer to have cfDNA screening rather than undergo definitive testing. This approach may delay definitive diagnosis and management and may fail to identify some fetuses with aneuploidy.

The Royal College of Obstetricians and Gynaecologists Guidelines on Noninvasive Prenatal Testing (Green Top)

There is no Green Top guideline yet. However, the scientific impact paper no. 15, March 2014 speculates this technology is likely to become the primary screen for chromosomal abnormalities in pregnancy. This will enhance the information available to pregnant women while greatly reducing the loss of uncomplicated pregnancies as a result of miscarriage caused by unnecessary invasive procedures.

Though, it is yet to become a part of NHS screening program.

International Society for Prenatal Diagnosis

The International Society for Prenatal Diagnosis (ISPD) 2014 considered the offer of NIPT as a first-tier screening test for all pregnant women to be an "appropriate" option.[10]

■ ACCURACY OF NONINVASIVE PRENATAL TESTING[11]

Accuracy of NIPT has been presented in **Table 1**.

SECTION 3: Fetal Evaluation

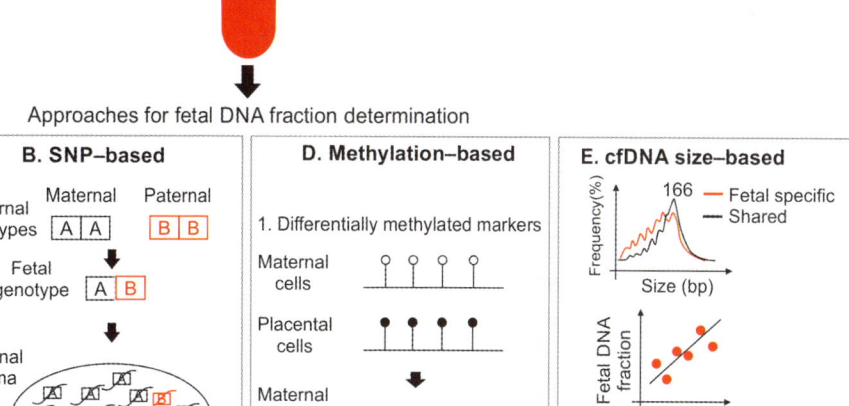
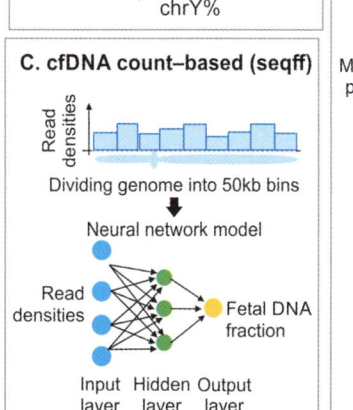
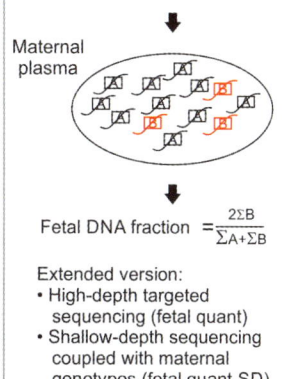
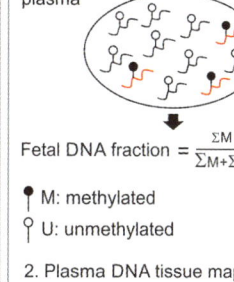
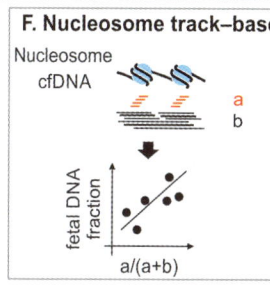

Figs. 4A to F: Schematic illustration of current approaches for the determination of fetal deoxyribonucleic acid (DNA) fraction in maternal circulating cell-free DNA (cfDNA). (A) Y chromosomal (chr) sequence-based fetal DNA fraction estimate. (B) Single-nucleotide polymorphism (SNP)-based approach. A direct way to estimate the fetal DNA fraction is to use the SNP loci, where both mother and father are homozygous but with different alleles. The resulting fetal genotype is obligately heterozygous. In maternal plasma, the fetal DNA fraction can be directly deduced by calculating the proportion of fetal specific alleles. Based on this concept, two extended versions of SNP-based methods for fetal DNA fraction estimate have been developed, namely *FetalQuant* and *FetalQuant*^{SD}, which can be used without the need of both paternal and maternal genotype information. (C) cfDNA count-based approach. Read densities across the genome-wide 50 kb windows are fitted into a neural network model to predict the fetal DNA fraction. (D) Differential methylation-based approaches. (E) cfDNA size-based approach. The proportion of short cfDNA molecules is correlated with fetal DNA fraction. (F) Nucleosome track-based approach. CfDNA distribution at the nucleosomal core and linker regions is correlated with fetal DNA fraction.[9]

TABLE 1: Accuracy of noninvasive prenatal testing.

Condition	Number of studies (tests)	Sensitivity (95% CI)	Specificity (95% CI)	Diagnostic odds ratio (95% CI)	Positive likelihood ratio (95% CI)	Negative likelihood ratio (95% CI)
Trisomy 21	31 (148,344)	0.994 (0.983–0.998)	0.999 (0.999–1.00)	285,903 (124,215–658,053)	1,720 (1,111–2,662)	0.006 (0.002–0.017)
Trisomy 18	24 (146,940)	0.977 (0.952–0.989)	0.999 (0.998–1.00)	68,110 (29,137–159,209)	1,569 (810–3,149)	0.023 (0.011–0.048)
Trisomy 13*	16 (134,691)	0.906 (0.823–0.958)	1.00 (0.999–1.00)	2,788 (285–27,252)	453 (26–7,864)	0.188 (0.080–0.44039)
Monosomy X	8 (6,712)	0.929 (0.741–0.984)	0.999 (0.995–0.999)	18,849 (2,277–156,069)	1,337 (213–8,407)	0.071 (0.017–0.292)

NB: All analyses performed by bivariate meta-analysis, apart from *, which indicates that univariate analysis was performed. (CI = confidence interval)

■ BENEFITS

- It is a noninvasive test and thus does not pose the risks of CVS or amniocentesis, such as pain, small risk of infection and the 0.22% [95% confidence interval (CI), 0.71 to 1.16%] and 0.11% (95% CI, 0.04 to 0.26%) procedure-related risk of miscarriage associated with CVS and amniocentesis, respectively.[12]
- Since cffDNA is cleared quickly from the maternal circulation, it is specific to that pregnancy. The test has a quick processing time, with the potential for results to be reported in 3–5 working days.

DISADVANTAGES AND LIMITATIONS

- Testing in monozygotic twins theoretically should be easier as they produce identical DNA molecules, but chorionicity must be certain. Another problem is that of single twin demise, as the effect that cffDNA from the demised twin has on the NIPT result is unknown. Because of these factors, various professional bodies do not currently recommend NIPT for aneuploidy in twin pregnancies.
- The most common reasons offered by authors for false and inconclusive results were:[13]
  - A low fetal DNA fraction in the blood sample, which is measured by specific markers of fetal DNA or algorithms applied to the sequencing data.
  - A "vanishing" twin that has disappeared prior to the woman's dating ultrasound scan, which if nonidentical may cause a false-positive result. This is likely to remain an issue even as technology advances.
  - Confined placental mosaicism, whereby the fetus and placenta have two different lineages. As the fetal DNA fragments originate from the placenta, NIPT is unable to distinguish between the two. This is also something that is unlikely to be overcome, despite continued advances in test technology, but it should be noted that this is an issue for invasive placental sampling (e.g., CVS) as well.
  - NIPT can detect maternal cancers and maternal copy number variants, which result in false positives and have ethical implications.
  - Testing in multiple pregnancies presents unique challenges. In dizygotic twins, aneuploidy discordance is a significant issue and there can be nearly a twofold intertwin difference in cffDNA fraction. This means that the affected fetus may have a cffDNA fraction below the threshold of 4% required for testing, while the unaffected twin may contribute a high cffDNA fraction; therefore, the total cffDNA fraction may appear sufficient and produce a false negative (low-risk) result.[13]
- Testing in monozygotic twins theoretically should be easier as they produce identical DNA molecules, but chorionicity must be certain. Another problem is that of single twin demise, as the effect that cffDNA from the demised twin has on the NIPT result is unknown. Because of these factors, various professional bodies do not currently recommend NIPT for aneuploidy in twin pregnancies, including the Royal College of Obstetricians and Gynaecologists (RCOG)[14] and the ACOG.[15]

ETHICAL VALUES

The development and increasing availability of NIPT raises a range of ethical issues, some of which are similar to those raised by prenatal screening itself.

CHOICE, AUTONOMY AND CONSENT

- One's ability to make free, informed choices about the medical tests and treatments they undergo is considered to be a key principle in modern healthcare. *Reproductive autonomy* refers to the capability a couple to make choices about when they become parents, how many children they have and whether or not to undergo screening tests such as prenatal testing.
- NIPT can facilitate the reproductive autonomy in many ways, including by allowing women and couples to prepare for a baby with a condition or trait, or decide to have a termination, potentially at an earlier stage of pregnancy.
- However, NIPT may also compromise autonomy and choice if reliable and appropriate information about the test and the conditions being tested for is not available, or when women and couples feel they are should to make a specific decision.

AVOIDING HARM

- The Government has an obligation to protect its citizens against harm. As part of this, it has a role to eliminate any harm that might be caused by medical interventions such as NIPT that are available through the government or the private healthcare sector.
- NIPT itself could also give anxiety if the information and support provided to women and couples is inadequate or misleading, or where there are incorrect or unreliable results. If NIPT results in a significant decrease in the number of people born with genetic conditions or impairments, it could lead to fewer resources being invested in research, healthcare, and education relating to and available to people affected by genetic conditions, and cause offence, social exclusion, and discrimination.

EQUALITY, FAIRNESS AND INCLUSION

- NIPT has the potential to contribute to women's ability to exert control over the circumstances of their pregnancies, with implications for their role in the workplace and wider society.
- This involves taking into account how policies such as a new health intervention might reduce or worsen existing inequalities. It also entails the duty to ensure that public money is spent fairly.
- However, NIPT has the potential to undermine equality, fairness, and inclusion for disabled people in a number of ways. For example, it may give rise to perceptions that people are to blame for having a baby with a disability, and make disabled people and their families more vulnerable to stigma and abuse.[16]

POSSIBLE FUTURE DEVELOPMENTS

This is a rapidly growing field and uses of NIPT for other single gene conditions, or "panel tests" for several related conditions, are likely to be developed in future. The availability of NIPT for significant medical conditions can enable pregnant women and couples to make informed decisions about their pregnancies regarding whether to continue and prepare for the birth of a disabled child or whether to have a termination.

If NIPT is ever to completely replace conventional cytogenetic analysis following CVS or amniocentesis, it will need to match the diagnostic accuracy as well as the scope of anomalies that can be detected.

It is also possible that NIPT could be developed in future to test fetuses for genetic conditions that are likely to affect them later in their adult life. Whole genome sequencing using NIPT might also become available to pregnant women and couples, where it is suspected that the fetus has a genetic condition but the origin is unknown.

Making decisions about whether NIPT should be offered for this kind of use and who it should be offered to will involve consideration of:
- How best to respect the autonomy and protect the interests of the future child or adult
- Whether the information being sought is medically useful
- What genetic counseling and support will be available to women and couples undergoing testing
- Whether NIPT might inadvertently reveal previously unknown genetic information about the pregnant woman or her partner.[16]

CONCLUSION

It is a noninvasive, relatively painless, and safe procedure without the related risk of miscarriage which is associated with amniocentesis and CVS. It should be noted that NIPT is not a diagnostic test and should be confirmed by invasive testing for the presence of any abnormal results. NIPT will change the face of prenatal testing; it is important that healthcare professionals counseling women on NIPT provide all the information required for them to make an informed decision regarding antenatal testing.

REFERENCES

1. Malone FD, Canick JA, Ball RH, Nyberg DA, Comstock CH, Bukowski R, et al. First-trimester or second-trimester screening, or both, for Down's syndrome. N Engl J Med. 2005;353:2001-11.
2. Driscoll DA, Gross S. Clinical practice. Prenatal screening for aneuploidy. N Engl J Med. 2009;360:2556-62.
3. Badeau M, Lindsay C, Blais J, Nshimyumukiza L, Takwoingi Y, Langlois S. Genomics-based non-invasive prenatal testing for detection of fetal chromosomal aneuploidy in pregnant women. Cochrane Database Syst Rev. 2017;11(11):CD011767.
4. Alberry M, Maddocks D, Jones M. Free fetal DNA in maternal plasma in anembryonic pregnancies: confirmation that the origin is the trophoblast. Prenat Diagn. 2007;27(5):415-8.
5. Hu P, Liang D, Chen Y, Lin Y, Qiao F, Li H, et al. An enrichment method to increase cell-free fetal DNA fraction and significantly reduce false negatives and test failures for non-invasive prenatal screening: a feasibility study. J Transl Med. 2019;17:124.
6. Pös O, Budiš J, Szemes T. Recent trends in prenatal genetic screening and testing. F1000Res. 2019;8:F1000.
7. Swanson A, Sehnert AJ, Bhatt S. Non-invasive Prenatal Testing: Technologies, Clinical Assays and Implementation Strategies for Women's Healthcare Practitioners. Curr Genet Med Rep. 2013;1:113-21.
8. Peng XL, Jiang P. Bioinformatics Approaches for Fetal DNA Fraction Estimation in Noninvasive Prenatal Testing. Int J Mol Sci. 2017;18(2):453.
9. Practice Bulletin No. 163: Screening for Fetal Aneuploidy. Obstet Gynecol. 2016;127(5):e123-37.
10. Benn P, Borrell A, Chiu RW, Cuckle H, Dugoff L, Faas B, et al. Position statement from the chromosome abnormality screening committee on behalf of the Board of the International Society for prenatal diagnosis. Prenat Diagn. 2015;35(8):725-34.
11. Mackie F, Hemming K, Allen S, Morris R, Kilby M. The accuracy of cell-free fetal DNA based non-invasive prenatal testing in singleton pregnancies: a systematic review and bivariate meta-analysis. BJOG. 2017;124:32-46.
12. Akolekar R, Beta J, Picciarelli G, Ogilvie C, D'Antonio F. Procedure-related risk of miscarriage following amniocentesis and chorionic villus sampling: a systematic review and meta-analysis. Ultrasound Obstet Gynecol. 2015;45:16-26.
13. Qu J, Leung T, Jiang P, Liao G, Cheng Y, Sun H, et al. Noninvasive prenatal determination of twin zygosity by maternal plasma DNA analysis. Clin Chem. 2013;59:427-35.
14. Royal College of Obstetricians and Gynaecologists. Non-invasive prenatal testing for chromosomal abnormality using maternal plasma DNA. Scientific Impact Paper No. 15. London: RCOG; 2014.
15. Committee opinion no. 640: Cell-free DNA screening for fetal aneuploidy. Obstet Gynecol. 2015;126:e31-7.
16. Nuffield Council on Bioethics 2017. Available at: https://www.nuffieldbioethics.org/assets/pdfs/NCOB-Annual-Report-2017.pdf

LONG QUESTIONS

1. What is the principal behind noninvasive prenatal testing?
2. What does NIPT screen for and what is its sensitivity and specificity?

SHORT QUESTIONS

1. When is NIPT performed? What are the conditions that can be screened?
2. What are the benefits of NIPT over the other prenatal tests?
3. What are the limitations or drawbacks of NIPT?
4. What is cffDna?
5. Who are the candidates for NIPT screening?

MULTIPLE CHOICE QUESTIONS

1. cffDNA originates from:
   a. Maternal RBCs
   b. Placental trophoblasts
   c. Fetal RBCs
   d. All of the above
2. cffDNA fragments are approximately base pairs (bp) in length:
   a. 20
   b. 12
   c. 100
   d. 200
3. Approximately how much percent of the cell-free DNA in maternal blood is of fetal origin?
   a. 40%
   b. 1–2%
   c. 25%
   d. 10%
4. NIPT provides the earliest testing available from as early as:
   a. 6–7 weeks
   b. 9–10 weeks
   c. 12 weeks
   d. 14–16 weeks
5. Following are the benefits of NIPT, except:
   a. It is specific to pregnancy and offer improved sensitivity and specificity for prenatal screening, and lower false-positive rates as compared with maternal serum analyte screening
   b. It is a diagnostic test
   c. It can be done early in pregnancy
   d. Processing time of the test results is less
6. What is the next best step after getting a positive screen test result via NIPT?
   a. Offer termination of pregnancy
   b. Repeat NIP testing
   c. Offer genetic counseling
   d. Offer diagnostic tests to confirm the results and then offer genetic counseling
7. Which of the following is not current indication(s) for preimplantation genetic screening?
   a. Advanced maternal age
   b. Repeated implantation failure
   c. Repeated pregnancy loss
   d. Sporadic miscarriage
8. The reason for false-positive results in NIPT are all, except:
   a. Vanishing twin
   b. Placental mosaicism
   c. Gestation age
   d. Low DNA
9. NIPT is increasingly used for detecting all, except:
   a. Trisomy 21
   b. Trisomy 13
   c. Trisomy 18
   d. Hemophilias
10. Least sensitivity of NIPT is for:
    a. Trismony 21
    b. Trisomy 13
    c. Trisomy 18

Answers

1. b 2. d 3. d 4. b 5. b 6. d
7. d 8. c 9. d 10. b

SECTION 4

Early Pregnancy Complications

4.1 ABORTION

Ranjana Desai

■ OVERVIEW

Abortion, also known in medical parlance as a spontaneous abortion, miscarriage, and pregnancy loss, is the loss of an embryo or fetus before it is able to survive independently **(Fig. 1)**. In fact miscarriage is the most common complication of early pregnancy.

Abortion may be classified as spontaneous or induced; Incidence of spontaneous abortion is between 15 and 22%. Etiology of abortion can be attributed to fetal causes, maternal causes, and paternal factors.

Pathologically abortion is hemorrhage occurring into the decidua basalis and is followed by necrosis of the tissues resulting in separation of the ovum from the uterine wall. Over the years, the evidence-based treatment has improved the outcome of various types of abortions but almost half of the abortions are treated empirically. This chapter includes definition, classification, etiology, pathology, and details of various types of spontaneous and induced abortions and their management.

Abortion has been the bane of womanhood since time immemorial. The term "Abortion" derives from the Latin word "*aboriri*" which means "*to miscarry.*" Abortion is the termination of pregnancy, either spontaneously or intentionally, before the fetus develops sufficiently to survive. In order to survive, the fetus must weigh 500 g corresponds to 22 weeks of pregnancy in developing country and 20 weeks in developed country.

Due to improvement of early neonatal management, the age of viability is considered to be 22 weeks as recommended by World Health Organization (WHO). But according to Royal College of Obstetricians and Gynaecologists (RCOG), the limit of viability is considered at 24 weeks of pregnancy. Hence, the definition of abortion varies according to state laws for reporting abortions, fetal death, and neonatal death.

■ INCIDENCE

The incidence of spontaneous abortion in clinically recognized pregnancy is between 15 and 22%, and the incidence of unrecognized abortion may be as high as 40–50%. More than 80% abortion occurs in the first 12 weeks and half of these is due to chromosomal anomalies. Maternal and fetal age and parity contributes to high incidence of abortion.

■ CLASSIFICATION

Depending upon various signs and symptoms abortion is classified into the following:
- *Spontaneous abortion:*
  - Threatened abortion
  - Inevitable abortion
  - Incomplete abortion
  - Complete abortion
  - Missed abortion

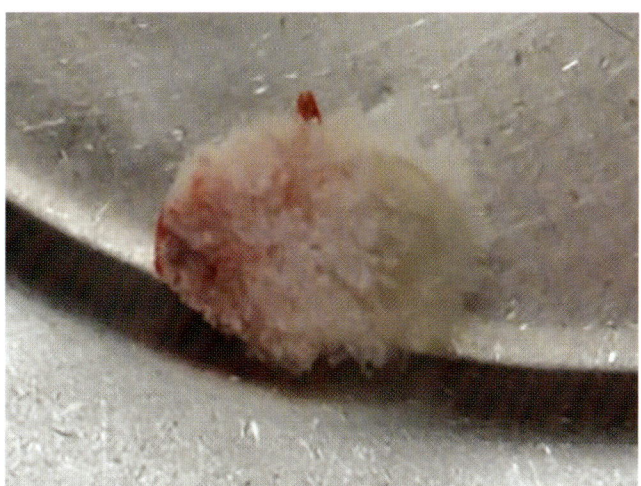

Fig. 1: Expelled products of conception.
(*Photo courtesy:* Dr R Desai)

- Septic abortion
- Recurrent abortion
- *Induced abortion:*
  - Legal [medical termination of pregnancy (MTP)]
  - Illegal (criminal)
  - Septic abortion.

ETIOLOGY OF ABORTION

- *Fetal causes:*
  - *Genetic factors*: 50% of abortions are due to chromosomal abnormality either numerical (aneuploidy) or structural. The most common chromosomal anomaly is trisomy 16 (7%) followed by monosomy X (45X) (8%). Others include triploidy, Robertsonian, and reciprocal translocations and mosaicism.
  - *Multiple pregnancy*: Spontaneous abortion is three times more common in multiple pregnancies and monochorionic abortus outnumber dichorionic abortus. In some cases, entire pregnancy is lost and in few only one pregnancy is lost or vanishes and patient delivers as singleton pregnancy. Usually occurs before the second trimester in 20–60% of twin pregnancy.
- *Maternal causes:*
  - Infections: Any acute infection can cause abortion. High fever may lead to fetal death. Malaria, septicemia, and viral infections such as rubella, cytomegalovirus, herpes simplex, variola, human immunodeficiency virus (HIV) are implicated as causes of abortion but remains inconclusive.
  - *Endocrine factors*: Contributes to 10–15% of abortions. Diabetes mellitus is an important reason where both spontaneous abortion and major congenital malformations may occur. Hyperthyroidism or hypothyroidism, polycystic ovarian disease (PCOD), excess of androgen, and luteal phase defects due to defective implantation and placentation are other factors.
  - *Systemic diseases*: Hypertension and chronic renal disease.
  - *Drug and environmental factors*: Many drugs, e.g., anesthetic agents, anticonvulsants, antimalarials, radiation in toxic doses, can induce abortion. Smoking, alcohol, caffeine in large amount, environmental toxins such as lead, formaldehyde, benzene, radiation, and intrauterine device (IUD) failure are associated risk factors.
  - *Uterine factors*: Asherman syndrome, cervical incompetence, Müllerian anomalies (bicornuate uterus) and septate uterus, and fibromyoma of the uterus, especially submucosal variety.
  - *Immunological factors*: Autoimmune defects such as antiphospholipid syndrome, alloimmune factors, and blood group incompatibility.
  - *Physical trauma*: Physical or surgical trauma
  - *Unexplained*: A large number (40–60%) of abortions have no identifiable etiological cause.
- *Paternal factors*: Chromosomal translocation in the sperm. *(First-trimester abortions are due to genetic causes, endocrinal cause, immunological cause, endocrinal and unexplained. Second-trimester abortions are caused by anatomical abnormality such as cervical incompetence, Müllerian defect, myoma uterus, and systematic illnesses such as infections and diabetes and autoimmune cause.)*

PATHOLOGY OF ABORTION

Hemorrhage occurring into the decidua basalis (subchorionic hemorrhage) is the pathogenetic mechanism of abortion. This hemorrhage is followed by necrosis of the tissues resulting in separation of the ovum from the uterine wall. If hemorrhage occurs <8 weeks into the pregnancy, there are greater chances of complete expulsion of the conceptus. If it happens in 8–14 weeks of gestation, there are chances of incomplete abortion rise manifold with retained products of conception. If the event occurs >14 weeks later, then the process of abortion behaves like a mini labor followed by complete expulsion of the immature fetus. Hence, the most dangerous period of abortion is between 8–14 weeks when the treatment is urgently needed to prevent complications, especially profuse hemorrhage.

Threatened Abortion

Threatened abortion is defined as hemorrhage from genital tract with a viable intrauterine pregnancy of <20 weeks gestation with os closed and cervix uneffaced irrespective of whether uterine contractions are present or not. On examination, the uterus feels soft and corresponds to the period of gestation and the signs of early pregnancy are evident.

Treatment is empirical and requires proper counseling, bed rest, sexual abstinence, and reassurance. Although there is no definite evidence that bed rest can affect the course of pregnancy, abstinence from physical activity and avoiding a dynamic family and social milieu for a couple of days may help women feel safer thus providing emotional relief. It is unlikely that progesterone improves outcome in women with threatened miscarriage. However, local application of a progestogen was found to subjectively decrease uterine cramping more rapidly than bed rest alone in one small study. Follow-up of fetal growth and cardiac activity by periodic ultrasound examination is mandatory in cases with threatened abortion. Anti-D prophylaxis should be given to an Rh negative mother. The condition is usually managed on an outdoor basis and the patient asked to report in case of excessive bleeding.

Inevitable Abortion

In this type of abortion, the expulsion of the product of conception is inevitable as evidenced by dilatation of the cervical os but as yet there has been no expulsion **(Fig. 2)**. The symptoms are the same as threatened abortion, i.e., bleeding per vaginum, except that the os is found open on examination. There is no chance of continuing the pregnancy.

Treatment

Requires admission and start intravenous crystalloids with 20 units of oxytocin. Patient should be prepared for evacuation immediately after taking consent. Intravenous antibiotics should be given if there is history of prolonged irregular bleeding. Blood transfusion is given in case of excessive blood loss.

Incomplete Abortion

This is the kind of abortion where part of the product of conception has been expelled. Incomplete expulsion of the products leads to excessive bleeding and uterine cramps **(Fig. 3)**.

Treatment

Same as inevitable abortion.

Complete Abortion

Here the pregnant patient has bleeding per vaginum and expulsion of all the products of conception. The uterus is well contracted on bimanual examination and smaller than the duration of pregnancy. The cavity is completely empty on ultrasonography (USG).

Treatment

No active treatment required. If the patient is bleeding, misoprostol tablets can be given. Anti-D should be given if patient is Rh negative. Antibiotics and hematinics to be prescribed.

Missed Abortion

In this type of abortion, the fetus is nonviable and retained inside the uterus for a variable period of time. The dead fetus undergoes maceration with absorption of liquor amnii **(Fig. 4)**. If the pregnancy products are retained for 4 weeks or more, then there are chances of serious coagulation defects. The signs and symptoms of pregnancy are regressed. Amenorrhea may persist and may be associated with spotting. Ultrasound is essential for confirmation of diagnosis.

Treatment

Requires admission:
- *Medical*: Misoprostol 800 µg vaginally in posterior fornix repeat after 24 hours if needed.
- *Surgical*: Manual vacuum aspiration (MVA), dilatation, and evacuation and suction evacuation under antibiotic cover

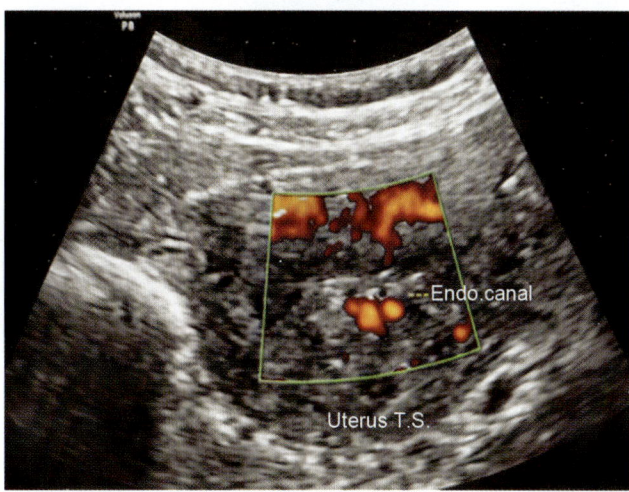

Fig. 3: Vascularized retained products of conception (RPOC). (*Photo courtesy:* Dr D Rajpurohit)

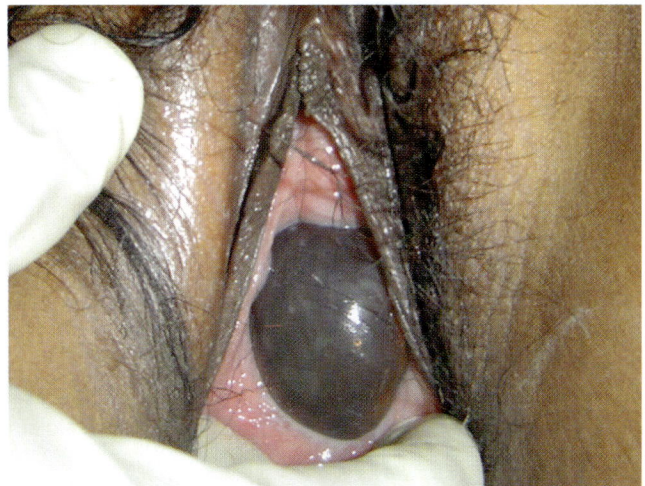

Fig. 2: Inevitable abortion. (*Photo courtesy:* Dr R Desai)

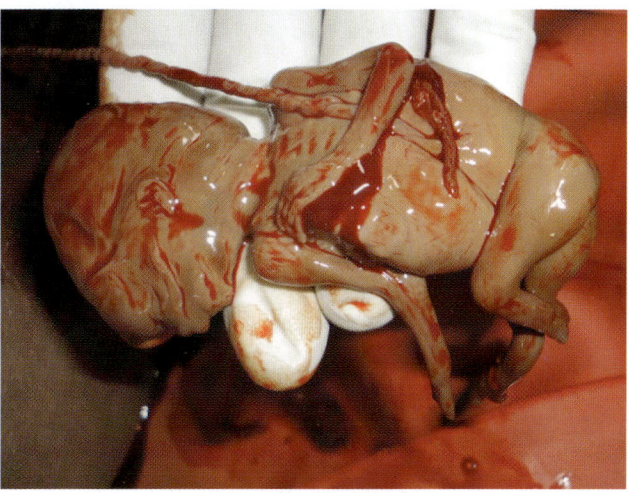

Fig. 4: Macerated fetus. (*Photo courtesy:* Dr R Desai)

Carneous Mole

Carneous mole is a type of missed abortion occurring before 12 weeks where repeated small hemorrhage in the choriodecidual space separates the fetus from the uterine wall and fetus usually dies and becomes rudimentary structure. Decidua capsularis remains intact and small repeated hemorrhage surrounding it makes the wall fleshy and becomes a mole-like structure.

Treatment

Same as missed abortion.

■ SEPTIC ABORTION

This is any type of abortion whether spontaneous or induced, if associated with signs of infection in the uterus and products of conception **(Figs. 5A and B)**. It is responsible for 10–12% admissions amongst abortion cases. The diagnosis is made when the patient has a temperature of at least 38°C with signs and symptoms of abortion. The diagnostic clinical triad of septic abortion are fever, foul-smelling discharge with lower abdominal pain and tenderness. The causative organisms are endogenous such as Gram-negative bacilli, Gram-positive cocci, and anaerobes.

Pathology

The etiopathogenic cause is endometritis in 80% of cases followed by endomyometritis in 15%. If left untreated, it can lead to general peritonitis, septicemia, and endotoxic shock. Abortion is clinically graded into five distinct types as shown in **Table 1**.

- *Grade I:* Most commonly associated with spontaneous abortion where the infection is restricted to the uterus.
- *Grade II:* Infection involves parametrium, tubes and ovaries, and pelvic peritoneum.

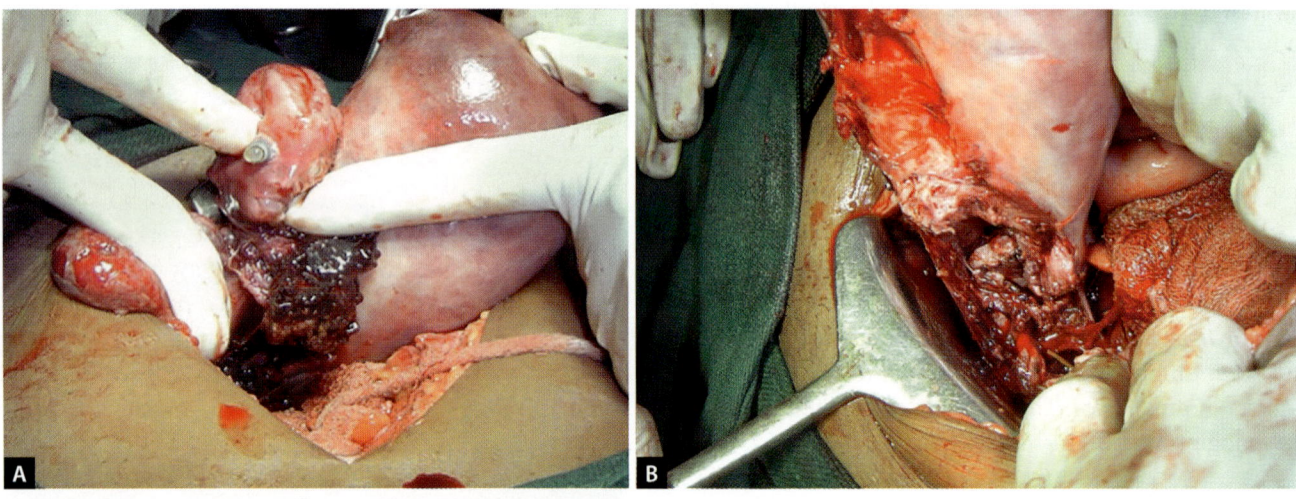

Figs. 5A and B: (A) Septic abortion showing decapitated head lying in abdomin cavity; (B) Perforation of uterus with bowel injury.
(*Photo courtesy:* Dr R Desai)

TABLE 1: Clinical grading of abortion.

	Threatened	Inevitable	Incomplete	Complete	Missed
Expulsion of products	Nil	Nil	History of expulsion	Complete expulsion	Nil
Vital signs	Stable	Features of shock may be present	Features of shock may be present	Stable	Stable
Pallor	Not marked	Moderate to severe	Moderate to severe	Not marked	Not marked
Per abdomen size of uterus	Same as of POG	Same as POG	<POG	Almost normal	<POG
Per vaginal examination	Os closed	Open and products felt	Open and product may be felt	Closed	Closed
USG	Cardiac activity present, perigestational hematoma	Distorted sac in the lower uterine segment	Gestational sac if present is collapsed, Echogenic debris present	Cavity empty, Echogenic line <4 mm	Deformed yolk sac, flattened fetus with absent cardiac activity
Treatment	Conservative	Evacuation	Evacuation	No treatment	Evacuation

(POG: period of gestation; USG: ultrasonography)

- *Grade III:* There is generalized peritonitis, septicemia, endotoxic shock, and multiple organ dysfunction syndrome (MODS).

Grade III type is associated with major complications such as acute respiratory distress syndrome (ARDS), disseminated intravascular coagulation (DIC), acute renal injury, bowel injury, and even maternal death. The mortality rate of these patients is between 0.4 and 0.6 per 100,000.

Septic Shock

Sepsis is the development of systemic inflammatory response syndrome in response to infection. It is severe when there is evidence of end-organ damage. Septic shock is defined as sepsis with hypotension (systolic blood pressure <90 mm Hg or a reduction of >40 mm Hg from baseline) despite volume replacement and use of vasopressors associated with perfusion abnormalities that may also include lactic acidosis, oliguria, or an acute alteration in mental status.

Investigations

- Complete blood count
- Urinalysis
- Coagulation profile
- Electrolyte panel
- Renal function test (RFT) and liver function test (LFT)
- Blood culture
- X-ray of chest
- USG.

The *1-hour bundle includes* serum lactate, blood cultures prior to antibiotics, broad-spectrum antibiotics, a 30 mL/kg crystalloid bolus for patients with hypotension or lactate ≥4 mmol/L, and vasopressors for persistent hypotension.

Management

- Notifying the police is mandatory if a criminal abortion is suspected.
- *Intravenous antibiotics*: Injection cefotaxime 1 g intravenous (IV) 12 hourly, injection metronidazole 500 mg IV 8 hourly and injection gentamicin 80 mg IV 12 hourly if renal failure is excluded.
- Intravenous fluid given at such a rate to maintain urine output of 30 mL per hour
- Tetanus toxoid injection
- Whole blood transfusion if needed
- Surgery in septic abortion
  - Evacuation of retained products of conception as soon as antibiotic therapy and fluid resuscitation has begun. Vacuum curettage is done under local anesthesia with minimal IV sedation.
  - Colpotomy in pelvic abscess
  - Laparotomy is needed if patient does not respond to medical therapy, in suspected uterine perforation or bowel injury and clostridial myometritis. A discolored woody appearance of uterus and adnexa, suspected clostridial sepsis, crepitation in the pelvic tissues and radiographic evidence of air within the uterine wall are indications for total hysterectomy and possible removal of both adnexa. Copious irrigation of purulent material is done and drainage with closed suction system is advised.

■ INDUCED ABORTION

As opposed to spontaneous abortion, an abortion which is brought about intentionally before the age of viability is called induced abortion. About 40% of unintended pregnancy ends in induced abortion. Before performing induced abortion, one must confirm pregnancy and gestational age by physical examination and USG. Common method of abortion are as follows:

First-trimester Abortion

- *Medical:* For pregnancy <9 weeks mifepristone 200 mg orally, followed by misoprostol 400 µg vaginally or buccally at 48 hours (WHO 2012). About 80% aborts within 24 hours of administration. The success rate is 90–98%.
- *Surgical*:
  - *MVA:* It is performed up to 7 menstrual weeks in an outpatient setting using a flexible vacuum cannula (6–12 mm) and 50 mL plastic syringe.
  - *Suction evacuation*: It consists of aspirating the products of conception with a plastic (Karman's) cannula fitted to a suction machine.
  - *Dilatation and evacuation*: It involves evacuating the products of conception by ovum forceps under IV sedation or paracervical block.
  - *Dilatation and curettage*: It consists of dilatation of cervix with dilators followed by uterine curettage with curette.

Second-trimester Abortion

- *Medical*: Various drugs can be used.
  - *Misoprostol as a single agent*: 200–800 µg as a single drug used orally, vaginally or buccally at an interval of 4 hours till expulsion of products of conception (maximum five to six doses). Success rate is 100%.
  - *Mifepristone and misoprostol combination*: Mifepristone 200 mg orally followed by 48 hours later misoprostol 800 µg vaginally further followed by 400 µg orally or vaginally 4 hours apart (maximum four doses). Success rate is 97%.
- *Surgical*:
  - *Dilatation and evacuation*: Not recommended.
  - *Hysterotomy*: May be required rarely in failed medical methods, large myoma blocking cervical access or in some cases of previous lower segment cesarean section (LSCS) or myomectomy scar.

The MTP Act of 1971 passed by the Parliament of India, enforced in April 1972 and revised in 1975 ensured the safeguard of health of mother undergoing abortion and the interest if the doctor performing the procedure. With the amendments, MTP Act, 2021 recognized the importance of safe, affordable, accessible abortion services to women who need to terminate pregnancy under certain specified conditions. With advancing technology [USG, computed tomography (CT) scan, magnetic resonance imaging (MRI)], there is scope for increasing upper gestational limit for terminating pregnancies in patient with fetal anomalies detected late in pregnancy. In order to reduce maternal mortality and morbidity due to unsafe abortions, there is need for access of women to legal and safe abortion services and exercising the reproductive rights.

UNSAFE ABORTION

Termination of pregnancy by people lacking the necessary skills, or in an environment lacking minimal medical standards or both, is termed unsafe abortion and it is a significant cause of maternal mortality and morbidity worldwide. Most unsafe abortions occur where abortion is illegal or in developing countries where affordable well-trained medical practitioners are not readily available, or where modern contraceptives are unavailable. About one in eight pregnancy-related deaths globally is associated with unsafe abortion **(Figs. 6A to C)**.

Differential Diagnosis

- *Ectopic pregnancy*: No intrauterine pregnancy on serial ultrasound and an extrauterine gestational sac, abnormal human chorionic gonadotropin (hCG), persistent pelvic pain, and bleeding
- *Ovarian torsion*: Beta-hCG negative, no intrauterine gestational sac, and USG findings suggested of ovarian mass
- *Gestational trophoblastic diseases*: Enlarged uterus, abnormally elevated hCG levels, and USG findings suggestive of molar pregnancy
- *Functional menstrual disorders*: Absent hCG and no gestational sac in USG.

RECURRENT ABORTION

Recurrent abortion is the occurrence of three or more consecutive spontaneous abortion before 20 weeks of gestation. It can be emotionally and physically traumatizing for the couple, as the risk of abortion increases with number of abortion. The incidence is 1% with the risk increasing to 10% with each abortion. The estimated risk is 24% after two clinically recognized losses, 30% after three losses, and 40–50% after four losses.

Miscarriage is often classified as either a clinical or a biochemical pregnancy loss. Clinical pregnancies are the ones that can be identified by ultrasound or histological evidence, while biochemical pregnancies occur earlier and can only be identified by a raised beta-hCG.

The incidence differs with definition of recurrent miscarriage (RM). The incidence of biochemical pregnancy loss in the general population may be as high as 60%, while the incidence of pregnancy loss after the detection of fetal cardiac activity is significantly lower.

Causes

First-trimester Recurrent Pregnancy Loss

- *Chromosomal anomalies*: Most common anomaly is balanced translocation contributing to 25% of cases. There is successful pregnancy outcome even without treatment in 50%.
- *Inherited thrombophilias*: Antithrombin III deficiency, protein C resistance, and hyperhomocysteinemia.
- *Endocrine causes*: Uncontrolled diabetes mellitus, thyroid dysfunction, luteal phase defects, and hyperprolactinemia
- *Immunological*: Antinuclear antibodies (ANAs), autoimmune factors such as antiphospholipid antibodies

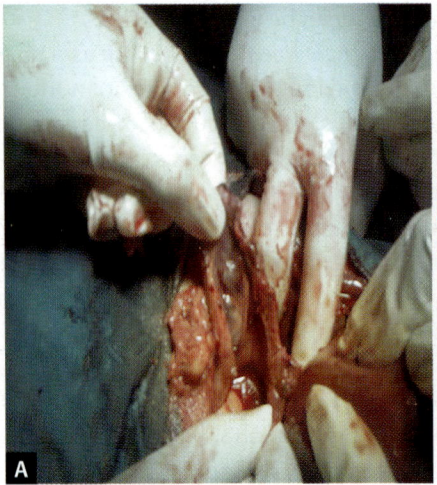
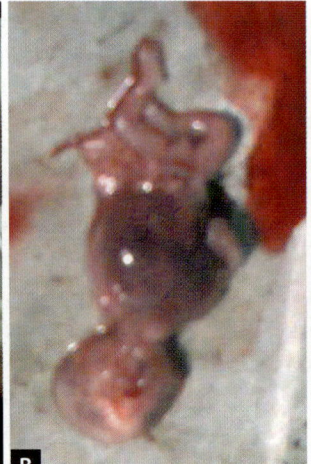
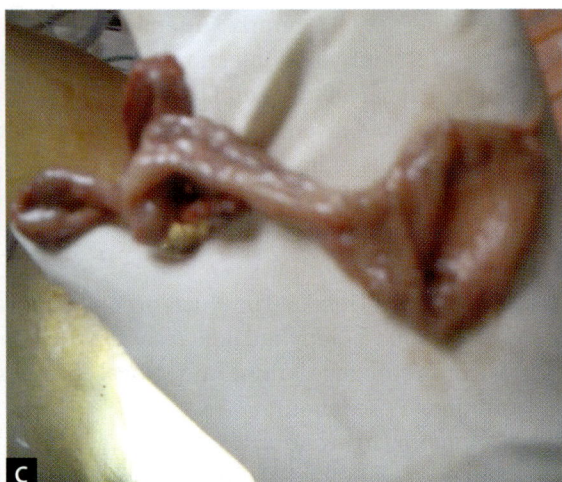

Figs. 6A to C: Criminal abortion showing fetus and totally detached bowel which was lying in vagina.
(*Photo courtesy:* Dr R Desai)

(APLA), lupus anticoagulant (LA), and anticardiolipin antibody (ACA). The cause of fetal demise is extensive thrombosis and infarction of placental vessels.
- *Unexplained*: Half of the patients do not have a conclusive diagnosis and fall into the category of unexplained recurrent pregnancy loss **(Table 2)**. It is again subdivided into two types.
  - *Unexplained RM type I*: One which has occurred by chance, in women with no specific underlying pathology. It has a good prognosis and there is no need of any intervention.
  - *Unexplained RM type II*: Refers to the RM that occurs due to an underlying pathology which cannot be identified by routine clinical investigations or due to significant environmental and lifestyle risk factors. This type has a poorer prognosis.

Typically type I unexplained RM is an older women (>40 years) with three or more biochemical or early losses, in whom the karyotype of fetus shows aneuploidy. A type II unexplained RM is a young women (<30 years), with four or more losses occurring after appearance of fetal heart beat and karyotyping shows a normal result.

Second-trimester Pregnancy Loss

The time span of mid-trimester abortion extends from the end of first trimester until the fetus weighs <500 g or gestational age reaches 20 weeks. Unlike first-trimester pregnancy losses, second-trimester spontaneous loss rate is 1.5–3% and it is due to a multitude of causes.

Etiology

- *Anatomical abnormalities*: Leading to 10–15% of miscarriages **(Fig. 7)**
  - *Congenital*:
    - Isolated weakness of cervix
    - Associated uterine anomalies
    - In utero exposure to diethylstilbestrol (DES)
  - Acquired due to cervical trauma in the past:
    - Forcible dilation and evacuation (D&E) during previous pregnancy
    - Cervical incompetence
    - Asherman syndrome
    - Uterine fibroids especially submucosal variety
- *Autoimmune factors*: Antiphospholipid antibody (APLA) syndrome
- *Maternal infections*: Toxoplasma and syphilis
- *Maternal disorders*: Uncontrolled diabetes, chronic renal disease, and systemic lupus erythematosus (SLE)
- Unknown.

Diagnosis

Diagnosis is arrived from detailed history and examination both general and systemic.

Investigations

Routine blood investigation including glucose tolerance test with 75 g glucose. Specific tests such as thyroid profile, anticardiolipin, antiphospholipid, lupus anticoagulant antibody, karyotyping, hysterosalpingography (HSG), and hysteroscopy.

Treatment

Reassurance and tender loving care is the keystone of treatment. Keeping that in mind, the underlying etiological causes must also be treated as summarized in **Table 3**.

CERVICAL INCOMPETENCE

Definition

Condition in which the cervix fails to retain the conceptus during pregnancy leading to premature painless dilatation of endocervical canal before the onset of labor. It constitutes 1% of total pregnant patients and 8% of recurrent mid trimester

TABLE 2: Unexplained recurrent miscarriage.

	Type I	Type II
Cause	By chance	Underlying pathology
Age	Older group	Younger group
Definition of RM	Biochemical pregnancy	Clinical pregnancy
Number of previous miscarriages	Lesser number	Higher number of miscarriages
Karyotype of products of conception	Sporadic fetal aneuploidy	Normal

(RM: recurrent miscarriage)

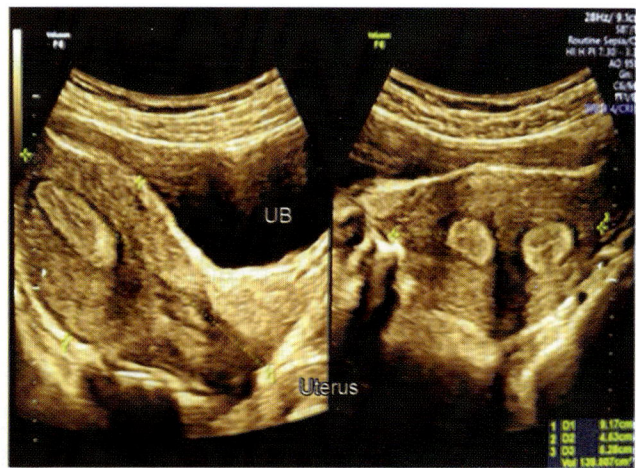

Fig. 7: Ultrasonography (USG) of patient with history of recurrent pregnancy loss (RPL) showing partial septate uterus.
(*Photo courtesy:* Dr D Rajpurohit)

TABLE 3: Etiology and treatment of 2nd trimester pregnancy loss.

Cause	Treatment
Genetic	Counseling
Endocrinological	• Insulin for diabetes mellitus • Treat hyper- or hypothyroidism • Natural micronized progesterone for LPD
Immunological	• Aspirin 75 mg daily • LMWH 40 mg daily up to 34 weeks
Anatomical	• Myomectomy • Synechiolysis • Septal resection • Cervical cerclage

(LMWH: low-molecular-weight heparin; LPD: luteal phase deficiency)

TABLE 4: Etiology of cervical incompetance.

Congenital	Acquired (Surgical trauma)
Isolated developmental weakness of cervix	Conization
Connective tissue disorder of cervix like Ehlers–Danlos syndrome	Fothergill operation in past
Associated Müllerian duct abnormalities such as septate uterus and bicornuate uterus	Forcible dilation during MTP procedure or D and C in past
DES exposure in utero	Vaginal delivery through incompletely dilated cervix

(D and C: dilation and curettage; DES: diethylstilbestrol; MTP: medical termination of pregnancy)

loss with the usual time of abortion ranging from 16 to 24 weeks.

Etiology

Cervical incompetence can be either congenital or acquired. **Table 4** enumerates and describes the various causes.

Pathogenesis

Alteration in connective tissue metabolism. There is decrease in total collagen content with increase in collagen stability and collagenolytic activity.

Diagnosis

- *History*: Typical of rupture of membranes followed by quick delivery of a preterm live fetus in the second or early third trimester.
- *Nonpregnant state*: Internal os may allow passage of No. 8 Hegar dilator without resistance. HSG shows typical funneling of internal os. Uterine anomalies such as bicornuate/septate uterus may be present.
- *Pregnancy*: Transvaginal ultrasound is ideal to detect early incompetence. Cervical length <25 mm, internal os diameter >8 mm, funneling of os and the lower uterine segment is V- or U-shaped instead of normal T or Y shape (T, Y, V, U is the order of change—*T*rust *Y*our *V*aginal *U*ltrasound). Sonographic serial evaluation (every 2 weeks) of the cervix for funneling and shortening in response to transfundal pressure has been found to be useful in the evaluation of incompetent cervix.
- *Cervical index:*
  - Cervical index = Funnel length + 1/endocervical length
  - Normally, it is 0.32. A cervical index of 0.52 or above is indicative of cervical insufficiency.

Management of Cervical Incompetence

Treatment is surgical which constitutes reinforcement of the weak cervix by a purse string suture which can be done transabdominally or vaginally. If there is well-documented history, encerclage is recommended. Otherwise follow-up with transvaginal scan (TVS) for early signs of cervical insufficiency and intervention if necessary.

Cervical encerclage makes the cervix competent by use of stitch that goes around the os and closes it. It is performed at around 12–14 weeks by which time the fetus is screened for anomalies and other causes of recurrent pregnancy loss (RPL) are ruled out. Cerclage can be prophylactic, therapeutic (salvage), and rescue/emergency/urgent.

Rescue Cerclage

Salvage measure in case of premature cervical dilatation with fetal membranes exposed to vagina. It can delay delivery by 5 weeks. It should only be done by an experienced obstetrician.
- *Vaginal cerclage*: There are choice of surgical operations to perform.
  - *McDonald's operation (1963)*: In this operation, a nonabsorbable suture of Mersilene tape or black silk is inserted in a purse string manner in the body of cervix near the internal os below the level of bladder **(Fig. 8)**. It is an easy surgery with little bleeding. The success rate is 85–90%. Since there is less scarring and fibrosis, hence chance of cervical dystocia is less. It is the most widely performed procedure because of its simplicity and ease.
  - *Modified Shirodkar operation (Dr V N Shirodhkar 1955)*: Done in spinal anesthesia or light general anesthesia (GA). The bladder is emptied, and the patient is put in lithotomy position and cervix is exposed by a posterior vaginal speculum. Lips of cervix are held with sponge holding forceps and a small transverse incision is given on the anterior lip of cervix at cervicovaginal junction. A vertical incision is made posteriorly at cervicovaginal junction. Bladder is pushed up and level of internal os is identified. A nonabsorbable Mersilene tape (5 mm) is passed through submucosa from anterior to posterior and posterior to anterior and tied up anteriorly by a

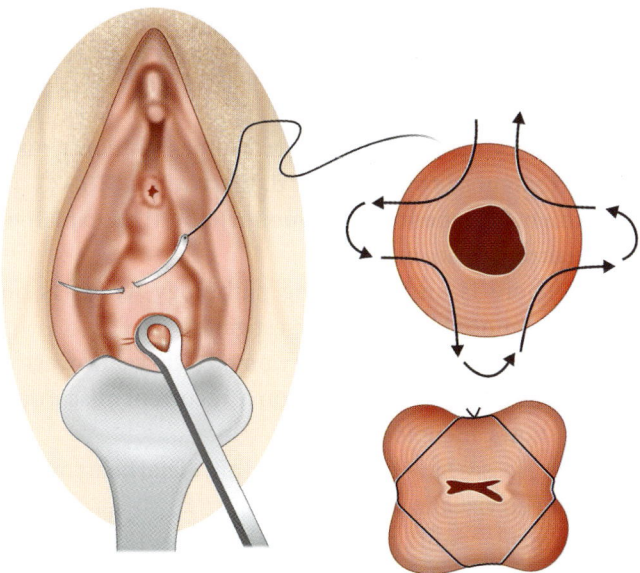

Fig. 8: Showing the placement of McDonald's suture.

reef knot. The mucosal incision is closed with chromic catgut to bury the suture. The Mersilene suture is removed at 37 weeks to allow normal vaginal delivery and stitch can be reapplied in a subsequent pregnancy. [Original Shirodkar operation was performed using fascia lata and knot was tied posteriorly. Shirodkar stitch can be left behind for future pregnancy and elective cesarean section (CS) can be done].

- *Others*: Wurm's stitch where two silk stitches are applied on cervix, one from right to left side and other from anterior lip to posterior lip. Usually applied in short effaced cervix.
- *Abdominal cerclage (Benson and Durfee cerclage)*: This is done for repeated failure of vaginal approach and inaccessible cervix. Stitches are placed at the level of internal os via a Pfannenstiel incision and are permanent. Delivery is by elective CS, even for abortion stitch has to be removed by laparotomy.
- *Others*: Laparoscopic, robotic cerclage, and Lash and Lash procedure are also used.

Complications

- Slipping or cutting of stitch through cervix
- Chorioamnionitis
- Rupture of membranes
- Preterm labor
- Abortions
- Cervical dystocia
- Rupture uterus
- Cervical necrosis

Contraindications

- Chorioamnionitis
- Preterm premature rupture of membranes
- Uterine contractions
- Cervical dilation >4 cm
- Congenital anomaly
- Fetal demise
- Active vaginal bleeding.

Postoperative Care

- Bed rest for 48 hours
- Micronized progesterone 200 mg daily or injection hydroxyprogesterone caproate 500 mg intramuscularly (IM) before surgery and the weekly until 37 weeks
- Antibiotics
- Stitch can be removed at 37 weeks or earlier if labor pains starts.

■ COVID-19 AND ABORTION

There are limited evidence for impact of Covid-19 during second and third trimesters and very scant data on first-trimester abortion. However, in a case control study of 225 pregnant patients, Covid-19 infection during the first trimester of pregnancy does not appear to predispose to abortion; its cumulative incidence did not differ from that of women with ongoing pregnancy.

■ CONCLUSION

Abortion is a significant problem in human reproduction and is defined as termination of pregnancy before fetal viability and it may be either spontaneous or induced. There are numerous causes for spontaneous abortion and the most common cause is chromosomal aneuploidy. Other contributing factors include diabetes, thyroid disorders, antiphospholipid syndrome, and incompetent os. Spontaneous abortion is classified according to clinical presentation. Septic abortion may follow either spontaneous or induced and carries high morbidity and mortality. The ability to successfully manage these entities and associated complications remains important for any gynecologist who gives care for the reproductive age women.

■ FURTHER READING

1. Aleman A, Althabe F, Belizán JM, Bergel E. Bed rest during pregnancy for preventing miscarriage. Cochrane Database Syst Rev. 2005;(2):CD003576.
2. American College of Obstetricians and Gynecologists. Cerclage for the management of cervical insufficiency. ACOG Practice bulletin no. 142. Obstet Gynecol. 2014;123(2 Pt 1):372-9.
3. Bricker L, Farquharson RG. Types of pregnancy loss in recurrent miscarriage: implications for research and clinical practice. Hum Reprod. 2002;17(5):1345-50.
4. Chard T. Frequency of implantation and early pregnancy loss in natural cycles. Bailliere Clin Obstetr Gynaecol. 1991;5(1):179-89.
5. Cosma S, Carosso AR, Cusato J, Borella F, Carosso M, Bovetti M, et al. Coronavirus disease 2019 and first-trimester spontaneous abortion: a case-control study of 225 pregnant patients. Am J Obstet Gynecol. 2021;224(4):391-e1.
6. Cunningham FG, Leveno KJ, Bloom SL, Dashe JS, Hoffman BL, Casey BM et al. Abortion. In: Williams Obstetrics, 25th edition. United States of America: McGraw-Hill Education; 2018. pp. 346-52.

7. Levy MM, Evans LE, Rhodes A. The surviving sepsis campaign bundle: 2018 update. Intensive Care Med. 2018;44(6):925-8.
8. Rinehart BK. Abortion. In: Rivlin M, Martin R (eds). Manual of Clinical Problems in Obstetrics and Gynecology, 5th edition. Philadelphia: Lippincott Williams & Wilkins; 2001. pp. 5-10.
9. Saade GR. Maternal sepsis. In: Foley MH, Strong TH Jr., Garite TJ. Obstetric Intensive Care Manual, 3rd edition. New Delhi: Tata McGraw Hill Education; 2011. pp. 111-6.
10. Saravelos SH, Li TC. Unexplained recurrent miscarriage: how can we explain it?. Human reproduction. 2012;27(7):1882-6.
11. Sharma JB. Early pregnancy hemorrhage. In: Textbook of Obstetrics, 2nd edition. Himachal Pradesh: Avichal Publishing Company; 2020. pp. 113-36.
12. Sotiriadis A, Papatheodorou S, Makrydimas G. Threatened miscarriage: evaluation and management. Bmj. 2004;329(7458): 152-5.
13. Stirrat GM. Recurrent miscarriage I: definition and epidemiology. Lancet. 1990;336(8716):673-5.
14. Stubblefield P, Averbach S. Septic abortion: Prevention and management. Glob Libr Women Med. 2014.
15. Wahabi HA, Fayed AA, Esmaeil SA, Bahkali KH. Progestogen for treating threatened miscarriage. Cochrane Database *Syst Rev.* 2018;(8):CD005943.
16. Yadav M. Critical Review of Recent Amendment in MTP Act, 2002 in India. Project-Medicoleagal Issues related to MTP in India. 2021.

LONG AND SHORT QUESTIONS

1. Discuss the causes of recurrent pregnancy loss. How will you manage a patient who is 30 years old with history of four consecutive abortions in first trimester of pregnancy?
2. Define abortion. Discuss the types and management of various types of abortion.

MULTIPLE CHOICE QUESTIONS

1. The most common viral infection which has been linked with fetal death is:
    a. Zika virus
    b. Herpes simplex virus
    c. Cytomegalovirus
    d. Parvovirus B19
2. Which statement is not true for type II unexplained recurrent miscarriage:
    a. There is an underlying pathology which is not diagnosed by routine investigation
    b. Usually seen in younger women (<30 years of age)
    c. The products of conception of recurrent miscarriage shows aneuploidy
    d. All losses have been occurred after fetal heart rate has been visualized
3. The incidence of late pregnancy loss (after 12 weeks) after antiretroviral therapy (ART) is:
    a. 1%
    b. 2–4%
    c. 4–6%
    d. 5%
4. Which investigation is not needed in recurrent spontaneous abortion?
    a. Test for antiphospholipid antibodies
    b. Glucose challenge test
    c. Thyroid function test
    d. TORCH test
5. McDonald's stitch is applied in all, except:
    a. Incompetent os
    b. Placenta previa
    c. Septate uterus
    d. Recurrent preterm labor

Answers
1. d   2. c   3. b   4. d   5. b

4.2 ECTOPIC PREGNANCY

K Aparna Sharma, Archana Kumari

INTRODUCTION

Ectopic pregnancy occurs when the blastocyst gets implants in tissue other than the endometrium. Although, the ampullary region of the fallopian tube is the most common site for ectopic implantation (70%), it may occur in other sites **(Fig. 1)**.

INCIDENCE

Ectopic pregnancy has been reported to occur in around 20 cases per 1,000 population and contributes significantly to the maternal mortality in first trimester.[1] In various reports from India, its contribution to maternal deaths has been 3.5–7.1% with an incidence of 0.91% without any maternal mortality.[2]

RISK FACTORS

Globally, the rising incidence of ectopic pregnancy can be attributed to increased incidence of salpingitis due to sexually transmitted infections, ovulation induction, surgeries on tubes as well as earlier detection through imaging. The various risk factors for ectopic gestations have been summarized in **Table 1**.

EVOLUTION AND POTENTIAL OUTCOMES OF ECTOPIC PREGNANCY

An ectopic implantation can evolve in various ways and have different outcomes. *Tubal rupture* can occur if the fertilized

SECTION 4: Early Pregnancy Complications

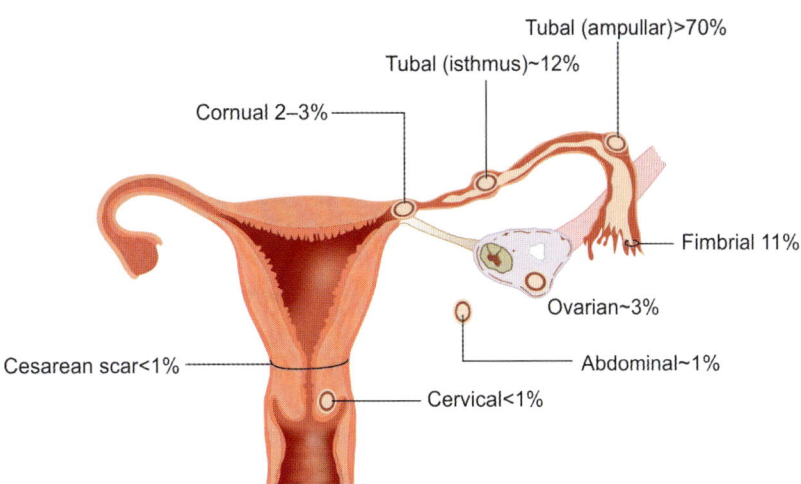

Fig. 1: Site of ectopic implantation.

TABLE 1: Risk factors for ectopic pregnancy.

	Risk factors	Remarks
1.	Previous ectopic pregnancy	Increase in risk after: • After one: 10–15% • After two: 30%
2.	Pelvic infection: • Chlamydia • Gonorrhea • Nonspecific salpingitis	Increase in risk after: • After one episode: 13% • After two episodes: 35% • After three episodes: 75%
3.	Tubal surgery: • Tubal reconstructive surgery • Tubal sterilization	7.3 per 1,000 sterilization procedures (10-year cumulative incidence)
4.	Infertility	4–40 times increase (depending on the etiology of infertility)
5.	ART can cause atypical implantations: • Cornual • Abdominal • Cervical • Ovarian • Heterotopic	1.6%
6.	IUD: • LNG IUD • Copper IUD	>50% of pregnancies with an IUD in situ are ectopic
7.	Tubal pathology: • Developmental anomalies • Salpingitis isthmica nodosa	
8.	Cigarette smoking	Dose-dependent manner

(ART: assisted reproductive technology; IUD: intrauterine device; LNG: levonorgestrel)

ovum comes to lie near or close to the muscularis after burrowing through the epithelium due to the invasion by the proliferating trophoblast. This happens because fallopian tube lacks submucosal layer. When the zygote gets extruded into the abdomen through the tubal ostium, it is termed as *tubal abortion*. In this, the bleeding may stop and symptoms may disappear. Bleeding may persist as long as products remain in tube leading to hemoperitoneum. If however, the fimbriated end of the tube is closed, hematosalpinx may form. In very rare conditions, aborted fetus can implant on any peritoneal surface leading to abdominal pregnancy. Sometimes, after spontaneous failure to thrive, *complete resorption* may occur. *Chronic ectopic* pregnancy may occur when abnormal trophoblast dies early. Beta-human chorionic gonadotropin (β-hCG) gradually becomes negative or static. It commonly forms complex pelvic mass which may later rupture.

■ CLINICAL FEATURES

History

The classic presentation of amenorrhea followed by pain and vaginal bleeding occurs in only 50% of patients, typically in those with ruptured ectopic pregnancy. Most common symptom presenting symptom of an ectopic gestation is abdominal pain. It may be continuous or intermittent, dull or sharp. Commonly, the presentation can be of two types depending on the hemodynamic stability as in **Table 2**.

Physical Examination

Mostly, prior to rupture, the diagnosis is made incidentally during an early dating scan. The patient is stable with normal vitals with nontender or mildly tender abdomen. The uterus may be just bulky. Cervical motion tenderness and adnexal mass may be present. But the mass may vary markedly in size, consistency, and tenderness.

When the ectopic pregnancy ruptures, hemoperitoneum occurs leading to features of hypovolemic shock such as tachycardia and hypotension. There is marked abdominal tenderness and rebound tenderness. Bowel sounds are decreased or absent. Cervical motion tenderness is present. A conclusive diagnosis may not be reached based on history and physical examination, requiring additional tests for differentiation between early viable intrauterine pregnancy, abnormal intrauterine pregnancy, and suspected ectopic pregnancy **(Flowchart 1)**.

TABLE 2: Clinical presentation based on hemodynamic status.

		Unstable hemodynamic status	Stable hemodynamic status
1.	History	Shoulder pain (due to hemoperitoneum irritating inferior surface of diaphragm)	
2.	Vital signs	• Signs of hypovolemic shock • Tachycardia • Hypotension	Normal
3.	Per abdomen	Signs of peritonism-guarding, rigidity, rebound tenderness, shifting dullness	Generalized abdominal tenderness
4.	Per vaginal	Palpable adnexal mass	Cervical motion tenderness may or may not be present

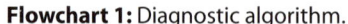

Flowchart 1: Diagnostic algorithm.

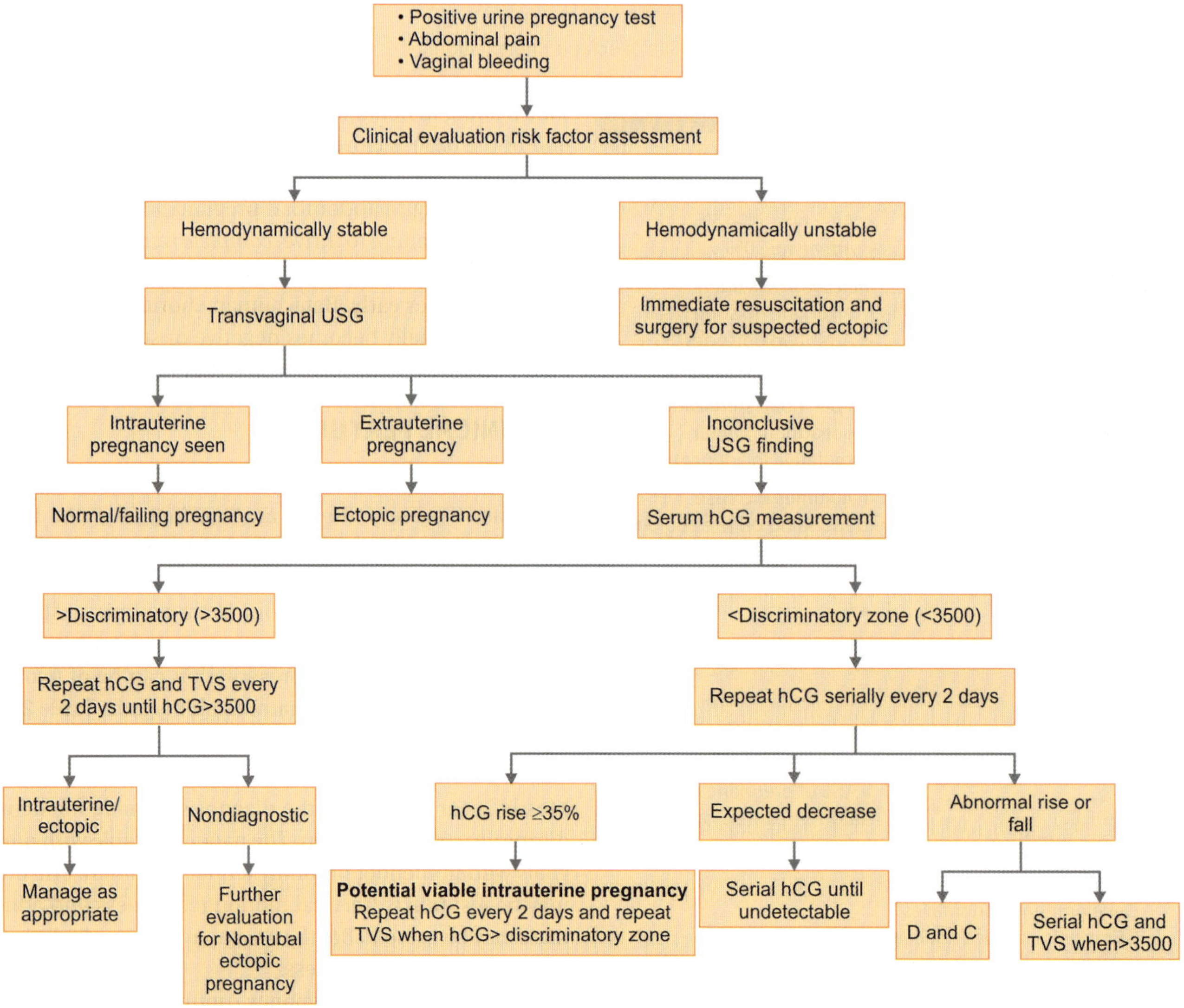

(D and C: dilation and curettage; hCG: human chorionic gonadotropin; TVS: transvaginal scan; USG: ultrasonography)

DIAGNOSIS

Transvaginal Ultrasonography

Diagnosis of ectopic pregnancy is made when the uterine cavity is empty and there is a visualization of a gestational sac in the adnexa **(Table 3)**. In most cases, however, there is an ill-defined mass which is seen in the adnexa in cases of early unruptured tubal ectopics with ovaries being visualized separately **(Fig. 2)**.[3,4]

Serum Beta-Human Chorionic Gonadotropin Measurement

Until the location of the pregnancy is confirmed, the diagnosis remains a pregnancy of unknown location (PUL).

TABLE 3: Ultrasound features of ectopic pregnancy.		
USG finding	Typical appearance	Approximate proportion
Blob sign	An inhomogeneous mass separate from ovary	60%
Bagel sign	A hypoechoic gestation sac within a mass	20%
Extrauterine gestational sac	Gestational sac with developing yolk sac or fetal pole with or without cardiac activity	20%
Free fluid in POD	Not seen until volume reaches 400–700 mL	
Intrauterine pseudo-gestational sac	Anechoic fluid collection in uterine cavity that conforms to shape of uterine cavity and is central in location	

(POD: pouch of Douglas; USG: ultrasonography)

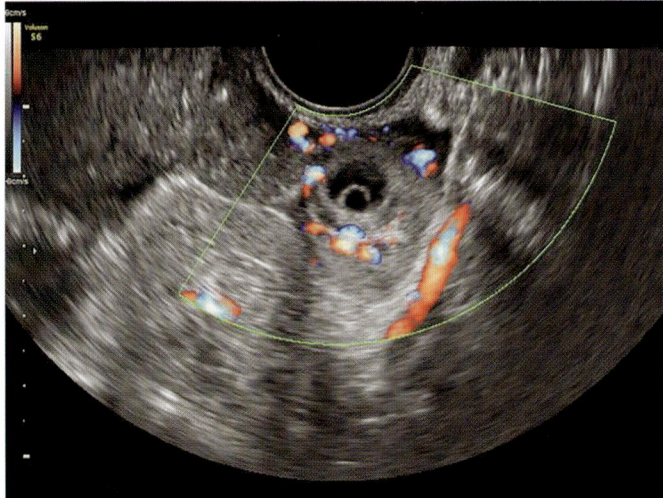

Fig. 2: Ultrasonography (USG) image of ectopic mass with ring of fire pattern in adnexa.

The intrauterine location of gestational sac with a yolk sac rules out ectopic pregnancy.[5,6]

However, quantitative serum β-hCG level can be used for diagnosis in the absence of such definitive finding. If the initial serum β-hCG level exceeds the set discriminatory level (level above which failure to visualize a uterine pregnancy indicates a failing pregnancy or an ectopic), diagnosis narrows to a failing intrauterine pregnancy, a recent complete abortion or an ectopic pregnancy or an early multifetal gestation.

However, recently[7] a case series reported intrauterine gestational sac on follow-up scan despite β-hCG level above the discriminatory level at initial scan, this raises a question on the utility of the discriminatory level.[8-10] Hence, the hCG discriminatory value should be kept high at 3,500 mIU/mL to avoid any misdiagnosis.[7,10]

Serial Serum Beta-Human Chorionic Gonadotropin Measurement

Because of the inability of a single β-hCG to confidently rule out ectopic pregnancy, serial hCG measurement can be employed.

The rise of serum β-hCG occurs in a curvilinear fashion until a plateau at 100,000 mIU/mL is reached by 10 weeks of gestation. Recently, it has been found that the minimum increase in hCG for a potentially viable intrauterine pregnancy occurs at a slower rate[11,12] and is dependent on the initial value.[13]

The rise on β-hCG may vary from 33% to up to 50% depending on the initial values and a rise below a minimal threshold raises the suspicion of an abnormal pregnancy either ectopic or an early pregnancy loss. However, even β-hCG patterns consistent with a growing or resolving gestation do not rule out an ectopic pregnancy.[14]

A failing pregnancy is suggested by decreasing β-hCG value. It should be monitored till spontaneous resolution to nonpregnant levels because rupture of an ectopic pregnancy can occur even while levels are decreasing or are very low.

Dilation and Curettage

Uterine curettage is performed for either a confirmed nonviable pregnancy or an undesirable pregnancy with unknown location.

Culdocentesis

Culdocentesis is now rarely used for diagnosis of ectopic pregnancy.

Laparoscopy

With the advances in ultrasound technology, more ectopic pregnancies are being diagnosed earlier allowing for medical interventions and reducing the need for surgical management. Hence, laparoscopy is no longer considered the gold standard for diagnosis.

■ DIFFERENTIAL DIAGNOSIS

Pregnancy should be ruled out in any sexually active woman of reproductive age who presents with abdominal pain or vaginal bleeding regardless of current history of contraceptive usage.[15,16]

Because of varied presentation ranging from asymptomatic to acute abdomen and shock, clinicians must have a high degree of suspicion in order to any delay in diagnosis. History, physical examination along with serum β-hCG estimation, and ultrasonography aid in making the final diagnosis of ectopic pregnancy and differentiating it from other causes of acute abdomen **(Table 4)**. Until the location of the pregnancy is confirmed, the diagnosis remains a pregnancy of unknown location.

MANAGEMENT OF ECTOPIC PREGNANCY

Depending on the hemodynamic status and clinical scenario, expectant, medical, or surgical management can be used for management of ectopic pregnancy (**Flowchart 2**).

Both laparoscopic surgery and medical management have equivalent safety and effectiveness for an unruptured ectopic pregnancy in clinically stable women. The decision should be made by the patient after discussion of benefits and risks of each approach in different clinical settings.

TABLE 4: Differential diagnosis of acute abdomen in early pregnancy.

S. No.	Diagnosis	Features
	Gynecologic conditions	
1.	Pelvic inflammatory disease	Urine pregnancy test is negative
2.	Threatened/incomplete miscarriage	Bleeding per vagina is usually heavier, no adnexal mass
3.	Ovarian torsion	Urine pregnancy test is negative, pain is intermittent initially and progresses to constant excruciating or dull pain, USG Doppler is helpful
4.	Ruptured ovarian cyst (corpus luteum or endometrioma)	Difficult diagnosis if pregnant
5	Degenerating or enlarging myoma	• USG localization of a myoma • Adnexa will be normal
	Nongynecologic condition	
6	Appendicitis/gastroenteritis/diverticulitis	Negative UPT with normal vaginal examination findings
7.	Urinary tract infection	
8.	Renal/ureteric calculus	

(UPT: urine pregnancy test; USG: ultrasonography)

Medical Management

Methotrexate (Mtx) is the first-line drug for medical management for ectopic pregnancy. Other drugs which can also be used are potassium chloride, prostaglandin (PGF2α), hyperosmolar glucose, and actinomycin. It is imperative to rule out all contraindications (listed in **Table 5**) before initiating Mtx therapy. The reported success rates with systemic Mtx are approximately 70–95%.[17,18] The protocol of single dose versus multiple dose is based on the initial levels of β-hCG with higher levels requiring multiple dose protocols (**Table 6**).

The patient should be counseled thoroughly regarding the following:
- Effects and side effects of Mtx
- Need for follow-up
- Need to report urgently—if severe abdominal pain and fainting attack
- Avoiding excessive sun-exposure, alcohol, vitamins, aspirin, and nonsteroidal anti-inflammatory drugs (NSAIDs).

Surgical Management

Laparoscopy is the preferred surgical treatment for ectopic pregnancy (**Figs. 3 and 4**) unless a woman is hemodynamically unstable. The choice between laparoscopic salpingectomy (when a part or whole of the tube is removed) and laparoscopic salpingostomy (when only the ectopic gestation is removed leaving the tube in situ) depends upon the future fertility desires of the patient and extent of fallopian tube damage. Following salpingostomy, a follow-up is required to ensure complete resolution of the ectopic mass, while this is not required following salpingectomy.[19]

Laparotomy is preferred in unstable patients, with massive hemoperitoneum (**Figs. 5 and 6**) or in patients in whom visualization is expected to be poor or compromised at laparoscopy.

NONTUBAL ECTOPIC PREGNANCY

Although they represent a minority of ectopic pregnancies, they pose significant diagnostic challenge and disproportionate

Flowchart 2: Prerequisites for various treatment options for ectopic pregnancy.

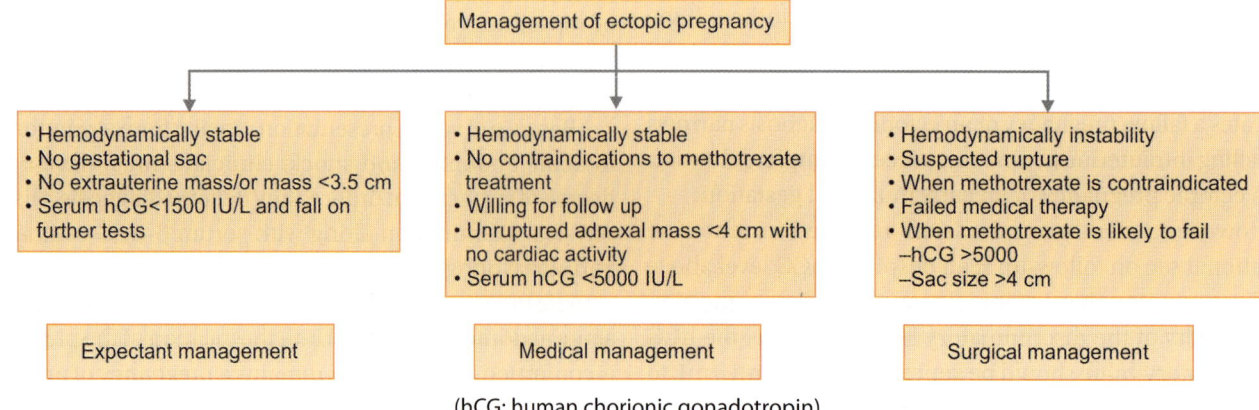

(hCG: human chorionic gonadotropin)

TABLE 5: Methotrexate therapy: Contraindications.	
Absolute contraindications	• Confirmed intrauterine pregnancy • Ruptured ectopic pregnancy • Known sensitivity to methotrexate • Immunodeficiency • Hematological disorders such as severe anemia, thrombocytopenia, or leukopenia • Active peptic ulcer disease • Hepatic/renal dysfunction • Active pulmonary disease • Breastfeeding mother • Unwilling for follow-up
Relative contraindications	• Presence of cardiac activity on transvaginal ultrasonography • Very high hCG concentration • Gestational sac more than 4 cm in size • Refusal to accept blood transfusion

(hCG: chorionic gonadotropin)

TABLE 6: Regimens for methotrexate treatment for ectopic pregnancy.		
	Single dose	**Multiple dose**
Dosing	One dose	Four doses
Schedule	50 mg/m² BSA D1	1 mg/kg (D1, 3, 5, 7) 0.1 mg (D2, 4, 6, 8)
Serum β-hCG	D1, 4, 7	D1, 3, 5, 7
Indication for additional dose	If fall in β-hCG is not 15% between D4 and D7	If fall in β-hCG is not 15%
Surveillance	Weekly	Weekly

(β-hCG: beta-human chorionic gonadotropin)

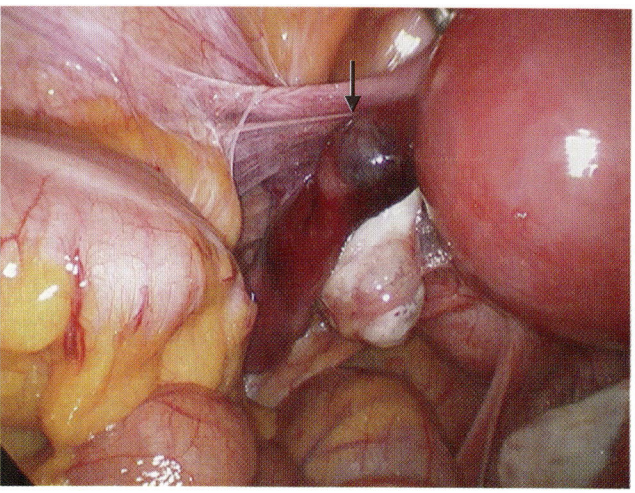

Fig. 4: Unruptured Left tubal ectopic pregnancy (black arrow) laparoscopic view.

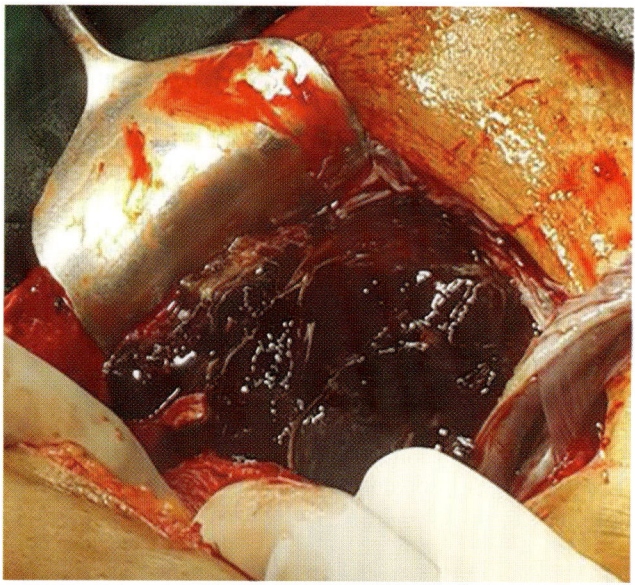

Fig. 5: Massive hemoperitoneum in a ruptured ectopic pregnancy.

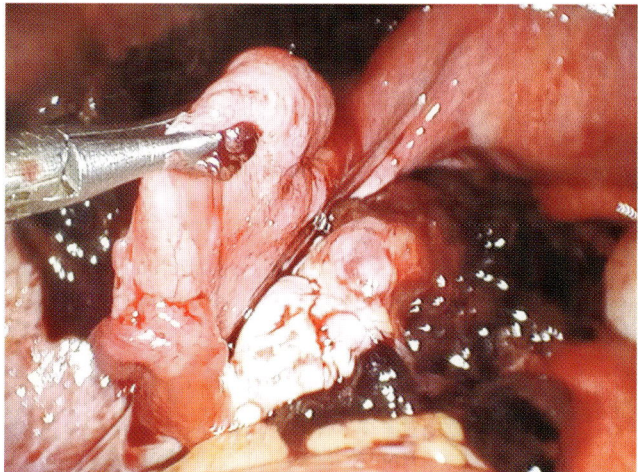

Fig. 3: Ruptured left tubal ectopic pregnancy with hemoperitoneum—laparoscopic view.

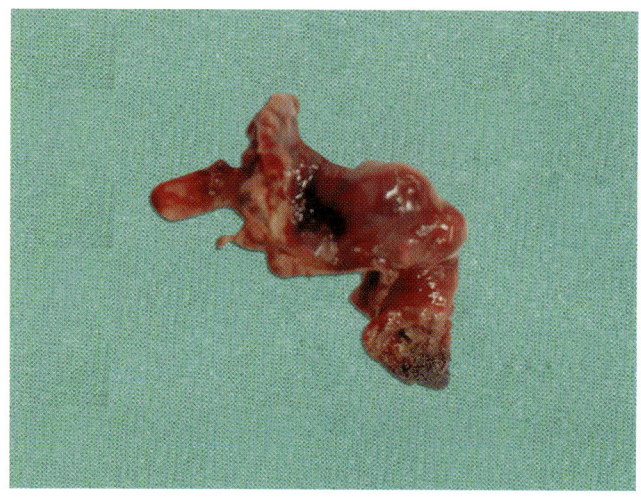

Fig. 6: Specimen of fallopian tube (salpingectomy) performed for ruptured ectopic pregnancy.

level of morbidity. These include interstitial, cesarean scar **(Fig. 7)**, cervical, heterotopic, and cornual and abdominal ectopic pregnancy. All these are discussed briefly in **Table 7**.

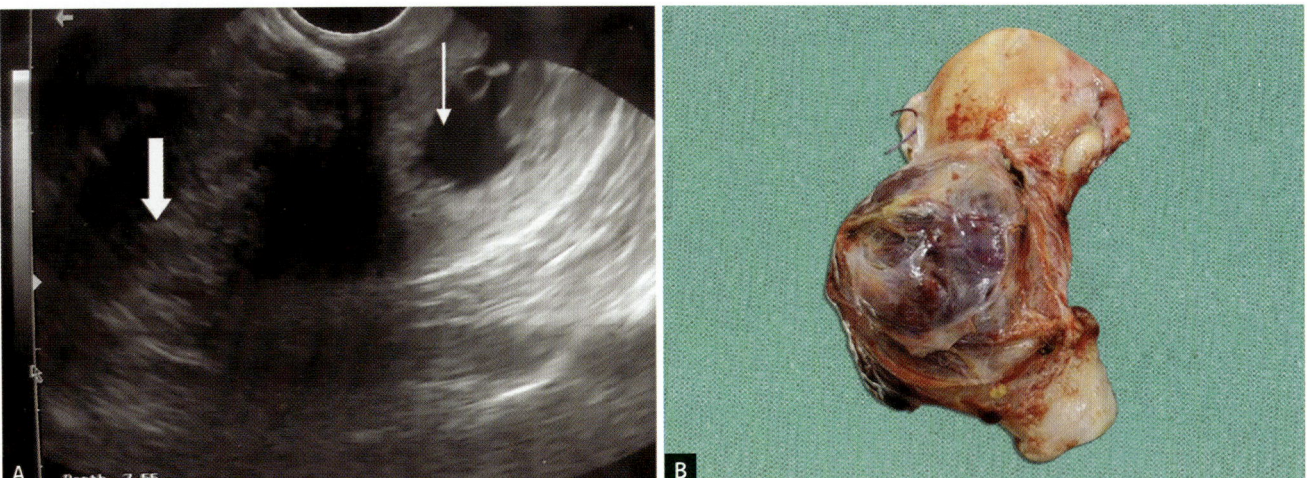

Figs. 7A and B: Scar ectopic pregnancy. (A) Ultrasound showing an empty endometrial cavity (white block arrow) and pregnancy (white plain arrow) in lower segment or scar; (B) Surgical specimen of hysterectomy performed for scar ectopic pregnancy of the same woman.

TABLE 7: Nontubal ectopic pregnancy.

Type of pregnancy	Incidence	USG features	Management
Cervical pregnancy	0.15%	• Empty uterus with gestational sac below the level of the internal cervical os • Barrel-shaped cervix • Absent "sliding sign" • Vascularity around the gestational sac in cervix	• Medical management with methotrexate • Chemoembolization • Intracardiac KCL injection
Interstitial pregnancy	1–6%	• Uterine cavity is empty • Gestational sac in the interstitial portion of tube surrounded by <5 mm of myometrium • The thin echogenic central uterine cavity echo can be seen extending to the edge of the interstitial sac and is referred to as the "interstitial line sign" (sensitivity 80%, specificity 98%)[20]	• Laparoscopic or open cornual excision • Local or systemic methotrexate • Hysteroscopic resection under laparoscopic or USG guidance
Cesarean scar pregnancy	1 in 2,000 pregnancies	• Uterus and cervix are empty • Gestational sac embedded into the scar site • Myometrium between the gestational sac and the bladder is thin or absent • Vascularity around the gestational sac[21-23]	• Local injection of methotrexate into the gestational sac under ultrasound guidance or systemic[24] • Suction evacuation or hysteroscopic resection or excision[25-29]
Abdominal pregnancy		• Uterus and adnexa are normal • Bowel loops seen surrounding the gestational sac, separated from them by peritoneum • Mobility noted toward the posterior cul-de-sac on pressure with transvaginal probe[30]	• Laparoscopic removal or systemic methotrexate with USG-guided feticide • Laparotomy for advanced pregnancy
Ovarian pregnancy		No specific criteria	Removal of POC by enucleation or wedge resection by laparoscopy or laparotomy
Heterotopic pregnancy		Co-existent gestational sac in uterine cavity along with an ectopic pregnancy	• The contents of the sac are aspirated • Local injection of KCL or hyperosmolar glucose given • Methotrexate to be given only if nonviable or undesirable pregnancy • Surgical management if vitals unstable

(KCL: potassium chloride; POC: products of conception; USG: ultrasonography)

KEY MESSAGES

- Diagnosis of ectopic pregnancy can be established by a comprehensive approach of history, examination, and use of transvaginal ultrasound.
- Serial serum β-hCG values may be needed to be performed and correlated with the clinical presentation and ultrasound findings for diagnosis of ectopic pregnancy.

- Medical or laparoscopic management can be offered if the woman has an unruptured ectopic and is hemodynamically stable. Single-dose Mtx is preferred if medical therapy is indicated and selected.
- The risk of subsequent ectopic pregnancy following an ectopic is approximately 15%.
- Surgical management and medical therapy have similar future reproductive outcome.

REFERENCES

1. Tenore JL. Ectopic pregnancy. Am Fam Physician. 2000; 61(4):1080-8.
2. Tahmina S, Daniel M, Solomon P. Clinical analysis of ectopic pregnancies in a tertiary care centre in southern India: A six year retrospective study. J Clin Diagn Res. 2016; 10(10):QC13-QC16.
3. Barnhart KT, Fay CA, Suescum M, Sammel MD, Appleby D, Shaunik A, et al. Clinical factors affecting the accuracy of ultrasonography in symptomatic first-trimester pregnancy. Obstet Gynecol. 2011;117(2 Pt 1):299-306.
4. Barnhart K, van Mello NM, Bourne T, Kirk E, Van Calster B, Bottomley C, et al. Pregnancy of unknown location: a consensus statement of nomenclature, definitions, and outcome. Fertil Steril. 2011;95(3):857-66.
5. Goldstein I, Zimmer EA, Tamir A, Peretz BA, Paldi E. Evaluation of normal gestational sac growth: appearance of embryonic heartbeat and embryo body movements using the transvaginal technique. Obstet Gynecol. 1991;77(6):885-8.
6. Rossavik IK, Torjusen GO, Gibbons WE. Conceptual age and ultrasound measurements of gestational sac and crown-rump length in in vitro fertilization pregnancies. Fertil Steril. 1988;49(6):1012-7.
7. Doubilet PM, Benson CB, Bourne T, Blaivas M, Barnhart KT, Benacerraf BR, et al. Diagnostic criteria for nonviable pregnancy early in the first trimester. Society of Radiologists in Ultrasound Multispecialty Panel on Early First Trimester Diagnosis of Miscarriage and Exclusion of a Viable Intrauterine Pregnancy. N Engl J Med. 2013;369(15):1443-51.
8. Doubilet PM, Benson CB. Further evidence against the reliability of the human chorionic gonadotropin discriminatory level. J Ultrasound Med. 2011;30(12):1637-42.
9. Mehta TS, Levine D, Beckwith B. Treatment of ectopic pregnancy: is a human chorionic gonadotropin level of 2,000 mIU/mL a reasonable threshold? Radiology. 1997;205(2):569-73.
10. Connolly A, Ryan DH, Stuebe AM, Wolfe HM. Reevaluation of discriminatory and threshold levels for serum beta-hCG in early pregnancy. Obstet Gynecol. 2013;121(1):65-70.
11. Seeber BE, Sammel MD, Guo W, Zhou L, Hummel A, Barnhart KT. Application of redefined human chorionic gonadotropin curves for the diagnosis of women at risk for ectopic pregnancy. Fertil Steril. 2006;86(2):454-9.
12. Morse CB, Sammel MD, Shaunik A, Allen-Taylor L, Oberfoell NL, Takacs P, et al. Performance of human chorionic gonadotropin curves in women at risk for ectopic pregnancy: exceptions to the rules. Fertil Steril. 2012;97(1):101-6.e2.
13. Barnhart KT, Guo W, Cary MS, Morse CB, Chung K, Takacs P, et al. Differences in serum human chorionic gonadotropin rise in early pregnancy by race and value at presentation. Obstet Gynecol. 2016;128(3):504-11.
14. Silva C, Sammel MD, Zhou L, Gracia C, Hummel AC, Barnhart K. Human chorionic gonadotropin profile for women with ectopic pregnancy. Obstet Gynecol. 2006;107(3):605-10.
15. Kirk E, Papageorghiou AT, Condous G, Tan L, Bora S, Bourne T. The diagnostic effectiveness of an initial transvaginal scan in detecting ectopic pregnancy. Hum Reprod 2007;22(11):2824-8.
16. van Mello NM, Mol F, Opmeer BC, Ankum WM, Barnhart K, Coomarasamy A, et al. Diagnostic value of serum hCG on the outcome of pregnancy of unknown location: a systematic review and meta-analysis. Hum Reprod Update. 2012;18(6):603-17.
17. Mavrelos D, Nicks H, Jamil A, Hoo W, Jauniaux E, Jurkovic D. Efficacy and safety of a clinical protocol or expectant management of selected women diagnosed with a tubal ectopic pregnancy. Ultrasound Obstet Gynecol. 2013;42(1):102-7.
18. Barnhart KT, Gosman G, Ashby R, Sammel M. The medical management of ectopic pregnancy: a meta-analysis comparing "single dose" and "multidose" regimens. Obstet Gynecol. 2003;101(4):778-84.
19. Cheng X, Tian X, Yan Z, Jia M, Deng J, Wang Y, et al. Comparison of the fertility outcome of salpingotomy and salpingectomy in women with tubal pregnancy: a systematic review and meta-analysis. PLoS One. 2016;11(3):e0152343.
20. Ackerman TE, Levi CS, Dashefsky SM, Holt SC, Lindsay DJ. Interstitial line: sonographic finding in interstitial (cornual) ectopic pregnancy. Radiology. 1993;189(1):83-7.
21. Godin PA, Bassil S, Donnez J. An ectopic pregnancy developing in a previous caesarian section scar. Fertil Steril. 1997;67(2):398-400.
22. Jurkovic D, Hillaby K, Woelfer B, Lawrence A, Salim R, Elson CJ. First-trimester diagnosis and management of pregnancies implanted into the lower uterine segment Cesarean section scar. Ultrasound Obstet Gynecol. 2003;21(3):220-7.
23. Seow KM, Hwang JL, Tsai YL. Ultrasound diagnosis of a pregnancy in a Cesarean section scar. Ultrasound Obstet Gynecol. 2001;18(5):547-9.
24. Timor-Tritsch IE, Monteagudo A, Santos R, Tsymbal T, Pineda G, Arslan AA. The diagnosis, treatment, and follow-up of cesarean scar pregnancy. Am J Obstet Gynecol. 2012;207(1):44.e1-13.
25. Yang Q, Piao S, Wang G, Wang Y, Liu C. Hysteroscopic surgery of ectopic pregnancy in the cesarean section scar. J Minim Invasive Gynecol. 2009;16(4):432-6.
26. Halperin R, Schneider D, Mendlovic S, Pansky M, Herman A, Maymon R. Uterine-preserving emergency surgery for cesarean scar pregnancies: another medical solution to an iatrogenic problem. Fertil Steril. 2009;91(6):2623-7.
27. Wang HY, Zhang J, Li YN, Wei W, Zhang DW, Lu YQ, et al. Laparoscopic management or laparoscopy combined with transvaginal management of type II cesarean scar pregnancy. JSLS. 2013;17(2):263-72.
28. He M, Chen MH, Xie HZ, Yao SZ, Zhu B, Feng LP, et al. Transvaginal removal of ectopic pregnancy tissue and repair of uterine defect for caesarean scar pregnancy. BJOG. 2011;118(9):1136-9.
29. Le A, Shan L, Xiao T, Zhuo R, Xiong H, Wang Z. Transvaginal surgical treatment of cesarean scar ectopic pregnancy. Arch Gynecol Obstet. 2013;287(4):791-6.
30. Gerli S, Rossetti D, Baiocchi G, Clerici G, Unfer V, Di Renzo GC. Early ultrasonographic diagnosis and laparoscopic treatment of abdominal pregnancy. Eur J Obstet Gynecol Reprod Biol. 2004;113(1):103-5.

LONG QUESTION

1. What is ectopic pregnancy? How will you manage a case of 24-year-old G2A1 female with 6-week pregnancy with pain in lower abdomen and slight vaginal bleeding?

SHORT QUESTIONS

1. Medical management of ectopic pregnancy
2. Diagnosis and management of cesarean scar pregnancy
3. Role of ultrasound for diagnosis of ectopic pregnancy
4. Surgical management of ectopic pregnancy

MULTIPLE CHOICE QUESTIONS

1. Which of the following is not a risk factor for an ectopic pregnancy?
    a. Prior tubal pregnancy
    b. Smoking
    c. A history of pelvic inflammatory disease
    d. In-vitro fertilization
    e. A prior ovarian pregnancy
2. The classic signs and symptoms of an ectopic pregnancy include all of the following, except:
    a. Vaginal bleeding
    b. Syncope
    c. Adnexal tenderness
    d. Adnexal mass
3. The discriminatory zone beyond which a gestational sac will be visualized in the uterus in 95% of cases is:
    a. 500 mIU/mL
    b. 1,000 mIU/mL
    c. 1,500 mIU/mL
    d. 3,000 mIU/mL
    e. 6,000 mIU/mL
4. Which of the following sonographic signs associated with an ectopic pregnancy is the most common?
    a. A pseudogestational sac
    b. An extrauterine gestation with cardiac activity
    c. An "echogenic ring"
    d. Debris-filled cul-de-sac fluid
    e. A complex adnexal mass
5. Which of the following ectopics will grow to the largest size before becoming symptomatic?
    a. Isthmus
    b. Fimbrial
    c. Cervical
    d. Cornual
    e. Ovarian
6. The medical management of an ectopic pregnancy requires that the β-hCG level drops by what percent between day 4 and 7 after therapy?
    a. 10%
    b. 15%
    c. 20%
    d. 25%
    e. 30%
7. The prevalence of a persistent ectopic pregnancy after linear salpingostomy at laparotomy is?
    a. 1%
    b. 2–5%
    c. 6–10%
    d. 11–15%
    e. 15%
8. In a case of ectopic pregnancy, medical treatment is contraindicated, if:
    a. Sac size is 3.0 cm
    b. Blood in pelvis is 70 mL
    c. Presence of fetal heart activity
    d. Previous ectopic pregnancy
9. Which of the following is not a radiological sign of cesarean scar pregnancy?
    a. Empty uterine cavity
    b. Empty cervical canal
    c. Thick myometrium between bladder and gestational sac
    d. Intrauterine mass seen in anterior part of the uterine isthmus
10. Which of the following is incorrect regarding management of cervical pregnancy?
    a. Chemoembolization has been tried with success
    b. Intracardiac injection of KCL can be done
    c. Intramuscular injection of methotrexate is best treatment modality
    d. Conservative management is feasible for many women

Answers

1. e 2. b 3. d 4. a 5. d 6. b
7. b 8. c 9. c 10. c

4.3 GESTATIONAL TROPHOBLASTIC DISEASE

VP Radhadevi, PK Sekharan

INTRODUCTION

Gestational trophoblastic disease (GTD) is a group of premalignant and malignant conditions resulting from abnormal trophoblastic proliferations. The benign lesions are complete and partial hydatidiform moles, resulting from abnormal fertilization of a defective ovum, and in both the conditions, there is an excess of paternal genome. The malignant lesions are gestational choriocarcinoma (CC), invasive mole (IM), placental site trophoblastic tumor (PSTT), and epithelioid trophoblastic tumor (ETT)—together grouped as gestational trophoblastic neoplasia (GTN). The atypical placental site nodule (APSN) is also added to the GTD spectrum as 10-15% APSN may coexist or develop into PSTT/ETT.[1] All types of GTN, except PSTT and ETT, produce large quantity of human chorionic gonadotropin (hCG), which serves as a very sensitive tumor marker. Even though there is a tendency for dissemination, GTN is a highly chemosensitive tumor. It has a high cure rate even when there is disease spread. Low-risk GTN can have nearly 100% cure with preservation of fertility. Almost 60% of GTN is following molar pregnancy and could be diagnosed early by clinical and hCG follow-up, but cases following delivery and abortion are diagnosed at an advanced stage. It is not essential for histological conformation of malignancy, but with rising or plateauing levels of hCG, GTN is diagnosed and treated with chemotherapy.

THE HISTORY OF TROPHOBLASTIC DISEASE

The history of the disease was reviewed by Ober in 1961.[2] As early as 400 BC, Hippocrates had described hydatidiform mole as "dropsy of the uterus." In 1600 AD, Aetius described the resemblance vesicles to drops of water and coined the term "hydatid" from the Greek word for drop. The story of the Countess of Hennberg, who was so cursed that she delivered 365 stillborn children (each a molar vesicle) on Good Friday in 1276 is the early anecdotal description of the molar pregnancy. The earlier understanding was that GTN originates from decidua and therefore sarcomatous. Marchand in 1894 established the origin from trophoblast and it is coined as carcinoma. Next major advance was the discovery by Ascheim and Zondek in 1928 of the secretion into urine of a gonadotropic substance during pregnancy. This was identified as the hCG and the various assay systems for diagnosis and follow-up of GTN were developed. Prior to 1956, surgery was the main treatment of GTN and even in patients with disease confines to uterus, the cure rate was <40%. In 1956, Roy Hertz and Min Chiu Li first reported the cure of a patient with metastatic CC using chemotherapy. This success was described by Arthur T. Hertig, Professor of Pathology, Harvard Medical school as "God's first cancer, man's first cure."[3]

Classification

The spectrum of GTD includes both the benign and the malignant lesions, the malignant conditions are grouped together as GTN.
- Hydatidiform mole:
  - Complete hydatidiform mole (CHM):
    - *Androgenetic complete hydatidiform mole (AnCHM)*: There is an inactivation of the maternal 23X set of haploid chromosomes. A single sperm with 23X enters this empty ovum. There is duplication and 46XX diploid karyotype results.
      - *Homozygous*: These are always 46XX. About 80% are of this variety. There is a duplication of the paternal haploid set of 23X and there is monospermic fertilization.
      - *Heterozygous*: These may be of 46 XX or 46XY Karyotype and are about 15-20%. They are formed as a result of dispermic fertilization.
    - *Biparental complete hydatidiform mole (BiCHM) or familial recurrent mole (FRIIM)*: In these conditions, there is a loss of maternal imprinting due to the effect of mutations of two maternal effect genes—*NLRP7* (75–80%) and *KHDC3L* (10–15%).
  - Partial hydatidiform mole (PHM):
    - When an ovum containing a haploid set of 23X is fertilized by two sperms (dispermy), the result is 69XXY/69XXX. It may also occur when there is a duplication of sperm with haploid set of 23X to result in 69XXX—triploid.
- *GTN:* Gestational trophoblastic neoplasia comprises a group of tumors with the potential for local invasion and metastases.
- Invasive mole (IM).
- Gestational carcinoma.
- Placental site trophoblastic tumor.
- Epithelioid trophoblastic tumor.
- In the absence of histopathological diagnosis, persistent elevation of hCG after evacuation of a molar pregnancy is also termed GTN.

GENETICS OF HYDATIDIFORM MOLE

Hydatidiform mole results from fertilization of an abnormal ovum. The CHM and PHM are different genetic entities. This has been demonstrated by the early work of Vassilakos, Szulman and Surti, and Lawler.[4,5] The genetically different entities also manifest differently in terms of phenotype, clinical outcomes, and malignant potential.

COMPLETE HYDATIDIFORM MOLE (FIG. 1)

As described above, CHM occurs due to fertilization of an "empty egg" (absent or inactivated maternal chromosomes). The varieties and means of fertilization are given above and represented below diagrammatically. The one karyotype that has not been observed is 46YY, since it is not compatible with early development. Heterozygous moles are at higher risk of developing malignancy. The nuclear DNA is paternal and the mitochondrial DNA is derived from the mother. CHM by dispermic fertilization (heterozygous) containing Y chromosome shows high malignant potential.[6]

PARTIAL HYDATIDIFORM MOLE (FIG. 2)

Partial hydatidiform mole are triploid and may have 69XXX, 69XXY, or 69XYY karyotype. This results from dispermic fertilization or diandric triploidy. Though it is thought to be of paternal origin, it can be hypothesized that the ovum is also abnormal, as a normal ovum will allow only one sperm to fertilize it.

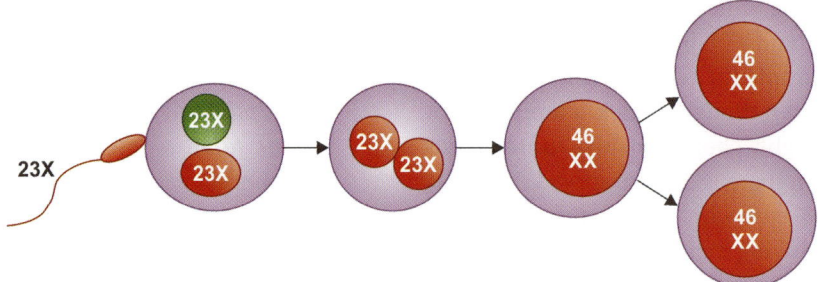

Fig. 1: Complete hydatidiform mole (CHM). An ovum whose haploid set of 23X chromosome is extruded or inactivated is fertilized by a sperm with its haploid set of 23X chromosome and duplicates to form 46XX chromosomes. About 15–20% of the CHM results by fertilization of an empty ovum by two sperms, 23X/23Y or 23X/23X—heterozygous, more malignant potential.

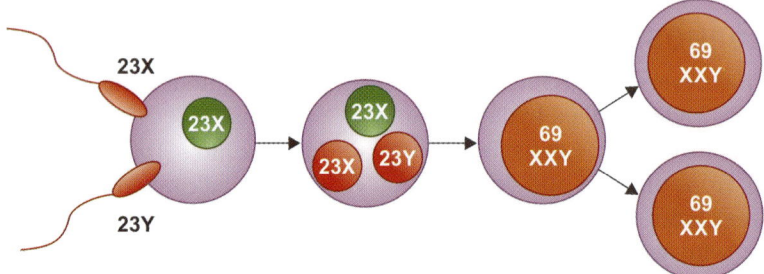

Fig. 2: Partial hydatidiform mole. Fertilization of an ovum containing 23X haploid set of chromosomes by two sperms with chromosome set of 23X and 23Y resulting in triploidy of 69XXY. Fertilization by two sperms with 23X can result in 69XXX.

BIPARENTAL COMPLETE HYDATIDIFORM MOLE (BiCHM) (FIG. 3)

Biparental complete mole is a rare condition seen in families with more than one member developing recurrent molar pregnancy. Both maternal and paternal genes are present, but failure of maternal imprinting causes only the paternal genome to be expressed. Familial recurrent biparental mole is an autosomal recessive condition associated with mutations of gene *NLRP7* in 70–80% of the cases and 5–10% results from mutations of *KHDC3L*. Genetic studies of such families has shown evidence of mutations in the Lucin-rich regions of *NLRP7* at chromosome *19q13.3.4*.[7]

Biparental complete hydatidiform mole seems to be a result of a defect in the methylation of paternal and maternal alleles of *H19* gene. The paternal allele is methylated and the maternal allele is not. The defect may be partial or may occasionally be overcome. This explains the very rare occurrence of a normal pregnancy in a woman with this defect, though theoretically, the risk of recurrence is 100%. Ovum donation in vitro fertilization (IVF) seems to be the option for such women to have a baby.

NORMAL TROPHOBLAST (FIG. 4)

Trophoblast is derived from the outer cell mass of the preimplantation embryo. The placental trophoblast consists of cytotrophoblast, syncytiotrophoblast, and intermediate trophoblast. Villous trophoblast covers the chorionic villi, the inner layer is the cytotrophoblast, and the outer layer is the syncytiotrophoblast. Cytotrophoblast is the stem cell from which the syncytiotrophoblast is formed by fusion. Syncytiotrophoblast secretes abundant hCG, some human placental lactogen (hPL), and placental alkaline phosphatase (PLAP). Inhibin-A is produced by syncytiotrophoblast, peaks in first trimester, declines in mid trimester, and rises again toward term. Production of hCG decreases, while hPL and PLAP increases as term advances. The amount of villous trophoblast also decreases near term. Trophoblast also synthesizes estrogen and progesterone. There are three types of intermediate trophoblast, the villous intermediate trophoblast located in the villous columns, implantation site intermediate trophoblast located in the placental site, and chorionic-type intermediate trophoblast located in the chorionic leave of the fetal membranes. The normal trophoblast is capable of invading into maternal decidua, blood vessels, and myometrium and can reach the pulmonary circulation. There is proliferation of both cytotrophoblast and syncytiotrophoblast in hydatidiform mole, IM, and CC and continues to secrete hCG.

The common trophoblastic stem cell develops along two lines of trophoblastic differentiation: villous and extravillous. Molar pregnancies and CC are derived from villous trophoblast and PSTT and ETT are derived from extravillous trophoblast.

Epidemiology

The incidence of trophoblastic disease is difficult to ascertain and varies widely in different parts of the world. Reports from

SECTION 4: Early Pregnancy Complications

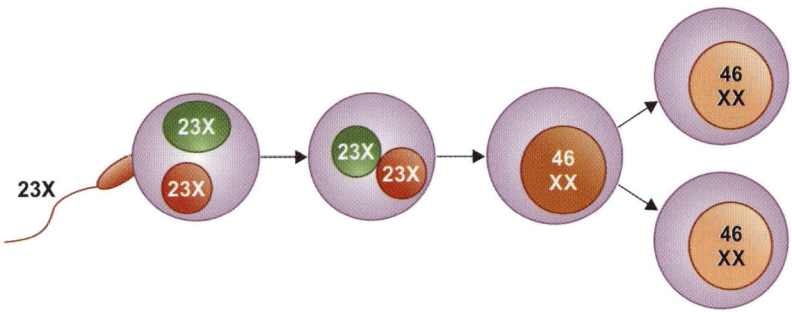

Fig. 3: Biparental complete hydatidiform mole (BiCHM). Biparental familial recurrent mole results from mutation of the gene *NLRP7* in >70% of the cases and in 5–10%, it may be mutation of KDC3L. An imprinting defect in maternal genome is silenced and the paternal genome is expressed.

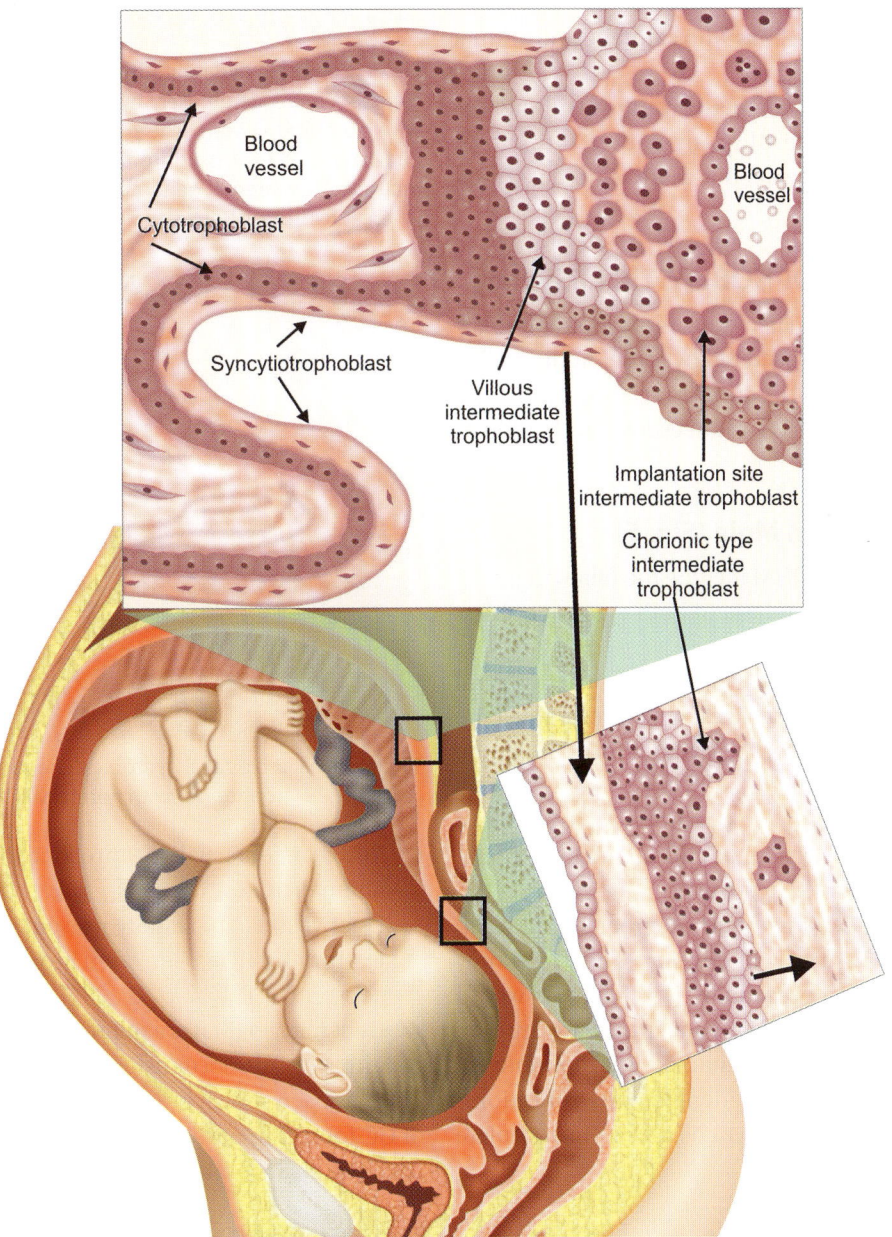

Fig. 4: Trophoblasts.

North America and Europe show a low incidence of 1 in 1,500 to 1 in 1,000 pregnancies. The reported incidence varies from 1 in 500 to 1 in 200 in some of the Latin American and Asian countries. The frequency ranges from 1 in 100 pregnancies in Indonesia to 1 in 200 in Mexico to 1 in 5,000 pregnancies in Paraguay. The difference may be due the differences in the population-based and institution-based studies. In the United Kingdom (UK), the reported incidence is 1 in 1,000 pregnancies for complete mole and 3 per 1,000 for partial mole.[8] In India, the reported incidence is 3-4 per 1,000 deliveries.

Risk Factors

The following risk factors may be considered significant:
- Previous history of molar pregnancy raises the risk to 10× the normal population. CC commonly develops after complete mole, rarely following partial mole and 2-7 per 100,000 after other pregnancies.
- *Age*: 2× the risk in teenage women and those over 35 years. 5-10× the risk in women over 40 years.[9]
- *Nutrition*: There are some links with carotene and animal fat deficiency.
- *Miscellaneous*: There are some associations with factors such as smoking, subfertility, ovulation induction, hormonal contraceptive use, but there is no described causative mechanism.

PATHOLOGY OF TROPHOBLASTIC LESIONS

The hallmark of all GTDs is proliferation of syncytiotrophoblast and cytotrophoblast. hCG is secreted by these. Additionally, placental-site trophoblastic tumor arising from the intermediate trophoblast cells produces low levels of hCG and hPL.

Complete Hydatidiform Mole (Fig. 5)

The histological features of CHM include the following:
- Generalized diffuse hyperplasia of both cytotrophoblast and syncytiotrophoblast
- Generalized edema of chorionic villi with central cistern formation of varying sizes, which resembles the macroscopic description of the hydatidiform mole, the "bunch of grapes"
- Absence of an embryo—resorption occurs before development of fetal circulation and no nucleated fetal erythrocytes are observed in the villi.

In modern practice, many moles are treated before all the pathognomonic features will develop. The pregnancy may be labeled as a failed pregnancy. The diagnosis would be missed unless the products of conception are studied by histopathology. Early CHM is marked by trophoblastic hyperplasia, which may not be evident in early conditions. Immunostaining using p57kip2 will be absent in complete mole.

Partial Hydatidiform Mole (Fig. 6)

The characteristics on pathology are as follows:
- Mild focal variable hydropic villi
- Mild trophoblastic hyperplasia, predominantly confined to syncytium

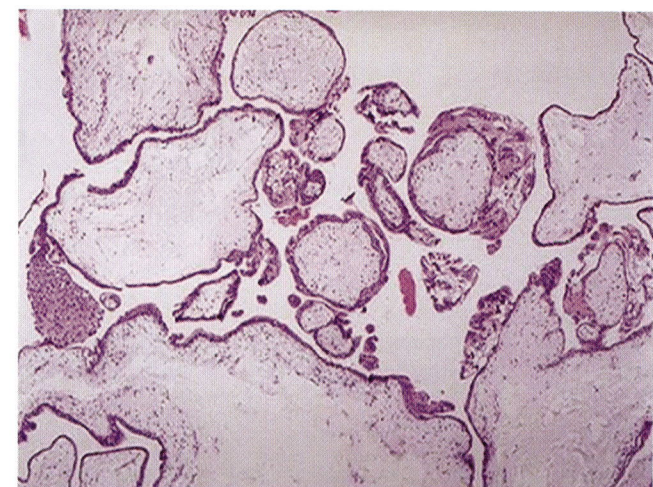

Fig. 5: Complete hydatidiform mole histology. The chorionic villi of complete mole are diffusely hydropic with central cistern formation with no blood vessels. The *p57kip2* gene (CDKN1C) is paternally imprinted and expressed from the maternal allele. Since complete moles lack a maternal genome, p57kip2 immunostaining is absent, whereas hydropic abortus and partial moles show positive staining.[12]

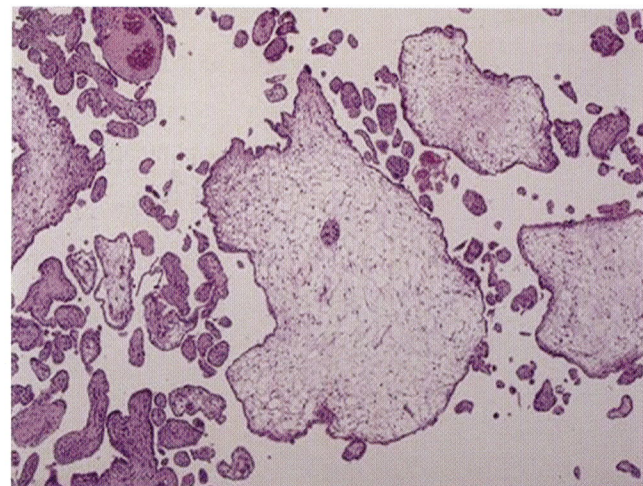

Fig. 6: Partial mole-focal hydropic degeneration with hyperplasia of trophoblast with normal villi in between.

- Embryo/fetus will be present often with congenital anomalies.
- Fetal vessels are usually present and contain nucleated fetal erythrocytes. Can often be misdiagnosed as a missed abortion

Generally, PHM has a milder clinical course. However, the belief that they do not transform into CC has not been borne out. This has been shown by Newlandes who reported three cases of CC following partial mole.[10] Subsequently, other authors have also corroborated these malignant sequelae after PHM.[11]

DISTINCTION BETWEEN COMPLETE HYDATIDIFORM MOLE AND PARTIAL HYDATIDIFORM MOLE

The important differences between CHM and PHM are described in **Table 1**.

TABLE 1: Distinction between complete hydatidiform mole (CHM) and partial hydatidiform mole (PHM).		
Feature	*Complete mole*	*Partial mole*
Karyotype	Diploid 46XX, 15% 46XY	Triploid 69XXX, 69XXY, rarely 69XYY
Fetal tissue	Absent	Present
Villi	Diffusely hydropic	Focal → hydropic → villi, → with normal villi and fetus
Trophoblastic proliferation	Diffuse, marked	Focal, mild
Size of uterus	Markedly enlarged in >50%	Normal/less for GA
Theca lutein cyst	Present in nearly 25%	Rare
Expression of p57kip2	Negative	Present
Malignant sequelae	7–15%	0.5–3%

(GA: gestational age)

INVASIVE MOLE (FIG. 7)

When there is an invasion of the molar villi into the myometrium or vessels of the uterus, the condition is called an invasive mole. The penetration may be of full thickness, causing massive bleeding into the abdominal cavity. The characteristic feature is trophoblast invasion of the myometrium with villous structures. The trophoblastic activity is moderate to marked. The gold standard of making a diagnosis is histopathology. However, this may not be clinically feasible, as a hysterectomy would be needed to make the diagnosis, but may not be warranted. Sonographic markers such as myometrial echogenicity in focal areas may raise suspicion. Doppler flow in these small fluid-filled heterogeneous areas show high vascularity patterns. The clinical presentation is usually one of heavy bleeding, subinvoluted, tender uterus, and rising hCG levels. These findings should be the basis of starting chemotherapy. Histopathological diagnosis is not mandatory.

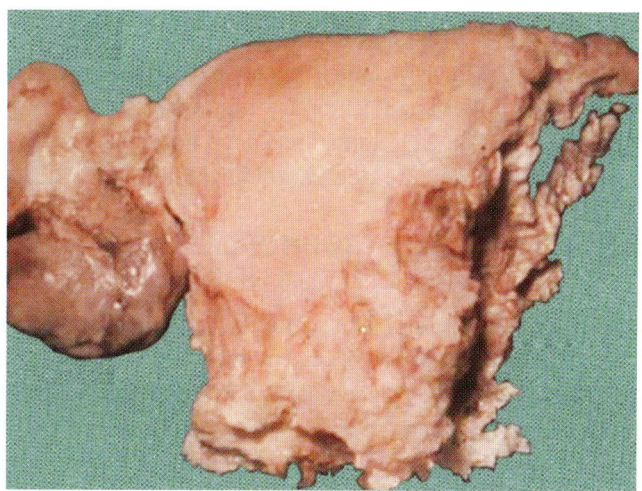

Fig. 7: Gross specimen of invasive mole. Subtotal hysterectomy done as a lifesaving procedure for spontaneous perforation of the uterus leading to intraperitoneal hemorrhage.

ECTOPIC HYDATIDIFORM MOLE

Rarely molar pregnancy may develop in the fallopian tube, presenting as tubal ectopic. The specimen on histopathological examination will show features of complete or partial mole and requires hCG follow-up.[13]

GESTATIONAL CHORIOCARCINOMA (FIG. 8)

Choriocarcinoma is a malignant neoplasm consisting of sheets of anaplastic cytotrophoblasts and syncytiotrophoblast without villous formation, with hemorrhage and necrosis and direct invasion to blood vessels leading to distant metastasis. Even though the absolute risk is low, CHM is an important risk factor for developing CC. It should be noted that any pregnancy (term, abortion, or ectopic) can also be followed by CC, but these are exceptionally rare. The histopathological picture is marked by a mixture of hemorrhage, necrosis, and scattered tumor cells **(Fig. 9)**. There is almost no stromal reaction. Since there is no intrinsic vasculature, the viable

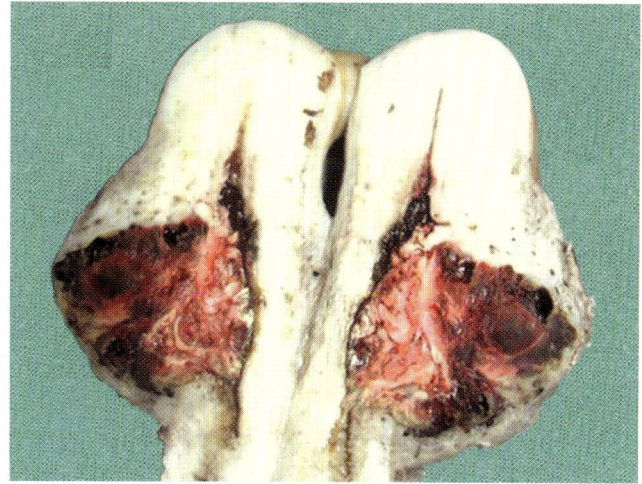

Fig. 8: Choriocarcinoma—hysterectomy, hemorrhagic and necrotic areas.

cells are seen at the edge of the neoplasm. This also causes widespread intravascular dissemination to lungs, brain, and other sites. At the metastatic sites, necrosis and hemorrhage

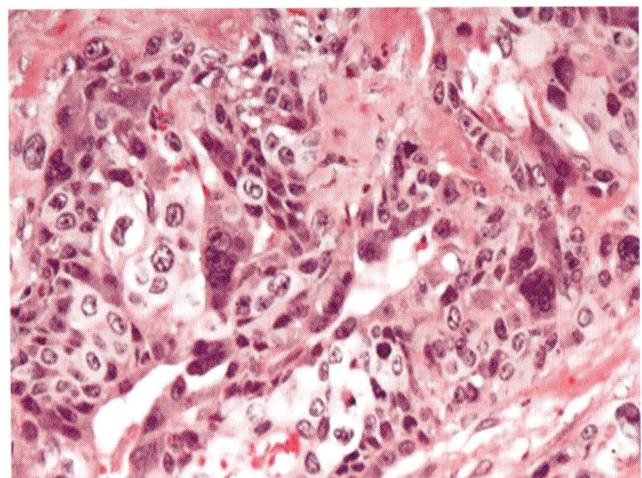

Fig. 9: Choriocarcinoma histology. Cytotrophoblastic and syncytiotrophoblastic hyperplasia and atypia are seen.

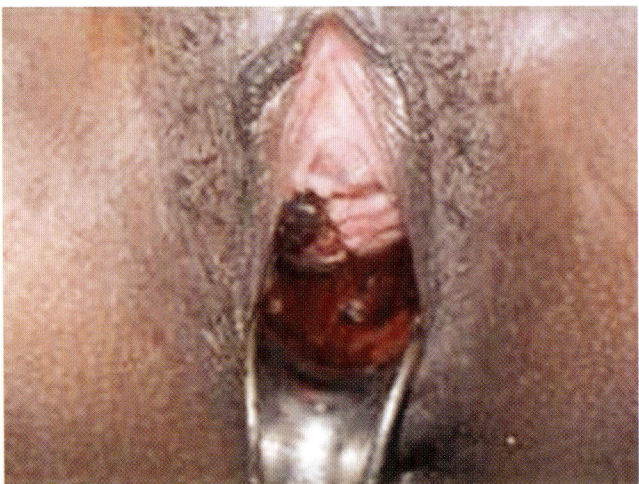

Fig. 10: Suburethral nodule causing vaginal bleeding in gestational trophoblastic neoplasia (GTN).

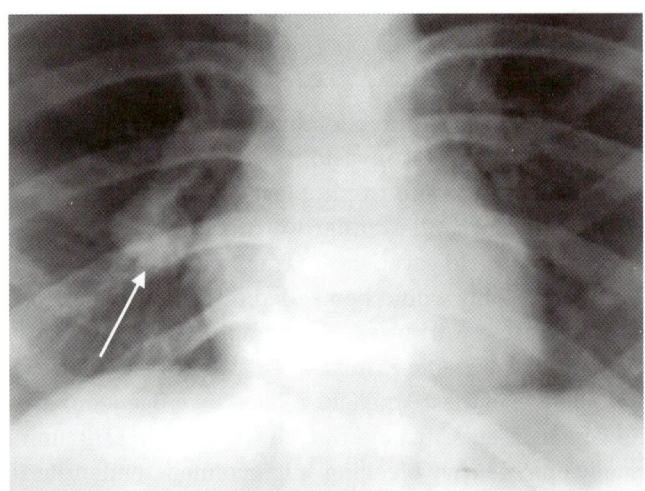

Fig. 11: X-ray of chest showing secondary nodules in the lung in gestational trophoblastic neoplasia (GTN).

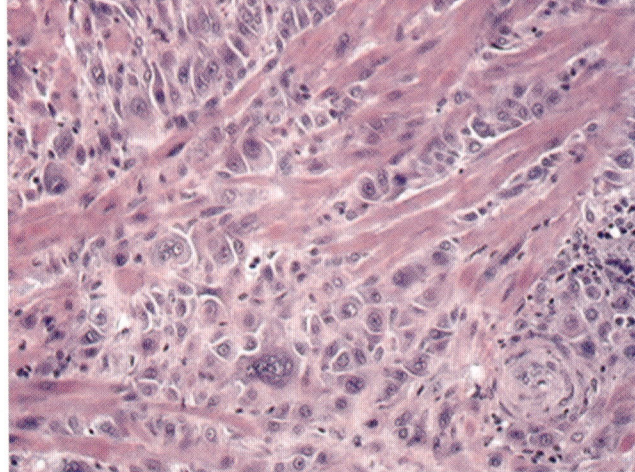

Fig. 12: Placental site trophoblastic tumor (PSTT) histology. Proliferation and atypia of extra villous trophoblasts splitting apart muscle fibers.

are common **(Fig. 10)**. This is because the mass outgrows its blood supply fast. Pulmonary metastasis is the most common site **(Fig. 11)**. Spread has been noted to the renal, gastrointestinal, hepatic, and neurological sites.

PLACENTAL SITE TROPHOBLASTIC TUMOR

A variant of gestational trophoblastic tumor was proposed in 1981 by Scully et al.[14] This is the PSTT.[14] This rare type of GTN is mainly composed of intermediate cytotrophoblastic cells arising from the placental implantation site. Vascular invasion and lymphatic spread are less. Histology shows less hemorrhage, necrosis, villous formation, and tumor infiltrates **(Fig. 12)**. PSTT produces more hPL than hCG. This is due to the lower syncytiotrophoblast reaction. hCG is therefore not a reliable tumor marker in this condition and the levels are lower than the clinically evident tumor mass. It is an indolent tumor and also slow to metastasize. The clinical presentation is of irregular vaginal bleeding or amenorrhea over a long course. The antecedent event may be any type of pregnancy.[15] As the proliferative component is low, response to chemotherapy is also muted. Stage I disease is best managed by hysterectomy. If there is systemic spread, multiagent chemotherapy is recommended. The prognosis depends on the interval from the antecedent pregnancy. If the interval is 4 years or less, the cure rates are better than with longer intervals.[16]

EPITHELIOID TROPHOBLASTIC TUMOR

Recently, epithelioid trophoblastic tumor, a rare entity, has been added to the group of GTN.[17] The antecedent may be a term pregnancy, abortion, or molar gestation. It is composed of chorionic-type intermediate trophoblast. The tumor is made of sheets and nests of mononuclear trophoblast with clear, eosinophilic, and vacuolated cytoplasm resembling "chorionic type" intermediate trophoblast **(Fig. 13)**. It resembles squamous cells carcinomas on histology. It is distinct from CC and PSTT, though it may coexist with other GTNs. On gross examination, it is a well-defined intrauterine solid to cystic, fleshy mass. It may be confused with a squamous

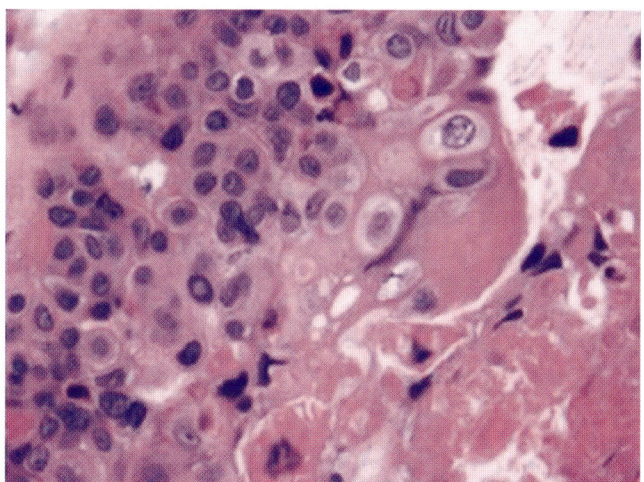

Fig. 13: Epithelioid trophoblastic tumor (ETT) showing epithelioid intermediate trophoblastic tumor cells and eosinophilic hyalinization (keratin-like material) within tumor nests, simulating invasive squamous cell.

cell carcinoma due to its predilection to affect the endocervix and lower uterine segment. The average interval between the antecedent pregnancy and development of the epithelioid trophoblastic tumor is about 5 years.

HUMAN CHORIONIC GONADOTROPIN IN GESTATIONAL TROPHOBLASTIC DISEASE

Human chorionic gonadotropin is a glycoprotein hormone secreted by the syncytiotrophoblast having an α-chain of 92 amino acids and a β-chain with 145 amino acids. The α-chain is similar to the α-chain of luteinizing hormone (LH), follicle-stimulating hormone (FSH), and thyroid-stimulating hormone (TSH), but the β-chain is unique to hCG. The sugar side chains comprise 30–40% of molecular weight of hCG. In pregnancy, the hCG present is mainly intact hCG and in early pregnancy, there is high level of hyperglycosylated hCG (hCG-H) which helps in invasion of the trophoblast.[18]

There are other types of hCG molecules produced by dissociation of intact hCG, hCG-free β subunit, and by cleavage, (nicked regular hCG, nicked hCG-H, nicked hCG-free β subunit, nicked hCG-H-free β subunit, nicked hCG missing the C-terminal peptide, nicked hCG-H missing the C-terminal peptide, nicked hCG-free β subunit missing the C-terminal peptide, nicked hCG-H-free β subunit missing the C-terminal peptide).

In complete and partial mole, regular hCG is produced in high levels by the syncytiotrophoblast. A small quantity of hCG-H is also produced by the extravillous cytotrophoblast. A serum hCG level of >100,000U/L in early pregnancy strongly suggests the possibility of a complete mole. Partial mole produces lesser amount of hCG. IM and CC produce very high levels of hCG. In PSTT, the level of hCG is low and usually it is β subunit.

In malignancy, all types of abnormal hCG are produced and the assay systems used in trophoblastic disease follow-up and diagnosis should be able to detect all forms of hCG. Unfortunately, most commercial assays fail to or variably detect all forms of hCG and therefore are prone to false-negative results in patients with cancer. Siemens immulite is the assay system that will pick up most abnormal types of hCG and is recommended for clinical use for diagnosis and management of GTN.[19]

CLINICAL PRESENTATION OF MOLAR PREGNANCY

The typical presentation with hydatidiform mole is marked by irregular bleeding vaginally and excessive vomiting with a period of amenorrhea. Early pregnancy ultrasound may not show the pathognomonic findings and the diagnosis may be given as an early failing pregnancy (missed abortion and blighted ovum).

In the early second trimester, if the diagnosis has not been made and pregnancy is continuing, the woman will have features of hyperthyroidism, early-onset preeclampsia, a uterus enlarged beyond the duration of gestation, and theca lutein cysts.

DIAGNOSIS OF HYDATIDIFORM MOLE

Ultrasound is the modality of choice in making a diagnosis. The classic appearance of a complete mole is called the "snowstorm appearance **(Fig. 14)**." The features are a heterogeneous mass with variably sized and shaped hypoechoic spaces. The elevated hCG level results in theca lutein cysts, often bilaterally in a third of women **(Fig. 15)**. These sonodiagnostic features become very evident with pregnancies beyond the first trimester. First trimester scans may not show all these typical features. The diagnostic accuracy at 10 weeks is about 50% in a series of 1,000 cases. The common misdiagnosis is of failed early pregnancy. The current gold standard of diagnosis is histopathological diagnosis.[20]

Partial moles present a variegated picture on ultrasound **(Fig. 16)**. The gestational sac transverse diameter is increased. There are focal cystic spaces in the placenta and the fetus is not adequately grown. There could be fetal structural anomalies due to the triploidy.

Immunostaining for p57kip2 may be done to differentiate early pregnancy failures from hydatidiform mole in some situations. P57kip2 is expressed by the maternal allele and is visible on histology as nuclear staining of cytotrophoblast and villous mesenchyme in placenta of all gestations apart from androgenetic complete mole.[21]

An unusual situation is a twin pregnancy with mole. This may be mistaken for a partial mole. The same misdiagnosis is also possible in cases of placental mesenchymal dysplasia. Three-dimensional (3D) ultrasound may be a useful modality for the diagnosis. The final diagnosis is possible with amniocentesis and karyotype, which will confirm a triploidy.

All products of conception from nonviable pregnancies should undergo histological examination irrespective of

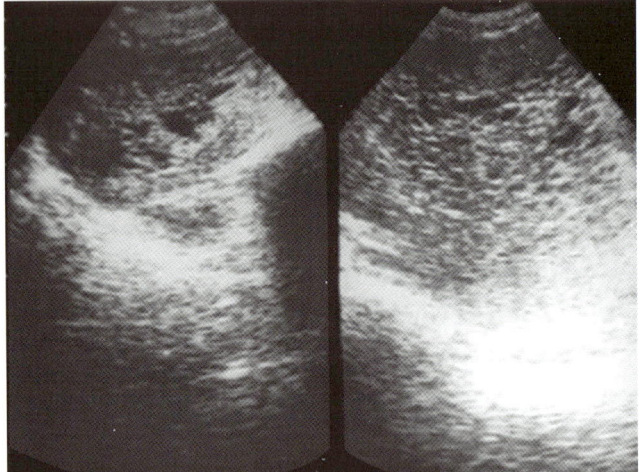

Fig. 14: Ultrasound showing complete mole.

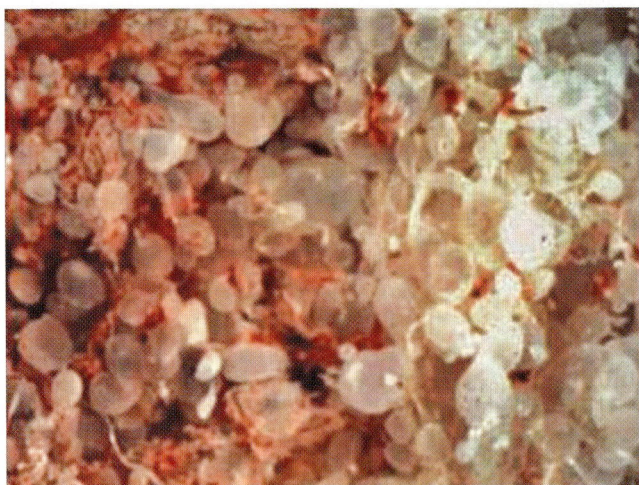

Fig. 17: Moles evacuated by suction.

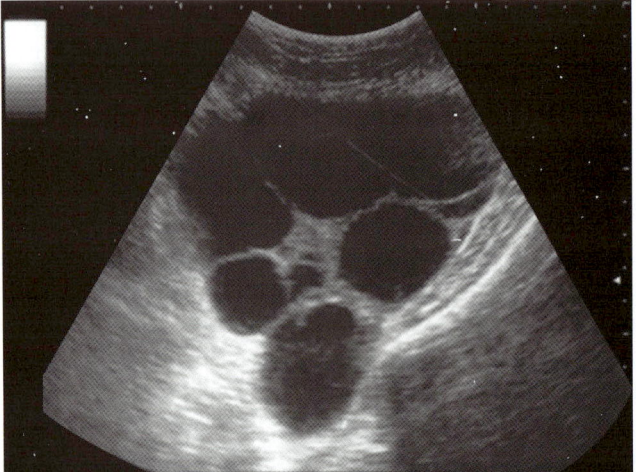

Fig. 15: Ultrasound showing theca lutein cysts in molar pregnancy.

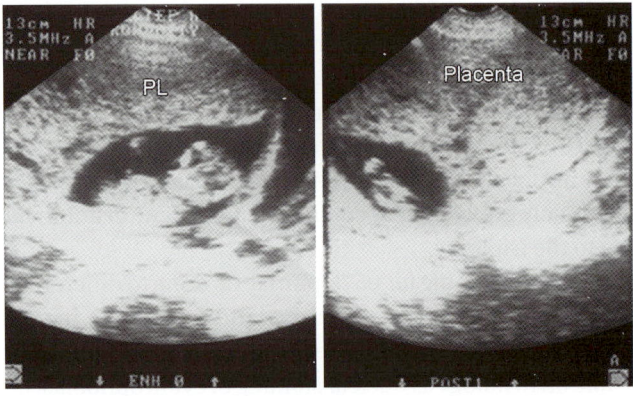

Fig. 16: Ultrasound showing fetus and partial mole.

ultrasonographic findings and all patients after medical termination of pregnancy should have urine hCG tested after 4 weeks to rule out any persistent trophoblastic activity.

MANAGEMENT OF HYDATIDIFORM MOLE

Suction curettage is the preferred method of primary management of hydatidiform mole.[22] Prior to evacuation, patient should be examined for evidence of anemia, hyperthyroidism, and pre-eclampsia. The laboratory investigations include complete blood count (CBC), hCG, liver function test (LFT), renal function test (RFT), thyroid function test (TFT), and serum electrolytes and chest X-ray. Cervical ripening with misoprostol 2–3 hours prior to planned evacuation is not contraindicated and the dilatation of the cervix will be made easy. Blood and blood products must be made available.

Suction evacuation using a 12–14 mm cannula under anesthesia is the primary management of hydatidiform mole irrespective of the size of the uterus.[23] The suction cannula is introduced slowly into the lower uterine cavity and with suction and gentle rotatory movements will make quick evacuation of the moles (**Fig. 17**) and the bleeding could be reduced starting a Pitocin infusion at this time. At the end of the procedure, a gentle curettage is done with blunt curette to make sure the uterine cavity is empty. Evacuation under ultrasound guidance may be preferable. Profuse bleeding and risk of perforation of the uterus are the complications that can occur during evacuation, especially if the uterus is 16 weeks and above. Starting a Pitocin infusion will help to control the bleeding in such cases. Patients who are Rh negative should receive anti-D.

For women who are above 40 years of age and have completed their families, hysterectomy with the mole in situ can be considered (**Fig. 18**). It reduces future CC and IM risk. At hysterectomy, theca lutein cysts can be drained by multiple needle punctures to prevent torsion. Even after a hysterectomy, regular follow-up is needed.

CHEMOPROPHYLAXIS

The practice of chemoprophylaxis as a primary co-intervention with evacuation of a hydatidiform mole is controversial. It can reduce the risk of postmolar GTN in high-risk cases. The benefits are not as remarkable in low-risk cases.[24] Women who develop GTN after primary chemoprophylaxis need more courses of chemotherapy. Correct identification of

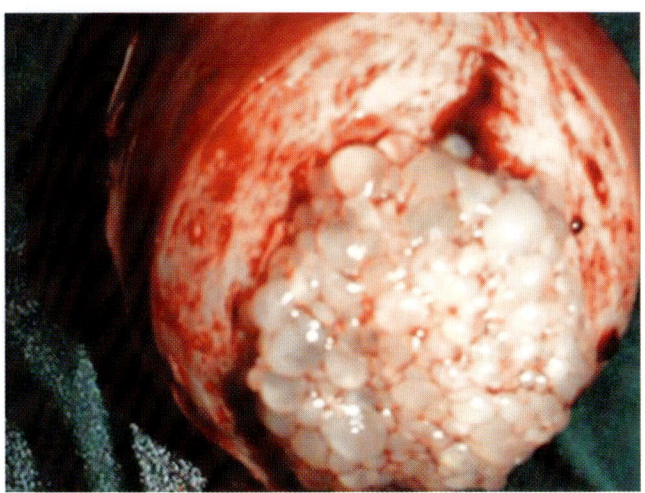

Fig. 18: Hysterectomy specimen with mole in situ.

cases for such an approach should be essential. Those who are considered to be high risk (>35 years of age, uterine size exceeds gestation age by 4 weeks, pre-evacuation hCG ≥100,000 IU/L, and bilateral theca lutein cysts) or those women where follow-up is likely to be unavailable or unreliable can be given chemoprophylaxis. The counterpoints to routine use of chemoprophylaxis are that only one out of five women will have persistent disease and they can be identified with proper follow-up. In case chemoprophylaxis is planned, it should be given as a complete course and hCG follow-up is necessary until it is negative.

Follow-up

Gestational trophoblastic neoplasia is a highly curable cancer if detected early. Without proper follow-up, patients who are generally young can come with advanced disease where morbidity and mortality are very high even with multiagent chemotherapy. There should be regional centers for trophoblastic disease where proper follow-up and management of this rare disease could be organized and can achieve good results.

Following evacuation, patients can be discharged the next day after taking blood for serum β-hCG. She should report after week for clinical examination to check for any bleeding. An ultrasonography is done at this time to rule out incomplete evacuation. A repeat curettage is done *only* if there is any retained products. Blood is sent for serum β-hCG with instruction to report every week till β-hCG is negative for three consecutive weeks.

As per our experience, it is enough to check the β-hCG once in 2 weeks till it is negative to pick up the cases of GTN early and to start chemotherapy for complete cure.[25]

Once the hCG becomes negative for 3 weeks, follow-up with monthly serum/urine hCG for 6 months is sufficient for complete moles. Patients who were having partial mole can have a shorter period of follow-up and once the hCG has become negative, only one more measurement of hCG is done after 1 month.[26]

During follow-up, patients should be advised to have contraception, and low-dose combined oral contraception (COC) is safe.[27] If any patient becomes pregnant during the follow-up period, it is safe to continue the pregnancy.

Normal regression of hCG is one log per week, that is the level of hCG will fall by one-tenth of the previous week. A rise in hCG is defined as 10% increase from the previous week and three such values over 2 weeks is considered as rise in hCG to diagnose GTN. Plateauing of hCG is a fall in hCG of <10% of the previous week and four such values over 3 weeks is considered as plateauing of hCG for diagnosis of GTN.

DIAGNOSIS OF GESTATIONAL TROPHOBLASTIC NEOPLASIA

Gestational trophoblastic neoplasia usually develops following hydatidiform mole, but can occur after any pregnancy including normal pregnancy, abortion, and ectopic pregnancy. Regular clinical and hCG follow-up after molar evacuation can diagnose GTN at an early stage, but cases following delivery and abortions are diagnosed at a later stage with metastasis. It is not essential to have histological conformation to start chemotherapy.

Development of GTN following molar pregnancy will be associated with irregular vaginal bleeding, subinvolution of the uterus, persistence or enlargement of theca lutein cysts with persistent rise, or plateauing of hCG. Doppler study may show highly vascular nodule in the myometrium in cases of IM. GTN following delivery and abortion will report with abnormal vaginal bleeding (AVB) with symptoms relating to metastasis such as dyspnea and hemoptysis, epilepsy, and hCG assay will diagnose the condition.

CRITERIA FOR THE DIAGNOSIS OF POSTMOLAR GESTATIONAL TROPHOBLASTIC NEOPLASIA AND INDICATION FOR CHEMOTHERAPY (TABLE 2)

About 20% of women after CHM evacuation will develop postmolar GTN. The reported range is 6–36%.[28,29] In our own series, of 1,569 cases of hydatidiform moles diagnosed and treated over a period of 15 years from June 1990, the incidence of GTN was 20.5%.[25] 60% of GTN develops after hydatidiform mole, 30% following abortions, and 10% following normal pregnancy or ectopic.

CHOICE OF CHEMOTHERAPY IN GESTATIONAL TROPHOBLASTIC NEOPLASIA

Most cases of GTN can be managed with chemotherapy to achieve remission and the choice of chemotherapy depends on the FIGO (International Federation of Gynecology and Obstetrics) stage and risk score. To accurately stage the disease and to allot the risk score, metastatic work up should be done in every case. FIGO stages I, II, and III with risk score ≤6 are

TABLE 2: Criteria for the diagnosis of postmolar gestational trophoblastic neoplasia (GTN) and indication for chemotherapy.	
Plateau of hCG	Fall in hCG of <10%, 4 values over a period of 3 weeks.
Rise of hCG	Rise in hCG of >10% every week of 3 values over 2 weeks.
Level of hCG	Remains elevated 6 months postmole irrespective of the level. (Present recommendation is to wait if there is falling level)
Serum hCG	>20,000 IU/L 4 weeks after evacuation. (Risk of perforation of the uterus) Histological evidence of choriocarcinoma
	Heavy vaginal bleeding or intraperitoneal bleeding
	Ultrasound evidence of invasive mole

(hCG: human chorionic gonadotropin)

TABLE 3: FIGO Staging—gestational trophoblastic neoplasia (GTN) 2002.	
Placental site trophoblastic tumor will be categorized separately from other gestational trophoblastic neoplasia. The staging is as for GTN but no risk scoring is done.	
Stage I	GTN strictly confined to the uterine corpus
Stage II	GTN extends to the adnexa or to the vagina but is limited to the genital structures (adnexa, vagina, and broad ligament)
Stage III	GTN extends to the lungs with or without genital tract involvement
Stage IV	All other metastatic sites

treated with single-agent chemotherapy. FIGO stage IV and risk score ≥7 are treated with multiagent chemotherapy. The response to single-agent chemotherapy in patients with risk score of 5 and 6 and with pathological diagnosis of CC is poor, but still can achieve 40–50% and can avoid the toxicity of multiagent chemotherapy. In these group of patients, there is a low threshold for multiagent chemotherapy and if there is poor response to single agent, patient should be started on multiagent chemotherapy. Risk score of ≥13 is grouped as ultrahigh risk with induction chemotherapy using etoposide and cisplatin before starting multiagent chemotherapy to avoid early death due sudden tumor collapse with severe bleeding and sepsis with multiorgan failure.

Gestational trophoblastic neoplasia is managed as per the staging and risk score adopted by FIGO in 2002.[30] Stages I, II, and III with risk score of ≤6 are low-risk GTN and are treated with single-agent chemotherapy. Stage IV and patients with risk score of ≥7 in stages I, II, and III are treated with multiagent chemotherapy. It is noticed that patients with risk score of 5 and 6 may not respond well with single-agent therapy. However, such cases showing resistance to single-agent therapy can achieve remission with multiagent chemotherapy. So it may be safe to start with single agent chemotherapy to patients with risk score of 5 and 6, and those showing resistance can be switched over to multiagent chemotherapy. This strategy will avoid the toxic effect of multiagent therapy to all patients of this group as many of them will respond to single-agent therapy and those who develop resistance can be managed by multiagent chemotherapy to achieve complete remission.

METASTATIC WORK-UP FOR STAGING AND RISK SCORE

Once GTN is diagnosed, metastatic work-up for staging and risk score is done. Chest X-ray/computed tomography (CT) of chest is done to diagnose lung metastasis, including the number and size of the lesion. Pelvic ultrasonography is to be done to diagnose lesions on the uterus, and hepatic and other intraabdominal involvement. GTN following molar pregnancy need not have further evaluation if there is no pulmonary secondaries. If there is evidence of pulmonary secondaries, and inpatients developing GTN following delivery or abortion should have CT of chest, magnetic resonance imaging (MRI) of brain, and pelvic ultrasonography and CT of the abdomen. Serum hCG measurement is also necessary for calculating the risk score. Additional imaging techniques—8-flurodeoxyglucose positron emission tomography (FDG-PET)—may be useful to localize the metabolically active viable tumor so that surgical removal of the resistant mass is possible. The common metastatic sites are lung (80%), vagina 30%, brain (10%), and liver (10%).

FIGO Staging—GTN 2002[30] (Table 3)
FIGO Risk Factor Scoring[30]

Bagshawe introduced a prognostic risk scoring system in 1976,[31] which was modified and adopted by World Health Organization (WHO)[32] and is now accepted in the FIGO risk scoring system. From the WHO scoring, ABO blood group has been omitted and liver metastasis has been given the maximum score of 4. PSTT has been classed separately. There is no intermediate risk group.

FIGO Risk Factor Scoring System (Table 4)

Management of GTN depends on the stage and risk scoring
- Low-risk GTN:
  • Stages I, II, and III, risk score ≤6: Single-agent chemotherapy
- High-risk GTN:
  • Stages I, II, and III with risk score ≥7 and stage IV: Combination chemotherapy
- Ultra-high-risk GTN:
  • Induction therapy with etoposide and cisplatin followed by multiagent chemotherapy

TABLE 4: FIGO risk factor scoring system.

FIGO scoring	0	1	2	4
Age	<40	>40		
Antecedent pregnancy	Mole	Abortion	Term	
Months from index pregnancy	<4	4 ≤ 7	7 ≤ 13	≥13
Pretreatment serum hCG (IU/l)	<1,000	1,000 ≤ 10,000	10,000 ≤ 100,000	≥100,000
Largest tumor size (cm)	<3	3 ≤ 5	≥5	
Site of metastasis	Lung	Spleen and kidney	GIT	Liver and brain
Number of metastasis	–	1–4	5–8	>8
Previous failed chemotherapy	–	–	Single drug	Two or more drugs

(hCG: human chorionic gonadotropin; GIT: gastrointestinal tract)

LOW-RISK GESTATIONAL TROPHOBLASTIC NEOPLASIA

Low-risk patients are started on single-agent chemotherapy, either methotrexate or actinomycin-D. In our experience, methotrexate with folinic acid (MTX/FA) regimen is less toxic and gives >80% cure rate with risk score of 1–4. If there is resistance to MTX/FA regimen, they are given alternate single-agent therapy with 5-day course of actinomycin-D. Only 5% of our patients required multidrug therapy.[25]

Methotrexate

Methotrexate is almost 100% curative in the treatment of low-risk nonmetastatic GTD. It is in use since 1956. Before treatment, blood count, renal and liver functions should be checked before every course. Anemia and infection increase the risk of toxicity. Methotrexate should be withheld in women where renal or hepatic biochemistry is abnormal because these are the routes of metabolism and excretion. Response is assessed by hCG levels done biweekly. Women should be counseled about possible side effects including gut ulceration (resulting in vomiting and diarrhea), bone marrow suppression, alopecia, and skin photosensitivity.

Methotrexate–Folinic Acid Regimen

Folinic acid is used as a co-treatment with methotrexate to rescue normal tissues from the dihydrofolate reductase block of methotrexate. This allows a higher dose of methotrexate to be used with fewer toxic effects. The regimen was proposed by Bagshawe and Wilde.[33,34]

The regimen is to use methotrexate at a dose of 1 mg/kg to a maximum of 50 mg given intramuscular (IM) on days 1, 3, 5, and 7. Folinic acid in a dose of 0.1 mg/kg is given on days 2, 4, 6, and 8. The folinic acid dose should be given 30 hours after the methotrexate dose. The cycle is repeated every 15 days. If there is resistance to these drugs, the next agent is actinomycin-D. If the hCG levels are >100 IU/L, multidrug chemotherapy is indicated and has been to effect a cure in almost all patients.[35] After hCG level is negative, a further 2–3 cycles are given as a consolidation to prevent recurrences. The overall complete remission rate in low-risk disease is close to 100%.[36]

Other single-agent chemotherapy schedule for low-risk GTN is as follows:
- Methotrexate 0.4 mg/kg IM for 5 days repeated every 2 weeks. This uses a lower doses of methotrexate in a bid to reduce side effects, but 10% of low-risk cases may need further treatment.
- Methotrexate 50 mg/m^2 IM given weekly is a convenient regiment but failure rate is higher than the daily dose regimen.
- Actinomycin-D 9-12 µg/kg intravenous (IV) daily for 5 days, repeated every 2 weeks. Actinomycin causes severe slough if extravasated and must be injected via a new free running IV infusion. If any extravasation does occur, the area should be infiltrated with 100 mg hydrocortisone and 2 mL of 1% xylocaine.
- Actinomycin-D pulse: Actinomycin-D 1.25 mg/m^2 intravenously every 2 weeks.

In a series of 321 low-risk cases treated by the author's group, using Methotrexate–Folinic Acid Regimen regimen, complete remission could be achieved in 92% of cases. Remission could be achieved in 3% cases with alternating course of actinomycin-D and 3.6% required multiagent chemotherapy [methotrexate, actinomycin-D, and cyclophosphamide (MAC) and etoposide, methotrexate, actinomycin-D, cyclophosphamide and vincristine (EMA-CO)].[25]

In one controlled randomized trial, it was reported that pulsed actinomycin-D is superior to weekly methotrexate, (not with MTX/FA regimen).[37] The study from the New England Trophoblastic Disease Center showed that 8-day methotrexate/folinic acid remains the treatment of choice at low-risk GTN.[38]

HIGH-RISK GESTATIONAL TROPHOBLASTIC NEOPLASIA

High-risk GTN may present months or years after the antecedent pregnancy with no menstrual irregularities.

The clinical features are those related to the organ of metastasis. This could be neurological (headaches, seizures, and hemiparesis) or pulmonary (pleuritic chest pain, hemoptysis, and breathlessness). The diagnosis may be elusive unless this possibility is kept in mind. hCG measurement usually prompts further work-up. This should be accompanied by appropriate imaging studies of the central nervous system (CNS), chest, and abdomen to stage the disease and calculate the risk score.

Women who have a high-risk GTN (FIGO stages I, II, and III with FIGO score 7 or greater or stage IV) are treated with multiagent chemotherapy. This is accompanied by surgery or radiation. Until the 1980s, the regimen used was MAC and reported cure rates ranged from 63 to 71%.[39]

After the 1980s, the regimen was modified to include etoposide, which is a highly effective agent for GTN. Newlands et al. formulated the EMA-CO regimen employing etoposide, high-dose methotrexate with folinic acid, actinomycin-D, cyclophosphamide, and vincristine with a complete clinical response of 80%.[40]

EMA-CO Regimen for High-risk GTN (Table 5)

Though the risk of teratogenicity after treatment is low, patients are advised to avoid pregnancy for 12 months after chemotherapy is completed.

The high response rates, good long-term survival, and the minimal acute and cumulative toxicity associated with EMA-CO protocol make it the current initial treatment of choice for high-risk metastatic gestational trophoblastic tumor. Granulocyte colony stimulating factor (G-CSF) 300 µg subcutaneously may be given on days 9–14 of each subsequent treatment cycles in patients who develop neutropenia. Prolonged courses of more than six cycles are rarely associated with secondary malignancy such as leukemia. After achieving complete remission, three more courses are given for consolidation.

TABLE 5: EMA-CO Regimen for high-risk gestational trophoblastic neoplasia (GTN).

Day	Drug	Dose
1	Etoposide	100 mg/m² IV over 30 minutes
	Actinomycin-D	0.5 mg IV bolus
	Methotrexate	100 mg/m² bolus and 200 mg/m² IV infusion in 1,000 mL of 5% dextrose over 12 hours
2	Etoposide	100 mg/m² IV infusion over 30 minutes
	Actinomycin-D	0.5 mg IV bolus
	Folinic acid	15 mg IM every 12 hours, for four doses beginning 24 hours after start of methotrexate
8	Cyclophosphamide	600 mg/m² IV
	Vincristine	1 mg/m² IV bolus

Repeat cycles on every 2 weeks.

For women with incomplete remission, the EMA-EP (etoposide, methotrexate, actinomycin-D–etoposide, cisplatin) regimen, substituting etoposide and cisplatin for cyclophosphamide and vincristine in the EMA-CO regimen, seems to be the most appropriate therapy. The BEP (bleomycin, etoposide, cisplatin) VIP (etoposide, ifosfamide, cisplatin), and ICE (ifosfamide, carboplatin, etoposide) protocols were also successful in patients who failed to respond to EMA-CO regimen. Several patients with drug-resistant tumor reported to have responded to gemcitabine or paclitaxel-based single-agent or combination therapy. An alternating combination of paclitaxel-cisplatin and paclitaxel-etoposide (TP-TE) every 2 weeks seems to be much better tolerated than is EMA-EP, and is effective in patients with relapsed or refractory neoplasia.

When CNS metastasis is present, whole brain irradiation (3000 cGy in 200 cGy fractions) is given simultaneously with initiation of chemotherapy. Brain irradiation has the dual purpose of being both tumoricidal and hemostatic. During radiotherapy, the methotrexate infusion dose in the EMA-CO protocol is increased to 1 g/m² and 30 mg folinic acid is given every 12 hour for 3 days, starting 32 hours after the infusion begins. As an alternative to brain irradiation, the Charring Cross Hospital Group recommended intrathecal as well as high dose IV methotrexate.

Liver metastases from CC are ominous as they tend to be associated with extensive disease at multiple sites. There is a significant risk of serious hepatic bleeding, especially during the first course of chemotherapy. Whole-liver irradiation with 2000 cGy over 2 weeks combined with chemotherapy is recommended to reduce the risk of bleeding.

Intensive multi-modality therapy with appropriate combination chemotherapy, adjuvant radiotherapy, and surgery has resulted in cure rates of 80–90% in patients with high-risk metastatic gestational trophoblastic tumor.

ULTRA-HIGH RISK GESTATIONAL TROPHOBLASTIC NEOPLASIA

Among the high-risk group defined by FIGO, patients with risk score of ≥13 are grouped as ultra-high-risk GTN. In these patients, starting with full-dose combination therapy will lead to tumor collapse with severe bleeding, metabolic acidosis, myelosuppression, septicemia, and multiorgan failure and can lead to early death.[1] To avoid this, start with gentle, induction therapy with etoposide 100 mg/m² and cisplatin 20 mg/m² on days 1 and 2 repeated weekly for 2–3 weeks before starting the full multiagent therapy. This will help to reduce such early deaths in ultra-high-risk cases.

Role of Surgery in the Management of Trophoblastic Disease

Surgery has an important role in the management of GTD. Molar pregnancies should be evacuated by suction curettage and medical methods are best avoided. Hysterectomy may be considered as part of primary treatment if other gynecological morbidity is present or the woman is above 35 years of age and do not want to conceive again. Additional surgical procedures, especially hysterectomy and thoracotomy, are of use in removing known foci of chemotherapy-resistant cases with persistent or recurrent high-risk metastatic disease. Prompt hCG regression within 1 or 2 weeks of surgical resection indicates a favorable outcome. In women with excessive vaginal bleeding, arterial embolization should be considered if maintenance of fertility is desirous. Hysterectomy may be required for the management of excessive uterine bleeding either at presentation or after the onset of chemotherapy and in the management of chemotherapy resistant disease localized in the uterus. Hysterectomy is the treatment of choice for the management of stage I PSTT. In cases of intraperitoneal bleeding due to perforation of the uterus by IM, resection and closure or even hysterectomy may be required.

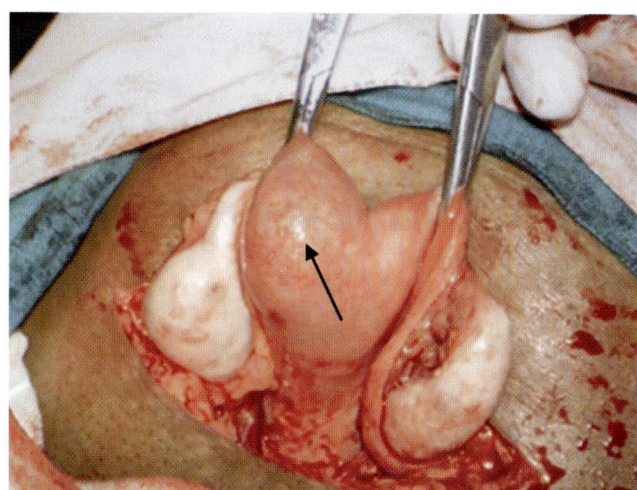

Fig. 19: Appearance of the uterus at hysterectomy of a 28-year-old lady who was diagnosed with PSTT in the curettage specimen

Follow-up after Treatment

The risk of relapse after treatment is about 3% and occurs within 1 year and careful clinical hCG follow-up is necessary during this period. Patients are advised to avoid pregnancy and to use contraception. Present day low-dose COC is safe to use. However, patients who conceive during this period can be assured a normal outcome, risk similar to the general population.[41]

After chemotherapy, hCG monitoring is done weekly for 6 weeks, once in 2 weeks for 6 months and then urine for hCG every month till 1 year. Follow-up can be continued for 5 years/lifelong with urine hCG once in 6 months. If the patient conceives, follow-up is stopped and hCG is checked 6 and 10 weeks after delivery. Elderly patients who want to conceive should be advised to attempt pregnancy after 1 year, especially if they were treated by EMA-CO, as they are at the risk of early menopause.

PLACENTAL SITE TROPHOBLASTIC TUMOR AND EPITHELIOID TROPHOBLASTIC TUMOR

Placental site trophoblastic tumor and ETTs are slow growing tumors and can present many years after term delivery, nonmolar abortion, or complete mole. They are primarily treated with surgery as they are less sensitive to chemotherapy. They may present as AUB and pregnancy test may be positive and diagnosis is possible with curettage. In PSST confined to uterus hysterectomy with pelvic and abdominal lymph node, sampling is the choice of treatment in stage I disease **(Figs. 19 and 20)**.

Metastatic disease and those seen after 4 years of the antecedent pregnancy are having poor prognosis and will require combination chemotherapy, preferably EMA-EP regimen. Residual tumor needs removal along with hysterectomy. ETTs are managed same way as PSTTs.

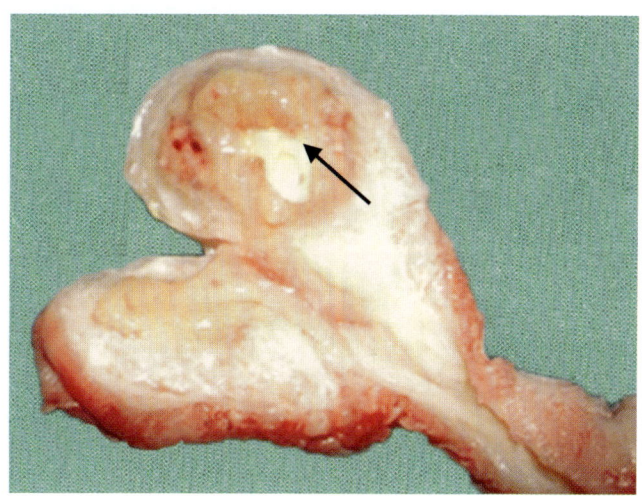

Fig. 20: Section of the uterus showing tumor in the myometrium (PSTT). Necrosis is present, hemorrhage is less.
(*Courtesy:* Dr Prasannakumari, MD)

PREGNANCY FOLLOWING GESTATIONAL TROPHOBLASTIC DISEASE

Patients who had GTD may be assured that they may expect a normal reproductive outcome. However, patients are advised not to become pregnant until 12 months after completion of chemotherapy to reduce the potential for teratogenicity. Patients who have had a prior molar pregnancy are at an increased risk of developing recurrent molar pregnancy, the reported risk being 1%. Risk of congenital anomalies is not increased by chemotherapy for GTN. An increased risk of placenta accrete was reported by some authors. All patients should have an ultrasound at 8–10 weeks in the subsequent pregnancy to rule out molar changes.

In our own series, out of the 262 pregnancies following hydatidiform mole, 224 had full term normal delivery, 17 had cesarean section, 16 ended in abortion and 2 developed ectopic pregnancy and 3 patients developed recurrent mole.[25]

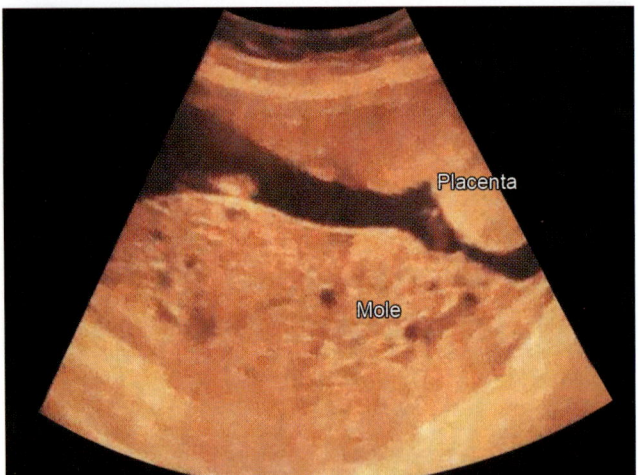

Fig. 21: 3D-Ultrasound showing molar tissue and normal placenta in a case of twin with one *mole*.

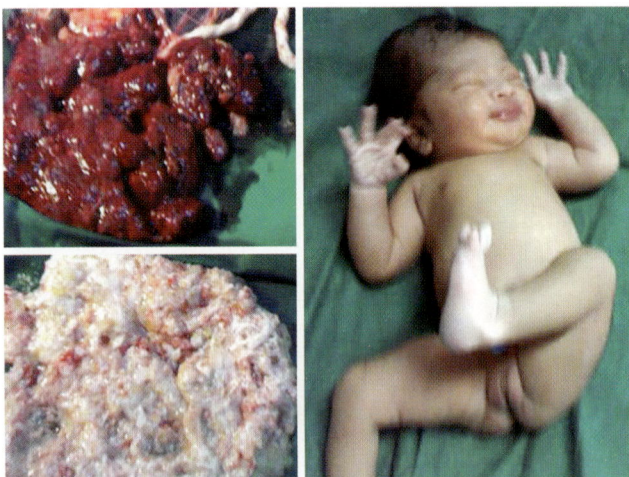

Fig. 22: Outcome of twin pregnancy with one CHM and other normal fetus (46XX) and placenta.

TWIN PREGNANCY WITH ONE MOLE AND COEXISTING NORMAL FETUS

This is a rare condition estimated to be 1 per 22,000–100,000 pregnancies.[42] Though complications such as bleeding, pre-eclampsia, need for operative interventions, and risk of malignancy are more, in 40–50% of cases, it is possible to have a normal baby. Careful repeated sonographic evaluation, especially by 3D ultrasound, will show that the molar tissue is separate from the normal placenta amniotic sac and normal appearing fetus **(Fig. 21)**. The couple should be counseled properly and if it is a wanted pregnancy, may be allowed to continue after confirming the normalcy of the fetus. The partial mole is triploidy and the baby will have abnormalities. Amniocentesis and karyotyping will make sure that the baby is normal. Careful monitoring for development pre-eclampsia, and frequent sonographic evaluation of fetal well-being has to be done **(Fig. 22)**. The good prognostic points are hCG level remaining static, the molar tissue getting regressed, and absence of any bleeding.

FALSE POSITIVE HUMAN CHORIONIC GONADOTROPIN

False positive or "phantom hCG" is now recognized as a problem where patients are treated inappropriately by curettage, laparoscopy, single-agent and multiagent chemotherapy, and even hysterectomy assuming they have trophoblastic tumor. These false positive tests are due to heterophilic antibodies in the blood mimicking hCG during assay. This is due to the presence of heterophilic antibodies in circulation. To differentiate, check urine for hCG which will be negative as heterophilic antibodies will not appear in urine. Serum by serial dilution should show the proportionate value of hCG.

QUIESCENT GESTATIONAL TROPHOBLASTIC DISEASE

While on treatment of GTN, some cases will show no response to treatment with persistent low levels of real hCG. The disease has gone into an inactive phase or quiescent state with no response to treatment, as the chemotherapy will be effective only on dividing cells. The importance is that such cases can remain on the quiescent phase for months or even for years, and it is important to keep the patient on hCG and clinical surveillance till it becomes active, evidenced by rise in hCG. In such cases, it is the hCG-H that will start rising and test kit that picks up hCG-H should be used. In this active phase, start chemotherapy, which will be effective.

CONCLUSION

Early detection by systematic follow-up is the main determinant of the outcome of GTD. In Western countries, centralized national referral centers have resulted in very high cure rates. We do not have such a well-structured program in developing countries, including ours. The follow-up is subject to the knowledge and enthusiasm of the practicing physician. Some degree of organization is seen at regional tertiary care centers and teaching hospitals with the establishment of follow-up clinics and disease registry. We at Calicut in the northern region of Kerala in South India have started such a center 25 years back and so far, have followed up >2,500 cases with excellent results. GTN is the most curable of all cancers if diagnosed and treated early, most often with preservation of fertility.

REFERENCES

1. Ngan HYS, Seckl MJ, Berkowitz RS, Xiang Y, Golfier F, Sekharan PK, et al. Update on the diagnosis and management of gestational trophoblastic disease. Int J Gynecol Obstet. 2018;143(9):79-85.
2. Ober WB, Fass RO. The early history of choriocarcinoma. J Hist Med Allied Sci. 1961;16:49-73.
3. Goldstein DP. Gestational trophoblastic neoplasia in the 1990s. Yale J Biol Med. 1991;64(6):639-51.

4. Szulman AE, Surti U. The syndromes of hydatidiform mole. I. Cytogenetic and morphologic correlations. Am J Obstet Gynecol. 1978;131(6):665-71.
5. Szulman AE, Surti U. The syndromes of hydatidiform mole. II. Morphologic evolution of the complete and partial mole. Am J Obstet Gynecol. 1978;132(1):20-7.
6. Wake N, Fujino T, Hoshi S, Shinkai N, Sakai K, Kato H, et al. The propensity to malignancy of dispermic heterozygous moles. Placenta. 1987;8(3):319-26.
7. Moglabey YB, Kircheisen R, Seoud M, El Mogharbel N, Van den Veyver I, Slim R. Genetic mapping of a maternal locus responsible for familial hydatidiform moles. Hum Mol Genet. 1999;8(4):667-71.
8. Seckl MJ, Sebire NJ, Berkowitz RS. Gestational trophoblastic disease. Lancet. 2010 Aug 28;376(9742):717-29.
9. Sebire NJ, Foskett M, Fisher RA, Rees H, Seckl M, Newlands E. Risk of partial and complete hydatidiform molar pregnancy in relation to maternal age. BJOG. 2002;109(1):99-102.
10. Seckl MJ, Fisher RA, Newlands ES, Salerno G, Rees H, Paradinas FJ, et al. Choriocarcinoma and partial hydatidiform mole. Lancet. 2000;356(9223):36-9.
11. Szulman AE, Surti U, Berman M. (1978) Patient with partial mole requiring chemotherapy. Lancet. 1978;312(8099):1099.
12. Samadder A, Kar R. Utility of p57 immunohistochemistry in differentiating between complete mole, partial mole & non-molar or hydropic abortus. Indian J Med Res. 2017;145(1):133-7.
13. Borah T, Raphael V, Panda S, Saharia P. Ectopic molar pregnancy: A rare entity. J Reprod Infertil. 2010;11(3):201-3.
14. Scully R, Young R. Trophoblastic pseudotumour: A reappraisal. Am J Surg Pathol. 1981;5(1):75-6.
15. Vardar MA, Altintas A. Placental-site trophoblastic tumor. Principles of diagnosis, clinical behaviour and treatment. Eur J Gynaecol Oncol. 1995;16(4):290-5.
16. Hancock BW, Seckl MJ. Placental site and epithelioid trophoblastic tumours. In: Hancock BW, Seckl MJ, Berkowitz RS. Gestational Trophoblastic Disease, 4th edition. 2015
17. Palmer JE, Macdonald M, Wells M, Hancock BW, Tidy JA. Epithelioid trophoblastic tumor: a review of the literature. J Reprod Med. 2008;53(7):465-75.
18. Cole LA, Dai D, Butler SA, Leslie KK, Kohorn EI. (2006) Gestational trophoblastic diseases: 1. Pathophysiology of hyperglycosylated hCG. Gynecol Oncol. 2006;102(2):145-50.
19. Cole LA. Human chorionic gonadotropin tests. Expert Rev Mol Diagn. 2009;9(7):721-47.
20. Fowler DJ, Lindsay I, Seckl MJ, Sebire NJ. Routine pre-evacuation ultrasound diagnosis of hydatidiform mole: experience of more than 1000 cases from a regional referral center, Ultrasound Obstet Gynecol. 2006;27(1):56-60.
21. Fisher RA, Hodges MD, Rees HC, Sebire NJ, Seckl MJ, Newlands ES, et al. The maternally transcribed gene p57(KIP2) (CDNK1C) is abnormally expressed in both androgenetic and biparental complete hydatidiform moles. Hum Mol Genet. 2002;11(26):3267-72.
22. Tidy J, Seckl M, Hancock BW, on behalf of the Royal College of Obstetricians and Gynaecologists. Management of gestational trophoblastic disease. BJOG. 2021;128(3):e1-27.
23. Lurain JR. Gestational trophoblastic disease I: epidemiology, pathology, clinical presentation and diagnosis of gestational trophoblastic disease, and management of hydatidiform mole. Am J Obstet Gynecol. 2010;203(6):531-9.
24. Kim O, Moon I, Kim KT, Moon YJ, Hwang YY. Effects of prophylactic chemotherapy for persistent trophoblastic disease in patients with complete hydatidiform mole. Obstet Gynecol. 1986;67(5):690-4.
25. Sekharan PK, Sreedevi NS, Beegam R, Radhadevi VP, Raghavan J, Beena G. Management of postmolar gestational trophoblastic diseases with methotrexate and folinic acid: 15 years of experience. J Reprod Med. 2006;51(10):835-40.
26. Coyle C, Short D, Jackson L, Sebire NJ, Kaur B, Harvey R, et al. What is the optimal duration of human chorionic gonadotrophin surveillance following evacuation of a molar pregnancy? A retrospective analysis on over 20,000 consecutive patients. Gynecol Oncol. 2018;148(2):254-7.
27. Berkowitz RS, Goldstien DP, Marean AR, Bernstein M. Oral contraceptives and postmolar trophoblastic disease. Obstet Gynecol. 1981;58(4):474-7.
28. Bagshawe KD. Trophoblastic neoplasia. In: Holland JF, Bast Jr R, et al. (eds). Cancer Medicine, 3rd edition. Baltimore: Williams & Wilkins; 1993. pp. 169-968.
29. Lurain JR, Brewer JI, Torok FE, Halpern B. Natural history of hydatidiform mole after primary evacuation. Am J Obstet Gynecol. 1983;145(5):591-5.
30. Ngan HY. The FIGO staging for gestational trophoblastic neoplasia 2000, FIGO Committee Report. Int J Gynecol Obstet. 2002;77(3):285-7.
31. Bagshawe KD. Risk and prognostic factors in trophoblastic neoplasia. Cancer. 1976;38(3):1373-85.
32. WHO. Scientific Group: Gestational trophoblastic diseases Technical report series no. 692. Geneva, Switzerland: World Health Organization; 1983.
33. Bagshawe KD, Dent J, Newlands ES, Begent RH, Rustin GJ. (1989). The role of low dose methotrexate and folinic acid in gestational trophoblastic tumour. Br J Obstet Gynecol. 1989;96(7):795-802.
34. Berkowitz RS, Goldstein DP, Bernstein MR. Ten years' experience with methotrexate and Folinic acid as primary therapy for gestational trophoblastic disease, Gynecol Oncol. 1986;23(1):111-8.
35. Mangili G, Lorusso D, Brown J, Pfisterer J, Massuger L, Vaughan M, et al. Trophoblastic disease review for diagnosis and management. Int J Gynecol Cancer. 2014;24(9 Suppl 3):S109-16.
36. Lurain JR. Gestational trophoblastic disease II: Classification and management of gestational trophoblastic neoplasia. Am J Obstet Gynecol. 2011;204(1):11-8.
37. Osborne RJ, Filiaci V, Schink JC, Mannel RS, Secord AA, Kelley JL, et al. Phase III trial of weekly methotrexate or pulsed dactinomycin for low-risk gestational trophoblastic neoplasia: a gynecologic oncology group study. J Clin Oncol. 2011;29(7):825-31.
38. Maesta I, Nitecki R, Horowitz NS, Goldstein DP, de Freitas Segalla Moreira M, Elias KM, et al. Effectiveness and toxicity of first-line methotrexate chemotherapy in low-risk postmolar gestational trophoblastic neoplasia. the New England Trophoblastic Disease Center experience. Gynecol Oncol. 2018;148(1):161-7.
39. Lurain JR, Brewer JI. Treatment of high-risk gestational trophoblastic disease with methotrexate, actinimycin D and cyclophosphamice chemotherapy. Obstet Gynecol. 1985;65(6):830-6.
40. Newlands ES, Bagshawe KD, Begent RH, Rustin GJ, Holden L. Results with the EMA/CO (etoposide, methotrexate,

actinomycin D, cyclophosphamide, vincristine) regimen in high risk gestational trophoblastic tumours, 1979 to 1989. Br J Obstet Gynaecol. 1991;98(6):550-7.
41. Williams J, Short D, Dayal L, Strickland S, Harvey R, Tin T, et al. Effect of early pregnancy following chemotherapy on disease relapse and fetal outcome in women treated for gestational trophoblastic neoplasia. J Reprod Med. 2014;59(5-6):248-54.
42. Newlands ES. Twin gestation comprising mole in Concert with normal fetus: Test, Treat, Abort or let go to term. For the study of Trophoblastic Disease. J Int Soc. 1999;3.

LONG QUESTIONS

1. Primary management of hydatidiform mole.
2. Follow-up after molar pregnancy and diagnosis of gestational trophoblastic neoplasia (GTN).
3. How will you manage a case of low-risk gestational trophoblastic neoplasia (GTN)?
4. Discuss the management options for a resistant case of gestational trophoblastic neoplasia (GTN).

SHORT QUESTIONS

1. Write briefly on invasive mole.
2. Diagnosis and management of placental site trophoblastic disease human chorionic gonadotropin and its role in gestational trophoblastic disease (GTD).
3. Biparental mole.
4. Write briefly on ultra-high risk gestational trophoblastic neoplasia (GTN).
5. What are the pros and cons of chemoprophylaxis in hydatidiform mole?
6. Write a brief note on pregnancy after gestational trophoblastic disease (GTD).

MULTIPLE CHOICE QUESTIONS

1. The chromosomal pattern of a complete hydatidiform mole can be:
   a. 46XX
   b. 46XY
   c. Either of the above
   d. Neither of the above
2. The chromosomal pattern of a partial hydatidiform mole can be:
   a. 46XX
   b. 69XXX
   c. Either of the above
   d. Neither of the above
3. The following statement is true about pathogenesis of hydatidiform mole:
   a. There is an excess of paternal chromosomes.
   b. There is an excess of maternal genes.
   c. There is no role for genomic imprinting.
   d. Dispermy is universally present.
4. The following statement about the normal trophoblast is false:
   a. Trophoblast is derived from the outer cell mass of the pre-implantation embryo.
   b. Cytotrophoblast is the stem cell from which the syncytiotrophoblast is formed.
   c. Inhibin-A is produced by syncytiotrophoblast.
   d. Human placental lactogen (hPL) and placental alkaline phosphatase (PLAP) levels decrease as term advances.
5. The following epidemiological risk factor increases the risk of GTD:
   a. Maternal age of 25 years
   b. Alcohol consumption
   c. History of molar pregnancy
   d. Previous cesarean birth
6. The following statement about partial hydatidiform mole is false:
   a. Karyotype is triploid
   b. Fetal tissue is never seen
   c. Theca lutein cysts are seen rarely
   d. Malignant sequelae are seen in <5% of women
7. The following statement about gestational choriocarcinoma is not true:
   a. It occurs only after a complete hydatidiform mole
   b. Chorionic villi are abundantly seen
   c. Necrosis and hemorrhage is rare
   d. Widespread intravascular dissemination to lungs, brain, and other sites is common
8. The following are known clinical associations of GTD, except:
   a. Hyperemesis
   b. Small for dates uterus
   c. Pre-eclampsia
   d. Early pregnancy bleeding
9. Regarding the evacuation of hydatidiform mole all are wrong, expect:
   a. Medical abortion using prostaglandins
   b. The method of evacuation is by hysterotomy when size is >20 weeks
   c. Patients who are Rh negative should receive Rh immunoglobulin
   d. Hysterectomy eliminates the risk of choriocarcinoma

Answers
1. c 2. c 3. b 4. a 5. d 6. c
7. b 8. d 9. b

4.4 PREGNANCY AFTER PREVIOUS FETAL LOSS

Sudha Gandhi, Savitri Verma

INTRODUCTION

Pregnancy loss (fetal death) is a tragedy which causes severe emotional distress to parents and brings about a feeling of failure to their obstetrician. Pregnancy loss may be the final common symptom of multiple pathological phenomena which may require a diagnosis. A clinical approach to determine the possible etiology will permit specific treatment and improve the outcome of future pregnancy. This chapter discusses the various investigations required to establish the cause of late fetal death after 20 weeks of gestation and outlines strategies to a successful outcome in subsequent pregnancy.

DEFINITION AND INCIDENCE

World Health Organization (WHO) recommended definition of stillborn (SB) is a baby born with no sign of life at or after 28 weeks. Many countries differ in opinion regarding gestational age for defining SB for legislative and statistical purpose. In the United States, it refers to death beyond 20 weeks, while in England, it refers to death after 24 weeks. Hence, the incidence also varies. In India [Ministry of Health and Family Welfare, Government of India (MoHFW)], late fetal death is defined as a fetal death weighing at least 1,000 g (or a gestational age of 28 completed weeks or a crown-heel length of 35 cm or more).

Stillbirth has been defined as complete expulsion or extraction of a baby from its mother where the fetus does not breathe or show any evidence of life such as beating of heart, crying, or movement of limbs.

In India, at least 6 lakh stillbirth occur every year. As per the Lancet (2011), the current stillbirth rate is 22/1,000 of total births. India also considers <28 weeks of gestation fetus es not viable; however, the reporting for stillbirths is done for 20 weeks onward.

ETIOLOGY

Discerning the cause of stillbirth is a challenge. Many causes overlap with the first trimester, but there are specific causes for late pregnancy loss. A number of risk factors directly and or indirectly are associated with stillbirth. With proper history and examination of mother and fetus and relevant investigations cause can be ascertained in two-third of the cases. Known causes of stillbirth fall into the following broad categories:

Maternal

- Anatomical causes
- Hypertensive disorders of pregnancy
- Diabetes
- Asthma
- Systemic lupus erythematosus (SLE)
- Renal disease
- Inherited/acquired thrombophilias
- Cholestasis of pregnancy
- Trauma
- Smoking, alcohol, and illicit drug use
- Infections:
  - Malaria
  - Syphilis
  - Parvovirus B19
  - Listeria
  - Brucellosis
  - HIV (human immunodeficiency virus)
  - Toxoplasmosis
  - Cytomegalovirus (CMV)
  - Rubella
  - Hepatitis B
  - Varicella
  - Mycoplasma and ureaplasma.

Fetal

- Rh negative
- Nonimmune hydrops fetalis (NIHF)
- Premature rupture of the fetal membrane (PROM) and chorioamnionitis
- Multiple gestations
- Intrauterine growth restriction (IUGR)
- Chromosomal anomalies and genetic diseases
- Congenital malformations.

Placenta and Cord

- Accidents (cord prolapse)
- Abruption
- Placenta previa, accreta, and circumvallate placenta
- Infarction
- Tight knot in cord and abnormal umbilical cord coiling.

Intranatal

- Birth asphyxia due to malpresentations such as breech, shoulder dystocia, and prolonged or obstructed labor
- Maternal shock or injudicious use of analgesic drugs may interfere with establishment of normal breathing pattern of the baby by depressing the respiratory center of the deaths when it is needed the most.

Unidentified

In a significant number of cases, the cause of fetal death remains unexplained in spite of extensive investigations.

RISK ASSESSMENT

There are many contributory factors which may or may not be modifiable which are as follows:
- Primipara and elderly gravidas have more chances of unexplained SB even without any known medical disorder.
- Obesity [body mass index (BMI) >30], advanced maternal age, and social deprivation may cause unexplained stillbirth.
- Assisted reproductive technology (ART) pregnancy and pregnancy in subfertile couples even if conceived without treatment have a higher chance of unexplained SB. These couples should be counseled regarding increased need for maternal and fetal monitoring which will require frequent visits to the healthcare facility.
- Presence of chronic medical disorders.

EVALUATION OF FETAL DEATH

Once a fetal death is identified, every possible effort should be taken to ascertain the etiology, so that the outcome of next pregnancy can be optimized. A detailed history should be undertaken and medical records should be reviewed to identify the possible cause. All events surrounding the fetal death must be clearly recorded in chronological order. When performing an evaluation, it is important to be systematic and not confuse association with casualty. Kortweg et al. analyzed laboratory studies obtained in the evaluation of 1,025 fetal deaths in Netherlands from 2002 to 2008. The most useful tests were placental examination, fetal autopsy, and fetal karyotyping, which added in assigning the cause of death in 96, 73, and 29% of cases, respectively. Systematic approach should include maternal and fetal evaluation.

MATERNAL EVALUATION

- Postmaturity and fetal growth restriction (FGR) should be ruled out by dating scans.
- Enquiry should be made about specific complaints such as fever, rash, hypertension, diabetes mellitus/gestational diabetes mellitus (GDM), prelabor rupture of membranes, vaginal bleeding, or genital tract infection.
- Standard maternal hematological tests, coagulation time, random blood glucose, thyroid function, serology and bacteriology, autoimmune disorders screening, urine for occult drug use to be requested, based on history, and examination. Any abnormal antenatal test results, medical records of any pre-existing disease should be obtained and noted. The list of investigations with their applicability is listed in **Table 1**.

TABLE 1: Maternal evaluation for late pregnancy loss.

Maternal evaluation at time of demise	• Complete blood count
	• Syphilis
	• Thyroid stimulating hormone
	• *Fetal-maternal hemorrhage screen:* Kleihauer test or comparable test for fetal cells in maternal circulation
	• Anti-red cell antibodies
	• Human parvovirus 8-19 immunoglobulin C and immunoglobulin M antibody
	• Lupus anti-coagulant
	• Anticardiolipin antibodies
	• *Thrombophilia (selected cases only):*
	  – Factor V-Leiden
	  – Prothrombin gene mutation
	  – Antithrombin II
	  – Fasting homocysteine
		• Routine testing for thrombophilia is controversial and may lead to unnecessary interventions
		• Consider in cases with severe placental pathology and a growth restriction, or in the setting of a personal or family history of thromboembolic disease

Postpartum	• Protein S and protein C activity (selected cases) • Parental karyotype (if appropriate)	
In selected cases	• Indirect Coombs test • Glucose screening [oral glucose tolerance test and hemoglobin A1c (HbA1c)] • Toxicology screen	• If not performed previously in pregnancy • In the large for gestational age baby • In case of placental abruption or when drug use is suspected
Unproven benefit	• Antinuclear antibody test • Serology for toxoplasmosis, rubella, cytomegalovirus, and herpes simplex virus	• Many times in an incidental finding and may lead to unnecessary interventions • Rarely helpful, infection causing death is made by history and examining the baby, placenta, and cord
Developing technology	• Comparative genomic hybridization • Testing for single-gene mutations • Testing for confined placental mechanisms and needle acid- based testing for infection	The value of these has not yet been established

- Family history of genetic, chromosomal, and congenital anomalies in both parents and any siblings should be elicited.
- Amniocentesis, if it has been done during the antenatal period, can yield a diagnosis in up to 80% cases.

When planning the mode of delivery for stillbirth, both partners should be sensitized for further evaluations such as fetal autopsy.

FETAL AUTOPSY

Once patient has delivered, a detailed examination of the stillborn should be performed with description of normal features and any obvious abnormality. Fetal autopsy and study of placenta and cord by a perinatal pathologist are most helpful. Consent should be taken for postmortem and the parents must be explained that this might be helpful for a better future pregnancy outcome. If the parents do not agree, photographs, X-rays, and magnetic resonance imaging (MRI) can also be helpful. A full postmortem examination should include fetal chromosome culture with or without DNA analysis along with gross microbiological and histological examination of fetus and placenta.

Some common postmortem findings include:
- Fetal abnormality
- Evidence of fetal infection in form of hepatosplenomegaly
- Fetal hypoxic injury
- Placental dysfunction, infection, or infarction
- Tumors
- *Genetic abnormalities*: Deletion of ≥1 megabyte (MB) and duplication of 2 MB or more may be considered as associated with fetal loss.

Fetal evaluation in late pregnancy loss is summarized in **Table 2**. Parents are advised for a post-natal follow-up at the time of discharge.

TABLE 2: Fetal evaluation for late pregnancy loss.

Key components	Details
Fetal autopsy	If patient declines external evaluation by a trained perinatal pathologist. Other options include photographs, X-ray imaging, ultrasound, magnetic resonance imaging, and sampling of tissues, such as blood or skin.
Fetal genetics	Amniocentesis before delivery provides the greatest yield (84%). Umbilical cord proximal to placenta if no amniocentesis or chorionic villus sampling (CVS) (30%). Fluorescence in situ hybridization may be useful if fetal cells cannot be cultured.
Placental examination	Includes evaluation for signs of viral or bacterial infection. Discuss available tests with pathologists. New technology for DNA sequencing may be useful.

POSTNATAL FOLLOW-UP

A postnatal visit is planned when all the results of investigations are available, while discussing postnatal results with the parents, it is important to explain the difference between specific cause for intrauterine fetal death (IUFD), any contributory factors and coincidental findings, as this will affect the recurrence risk estimate and care to be planned in subsequent pregnancies. Parents should be given time to discuss their concerns, feelings, and expectations. Parents and particularly mothers should be assured that there was very likely nothing that they could have done to change the outcome unless there is a compelling evidence contrary (for example, drug abuse causing placental abruption and fetal demise).

Normal bereavements usually resolve within 6–12 months. Adequate health support is associated with lower levels of depression and anxiety but family support is most important. Grief is pathological when there is prolonged response usually longer than 6 months and if it interferes with daily activities. Patient characteristics that affected the intensity of grief were advanced gestational age at the time of fetal loss, lack of children in home, older age, preloss neurotic personality, and preloss psychiatric symptoms.

There is no specific time to plan for future pregnancy. Couples should be advised to try for the next conception, when they feel emotionally capable of undertaking it.

Acknowledge that a future pregnancy is likely to be stressful, but emphasize that there will be support to ensure the couple's and baby's health.

PREPREGNANCY MANAGEMENT STRATEGIES

History of previous unexplained fetal death confers a two- to tenfold risk of repeat fetal death. Such high risk women will therefore need specialist care and close supervision in subsequent pregnancies. The therapeutic approach should be specific to diagnosis. The risk of recurrence in a specific patient is related to the underlying pathophysiologic cause of the initial IUFD, and how that cause was addressed. For example, a patient who experienced an IUFD believed to be the result of uncontrolled diabetes can expect to have an improved outcome if her diabetes is brought under control before conceiving and she maintains control throughout the pregnancy. On the contrary, a patient who experienced an IUFD that was believed to be secondary to a nonmodifiable risk factor, such as lupus-induced chronic kidney disease, will continue to have a significant risk of recurrence of IUFD in the subsequent pregnancy.

It is important, as with any pregnancy, to optimize the woman's health prior to a pregnancy.

This can be targeted around addressing the key modifiable risk factors.

General Measures

- Obese patients should be motivated to obtain an optimum BMI for a better pregnancy outcome.
- Smoking (active and passive) and the use of illicit drugs should be discouraged.
- Women susceptible to rubella, varicella, and hepatitis B should be vaccinated.
- Folic acid supplementation can be started to reduce the risk of neural tube defects. Vitamin D supplements can also be added.

Specific Measures

- Anatomical causes can be diagnosed with three-dimensional (3D) ultrasonography (USG) or salpingography in pre pregnancy period. They usually lead to a preterm delivery of a nonviable fetus. Correction of a particular defect such as septate uterus can be done but literature does not support prophylactic resection in the absence of previous miscarriage.
- If a woman is diagnosed with a treatable condition that may have contributed to her previous stillbirth, e.g., diabetes, hypertension, thyroid disease or chronic renal disease, this disorder must first be optimized. Achieving good glycemic control in diabetic mothers is crucial during the period of organogenesis to prevent malformations.
- Most infections are acute, but it is still important to exclude and treat chronic infections such as urinary tract infections and malaria prophylaxis in endemic areas.
- Genetic testing and counseling can be advised if there is evidence of fetal chromosomal abnormalities, fetal structural malformations, or suspicion of genetic disorder. Genetic counseling should be done by an expert geneticist to discuss chances of recurrence of a specific trait and future reproductive options such as prenatal genetic screening, donor gamete, and even adoption.

MANAGEMENT IN SUBSEQUENT PREGNANCY

- Antenatal protocols to be followed which include dating scan, screening for trisomies, anomaly scan, oral glucose tolerance test (OGTT), and fetal growth monitoring.
- Daily administration of low-dose aspirin (75–150 mg) in pregnancy is now considered safe and is accepted as a preventive measure for prevention of preeclampsia and related fetal death.
- When the diagnosis is a specific autoimmune disease such as SLE or antiphospholipid antibody syndrome (APLA), there are standard guidelines based on literature for the treatment. Low-dose aspirin (75–200 mg) plus heparin unfractionated or low-molecular weight (LMW) (enoxaparin 1 mg per kg body weight or dalteparin 100 U/kg bodyweight subcutaneous) is an accepted regime. Postpartum anticoagulation should be continued with adjustments and gradual tapering off.
- Serial third trimester ultrasound with color Doppler in selective cases may identify poor fetal growth which may precede fetal death and also help in reassuring the parents.
- For intrapartum loss, pelvic assessment, vigilant fetal monitoring during labor, and a balanced decision regarding trial of labor are important. In the previous event of a difficult labor or instrumental delivery, lower segment cesarian section (LSCS) at 39 weeks is a justified option.
- Elective induction at term in subsequent pregnancies does not increase the live birth rate. However, many obstetricians offer elective delivery, frequently a cesarean after 37 weeks to allay parental anxiety and also to avoid the risk of sudden fetal death.

Intrauterine fetal death is associated with post-traumatic stress disorder (PTSD) and anxiety in subsequent pregnancies. Risk factors for PTSD and anxiety were conceived within 1 year of IUFD and a perceived lack of support at the time of loss. Physicians should be aware that there may be "false alarms" during the course of these pregnancies.

A balanced approach toward decision-making for future pregnancy based on facts and the patient's concern is important for a good outcome.

CONCLUSION

There is no universally accepted gestational age to define fetal death. Etiology can be determined in most cases by proper history taking, review of records, maternal investigation, and examination of fetus. The optimal approach for diagnosis is at the time of loss or before the next pregnancy so that a plan can be instituted in subsequent pregnancy for better outcome.

KEY MESSAGES

- Late pregnancy loss requires evaluation for better outcome in subsequent pregnancies.
- Common causes of pregnancy loss are medical disorder, infection, anatomical abnormalities, and genetic or abnormalities of placenta and cord.
- Examination of fetus and placenta after a stillbirth is important to ascertain the etiological factors.
- Prepregnancy strategies include optimization of weight, good glycemic control in diabetic patients, and normalization of medical disorders.
- When diagnosis is not certain for any specific disorder, management options are close monitoring of fetal growth and appropriate interventions according to fetal maturity.

FURTHER READING

1. ACOG. (2020). Management of Stillbirth Obstetric Care Consensus, No. 10. [online] Available from: https://www.acog.org/clinical/clinical-guidance/obstetric-care-consensus/articles/2020/03/management-of-stillbirth. [Last accessed October 2021].

2. ACOG Committee Opinion. Committee on Genetics. Genetic Evaluation of stillbirths and neonatal deaths. Obstetrics and Gynaecology. 2020;2991(97):1-3.
3. ACOG Committee Opinion. Low Dose Aspirin Use During Pregnancy. No. 743; 2018. [online] Available from: https://www.acog.org/clinical/clinical-guidance/committee-opinion/articles/2018/07/low-dose-aspirin-use-during-pregnancy. [Last accessed October 2021].
4. Badenhorst W, Hughes P. Psychological aspects of perinatal loss. Best Pract Res Clin Obstet Gynaecol. 2007;21(2):249-59.
5. Child Health Division of Ministry of Health and Family Welfare, Government of India. (2016). Operational Guidelines for Establishing Sentinel SB Surveillance System. [online] Available from: https://www.nhm.gov.in/images/pdf/programmes/RBSK/Operational_Guidelines/Operational_Guidelines_for_establishing_Sentinel_Stillbirth_Surveillance_System.pdf. [Last accessed October 2021]
6. Chung TKH, (ed). Clinical Obstetrics and Gynaecology: Psychological Issues in Obstetrics and Gynaecology, Volume 21, Number 21. Netherlands: Elsevier Limited; 2007.
7. Dudley DJ, Goldenberg R, Conway D, Silver RM, Saade GR, Varner MW, et al. Stillbirth Research Collaborative Network. A new system for determining the causes of stillbirth. Obstet Gynecol. 2010;116(2 pt 1):254-60.
8. Fretts RC. Etiology and prevention of stillbirth. Am J Obstet Gynecol. 2005;193(6):1923-35.
9. Huang DY, Usher RH, Kramer MS, Yang H, Morin L, Fretts RC. Determinants of unexplained antepartum fetal deaths. Obstet Gynecol. 2000;95(2):215-21.
10. Hughes PM, Turton P, Evans CD. Stillbirth as risk factor for depression and anxiety in the subsequent pregnancy: cohort study. BMJ. 1999;318(7200):1721-4.
11. Janssen HJ, Cuisinier MC, de Graauw KP, Hoogduin KA. A prospective study of risk factors predicting grief intensity following pregnancy loss. Arch Gen Psychiatry. 1997;54(1):56-61.
12. Korteweg FJ, Bouman K, Erwich JJ, Timmer A, Veeger NJGM, Ravisé JM, et al. Cytogenetic analysis after evaluation of 750 fetal deaths: proposal for diagnostic workup. Obstet Gynecol. 2008;111(4):865-74.
13. Korteweg FJ, Erwich JJ, Timmer A, van der Meer J, Ravisé JM, Veeger NJGM, et al. Evaluation of 1025 fetal deaths: proposed diagnostic workup. Am J Obstet Gynecol. 2012;206(1):53.e1-12.
14. Lancet. (2011). [online] Available from: Stillbirth 2011. [Last accessed October 2021].
15. Royal College of Obstetricians & Gynaecoloists. (2010). Late intrauterine fetal death and stillbirth. Green-top Guideline No. 55. [online] Available from: https://www.rcog.org.uk/en/guidelines-research-services/guidelines/gtg55/. [Last accessed October 2021].
16. Silver RM, Varner MW, Reddy U, Goldenberg R, Pinar H, Conway D, et al. Work-up of stillbirth: a review of the literature. Am J Obstet Gynecol. 2007;196(5):433-44.
17. Sims MA, Collins KA. Fetal death. A 10-year retrospective study. Am J Forensic Med Pathol. 2001;22(3):261-5.
18. SJ Gordin, JJ Erwich, TY Khong. Value of the perinatal autopsy: Critique. Pediatr Dev Pathol. 2005;5(5):480-8; 2005.
19. Smulian JC, Ananth CV, Vintzileos AM, Scorza WE, Knuppel RA. Fetal deaths in the United States. Influence of high-risk conditions and implications for management. Obstet Gynecol. 2002;100(6):1183-9.
20. Turton P, Evans C, Hughes P. Long-term psychosocial sequelae of stillbirth: phase II of a nested case-control cohort study. Arch Womens Mental Health. 2009;12(1):35-41.
21. Turton P, Hughes P, Evans CD, Fainman D. Incidence, correlates and predictors of post-traumatic stress disorder in the pregnancy after stillbirth. Br J Psychiatry. 2001;178:556-60.
22. Walsh CA, McMenamin MB, Foley ME, Daly SF, Robson MS, Geary MP. Trends in intrapartum fetal death, 1979-2003. Am J Obstet Gynecol. 2008;198(1):47.e1-47.e7.
23. Williams B, Datta S. Previous fetal death. In: Preconception Medicine and Management, Section 3. 2012. pp. 241-50.
24. World Health Organization. Stillbirths. [online] Available from: www.who.int. [Last accessed October 2021].
25. Young BK. Late pregnancy loss. In: Arora M, Mukhopadhaya N, (eds). Recurrent Pregnancy Loss, 3rd edition. New Delhi, London, Panama: The Health Sciences Publisher; 2019. pp. 196-201.

LONG QUESTION

1. Define stillbirth and enumerate its causes. How will you evaluate an intrauterine death at 28 weeks?

SHORT QUESTIONS

1. Discuss prepregnancy evaluation of mother who 6 months ago had a fetal demise at 32 weeks of gestation.
2. Discuss common infections associated with fetal death.

MULTIPLE CHOICE QUESTIONS

1. Following are causes of late still birth, except:
   a. Thyroid disorder
   b. Diabetes
   c. Cholestasis of pregnancy
   d. Trauma
2. Following infections may cause stillbirth in early third trimester, except:
   a. Malaria
   b. Syphilis
   c. Parvovirus B19
   d. Herpes simplex
3. Intrapartum causes of fetal death are all, except:
   a. Breech
   b. Shoulder dystocia
   c. Use of analgesia to mother
   d. Rh-negative pregnancy
4. Postmortem examination of fetus should include all, except:
   a. X-ray
   b. Photograph
   c. Computed tomography (CT) scan
   d. Magnetic resonance imaging (MRI)
5. Mandatory test for maternal evaluation after fetal death are all, except:
   a. Serology for syphilis
   b. Parental chromosome and DNA analysis
   c. Hemoglobin A1c (HbA1c)
   d. Kleihauer test

6. Maternal thrombophilia screen includes all, except:
   a. Lupus anticoagulant
   b. Antithrombin III
   c. Protein C and S deficiency
   d. Prothrombin time
7. Appropriate time for a conception after a previous loss should be:
   a. After 3 months
   b. After 6 months
   c. After 2 years
   d. Anytime couple feels comfortable
8. Preferred treatment in antiphospholipid antibody (APLA) syndrome is:
   a. Aspirin
   b. Aspirin and heparin
   c. Heparin and steroid
   d. Steroid and aspirin
9. A woman presenting for prenatal counseling after a late fetal death should have all vaccinations, except:
   a. Hepatitis
   b. Rubella
   c. Pneumococcal
   d. Varicella
10. Findings detected during autopsy of stillborn:
    a. Hepatosplenomegaly
    b. Placental infarction
    c. Genetic abnormalities
    d. All of the above

Answers									
1. a	2. d	3. d	4. c	5. b	6. d				
7. d	8. b	9. c	10. d						

SECTION 5

Pregnancy with Pre-existing Morbidities

5.1 CHRONIC HYPERTENSION IN PREGNANCY

Ragini Verma, Vijeta Jagtap

INTRODUCTION

Hypertension is an indisputable leader among risk factors of noncommunicable diseases with ever-increasing burden on healthcare globally. To this, pregnancy is no exception. Hence, hypertensive disorder is the most common medical condition complicating pregnancy and is directly proportional to maternal and perinatal morbidity and mortality worldwide.

Around 1.13 billion people are affected with hypertensive disorders worldwide including 20% of all women.[1] Incidence of chronic hypertension in pregnancy is variable and differs based on epigenetic factors. Nearly 5% of all pregnancies are affected.[2]

Early detection preferably prior to conception **(Fig. 1)** and timely management of chronic hypertension are important as diagnosis is often delayed during pregnancy due to decreased peripheral vascular resistance and fall in mean blood pressure (BP) in early and mid-pregnancy. Further, there is often superimposition of preeclampsia in cases of chronic hypertension during pregnancy which increases the proportion of adverse maternal and fetal outcomes. Also there is increased risk of lifelong morbidity and mortality due to end-organ damage to cardiovascular, cerebrovascular, and renal systems.

Chronic hypertension as per definition given by the American College of Obstetricians and Gynecologists (ACOG) 2001 is BP ≥140 mm Hg systolic and/or 90 mm Hg diastolic before pregnancy or before 20 weeks of gestation, use of antihypertensive medications before pregnancy, or persistence of hypertension for >12 weeks after delivery **(Fig. 2)**.[3]

Considering short-term and long-term complications and clinical management, chronic hypertension in pregnancy has been categorized into:

- Mild hypertension when systolic BP measures between 140 and 159 mm Hg or diastolic pressure measures between 90 and 109 mm Hg.
- Severe hypertension when systolic BP measures ≥160 mm Hg or diastolic pressure measures ≥110 mm Hg.[4]

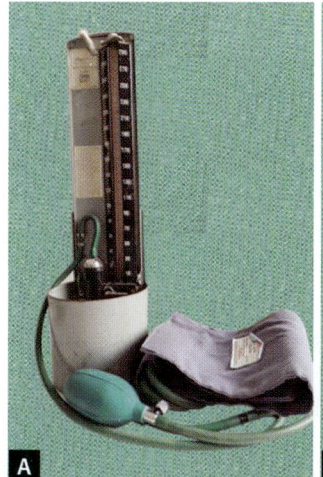
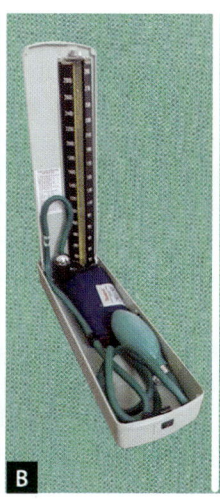
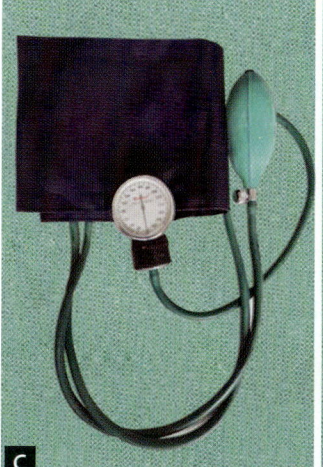
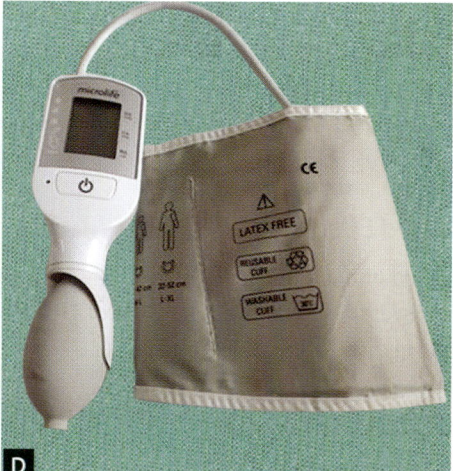

Figs. 1A to D: Blood pressure measurement apparatus. (A) Manual, wall mounted; (B) Manual, table top; (C) Manual, dial; (D) Electronic.

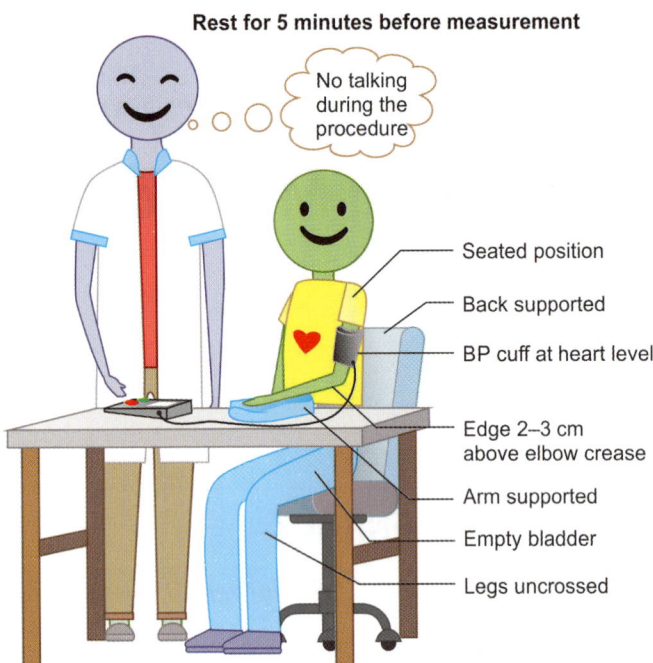

Fig. 2: Correct technique to measure blood pressure.

TABLE 1: Secondary causes of chronic hypertension.	
Secondary causes	
Renal	Parenchymal diseases, polycystic kidney disease, renal tumors, and obstructive uropathy
Renovascular	Renal artery stenosis (atherosclerotic or fibromuscular dysplasia)
Adrenal	Hyperaldosteronism, Cushing syndrome, pheochromocytoma, and hydroxylase deficiency
Other endocrine causes	Hypothyroidism, hyperthyroidism, hypercalcemia, and acromegaly
Collagen vascular diseases	Systemic lupus erythematosus, scleroderma, and Takayasu arteritis
Miscellaneous	Aortic coarctation, obstructive sleep apnea, medications, and increased intracranial pressure

■ TYPES

Chronic hypertension can be classified into the following types:[5]
- *Primary or essential hypertension* in 90% cases of chronic hypertension in pregnancy
- *Secondary hypertension* due to some underlying cause in remaining 10% cases.

Transient Hypertension

Transient hypertension is defined as an office systolic BP ≥140 mm Hg or a diastolic blood pressure (DBP) ≥90 mm Hg that is not confirmed after rest, on repeat measurement, on the same or on subsequent visits.

White Coat Hypertension

White coat hypertension is defined as elevated BP in office where systolic ≥140 mm Hg or diastolic ≥90 mm Hg but systolic <135 mm Hg and diastolic <85 mm Hg on ambulatory blood pressure monitoring (ABPM) or home blood pressure monitoring (HBPM).

Masked Effect Hypertension

Masked effect hypertension is defined as normal BP in office but elevated BP readings on ABPM or HBPM, i.e., systolic ≥135 mm Hg or diastolic ≥85 mm Hg.

■ ETIOLOGY

Essential hypertension is a polygenic disorder. Various combinations of genes, risk factors, and environmental exposures contribute to it. Mendelian form of hypertension is rare, seen mostly in cases of secondary hypertension due to endocrine or renal causes **(Table 1)**. Few studies have identified a rare autosomal dominant condition where there is missense mutation with substitution of serine with leucine at codon 810 (MR S810L) of mineralocorticoid receptor leading to exacerbation of hypertension or severe hypertension in early pregnancy.[6]

In 30–40% cases, family studies have shown heritability of BP. Epigenetic dysregulation is the hallmark in majority of cases. Ethnicity plays an important role in determination of incidence of hypertension. Africans and Asians are at highest risk followed by Whites and then Mexican Americans.

Increasing age, sedentary lifestyle, smoking, alcohol intake, obesity and increased body mass index, dyslipidemia, metabolic syndrome, and diabetes mellitus are significant risk factors predisposing to hypertension.

■ PATHOGENESIS

Increased cardiac output due to increased intravascular volume leads to raised BP. Increased peripheral vascular resistance leading to "pressure natriuresis", thus tries to revert back cardiac output to normal and eventually helps in maintaining blood pressure. In pregnancy due to hormonal effects, peripheral vascular resistance is low and cardiac output is high due to volume expansion. Hence, the balance is lost.

Sodium chloride (NaCl)-dependent hypertension is seen in renal and adrenal diseases. There is increase in circulating levels and physiological responsiveness to catecholamines. Increase in receptor affinity and density are also known to raise BP.

Hyperactivity of renin–angiotensin–aldosterone axis leads to sodium and water retention causing raised BP. Angiotensin II, a potent vasopressor, is also known to cause atherosclerosis, cardiac hypertrophy, and renal failure.

Altered vascular mechanisms leading to decreased lumen and elasticity of blood vessels and vascular endothelial dysfunction play an important role in mechanisms leading to raised BP.

Studies have also shown role of altered immune response, low-grade inflammation, and oxidative stress in etiopathogenesis of chronic hypertension.

INFLUENCE OF PREGNANCY ON CHRONIC HYPERTENSION AND VICE VERSA

Due to fall in peripheral vascular resistance and lowered BP, often the diagnosis of chronic hypertension is masked in early pregnancy or assessment of severity is hampered in already diagnosed cases.

Transient hypertension and white coat hypertension are associated with 40% risk of becoming gestational hypertension and 20% risk of preeclampsia. Masked hypertension should be considered when patient presents with unexplained end-organ damage such as chronic kidney disease, left ventricular hypertrophy, or retinopathy.[7]

Chronic hypertension carries a risk of progressing to severe hypertension or hypertensive crisis in pregnancy. There is a variable risk ranging from 25 to 50% for developing superimposed preeclampsia depending upon severity, duration, and associated end-organ damage leading to increased maternal morbidity and mortality. There is increased risk of abruptio placentae (5%) with worsened outcome in form of intrauterine fetal demise and disseminated intravascular coagulation. Acute renal failure may occur due to acute tubular necrosis or bilateral cortical necrosis. Chances of cesarean section are also increased. Adverse perinatal outcomes also include intrauterine growth restrictions (20%), preterm births (35–40%), and increased neonatal intensive care unit (NICU) admissions. Studies have shown increased risk of mid-trimester loss with inadequate or delayed treatment.[8]

Hypertensive patients are also at risk developing pulmonary edema, left ventricular dysfunction, and cerebrovascular accidents.

PRECONCEPTIONAL COUNSELING

Preconceptional counseling provides adequate time for risk assessment and interventions based on duration and control of disease, modifications in current therapy if required, baseline investigations for end-organ damage, and to take multidisciplinary (medical specialist, obstetrician, and fetal medicine specialist) approach to avoid pregnancy-related complications **(Table 2)**.

Dietary modifications as per DASH (Dietary Approaches to Stop Hypertension) including intake of vegetables, fruits and whole grains, high protein and low fat, and lowered sodium intake(≥2.4 g/day) is advisable. Very low sodium diet should be avoided in pregnancy.

Pregnancy outcomes improve with lifestyle modifications such as weight loss, avoiding smoking, alcohol, caffeine intake,

TABLE 2: Investigations for chronic hypertension.

Blood	Full counts with platelets
Urine analysis	• Routine, microscopy, culture • 24-hour urinary protein measurement (gold standard) (≥300 mg/day is significant in pregnancy) • *Others*: Spot urine protein/creatinine ratio (≥30 mg/mmol or +1 by dipstick) • Albumin/creatinine ratio >8 mg/mmol
Liver test	• Aspartate aminotransferase and alanine aminotransferase (>40 IU/L) • Raised lactate dehydrogenase • Serum proteins (especially albumin) • Serum bilirubin • Prothrombin time and international normalized ratio.
Renal function tests	• Serum creatinine (>1 mg/dL) • Serum electrolytes, serum uric acid, and BUN
Cardiac evaluation	Electrocardiography and echocardiography
	Oral glucose tolerance test, thyroid function tests, lipid profile
Ophthalmic evaluation	Hypertensive retinopathy signs
Renal pathology	Renal ultrasound (KUB) and renal artery Doppler, CT angiography or Gd-MRA
Pheochromocytoma Adrenal tumor	Labile blood pressure, orthostatic hypotension, palpitation, flushing, sweating and syncope 24-hour urinary fractioned metanephrines and normetanephrines (VMA) CT/MRI
Coarctation of aorta	• Absent/delayed femoral pulse • Systolic pressure difference >20 mm Hg in upper and lower limb • MR angiography or transthoracic echocardiography
Hyperaldosteronism Cushing syndrome	Renin-to-aldosterone ratio 24-hour urinary free cortisol Dexamethasone challenge test
Collagen vascular diseases Systemic lupus erythematosus	• Difference in BP in two limbs, absence of peripheral pulse, abnormal bruits on auscultation • Rheumatoid factor, antiphospholipid / antibody profile (LA/ACLA), ANA, ANCA, ESR, CRP • SLICC criteria and ANA
Obstructive sleep apnea syndrome	Polysomnography

(ACLA: anticardiolipin antibody; ANA: antinuclear antibody; ANCA: antineutrophil cytoplasmic antibody; BP: blood pressure; BUN: blood urea nitrogen; CRP: C-reactive protein; CT: computed tomography; ESR: erythrocyte sedimentation rate; Gd-MRA: gadolinium-enhanced magnetic resonance angiography; KUD: kidney, ureter, and bladder; LA: lupus anticoagulant; MR: magnetic resonance; MRI: magnetic resonance imaging; VMA: vanillylmandelic acid)

and simple aerobic exercises and brisk walking for 40 minutes per day, at least 4 days a week.

Diuretics, angiotensin-converting enzyme inhibitors (ACEIs), angiotensin receptor blockers (ARBs), and atenolol should be stopped either preconceptionally and if not then as soon as pregnancy is confirmed. Thiazides and diuretics are usually not associated with major birth-defects. Concern is about compromised placental circulation due to maternal volume depletion. Atenolol increases risk of intrauterine fetal growth restriction. ACEIs [Food and Drug Administration (FDA) class D] in pregnancy are contraindicated. They cause fetal growth restriction, fetal renal dysgenesis, anuresis, proximal tubular necrosis, pulmonary hypoplasia, reduced amniotic fluid and skull hypoplasia, thus increasing the risk of fetal and neonatal mortality. ARBs have also been associated with renal defects, dysmorphia, miscarriage, and neonatal deaths.[9]

Couple should be counseled regarding increased risk and worsening of end-organ damage, cardiovascular, cerebrovascular accidents, and renal failure in uncontrolled cases.

In cases with hypertension leading to myocardial infarction, chronic cardiac failure, stroke, and end-stage renal disease, pregnancy may better be avoided.

■ DIAGNOSIS

Definitive diagnosis and optimal management of chronic hypertension prior to conception is ideal, specifically in cases of secondary hypertension, assessment of end-organ damage, and having baseline investigations for early detection of complications. However, often reproductive age-group women seek healthcare facility only after few weeks of pregnancy which delays the definitive diagnosis until 6–12 weeks of postpartum.

Evaluation should begin with meticulous history and clinical systemic examination including assessment of all risk factors, associated comorbid condition, any earlier obstetric events, end-organ damage, duration, progress, and drugs and control in already diagnosed cases.

Mercury sphygmomanometer is the gold standard for recording BP. Calibrated automated devices may be used by patients with adequate training for ABPM or HBPM which is particularly useful in conditions such as masked hypertension or white coat hypertension in early pregnancy. Systolic BP ≥135 mm Hg and diastolic BP ≥85 mm Hg on ABPM/HBPM require further evaluation.[10]

■ ANTENATAL CARE AND FETAL SURVEILLANCE

Well-controlled mild hypertension in pregnancy has same obstetric outcomes as general population. Adverse maternal and perinatal outcomes are seen in cases with severe uncontrolled hypertension, superimposed preeclampsia/HELLP (hemolysis, elevated liver enzyme levels, and low platelet levels) or with end-organ damage. Previous adverse obstetric event is also associated with increased risk in current pregnancy. Hence, severity assessment should be done at each visit to antenatal clinic and especially at term.

Ideally these patients should visit antenatal clinic every 2 weeks till 32–34 weeks and then weekly till delivery. Complicated and severe cases may be called more frequently, i.e., weekly or as per need.

Blood pressure, weight, symphysiofundal height, and urinary proteins should be checked on each visit. HBPM is useful in masked hypertension and white coat hypertension.

Baseline investigations should be done as early in pregnancy as possible along with early and accurate gestational age estimation by ultrasonography. Complete blood counts, complete urine analysis, and liver and renal function tests should be done in each trimester.

Fetal Surveillance

Accurate dating scan should be done as soon as pregnancy is diagnosed. Auscultation of fetal heart should be done at each visit. A detailed anomaly scan is recommended at 18–20 weeks of gestation.

Early evaluation includes bilateral uterine artery Doppler study at 24 weeks. Diastolic notching may predict uteroplacental insufficiency and growth restriction in fetus.

Ultrasonographic assessment of fetal growth and measurement of deepest amniotic fluid pocket to check for oligohydramnios is to be undertaken once in every 3–4 weeks in uncomplicated and well-controlled cases. In case of intrauterine growth restriction where fetal weight is <10th centile, umbilical artery Doppler to look for increased resistance and absent or reversal of end-diastolic flow, ductus venosus Doppler, and middle cerebral artery Doppler for brain-sparing effect should be done at least once in 2 weeks. If umbilical artery Doppler shows increased resistance, monitoring is done on weekly basis and in case of absent or reversal of flow, it is done twice or thrice in a week, respectively, including cardiotocography beyond 26 weeks of gestation until delivery.[11,12]

■ TREATMENT OF CHRONIC HYPERTENSION

Nonpharmacologic Lifestyle Interventions

Bed Rest

Bed rest in left lateral position improves placental circulation due to increased venous return by releasing pressure by gravid uterus. It may lower the BP to some extent and improve diuresis. But absolute bed rest and restricted mobilization is more harmful than useful as it predisposes pregnant women to venous thrombosis, infection, psychosocial adverse effects, and weakening of bones and muscles. Hence, absolute bed rest is not recommended.

De-addiction

Ideally to be undertaken prior to conception. Addiction to smoking, alcohol, opioids, and caffeine, all are linked with adverse pregnancy outcomes.

Dietary Modifications and Salt Restriction

Dietary modifications as per DASH are useful in general population. However, there is no evidence so far about its protective role in hypertensive disorders of pregnancy and adverse outcomes.[13] Salt restriction is not recommended in pregnancy as physiological volume expansion is required.

Exercise and Weight Management

Strenuous physical activity and weight loss are not recommended during pregnancy. Obese women should lose weight preconceptionally. Body mass index of <25 kg/m² is desirable.

Pharmacotherapy

There has always been discrepancy in recommendations and dilemma for obstetricians treating hypertensive disorders in pregnancy with respect to when to start antihypertensives and what is the ideal control of BP. Tight control of pressure is required to prevent severe hypertension, superimposed preeclampsia, and abruption placentae and too tight control may lead to fetal growth restriction due to compromised placental circulation.[14]

However, after the CHIPS trial (Control of Hypertension in Pregnancy Study), recommendations have shifted from "less tight" control (target DBP of up to 100 mm Hg) to "tight" control (target DBP of 85 mm Hg) of BP during pregnancy to prevent severe hypertension, stroke, and other serious maternal complications, adverse perinatal outcomes independent of those with co-occurrence of preeclampsia.[15]

As per National Institute for Health and Care Excellence (NICE) 2019 guidelines, all antenatal women with chronic hypertension and with sustained BP ≥140/90 mm Hg should be offered antihypertensives if already not taking. Aim of treatment should be a target pressure of 135/85 mm Hg.

Choosing a single best antihypertensive for monotherapy depends upon multiple factors including patient profile, cause and degree of hypertension, and the extent of end-organ damage. If adequate control is not achieved despite of three different drugs, it is called as resistant hypertension.

In nonpregnant individuals, ARBs (such as losartan and telmisartan), ACEIs (such as captopril and ramipril), and diuretics (thiazides and loop diuretics such as furosemide) are mainstay of treatment for hypertension. But these drugs are contraindicated in pregnancy as discussed earlier.

As per current guidelines and recommendations, labetalol is the drug of choice for treatment of chronic hypertension in pregnancy. When labetalol is contraindicated or in case of inadequate control, nifedipine may be used, while methyldopa is to be used as an adjunct or when both of the above are not tolerated by patient.[16]

Peripherally Acting Adrenergic Receptor Blockers

β-blockers

β-blocking agents lower BP by reducing heart rate and contractility which reduces cardiac output. Also, they affect the central nervous system and inhibit release of renin.

Propranolol (nonselective β-blocker) and atenolol (cardioselective $β_1$-blocker) have been used in pregnancy previously. Though nonteratogenic, they are known to cause fetal growth restriction, decreased placental weight, and fetal bradycardia.

Labetalol

Labetalol is the drug of choice for treating hypertension in pregnancy. It is safe, nonteratogenic, no fetal bradycardia with oral therapy, improved maternal outcomes due to decreased progression to severe hypertension, and improved neonatal outcomes by preventing preterm births.[17]

- *Mechanism of action*: Adrenergic $α_1$ and nonselective $β_1$ + $β_2$ blocker. In addition to antihypertensive effect such as other β-blockers, labetalol also blocks the α-mediated peripheral vasoconstriction.
- *Metabolism*: Hepatic first pass metabolism.
- *Side-effects*: Fatigue, lethargy, muscle weakness, and bronchoconstriction. Very high doses and intravenous (IV) therapy in labor is occasionally associated with fetal bradycardia and neonatal hypoglycemia.
- *Contraindications*: Asthma, chronic obstructive pulmonary disease (COPD), heart blocks, and sick-sinus syndrome.
- *Dose*: 200–1,200 mg/d in two or three divided doses orally.

In acute severe hypertension, 20 mg of IV bolus loading dose over 10 minutes, repeat dose of 20–80 mg after 10–20 minutes or IV infusion of 1–2 mg/min can be given. Maximum dose is 300 mg.

Prazosin

Prazosin is a postsynaptic selective α-adrenergic antagonist. It is useful in secondary hypertension due to pheochromocytoma. Along with diuretics, it is highly effective in refractory severe hypertensive crisis. However, routine use is not recommended.

- *Mechanism of action*: Lowers BP by decreasing peripheral vascular resistance
- *Side effects*: Postural hypotension, dizziness, flushing, and light headedness
- *Dose*: 0.5–5 mg maximum, divided into three doses.

Calcium Channel Blockers
Nifedipine
Nifedipine is usually a second-line drug for management of hypertension in pregnancy. It is safe for the fetus.
- *Mechanism of action*: It causes smooth muscle relaxation and lowers BP by reducing peripheral vascular resistance by calcium-gated L-channel blockade.
- *Metabolism*: Metabolized by liver followed by renal elimination
- *Dose*: 30–120 mg/day in three/four divided doses orally. In severe hypertension, 10–30 mg can be given orally. Repeated after 45 minutes, if required. Sublingual route is no longer preferred as it may cause sudden maternal hypotension, myocardial infarction in cases of coronary artery disease, and fetal bradycardia.
- *Side effects*: Headache, dizziness, facial flushing, tachycardia, palpitations, and postural hypotension.

There were concerns raised in some cases of preeclampsia when nifedipine was used along with magnesium sulfate leading to cardiorespiratory depression, collapse, and neuromuscular blockade. As per recent evaluations, such risk appears to be more theoretical.

Centrally Acting Sympatholytic Agents
Methyldopa
For decades before labetalol, methyldopa was the first-line drug for management of hypertension in pregnancy due to its safety profile.
- *Mechanism of action*: Centrally acting α_2-sympathetic agonists, decreases peripheral vascular resistance by inhibiting central sympathetic outflow
- *Metabolism*: Hepatic metabolism followed by renal excretion
- *Dose*: 500 mg to 2 g maximum in divided doses
- *Side effects*: Dizziness, headache, drowsiness, and nasal stuffiness are temporary side effects. Serious side effects include fainting due to postural hypotension, muscle spasms, allergic reaction, sudden weight gain, fluid retention, mood changes, and depression. Rare but fatal side effects include rebound hypertension, hepatitis, hepatic necrosis, and hemolytic anemia.

Clonidine
Another centrally acting α_2-sympathetic agonists, not used routinely in pregnancy due to possibility of sleep disturbances in exposed neonates. It may be useful in cases of refractory hypertension.

Peripheral Vasodilators
Hydralazine
Hydralazine is a directly acting smooth muscle relaxant for arterial fibers reducing BP. It has nitric oxide (NO) enhancing action.
- *Dose*: 50–300 mg/day in two–four divided doses
Hydralazine is usually recommended for hypertensive crisis management in dose of 5 mg IV or intramuscular (IM), then 5–10 mg every 20–40 minutes. Once BP is controlled, it may be repeated every 3 hourly or for infusion at the rate of 0.5–10.0 mg/h for persistent severe hypertension. Maximum dose is 30 mg.
- *Side effects*: Nausea, vomiting, headache, facial flushing, tachycardia, palpitations, and sudden hypotension

Other rare but significant adverse effects include polyneuropathy responsive to pyridoxine and drug-induced lupus syndrome. Sudden hypotension in mother may lead to fetal distress and rarely abruption of placenta. Neonatal side effects such as thrombocytopenia and lupus have also been noted.[18]

Sodium nitroprusside is rarely used in pregnancy. Infusion form is considered as the last resort in life-threatening refractory hypertension. Risk of fetal cyanide intoxication still remains unknown.

Diuretics
Thiazides
Thiazides is often used as a monotherapy or in combination with other antihypertensives for essential hypertension. It inhibits NaCl pump in the distal convoluted tubule and promotes sodium excretion. Hyperglycemia, hyperuricemia, hypokalemia, and neonatal thrombocytopenia are some of the side effects of thiazides.

Diuretics in pregnancy may cause volume contraction and compromise placental perfusion. The National High Blood Pressure Education Program (NHBPEP) has concluded that thiazides in dose of 12.5–25 mg/day may be continued in pregnancy, especially for women having salt-sensitive hypertension.[2] Thiazides, triamterene, and amiloride are nonteratogenic. Spironolactone has anti-androgenic potential.

Loop diuretic such as furosemide is to be reserved for specific indications during pregnancy such as pulmonary edema, congestive cardiac failure, renal insufficiency, or severe hypertensive crisis.

Adjuncts to Antihypertensive Agents
Aspirin
Aspirin in low doses selectively inhibits thromboxane α_2, a potent vasoconstrictor produced by platelets. Imbalance between thromboxane α_2 and prostacyclin increases response to vasopressors and is implicated in pathophysiology of preeclampsia. Aspirin is known to reduce risk of superimposed preeclampsia and adverse perinatal outcomes without increasing antepartum and postpartum hemorrhage. Hence, all antenatal women with chronic hypertension should be offered aspirin in oral dose of 75–150 mg/day from 12 weeks of gestation.[19]

Calcium

Calcium reduces the level of parathormone which reduces its intracellular concentration leading to decreased contractility of vascular smooth muscles. High doses of calcium (≥1 g/day) may have some protective role in reducing risk of preeclampsia and preterm birth, especially in women taking low-calcium diet.[20]

Specific Clinical Conditions

Severe Chronic Hypertension

Systolic BP ≥160 mm Hg and diastolic pressure ≥110 mm Hg is labeled as severe hypertension in pregnancy. If left uncontrolled, it may lead to life-threatening complications such as hypertensive encephalopathy, stroke, acute left ventricular failure and myocardial infarction, pulmonary edema, acute renal failure, and rarely aortic dissection.

Hypertensive encephalopathy is usually seen when BP rises above 200/130 mm Hg. There is loss of autoregulation of cerebral arterioles due to raised cerebral perfusion pressures. Pathological features include cerebral edema, necrotizing arteriolitis, microinfarcts or petechial hemorrhages, and small multiple thrombi. Clinical features include severe generalized headache, nausea and vomiting, papilledema or retinal infarcts leading to blurring or loss of vision, convulsions, and altered level of consciousness or even coma. Impaired coronary blood flow leads to altered myocardial contractility and systolic dysfunction. Hypertrophic left ventricle leads to diastolic dysfunction. Pulmonary edema may be cardiogenic or due to iatrogenic fluid-overload, hypoproteinemia, or due to renal failure. Acute renal failure is commonly seen in cases of abruptio placentae with disseminated intravascular coagulopathy.

Treatment requires admission at a critical-care facility with multidisciplinary approach. Aim should be to lower mean BP by 25%, systolic pressure of 140–160 mm Hg and diastolic pressure of 100 mm Hg within few minutes to few hours. IV labetalol is usually the first-line drug to be used followed by oral nifedipine. Hydralazine is considered when there is inadequate control in spite of their use. Sodium nitroprusside is the last resort in refractory cases. During treatment, BP should be measured every 15–30 minutes. Overzealous treatment and sudden hypotension should be avoided in antenatal patients as there is risk of fetal distress due to reduced placental blood flow.

In diagnosed and indicated cases with raised intracranial pressure, IV mannitol 20% solution 250–500 mL can be given. Intubation-hyperventilation and cerebrospinal fluid drainage should be considered in nonresponsive cases but only after expert opinion. Magnesium sulfate is the drug of choice for prophylaxis and management of convulsions in cases of hypertensive disorders of pregnancy. It also reduces cerebral edema. Phenytoin may be used in seizures refractory to magnesium sulfate in pregnancy.

Pulmonary edema is treated with fluid restriction, oxygen therapy, and furosemide 20–40 mg intravenously 6–12 hourly. Acute renal failure is managed by giving fluid challenge, diuretics, vasodilators, and hemodialysis in nonresponsive cases with severe metabolic and electrolyte imbalance.

Superimposed Preeclampsia and HELLP

Seen in about 25% cases of chronic hypertension in pregnancy and adverse maternal and perinatal outcomes may be associated with 50% of severe cases. Superimposed preeclampsia is often associated with resistant hypertension, new-onset or worsening of pre-existing proteinuria, and one or more severe complications which are given in **Table 3**.

HELLP Syndrome

Hemolysis, elevated liver enzymes, and low platelets. This is usually a severe condition requiring immediate termination of pregnancy.[21]

Timing of Delivery

Women with mild chronic hypertension well-controlled with or without medication do not require early termination of pregnancy. Induction of labor can be done at 38 or 39 weeks of gestation to prevent development of severe hypertension and superimposed severe preeclampsia without causing increased risk of cesarean section.[22,23] Women with BP ≤160/110 mm Hg with or without medication should not be offered induction of labor before 37 weeks.

In women with severe hypertension or new-onset preeclampsia at ≥37 weeks of gestation, induction of labor is recommended. In women with chronic hypertension and previous pregnancy loss, uncontrolled hypertension and superimposed severe preeclampsia may require early delivery.[24] If BP is uncontrolled or dose of antihypertensives needs to be increased frequently, then pregnancy should be terminated between 36 and 37 weeks.[25]

TABLE 3: Complications associated with severe preeclampsia.	
Cardiorespiratory	Resistant/severe hypertension, pulmonary edema, anasarca, respiratory distress, and left ventricular dysfunction
Renal	Proteinuria, acute tubular necrosis, glomeruloendotheliosis, acute renal failure
Hepatic	Hepatic dysfunction, acute liver failure, hepatic hematoma, and rupture
Neurological	Eclampsia, stroke, and posterior reversible encephalopathy syndrome
Hematological	Microangiopathic hemolytic anemia, thrombocytopenia, and disseminated intravascular coagulation

Role of Antenatal Steroids

Antenatal corticosteroids for fetal lung maturation should be considered between 24 and 34 weeks of gestation when early delivery is anticipated. It may be administered until 39 weeks for elective cesarean delivery. Multiple repeated courses of steroids are not recommended. However, a single course may be repeated in cases where delivery is anticipated in next 7 days and previous steroid course was before 7-14 days.[26]

Role of Magnesium Sulfate for Fetal Neuroprotection

$MgSO_4$ for fetal neuroprotection should be administered if delivery is planned before 32 weeks of gestation.[27] Recommendation is to give 6 g loading dose over 20 minutes followed by 2 g/hour for at least 12 hours or until delivery.

Intrapartum Care

Mode of delivery is decided on individual basis depending upon maternal condition, severity, and cause of disease and fetal compromise, if any. Vaginal delivery is preferred unless there is any obstetric indication for cesarean section.

Antihypertensive medications should be continued during labor and BP should not be allowed to cross 160/110 mm Hg. BP monitoring every 15-30 minutes with continuous fetal monitoring is recommended. Absolute fluid restriction is not advisable. Fluid intake up to 60-80 mL/hour can be allowed safely. Magnesium sulfate in recommended doses for convulsion prophylaxis in mother should be given in severe hypertension and severe superimposed preeclampsia.

Epidural analgesia can be offered to women with chronic hypertension. If any operative intervention is required, regional anesthesia (spinal/epidural) is preferred over general anesthesia, unless it is contraindicated.[28]

Central venous catheter for pressure monitoring is currently not recommended in all cases. Invasive arterial catheter for BP monitoring may be used in severe uncontrolled hypertension in intensive care unit only, though not routinely recommended.

Postpartum Care: Within 6 Weeks of Postpartum

Postpartum period should not be taken lightly as BP is labile with frequent fluctuations. Movement of extracellular fluid and intravascular volume expansion causes deterioration in up to 25% of cases. About 30-40% women with severe superimposed preeclampsia may develop life-threatening complications such as eclampsia and stroke.[29]

Blood pressure should be monitored everyday at least three to four times till discharge from hospital. In uneventful pregnancy and early discharge, BP should be checked on day 3, then at 7-14 days, and at 6 weeks of postpartum. Frequent follow-up may be required as per maternal condition. Target of treatment should be 140/90 mm Hg in uncomplicated cases and 130/80 mm Hg in mothers with other comorbidities such as diabetes.

Few women who had discontinued antihypertensive treatment in pregnancy due to fall in BP may require medication now. All antihypertensives including ACEIs can be safely continued during breastfeeding. Although these drugs are excreted in breast milk, clinical implications are seen rarely in cases of preterm infants with low birth weight. Atenolol and diuretics should be avoided in breastfeeding mothers.

Nonsteroidal anti-inflammatory drugs (NSAIDs) should be avoided due to increased risk of acute kidney injury. Thromboprophylaxis should be offered as per individual risk assessment.

Posttraumatic stress disorder may be seen in cases of adverse neonatal outcome or when there is chronic morbidity. Necessary counselling, support, and medical treatment should be given according to the condition.

Contraception

Any unintended pregnancy in a woman with chronic hypertension would be detrimental for her health and burden to the healthcare system. Hence, no opportunity for contraceptive counselling should be missed **(Table 4)**.

Combined oral contraceptives (COCs) increase BP, risk of myocardial infarction, and stroke in a dose-dependent manner. Hence, COCs are better avoided in patients having chronic hypertension.[31]

Women who desire permanent contraception should be offered tubal ligation if their clinical condition permits or their partners may be offered vasectomy.

Extended Postpartum Care: Beyond 6 Weeks Following Birth

Women should be referred to concerned specialist for further evaluation and definitive diagnosis for suspected secondary hypertension as all the physiological changes of pregnancy have now reverted back.

TABLE 4: Contraception in women with chronic hypertension.

	Well-controlled hypertension or BP <160/100 mm Hg	BP ≥160/100 mm Hg or any vascular disease
Barrier contraception or copper containing IUD	1	1
LNG-IUS or LNG implant	1	2
POP	1	2
DMPA	2	3
COC	3	3/4*

(BP: blood pressure; COC: combined oral contraceptive pills; DMPA: depot medroxyprogesterone acetate; IUD: intrauterine device; IUS: intrauterine system; LNG: levonorgestrel; POP: progesterone only pills) *WHO-MEC/US-MEC[30]

Uncontrolled BP in any age-group or ethnicity has been directly associated with 40% increased risk of developing ischemic heart disease, cardiomyopathy, hemorrhagic and ischemic stroke, peripheral artery disease, and end-stage renal disease and increase in mortality risk by two times.[32] Risk increases up to 70% in those with severe superimposed preeclampsia.[33] Risk is further increased by other comorbidities such as diabetes, obesity, and dyslipidemia.

Lifestyle modifications such as healthy diet, salt restriction, weight loss in obese women, regular exercise, and stress management should be followed. Necessary changes in medication such as use of cardioprotective antihypertensives and annual medical review for end-organ damage should be done.

Studies have shown that women who were preterm at birth and whose mothers had complicated hypertensive disorders of pregnancy are themselves at risk of developing hypertension and stroke at an early age along with increased risk of severe preeclampsia/HELLP syndrome and gestational diabetes.[34]

Counseling for creating awareness and motivating them to maintain a healthy lifestyle and to undertake screening and medical review for their daughters in future is necessary to ensure quality maternal and child healthcare in the long run.

MISCELLANEOUS TOPICS

Apparatus and Blood Pressure Measurement Method

Mercury sphygmomanometers are the gold standard for BP measurement in pregnancy. Automated devices should be calibrated with mercury sphygmomanometer first.

In clinics, BP should be measured in a comfortable seating position with legs resting on a flat surface and arms resting at the level of heart. Intrapartum BP measurement should be done in lateral recumbent position to avoid supine hypotension.

Systolic BP is noted at the first Korotkoff sound heard (K1) and the DBP at the disappearance of sounds completely (K5). K4, i.e., muffling sound should be noted only when K5 is absent. Inflatable bladder cuff should cover 80% of arm circumference. Cuff size should be used as per patient's arm circumference.[35]

Screening for Preeclampsia

Pathogenesis of preeclampsia has been related to imbalance between angiogenic factors such as vascular endothelial growth factor or placental growth factor (PlGF) and antiangiogenic factors such as soluble fms-like tyrosine kinase 1 (sFlt-1). In normal pregnancies, the level of sFlt-1 starts to rise after 30–32 weeks of gestation and PlGF level starts to decrease after 30 weeks of gestation.

Few recent studies suggest that increased sFlt1/PlGF ratio is a better marker compared to measuring sFlt1 or PlGF separately for early diagnosis of PE.[36] Though this is not routinely recommended, NICE guidelines suggest that PlGF-based testing should be offered between 20 and 35 weeks of gestation, to women with chronic hypertension, suspected to develop preeclampsia.

Role of Supplementary Therapy

None of the guidelines recommend use of progesterone, multivitamins (C/D/E), micronutrients such as zinc, magnesium, copper, iodine or selenium, fish oils, or garlic for preventing hypertension in pregnancy.

Numbers indicate Medical Eligibility Criteria category. 1—safe, no restriction for use; 2—advantage outweighs risks; 3—risks outweigh advantages, not recommended usually; 4—unacceptable health risk hence contraindicated.

REFERENCES

1. NCD Risk Factor Collaboration. Worldwide trends in blood pressure from 1975 to 2015: a pooled analysis of 1479 population-based measurement studies with 19.1 million participants. Lancet. 2017;389(10064):37-55.
2. Report of the National High Blood Pressure Education Program Working Group on High Blood Pressure in Pregnancy. Am J Obstet Gynecol. 2000;183(1):S1-22.
3. Committee on Hypertension in Pregnancy. Hypertension in Pregnancy. Washington, DC: American College of Obstetricians and Gynecologists; 2013.
4. NICE guidelines. (2019). Hypertension in Pregnancy: Diagnosis and Management. [online] Available from: www.nice.org.uk/guidance/ng133. [Last accessed October 2021].
5. Magee LA, Pels A, Helewa M, Evelyne Rey 4, von Dadelszen P; Canadian Hypertensive Disorders of Pregnancy Working Group. Diagnosis, evaluation, and management of the hypertensive disorders of pregnancy: Executive summary. SOGC Clinical Practice Guideline. 2014;36(5):416-38.
6. Schmider-Ross A, Wirsing M, Büscher U, Neitzel H, Krause M, Henrich W, Reles A, et al. Analysis of the S810L point mutation of the mineralocorticoid receptor in patients with pregnancy-induced hypertension. Hypertens Pregnancy. 2004;23(1):113-9.
7. Brown MA, Mangos G, Davis G, Homer C. The natural history of white coat hypertension during pregnancy. BJOG. 2005;112(5):601-6.
8. Redman CW. Fetal outcome in trial of antihypertensive treatment in pregnancy. Lancet. 1976;2(7989):753-6.
9. Serreau R, Luton D, Macher MA, Delezoide AL, Garel C, Jacqz-Aigrain E. Developmental toxicity of the angiotensin II type 1 receptor antagonists during human pregnancy: a report of 10 cases. BJOG. 2005;112(6):710-2.
10. Brown MA, Roberts LM, Mackenzie C, Mangos G, Davis GK. A prospective randomized study of automated versus mercury blood pressure recordings in hypertensive pregnancy (PRAM Study). Hyperten Pregnancy. 2011;31(1):107-19.
11. American College of Obstetricians and Gynecologists' Committee on Practice Bulletins—Obstetrics. ACOG Practice Bulletin No. 203: Chronic Hypertension in Pregnancy. Obstet Gynecol. 2019; 133(1):26-50.

12. Brown MA, Magee LA, Kenny LC, Karumanchi SA, McCarthy FP, Saito S, et al. Hypertensive disorders of pregnancy. ISSHP classification, diagnosis, and management recommendations for international practice. Hypertension. 2018;72(1):24-43.
13. Fulay AP, Rifas-Shiman SL, Oken E, Perng W. Associations of the dietary approaches to stop hypertension (DASH) diet with pregnancy complications in project viva. Eur J Clin Nutr. 2018;72(10):1385-95.
14. Abolas E, Duley L, Styen DW, Gialdini C. Antihypertensive drug therapy for mild to moderate hypertension during pregnancy. Cochrane Database Syst Rev. 2007;(1):CD002252.
15. Magee LA, Dadelszen PV, Singer J, Lee T, Rey E, Ross S, et al. The CHIPS Randomized Controlled Trial (Control of Hypertension in Pregnancy Study). Is Severe Hypertension Just an Elevated Blood Pressure? Hypertension. 2016;68(5):1153-9.
16. Regitz-Zagrosek V, Roos-Hesselink JW, Bauersachs J, Blomström-Lundqvist C, Cífková R, De Bonis M, et al. ESC Scientific Document Group. 2018 ESC Guidelines for the management of cardiovascular diseases during pregnancy. Eur Heart J. 2018;39(34):3165-241.
17. Magee LA, Helewa M, Moutquin JM, von Dadelszen P; Canadian Hypertensive Disorders of Pregnancy Working Group. Diagnosis, evaluation, and management of the hypertensive disorders of pregnancy. J Obstet Gynecol Can. 2008;30(3 Suppl 1):S9-15.
18. Magee LA, Cham C, Waterman EJ, Ohlsson A, von Dadelszen P. Hydralazine for treatment of severe hypertension in pregnancy: Meta-analysis. BMJ. 2003;327(7421):955-60.
19. Askie LM, Duley L, Henderson-Smart DJ, Stewart LA; PARIS Collaborative Group. Antiplatelet agents for prevention of pre-eclampsia and its complications. A meta-analysis of individual data. Lancet. 2007;369(9575):179-80.
20. Hofmeyr G, Lawrie TA, Atallah ÁN, Torloni M. Calcium supplementation during pregnancy for preventing hypertensive disorders and related problems. Cochrane Database Syst Rev. 2018;10:CD001059.
21. Von Dadelszen P, Payne B, Li J, Ansermino JM, Pipkin FB, Côté, AM, et al. Prediction of adverse maternal outcomes in pre-eclampsia: development and validation of the full PIERS model. Lancet. 2011;377(9761):219-27.
22. American College of Obstetricians and Gynecologists. ACOG Practice Bulletin No.125: Chronic hypertension in pregnancy. Washington DC. Obstet Gynecol. 2012;119(2 Pt 1):396-407.
23. Ram M, Berger H, Geary M, McDonald SD, Murray-Davis B, Riddell C, et al. Timing of delivery in women with chronic hypertension. Obstet Gynecol. 2018;132(3):669-77.
24. Harper LM, Biggio JR, Anderson S, Tita AT. Gestational age of delivery in pregnancies complicated by chronic hypertension. Obstet Gynecol. 2016;127(6):1101-9.
25. Spong CY, Mercer BM, D'Alton M, Kilpatrick S, Blackwell S, Saade G. Timing of indicated late-preterm and early-term birth. Obstet Gynecol. 2011;118(2 Pt 1):323-33.
26. FIGO Working Group on Good Clinical Practice in Maternal-Fetal Medicine. Good clinical practice advice: Antenatal corticosteroids for fetal lung maturation. Int J Gynecol Obstet. 2019;144(3):352-5.
27. Doyle LW, Crowther CA, Middleton P, Marret S, Rouse D, et al. Magnesium sulphate for women at risk of preterm birth for neuroprotection of the fetus. Cochrane Database Syst Rev. 2009;1:CD004661.
28. Sia AT, Fun WL, Tan TU. The ongoing challenges of regional and general anaesthesia in obstetrics. Best Pract Res Clin Obstet Gynaecol. 2010;24(3):303-12.
29. Cairns AE, Pealing L, Duffy JMN, Roberts N, Tucker KL, Leeson P, et al. Postpartum management of hypertensive disorders of pregnancy: a systematic review. BMJ Open. 2017;7(11):e018696.
30. Altshuler A, Berry-Bibee E, Curtis K, et al. WHO. Medical Eligibility Criteria Wheel for Contraceptive Use-2015 Update. WHO; 2015. http://www.who.int/reproductivehealth/en/.
31. Curtis KM, Mohllajee AP, Martins SL, Peterson HB. Combined oral contraceptive use among women with hypertension: a systematic review. Contraception. 2006;73(2):179-88.
32. Williams B, Mancia G, Spiering W, Rosei EA, Azizi M, Burnier M, et al. 2018 ESC/ESH Guidelines for the management of arterial hypertension. Eur Heart J. 2018;39(33):3021-04.
33. Wu P, Haththotuwa R, Kwok CS, Babu A, Kotronias RA, Rushton C et al. Preeclampsia and future cardiovascular health: A systematic review and meta-analysis. Circ Cardiovasc Qual Outcomes. 2017;10(2):e003497.
34. Boivin A, Luo ZC, Audibert F, Mâsse B, Lefebvre F, Tessier R, et al. Pregnancy complications among women born preterm. Can Med Assoc J. 2012;184(16):1777-84.
35. Lowe SA, Bowyer L, Lust K, McMahon LP, Morton M, North RA, et al. SOMANZ guidelines for the management of hypertensive disorders of pregnancy 2014. Aust N Z J Obstet Gynaecol. 2015;55(5):e1-29.
36. Nikuei P, Rajaei M, Roozbeh N, Mohseni F, Poordarvishi F, Azad M, et al. Diagnostic accuracy of sFlt1/PlGF ratio as a marker for preeclampsia. BMC Pregnancy Childbirth. 2020;20(1):80.

LONG QUESTIONS

1. A 25-year-old primigravida was diagnosed with hypertension on her booking visit at 8 weeks of gestation. Describe the possible etiology of hypertension and investigations for the same in this condition. How will you provide antenatal care to this lady?
2. How will you manage a case of severe hypertension in pregnancy at term?

SHORT QUESTIONS

1. How will you offer preconceptional counselling to a lady with chronic hypertension?
2. Describe intrapartum management of a patient with hypertensive disorder of pregnancy.
3. Discuss various contraceptive methods with benefits and risks for a woman with chronic hypertension.
4. How will you provide postpartum care to a woman with chronic hypertension who had a cesarean delivery today?

MULTIPLE CHOICE QUESTIONS

1. Incidence of chronic hypertension in pregnancy is:
   a. 3%   b. 5%
   c. 15%   d. 20%

2. When a patient's systolic blood pressure ≥140 mm Hg or a diastolic blood pressure ≥90 mm Hg in clinic but normal otherwise on subsequent visits, then it is called as:
   a. White coat hypertension
   b. Mild chronic hypertension
   c. Transient hypertension
   d. Masked effect hypertension
3. Diastolic blood pressure is noted at:
   a. Appearance of Korotkoff sound K4
   b. Disappearance of K4
   c. Appearance of K5
   d. Disappearance of K5
4. Risk of developing superimposed preeclampsia in a pregnant woman with chronic hypertension is:
   a. 10–20%   b. 25–50%
   c. 50–60%   d. 70–80%
5. In a pregnant woman with chronic hypertension, superimposed preeclampsia is characterized by all of the following, except:
   a. New onset proteinuria
   b. Increase in systolic blood pressure by 30 mm Hg or diastolic blood pressure by 15 mm Hg
   c. Blurring of vision
   d. Increasing levels of serum lactate dehydrogenase (LDH)
6. Secondary chronic hypertension is seen in all, except:
   a. Hyperaldosteronism   b. Hypothyroidism
   c. Renal tubular acidosis   d. Hypercalcemia
7. Assessment of fetal growth by ultrasonography, in as case of chronic hypertension, is done:
   a. Twice in a week   b. Once in a week
   c. Every 15 days   d. Every 3–4 weeks
8. Aim of pharmacotherapy in chronic hypertension in pregnancy is:
   a. Target pressure of 130/80 mm Hg
   b. Target pressure of 135/85 mm Hg
   c. Target pressure of 140/90 mm Hg
   d. Target pressure of 145/95 mm Hg
9. Which of the following drug is never used in pregnancy to treat hypertension?
   a. Diazoxide   b. Sodium nitroprusside
   c. Hydralazine   d. Clonidine
10. A 24-year-old primigravida was diagnosed with chronic hypertension on her booking visit. After a few weeks, she was started on oral labetalol due to inability to control blood pressure by nonpharmacological methods. Her labetalol dose was increased twice during subsequent weeks. What is the ideal time of delivery for her?
    a. 35 weeks   b. 37 weeks
    c. 39 weeks   d. 40 weeks

Answers

1. b   2. c   3. d   4. b   5. b   6. c
7. d   8. b   9. a   10. b

5.2 HEART DISEASE IN PREGNANCY

Vanita Raut, Shruti Panchbudhe, Anahita Chauhan

INTRODUCTION

Cardiac disease is an important cause of maternal morbidity and mortality, both in the antepartum and postpartum period. Heart diseases of variable types complicate 1–3% of all pregnancies both in developed and developing countries, and in fact may be diagnosed for the first time when patient presents for antenatal care.[1] Cardiac disease can be broadly divided into congenital and acquired types. Rheumatic heart disease is still a major problem in developing countries; MS accounts for nearly three quarter of the cases, while aortic lesions are less common and account for <5% of cases. Cardiomyopathy and congenital heart disease are predominant in developed countries.

HEMODYNAMIC CHANGES DURING PREGNANCY

Pregnancy causes important anatomical and physiological changes in the cardiovascular system. The rise in cardiac output begins during the first 5–8 weeks of pregnancy and reaches its peak late in the second trimester and continues up to 32 weeks, after which it plateaus. Patients with existing cardiac disease and cardiac decompensation often coincides with this peak. These hemodynamic changes return to the prepregnant baseline within 2–4 weeks following vaginal delivery and within 4–6 weeks after cesarean section. These changes are outlined in **Table 1**.[2,3]

EFFECTS OF PREGNANCY ON MATERNAL CARDIAC DISEASE

The normal hemodynamic changes of pregnancy seen in **Table 1** have a profound impact on patients with cardiac problem. The dangerous periods in pregnancy when the risk of cardiac decompensation is greatest are:

- Between 12 and 16 weeks when hemodynamic changes of pregnancy begin
- 28–32 weeks when these changes peak

TABLE 1: Normal hemodynamic changes during pregnancy.[5,6]

Hemodynamic parameter	Changes during normal pregnancy	Change during labor and delivery	Change during postpartum
Blood volume	Increases by 40–50%	Further increases	Decreases (autodiuresis)
Heart rate	Increases by 10–15 beats/min	Further increases	Decreases
Cardiac output	Increases 30–50% above baseline due to: • Increase in preload due to greater blood volume • Decrease in afterload due to decrease in systemic vascular resistance • Increase in maternal heart rate by 10–15 beats/min	Increases by additional 50% (Labor pains, uterine contraction, relief of caval compression after delivery and autotransfusion of blood from emptied and contracted uterus contribute to increase cardiac output)	Decreases
Blood pressure	Decreases by 10 mm Hg in mid trimester due to decrease in systemic vascular resistance	Increases	Decreases
Stroke volume	Increases in first and second trimesters; decreases in third trimester due to compression by gravid uterus	Increases (300–500 mL/contraction)	Decreases
Systemic vascular resistance	Decreases (smooth muscle relaxing effect of progesterone, nitrous oxide, prostaglandins)	Increases	Decreases

- During labor as each uterine contraction pumps 300–500 mL of blood from the uteroplacental circulation into maternal circulation, further aggravated by maternal bearing down efforts in the second stage
- Immediately after delivery due to autotransfusion and also removal of pressure effect of the gravid uterus on the inferior vena cava.

EFFECTS OF MATERNAL CARDIAC DISEASE ON PREGNANCY

The risk of spontaneous miscarriage and therapeutic abortion is increased in women with heart disease. The offspring of a mother with congenital heart disease is at increased risk of inheriting a congenital heart disease and the risk of the offspring inheriting polygenic cardiac disease is quoted as 3–5%, compared with a 1% risk in the general population.[4] Fetal morbidity is secondary to preterm delivery and complications of prematurity, and intrauterine growth restriction. Certain cardiac medications can adversely affect the fetus [e.g., angiotensin-converting enzyme (ACE) inhibitors, warfarin, and statins]. Neonatal complications are particularly high in women with cyanotic heart disease; fetal death occurs in these patients due to maternal polycythemia, which in turn leads to chronic hypoxia.

CARDIOVASCULAR EVALUATION DURING PREGNANCY

The history is an essential part of the initial risk assessment and should include information on the baseline functional status and previous cardiac events, as these are strong predictors of peripartum cardiac events. Certain changes of pregnancy can mimic or mask cardiac disease and therefore it is important to be aware of both signs and symptoms of normal pregnancy and those that may herald underlying heart disease are mentioned in **Table 2**. However, angina, resting dyspnea, paroxysmal nocturnal dyspnea, or a sustained arrhythmia are not expected with pregnancy and need a further diagnostic workup.

The most important predictors for primary cardiac events or complications during pregnancy were first analyzed by Siu and Colman (2004). They describe "The Cardiac Disease in Pregnancy (Carpreg) Risk Score"[5] which calculates a woman's cardiac risk during pregnancy (**Box 1**). To assess

TABLE 2: Normal clinical findings that mimic heart disease in pregnancy.

Symptoms	Signs
Palpitations	Tachycardia
Fatigue	Premature atrial/ventricular beats
Dyspnea on exertion	Raised jugular venous pressure (prominent "a" and "v" waves, brisk "x" and "y" descents)
Lower extremity edema	Basal crepitations
Orthopnea	Displacement of the apex beat upward and outside the midclavicular line
	Exaggerated first heart sound with splitting
	Midsystolic murmur at the left base (flow murmur)
	Continuous murmur (mammary souffle)
	Lower extremity edema

> **BOX 1:** Cardiac disease in pregnancy (CARPREG) risk score (adapted from Siu[8]).
>
> *One point for each:*
> - History of prior cardiac event (stroke, transient ischemic attack, heart failure, or arrhythmias)
> - New York Heart Association (NYHA) functional class >II or cyanosis
> - Left heart obstruction (mitral valve area <2 cm^2, aortic valve area <1.5 cm^2, or left ventricular outflow tract gradient >30 mm Hg)
> - Left ventricular ejection fraction <40%
>
> *Chance of cardiac complication:*
> - 0 points = 5%
> - 1 point = 27%
> - ≥2 points = 75%

TABLE 3: Estimated fetal and maternal effective doses of various diagnostic and interventional radiological procedures.

Procedure	Fetal exposure	Maternal exposure
Chest radiograph [Posteroanterior (PA) and lateral]	<0.01 mg	0.1 mg
Computed tomography (CT) chest	0.3 mg	7 mg
Coronary angiography	1.5 mg	7 mg
Percutaneous coronary intervention (PCI) or radio-frequency catheter ablation	3 mg	15 mg

> **BOX 2:** New York Heart Association functional classification of heart failure.[9]
>
> *Class I:* Patients with cardiac disease but without resulting limitations of physical activity. Ordinary physical activity does not cause fatigue, palpitations, dyspnea, or angina
> *Class II:* Patients with cardiac disease resulting in slight limitation of physical activity. They are comfortable at rest. Ordinary physical activity results in fatigue, palpitations, dyspnea, or angina
> *Class III:* Patients with cardiac disease resulting in marked limitation of physical activity. They are comfortable at rest. Less than ordinary physical activity results in fatigue, palpitations, dyspnea, or angina
> *Class IV:* Patients with cardiac disease resulting in an inability to carry on any physical activity without discomfort. Symptoms of cardiac insufficiency may even be present at rest. If any physical activity is undertaken, discomfort is increased

the functional status, the New York Heart Association classification **(Box 2)** is universally accepted but is limited by wide individual variation, subjective nature, and some limitations of activity due to pregnancy itself.[6]

SPECIAL INVESTIGATIONS

Electrocardiography

Electrocardiography is a cost-effective screening and if abnormal, may identify the need for further study.

Echocardiography

Echocardiography is the best method to detect structural abnormality of the heart in all types of cardiac lesions, severity of lesion, degree of pulmonary hypertension, and left ventricular function.

Chest X-ray

Chest X-ray is usually avoided in pregnancy but if required, an abdominal shield can be used.

Coronary Angiography

Coronary angiography helps in the diagnosis and potential treatment in acute myocardial infarction (AMI). This procedure is reassuring and there is no evidence to suggest an increased risk of congenital malformations, intellectual disability, growth restriction, or pregnancy loss at doses of radiation of <50 mGy to the pregnant woman **(Table 3)**.

Magnetic Resonance Imaging

Magnetic resonance imaging is used in special cases of congenital heart disease and aortic dissection. It is safe in pregnancy and should be advised if other noninvasive diagnostic measures are not sufficient for definitive diagnosis.

MANAGEMENT DURING PREGNANCY: GENERAL GUIDELINES

Preconceptional Counseling

Prepregnancy counseling has a major preventive role in ensuring an optimal pregnancy outcome and includes the following:

- Obstetrician and cardiologist collaboration
- Optimal control of disease, medically or surgically
- Discussion of maternal and fetal risks
- Evaluation of current cardiac status
- Discussion of safe and effective contraception until pregnancy desired
- Modifications/alterations of drugs known to cause fetal effects (ACE inhibitors and warfarin)
- Specialist geneticist referral for patients with inherited cardiac lesions
- Advice against pregnancy with certain cardiac conditions.

ANTEPARTUM MANAGEMENT

The risk assessment of any woman with a heart murmur or a history of any cardiac disease should be carried out early in pregnancy in a multidisciplinary clinic. The pregnancy heart team has been put forward in the new European Society of Cardiology (ESC) 2018 guidelines and evolved from the multidisciplinary management team of the 2011 guidelines. The minimum team requirements are a cardiologist, an obstetrician, and an anesthetist, the other additional experts depending on the condition are a geneticist, cardiothoracic surgeon, pediatric cardiologist, fetal medicine specialist, neonatologist, hematologist, nurse specialist, pulmonary specialist, and others where required. In this team, patients from other centers can also be discussed, so not every hospital needs to have its own pregnancy heart team. Though not exhaustive, following are some important management guidelines during the antenatal period:

- General measures such as intake of healthy diet, hematinics, calcium supplementation, and bed rest should be followed.
- Assessment of functional class of heart disease.
- *Advice regarding antenatal visits*: Patients with mild valvular disease should be followed up every month till 28–30 weeks, after which they may require monitoring every 2 weeks.
- Change to necessary medications that are not contraindicated in pregnancy
- Anticoagulation for certain conditions; discuss the risks and benefits of continued warfarin therapy versus changing to subcutaneous heparin
- Detection of conditions which can precipitate heart failure which includes anemia, infections, arrhythmias, noncompliance with medications, preeclampsia, and hyperthyroidism
- Frequent monitoring if new symptoms develop or changes in functional class
- Most tocolytic agents are contraindicated in cardiac pregnant patients due to potential side effects. **Table 4** lists tocolytic agents which can be used in these cases.
- Fetal two-dimensional (2D) echocardiography in second trimester for patients with congenital heart disease and if fetal cardiac anomaly is suspected, it is mandatory to obtain the following:
  - Full fetal echocardiography
  - Detailed scanning to identify associated anomalies (digits and bones)
  - Family history
  - *Maternal medical history*: Medical disorders, viral illness, or teratogenic medication
  - Fetal karyotype (e.g., deletion in 22q11.2 with conotruncal anomalies)
  - Referral to a fetal medicine specialist, pediatric cardiologist, geneticist, and neonatologist
  - Delivery at an institution that can provide neonatal cardiac care
- Fetal surveillance for growth and development
- Digitalization in cases with rapid pulse rate or atrial fibrillation and left ventricular systolic dysfunction.
- Valvuloplasty or valve replacement surgery in patients refractory to medical treatment.

LABOR AND DELIVERY

Patients should be managed in tertiary care centers with high-dependency and intensive care units. Consultation with an anesthetist experienced in obstetrical care is recommended, usually in the third trimester. Patients may await spontaneous labor and are counseled that the rate of cesarean section is not increased because of heart disease alone. Vaginal delivery is safe and well-tolerated in most patients with cardiovascular disease and is associated with less bleeding, decreased risk of infection, venous thrombosis, and embolism. Previously induction of labor had a little place in the management of cardiac patients as a prolonged induction-delivery interval may result in infection; failure of induction may need cesarean section which might otherwise not have been required and anxiety associated with induction will worsen cardiac condition. But the ESC 2018 recommends that induction of labor should be considered at 40 weeks of gestation in all women with cardiac disease; this reduces the risk of emergency cesarean section by 12% and the risk of stillbirth by 50% in women without heart disease, and this benefit is likely to be greater for women with heart disease who have higher rates of obstetric complications.

If the progression of labor is adequate, no intervention will be required in the second stage but if there is the slightest delay, it is wiser to proceed with assisted vaginal delivery

TABLE 4: Tocolytic agents in heart disease in pregnancy.[12]

Drug	Category	Maternal cardiovascular side effects	Safety in cardiac patients
• Terbutaline • Isoxsuprine • Ritodrine	β-agonists	Cardiac arrhythmias, pulmonary edema, myocardial ischemia, tachycardia, and death	Contraindicated
Nifedipine	Calcium channel blocker	Hypotension and tachycardia	Contraindicated
Indomethacin	NSAIDs	No cardiac effects	Safe
Atosiban	Oxytocin receptor antagonist	No cardiac effects	Safe

(NSAIDs: nonsteroidal anti-inflammatory drugs)

(forceps or vacuum) with a wide episiotomy. Cesarean section should be considered for obstetric indications, patients in labor on oral anticoagulants, with aggressive aortic pathology, and in acute intractable heart failure and severe forms of pulmonary hypertension (including Eisenmenger syndrome). Perimortem cesarean section should be considered for acute life-threatening maternal event where immediate delivery is required as it improves the chance of successfully resuscitating the mother and only secondarily, of improving fetal survival. It should be considered from 24 weeks of gestation, as before this time the degree of uterine vena cava compression is minimum and the baby is not considered to be viable and the delivery should be performed within 4 minutes of the cardiac arrest. Third stage of labor should never be hurried and routine use of ergometrine is barred as it increases the cardiac load by causing additional blood squeeze from the uterus into the circulation. Oxytocin in an intravenous (IV) drip is preferred for third-stage bleeding and furosemide 40 mg IV is given to relieve the heart from volume overload. **Box 3** outlines the general management of labor.

Infective endocarditis is a rare but life-threatening complication of pregnancy with a reported incidence in pregnancy of 0.006%. The American College of Cardiology (ACC) and the American Heart Association (AHA) have advised that prophylaxis is recommended in women with moderate- and high-risk lesions in the setting of possible bacteremia. Vaginal delivery without any infection of the vagina and clean cesarean section do not require prophylaxis as per the latest recommendations.[7,8] Recommendations are given in **Table 5**.

> **BOX 3:** General management of cardiac patients in labor.
>
> *Management team:*
> - Cardiologist
> - Obstetrician
> - Neonatologist/pediatrician
> - Anesthetist
>
> *Patient care:*
> - Semi-recumbent positioning/left lateral tilt
> - Strict input and output charting (restriction of intravenous fluids to 75 mL/hour)
> - Continuous electrocardiogram (ECG) monitoring
> - Oxygen supplementation
> - Pulse oximetry
> - Fetal monitoring
> - Arterial line
> - Adequate pain control
> - Infective endocarditis prophylaxis (moderate and high risk lesions—see **Table 5**)
> - Thrombosis prophylaxis (see **Table 7**)
> - Oxytocin: Concentrated drip or via infusion pump for induction and augmentation of labor (to avoid fluid overload due to antidiuretic effect of oxytocin)
> - Cut short second stage of labor with prophylactic forceps or vacuum
> - Avoid ergot alkaloids in the third stage
> - Control hemorrhage

TABLE 5: Antibiotic prophylaxis for the prevention of infective endocarditis.[16-18]

Cardiac lesion	Prophylaxis- uncomplicated delivery	Prophylaxis- infective endocarditis	Regimen
Negligible risk: • Mitral valve prolapse without regurgitation • Prior rheumatic fever—no valvular dysfunction • Kawasaki disease—no valve dysfunction • Pacemaker • Prior coronary bypass surgery • Surgically corrected ASD, VSD and PDA without prosthesis	None None None None None None	None None None None None None	None None None None None None
Moderate risk: • Mitral valve prolapse with regurgitation • Acquired valve dysfunction • Unrepaired ASD, VSD, PDA • Hypertrophic cardiomyopathy	None None None None	Recommended Recommended Recommended Recommended	Ampicillin 2 g IV/ IM or Amoxicillin 2 g PO or if Penicillin allergies: Vancomycin 1 g IV over 1–2 hours
High risk: • Prosthetic valves • Prior infective endocarditis • Cyanotic malformation • Surgically corrected systemic pulmonary shunts	Discretionary Discretionary Discretionary Discretionary	Recommended Recommended Recommended Recommended	Ampicillin 2 g IV/ IM plus Gentamicin 1.5 mg/kg IV (max. 120 mg) loading dose, followed 6 hours later by ampicillin 1 g IV or Amoxicillin 1 g PO. If penicillin allergies: Vancomycin 1 g IV over 1–2 h; Gentamicin 1.5 mg/kg IV (max. 120 mg)

(ASD: atrial septal defect; IM: intramuscular; IV: intravenous; PDA: patent ductus arteriosus; VSD: ventricular septal defect)

POSTPARTUM CARE

Close monitoring should be continued while the cardiac output remains elevated; that is, for at least 48 hours. Most patients can breastfeed, including those on warfarin as the quantity of drug secreted in the breast milk is extremely small.

CONTRACEPTION

This is an important part of the complete care of the patient with cardiac disease, especially true in cases in which pregnancy is contraindicated or its timing is critical. Male sterilization carries the least risk for those who have completed their family. Barrier methods when used consistently and properly are usually effective, with a failure rate of 2–18%. Combined oral contraceptive pills are contraindicated as thrombosis and paradoxical embolism can occur. Progestin-only oral contraceptives or depot medroxyprogesterone acetate may be used by these women, as the thromboembolic risk of oral contraceptives is thought to be due to the estrogen component and failure rate is <1%. For emergency contraception, a copper intrauterine device is effective and also provides ongoing contraception or a single dose of 1.5 mg levonorgestrel is effective if taken within 72 hours. The progesterone receptor modulator ulipristal acetate has been shown to be more effective than levonorgestrel and is not associated with increased risk of thrombosis.

SPECIFIC CARDIAC CONDITIONS AND MATERNAL CARDIOVASCULAR RISK

The ESC 2011 guidelines have classified maternal cardiovascular risk based on various cardiac conditions, modified from World Health Organization (WHO) guidelines of 2006 (**Table 6**).[9] This ESC guideline was updated in 2018 based on the previously published ESC (2011), the literature systematic search from 2011 to 2016 in the National Institutes of Health database (PubMed), and on recent publications and recommendations from the American Heart Association and the ACC (**Tables 7 and 8**).

This section outlines the common cardiac conditions and describes the salient diagnostic and management features of each condition.

Stenotic Lesion

Mitral Stenosis

Mitral stenosis is the most common rheumatic valvular lesion encountered during pregnancy. The normal mitral valve area is 4.0–5.0 cm^2. Mild MS corresponds to a valve area of 2–2.5 cm^2, moderate 1.5–2 cm^2, severe 1–1.5 cm^2, and critical <1 cm^2 and narrowing to 2.5 cm^2 must occur before development of symptoms. The hypervolemia and tachycardia associated with pregnancy exacerbate the impact of mitral valve obstruction and result in increase in left atrial pressure and

TABLE 6: Modified World Health Organization (WHO) classification of maternal cardiovascular risk (adapted from ESC Guidelines 2011[21] and Thorne[22]).

Risk class	Risk of pregnancy	Conditions
I	No detectable increased risk of maternal mortality; no/mild increase in morbidity	• Uncomplicated, small or mild PS, PDA, MV prolapse • Successfully repaired simple lesions (ASD, VSD, PDA)
II	Small increased risk of maternal mortality or moderate increase in morbidity	• Unoperated ASD and VSD • Repaired tetralogy of Fallot • Mild left ventricular impairment • Hypertrophic cardiomyopathy • Native or tissue valvular heart disease not considered WHO I or IV • Marfan syndrome without aortic dilatation • Repaired coarctation
III	Significantly increased risk of maternal mortality or severe morbidity. Expert counseling required. If pregnancy is decided upon, intensive monitoring needed throughout pregnancy, childbirth, and the puerperium	• Mechanical valve • Systemic right ventricle • Cyanotic heart disease (unrepaired) • Complex congenital heart disease • Aortic dilatation 40–45 mm (Marfan) • Aortic dilatation 45–50 mm in aortic disease associated with bicuspid aortic valve
IV	Extremely high risk of maternal mortality or severe morbidity; pregnancy contraindicated. If pregnancy occurs termination should be discussed. If pregnancy continues, care as for class III	• Pulmonary arterial hypertension; any cause • Severe systemic ventricular dysfunction (LVEF <30%, NYHA III–IV) • Previous peripartum cardiomyopathy with residual impairment of LV function • Severe mitral stenosis, severe symptomatic aortic stenosis • Marfan syndrome, aorta dilated >45 mm • Aortic dilatation >50 mm in aortic disease associated with bicuspid aortic valve • Native severe coarctation

(ASD: atrial septal defect; ESC: European Society of Cardiology; LV: left ventricular; LVEF: left ventricular ejection fraction; MV: mitral valve; NYHA: New York Heart Association; PDA: patent ductus arteriosus; PS: pulmonary stenosis; VSD: ventricular septal defect)

TABLE 7: Modified World Health Organization (mWHO) classification of maternal cardiovascular risk adapted from ESC 2018.

	mWHO I	*mWHO II*	*mWHO II–III*	*mWHO III*	*mWHO IV*
Diagnosis (if otherwise well and uncomplicated	Small or mild • Pulmonary stenosis • Patent ductus arteriosus • Mitral valve prolapse, Successfully repaired simple lesions (atrial or ventricular septal defect, patent ductus arteriosus, and anomalous pulmonary venous drainage) and atrial or ventricular ectopic beats, isolated	Unoperated atrial or ventricular septal defect, repaired tetralogy of Fallot, most arrhythmias (supraventricular arrhythmias) and Turner syndrome without aortic dilatation	Mild left ventricular impairment (EF >45%), hypertrophic cardiomyopathy, native or tissue valve disease not considered WHO I or IV (mild mitral stenosis and moderate aortic stenosis), Marfan or other HTAD syndrome without aortic dilatation, aorta <45 mm in bicuspid aortic valve pathology, repaired coarctation and atrioventricular septal defect	Moderate left ventricular impairment (EF 30–45%), previous peripartum cardiomyopathy without any residual left ventricular impairment, mechanical valve, systemic right ventricle with good or mildly decreased ventricular function, and Fontan circulation. If otherwise the patient is well and the cardiac condition uncomplicated, unrepaired cyanotic heart disease, other complex heart disease, moderate mitral stenosis, severe asymptomatic aortic stenosis, moderate aortic dilatation (40–45 mm in Marfan syndrome or other HTAD; 45–50 mm in bicuspid aortic valve, Turner syndrome ASI 20–25 mm/m^2, tetralogy of Fallot <50 mm) ventricular tachycardia	Pulmonary arterial hypertension, severe systemic ventricular dysfunction (EF <30% or NYHA class III–IV), previous peripartum cardiomyopathy with any residual left ventricular impairment, severe mitral stenosis, severe symptomatic aortic stenosis, systemic right ventricle with moderate or severely decreased ventricular function, severe aortic dilatation (>45 mm in Marfan syndrome or other HTAD, >50 mm in bicuspid aortic valve, Turner syndrome ASI >25 mm/m^2, tetralogy of Fallot >50 mm) vascular Ehlers–Danlos severe (re) coarctation Fontan with any complication
Risk	No detectable increased risk of maternal mortality and no/mild increased risk in morbidity	Small increased risk of maternal mortality or moderate increase in morbidity	Intermediate increased risk of maternal mortality or moderate-to-severe increase in morbidity	Significantly increased risk of maternal mortality or severe morbidity	Extremely high risk of maternal mortality or severe morbidity
Maternal cardiac event rate	2.5–5%	5.7–10.5%	10–19%	19–27%	40–100%
Counseling	Yes	Yes	Yes	Yes: Expert counseling required	Yes: Pregnancy contraindicated: If pregnancy occurs, termination should be discussed
Care during pregnancy	Local hospital	Local hospital	Referral hospital	Expert center for pregnancy and cardiac disease	Expert center for pregnancy and cardiac disease
Minimal follow-up visits during pregnancy Once or twice Once per trimester bimonthly monthly or bimonthly monthly	Once or twice	Once per trimester	Bimonthly	Monthly or bimonthly	Monthly
Location of delivery	Local hospital	Local hospital	Referral hospital	Expert center for pregnancy and cardiac disease	Expert center for pregnancy and cardiac disease

(ASI: aorta size index; EF: ejection fraction; ESC: European Society of Cardiology; HTAD: heritable thoracic aortic disease; NYHA: New York Heart Association)

TABLE 8: Selected revised recommendations and selected new recommendations Comment/comparison with 2011 version 2018 of European Society of Cardiology.

2011	2018
Strengthening mWHO classification of maternal risk	It is recommended to perform risk assessment in all women with cardiac diseases of childbearing age and before conception, using the modified World Health Organization (mWHO) classification of maternal risk (IC)
Upgrade in class of recommendation; patients with severe MS should undergo intervention before pregnancy Intervention is recommended before pregnancy in patients with MS and valve area <1.0 cm² (IC)	Intervention is recommended before pregnancy in patients with MS and valve area <1.0 cm² (IC)
In 2011, OACs were recommended during the second and third trimesters until the 36th week. Now, separate recommendations for women with low and high dose are given for vitamin K antagonist (VKA) use during the second and third trimesters	During the second and third trimesters until the 36th week, VKAs are recommended in women needing a low dose (low-dose VKA: warfarin <5 mg/day, phenprocoumon <3 mg/day, or acenocoumarol <2 mg/day) (IC)
Sotalol deleted	Flecainide or propafenone are recommended for prevention of SVT in patients with WPW syndrome[12] (IC)
Changed in high-risk patients from unfractionated heparin (UFH) to low molecular weight heparin (LMWH). Dosing based on body weight introduced	LMWH is the drug of choice for the prevention and treatment of venous thromboembolism (VTE) in all pregnant patients[13] (IB). It is recommended that the therapeutic dose of LMWH is based on body weight[14] (IC)
Changes: dose adjustment of UFH or LMWH dose within 36 hours now recommended	In pregnant women on LMWH or UFH, it is recommended to perform weekly anti-Xa level monitoring or aPTT monitoring with dose adjustment (within 36 hours) (IC)
Upgrade of recommendation: IIb to IIa	Catheter ablation with electroanatomical systems should be considered in experienced centers in case of drug-refractory and poorly tolerated supraventricular tachyarrhythmia (SVT)[15] (IIaC)
Change from D-dimers to imaging as the first line of investigation, as D-dimers are unreliable in pregnancy	If compression ultrasound is negative, magnetic resonance venography should be considered to diagnose VTE (IIaC)
Food and Drug Administration (FDA) categories A–X were used for all drugs in 2011	Decision-making based on former FDA categories is no longer recommended (IIIC)
Pre-pregnancy surgery is now deleted. Now also information on Turner syndrome with aortic diameter corrected for body surface area (BSA)	Pregnancy is not recommended in patients with severe dilatation of the aorta (heritable thoracic aortic disease such as Marfan syndrome >45 mm, bicuspid aortic valve >50 mm, >27 mm/m² BSA, or Turner syndrome ASI >25 mm/m² BSA) (IIIC)

Selected new recommendations

- Right heart catheterization is recommended to confirm the diagnosis of pulmonary arterial hypertension (PAH). This can be performed during pregnancy but with very strict indications[10] (IC). LMWH in therapeutic dose is recommended in pregnant patients with chronic thromboembolic pulmonary hypertension (IC). In patients with pulmonary embolism, thrombolytic therapy is recommended only in severe hypotension or shock (IC). In women at high risk for thromboembolism, it is recommended to convert LMWH to UFH at least 36 hours prior to delivery and stop the UFH infusion 4–6 hours prior to anticipated delivery. Activated partial thromboplastin time (aPTT) should be normal before regional anesthesia (IC). In women at low risk for thromboembolism on therapeutic LMWH, induction or cesarean section is recommended to be performed 24 hours after the last dose of LMWH (IC)
- In treatment-naive pregnant PAH patients, initiating treatment should be considered (IIaC). In patients with (history of) aortic dissection, cesarean delivery should be considered (IIaC). Beta-blocker therapy throughout pregnancy should be considered in women with Marfan syndrome and other heritable thoracic aortic diseases (IIaC). Induction of labor should be considered at 40 weeks of gestation in all women with cardiac disease (IIaC)
- In patients with PPCM, bromocriptine treatment may be considered to stop lactation and enhance recovery (LV function) (IIbB)
- Pregnancy is not recommended in patients with vascular Ehlers–Danlos syndrome (IIIC). Breastfeeding is not recommended in mothers who take antiplatelet agents other than low-dose aspirin (from section 7, see section 12) (IIIC)

New concepts

- Enforcing mWHO classification of maternal risk Introduction of the pregnancy heart team
- More attention for assisted reproductive therapy
- Discussion of the use of bromocriptine in peripartum cardiomyopathy (PPCM)
- Introduction of specific levels of surveillance based on low/medium/high risk for arrhythmia with hemodynamic compromise at delivery
- New information on pharmacokinetics in pregnancy, more detailed information on pharmacodynamics in animal experiments on all drugs (Supplementary Data)
- Perimortem cesarean section is discussed
- Advice on contraception and the termination of pregnancy in women with cardiac disease is now provided

(ASI: aorta size index; LV: left ventricular; OAC: oral anticoagulant)

atrial fibrillation. Thus, patients with mild-to-moderate MS, who are asymptomatic before pregnancy, may develop atrial fibrillation and heart failure during the ante and peripartum periods. Patients with moderate or severe MS can be managed with medical therapy, which includes control of heart rate, volume status, and frequent monitoring. The two goals of medical therapy are to reduce the heart rate and reduce the left atrial pressure. Treatment with β-blockers, diuretics, and digitalization are the mainstay of therapy in conjunction with general management outlined earlier. Closed mitral valvotomy which was for a long time the procedure of choice has now been replaced by balloon mitral valvuloplasty. Open heart surgery and valve replacement surgery during pregnancy have a high fetal loss rate but can be performed in expert hands if indicated.

Aortic Stenosis

Congenital bicuspid aortic valve is the most common cause of aortic stenosis (AS) in pregnancy, but in some cases, the aortic valve is narrowed due to rheumatic heart disease. Mild-to-moderate AS with preserved left ventricular function is well-tolerated during pregnancy. In severe AS (aortic valve area <1.0 cm^2, mean gradient >50 mm Hg), the left ventricle fails to overcome resistance to flow and patients develop congestive cardiac failure (CCF). Symptoms such as dyspnea, angina pectoris, or syncope become apparent late in the second trimester or early in the third trimester.

Women with severe AS should be referred to a cardiologist and ideally undergo correction of the valvular abnormality before conception. Treatment options include surgical repair, surgical valve replacement, and percutaneous balloon valvotomy. When severe symptomatic AS is diagnosed during pregnancy, maximal medical therapy is preferred over any intervention, but in patients with refractory symptoms and hemodynamic deterioration, percutaneous balloon valvotomy or surgery may be performed; if patient presents in earlier trimester, medical termination should be offered. The cornerstone for management is bed rest as due to fixed stroke volume, any activity will increase heart rate and demand on left ventricle. Epidural and spinal anesthesia should be avoided as they decrease the systemic vascular resistance, which is poorly tolerated in patients with AS; general anesthesia remains the preferred technique for cesarean section in patients with AS. In contrast to most cardiac patients, patients with AS should be kept on the "wet" side during labor and delivery with respect to IV fluids, i.e., infusion at the rate of 125–150 mL/hour.

Pulmonary Stenosis

The etiology of pulmonary stenosis is mostly congenital and valvular. The prognosis depends upon the degree of obstruction to flow: When the gradient is small, pregnancy is well tolerated and when the gradient is >50 mm of Hg, it is severe, and consideration for balloon valvuloplasty should be given.

Regurgitant Lesions

Mitral Regurgitation

The most common etiologies of mitral regurgitation (MR) in pregnancy are mitral valve prolapse and rheumatic heart disease. Pregnancy is generally well-tolerated by patients with MR, and it has been theorized that MR may actually improve in pregnancy because of the physiologic reduction in systemic vascular resistance. Asymptomatic patients do not require treatment during pregnancy. Those patients who develop left ventricular dysfunction with hemodynamic abnormalities and symptoms of heart failure require the use of diuretics and digoxin.

Aortic Regurgitation

Aortic regurgitation may be due to a congenital bicuspid valve, rheumatic heart disease, or aortic annular dilatation. The condition is well-tolerated during pregnancy and symptomatic patients respond well to afterload reduction, diuretics, and digoxin.

Tricuspid Regurgitation

Secondary tricuspid regurgitation (TR) is more common than primary TR, which may be due to endocarditis or Ebstein anomaly. Severe TR with heart failure is managed conservatively during pregnancy. When surgery for left-sided valve lesions is performed, additional tricuspid repair is indicated in severe TR and should be considered in moderate TR with annular dilatation (≥40 mm).

Women with Prosthetic Heart Valves

In women of childbearing age, the selection of a prosthetic heart valve is challenging and needs to be individualized. The bi-leaflet mechanical valves have a superior durability, an excellent hemodynamic profile, and a small risk of bleeding and thromboembolic complications with careful anticoagulation. On the other hand, biological valves have limited durability (which is a major factor in young patients) because of structural valve deterioration (SVD), i.e., thickening, progressive calcification, mechanical wear, and tear/rupture of the valve; however, their important advantage is that they do not require anticoagulation.

Anticoagulation is particularly important in patients with mechanical heart valves and atrial fibrillation. The ACC/AHA Task Force report of 2006[10] divides patients into higher risk (history of thromboembolism or an older generation mechanical prosthesis in the mitral position) and low risk (no history of thromboembolism, newer generation mechanical prosthesis) categories for anticoagulation. They recommend:

- Low molecular weight heparin (LMWH) or unfractionated heparin (UFH) between 6 and 12 weeks, warfarin [maintaining a target international normalized ratio (INR) of 2–3] between weeks 12 and 36, and then switching to LMWH or UFH after 36 weeks; or
- Dose-adjusted UFH throughout pregnancy (intravenously continuous or subcutaneously); or
- Dose-adjusted LMWH throughout pregnancy.

Table 9 lists combined approach for anticoagulation prophylaxis in women with prosthetic heart valves during pregnancy.[10-12]

Warfarin achieves good anticoagulation but crosses the placental barrier. The incidence of warfarin embryopathy is 4–10%, and the risk is highest when it is administered during 6–12 weeks. Risks include fetal abnormalities such as nasal hypoplasia, hypertelorism, prominence of frontal bones, short stature, and abnormalities of central nervous system, mental retardation, and stippling of epiphysis of long bones (chondrodysplasia punctata).

Unfractionated heparin does not cross the placenta and is safer for the fetus but is associated with maternal osteoporosis, hemorrhage, and thrombocytopenia. UFH can be administered parenterally or subcutaneously throughout the duration of pregnancy; dose adjustment is based on an activated partial thromboplastin time (aPTT) of 2.0–3.0 times the control level.

Low molecular weight heparin produces a more predictable anticoagulant response than UFH and is less likely to cause heparin induced thrombocytopenia (HITT) and osteoporosis and has a superior subcutaneous absorption, bioavailability, and a longer half-life. Postdelivery when the risk of hemorrhage has passed, heparin is restarted after 6 hours of normal delivery and 12 hours after cesarean section. Warfarin is restarted as it is safe in breastfeeding with overlap with heparin, till the desired INR of 2–3 is attained with warfarin.

Cardiomyopathies

Peripartum Cardiomyopathy

Peripartum cardiomyopathy (PPCM) is a form of idiopathic dilated cardiomyopathy diagnosed by unexplained left ventricular systolic dysfunction, confirmed echocardiographically, presenting during the last antepartum month or in the first five postpartum months. The exact etiology of PPCM is not known, but viral myocarditis and autoimmune phenomena have been proposed as possible causes. Clinical definition of PPCM includes the following:[13]

- Heart failure within last month of pregnancy or 5 months postpartum
- Absence of prior heart disease
- No determinable cause for cardiac failure
- Strict echocardiographic indication of left ventricular dysfunction:
  - Ejection fraction (EF) <45% or fractional shortening <30% or both
  - End-diastolic dimension >2.7 cm/s/m^2 body surface area.

Peripartum cardiomyopathy usually manifests as heart failure, arrhythmias and embolic events also occur. Diagnosis rests on the echocardiographic identification of new left ventricular systolic dysfunction during a limited period around parturition, when other causes of cardiomyopathy have been excluded. Bed rest, dietary salt restriction, diuretics, digitalis, and anticoagulant are important interventions in the management of PPCM. More than half of women with PPCM

TABLE 9: Guidelines for anticoagulation in women with cardiac lesions.

Anticoagulation	Higher risk	Lower risk
Clinical factors	• First-generation PHV (e.g., Starr–Edwards, Björk–Shiley) in the mitral position • Atrial fibrillation • History of TE on anticoagulation	Second-generation PHV (e.g., St. Jude Medical, Medtronic-Hall) and any mechanical PHV in the aortic position
Option 1	Warfarin (INR 2.5–3.5) for 35 weeks, followed by IV UFH (mid-interval aPTT >2.5) or LMWH (pre-dose anti-Xa ~0.7) + ASA 80–100 mg daily, or	SC UFH (mid-interval aPTT 2.0–3.0) or LMWH (pre-dose anti-Xa ~0.6) for 12 weeks, followed by warfarin (INR 2.5–3.0) for 35 weeks, then SC UFH (mid-interval aPTT 2.0–3.0) or LMWH (pre-dose anti-Xa level ~0.6), or
Option 2	UFH (aPTT 2.5–3.5) or LMWH (pre-dose anti-Xa ~0.7) for 12 weeks, followed by warfarin (INR 2.5–3.5) to 35th week, then UFH (aPTT>2.5) or LMWH (pre-dose anti-Xa~0.7) + ASA 80–100 mg daily	SC UFH (mid-interval aPTT 2.0–3.0) or LMWH (pre-dose anti-Xa ~0.6) throughout pregnancy

(aPTT: activated partial thromboplastin time; ASA: acetylsalicylic acid; INR: international normalized ratio; IV: intravenous; LMWH: low molecular weight heparin; PHV: prosthetic heart valve; SC: subcutaneous; TE: thromboembolism; UFH: unfractionated heparin)

completely recover normal heart size and function, usually within 6 months of delivery. Complete recovery is likely in women with a left ventricular EF of >30% at diagnosis. The relapse rate during subsequent pregnancies is substantial in women with evidence of persisting cardiac enlargement or left ventricular dysfunction. The EurObservational Research Programme international PPCM registry has provided new information on PPCM in which the predisposing factors include multiparity, African ethnicity, smoking, diabetes, prior PPCM, eclampsia, malnutrition, advanced age, and teenage pregnancy. The cause is uncertain but probable etiologies are inflammation and vascular damage due to biologically active 16-kDa prolactin and other factors, such as soluble fms-like tyrosine kinase 1 (sFlt1), which may initiate and drive the process. Based on these reports, bromocriptine (2.5 mg once daily) for at least 1 week may be used in uncomplicated cases, whereas prolonged treatment (2.5 mg twice daily for 2 weeks, then 2.5 mg once daily for 6 weeks) may be considered in patients with EF <25% and/or cardiogenic shock.[14] Bromocriptine treatment is accompanied by anticoagulation with heparin, LMWH, or unfractionated heparin, at least in prophylactic dosages. The important steps of treatment for patients with acute PPCM have been summarized as bromocriptine, oral heart failure therapies, anticoagulants, vasorelaxing agents, and diuretics (BOARD).

Hypertrophic Cardiomyopathy

The observed incidence of hypertrophic cardiomyopathy (HCM) in pregnancy is <1:1000 and the same risk stratifications as for nonpregnant women are recommended. In patients with HCM, it is recommended that β-blockers are continued in women who used them before pregnancy. Cardioversion should be considered for persistent atrial fibrillation in patients with hypertrophic obstructive cardiomyopathy (HOCM).

Arrhythmias in Pregnancy

Premature atrial or ventricular complexes, or both, are the most common arrhythmias during pregnancy. They are not associated with adverse maternal or fetal outcomes and do not require antiarrhythmic therapy. Supraventricular tachyarrhythmia (SVT) is also common and can be terminated by vagal maneuvers (carotid sinus massage) or IV drugs such as adenosine, verapamil, or diltiazem **(Table 10)**. Women with a history of prepregnancy tachyarrhythmias have a high likelihood of recurrence during pregnancy and also

TABLE 10: Characteristics of antiarrhythmic drugs in pregnancy.

Drug	Vaughan–Williams class	FDA risk category*	Potential adverse effects	Teratogenic	Use during lactation
Quinidine	IA	C	Thrombocytopenia, ototoxicity, and torsades de pointes	No	Compatible but caution advised
Procainamide	IA	C	Drug-induced lupus and torsades de pointes	No	Compatible for short-term use
Disopyramide	IA	C	Uterine contractions	No	Compatible
Lidocaine and mexiletine	IB	B	Bradycardia, CNS adverse effects	No	Compatible
Flecainide	IC	C	Well tolerated in structurally normal hearts	No	Compatible
Propafenone	IC	C	Same as flecainide	No	Not known
Propranolol and metoprolol	II	C	Bradycardia, growth retardation, and apnea	No	Compatible
Atenolol	II	D	Hypospadias (first trimester), birth defects, low birth weight, bradycardia and hypoglycemia in fetus (second and third trimesters)	No	No
Amiodarone	III	D	Fetal hypothyroidism, growth retardation, prematurity	Yes	Avoid
Dronedarone	III	X	Vascular and limb abnormalities, cleft palate	Yes	Contraindicated
Verapamil and diltiazem	IV	C	Maternal hypotension, fetal bradycardia	No	Compatible
Adenosine	N/A	C	Dyspnea, bradycardia	No	Unknown
Digoxin	N/A	C	Low birth weight	No	Compatible

(CNS: central nervous system; FDA: Food and Drug Administration)

an increased risk of adverse fetal complications, including premature birth, low birth weight, respiratory distress syndrome, and death.

Congenital Heart Disease

Most women who enter pregnancy with congenital heart disease can be reassured that pregnancy will not significantly increase their risk of morbidity or mortality. Only women with complex heart disease will require very close monitoring by both obstetricians and cardiologists. Women with any type of congenital heart disease should be advised of the risk that their offspring may also be affected, and fetal echocardiography is recommended. The heart can usually be visualized at 16–18 weeks and abnormalities can be detected as early as 18–20 weeks.

Left-to-Right Shunts

These shunts are well-tolerated in pregnancy but the main problem is that these shunts may cause pulmonary hypertension with reversal of shunt and production of cyanosis. Therefore, these patients should be evaluated by echocardiography before or during pregnancy to rule out pulmonary hypertension.

- *Atrial septal defect (ASD)* is the most common congenital lesion recognized in adult life. Pregnancy is generally well-tolerated. Secondary pulmonary hypertension may develop in a small subset of these patients by the time they reach adulthood. This, in turn, could lead to reversal of the shunt, cyanosis, and increased morbidity and mortality.
- *Ventricular septal defect (VSD)* is present in 1.5–2.5 of 1,000 women with a pregnancy resulting in a live birth. Many of these defects close spontaneously or are surgically corrected before childbirth. Pregnancy is usually well-tolerated in women with corrected VSD, although thorough evaluation for evidence of pulmonary hypertension is needed in patients with delayed closure or no closure of VSD.
- *Patent ductus arteriosus (PDA)* is rarely seen during pregnancy because most of these cases are corrected during childhood; the outcome of pregnancy is determined by presence or absence of pulmonary hypertension.

Right-to-Left Shunts

These shunts are characterized by passage of deoxygenated blood into the systemic circulation resulting in cyanosis and require surgical correction in childhood to permit survival. Pregnancy outcome in uncorrected cyanotic heart disease is poor as severe maternal hypoxemia is likely to lead to miscarriage, preterm delivery, or fetal deaths.

- *Tetralogy of Fallot (TOF)* is the most common cyanotic heart lesion that permits survival into adulthood. The severity of this condition is inversely proportional to the systemic vascular resistance and therefore it worsens in pregnancy due to decrease in systemic vascular resistance. This leads to further cyanosis which causes a compensatory rise in hematocrit, and a corresponding decrease in arterial oxygen saturation. Prognosis is poor for patients whose shunting is of such a degree as to result in a hematocrit 60% or more or an arterial oxygen saturation of <80%.
- *Ebstein anomaly* is an uncommon and represents approximately 1% of all congenital cardiac lesions. Cases with Ebstein anomaly of the tricuspid valve may reach the reproductive age group. In these patients, right ventricular failure from volume overload and appearance or worsening of cyanosis are common during pregnancy; in the absence of cyanosis, pregnancy is well-tolerated.
- *Eisenmenger syndrome*: It is an acquired elevation of pulmonary vascular resistance and pulmonary artery pressure (PAP) as a result of a left-to-right intracardiac shunt, which eventually results in a right-to-left or bidirectional shunt, with subsequent cyanosis and polycythemia.[15] It is usually associated with congenital abnormalities but can also occur as a consequence of pulmonary hypertension secondary to any etiology. Miscarriage, intrauterine growth restriction, premature labor, and high perinatal mortality rate is seen in these patients. Despite advances in cardiology, the mortality rate in women affected with Eisenmenger syndrome has shown little improvement, and pregnancy is contraindicated in these patients. Preconception discussion with a pulmonary hypertension specialist regarding pulmonary vasodilator therapy during pregnancy is important if women conceive, as some vasodilators are teratogenic (Bosentan). Pregnant woman with Eisenmenger syndrome should receive coordinated care which includes a congenital heart disease specialist, pulmonary hypertension specialist, high-risk obstetrician, and an obstetric anesthetist. Management of volume status is extremely important as hypovolemia can lead to increased right-to-left shunting, reduced cardiac output, and refractory hypoxemia. Similarly, hypervolemia should also be avoided as it cannot be accommodated by the compromised pulmonary vascular bed and/or right ventricle and can result in heart failure and increasing right-to-left shunt. Underlying pulmonary thromboembolic disease is common, even in nonpregnant women and thromboprophylaxis is essential if the patient is relatively immobile. Successful vaginal and cesarean deliveries have been reported and decision regarding mode of delivery should be based on the individual patient and the local obstetrical experience. Isolated case reports have suggested a more favorable maternal outcome with the use of pulmonary vasodilators such as IV epoprostenol (Prostaglandin I$_2$) and inhaled nitric oxide.

The primary anesthetic goal is to avoid hemodynamic changes that might increase the right-to-left shunt and thereby increase hypoxemia. The risk of mortality risk is high in the postpartum period and many experts advise an extended postpartum period of monitoring in hospital.

Primary Pulmonary Hypertension

Primary pulmonary hypertension is defined clinically by a persistently elevated PAP, mean pressure >25 mm Hg at rest, without an obvious etiology. The maternal mortality associated with primary pulmonary hypertension ranges from 30 to 56%. Preterm delivery is indicated for maternal reasons in the majority of cases, and associated neonatal morbidity and mortality is high. Maternal deaths occur in the last trimester and in the postpartum period due to sudden cardiac collapse. These patients should be advised against getting pregnant and should be treated in the similar way as patients with Eisenmenger syndrome.

Coronary Artery Disease

Ischemic heart disease during pregnancy is rare, occurring in 1 in 10,000 pregnancies. The various independent predictors of AMI during pregnancy include chronic hypertension, maternal age, diabetes, and preeclampsia. The various differential diagnosis of ischemic chest pain must include hemorrhage, sickle cell crisis, preeclampsia, acute pulmonary emboli, and aortic dissection. Maternal mortality is considered highest in the antepartum and intrapartum periods. **Table 11** lists the electrocardiogram (ECG) changes in normal pregnancy and in myocardial infarction. Cardiac-specific troponin I and troponin T are the biomarkers of choice for diagnosing myocardial infarction, however, a negative troponin at presentation does not exclude cardiac damage as it can take 12 hours for the level to peak. However, other cardiac markers—myoglobin, creatinine kinase, creatinine kinase isoenzyme MB—can be increased significantly in labor. Treatment of myocardial infarction is similar to that of nonpregnant patients and drugs such as streptokinase and tissue plasminogen activator can be used. Although reports of abruption and neonatal intracranial bleeding are seen with these drugs but maternal well-being is more important than fetal well-being. The administration of intramuscular or IV ergometrine to induce uterine contractions postpartum is associated with myocardial infarction due to coronary artery spasm and should be avoided. The various percutaneous coronary interventions using both balloon angioplasty and stenting have been successfully performed in pregnant patients with AMI, with the use of lead shielding to protect the fetus. If permissible, delivery should be delayed by 2–3 weeks following AMI because of the increased risk of maternal mortality during this time.

Diseases of the Aorta

Coarctation of the Aorta

Coarctation of the aorta has a prevalence of 0.3–1 in 1,000 in the female population. Uncomplicated, uncorrected aortic coarctation carries a low maternal mortality risk (3%), but this risk is higher with coexisting hypertension or other cardiac anomalies. Typical findings include hypertension in the upper extremities but normal or reduced pressure in the lower extremities. The most severe complication is aortic dissection and rupture, particularly in the third trimester; other complications include congestive heart failure and bacterial endocarditis.

Aortic Dissection

Aortic dissection may occur acutely in pregnancy in association with severe hypertension due to preeclampsia, coarctation of the aorta, or connective tissue diseases such as Marfan syndrome, Ehlers–Danlos syndrome, Turner syndrome, and Noonan syndrome. Although rare, aortic dissection occurring during pregnancy accounts for 50% of all dissections in women under the age of 40 years. The mother typically presents with severe chest or interscapular pain associated with end-organ ischemia and/or acute heart failure secondary to acute aortic incompetence or hemopericardium and tamponade. Diagnosis is made by transthoracic echocardiography and computed tomography (CT). The maternal mortality is as high as 25% and fetal mortality is still higher.

Specific Syndromes

Marfan Syndrome

Marfan syndrome is rare, with an incidence of 5/100,000. It is inherited as an autosomal dominant trait with a high degree of penetrance. Aortic dilatation and dissecting aneurysm are the most serious abnormalities and death is due to valvular insufficiency and heart failure or due to dissecting aneurysm. Prenatal diagnosis is possible by genetic linkage and patients should be counseled regarding the risk of autosomal dominant

TABLE 11: Electrocardiogram (ECG) changes in pregnancy and acute myocardial infarction.

Normal changes in pregnancy	Acute myocardial infarction
• 15–20° left axis shift • ST segment depression • T-wave inversion in inferior and lateral leads • Small Q wave • Inverted T wave in lead III Q wave in lead aVF inverted T waves in V1, V2, and occasionally V3	• ST elevation • ST depression • Symmetrical T wave inversion • Newly developed Q waves

inheritance and the need for follow-up for their offspring. The management of patients should start preconceptionally and current recommendations call for prophylactic surgery in cases of ascending aortic dilatation >50 mm for patients with Marfan syndrome. Vaginal delivery is safe in those patients who have no significant cardiovascular involvement and normal aortic diameter (<40 mm). Patients with aortic dilatation ≥40 mm, progressive dilatation of the aorta during pregnancy, or a history of aortic repair for prior dissection are at high risk for aortic dissection and should therefore have an elective cesarean section with epidural or general anesthesia to minimize hemodynamic changes associated with vaginal delivery. In case of an urgent need for surgery and to prevent unfavorable fetal outcome, an immediate cesarean section followed by cardiac surgery is recommended.

Bicuspid Aortic Valve

Aortic dilatation occurs in ≤50% of patients with a bicuspid aortic valve and occurs in the distal ascending aorta. This is visualized by echocardiography or if not visualized, then magnetic resonance imaging (MRI) or CT should be performed prepregnancy. The risk of dissection is small and the risk factors are the type of bicuspid aortic valve morphology, aortic dilatation, and coarctation of the aorta. Pregnancy should be avoided when the aorta diameter is >50 mm.

Vascular Ehlers–Danlos Syndrome

The IV Ehlers–Danlos syndrome (vascular) is associated with serious vascular complications. With significant maternal mortality, and is also associated with uterine rupture and dissection of major arteries and veins. Pregnancy is therefore considered as a very high risk and is not advised.

Turner Syndrome

Turner syndrome is associated with an increased risk of congenital heart disease, aortic dilatation, hypertension, diabetes, and atherosclerotic events. Turner's mosaics patients can conceive spontaneously (0.5–10%), but pregnancy is now most commonly secondary to assisted fertility techniques. Cardiovascular evaluation is recommended before starting fertility treatment.

Cardiac Transplantation

Women who underwent cardiac transplantation tolerate pregnancy well provided the function of the transplant was stable before pregnancy. A transplanted heart is denervated and thus free from the control of the autonomic nervous system. Therefore, the transplant responds to pregnancy-related hemodynamic changes through atypical adaptive mechanisms. Complications in such pregnancies are related to the immunosuppressive therapy and include hypertension, preeclampsia, infections, and episodes of acute rejection in the mother, and fetal risks related to immunosuppressive therapy includes spontaneous abortions, stillbirth, congenital malformations, prematurity, low birth weight, and infection. A cardiac transplant in a pregnant woman is not in itself an indication for cesarean section. The choice between spontaneous delivery and cesarean section is made on the basis of both maternal and fetal status.

Cardiac Valve Surgery

Cardiac valve surgery is a difficult and complex undertaking in the pregnant patient. Although the use of cardiopulmonary bypass techniques promotes high flow rates and warm perfusion temperatures, there is still a high incidence of fetal distress, growth retardation, or wastage. If possible, surgery should be delayed until the fetus is viable and a cesarean section can be performed as part of a concomitant procedure. Surgery is recommended only in the setting of medically refractory symptoms.

Assisted-reproductive Therapy in Cardiac Patients

Assisted reproductive techniques in cardiac patients entail additional risks on top of the underlying risk of pregnancy. Ovarian hyperstimulation syndrome (OHSS) leads to significant fluid shifts and an increased risk of thrombosis. Single embryo transfer is the preferred technique in women with heart disease because multiple pregnancies are associated with significantly more complications than singleton pregnancies.[16] Fertility treatment is contraindicated in women with modified World Health Organization (mWHO) class IV.

■ CONCLUSION

The pathways for early detection, appropriate referral to specialist centers, and timely delivery with multidisciplinary support can minimize the serious consequences of poorly controlled heart disease in pregnancy. A close collaboration between the maternal-fetal medicine specialist and the cardiologist is important in order to optimize best maternal and neonatal outcome. Labor, delivery, and the immediate postpartum period are associated with significant hemodynamic challenges and patients should be monitored throughout. Although minority of patients with severe disease requires medical or surgical therapy before pregnancy, and for those with lesions where pregnancy is contraindicated, pregnancy usually has a successful outcome.

■ KEY MESSAGES

Cardiac disorders complicate 1–4% of pregnancies, and are responsible for significant maternal morbidity and mortality. Patients with preexisting cardiac lesions should be counseled in advance about the risk of pregnancy. Risk stratification should use available scores; pregnancy is contraindicated in severe pulmonary hypertension, Eisenmenger syndrome, severe uncorrected valvular stenosis, and Marfan syndrome with abnormal aorta. Mitral stenosis (MS) is the most common valvular lesion seen in India; patients may present for the first time in pregnancy. Antibiotic prophylaxis, anticoagulation, and cardiac interventions in pregnancy should follow current recommendations. Close collaboration between obstetrician, cardiologist, anesthesiologist, and neonatologist is important in order to optimize maternal and neonatal outcomes.

REFERENCES

1. Montoya ME, Karnath BM, Ahmad M. Endocarditis during pregnancy. South Med J. 2003;96(11):1156-7.
2. Adams JQ, Alexander AM Jr. Alterations in cardiovascular physiology during labour. Obstet Gynecol. 1958;12(5):542-9.
3. Lee W. Cardiorespiratory alterations during normal pregnancy. Crit Care Clin. 1991;7(4):763-75.
4. Gelson E, Johnson M. Pregnancy outcomes: effect of maternal heart disease: Effect of heart disease on pregnancy outcomes. Expert Rev Obstet Gynecol. 2010;5(5):1-13.
5. Siu SC, Sermer M, Colman JM, Alvarez AN, Mercier LA, Morton BC, et al. Prospective multicenter study of pregnancy outcomes in women with heart disease. Circulation. 2001;104(5):515-21.
6. The Criteria Committee of the New York Heart Association. Diseases of the Heart and Blood Vessels: Nomenclature and Criteria for Diagnosis, 6th edition. Boston: Little, Brown; 1964.
7. American College of Obstetricians and Gynecologists. ACOG practice bulletin number 47, October 2003: Prophylactic antibiotics in labor and delivery. Obstet Gynecol. 2003;102(4): 875-82.
8. ACC/AHA guidelines for the management of patients with valvular heart disease: A report of the ACC/AHA Task Force on Practice Guidelines (Committee on Management of Patients with Valvular Heart Disease). J Am Coll Cardiol. 1998;32(5):1486-588.
9. European Society of Gynecology (ESG); Association for European Paediatric Cardiology (AEPC); German Society for Gender Medicine (DGesGM); Regitz-Zagrosek V, Lundqvist CB, et al. ESC Guidelines on the management of cardiovascular diseases during pregnancy, The Task Force on the Management of Cardiovascular Diseases during Pregnancy of the European Society of Cardiology (ESC). Eur Heart J. 2011;32(24):3147-97.
10. Bonow RO, Carabello B, DeLeaon AC, Edmunds Jr LH, Fedderly BJ, Freed MD, et al. ACC/AHA guidelines for the management of patients with valvular heart disease. J Am Coll Cardiol. 1998;32(5):1486-588.
11. Bates SM, Greer IA, Hirsh J, Ginsberg JC. Use of antithrombotic agents during pregnancy: the seventh ACCP conference on antithrombotic and thrombolytic therapy. Chest. 2004;126:627S-44S.
12. Elkayam U, Singh H, Irani A, Akhter MW. Anticoagulation in pregnant women with prosthetic heart valve. J Cardiovasc Pharmacol Ther. 2004;9(2):107-15.
13. Hibbard JU, Lindheimer M, Lang RM. A modified definition for peripartum cardiomyopathy and prognosis based on echocardiography. Obstet Gynecol. 1999;94(2):311-6.
14. Arrigo M, Blet A, Mebazaa A. Bromocriptine for the treatment of peripartum cardiomyopathy: welcome on BOARD. Eur Heart J. 2017;38(35):2680-2.
15. Wood P. The Eisenmenger syndrome or pulmonary hypertension with reversed central shunt. I. Br Med J. 1958;2(5099):755-62.
16. Sliwa K, Mebazaa A, Hilfiker-Kleiner D, Petrie MC, Maggioni AP, Laroche C, et al. Clinical characteristics of patients from the worldwide registry on peripartum cardiomyopathy (PPCM): EURObservational Research Programme in conjunction with the Heart Failure Association of the European Society of Cardiology Study Group on PPCM. Eur J Heart Fail. 2017;19(9): 1131-41.

LONG QUESTIONS

1. Describe the hemodynamic changes in the cardiovascular system in pregnancy.
2. A 24-year-old primigravida, known case of rheumatic heart disease with severe mitral stenosis with mitral valve replacement done 2 years ago, presents to the antenatal outpatient department (OPD) at 7 weeks of gestation. Describe anticoagulation during the course of her pregnancy till the postpartum period, monitoring during treatment, and warfarin embryopathy.
3. Describe the role of infective endocarditis prophylaxis in pregnancy.
4. A 28-year-old G2P1 A0L1 with 9 months amenorrhea, known case of moderate mitral stenosis with mitral valve area of 1.8 cm^2 presents to the emergency department in true labor. Describe the management of this patient in labor. What contraceptive advice will you give her postdelivery?
5. Define peripartum cardiomyopathy. What are the clinical features, diagnostic criteria, and management of a case of peripartum cardiomyopathy?

SHORT QUESTIONS

1. Peripartum cardiomyopathy.
2. Warfarin embryopathy.
3. Role of anticoagulation in pregnant patients with prosthetic heart valves.
4. Eisenmenger syndrome in pregnancy.
5. Describe diseases of the aorta in pregnancy.
6. Briefly describe the symptomatology and evaluation of cardiac disease in pregnancy.
7. What is the importance and role of preconceptional counseling in cardiac patients?
8. Coronary artery disease in pregnancy.
9. Arrhythmias in pregnancy.

MULTIPLE CHOICE QUESTIONS

1. Maximum strain to the parturient heart occurs during:
   a. At term
   b. Immediate postpartum
   c. First trimester
   d. Second trimester
2. In a pregnant woman with heart disease all of the following should be done, except:
   a. Cut short second stage of labor
   b. Infective endocarditis prophylaxis
   c. IV methergin after delivery
   d. IV furosemide postpartum

3. Normal pregnancy can be continued in:
   a. Primary pulmonary hypertension
   b. Eisenmenger syndrome
   c. Tachyarrhythmias
   d. Marfan syndrome with aortic root dilatation >45 mm
4. Most common heart disease associated with pregnancy is:
   a. Mitral stenosis
   b. Mitral regurgitation
   c. Atrial septal defect
   d. Tetralogy of Fallot
5. Most common heart lesion in developed countries is:
   a. Congenital heart disease
   b. Rheumatic heart disease
   c. Ischemic heart disease
   d. Arrhythmias
6. All are correct about management of heart disease during labor, except:
   a. Minimal trial of labor
   b. Cut short the second stage of labor
   c. Lower segment caesarian section (LSCS) for obstetric indication
   d. Elective induction at 38 weeks
7. A para 2, poorly compensated cardiac patient has delivered 2 days ago. Contraception advice to her will be:
   a. Undergo immediate puerperal tubal ligation
   b. To insert intrauterine contraceptive device (IUCD) after 6 weeks
   c. Take combined oral contraceptive pills after 6 months
   d. Counsel the husband to undergo vasectomy
8. A 24-year-old pregnant woman is detected with a diastolic murmur in the mitral area. Echocardiography reveals a valve area of 0.8 cm². The most likely cause of her murmur is:
   a. Mild mitral stenosis
   b. Severe mitral stenosis
   c. Functional murmur
   d. Mammary soufflé
9. Normal mitral valve area is:
   a. 6–7 cm²
   b. 2–3 cm²
   c. 4–5 cm²
   d. 1–2 cm²
10. A pregnant patient with a prosthetic valve who is on oral anticoagulant therapy should be switched over to heparin at:
    a. 28 weeks
    b. 32 weeks
    c. 36 weeks
    d. 40 weeks
11. Infective endocarditis prophylaxis is required in:
    a. Mitral valve prolapse without regurgitation
    b. Surgically corrected ASD
    c. VSD
    d. Prosthetic valves
12. Incidence of heart disease in pregnancy is:
    a. 1–3%
    b. 4–6%
    c. 6–8%
    d. 8–10%

Answers
1. b 2. c 3. c 4. a 5. a 6. d
7. d 8. b 9. c 10. c 11. d 12. a

5.3 DIABETES MELLITUS

Sujata Misra

■ INTRODUCTION

Diabetes is a metabolic disorder marked by high levels of blood glucose due to defects in insulin production, insulin action, or both. Its incidence is 2–5% of all pregnancies. 90% of these are detected during pregnancy (gestational diabetes mellitus/GDM), the rest are pregestational and referred to as pregnancy with pregestational diabetes mellitus (PGDM). Gestational diabetes is covered in another chapter in the textbook.

■ CLASSIFICATION

Women with diabetes prior to conception are designated as pregestational/overt diabetics.

Diabetes in pregnancy is classified in **Box 1**.

■ CARBOHYDRATE METABOLISM DURING PREGNANCY

Maternal Physiology

Major hormonal changes occurring in pregnancy readjust the carbohydrate metabolism in order to maintain a supply of nutrients to the developing fetus. This results in reduced blood levels of fasting blood sugar and amino acids, and raised postprandial blood sugar, free fatty acids, ketones, and triglyceride with increased insulin secretion in response to glucose in normal nondiabetic pregnant women. This diabetogenic state of pregnancy is due to the production of placental somatomammotropins; increased production of cortisol, estriol and progesterone, and increased destruction of insulin by the placental insulinase. Increased lipolysis and altered neoglucogenesis too add to it.

> **BOX 1:** Diabetes in pregnancy.
>
> *Type 1 diabetes* [previously called insulin-dependent diabetes mellitus (IDDM) or juvenile-onset diabetes], It is characterized by β-cell destruction and an absolute insulin deficiency:
> - Immune mediated
> - Idiopathic
> - Immune mediated
> - Idiopathic
>
> *Type 2 diabetes* (previously called noninsulin-dependent diabetes mellitus—NIDDM or adult-onset diabetes). The defect may be in insulin secretion or due to increased insulin resistance
>
> *Gestational diabetes* (glucose intolerance diagnosed during pregnancy)
>
> Gestational diabetes can be further subdivided into A_1 or A_2 depending on their fasting and 2-hour plasma glucose levels
>
> A_1 Fasting plasma glucose level <105 mg/dL and 2-hour plasma glucose < 120 mg/dL
>
> A_2 Fasting plasma glucose level >105 mg/dL and 2-hour plasma glucose > 120 mg/dL
>
> *IV other types* of diabetes resulting from specific genetic conditions (such as maturity-onset diabetes of youth), surgery, medications, infections, pancreatic disease, and other illnesses

TABLE 1: Effect of maternal diabetes on the mother and fetus.

Fetus	Mother
Still birth	Miscarriage
Macrosomia	Polyhydramnios
Congenital abnormalities	Infection—pyelonephritis, UTI, *Monilia*
Hypoglycemia	Preeclampsia
Vaginitis	Preterm labor
Hyperviscosity syndrome	Intraoperative interference
Hyaline membrane disease	Puerperal sepsis
Hypercalcemia	Failing lactation
Increased perinatal morbidity/mortality	Medical complication—hypoglycemia, nephropathy, retinopathy, and neuropathy

(UTI: urinary tract infection)

In early pregnancy (till 20 weeks), the rising estrogen level stimulates pancreatic insulin secretion, improves peripheral utilization of glucose resulting in a decrease in fasting glucose levels, improved glucose tolerance, and an increase in tissue glycogen storage. In later pregnancy, increased production of insulin antagonists (human placental lactogen, prolactin, cortisol, human growth hormone, and progesterone) leads to increased blood glucose levels and increased levels of basal levels of insulin in the second half of pregnancy. In addition, the increased binding of insulin to adipocytes and hepatocytes results in insulin resistance due to postreceptor mechanism. Women unable to cope with these changes develop gestational diabetes.

As a result of these physiologic changes in pregnancy, the normal fasting blood glucose is 65 ± 9 mg/dL and the mean nonfasting levels are 80 ± 10 mg/dL. Postprandial elevation usually never exceeds 140 mg/dL.

Fetal Physiology

Fetal pancreatic insulin secretion commences between 9 and 11 weeks of gestation in response to glucose and amino acid stimulation. While glucose is transported across the placenta by facilitated diffusion, amino acids are actively transported. The fetus preferentially uses alanine, and this deprives the mother of a major neoglucogenic substrate. Ketones readily diffuse across the placenta while free fatty acids undergo gradient-dependent diffusion. The fetal brain and liver oxidize ketones for use. Free insulin and glucagon in maternal circulation do not cross the placental barrier, but glucose crosses in a gradient-dependent manner: higher the maternal blood glucose level, greater is the transplacental transport to the fetus.

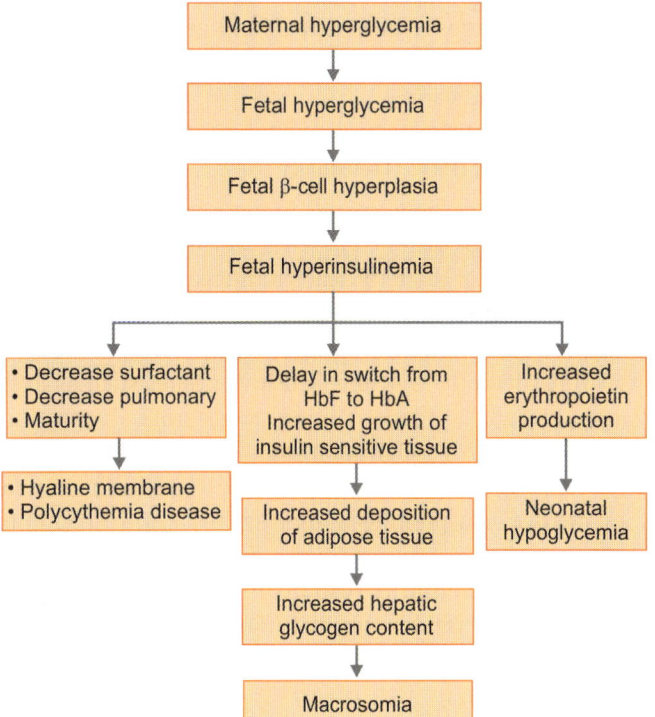

Flowchart 1: Complications of fetal hyperinsulinemia.

■ EFFECT OF DIABETIC STATE ON PREGNANCY

The effect of uncontrolled diabetic state on pregnancy is multifold **(Table 1)** due to a tendency toward metabolic instability and hence needs frequent monitoring, strict therapy and a well-regulated life style. The importance of maintaining a euglycemic state of pregnancy is mandatory to prevent fetal hyperinsulinemia and its attendant complications **(Flowchart 1)**.

TABLE 2: Factors influencing congenital malformations.

Glucose control	Incidence of congenital malformations
Normoglycemia at conception	2–3%
Hypercalcemia at conception	6–12%
HbA1c < 8.5%	2.4
HbA1c > 8.5%	22.4%
Overt diabetics without vascular disease	1.6%
Overt diabetes with vascular disease	6.8%

First Trimester

Hyperglycemia in the mother leads to fetal hyperglycemia, which if present at the time of organogenesis (2-8 weeks) is associated with increased prevalence of congenital malformations. Major defects include anencephaly, spina bifida, and caudal regression. Malformation rate is related to the severity of maternal hyperglycemia, early onset of disease, vasculopathy, genetic susceptibility, ketoacidosis, hypoxia, generation of free oxygen radical, and genotoxicity in the teratogenic 1 period **(Table 2)** and tight glycemic control can reduce this significantly.

Second and Third Trimester

Poor control of diabetes results in increased transportation of glucose and other nutrients across the placenta. Hyperglycemia in the fetus leads to increased β-cell insulin secretion resulting in fetal hyperinsulinemia. Hyperglycemia along with other nutrients is responsible for accelerated fetal growth particularly in insulin sensitive tissues such as liver, muscle, and adipose tissue causing macrosomia. Macrosomia is defined as birth weight that exceeds 90th percentile for gestational age or >4,000 g. It predisposes to birth trauma, shoulder dystocia, prolonged labor, asphyxia, and meconium aspiration.

Hyperinsulinemia is responsible for neonatal hypoglycemia as well as poor lung maturation causing respiratory distress in the newborn. The other fetal and neonatal effects are intrauterine growth retardation (20%), intrauterine death (last 4 weeks), hyperbilirubinemia, and polycythemia (33% of neonates). Uncontrolled diabetes also causes hypomagnesemia and hypocalcemia in the neonate.

EFFECT OF PREGNANCY ON DIABETES

The effect of pregnancy on diabetes is largely dependent upon the optimal control of blood glucose levels. Uncontrolled glucose levels result in an increased risk of complications such as diabetic cardiomyopathy, nephropathy, and retinopathy. The association of proteinuria, raised serum creatinine (>1.5 mg/dL), hypertension, and ketoacidosis prior to 20 weeks of gestation too have an adverse effect on perinatal outcome.

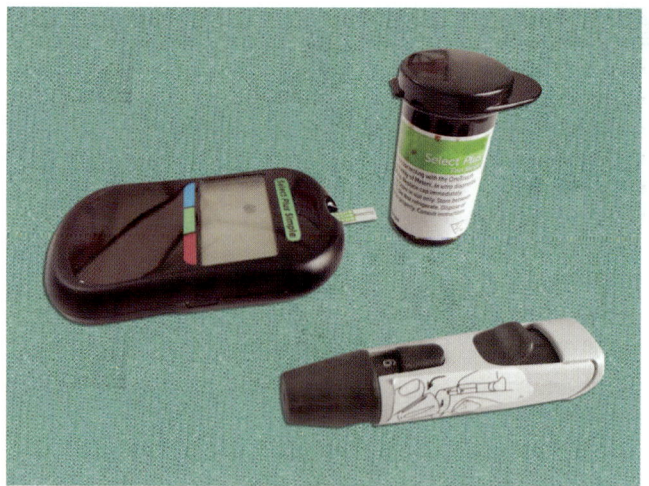

Fig. 1: Glucometer.

PRECONCEPTIONAL COUNSELING AND CARE

Good metabolic control is the key to prevent adverse outcome and in PGDM, this has to be achieved prior to planning pregnancy. It is important to inform and counsel diabetic women planning a pregnancy, about the importance of maintaining good blood glucose control **(Fig. 1)** before conception and throughout pregnancy.

- Diabetic women should be counseled regarding the role of diet, body weight, exercise, and good blood glucose control.
- Dietary advice should be individualized along with the required supplementations (especially folic acid 5 mg/day to reduce the risk of a neural tube defect in the baby).
- Women with uncontrolled diabetes, planning a pregnancy, should be assessed for diabetic retinopathy and diabetic nephropathy in addition to controlling blood sugar before becoming pregnant. Their glycated hemoglobin (HbA1C) levels should be monitored and aimed to be below 6.5% prior to planning pregnancy.
- Diabetic women with a body mass index (BMI) above 27 kg/m^2 should be advised to lose weight before planning pregnancy. Advise diabetic women, who are planning a pregnancy, to take folic acid (5 mg/day) until 12 weeks of gestation to reduce the risk of having a baby with a neural tube defect.
- While insulin and metformin are used during pregnancy, a suitable alternative to other hypoglycemic drugs should be advised.

MANAGEMENT OF THE PREGNANT DIABETIC WOMAN

Every effort should be made to achieve euglycemia throughout pregnancy to. This requires a multidisciplinary approach with a healthcare team **(Box 2)**.

> **BOX 2:** Healthcare team for diabetic pregnancy.
> - Diabetologist
> - Obstetrician
> - Diabetes specialist nurse
> - Dietitian
> - Neonatal pediatrician
> - Motivated patient

The main principles of management are:
- Good glycemic control
- Prevention of obstetric complications
- Early detection and prompt treatment of medical problems
- Optimal time and mode of delivery
- Arrangement for the care of the newborn
- Advice on contraception
- Postpartum check of glucose levels

GLYCEMIC CONTROL DURING PREGNANCY

Glycemic control during pregnancy is achieved by modifications in the diet, insulin dose and regimen, and appropriate advice on exercise. A carefully selected insulin regimen and home blood glucose monitoring have revolutionized the achievement and maintenance of euglycemia. Capillary blood glucose should be measured before and 90–120 minutes after each meal and occasionally at 3 AM to detect asymptomatic hypoglycemia. The 7-point monitoring is helpful though not very convenient for all. Targets of premeal capillary glucose should be between 60 and 90 mg/dL and about 120 mg/dL after meal.

Diet

A regulated diet is a prerequisite to allow predictable and smooth glycemic control. The diet should consist of approximately 40% of complex carbohydrates, 30% of fats with saturated fats restricted to 10%.

Exercise

Exercise improves both hepatic glucose output and peripheral glucose utilization and is particularly useful in overweight pregnant diabetics. Most advice of exercise in diabetic pregnancies has to be supervised closely. Diet and exercise may obviate the need for insulin treatment in many patients with GDM.

Insulin

Insulin therapy is still the gold standard. Due to a decrease in insulin sensitivity, the insulin requirement goes up especially during later-half of pregnancy. Requirements may range from 0.7 μ/kg/day in the first trimester to about 1.0 μ/kg/day in the third trimester. A split-mix regimen may be sufficient for few patients while most patients require multiple dose injections (MDI), i.e., intermediate- or long-acting insulin at bedtime and regular insulin before each meal. Patients of GDM may be controlled with simpler regimens.

Pharmacotherapy: Use of Oral Hypoglycemic Agents

Among the oral hypoglycemic agents, glibenclamide and metformin are the two drugs which have been extensively studied for management of GDM. The added risk of these drugs in the pregnant state are determined by the transplacental passage, association with fetal anomalies, potential for maternal adverse effects; and the safety of the medications during breastfeeding.

Glibenclamide (Category C in Pregnancy)

Glibenclamide is a second-generation oral sulfonylurea, which acts by enhancing the release of insulin from the pancreatic beta cells in normal and diabetic patients. While 1–5% of cases may have hypoglycemia with glibenclamide, the most common adverse effects are gastrointestinal (nausea, vomiting, and dyspepsia) and dermatologic (pruritus, urticaria, erythema, and maculopapular eruptions). Though elevations of liver function tests have been reported, the incidence of jaundice is rare. It is well absorbed, independent of food intake and is metabolized by the liver and time to peak concentration is 2–3 hours with a half-life of 7–10 hours.

The initial dose of glibenclamide is 2.5 mg once or twice a day and can be increased after titration with blood glucose values up to a maximum of 20 mg/day. Care should be taken that no >7.5 mg should be taken at each time. Unlike other sulfonylureas, there is substantial evidence demonstrating the lack of transplacental passage of glibenclamide to the fetus suggesting insignificant fetal exposure with this drug and its safety in pregnancy. Possible explanations for such lack of placental transport include the extensive plasma protein binding and short elimination half-life.

Metformin (Category B Medication in Pregnancy)

Metformin is a biguanide that improves insulin sensitivity and reduces both fasting and postprandial plasma glucose. It functions by decreasing hepatic glucose output by inhibition of gluconeogenesis and enhances peripheral glucose uptake in the muscles and adipose tissues. It also decreases intestinal glucose absorption and increases insulin sensitivity. It is metabolized by the CYP 450 pathway with a half-life of 6 hours and is excreted in urine. Metformin is available in 250 mg, 500 mg, 850 mg, and 1,000 mg tablets in both regular-release and extended-release forms. The usual starting dose is 500–1,000 mg/day, which can be increased gradually to a maximum dose of 2,500 mg/day. The frequently observed gastrointestinal adverse effects include diarrhea, flatulence, nausea, and vomiting, with the incidence ranging from 2 to 63%. Hence, metformin is started at a low dose and increased gradually. Hypoglycemia related to metformin may occur in 0–21% of pregnant women.

Metformin is considered to be absolutely safe for breast fed infants. The mean infant exposure to the drug is >1% of the weight-normalized maternal dose, which is much below the 10% level of concern for breastfeeding.

OTHER ORAL HYPOGLYCEMIC AGENTS

Other oral hypoglycemic agents are given in **Table 3**.

Fetal Monitoring

Fetal monitoring is essential in both GDM and pregestational diabetes. The frequency and type of testing depend upon the severity of glucose intolerance, associated medical complications, and patient compliance **(Table 4)**.

American College of Obstetricians and Gynecologists (ACOG) recommends the need of antenatal fetal monitoring in patients with pregestational diabetes, gestational diabetes with poor glycemic control, and patients with other obstetrical

TABLE 3: Other oral hypoglycemic agents.

Drug	Status
Alpha-glucosidase inhibitor, thiazolidinediones, glinides, and glucagon-like DPP4 inhibitor agonists	Considered experimental during pregnancy
Alpha-glucosidase inhibitor (acarbose)	• Delays the absorption of carbohydrate in the gut • Zarate has done a small study with 6 different pregnant women, showing efficacy of acarbose in blood sugar control without any complications • Though reported to be safe, it lacks randomized study
Glitazones	• Cause of growth restriction and fetal death in animal • Not recommended in pregnancy
Glinides have	Not been approved for use in pregnancy
DPP4 inhibitors	Have not been approved for use in pregnancy

(DPP4: dipeptidyl-peptidase 4)

TABLE 4: Fetal monitoring.

Method	Analysis
Fetal kick counting	Daily fetal movement counting is the simplest, subjective, and least expensive method for monitoring fetal well-being in second half of pregnancy. The "count 10 method" is the most commonly used one
Fetal nonstress test (NST)	NST is started at the gestational age of 32 weeks in diabetic women and done on a twice weekly basis. It should be started at 28 weeks in patients with hypertension, renal disease, and intrauterine growth restriction (IUGR). The negative predictive value of NST is 90%, but the positive predictive value varies from 50 to 70%. False positive rate of NST varies from 45 to 70% thus increasing the possibility of unnecessary and sometimes preterm delivery of a normal fetus. The test can better rule out rather than predicting fetal compromise
Biophysical profile (BPP)	Biophysical profile helps in prediction of acute and chronic tissue hypoxia. The parameters of BPP include NST, fetal gross body movements, fetal tone, breathing movements, and amniotic fluid index detected on ultrasound. Each parameter of BPP is given score of 0 or 2 depending upon the finding. Twice weekly NST and amniotic fluid index assessment can be used to prevent stillbirth in diabetic pregnancy
Ultrasonography	A detailed level II scan in second trimester is essential to rule out congenital anomalies in the fetus.[47] Fetal echo is also recommended in all patients with pregestational diabetes or gestational diabetes mellitus diagnosed in first trimester. In the third trimester, ultrasonography plays an important role for assessment for fetal growth and well-being. The main drawback of ultrasonography is the limited sensitivity to detect macrosomia. The sensitivity of ultrasonography for weight estimation in third trimester varies from 24 to 97% and specificity varies from 82 to 98%. Another method to predict weight in a macrosomic baby is serial abdominal circumference estimation.[49] Miller et al. introduced another formula to detect fetal macrosomia. The difference between fetal abdominal circumference and biparietal diameter is calculated, if it is ≥2.6 cm is diagnostic of macrosomia. Macrosomia occurs in 88% of pregnancies if estimated fetal weight and abdominal circumference both exceed 90th percentile. USG also helps in amniotic fluid assessment and dynamic fetal assessment by biophysical profile and Doppler studies. IUGR (fetal weight <10th percentile) is also seen in patients with advanced pregestational diabetes with vascular complications
Contraction stress test	This test has been used for a long time to detect fetal distress. As the test evaluates the fetal heart response to uterine contractions, it can also diagnose a chronic condition and placental perfusion. The test is performed weekly and has high negative predictive value. There are some limitations of the test. The false positive rate of test is 50–60%. It results in unnecessary preterm delivery of a normal fetus. Overall, the test is more expensive, less convenient, and less efficient than NST. So it is not used widely these days for fetal surveillance
Doppler velocimetery	Doppler studies are important especially in patients with pregestational diabetes. They are more prone to develop intrauterine growth restriction, preeclampsia, and further decreased placental perfusion. Doppler changes are calculated in terms of increased systolic diastolic ratio (S/D ratio). With increasing fetal compromise, there occurs increased S/D ratio, absent diastolic flow, and ultimately reversal of diastolic flow. Absent end-diastolic flow necessitates daily Doppler, anytime reversal of diastolic flow indicates the need of immediate termination of pregnancy

complications. Twice weekly nonstress test (NST) should be started at a gestational age of 32 weeks. In patients with IUGR and preeclampsia, testing should be started at 28 weeks of gestation.

Gestational diabetics controlled on diet alone, can be managed by fetal kick counting only starting at 32 weeks POG. NST is optional and it can be started any time between 32 and 40 weeks of gestation. Patients on oral hypoglycemia often face complications of fetal macrosomia and induction is advised at 38 completed weeks. Patients controlled on diet only with no other complication can be managed by expectant management until term.

Management during Labor and Postpartum

Patients with good metabolic control can be carried to term and a normal vaginal delivery. Patients who did not have good control can be delivered at 38 completed weeks after assessment of fetal well-being. It is advisable to deliver insulin-dependent diabetics at 38 weeks of gestation as there is little fetal benefit after 38 weeks in utero (FOGSI). The major disadvantage is the risk of failure of induction due to unfavorable cervix. Spontaneous vaginal delivery may be contemplated in the absence of other obstetric indications and fetal macrosomia. The risk of shoulder dystocia is 0.07% in vaginal deliveries of infants weighing <4,000 g and 23% in infants weighing >4,000 g.

Patients who are to be induced should not receive the morning dose of insulin or 6–10 units of an intermediate acting insulin may be given subcutaneously. Intravenous line is placed for administering oxytocin and fluids. Generally, Ringer's lactate is administered at 100 mL/h through a controlled infusion pump. Maternal capillary blood sugar should be checked hourly, and if the value is above 120 mg/dL intravenous insulin infusion can be initiated. Usually, 10 units of regular insulin is added to 100 mL of normal saline and infused in a controlled manner. Bolus dose of glucose (5 g/h of glucose) solution should be avoided. The aim is to maintain a blood glucose around 100 mg/dL.

Prior to elective cesarean section, approximately one-third of the patient's prepregnancy dose of insulin is given as intermediate-acting insulin in the morning of the day of surgery. Infusion of glucose solutions should be avoided during surgery unless there is a delay between insulin administration and surgery. In the latter event, a glucose infusion drip, as described previously, should be instituted. A neonatal pediatrician should be present to take care of newborn.

Postpartum insulin resistance is decreased and insulin requirement goes down suddenly in pregestational diabetes while GDM women may not require insulin at all. The insulin dose should be adjusted accordingly. These patients should be advised to undergo an oral glucose tolerance test (OGTT) at 6 weeks and also counseled regarding recurrence in subsequent pregnancy and increased risk of developing diabetes mellitus in later life.

The outlook for pregestational diabetics who are free of complications has improved considerably with meticulous metabolic control from preconception stage and throughout the duration of pregnancy.

Management of Diabetic Complications in Pregnancy

Pregnancy may worsen renal function in women with diabetic nephropathy. Hence, blood pressure must be kept under optimal control. Retinopathy, particularly preproliferative and proliferative may rapidly deteriorate during pregnancy especially once glycemic control is suddenly improved. Prophylactic photocoagulation should be done in such patients before planning pregnancy or early in pregnancy. Coronary heart disease also manifests more frequently in diabetic pregnancies. If known before conception, the patient should be advised against pregnancy. If detected during pregnancy, appropriate management strategies should be followed.

Management on the Infant Born from a Diabetic Pregnancy

A neonatologist should be actively involved in the management of the infant born to diabetic mothers. Broad outlines of management are summarized in **Table 5**.

Puerperal and Neonatal care

Irrespective of the women being a pregestational diabetic or gestational diabetic, appropriate puerperal and neonatal care is mandatory. Following delivery, the insulin sensitivity returns to the normal state within minutes in women with gestational diabetes. For the neonate, blood glucose should be measure within 2–4 hours of birth. If the woman was only

TABLE 5: Management of the infant of diabetic mother.

Problem	Management
Day 1	
Congenital malformations	Early detection, supportive measures, specific corrective treatment
Birth asphyxia	Supportive measures including ventilator support
Birth trauma	Early detection, specific and supportive measures
Macrosomia	Avoid birth trauma
Cardiomyopathy	Confirmation by echocardiography, supportive measures
Hypoglycemia	Intravenous glucose, glucagon/epinephrine
RDS	Prevention (avoid prematurity, corticosteroids, and surfactant therapy) supportive and ventilatory therapy
Day 2 and 3	
Hypocalcemia	Calcium and magnesium supplementation
Hyperbilirubinemia	Phototherapy, exchange transfusion
Polycythemia	Hydration, partial exchange transfusion
Renal vein thrombosis	Supportive measures, heparin (to be considered)
Long term	Increased incidence of DM
	Increased incidence of obesity

on diet control, random blood glucose is tested the day after the birth and four blood glucose levels (fasting and 2 hours postmeals for three meals) done 1 day prior to discharge. If the levels are within the normal range, blood glucose monitoring is not required further. The patient is advised regarding the diet and lifestyle modification factors (planned physical activity, weight control, and smoking cessation) and called for review after 6 weeks following delivery for a glucose challenge test.

According to American Diabetes Association (ADA) 2011, screening for diabetes should be done at 6–12 weeks postpartum according to the OGTT criteria for nonpregnant women using a 2-hour 75-g OGTT. Because women with GDM are at a considerably increased risk of developing diabetes later, lifelong screening for diabetes should be performed at least every 3 years. Diabetes in Pregnancy Study Group of India (DIPSI) group advocates the DIPSI test at 6 weeks postpartum. The longer-term risks for babies born to mothers with GDM include a doubling of the risk of developing childhood obesity and an increased risk of the child developing T2DM in adult life.

PREVENTION AND ASSESSMENT OF NEONATAL HYPOGLYCEMIA

Clinical hypoglycemia in the newborn is a complication of GDM. In Hyperglycemia and Adverse Pregnancy Outcome (HAPO) only (2.1%) infants had clinical hypoglycemia. In Australian Carbohydrate Intolerance Study in Pregnant Women (ACHOIS), the prevalence of clinical hypoglycemia was 7% in GDM receiving intervention and 5% in GDM not receiving intervention, a nonsignificant difference.

Glycemia monitoring is recommended for newborns of mothers with GDM treated with insulin or in whom the birth weight is <10th or >90th percentile. In the absence of clinical signs, glycemia monitoring must start only after the first feed or just before the second. The presence of clinical signs indicates that glycemia monitoring should be started earlier.

Blood glucose monitoring should be commenced, using accurate method, at 2–4 hours after birth. Observational data indicate that testing blood glucose within the first 2 hours of life is very likely to yield low values. It is recommended that hypoglycemia readings identified with glucose test strips be confirmed by laboratory measurement.

Breastfeeding

All women, including those with PGDM and GDM should be encouraged to exclusively breastfeed to the greatest extent possible during the first year of the infant. It encourages weight loss, is associated with better glucose tolerance and reduced incidence of future metabolic syndrome. It is associated with a lower risk of overweight and obesity during childhood.

LONG-TERM RISKS FOR BABY

The longer-term risks for babies born to mothers with diabetes include a doubling of the risk of developing childhood obesity and an increased risk of the child developing type 2 diabetes mellitus (T2DM) in adult life. Genetic predisposition for T2DM and obesity may also be inherited from one or both parents by offspring of diabetic mothers.

There is also evidence that the children of mothers with diabetes have a worse attention span, perform less well in tests of motor function and have increased risk of language impairment. The extent to which strict control of maternal blood sugars or postnatal modification in diet such as breastfeeding or bottle-feeding modifies childhood risks is unknown.

A study has found that children of diabetic mothers who were breastfed for >3 months had a 45% decrease in rates of being overweight (BMI > 90th percentile) at 2–8 years compared with those who were bottle-fed.

Contraception

Contraceptive options should be tailored to individual lifestyle and preference. The NICE postnatal care guideline 37 recommends that contraception should be discussed within the first week of birth. Diabetic women are encouraged to use copper containing intrauterine devices. The use of oral contraceptive pill is controversial as it may increase the risk of cardiovascular accidents. However, the low-dose pills can be prescribed to women who do not suffer from microvascular disease. If the woman has completed her family, she should be advised laparoscopic sterilization.

CONCLUSION

From the days of being a contraindication to having children, the overall approach and outlook to women who have diabetes has changed remarkably over the last few decades. The St Vincent declaration in 1989 stated that healthcare should be geared to realize similar pregnancy outcomes for diabetic women as their nondiabetic counterparts. There has been remarkable progress toward this goal. As a public health issue, government policies and infrastructure recognize diabetes as an important determinant and target condition for intervention. The importance of glycemic control and fetal monitoring is paramount.

FURTHER READING

1. American College of Obstetricians and Gynaecologists. Management of diabetes mellitus in pregnancy. Am Coll Obstetr Gynaecol, Technical Bulletin. 1986;92:1.
2. American diabetes association. Clinical practice recommendations 2000. Gestational Diabetes Mellitus. Diabetes care. 2000;23:77-9.
3. Bresnick G, Palta M. Predicting progression to severe proliferative diabetic retinopathy. Arch Ophthalmol. 1987;105:810.
4. Brinchmann-Hanson O, Dahl-Jorgensen K, Hanssen KF, Sandvik L. Effects of intensified insulin treatment on various lesions of diabetic retinopathy. Am J Ophthalmol. 1985;100:644.
5. Buckshee K, Rohatgi TB. Diabetes in pregnancy: Current Concepts. In: Saraiya UB, Rao KA, Chatterjee A (Eds). Principles and practice of obstetrics and gynaecology for postgraduates. New Delhi: FOGSI Publication. New Delhi: Jaypee Publishers; 2014.
6. Chang S, Fuhrmann K, Javanovic L. The diabetes in early pregnancy study group (DIEP): Pregnancy, retinopathy, normoglycaemia: A preliminary analysis. Diabetes. 1985;35(Suppl):3A.
7. Clapp JF, Rokey R, Treadway JL, Carpenter MW, Artal RM, Warrnes C. Exercise in pregnancy. Med Sci Sports Exerc. 1992;24:S294.

8. Combs CA, Cavin LA, Gunderson E, Gavin LA, Main EK. Relationship of fetal macrosomia to maternal postprandial glucose during pregnancy. Diabetes Care. 1992;15:1251.
9. Fauci AS, Braunwald E, Kasper DL, Hauser S, Longo D, Jameson JL, et al. Diabetes mellitus. In: Powers PE (Ed). Harrison's Principles of Internal medicine, 17th edition. New York: McGraw Hill Education; 2008. pp. 2275-304.
10. Fuhrmann K, Ruher H, Semmler K, Fischer F, Fischer M, Glöckner E. Prevention of congenital malformations in infants of insulin dependent diabetic mothers. Diabetes Care. 1983;6:219.
11. Girling JC, Dornhrost A. Pregnancy and diabetes mellitus. In: Pickup JC, Williams G (Eds). Textbook of Diabetes, 2nd edition. London: Blackwell Scienctific: 1997. pp. 72.1-72.34.
12. Healy K, Peterson LJ, Peterson MC. Pancreatic disorders of pregnancy-pregestational diabetes. Endocrine Metab Clin North Am. 1995;24:74-101.
13. Javonovic-peterson L, Petersonm CM, Reed G, Metzger BE, Mills JL, Knopp RH, et al. Maternal post prandial glucose levels and infant birthweight. The Diabetes in early pregnancy study. Am J Obstet Gynecol. 1991;164:103-11.
14. Jovanovic-peterson L, Peterson CM. Insulin and glucose requirements during the first stage of labour in insulin dependent diabetic women. Am J Med. 1983;75:607-12.
15. Jovanovic-peterson L. Medical management of pregnancy complicated by Diabetes. Alexandria, VA: American Diabetes Association; 1993.
16. Kitzmiller JL, Gavin LA, Gin GD, Jovanovic-Peterson L, Main EK, Zigrang WD. Preconceptual care of diabetes: Glycaemic control prevents congenital anomalies. JAMA. 1991;265:560-80.
17. Misra S. (2008). Diabetes and Pregnancy. Complication of Diabetes in Indian Scenario. [online] Available from: https://www.researchgate.net/publication/268810666_Diabetes_in_pregnancy [Last accessed December, 2021].
18. National Institute for Health and Care Excellence: Guidelines. Diabetes in pregnancy: management from preconception to the postnatal period. NICE. 2020.
19. Peterson LJ, Peterson CM. Pregnancy in the diabetic woman. Endocrine Metab Clin North Am. 1992;21:433-54.
20. Reece EA, Homko C. Management of pregnant women with diabetes. In: Lebovitz HE, DeFronzo RA, Genuth S, Kreisberg RA, Pfeifer MA, Tamborlane WV (Eds). Therapy for diabetes mellitus and related disorders, 2nd edition. Virginia: American Diabetes Association; 1994. pp. 17-24.
21. Tamas G, Kerenyi Z. Current controversies in the mechanisms and treatment of gestational diabetes mellitus. Current Diabetes Rep. 2002;2(4):337-46.

LONG QUESTIONS

1. Discuss the pathogenic effects of maternal hyperglycemia on the fetoplacental unit.
2. Discuss the management of labor and delivery in diabetic women.

SHORT QUESTIONS

1. What is the appropriate dietary distribution of macronutrients for diabetic women?
2. Which oral hypoglycemic agents can be used in pregnancy for diabetic women?
3. Name the rationale indications for cesarean section in diabetic women.
4. What are the highlights of postpartum care for diabetic women?
5. What contraceptive methods are appropriate for diabetic women?

MULTIPLE CHOICE QUESTIONS

1. Pregnancy is a diabetogenic state because of the following factors, except:
    a. Placental somatomammotropins
    b. Increased cortisol production
    c. Placental insulinase
    d. Placental estriol
2. Poor maternal glycemic control leads to:
    a. Decreased glucose transport to the fetus
    b. Increased insulin production in the fetus
    c. Future neonatal hyperglycemia
    d. Future neonatal hypercalcemia
3. The following obstetric conditions are usually associated with maternal diabetes, except:
    a. Oligohydramnios   b. Pre-eclampsia
    c. Fetal macrosomia   d. Shoulder dystocia
4. The risk of congenital anomalies in the fetus is best correlated to:
    a. Random blood sugar at first antenatal visit
    b. HbA1c in the first trimester
    c. Creatinine level in second trimester
    d. Presence of forward flow in ductus venosus at 12 weeks
5. Appropriate diabetic diet should have the following proportion of contributing macronutrients:
    a. 10% as protein   b. 50% as fat
    c. 30% as carbohydrate   d. 30% as saturated fats
6. Which one of the following group of oral hypoglycemic agent is associated with fetal growth restriction and fetal death?
    a. Glibenclamides   b. Glitazones
    c. Glinidies   d. DPP4 inhibitors
7. According to ACOG, fetal monitoring should be started in diabetic women from:
    a. 20 weeks   b. 24 weeks
    c. 28 weeks   d. 34 weeks
8. Insulin-dependent diabetes is an indication for delivery at the following gestational age:
    a. 34 weeks   b. 36 weeks
    c. 38 weeks   d. 40 weeks
9. Regarding postdelivery care of a diabetic woman the following statement is true:
    a. Breastfeeding should not be initiated early
    b. Insulin requirement will increase
    c. Risk of puerperal sepsis is higher
    d. Postpartum intrauterine device is contraindicated
10. Which one of the following declaration was made in relation to outcomes of pregnancies in diabetic women?
    a. Innocenti declaration   b. St. Vincent declaration
    c. St. Winfred declaration d. WHO declaration

Answers
1. d   2. b   3. a   4. b   5. c   6. b
7. c   8. c   9. c   10. b

5.4 THYROID DISORDERS IN PREGNANCY

Kanan Yelikar, Sonali Deshpande, Ashwini Kale

INTRODUCTION

It has been observed that thyroid disorders have increased in the recent past in India. Due to insufficient production of thyroid hormones by the thyroid gland, the bodily needs are not met leading to hypothyroidism. The prevalence is 10% amongst Indian adults. Pregnancy-related thyroid disorders are not unusual. Failure to evaluate and treat may have adverse impact on the mother and the fetus. Pregnancy is a time of complex hormonal changes. Thyroid hormones have profound variation and are associated with severe health impacts.[1] During the first trimester of pregnancy, in pregnant women with normally functioning thyroid gland, physiological rise in thyroxine (T_3) and triiodothyronine (T_4) causes inhibition of thyrotropin [thyroid-stimulating hormone (TSH)] owing to a high human chorionic gonadotropin (hCG) level that stimulates the structurally similar TSH receptor.[2,3] The demand for thyroxine increases in the hyperestrogenic state of pregnancy owing to the expanded plasma volume leading to altered distribution of hormone, accelerated metabolism of hormone, increased renal clearance of iodide, and elevated hepatic production of thyroid binding globulin (TBG).[4] It must be emphasized that the true biochemical function of thyroid gland is determined by "free" thyroid hormone levels as the total hormone level will always be higher even if the patient is euthyroid. Total prevalence of hypothyroidism is 12% in India, while 1.25% of pregnant women have hyperthyroidism.[5]

PHYSIOLOGICAL ADAPTATION DURING PREGNANCY

Pregnancy has significant effect on thyroid physiology. Increased basal metabolic rate as a result of increased metabolism in pregnancy causes increased secretion of thyroid hormones because of actions of hCG and human chorionic thyrotropin (HCT), which are similar in molecular structure and also share cross-reactivity with TSH receptor.[6] Although hCG is 1/4,000th potent compared to TSH to stimulate thyroid activity, very increased levels of hCG in normal pregnancy are sufficient to lead to physiological thyrotoxicosis, while T_4 levels are higher with conditions with excess hCG titers, e.g., molar pregnancy and multiple pregnancies. Placental transfer of thyroid hormone, albeit limited, can provide protection, especially to fetal brain.[6,7]

THYROID HORMONE PHYSIOLOGY (TABLE 1)

Screening for Thyroid Disease in Pregnancy

Identification and treatment of subclinical hypothyroidism (SCH) in pregnancy has not shown promising results in

TABLE 1: Thyroid hormone physiology.

Maternal physiology	Fetal and neonatal physiology
• High basal metabolic rate (BMR) • Increased iodine uptake • Increased size of gland—hyperplasia and hypervascularity • Iodide clearance increased • Iodide loss to fetus reduces iodide levels • Transfer of TSH, T_3, and T_4 across placenta but sufficient for neuroprotection is limited hCG peak at 10 weeks corresponding to nadir of TSH • Marked increase in thyroid-binding globulin (TBG) peak at 15 weeks • Increased activity of thyroid gland due to direct stimulation by hCG and HCT • Decreased free T_3 and free T_4 levels but within normal range • Hyperemesis gravidarum and transient hyperthyroidism due to high specific subgroup of hCG with reduced sialic acid content	• TSH and T_4 appear in the fetus at 10–13 weeks and rise abruptly at 20 weeks • T_4 rises rapidly and exceeds maternal values at term but very low T_3 levels • Reverse T_3 (RT_3) levels exceed normal adult levels • TSH peaks at 30 minutes of age • T3 peaks at 24 hours • T4 peaks at 24–48 hours • High RT_3 reaches normal values by 2 weeks

improving neurocognitive function in offspring; hence universal screening for thyroid disorder in pregnancy is not recommended. Those having history of thyroid disorder or with signs and symptoms of thyroid disease should be tested for thyroid function. An increase in plasma volume and extracellular fluid in the third trimester leads to increased thyroid volume by 10–30% in pregnancy. In the absence of significant history, signs, and symptoms of thyroid disease, an increase in the size of thyroid gland solely does not indicate screening for thyroid disease.[8] Maternal SCH in pregnancy can cause various adverse outcomes. This warranties early pregnancy screening of thyroid disorders, which will aid earlier detection of cases and timely intervention to prevent adverse perinatal outcomes Regardless, universal screening of thyroid function in early pregnancy is controversial and no country recommends universal thyroid screening due to lack of data but advocate screening of high-risk pregnant women.

Protocol for Screening and Management of Hypothyroidism in Pregnancy

High Risk Factors for Hypothyroidism[9]

- Living in a known moderate-to-severe iodine insufficiency residential area (as per area mapping)

- Obesity [prepregnancy or first trimester body mass index (BMI) ≥30 kg/m^2] (BMI = weight in kg/height in m^2)
- Pregnant women with thyroid dysfunction or history of thyroid surgery, signs, and symptoms of thyroid dysfunction or goiter
- Having first-degree relative (parents/siblings/children) with thyroid dysfunction. Having diagnosed mental retardation in family or previous births
- Pregnant women with autoimmune diseases such as type I diabetes/systemic lupus erythematosus (SLE)/rheumatoid arthritis (RA)/Addison disease/celiac disease
- Women with recurrent pregnancy loss, preterm delivery, intrauterine fetal demise (IUFD), preeclampsia/eclampsia, and abruptio placentae
- Infertility (inability to conceive after 1 year of unprotected intercourse)
- Use of amiodarone or lithium, or recent administration of iodinated radiologic contrast.

Types of Hypothyroidism Encountered in Pregnancy

Hypothyroidism in pregnancy is of two types: Overt hypothyroidism (OH) or SCH.
- *OH*: Serum (Sr.) TSH levels are elevated and low Sr. T_4/free T_4 (FT_4) levels. Sr. TSH ≥10 mIU/L is taken as OH, irrespective of FT_4 levels.
- *SCH*: Raised Sr. TSH level (≤10 mIU/L) with normal Sr. T_4/FT_4.[9]

Causes of Hypothyroidism
- Iodine deficiency
- *Autoimmune thyroiditis (Hashimoto thyroiditis)*: Most common cause and diagnosed by elevated titers of thyroid peroxidase antibody (TPO) antibody.

Consequences of Hypothyroidism in Pregnancy

Consequences of hypothyroidism in pregnancy include low birth weight baby, hypertension, or convulsions during pregnancy, miscarriage, IUFD, preterm birth, and chances of congenital anomaly or baby with low intelligence quotient (IQ).

If left untreated, hypothyroidism in pregnancy may lead to adverse maternal effects. It is known to lead to various complications during pregnancy: miscarriages (in early pregnancy), recurrent pregnancy losses, anemia, preeclampsia, gestational diabetes mellitus (GDM), abruptio placentae, postpartum hemorrhage (PPH), increased cesarean sections as a consequence of fetal distress, and infrequently myopathy and even congestive cardiac failure (CCF) in severe cases. Maternal hypothyroidism may result in preterm births, fetal growth restriction (FGR), IUFD, respiratory distress, and increased perinatal mortality (PNM). Thyroid hormone is vital for fetal brain development; its deficiency may result in cognitive, neurological, and developmental impairment in newborns.[9]

Diagnostic Criteria of Hypothyroidism in Pregnancy[9] (Table 2)

In pregnancy, levels of TSH are lower compared to nonpregnant state. Trimester-wise reference levels for TSH in pregnancy are as follows:
- SCH: Sr. TSH—2.5–10 mIU/L with normal FT_4 levels
- OH: Sr. TSH >2.5–3 mIU/l with low FT_4 levels. TSH >10 mIU/l irrespective of T4 levels is OH.

Effect of Hypothyroidism on Pregnancy[10]

Several studies have shown that there is twofold increase in the rate of miscarriage in women with elevated Sr. thyroid antibodies level even being euthyroid; but is not universally confirmed. Thyroid antibodies [antiperoxidase (TPO), antimicrosomal antibody (AMA), and antithyroglobulin (ATG)] can cross placenta and result in neonatal hypothyroidism; if untreated, may lead to serious cognitive deficiencies. Even in children of very mildly hypothyroid women, lower IQs have been reported. There is an increased risk of preeclampsia, placental abruption, intrauterine growth restriction, prematurity, and intrauterine fetal demise. Increase in severity of hypothyroidism is directly related to the severity of hypertension and other perinatal complications. Thus, early identification, treatment, and vigilant monitoring to ensure euthyroidism will prevent or decrease perinatal complications.

Protocol for Management of Hypothyroidism in Pregnancy[9]

- Treatment of choice in pregnancy is levothyroxine sodium. It is a "category A" drug for pregnancy and can be used safely during pregnancy and lactation with no adverse effects on mother or fetus. Levothyroxine should be taken orally, empty stomach in the morning and patient should refrain from taking anything orally for half an hour after taking the drug. On missing out on a dose, the woman should take it as soon as she remembers and refrain from eating anything for next half an hour. If entire tablet is missed altogether, she should take double the dose the next morning. While prescribing, a whole bottle of levothyroxine tablets (25/50/75/100 µg) is to be provided to patients.

Treatment steps as per Sr. TSH levels:
- TSH level <2.5 in I trimester and <3 in II and III trimesters: No further management; continue routine pregnancy care

TABLE 2: Diagnostic criteria of hypothyroidism in pregnancy.[9]

First trimester	0.1–2.5 mIU/L
Second trimester	0.2–3 mIU/L
Third trimester	0.3–3 mIU/L

Flowchart 1: Dose of levothyroxine based on Sr. thyroid-stimulating hormone (TSH) levels in pregnancy and postpartum period.

```
1: <2.5 mIU/l (1st trimester) or <3 mIU/l (2nd or 3rd trimester) → No treatment

2: 2.5–10 mIU/l (1st trimester) or 3–10 mIU/l (2nd or 3rd trimester) → 25 μg L-thyroxine/day during pregnancy → No treatment required in postpartum period

3: ≥10 mIU/L (any trimester) → 50 μg L-thyroxine/day → Same dose to be continued in postpartum period

4: Pregnant women on treatment for hypothyroidism before pregnancy → L-thyroxine dose to be modified according to 2 and 3 → Pre-pregnancy dose of L-thyroxine to be continued in postpartum

Repeat TSH 6 weeks postpartum. Further treatment will be as required
```

- TSH—2.5/3–10: Start 25 μg of levothyroxine daily
- TSH >10: Start 50 μg of levothyroxine daily
- Treatment to be stopped after delivery if first TSH level was <10; if >10, same dose continued
- If patient is already on treatment even before pregnancy, continue same treatment with required target range
- TSH levels should be repeated after 6 weeks of starting date of treatment.

Treatment of Hypothyroid Woman based on TSH Level[9]

The treatment algorithm of hypothyroid woman based on TSH level is shown in **Flowchart 1**.

Dose Modification According to TSH Level[9]

According to TSH level, dose modification is listed in **Table 3**.

■ HYPERTHYROIDISM IN PREGNANCY

Hyperthyroidism can likewise complicate pregnancies, although its incidence is lesser than hypothyroidism. The prevalence of hyperthyroidism (also known as thyrotoxicosis) is between 0.05 and 0.2% in pregnancy. The most common cause for hyperthyroidism in pregnancy is Graves' disease. Graves' disease occurs due to formation of thyroid-stimulating antibody (TSAb) belonging to the immunoglobulin G (IgG) class, which binds with high affinity to the TSH receptor. TSAb has potential to cross placenta and bind fetal TSH receptors leading to fetal or neonatal hyperthyroidism. However, only those with very high titers may get affected as placenta acts as a partial barrier. Other causes of hyperthyroidism include thyroiditis, thyroid adenoma, and multinodular goiter.[10]

Essential of Diagnosis

- Raised free T_4 and T_3 levels; decreased TSH levels
- Signs and symptoms of hyperthyroidism include heat intolerance, fatigue, anxiety, diaphoresis, tachycardia, and a widened pulse pressure.[10]

TABLE 3: Dose modification according to thyroid-stimulating hormone (TSH) level.[9]

TSH level	Current dose	Increase to
First trimester		
>2.5	25	50
>2.5	50	75
>2.5	75	100
>2.5	100	125
Second/third trimester		
>3	25	50
>3	50	75
>3	75	100
>3	100	125

Clinical Features of Hyperthyroidism

The signs and symptoms of hyperthyroidism—heat intolerance, fatigue, anxiety, diaphoresis, tachycardia, and a widened pulse pressure—can all be features of a normal pregnancy. Specific signs of hyperthyroidism are as follows: pulse >100 beats per minute, goiter, and exophthalmos, but these may not be present. Patients may also present with severe nausea and vomiting as gastrointestinal symptoms but these may be due to elevated β-hCG levels in pregnancy. Confirm elevated T_4, fT_4, T_3, and free T_3 (fT_3) levels and a suppressed or undetectable TSH level by testing. Thyroid-stimulating antibody (TSAb) titers will be elevated in a significant number of patients. Other findings may be found—a normocytic normochromic anemia, mild neutropenia, and elevated liver enzymes.

Subclinical Hyperthyroidism

Subclinical hyperthyroidism is a condition in which there are decreased level of TSH and normal T_4 and T_3 levels can present in pregnancy; subclinical disease was reported in 1.7% of screened women. There is no effect of subclinical hyperthyroidism in pregnancy, so screening and treatment for this entity are not warranted.[11]

Effect of Hyperthyroidism in Pregnancy

Maternal Complications

Maternal complications includes preeclampsia, miscarriages, preterm delivery, congestive heart failure and severe cases of arrhythmia, placental abruption, thyroid storm, anemia, and higher susceptibility to infections.

Fetal Complications

Fetal complications include low birth weight, FGR, prematurity, stillbirth, fetal hyperthyroidism, increased PNM, and neonatal thyrotoxicosis.

Treatment of Hyperthyroidism

Antithyroid medications form the basis for management of hyperthyroidism in pregnancy. Exceptional situations, e.g., allergies to all or any drugs available or lack of response to very large doses (drug resistance), warrant surgery. The treatment aims at achieving and maintaining euthyroid levels with minimum amount of medication, provide symptomatic relief, and maintain fT_4 levels within upper third of normal.

- Thionamides [propylthiouracil (PTU) and methimazole] are the first line and most common prescribed class of medications for the treatment of hyperthyroidism in pregnancy. The initial methimazole dose is 20–40 mg/d; the initial PTU dose is 200–400 mg/d.
- Severe, uncontrolled cases within third trimester may warrant hospitalization due to increased risk of complications.
- Women who have remained euthyroid while taking small amounts of PTU (≤100 mg/d) or methimazole (≤10 mg/d) for 4 weeks or longer can stop taking the medication altogether by 32–34 weeks' gestation under close surveillance. This is to minimize the risk of fetal/neonatal hypothyroidism, which is otherwise uncommon with PTU doses ≤200 mg/d or methimazole ≤20 mg/d. The therapy is resumed if symptoms recur.
- A white blood corpuscle (WBC) count is mandatory before treatment is started; as agranulocytosis is the most severe complication.
- Irreversible liver damage, leading potentially to liver failure, is found to be associated with PTU. However, methimazole features a stronger association with teratogenic effects on the fetus.

TREATMENT OF THYROID DISORDERS IN PREGNANCY (FLOWCHART 2)

Manifestations of Hyperthyroidism in Pregnancy

- Thyrotoxicosis during pregnancy
- Cardiac failure with thyroid storm

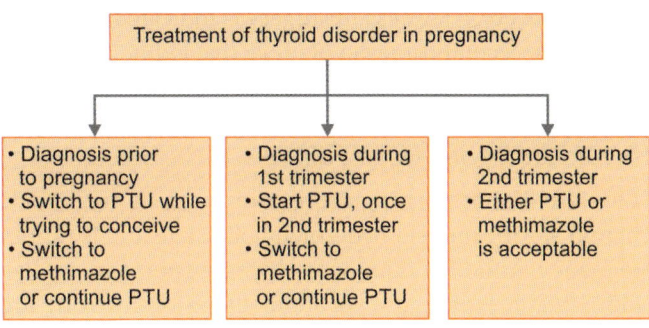

Flowchart 2: Treatment of thyroid disorders in pregnancy.

(PTU: propylthiouracil)

- Hyperemesis gravidarum and gestational transient thyrotoxicosis
- Thyrotoxicosis and gestational trophoblastic disease
- Subclinical hyperthyroidism.

Thyrotoxicosis in Pregnancy/Graves' Disease

Graves' disease is due to autoimmune process wherein TSH receptor antibodies stimulate the thyroid gland, affecting 0.2% of pregnant women. Graves' disease in pregnancy is associated with initial hyperthyroid symptoms due to hCG stimulation, but this wears off once β-hCG levels fall in the second trimester. Neonatal hypothyroidism is seen to occur in women with past history of Graves' disease or active disease. The incidence is 1–5%. This is known to cause increased fetal morbidity if left untreated.[10]

Preconceptional counseling: All women with Graves' disease must receive preconceptional counseling. Women with Graves' hyperthyroidism should be advised to delay conception and use contraception until Graves' hyperthyroidism is controlled. Women with uncontrolled hyperthyroidism should be offered definitive treatment of radioactive iodine ablation or thyroidectomy.[10]

Clinical features: Signs and symptoms of Graves' disease in pregnancy are no different than that of nonpregnant patient. Graves' disease must be suspected in a hyperthyroid pregnant woman who:
- was having symptoms from even before pregnancy
- had a previous diagnosis of hyperthyroidism
- had previously given birth to an infant with thyroid dysfunction.[12]

Treatment: Thionamides are the treatment of choice for Graves' disease in pregnancy.

We start with 300 or 450 mg of PTU daily in three divided doses for pregnant women. Occasionally, daily doses of 600 mg are necessary. Generally, methimazole is not required to be shifted to during the third trimester. The goal of treatment is to use lowest possible thionamide dose to take care of hormone levels slightly above or within the high normal range while TSH levels remain suppressed. Sr. free T_4 concentrations are tested every 4–6 weeks. If surgery is indicated, it is to be done in the second trimester. Radioactive iodine ablation is contraindicated during pregnancy.[11]

Thyroid Storm and Heart Failure

These are life-threatening acute conditions in pregnancy. Thyroid storm can be a hypermetabolic state and is rare in pregnancy. Although pulmonary hypertension and cardiac failure due to profound myocardial effects of thyroxine are encountered commonly in pregnant women.[13] With already less cardiac reserve, conditions such as preeclampsia, anemia, sepsis, or a combination of the same, decompensation may be precipitated in a pregnant woman. Fortunately, thyroxine-induced cardiomyopathy and pulmonary hypertension are usually reversible.[12-14]

Treatment of thyroid storm[2] (Flowchart 3): Treatment of severe preeclampsia, infection, or anemia should be done prior to delivery.

Hyperemesis Gravidarum and Gestational Transient Thyrotoxicosis

Transient biochemical features of hyperthyroidism could also be observed in 2–15% of girls in early pregnancy.[15] Women with hyperemesis gravidarum generally present with low TSH and extremely high Sr. thyroxine levels.[16] This occurs due to stimulation of TSH receptor by β-hCG secreted during pregnancy. It is also known as gestational transient thyrotoxicosis. Antithyroid medication is not indicated even if the woman has hyperemesis.[8] The hCG normalizes by mid-pregnancy and hence normalizes the previously deranged thyroid values.[17]

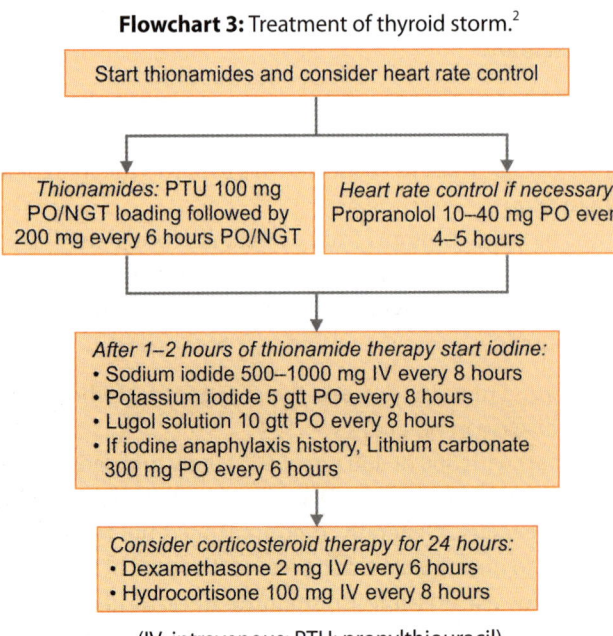

Flowchart 3: Treatment of thyroid storm.[2]

(IV: intravenous; PTU: propylthiouracil)

Subclinical Hyperthyroidism

Third-generation TSH assays with an analytical sensitivity of 0.002 mU/mL permit identification of subclinical thyroid disorders. Subclinical hyperthyroidism has not been associated with adverse impact on pregnancy. Hence, its treatment is uncalled for since the antithyroid drugs may negatively impact the fetus. They can be periodically monitored for symptoms and by assessing Sr. TSH levels; since almost 50% are seen to have normal levels eventually.

Postpartum thyroiditis: Also known as transient autoimmune thyroiditis.

Painless thyroiditis within 1 year after child birth (5–10%), may occur after abortions, either induced or spontaneous.[18] Propensity for postpartum thyroiditis is higher in women with thyroid-antibody positive in first trimester (up to 50%), women with type 1 diabetes.[19]

Clinical presentation
- Temporary hyperthyroidism alone (32% of patients)
- Temporary hypothyroidism alone (43% of patients)
- Hypothyroidism which is preceded by transient hyperthyroidism that generally tends to recover in a matter of time (25% of patients).[16,20]

Pathophysiology
Presence of thyroid peroxidase antibodies (TPO antibodies) in cases of autoimmune disorder. It is referred to as destructive thyroiditis with lymphocytic infiltration within thyroid gland.
- Inflammatory process initiated in the presence of TPO antibodies
- Complement cascade activation
- Lymphocyte abnormalities with increased IgG1 levels
- NK cells activity along with certain specific human leukocyte antigen (HLA) haplotypes
- Proteolytic destruction of thyroglobulin
- Follicles within thyroid gland are destroyed
- Release T_3 and T_4 into blood (hyperthyroid state)
- Transient till no thyroglobulin storage left
- Later develop hypothyroid state.

Clinical symptoms: Two clinical phases (Classic)[8]
1. In destruction-induced thyrotoxicosis, women present with fatigue and palpitations and painless goiter which lasts for few months.
2. Hypothyroid state presents between 4 and 8 months postpartum, thyromegaly common feature
3. Autoimmune disease leading to subclinical thyroid in pregnancy and postpartum
4. Permanent hypothyroidism (associated with higher TSH values and the anti-TPO antibodies titer in the initial hypothyroid state). Levothyroxine dose can be altered 1 year after delivery. This should be done gradually with regular monitoring of Sr. TSH every 6 weeks.[21]

Postpartum surveillance with Sr. TSH, free T_4, and anti-TPO antibody at 6 and 12 months.[19]

Differential diagnosis
- *Graves' disease*: Hyperthyroidism is mild clinically and biochemically in postpartum thyroiditis, thyroid is enlarged minimally, Graves' ophthalmology is not apparent, usually resolves in 3–4 weeks)
- *Lymphocytic hypophysitis*: Sr. TSH is low or maybe normal, along with low free T_4. In postpartum thyroiditis, Sr. free T_4 is decreased along with a high Sr. TSH level
- Hashimoto thyroiditis
- Postpartum mood disorder.

Treatment: In hyperthyroid state, if symptoms are severe, β-blocking agents are effective.

In hypothyroid state, thyroxine replacement (25–75 µg) given for 6–12 months. There is an association between postpartum depression and postpartum thyroiditis.[8]

ROLE OF MEDICAL TERMINATION OF PREGNANCY JUST IN CASE OF THYROID DISORDER

Overt hypothyroidism is not an indication for medical termination of pregnancy (MTP) as per MTP guidelines.[22] However, the definition of "serious mental abnormalities so on be handicapped in life" has not been elaborated and is open to individual interpretation. In the present era of patient-centered care, the mother's opinion about possible neurological damage of fetal brain should be considered and her decision for MTP should be taken into account graciously. Considering the fact that women with uncontrolled diabetes mellitus who came to our outpatient departments (OPDs) with unplanned conception can be offered MTP, but there are no predefined values of hemoglobin A1c (HbA1c) at which MTP is strongly recommended. The decision differs from case to case and applies for women with OH. In later pregnancy, the triple marker test can be applied to assess the risk of Down syndrome, trisomy 18, and neural tube defects. However, there is no definite value at which to enforce an MTP: The results can at the best be considered implicational the fetal risk. Similarly, in pregnancy complicated by OH, the decision to continue or terminate pregnancy will vary from case to case based on multiple factors.

Role of Medical Termination of Pregnancy in Hypothyroidism Complicated Pregnancy

Severity of hypothyroidism, gestation gravity, iodine nutrition status, past h/o infertility, past h/o miscarriage/fetal loss, past h/o congenital malformation, past h/o offspring with intellectual impairment, patient's attitudes and beliefs regarding MTP, family h/o congenital malformation, and family h/o intellectual impairment.

Keeping the above discussion in mind, management of women should be as follows:
- *SCH, at any trimester*: Treat with levothyroxine. MTP is not recommended.
- *OH >20 weeks of gestational age*: Treat with levothyroxine. MTP is not recommended.
- *OH <20 weeks of gestational age*: Treat with levothyroxine. MTP is not recommended. MTP can be done only if requested by the patient after adequate counseling.

Maternal hypothyroidism may go undiagnosed in pregnancy and postpartum. There are no studies so far, analyzing the severity of detrimental effects of the disease in the neonate. The consequences of maternal hypothyroidism on the fetus or neonate are probably the results of interplay of several factors acting, like decreased availability of maternal thyroid hormones at crucial times in fetal brain development, obstetric events related to maternal hypothyroidism, and possibly prolonged concealed maternal hypothyroidism during pregnancy. Ethically important but debatable issue is whether or not clinicians should recommend terminating pregnancy when severe hypothyroidism is diagnosed late in gestation. Undiagnosed hypothyroidism throughout pregnancy may have dilapidating effects on fetal brain, despite treatment with thyroxine. However, there is no surety of its occurrence and hence obstetricians and endocrinologists do not recommend abortion. It is highly unlikely for randomized clinical trial to be conducted in order to determine the criteria of TSH values for undergoing MTP given the nature of the disease. Any discussion regarding this may necessarily court controversy, skirting with the grey zones of eugenics, ethics, public health, obstetrics, and endocrinology. Due to the varied nature of the disease, depending upon the region, levels of iodine in diet and intensity of OH in pregnancy will differ. Also, as per the personal experience of clinicians in regards of obstetric outcome related to the disease, the decision for abortion will differ. Most of the time, clinicians may consider non-endocrine issues as the cause for aborting a viable pregnancy with OH which may only be a contributory factor for performing MTP.

KEY MESSAGES

- Universal screening for thyroid in pregnancy is not recommended.
- Testing for thyroid function should be done only if indicated; like in women with history if thyroid disorder or having symptoms of the disease.
- Thyroid status of women is assessed by measuring TSH level as the first-line investigation.
- Both Sr. TSH and free T_4 levels are necessary to diagnose thyroid diseases in pregnancy.
- Thyroid hormone treatment should be given to pregnant females with hypothyroidism to prevent its adverse effects.
- Dose of levothyroxine is altered as per the serial Sr. TSH levels after commencing treatment.
- Thionamide is used for treating women with OH in order to prevent complications related to the disease.
- Pregnant women on thionamide should have regular monitoring of free T_4 levels and the dose altered accordingly.

- Both PTU and methimazole can be used to manage overt hyperthyroidism in pregnancy as single-agent therapy.

REFERENCES

1. Zadeh-Vakili A, Ramezani Tehrani F, Hashemi S, Amouzegar A, Azizi F. Relationship between sex hormone binding globulin, thyroid stimulating hormone, prolactin and serum androgens with metabolic syndrome parameters in Iranian women of reproductive age. J Diabetes Metab. 2012; S2.
2. Williams GR. Neurodevelopmental and neurophysiological actions of thyroid hormone. J Neuroendocrinol. 2008;20(6):784-94.
3. Glinoer D. The regulation of thyroid function in pregnancy: Pathways of endocrine adaptation from physiology to pathology. Endocr Rev. 1997;18(3):404-33.
4. Krajewski DA, Burman KD. Thyroid disorders in pregnancy. Endocrinol Metab Clin N Am. 2011;40(4):739-63.
5. Ajmani SN, Aggarwal D, Bhatia P, Sharma M, Sarabhai V, Paul M. Prevalence of overt and subclinical thyroid dysfunction among pregnant women and its effect on maternal and fetal outcome. J Obstet Gynecol India. 2014;64(2):105-10.
6. Khadilkar S. Thyroid-stimulating hormone values in pregnancy: Cutoff controversy continues? J Obstet Gynecol India. 2019;69(5):389-94.
7. Fritz MA, Sperof L. Reproduction and thyroid. Chapter 20, Clinical gynecologic endocrinology and infertility, 8th edition. Philadelphia: Wolters Kluwer Health Lippincott Williams and Wilkins; 2010. pp. 340-2.
8. Practice Bulletin No. 148: Thyroid disease in pregnancy. Obstet Gynecol. 2015;125(4):996-1005.
9. Maternal Health Division. Ministry of Health & Family Welfare Government of India. (2014). National Guidelines for Screening of Hypothyroidism during Pregnancy. [online] Available from: http://www.nrhmorissa.gov.in/writereaddata/Upload/Documents/National_Guidelines_for_Screening_of_Hypothyroidism_during_Pregnancy.pdf. [Last accessed October 2021].
10. Bannerman CG. Thyroid and other endocrine disorders during pregnancy. In: LANGE Diagnosis and Treatment: Obstetrics and Gynecology, 12 edition. New York: McGraw-Hill Education; 2019.
11. Leveno KJ, Spong CY, Dashe JS, Casey BM, Hoffman BL, Cunningham FG, et al. William's Textbook of Obstetrics, 25th edition. New York: McGraw-Hill Education; 2018. pp. M0412-1344.
12. Nguyen CT, Sasso EB, Barton L, Mestman JH. Graves' hyperthyroidism in pregnancy: a clinical review. Clinical diabetes and endocrinology. 2018;4(1):4.
13. Sheffield JS, Cunningham FG. Thyrotoxicosis and heart failure that complicate pregnancy, Am J Obstet Gynecol. 2004;190:211-7.
14. Siu CW, Zhang XH, Yung C, Kung AWC, Lau CP, Tse HF. Hemodynamic changes in hyperthyroidism-related pulmonary hypertension: a prospective echocardiographic study. J Clin Endocrinol Metab. 2007;92(5):1736-42.
15. DeGroot L, Abalovich M, Alexander EK, Amino N, Barbour L, Cobin RH, et al. Management of thyroid dysfunction during pregnancy and postpartum: an Endocrine Society clinical practice guideline. J Clin Endocrinology Metabolism. 2012;97(8):2543-65.
16. Muller AF, Drexhage HA, Breghout A. Postpartum thyroiditis and autoimmune thyroiditis in women of childbearing age: recent insights and consequences for antenatal and postnatal care. Endocr Rev. 2001;22(5):605-30.
17. Yoshihara A, Noh JY, Mukasa K, Suzuki M, Ohye H, Matsumoto M, et al. Serum human chorionic gonadotropin levels and thyroid hormone levels in gestational transient thyrotoxicosis: is the serum hCG level useful for differentiating between active Graves' disease and GTT? Endocr J. 2015;62(6):557-60.
18. Stagnaro-Green A. Overt hyperthyroidism and hypothyroidism during pregnancy. Clin Obstet Gynaecol. 2011;54(3):478-87.
19. Nathan N, Sullivan SD. Thyroid disorders during pregnancy. Endocrinol Metabol Clin North Am. 2014;43(2):573-97.
20. Vydt T, Verhelst J, De Keulenaer G. Cardiomyopathy and thyrotoxicosis: tachycardiomyopathy or thyrotoxic cardiomyopathy? Acta Cardiol. 2006;61(1):115-7.
21. Alexander EK, Pearce EN, Brent GA, H, Dosiou Brown RS, Chen C, et al. 2017 Guidelines of the American Thyroid Association for the diagnosis and management of thyroid disease during pregnancy and the postpartum. Thyroid. 2017;27(3):315-89.
22. The Medical Termination of Pregnancy Act, 1971 (Act No. 34 of 1971). [online] Available from: http://bhind.nic.in/Sparsh_MTP-Act-1971. [Last accessed October 2021].

LONG QUESTIONS

1. Define hypothyroidism in pregnancy. Elaborate diagnostic criteria of hypothyroidism in pregnancy. Describe maternal and fetal effects of hypothyroidism in pregnancy.
2. Describe clinical features and defects of hyperthyroidism in pregnancy. What is the management of hyperthyroidism in pregnancy?

SHORT QUESTIONS

1. Screening of thyroid disorders in pregnancy.
2. Management of hypothyroidism in pregnancy.
3. Write a short note on postpartum thyroiditis.

MULTIPLE CHOICE QUESTIONS

1. Drug of choice for thyrotoxicosis in pregnancy:
   a. Propylthiouracil
   b. Methimazole
   c. Carbimazole
   d. Propranolol
2. Uncontrolled maternal hyperthyroidism has been linked to which of the following effects in the offspring:
   a. Cretinism
   b. Dwarfism
   c. Hypogonadism in child
   d. Limb reduction deformities
3. Which of the following is false in hyperthyroidism in pregnancy?
   a. In most cases, the perinate is euthyroid
   b. Goiter can occur in the perinate
   c. Preterm delivery can occur in women with hyperthyroidism
   d. Preeclampsia is not a common complication of uncontrolled thyrotoxicosis

4. Most common cardiac complication seen in uncontrolled thyrotoxicosis:
   a. Dilated cardiomyopathy
   b. Hypertrophic obstructive cardiomyopathy (HOCM)
   c. Restrictive cardiomyopathy
   d. Ventricular dysplasia
5. In OH:
   a. TSH level is elevated, free T_4 levels are low
   b. TSH levels are low, free T_4 levels are low
   c. TSH levels are elevated, free T_4 levels are elevated
   d. TSH levels are low, free T_4 levels are elevated
6. Subclinical hypothyroidism is associated with:
   a. Elevated Sr. TSH with normal Sr. thyroxine
   b. Elevated Sr. TSH with elevated Sr. Thyroxine
   c. Elevated Sr. TSH with low Sr. thyroxine
   d. Normal TSH with normal Sr. thyroxine
7. Most common cause of hyperthyroidism in pregnancy:
   a. Graves' disease
   b. Hashimoto thyroiditis
   c. Thyroid nodules
   d. Autoimmune thyroiditis
8. Most common complication seen with hypothyroidism:
   a. Preeclampsia
   b. Preterm delivery
   c. Placental abruption
   d. Stillbirth
9. Daily iodine intake recommended in pregnancy:
   a. 250 µg
   b. 350 µg
   c. 450 µg
   d. 550 µg
10. Most common cause of congenital hypothyroidism:
    a. Maternal hypothyroidism
    b. Hypoplasia of the thyroid gland
    c. Exposure to antithyroid drugs
    d. Maternal hyperthyroidism
11. The following is contraindicated in treatment of Graves' disease in pregnancy:
    a. Methimazole
    b. Propylthiouracil
    c. Iodine ablation
    d. Surgical management
12. False about hCG:
    a. It has thyrotropic activity
    b. It peaks at 10–12 weeks
    c. It causes decrease in TSH levels
    d. It causes increase in TSH levels
13. Which of the following is not a common complication of hypothyroidism in pregnancy?
    a. Abortion
    b. Abruptio placenta
    c. Gestational hypertension
    d. Prolonged pregnancy
14. Thyroxine is required by the fetus for:
    a. Normal neurological development
    b. Kidney development
    c. Lung function
    d. Development of the liver
15. TSH is closely related to which of the following hormones?
    a. β-hCG
    b. Inhibin
    c. Human placental lactogen
    d. Luteinizing hormone

Answers

1. a	2. a	3. d	4. a	5. a	6. a
7. b	8. a	9. a	10. b	11. c	12. d
13. d	14. a	15. a			

5.5 ANEMIA

Hema Divakar, Arulmozhi Ramarajan

WHAT IS ANEMIA?

Anemia is the decreased ability of the red blood cells to provide adequate oxygen to body tissues. This can lead to disease, disability, or death. It is a condition rather than a disease, and the underlying cause must always be identified. The presentation of anemia varies from an emergency, in cases of acute blood loss, to asymptomatic, in cases of mild iron deficiency. Signs and symptoms include pallor, fatigue, irritability, shortness of breath, and cardiac failure. This variability in the spectrum of presentation is dependent on the abruptness of onset, the severity of anemia, and the ability of the cardiopulmonary system to compensate.

The normal hemoglobin varies with the age and sex of the individual and is given in **Table 1**. Anemia is said to be present when the level of hemoglobin falls below these levels (**Table 2**).[1]

TABLE 1: Normal hemoglobin level.

Population group	Normal hemoglobin (g/dL)
Adult female (nonpregnant)	12
Adult female (pregnant)	11
Children 6–59 months of age	11
Children 12–14 years of age	12

TABLE 2: Severity of anemia.

Severity	Hemoglobin (g/dL)
Mild	10 and above
Moderate	7–9.9
Severe	Below 7
Very severe	Below 4

WHAT ARE THE COMMON CAUSES OF ANEMIA?

- Nutritional anemia
- Anemia due to infections and infestations
- Anemia due to hemoglobin disorders
- Anemia due to acute blood loss.

WHAT ARE THE OTHER CAUSES OF ANEMIA?

- Anemia of chronic disease
- Anemia due to endocrine disorders
- Anemia due to heavy metal poisoning
- Hemolytic anemia
- Aplastic anemia.

WHAT ARE THE CONSEQUENCES OF IRON DEFICIENCY?[2]

- *Effects on the developing central nervous system*: Iron deficiency results in impaired cognitive performance, diminished IQ, overall decrease in scholastic performance, and behavioral abnormalities including attention deficit disorder (ADD). The tragedy of this is that the deleterious effects of iron deficiency on the cognitive performance in infancy and childhood are not correctable by subsequent iron therapy. This impairment in cognitive performance is irreversible.
- *Effects of iron deficiency on scholastic achievement in older children*: Iron deficiency results in poor learning ability even among older children and adolescents. Numerous studies have demonstrated poor learning scores in older children and adolescents with iron deficiency including those with iron deficiency without anemia.[3,4]
- *Compromised cardiovascular response to physical exercise*: The cardiovascular response to physical exercise is compromised in children with nutritional anemia even when it is mild, and hence these children may never attain their full potential in various school activities.[5]
- *Impaired immune status*: Iron deficiency causes increased mortality and morbidity from infections *in all age groups.* This is because iron deficiency results in impaired intracellular killing in the leukocytes, decreased ability of the lymphocytes to replicate, and lowered concentration of cells responsible for cell-mediated immunity.[6] In one study in India, it was found that anemic children were 5.75 times more susceptible to lower respiratory infections compared with their nonanemic counterparts. The authors concluded that prevention of anemia will reduce the incidence of lower respiratory tract infection (LRTI).[7]
- *Suboptimal utilization of energy sources by the muscle cells*: Iron deficiency causes impaired work performance in adults and adolescents with even mild iron deficiency without anemia.
- *Breath-holding spells and febrile seizures*: Iron deficiency is implicated in the causation of breath-holding spells in infants and young children. Iron supplementation results in a decrease in the frequency of breath-holding spells.[8] Children with iron deficiency have a greater chance of having febrile seizures than their non-iron-deficient counterparts.[9]
- *Cold intolerance*: Chronic iron deficiency causes cold intolerance in one-fifths of the patients by interfering with thyroxin and catecholamine metabolism. This may manifest as neuralgia, tingling and numbness, and vasomotor disturbances.
- *Increased heavy metal absorption*: Divalent metals, such as zinc and cadmium, are absorbed excessively in the presence of iron deficiency leading to their toxicity.[10,11]
- *Iron deficiency in pregnancy*: Iron deficiency increases the maternal mortality and morbidity, perinatal mortality, and prematurity. Infants of iron-deficient mothers develop anemia earlier and require more iron than that available in breast-milk **(Flowchart 1)**.

WHAT ARE THE TESTS TO DIAGNOSE ANEMIA AND IRON DEFICIENCY?

Tests to diagnose anemia: Hemoglobin estimation, peripheral blood smear, and reticulocyte count **(Fig. 1)**.

Tests to diagnose iron deficiency: The important tests that are used to diagnose iron deficiency are serum ferritin, serum transferrin (total iron-binding capacity), and serum transferrin receptor (sTfR) levels.

Serum ferritin: This is the best single test for diagnosing iron deficiency. The only disadvantage is that ferritin is an acute-phase reactant and is therefore elevated in chronic inflammatory states. Thus, while a low serum ferritin level is diagnostic of iron deficiency, a normal level in the presence of chronic inflammation does not exclude iron deficiency. A level < 15 µg/L is diagnostic of iron deficiency.

sTfR: It is a sensitive test and is not affected by chronic inflammation. The normal range is 3–9 mg/L.

Another useful test to diagnose iron deficiency anemia (IDA) in its early stages is the red cell distribution width (RDW). This is an index of the variation of red cell size and

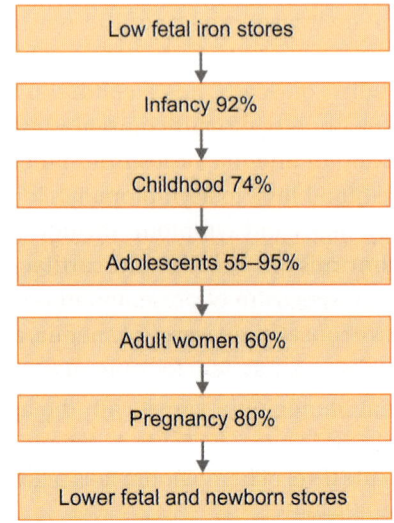

Flowchart 1: Anemia cycle.

SECTION 5: Pregnancy with Pre-existing Morbidities | **275**

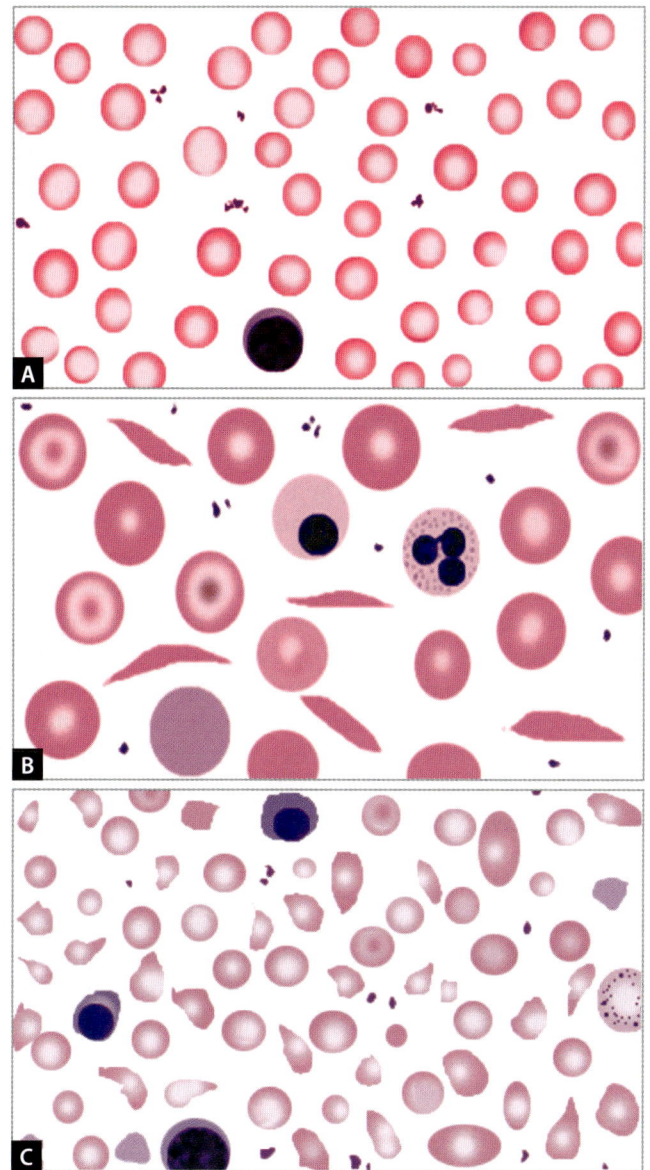

Figs. 1A to C: Peripheral smear. (A) Iron deficiency anemia: Peripheral blood smear in iron deficiency anemia. Compare the size of red cells with the nucleus of a small lymphocyte; (B) Thalassemia: Blood smear in thalassemia major showing microcytic hypochromic red cells, nucleated red cells, anisopoikilocytosis, target cells, basophilic stippling, and polychromasia; (C) Sickle cell anemia: Blood smear in sickle-cell anemia.

can detect subtle degrees of anisocytosis. Elevated RDW is the earliest sign of IDA and is more sensitive than a peripheral blood smear in the diagnosis of IDA.[12] The normal range of RDW is 11.5–14.5.

A practical and inexpensive method of diagnosing iron deficiency is to assess the response to iron therapy. Iron deficiency is confirmed if the hemoglobin rises by 1 g/dL or the hematocrit rises by 3% following a 4-week course of iron therapy in the dose of 3 mg/kg/day of elemental iron.

■ ANEMIA ERADICATION, A CHALLENGE

As primary care physicians for women, we are seriously concerned about maternal mortality and morbidity caused by anemia. Anemia is the chief contributor to maternal death and disability that is entirely preventable. Although the causes of anemia are known and specific treatment is also available, eradication of anemia remains a challenge. *The devastating effects on health, physical, and mental productivity translate into significant economic losses for the nation.*

Anemia gets worse with each generation: Iron deficiency is intergenerational. It is a vicious cycle that perpetuates through generations. Therefore, unless the chain is broken at some point in the current population, anemia is bound to prevail in the years to come, in the coming generations.

Let us target adolescent anemia—preparatory (ideal): Anemia in the developing years has a severe impact on all the organ systems. The chief causes are malnutrition and worm infestation. Notable effects include impaired gastrointestinal function, impaired cognitive performance, reduction of physical work capacity and productivity, increased morbidity from infectious diseases, altered patterns of hormone production, impaired DNA replication and tissue repair, damage to immune mechanisms, and impaired performance in tests of language skills, motor skills, and coordination, equivalent to a 5–10-point deficit in IQ.

Continuing malnutrition, faulty food habits of teenagers, and menstrual losses are the chief causes of anemia in adolescence. FOGSI's 12 × 12 initiative aimed at achieving at least 12 g% hemoglobin by 12 years of age, so that the system is geared up to face the challenge of menstrual losses and accelerated physical growth. Early marriage and teenage pregnancies add insult to injury and significantly increase the morbidity.

Gestational anemia—do not lose an opportunity (desirable): Anemia antedates pregnancy, pregnancy perpetuates it, and delivery depletes the woman further. The effects of anemia on pregnancy include abortions, preterm labor, and life-threatening obstetric hemorrhage. Perinatal outcome is also challenged because of intrauterine growth restriction and small-for-gestational age babies. Babies born to anemic women have low iron stores at birth. Correction of anemia in pregnancy should be done on a war-footing, to avert maternal morbidity and mortality. If the woman is unable to tolerate oral iron or if her response to oral iron is poor, intravenous iron sucrose must be given. It has been tested to be safe in the second and third trimesters of pregnancy.[13,14]

Postpartum anemia—yet another chance (at least): Delivery, however "normal," entails some blood loss because human beings have a hemochorial placenta. Therefore, every postpartum woman is hungry for iron. Also, in the postpartum period, the erythropoietin levels are about five times higher, and the utilization of iron and its incorporation into heme is that much higher. Thus, the postpartum period is a very fine time to provide iron, to improve the hemoglobin status of the woman while she is still under our care after delivery. While oral iron is the first-line measure in the management of anemia, intravenous iron sucrose can be administered in divided doses of 200 mg on alternate days.[15]

In a further step forward, the single-dose intravenous iron, namely ferric carboxymaltose (FCM), may be even more appropriate. This is available in 2- and 10-mL vials with 50 mg of FCM per milliliter. Studies have shown that it is safe to administer 1,000 mg of the drug as a single dose. As of now, this molecule is accepted for postpartum use but not for use during pregnancy. In some women with severe anemia and blunted erythropoiesis due to infection and/or inflammation, additional recombinant human erythropoietin may be considered.[16]

Certainty, compliance, efficacy, and safety make intravenous iron a powerful tool in our armamentarium to fight anemia.

TREATMENT OF ANEMIA

Oral Iron

The absorption of iron from the gut depends upon various parameters of which the following are of clinical importance having therapeutic implications:

- *Inhibitors of iron absorption*: Many factors that are commonly found in the diet are potent inhibitors of iron absorption. Some of the common inhibitors are phytates (present in cereals, legumes, nuts, and seeds), calcium (found in milk and milk products), and tannins (present in tea, coffee, and cocoa).
- *Enhancers of iron absorption*: Hemoglobin iron is present in the meat and poultry, Vitamin C found in fruits, juices, potatoes, and vegetables, such as green leaves, cauliflower, and cabbage, and condiments such as soya sauce enhance the absorption of iron several fold.

Elemental iron 120–180 mg/day is the therapeutic dose of iron. It should preferably be taken on an empty stomach, at least 2 hours before or after coffee/tea. It can be taken with fresh fruit juice for better absorption. If this causes gastrointestinal disturbance, it can be taken after food or in split dosage.

Intravenous Iron Sucrose

Iron sucrose complex therapy is a valid first-line option for the safe and rapid reversal of IDA.[17] Response to IV iron is not greater or faster but is more certain. Iron sucrose injection is a brown, sterile, aqueous complex of polynuclear iron hydroxide in sucrose for intravenous use. It has a molecular weight of approximately 60,000 Daltons. The low molecular weight and absence of biological polymers and preservatives make the molecule safe for use, even in pregnancy. The drug has a half-life of 5.2 hours, and repeat doses can be administered after 48 hours.

> **Calculation of dose of IV iron:**
> Iron deficit in mg = Prepregnancy body wt in kg × Hb deficit in g/dL × 2.4 + 500 mg for stores.
> The total deficit is given in divided doses of 200 mg per dose, with a spacing of at least 48 hours between doses.

Intravenous iron sucrose can be administered undiluted as an IV bolus in a dose of 100–200 mg over 2–5 minutes or as an intravenous infusion in normal saline in a dose of 100–200 mg in 100 mL NS over 15–20 minutes. Cost analysis revealed that the slow infusion was seven times more expensive than the bolus push technique (200 vs. 30 INR).[18] Response to therapy can be noticed in as early as 7 days of starting treatment. Patients report a feeling of wellness; reticulocytosis, improvement in red cell indices, and rise in hemoglobin also become evident.

Intravenous Ferric Carboxy Maltose

Ferric carboxymaltose complex is a novel iron dextran-free intravenous iron preparation that addresses the limitations of current intravenous iron therapies.[19] It can be administered in doses of up to 1,000 mg of iron given over a time period of 15–20 minutes. Unlike iron dextran, anaphylaxis is virtually unknown in association with its use. Thus, FCM is a promising intravenous iron preparation that is highly suited to low-resource settings. However, cost remains an issue and in this study, we sought to evaluate the noninferiority of a 500-mg dose versus the usual 1,000 mg; if 500 mg could be shown to be as efficacious as 1,000 mg, two women can effectively be treated in place of one.

Numerous clinical trials involving over 2,000 patients have demonstrated the unequivocal effectiveness of a 1,000-mg FCM dose in raising hemoglobin levels and replenishing iron stores, and this dose has been shown to be safe and well tolerated. In India, the single dose of 1,000 mg costs approximately INR 5,000 (85 USD) while a 500-mg dose costs less than half at INR 2,000 (35 USD). The demand for always seeking affordable yet effective therapy compelled us to investigate the noninferiority of a 500-mg dose versus the 1,000-mg dose in a postpartum population of anemic women. A prior pilot study had suggested that the 500-mg dose could be just as efficacious as the 1,000-mg dose and given the significantly lower cost of the 500-mg dose, it became imperative to conduct a definitive evaluation. The immediate postpartum period was the ideal time to target a vulnerable population of women with an unmet need, since they are immediately captive following delivery. Prior experience informs us that such women are difficult to follow up once they leave the maternity unit, and therefore a single "total dose" infusion is ideal for such a population.

Dose of FCM: The standard approach as recommended by manufacturers is that the total dose of FCM is calculated on the basis of hemoglobin deficit and body weight using the Ganzoni formula: Total iron deficit (mg) = Body weight (kg) × [target Hb – actual Hb (g%)] × 0.24 + Depot iron (mg). Depot iron = 15 mg/kg in case body weight <35 kg and 500 mg in case of weight >35 kg. In practice, the prevalence and severity of pregnancy-related IDA in India are such that a majority of women will require at least 1,000 mg, which is the recommended maximum safe dose that can be administered at one sitting. We can also take the pragmatic decision based on extensive practices in India to administer a single fixed dose, either 500 or 1,000 mg, without applying the Ganzoni formula, since this is what actually happens on the ground.

This offers a window of opportunity to treat postpartum anemia, but not using conventional approaches such as oral iron or IV iron sucrose since the former requires compliance and effectiveness is hampered by chronic disease and worm infestation, while the latter requires multiple visits over a course of weeks, which simply would not happen. We support the concept of using a single, efficacious, cost-effective therapy such as FCM at a lower and cheaper dose allowing for the scale-up of anemia eradication programs.

IMPACT ON NEONATE (KNOWN AND UNKNOWN)

A basic principle of fetal/neonatal iron biology is that iron is prioritized to red cells at the expense of other tissues, even including the brain.[20] Thus, when iron supply does not meet iron demand, the fetal brain may be at risk even if the fetus/infant is not anemic. Maternal iron deficiency causes reduced fetal iron supply and stores. The degree of reduction in brain iron concentrations in infants born to IDA mothers is not known, since brain iron can only be determined at autopsy. Neonates born to mothers with IDA have lower ferritin concentrations and may even have IDA if the mother is severely anemic. The sequalae of ID and IDA such as impaired cognitive function in the neonate presumably have their origins in the deprivation of iron of the fetal brain in utero.

Infants of mothers with IDA in the peripartum period have been shown to have lower scores for hand–eye movement at 10 weeks and locomotion at 9 months. A longitudinal study found that lower cord ferritin levels predicted poorer behavior/development at 5 years, specifically poorer auditory comprehension of language, fine motor skills, and self-regulation. This is additional evidence, linking maternal prenatal iron status to ID and IDA in neonates and infants. IDA delays psychomotor development and impairs cognitive performance in infants and children, and a majorly worrying aspect of this is that subsequent iron supplementation may not correct the effects of the earlier deficiency.

There is now strong evidence that iron is important in the development of the immune system as well as the immune response itself. Thus, morbidity from infectious disease is increased in iron-deficient populations. Iron is also important in other metabolic pathways in the body including those involving the endocrine and nervous systems. IDA results in an increased capacity for iron absorption—this is a physiological response aimed at correcting the iron deficiency. Unfortunately, this increased absorption capacity is not confined to iron but includes increased absorption capacity for other divalent metals that include toxic metals. Thus, an important consequence of ID is an apparent increased risk of heavy metal poisoning in children, including lead poisoning.

NEWER THOUGHTS AND STRATEGIES (WHAT WORKS FOR US)

Eradication of anemia will directly translate into a marked reduction in maternal mortality. Effective correction of anemia not only saves lives but also adds life to years. It averts the need for blood transfusion.

Strategies to prevent anemia would include the following:
- Health education, improved nutrition, iron enrichment of staple foods
- Improved hygiene, good sanitation, periodic deworming
- Antimalaria measures
- Empowerment of the girl child, delaying marriage and first pregnancy, building contraceptive choices for spacing, and limiting family size
- Screening of children, adolescents, and women planning pregnancy or already pregnant; targeted iron therapy in the postpartum period
- Reassessment of hemoglobin after treatment, identification of nonresponders, and appropriate management
- Liberal use of intravenous iron sucrose in the management of moderate-to-severe anemia caused by iron deficiency.

KEY MESSAGES

- ID is a universal problem in children and women of child-bearing age.
- ID is a systemic disease and not merely a hematological disease.
- Impairment of cellular functions occurs in ID even when there is no anemia.
- ID can cause irreversible cognitive and learning disabilities with an overall reduction in the IQ.
- ID being a public health problem in India, all children and women in the reproductive age group require prophylactic low-dose medicinal iron to prevent iron deficiency.
- Intravenous iron therapy is now the way forward in anemia management.

REFERENCES

1. World Health Organization. Iron Deficiency Anemia: Assessment, Prevention and Control—A Guide for Program Managers. Geneva: WHO; 2001.
2. Bangalore Society of Obstetrics and Gynecology. (2007). Anemia: a monograph. [online] Available from: https://cupdf.com/document/anemia-monograph.html [Last accessed December, 2021].
3. Halterman JS, Kaczorowski JM, Aligne CA, Auinger P, Szilagyi PG. Iron deficiency and cognitive achievement among school-aged children and adolescents. Pediatrics. 2001;107:1381-6.
4. Sen A, Kanani SJ. Deleterious functional impact of anemia on young adolescent school girls. Indian Pediatr. 2006;43(3):219-26.
5. Mani A, Singh T, Calton R, Chacko B. Cardiovascular response in anemia. Indian J of Pediatr. 2005;72:297-300.
6. Mullick S, Rusia U, Sikka M, Faridi MA. Impact of iron deficiency anaemia on T lymphocytes and their subsets in children. Indian J Med Res. 2006;124(6):647-54.
7. Ramakrishnan K, Harish PS. Hemoglobin level as a risk factor for lower respiratory tract infections. Indian J Pediatr. 2006;73(10):881-3.

8. Daoud AS, Batieha A, al-Sheyyab M, Abuekteish F, Hijazi S. Effectiveness of iron therapy on breath-holding spells. J Pediatr. 1997;130:547-50.
9. Naveed-ur-Rehman, Billoo AG. Association between iron deficiency anemia and febrile seizures. J Coll Physicians Surg Pak. 2005;15(6):338-40.
10. Goyer RA. Nutrition and metal toxicity. Am J Clin Nutr. 1995;61(3 Suppl):646S-650S.
11. Peraza MA, Ayala-Fierro F, Barber DS, Casarez E, Rael LT. Effects of micronutrients on metal toxicity. Environ Health Perspect. 1998;106(Suppl 1):203-16.
12. Vishwanath D, Hegde R, Murthy V, Nagashree S, Shah R. RDW in the diagnosis of IDA. Indian J Pediatr. 2001;68(12):1117-9.
13. Perewunsnyk G, Huch R, Huch A, Breymann C. Parenteral iron therapy in obstetrics: 8 years experience with iron-sucrose complex. Br J Nutr. 2002;88(1):3-10.
14. Divakar H, Nandakumar BS, Manyonda IT. (2009). Iron deficiency anemia in pregnancy: is intravenous iron sucrose an alternative to the oral iron-folate supplementation program in India? [online] Available from http://www. abcofobg. com/IDA/docs [Last accessed December, 2021].
15. Kharde PS, Bangal VB, Panicker KK. Comparative study of intravenous iron sucrose versus oral iron therapy in iron deficiency anemia during postpartum period. Int J Biomed Adv Res. 2012;3(4):238-43.
16. Milman N. Postpartum anemia II: prevention and treatment. Ann Hematol. 2012;91(2):143-54.
17. Perewusnyk G, Huch R, Huch A, Breymann C. Parenteral iron therapy in obstetrics: 8 years experience with iron-sucrose complex. Br J Nutr. 2002;88:3-10.
18. Divakar H, Gautham M S, Manyonda IT. Rapid versus slow intravenous iron sucrose administration: efficacy, safety and potential cost-savings in an Indian rural pregnant population with iron deficiency anemia.
19. Van Wyck DB, Martens MG, Seid MH, Baker JB, Mangione A. Intravenous ferric carboxymaltose compared with oral iron in the treatment of postpartum anemia: a randomized controlled trial. Obstet Gynecol. 2007;110(2 Pt 1):267-78.
20. Divakar H, Manyonda IT. Management of gestational anemia. Fresh thinking and new frontiers in India. Macmillan Medical Communications; 2011.

LONG QUESTIONS

1. Elaborate the causes and management of severe anemia in the third trimester.
2. What is the management of iron deficiency anemia in a pregnant woman? What are the investigations to be done in a nonresponder to iron therapy?
3. Discuss the hematological changes in normal pregnancy. What is the iron requirement in pregnancy?
4. Discuss the importance of hemoglobin indices and peripheral smear in the diagnosis of anemia.
5. "Anemia is an intergenerational problem"—discuss. What are the effects of anemia on the fetus/neonate/infant?
6. Discuss the prevalence of anemia in our women and its implications on the maternal mortality rate (MMR). Enumerate the complications of anemia in pregnancy and their management.

SHORT QUESTIONS

1. Name the common types and etiologies of anemia.
2. What are ferrokinetic studies?
3. Name the tests to assess the response to iron therapy.
4. Name the commonly found inhibitors and enhancers of iron absorption.
5. What is the relationship of infectious diseases and anemia?

MULTIPLE CHOICE QUESTIONS

1. Iron-rich foods include:
   a. Pulses and cereals   b. Coffee, tea
   c. Green leafy vegetables   d. Jaggery
2. Causes of anemia include:
   a. Nutritional deficiency   b. Malaria
   c. Worm infestation   d. HIV and HPV infection
3. Tests to diagnose iron deficiency anemia are:
   a. Hemoglobin   b. Peripheral smear
   c. Electrophoresis   d. Serum ferritin
4. Manifestations of anemia include:
   a. Fatigue   b. Weakness
   c. Cardiac failure   d. Infertility
5. Oral iron therapy for anemia is:
   a. Elemental iron 60 mg/day
   b. 100 mg for 100 days
   c. 120–180 mg/day
   d. 90 mg/day with 5 mg folic acid
6. Nonresponse to iron therapy may be due to:
   a. Poor compliance   b. Malabsorption
   c. Non-IDA   d. Hypothyroidism
7. Anemia in pregnancy can cause any of these, except:
   a. Early miscarriage
   b. Preterm labor
   c. Intrauterine growth restriction (IUGR)
   d. Postpartum hemorrhage (PPH)
8. Intravenous iron therapy is indicated in pregnancy:
   a. As first line therapy of anemia
   b. In those who do not respond to oral iron
   c. To avoid blood transfusion
   d. To build up iron stores
9. Inj. Iron sucrose may be safely administered as:
   a. Intramuscular injection of 100 mg
   b. Intravenous bolus of 200 mg
   c. Total dose IV infusion of up to 400 mg
   d. IV infusion over 20 minutes
10. The prevalence of anemia in women of reproductive age in India is:
    a. 40%   b. 45%
    c. Up to 90%   d. 20%

Answers

| 1. | b | 2. | d | 3. | c | 4. | d | 5. | c | 6. | d |
| 7. | a | 8. | a | 9. | a | 10. | c | | | | |

5.6 OTHER ANEMIAS IN PREGNANCY

Jyothika Desai, Megha Chauhan

INTRODUCTION

According to etiology, anemias can be classified into hereditary anemias and acquired anemias. This chapter will deal only with hereditary anemias, *otherwise known as hemoglobinopathies*. These are due to intrinsic defects in the erythrocyte membrane, glycolytic pathway, glutathione metabolism, or hemoglobin molecule.

HEMOGLOBINOPATHIES

The hemoglobinopathies are inherited disorders of hemoglobin *synthesis* (thalassemia) or *structure* (sickle cell disorders). They are seen mostly in people from Africa, the Mediterranean region, Far-East, and Asia. Since people from all parts of the world migrate, we see it in most parts of the world today. They are one of the most common monogenic inherited diseases. The prognosis varies with access to medical care. However, with modern care, more than 90% of those who have it survive into adulthood. It is of interest to know that more than 7% of the world's population is in the carrier state.[1]

Classification of Hemoglobinopathies

Hemoglobin disorders can be broadly classified into two main categories:

1. Those in which there is a *quantitative defect* in the production of one of the globin subunits, either total absence or marked reduction - the thalassemia syndromes.
2. Those in which there is a *structural defect* in one of the globin subunits.
    I. *Quantitative disorders of globin chain synthesis* - the thalassemia syndromes which are broadly classified into:
        i. β thalassemia—clinical classification:
            a. β-thalassemia minor or trait
            b. β-thalassemia major
            c. β-thalassemia intermedia
        Biochemical/genetic classification:
            a. β0-thalassemia
            b. β+-thalassemia
            c. δ-thalassemia
            d. γ-thalassemia
        β-thalassemia with other variants:
            a. HbS/β-thalassemia
            b. HbE/β-thalassemia
        ii. α Thalassemia:
        A. *Due to deletions of α-globin genes:*
            a. One gene: α+-thalassemia
            b$_1$. Two genes in cis: α0-thalassemia—seen more in Asians
            b$_2$. Two genes in trans: homozygous α+-thalassemia (phenotype of α0-thalassemia) - seen more in Africa
            c. Three genes: HbH disease
            d. Four genes: Hydrops fetalis with Hb Bart's
        B. *Non-deletion mutants:*
            a. Hb constant spring
            b. Others
        C. *De novo and acquired α-thalassemia*
            a. α-thalassemia with mental retardation syndrome (ATR)
            b. α-thalassemia (HbH disease) associated with myelodysplastic syndromes (ATMDS)
    II. *Qualitative disorders of globin structure: structural variants of hemoglobin*
        A. *Sickle cell disorders*
            a. SA, sickle cell trait
            b. SS, sickle cell anemia/disease
            c. SC, HbSC disease
            d. S/β thalassemia, sickle β-thalassemia disease
            e. S with other Hb variants: D, O-Arab, other
            f. SF, Hb S/HPFH
        B. *Hemoglobins with decreased stability (unstable hemoglobin variants)*
            a. Mutants causing congenital Heinz body hemolytic anemia
            b. Acquired instability—oxidant hemolysis: drug-induced, G6PD deficiency
        C. *Hemoglobins with altered oxygen affinity*
            a. High/increased oxygen affinity states:
            b. Fetal red cells
            c. Decreased RBC 2,3-BPG
            d. Carboxyhemoglobinemia, HbCO
        D. *Methemoglobinemia*
            a. Congenital methemoglobinemia:
            b. Acquired (toxic) methemoglobinemia
        E. *Post-translational modifications*[2]

Sickle cell disease (SCD) or *Sickle cell anemia (SCA)* is an autosomal recessive genetic disorder with over-dominance, characterized by RBCs that assume an abnormal, rigid, sickle shape. Sickling occurs due to a mutation in the *Hb* gene and reduces the cell's flexibility resulting in various complications **(Fig. 1)**. Earlier, SCD was considered as a disease of children. But today, due to advances in immunization, screening and management, the average survival age is about 50 years in individuals with SCD while patients with HbSC or HbS/ß+-thalassemia genotypes have an almost normal lifespan.[3] SCD is commonly seen in sub-Saharan Africa, South-East Asia, and parts of India; geographical areas where malaria is endemic.[4]

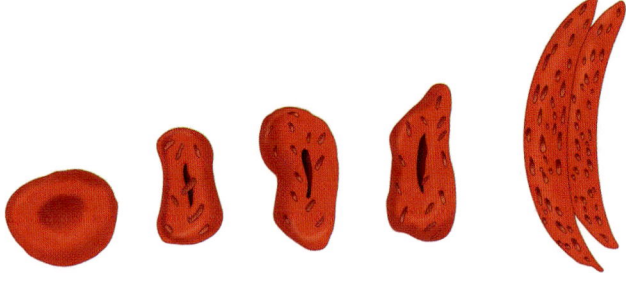

Fig. 1: Stages in the sickling process.

Hemoglobin usually exists in a soluble form, but here, it is precipitated as insoluble crystals, leading to RBCs of abnormal shape and size, which get phagocytosed.[5,6]

Sickle cell diseases occur in 3 different forms[7]
1. *Homozygous state*: Sickle cell anemia- Hb SS
2. *Heterozygous state*: Sickle cell trait- Hb SA- point mutation of only one of the β-globin chains, carrier state. Such patients do not suffer from the disease
3. *Double heterozygous states*: One copy of Hb S and one copy of other abnormal forms:
   - Sickle cell C disease – Hb SC
   - Sickle cell D disease – Hb SD
   - Sickle cell E disease – Hb SE
   - Sickle cell O Arab disease – Hb SO Arab
   - Sickle cell thalassemia disease – Hb S/B° or Hb S/B⁺
   - Unstable hemoglobinopathies

Maternal and perinatal morbidity and mortality are high in all.

Pathophysiology

Hemoglobin A: 2 alpha and 2 beta chains, 96–97% of adult Hb

Hemoglobin A2: 2 alpha and 2 delta chains

Hemoglobin F: 2 alpha and 2 gamma chains

Hemoglobin S: 2 wild type α-globin subunits and 2 mutant β-globin subunit forms.

- Sickle cell anemia is caused by a point mutation in the β-globin chain of Hb, causing the hydrophilic amino acid glutamic acid to be replaced by the hydrophobic amino acid valine at the 6th position. The β-*globin* gene is found on the short arm of chromosome 11.
- Under low oxygen conditions, the absence of a polar amino acid at position 6 of the β-globin chain, promotes the noncovalent polymerization of Hb, resulting in distortion of the RBCs into a sickle shape decreasing their elasticity. Normal hemoglobin is soluble, and it does not precipitate in the presence of hypoxia, low pH, and dehydration.
- The deoxygenated HbS aggregates to form rod-like polymers which align together and distort the red cells.
- The loss of RBC elasticity is central to the pathophysiology of sickle cell disease. Normal red cells are quite elastic thus allowing the cells to distort to pass through capillaries. In sickle cell disease however, low oxygen tension promotes sickling and repeated episodes of sickling and desickling damage cell membranes and further decrease the cell's elasticity
- These cells fail to return to their normal shape on restoration of normal oxygen tension. As a result, the rigid RBCs are unable to distort while passing through capillaries leading to vessel occlusion and ischemia. Any slowing of RBC passage through the microcirculation can contribute to vaso-occlusion. Some of the conditions that can contribute to this are—vasomotor dysregulation, endothelial cell adhesion, and RBC dehydration. These can lead to ischemia and infarction in various organs causing sometimes very severe pain called a sickle cell crisis.
- The actual anemia is caused by hemolysis due to phagocytosis of the misshapen RBCs in the spleen by macrophages. The bone marrow tries to compensate by producing new RBCs, but it cannot match the rate of destruction.
- Normal RBCs have a lifespan of about 90–120 days, while sickle or Holly leaf-shaped cells survive only for 10–12 days.
- Factors which determine the rate at which polymerization of HbS and the consequent sickling are
  - *Presence of non-HbS hemoglobins:* RBCs with HbF are protected from sickling
  - Intracellular concentration of HbS
  - Total Hb concentration
  - Extent of deoxygenation
  - Presence of acidosis and dehydration
  - Increase in concentration of 2,3DPG in RBCs.
- *Inheritance:* Seen more often in people from tropical or subtropical regions where malaria is or was more common. It is part of the newborn screening protocol in USA since 2006. One-third of all indigenous inhabitants of sub-Saharan Africa carry the gene. Sickle cell disease is prevalent in many parts of India in the range of 9.4–22.2%.
- *Sickle cell trait:* Inheritance of one gene for Hb S and one for normal Hb A from each parent. Seen in 1 in 12 African-Americans.
- *Sickle cell anemia*: Inheritance of gene for HbS from each parent. Computed incidence is 1 in 576 in African Americans. Rarely seen in pregnancy as mortality is high in childhood.
- Hemoglobin gene in Hb C is seen in 1 in 40 African-Americans.
- *Sickle cell Hb C disease:* Inheritance of one gene for Hb S and another for Hb C seen in 1 in 2,000 African-Americans.
- *Sickle cell β thalassemia disease:* Incidence is 1 in 2,000.

If one parent has sickle cell anemia (SS) and the other has sickle cell trait (AS), there is a 50% chance of a child having sickle cell disease (SS) and a 50% chance of a child having sickle cell trait (AS). When both parents have sickle cell trait (AS) then a child has only 25% chances of getting sickle cell disease (SS).

Clinical Features

Symptoms appear after the 6th month of life when most of the HbF has been replaced.

Sickle cell crisis: This term is used to describe several independent acute conditions occurring in patients with sickle cell disease. Most episodes of sickle cell crises last for 5 to 7 days. Sickle cell crisis can be of many types:
- Vaso-occlusive crisis
- Aplastic crisis
- Sequestration crisis
- Hemolytic crisis.

Vaso-occlusive crisis (VOC) is caused by sickle-shaped RBCs that obstruct capillaries and restrict blood flow to organs, resulting in ischemia, pain, necrosis, and often organ damage. The severity, duration, and frequency vary considerably. Severe painful crises are treated with analgesics, hydration, and blood transfusion and may even require admission. Vaso-occlusive crises involving the lungs are considered an emergency and packed cell transfusion given. Incentive spirometry is recommended in such cases.

Infarcts are of two types:
1. *Microinfarcts:* Involving abdomen, spine, and joints causing recurrent painful crises in SS
2. *Macroinfarcts:* Involving spleen, lungs, kidneys, liver, bones, and skin resulting in their anatomical and functional damage.

Splenic sequestration crisis: The spleen is frequently affected because of its narrow vessels and its function of clearing defective RBCs. It is infarcted in childhood in sickle cell anemia. The resulting autosplenectomy increases the risk of infection from organisms like *Streptococcus pneumoniae*, *Haemophilus influenza* B, etc. and prophylactic antibiotics and vaccinations (pneumococcal, meningococcal, and influenza) are recommended for patients with asplenia. The splenic sequestration crises lead to acute, painful enlargement of the spleen. Sudden pooling of blood occurs in the spleen leading to systemic hypovolemia. The abdomen becomes distended and hard and if not treated as an emergency, the patient can die within 1–2 hours of circulatory failure. Management is supportive, sometimes with blood transfusions. Milder ones are transient and may last for 3–4 hours and rarely for a day.

Aplastic crisis is acute worsening of the baseline anemia leading to pallor and tachycardia. It is usually triggered by infection with parvovirus B19, which invades the RBC precursors, multiplies in them and destroys them, thereby directly affecting erythropoiesis for 2–3 days. In normal people, this is of no consequence, but in sickle cell patients, the lifespan of the RBC being shortened, this results in a life-threatening situation. This crisis takes about 4–7 days to disappear. Most patients can be managed conservatively, though some may require transfusions.

Hemolytic crises are acute accelerated drops in Hb level due to breaking down of RBCs at a faster rate. It is seen particularly in patients with G6PD deficiency. Management as usual is supportive with an occasional transfusion.

Other crises, dactylitis, one of the earliest manifestations can present itself as early as 6 months postnatally and can be seen in children with sickle trait too. It may last up to a month. *Acute chest syndrome* characterized by fever, chest pain, difficulty in breathing, and parenchymal infiltration. It is usually caused by atelectasis, marrow emboli, thromboembolism, and infection with atypical bacteria and viruses. With improved ventilator care, which is needed in 15% of cases, the mortality of acute chest syndrome has come down to 1%, with a perinatal mortality of 9%.

Complications
- *Overwhelming post (auto) splenectomy infection (OPSI):* Due to functional asplenia caused by streptococcus pneumoniae and hemophilus influenza. Indefinite daily penicillin prophylaxis was the treatment in the past. Not seen often today due to vaccination against *H. influenzae*, *S. pneumoniae*, and *N. meningitidis*.
- *Stroke:* Resulting from a progressive narrowing of cerebral blood vessels and seen as cerebral infarction in children and cerebral hemorrhage in adults.
- *Silent stroke* is probably five times as common as symptomatic stroke. It is usually asymptomatic but is associated with brain damage. About 10–15% of children with sickle cell disease suffer from strokes of the silent type.
- *Cholelithiasis and cholecystitis* resulting from prolonged hemolysis.
- *Avascular necrosis* (aseptic bone necrosis, osteonecrosis) of the hip and other major joints due to ischemia causing a limp.
- *Decreased immune reactions* due to malfunctioning of the spleen (hyposplenism).
- *Osteomyelitis:* Commonly due to atypical Salmonella (*S. typhimurium, S. enteritidus, S. choleraesuis,* and *S. paratyphi* B), followed by infection with *Staph. aureus* and gram-negative enteric bacilli probably as a result of patchy ischemia due to intravascular sickling of the bowel.
- *Acute papillary necrosis in the kidneys and chronic renal failure* as a result of sickle cell nephropathy manifest with hypertension, proteinuria, hematuria, and worsening anemia with a poor prognosis.
- *Pulmonary hypertension* can lead to heart failure with typical symptoms of breathlessness, decreased exercise tolerance, and episodes of syncope.
- *Progressive retinopathy, vitreous hemorrhages, and retinal detachment* can lead to blindness.

DIAGNOSIS: HbSS
- *Hb:* Usually in the range of 6–8 g%. In other forms of sickle cell disease, Hb level tends to be higher.
- *Peripheral blood smear:* May show a
  - Normocytic normochromic picture
  - Fragmented RBCs
  - Anisopoikilocytosis
  - Reticulocytosis
  - Target cells and Howell–Jolly bodies (features of hypersplenism)

- *Reticulocyte count*: Increased (as the bone-marrow compensates for the destruction of sickle cells by producing more RBCs)
- *Mean corpuscular volume (MCV)/mean corpuscular hemoglobin (MCH)*: Normal, *mean corpuscular hemoglobin concentration* (*MCHC*): Increased
- *Erythrocyte sedimentation rate (ESR)*: Decreased due to reduced RBC count
- *Bone-marrow*: Erythroid hyperplasia
- *Osmotic fragility*: Decreased
- *Sickling test*: Positive, rapid, and reliable test, HbS is precipitated to deoxygenated HbS. Sickling can be induced by the addition of sodium met bisulfite (sickledex) or ascorbic acid to a blood film
- *Sickling solubility test*: A mixture of HbS and a reducing solution-like sodium dithionite gives a turbid result in contrast to HbA which remains clear
- *Lifespan of RBCs*: Reduced to only 10–12 days
- Acute sickle cell crisis is often precipitated by infection. Hence, *urine analysis* to detect occult urinary tract infection and a *chest X-ray* to look for occult pneumonia should be routinely done
- *Gel electrophoresis*: Abnormal Hb forms move at different speeds and can be identified, especially HbS, and HbSC
- *High performance liquid chromatography (HPLC)*: Diagnosis further confirmed
- *Genetic testing*: Rarely needed as other tests are highly specific for HbS and HbC
- *Genetic counseling*: For known carriers of the disease before undertaking a pregnancy
- If the mother has a trait and the father carries a gene for any abnormal Hb, be it S, C and D, or for the β-thalassemia trait, prenatal diagnosis through *amniocentesis* or *chorionic villus sampling* (*CVS*) and *preimplantation genetic screening* can be offered.

Treatment: General Management

- Penicillin to prevent and treat infections, especially in children till the age of 5 years.
- Folic acid supplementation for life, 1 mg daily to grow new RBCs.
- *Malaria prophylaxis:* Patients with sickle cell disease are uniquely vulnerable to malaria which may be the most common cause of painful crises, unlike patients with sickle cell trait who have a protective effect. Affected people living in countries where malaria is endemic should take antimalarial chemoprophylaxis for life.
- *Pain medication for vaso-occlusive crises:* Analgesics, nonsteroidal anti-inflammatory drugs (NSAIDs), opioids, etc. For more severe crises, patient controlled analgesia (PCA) may be used.
- *Blood transfusion:* To maintain hematocrit above 30%.
- Thromboprophylaxis in patients admitted with severe crises.
- Others:
  - *Recombinant human erythropoietin.*
  - *Induction of HbF* by stimulating gamma-chain synthesis inhibits polymerization of HbS and resultant sickling. Hydroxyurea, a ribonucleotide reductase inhibitor with dose-dependent cytotoxic effects, increases HbF production with fewer sickling episodes. It also reduces RBC membrane and vessel wall is damaged by decreasing the adherence of RBC to the endothelium.[8] Its teratogenic potential and whether it improves long-term survival are still not known. Decitabine, an antineoplastic drug, has been used when there was no response to hydroxyurea.[9] Hydroxyurea should be stopped at least 3 months before conception as its teratogenic potential is not known. Sudden cessation of hydroxyurea can lead to complications in an already jeopardized pregnancy. Since there are no reports of teratogenesis in humans with the dose given, it is debatable whether it should be stopped before or during conception. However, the inserts carry the warning that it is contraindicated in pregnancy and during lactation.[10]
  - *Inhaled nitric oxide* has been tried with some success in acute vaso-occlusive crises.
  - *Arginine butyrate infusions.*
  - *Zinc* prevents vaso-occlusive episodes and decreases infection.
  - *Hemopoietic cell transplantation*, bone marrow transplantation, and cord blood stem cell transplantation have been tried with varying degrees of success.[11] In utero, stem cell therapy with HbA cells, prenatally diagnosed and extracted cells conditioned to produce only HbA, and gene therapy using a modified β *globin* gene that encodes a sickling resistant protein are some of the therapies tried out for both sickle cell anemia and thalassemia.
  - *Erythrocytapheresis*: RBC exchange has been found to be safe, without the danger of iron overload, especially in those who are sensitive to hydroxyurea.[12]
  - *Chelation therapy*: As a result of multiple transfusions, iron gets deposited in various organs. Iron chelators—deferasirox (oral), deferoxamine (parenteral), deferiprone (oral, off-label) are given at the same time to remove this extra iron.[13]

Pregnancy and sickle cell syndrome: Pregnancy is risky in women with any of the major sickle hemoglobinopathies, especially HbSS disease. Pregnancy is a serious burden on the already compromised hematological system. Maternal mortality (1%) is usually due to acute chest syndrome, pneumonia, pulmonary infarction, and pulmonary embolism.[14]

Maternal Complications

Pre-existing medical disorders like the following can further complicate the pregnancy
- Pulmonary hypertension

- Cardiomyopathy
- Asymptomatic bacteriuria
- Renal failure.

Pregnancy complications:
- Cerebral vein thrombosis
- Acute chest syndrome: Appearance of new pulmonary infiltrates involving at least one complete segment, accompanied by fever, cough, chest pain, wheezing, tachypnea decreased oxygen tension and abnormal pulmonary function tests. Multilobar involvement is common and four precipitants are usually involved: (1) infection, (2) marrow emboli, (3) thromboembolism, and (4) atelectasis[15]
- Pyelonephritis
- Deep vein thrombosis (DVT)—pulmonary embolism
- Sepsis syndrome
- Pre-eclampsia.

Complications during labor:
- Placental abruption
- Stillbirth.

Fetal risks:
- Miscarriage (20%)
- Intrauterine growth restriction (IUGR) (37.5%)
- Prematurity
- Increased perinatal morbidity and mortality (11–22%).

Pregnancy and sickle cell HbC disease: These patients tolerate pregnancy better than patients with HbSS. However, severe bone pain and acute chest syndrome are seen both during pregnancy and the puerperium. The perinatal mortality is also less.[16,17]

Management during pregnancy:
- Prenatal folic acid 4 mg daily recommended to support the rapid turnover of RBC. (ACOG, 2007).[18]
- Before prescribing hematinics, the serum ferritin should be checked. If high, iron should not be given.
- About hydroxyurea continuation, the woman should consult a maternofetal medicine specialist about the pros and the cons. She can stop it during the first trimester and restart later.
- Close monitoring is advocated to compensate for the shortened lifespan of RBC. Hemopoiesis is increased during pregnancy and any condition that interferes with the production of RBC, or causes increased destruction can aggravate the anemia.
- Sickle cell crisis may mimic other acute conditions associated with pain, for example, ectopic pregnancy, appendicitis, abruption, pyelonephritis, etc. and it should be diagnosed only after excluding other conditions associated with pain, fever, and anemia. Sickling in the bone can be managed with:
  - Intravenous fluids, narcotics, and oxygen inhalation to reduce capillary sickling.
  - Prophylactic RBC transfusions can prevent further sickling crises.[19] Therapeutic transfusions are not advocated. Partial volumetric transfusions are given to maintain the Hct >35%, HbA 1 at 40%.

- Monthly urine cultures to be done and any infection promptly treated as pyelonephritis can cause increased destruction of RBC along with suppression of erythropoiesis by endotoxins.
- Pneumonia caused by *Streptococcus pneumoniae* is seen often and needs to be tackled energetically.
- CDC 2008[20] recommends the following vaccines for sickle cell patients: Polyvalent pneumococcal, *H. influenzae* type B and meningococcal vaccines.
- About 40% suffer from acute chest syndrome which can be recurrent and lead to pulmonary hypertension and restrictive lung disease later on. Pre-existing ventricular hypertrophy and cardiac dysfunction are seen in patients with HbSS anemia can be worsened by pulmonary embolism and can result in ventricular failure.[21]
- Since pre-eclampsia is more common, there could be a role for low-dose aspirin.

Fetal surveillance: Since there is a high incidence of FGR and increased PNM, serial growth scans to monitor growth and volume of amniotic fluid are recommended from 26 to 28 weeks gestation. Nonstress tests should be done in the presence of FGR from 32 weeks onward. The nonstress tests are usually nonreactive during a crisis and become reactive once the crisis is over.

Management of Labor and Delivery

This is very similar to that of a patient with cardiac disease. A comfortable position during labor with epidural analgesia for pain relief and packed cell transfusion if the hematocrit goes below 20.[22] Circulatory overload and pulmonary edema from ventricular failure should be prevented. For those on opioids, the neonate has to be monitored for withdrawal. To prevent venous thromboembolism (VTE), the woman will have to be on low-molecular-weight heparin (LMWH) for 6 weeks after delivery.

Prophylactic RBC transfusion: Indicated in sickle cell syndromes perioperatively and during pregnancy to decrease morbidity, to maintain the hematocrit above 25%, and HbS below 60%. The frequency of stroke is also seen to be reduced with transfusions. A significant reduction in maternal morbidity and need for hospitalization are seen with decreased fever, pain, and suppression of erythropoiesis. Some studies however have not shown any benefit with prophylactic transfusions. A delayed hemolytic reaction (DHTR) is seen in 10% of cases with iso-immunisation in 25% of chronically transfused sickle cell patients. The American Hematologic Society (AHS) has come out with 10 recommendations before transfusions in patients with SCD.[23]

Contraception: Issues like chronic debility, pregnancy-related complications, and a shortened lifespan make contraception, temporary or permanent very relevant. Combined oral contraceptives (COCs) are not recommended due to their adverse vascular and thrombotic effects precipitating VTE or stroke. Progesterone containing pills or implants are favored because of their role in reducing painful sickling crises. Injectable depot medroxyprogesterone acetate (DMPA) is not advised as it can cause VTE in these patients. Intrauterine contraceptive devices are not advised because of their potential to cause infection. Condoms though safe are not promoted because of high failure rate. Sterilization is a safe option.

Sickle cell trait: Heterozygous inheritance of the gene for HbS results in sickle cell trait. Almost 8% of African-Americans have it. HbS averages about 30% in each RBC. Though there are reports stating that sickle cell trait is associated with occasional hematuria and renal papillary necrosis, it has no adverse effects on pregnancy. There is no increased incidence of abortions, FGR, pre-eclampsia, or perinatal deaths. However, there is an increased incidence of asymptomatic bacilluria and urinary infection. Pregnancy is therefore not risky in women with sickle cell trait and should not be discouraged. A higher incidence of VTE has been noted in African-American women on COCs. More evidence is needed before withholding COCs from women with the trait.

■ OTHER HEMOGLOBINOPATHIES
Hemoglobin C and C-β-Thalassemia

Hemoglobin C is produced by the single β-chain substitution of glutamic acid by lysine at position 6. About 2% of African-Americans have the C trait which does not adversely affect pregnancy, nor does it cause anemia.[24] But when it coexists with the sickle cell trait, HbSC, and then all problems occur. Homozygous HbCC disease and HbC-β-thalassemia produce only mild-to-moderate anemia in pregnancy and are relatively benign. Iron and folate should be supplemented in pregnancy.

Hemoglobin E: Results when a single β-chain substitution of lysine for glutamic acid occurs at codon 26. It is the second most common Hb variant and is particularly susceptible to oxidative stress. The homozygous HbE, HbE plus β-thalassemia, and the Hb C trait are seen in one-third of Cambodians and one-fourth of Laotians and are associated with minimal anemia, hypochromia, microcytosis, and target cells. Heterozygous E trait is common in south-east Asia. The doubly heterozygous HbE-β-thalassemia is commonly associated with FGR, preterm delivery, and childhood anemia.

Prenatal diagnosis: Most of the tests are DNA based and are done on CVS or amniotic fluid samples. Polymerase chain reaction (PCR)-based techniques and targeted mutation analyses are used to detect mutant or abnormal hemoglobins.

Hemoglobinopathy in the newborn: The MCH Bureau (2005) recommendation that all newborns be tested for sickle-cell disease by cord blood electrophoresis, has decreased mortality rates in identified infants.

Thalassemia is the most common autosomal recessive, genetic blood disorder that affects the production of hemoglobin and is due to impaired synthesis of one or more of the globin peptide chains resulting in ineffective erythropoiesis, hemolysis and varying degrees of anemia **(Fig. 2)**. The name was coined at the University of Rochester, New York, by George Whipple and William Bradford. The Greek words- "thalassa" means sea and "emia" blood. Several hundred syndromes have been identified and classified according to the deficient globin chain. The two major types are the α-thalassemia, when the α peptide chain is involved and β-thalassemia when the β peptide chain is impaired. Rarer types where there is impaired synthesis of γ and δ peptide chains and combinations thereof are also seen but are clinically insignificant. Though the molecular basis of the different types of thalassemia is different, the clinical phenotypes are almost homogeneous.

Incidence: It is estimated that there are about 200,000 thalassemics in the world, among who 5,000 to 8,000 are in India. It is most commonly seen in Italy, Greece, Middle East, South Africa, and South Asia. About 100,000 babies worldwide are born with severe forms of thalassemia every year. These are seen to occur in 1 in 300 to 500 of all pregnancies. The reason that the gene for β-thalassemia is relatively common in Italy and Greece is because parts of Italy and Greece were once endemic for malaria. The presence of thalassemia minor (like sickle cell trait in Africa) afforded protection against malaria and therefore this gene thrived. In India too, thalassemia is common in areas like the Kutch where malaria was once endemic.

Classification
- α-thalassemia
- β-thalassemia

Results from impaired production or instability of α or β-globin chains along with lack of a part of an oxygen carrying protein in the RBCs.

Globin chain composition of normal and abnormal hemoglobins

Hb A – α2β2
Hb A2– α2δ2
Hb F – α2γ2
Hb H – β4
Hb Bart – γ4

Inheritance: Both types of thalassemia are inherited in the same manner. The disease is passed to children by parents who carry the mutated thalassemia gene. A child who inherits one mutated gene is a carrier, thalassemia trait or thalassemia minor. Most carriers lead completely normal lives. A child who inherits two thalassemia genes, one from each parent, will have the disease-thalassemia major. A child of two carriers has a 25% chance of receiving two trait genes and developing the disease and a 50% chance of being a thalassemia carrier. If one of the parents is a carrier, the offspring has no risk of being a thalassemic major, but has 50% chance of being a carrier.

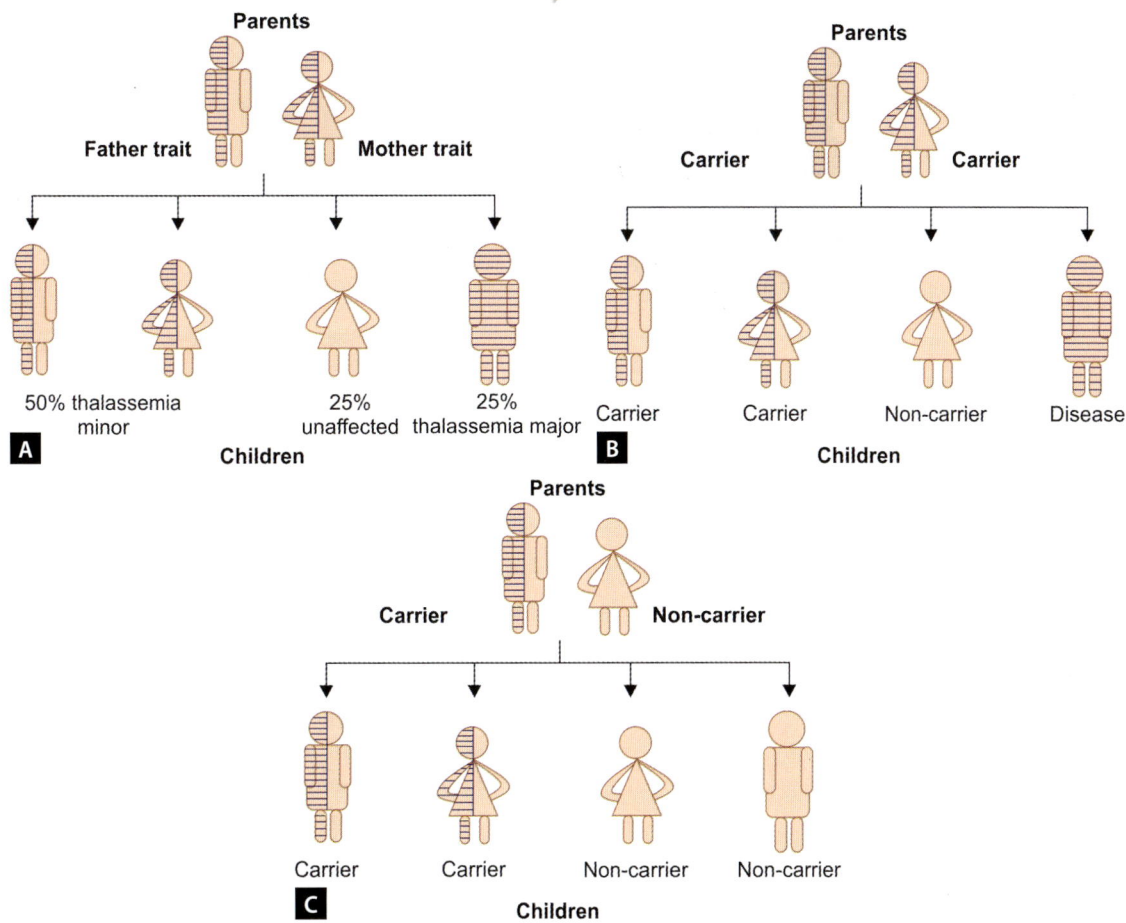

Figs. 2A to C: Autosomal recessive pattern of inheritance.

Two new terminologies are being used more often in clinical settings today are transfusion requiring and nontransfusion requiring thalassemia, depending on the requirement of frequent blood transfusions or not.[25-27]

α-thalassemia: The inheritance of α-thalassemia is complicated because of the presence of 4 α-globin chains.[28] There is a close correlation between clinical severity and the degree of impairment of α-globin chain synthesis. The α-globin chain gene loci are doubled on chromosome 16 as αα/αα genotype. The following types can be seen:

1. Deletion of all four globin chain genes **(--/--)**, characterizes *homozygous α-thalassemia.* Since none of the four genes are expressed, there are no α-globin chains, and Hb Bart (γ4) and Hb H (β4) are formed as abnormal tetramers. Hb Bart has increased affinity for oxygen, is not very good as an oxygen transporter; hence does not release oxygen to the tissues normally. This results in Hb Bart disease which is characterized by nonimmune hydrops fetalis and stillbirths **(Fig. 3)**. Ultrasound at 12–13 weeks is 100% sensitive in identifying affected fetuses by measuring the cardiothoracic ratio whereas Doppler flow measurement of the middle cerebral artery velocity can detect fetal anemia. Occasionally, these fetuses can be saved by intrauterine transfusions, but the child has to have transfusions throughout life as in β-thalassemia major **(Fig. 4)**.

2. *A compound heterozygous state* with deletion of three of four genes **(--/-α)**, with only one functional α-globin gene called *Hb H disease* (β4) is compatible with extrauterine life. The abnormal RBCs at birth contain a mixture of Hb Bart (γ4), Hb H (β4), and HbA. The disease is characterized by hemolytic anemia which develops postnatally due to replacement of Hb Bart by HbH. The anemia worsens in pregnancy.

3. A deletion of two genes results in *α-thalassemia minor* which may be the result of α0-thalassemia or α+-thalassemia traits with the genotype being either(-α/-α) or (--/αα), the two being differentiated only by DS-DNA analysis. Except for mild anemia with hypochromic and microcytic RBCs, pregnancy is usually uneventful. Except for anemia, hemolysis is not seen unlike in Bart's disease and Hb H disease.

4. The single gene deletion (-α/αα) is the *silent carrier state* without any clinical abnormality.

Frequency: The frequency of α-thalassemia minor, Hb Bart disease, and Hb H disease vary among different races. All three are seen in Asians. Among Africans, Hb Bart and Hb H are unreported and α-thalassemia is seen in< 2% of women.

Diagnosis: α-thalassemia minor and major can be diagnosed in utero by:

a. Prenatal diagnosis with chorionic villi sampling at 8–10 weeks or

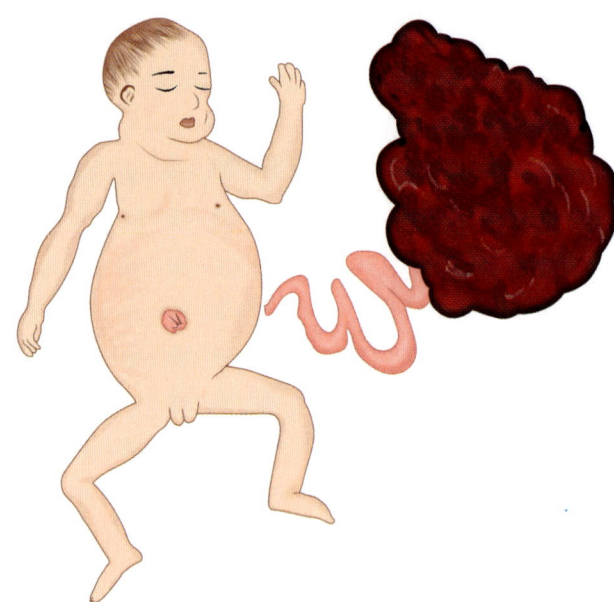

Fig. 3: Hemoglobin Bart disease.

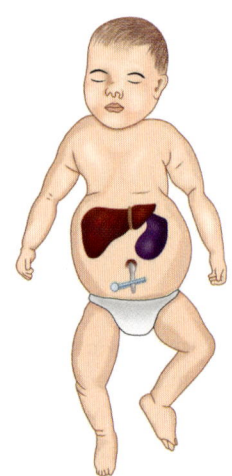

Fig. 4: Beta-thalassemia major with gross hepatosplenomegaly.

b. By amniocentesis at 14–20 weeks' gestation in high-risk families.[29,30]

β-thalassemia: This is the more familiar type of thalassemia. It involves decreased production of normal adult Hb (Hb A), the predominant Hb which is seen soon after birth and continues until death. The globin part of Hb A has four protein sections called polypeptide chains-2 identical α chains and 2 also identical β chains. In β-thalassemia there is reduced or absent synthesis of the β-chains. So there is impaired synthesis of β-globin chains, with precipitation of excess α chains or instability of α-globin chains causing damage to cell membrane. Also mutations in the α-Hb stabilizing protein (AHSP) may modify the clinical picture of β-thalassemia. So, we have homozygous β-thalassemia major and heterozygous β-thalassemia minor. The hallmark of β-thalassemia is the presence of elevated HbA2.

Types: There are two forms of β-thalassemia—thalassemia major or Cooley's anemia and thalassemia minor or trait.

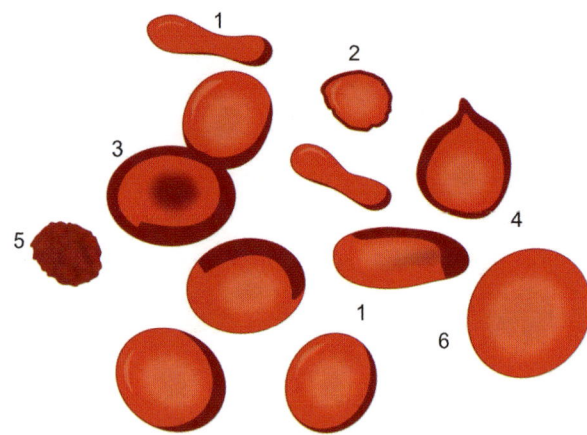

Poikilocytic red cells (1 elliptocytes, 2 schistrocytes, 3 target cells, 4 tear drop, 5 spherocytes and 6 hypochromic usually present in thalassemia major)

Fig. 5: Peripheral smear in thalassemia major.

Thalassemia minor: Persons with thalassemia minor have only one copy of the thalassemia gene along with another normal β-chain and are said to be heterozygous for β-thalassemia.

- *Diagnosis*: As thalassemia minor is a carrier state, it is typically asymptomatic
- Mild anemia is seen similar to mild iron deficiency anemia. Low Hb% and low MCV
- *Iron indices*: Serum iron level is normal to raised, serum ferritin- 300–3000 ng/dL, TIBC- 70%
- *Mentzer index* (MCV divided by RBC count) <13 – probably thalassemia, >13 - iron deficiency anemia[29]
- *Low RDW* unlike in Iron deficiency and Sideroblastic anemia where it is high
- *Peripheral smear*: Hypochromic and microcytic RBCs, with poikilocytes, anisocytes, Heinz bodies, target cells, tear drop cells, granular cytoplasmic inclusion bodies, polychromasia and marked reticulocytosis >10% **(Fig. 5)**
- *Hemoglobin electrophoresis (Fig. 6)*: Normal- 95–98% of Hb A, Hb A2- <2–3% and Hb F- <2%
- β-thalassemia major- higher Hb A2 and Hb F, less Hb A
- β-thalassemia minor- Hb A2 (2α + 2δ-globin chains) >3.5%, Hb F (2α + 2γ-globin chains) >2%.

A common confounding factor in HPLC is a coexisting iron deficiency that masks β-thalassemia minor giving a normal report. Iron deficiency makes the HbA2 percentage normal- the key finding in β-thalassemia minor. HbA2 may be raised in antiretroviral therapy, B12/folate deficiency and hyperthyroidism. HPLC can also unmask coexisting hemoglobinopathies too.[31]

Bone marrow micronormoblastic reaction, erythroid hyperplasia, striking basophilic stippling, increased iron deposition, and ring sideroblasts.

Decreased Osmotic Fragility

Alkali denaturation tests: HbA gets denatured with alkali but HbF is resistant and not destroyed. If HbF is high then it is thalassemia major.

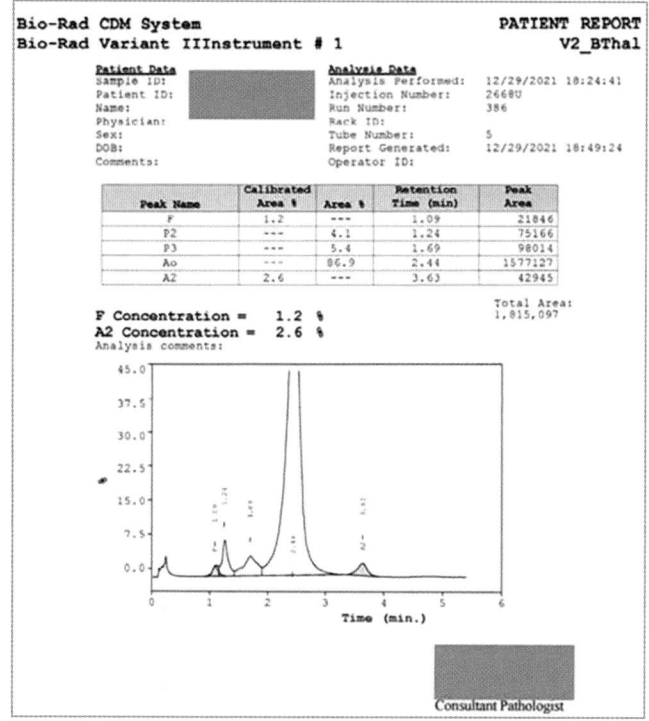

Fig. 6: Normal hemoglobin electrophoresis report.

DNA analysis: To confirm mutations in the alpha and beta globin-producing genes. It is not a routine procedure but can be used to help diagnose thalassemia and to determine carrier status, if genetic testing of amniotic fluid is indicated if both the parents are carriers.

Erythrocyte porphyrin levels rarely indicated to distinguish between β-thalassemia minor and iron-deficiency anemia and lead poisoning. Porphyrin levels are normal in thalassemia, but elevated in the other two.

The *ZPP test* is used to differentiate true iron-deficiency anemia from thalassemia. In the final stage of hematopoiesis, if iron is deficient, zinc instead of iron is incorporated into the protoporphyrin ring of the heme molecule in the bone marrow and accumulates in the blood.[32]

Dichlorophenolindophenol (DCIP) and one-tube osmotic fragility (OF) tests are also used to diagnose thalassemia when the iron indices are low.

There is usually pregnancy-induced augmentation of erythropoiesis, normal blood volume expansion, and subnormal red cell expansion.

Treatment: Mild thalassemia (Hb: 6–10 g/dL): Signs and symptoms are generally mild and little or no treatment is needed. Rarely, patients may need a transfusion following surgery, etc. There is no specific treatment for β-thalassemia minor during pregnancy. Prophylactic iron and folic acid are given. Fetal growth restriction and oligohydramnios are increased two-fold in affected women.

β-*thalassemia major (Cooley's anemia):* The child with this disorder is homozygous for β-thalassemia with a striking deficiency in β-chain and Hb A production, resulting in a serious disease. At birth the baby with thalassemia major seems entirely normal. This is because the predominant Hb at birth is still Hb F which has 2 α-chains (like Hb A) and 2γ-chains (unlike Hb A). It has no β-chains, so the baby is protected at birth from the effects of thalassemia major. Within the first month of birth, anemia develops and becomes progressively more severe. The infant fails to thrive and has feeding problems (due to easy fatigue from lack of oxygen), bouts of fever (due to infections), diarrhea as a direct consequence of anemia, and other intestinal problems.

Complications[33,34]

- Increased extramedullary hematopoiesis may result in brittle and thin bones with deformed facial bones and an appearance known as chipmunk face
- Bronze color skin due to iron deposition in the skin
- Arrhythmia, cardiomyopathy, and heart failure may ensue due to iron deposition in myocytes following multiple transfusions leading to high mortality
- Cholelithiasis, hepatosplenomegaly, jaundice, cirrhosis, and chronic liver failure may result either because of the disease itself or the treatment
- Neurological complications such as peripheral neuropathies
- Slow growth rate and delayed puberty
- Increased risk of parvovirus B19 infection
- Diabetes and hypothyroidism also are more commonly seen.

Without treatment, the spleen, liver, and heart enlarge and death follows infection and heart failure. With treatment and adequate transfusions, the child develops normally until the end of the first decade. Then effects of iron loading become apparent. Prognosis improves with iron chelation therapy.

Treatment: Moderate-to-severe thalassemia (Hb < 5–6 g/dL):
- *Blood transfusions:* Frequently needed sometimes every couple of months, to keep the Hb% around 9–10 g% for a feeling of wellbeing and to suppress extramedullary erythropoiesis. Packed RBC at the rate of 8–15 mL/kg body weight over 1–2 hours is recommended.
- *Chelation therapy:* As a result of multiple transfusions, iron gets deposited in various organs. Iron chelators—deferasirox (oral), deferoxamine (parenteral), deferiprone (oral, off-label) are given at the same time to remove this extra iron **(Fig. 7)**.[13]
- *Stem cell transplant:* Bone marrow transplant can be considered in children with severe disease to avoid repeated blood transfusions and the ensuing problems.[35] However, the complications following stem cell transplant like chronic immunosuppressive therapy, GVHD, graft failure, etc. are also to be considered.[36]
- *Gene therapy:* It is the latest advancement in severe thalassemia management. It involves harvesting the patient's hematopoietic stem cells (HSCs) and modifying

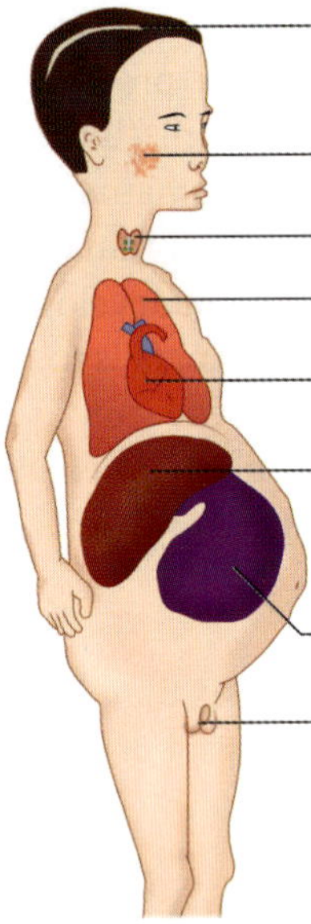

Fig. 7: Thalassemia major after multiple transfusions.

them genetically with normal genes expressing vectors, which are then reinfused to the patients after they have been conditioned to destroy the existing HSCs. The genetically modified HSCs produce normal hemoglobin chains with normal erythropoiesis ensuing.

Genome Editing Techniques[37]

- *Splenectomy* indicated in thalassemia major to reduce the number of transfusions and to limit extramedullary erythropoiesis. Done especially when the transfusion rate exceeds 200–220 RBCs/kg/year with a hematocrit above 70%. However, postsplenectomy, infections are common, hence immunizations are necessary. Done only after the age of 6–7 years; followed by penicillin prophylaxis for several years.
- *Cholecystectomy* due to Hb breakdown, bilirubin may accumulate in the gall bladder as gall stones. Cholecystectomy can be done at the time of splenectomy, if symptomatic.
- *Diet:* Tea helps in reducing iron absorption from the intestine and vitamin C in increasing iron excretion from the intestine. Can be combined with deferoxamine too.[37]

Differential Diagnosis

It can rule out the following by doing:
- *Iron-deficiency anemia:* Iron studies and Mentzer index
- *Anemia of chronic disease and renal failure:* Raised inflammatory markers (CRP, ESR)
- *Sideroblastic anemias:* Iron studies and peripheral blood smear
- *Lead poisoning:* Serum protoporphyrin level.

Thalassemia and pregnancy: Pregnancy with β-thalassemia is now possible because of transfusions and chelation therapy.
- A multidisciplinary team approach with a hematologist, perinatologist, and a genetic counselor is needed.
- In pregnancy, the need for transfusion increases.
- No iron is given for fear of overload.
- Folic acid is advocated preconception and till 12 weeks gestation to facilitate cell division.
- Vitamin C 100–150 mg daily helps to remove excess iron from the gut.
- Pregnancy is recommended only if there is normal cardiac function and Hb is maintained at 10 g%.
- Risk of developing insulin-dependent diabetes mellitus high.
- Genetic counseling is necessary to assess fetal risk.
- Prenatal diagnosis of β-thalassemia major is difficult because of many mutations.
- Targeted mutation analysis has to be done after identifying the disease causing mutation for that family.
- These can be done by CVS, preimplantation blastomere biopsy and testing of nucleated RBCs from the maternal circulation.

Screening: Universal screening is not recommended. Screening is done only in selected races, and when the Hb is low, MCV <80 and iron study is normal. Hb electrophoresis is usually sufficient. Test is offered to the partner of a carrier of hemoglobinopathies or any woman with a HBA2 >3.5% to assess fetal risk. If both parents are carriers, then fetal DNA based tests are done.

Prenatal diagnosis includes
- PCR of fetal DNA is extracted from amniotic cells or trophoblasts from CVS at 10–12 weeks or fetal RBCs from cordocentesis at 19 weeks
- Isolation of single nucleated RBCs from maternal circulation is being explored for prenatal diagnosis of β-thalassemia[38]
- PGD and DNA analysis of embryos
- Genomic study of DNA by southern blotting of endonucleases is a useful test.

Patient Education

Patients have to be counseled on healthy eating and safe living to avoid complications
- To avoid excess iron: Not to have vitamin tablets which contain iron unless prescribed
- To eat a healthy diet: A good nutritious diet with folic acid helps natural erythropoiesis
- To avoid infections: Especially postsplenectomy. All routine immunizations are to be strictly followed
- To be counseled about the inheritance patterns and to seek genetic counseling preconception.[39]

■ KEY MESSAGES

- Sickle cell disease or sickle cell anemia is an autosomal recessive genetic disorder characterized by rigid, sickle shaped RBCs which reduce its flexibility resulting in various complications.

- Sickle cell crisis can be of many types: The vaso-occlusive, aplastic, sequestration, and the hemolytic types.
- Some of the common complications are aseptic bone necrosis, chronic renal failure, pulmonary hypertension, etc.
- Diagnosis is based on a low Hb%, peripheral smear, sickling test, and gel electrophoresis.
- There is no specific treatment for sickle cell anemia. Supportive therapy includes antibiotics, blood transfusion, folic acid supplementation, analgesics, etc.
- Sickle cell trait is however not a contraindication for pregnancy.
- *Thalassemia* is the most common autosomal recessive, genetic blood disorder that affects the production of hemoglobin resulting in ineffective erythropoiesis, hemolysis, and varying degrees of anemia.
- There are 2 types—alpha and beta thalassemia. The frequency of α-thalassemia minor, Hb Bart disease, and Hb H disease vary among different races.
- *β-thalassemia* is the more familiar type of thalassemia due to decreased production of normal adult Hb (Hb A). There are two forms of β-thalassemia—thalassemia major or Cooley's anemia and thalassemia minor or trait.
- There is no specific treatment for β-thalassemia minor during pregnancy. Prophylactic iron and folic acid are given. Fetal growth restriction and oligoamnios are increased two-fold in affected women.
- Iron overload may occur and cause damage to heart, liver and other organs. Iron chelation treatment with deferoxamine may be required.

REFERENCES

1. Chakravorty S, Dick MC. Antenatal screening for haemoglobinopathies: current status, barriers and ethics. Br J Haematol. 2019;187(4):431-40.
2. Forget BG, Bunn HF. Classification of the disorders of hemoglobin. Cold Spring Harb Perspect Med. 2013;3(2):a011684.
3. Gardner K, Douiri A, Drasar E, Allman M, Mwirigi A, Awogbade M, et al. Survival in adults with sickle cell disease in a high-income setting. Blood. 2016;128(10):1436-8.
4. Mangla A, Ehsan M, Maruvada S. Sickle cell anemia. Treasure Island (FL): StatPearls Publishing; 2020.
5. Porter M, Rapid fire: sickle cell disease. Emerg Med Clin North Am. 2018;36(3):567-76.
6. Badawy SM, Cronin RM, Hankins J, Crosby L, DeBaun M, Thompson AA, et al. Patient-centered ehealth interventions for children, adolescents, and adults with sickle cell disease: systematic review. J Med Internet Res. 2018; 20(7):e10940.
7. Stuart MJ, Nagel RL. Sickle cell disease. Lancet. 2004;364:1343.
8. Platt OS. Hydroxyurea for the treatment of sickle cell anemia. New Engl J Med. 2008;358:1362.
9. DeSimone J, Koshy M, Dorn L, Lavelle D, Bressler L, Molokie R, et al. Maintenance of elevated hemoglobin levels by decitabine during dose interval treatment of sickle cell anemia. Blood. 2002;99:3905.
10. Clinical Trials. Hydroxyurea Exposure Limiting Pregnancy and Follow-Up Lactation (HELPFUL). [online] Available from: https://clinicaltrials.gov/ct2/show/NCT04093986. [Last Accessed November, 2021].
11. Pinto FO, Roberts I. Cord blood stem cell transplantation for hemoglobinopathies. Br J Haematol. 2008;141:309.
12. Masera N, Tavecchia L, Pozzi L, Riva F, Vimercati C, Calabria M, et al. Periodic erythroexchange is an effective strategy for high risk paediatric patients with sickle-cell disease. Transfus Apher Sci. 2007;37(3):241-7.
13. Vichinsky E, Torres M, Minniti CP, Barrette S, Habr D, Zhang Y, et al. Efficacy and safety of deferasirox compared with deferoxamine in sickle cell disease: two-year results including pharmacokinetics and concomitant hydroxyurea. Am J Hematol. 2013;88(12):1068-73.
14. Chakravarthy EF, Khanna D, Chung L. Pregnancy outcomes in systemic sclerosis, primary pulmonary hypertension and sickle cell disease. Obstet Gynecol. 2008;111:927.
15. Medoff BD, Shepard JO, Smith RN, Kratz A. Case 17- 2005: A 22 year old woman with back and leg pain and respiratory failure. N Engl J Med. 2005;352:2425.
16. Tita ATN, Biggio JR, Chapman V, Neely C, Rouse DJ. Perinatal and maternal outcomes in women with sickle or Hb C trait. Obstet Gynecol. 2007;110:1113.
17. Pritchard JA, Scott DE, Whalley PH, Cunningham FG, Mason RA. The effects of maternal sickle cell hemoglobinopathies and sickle cell trait on reproductive performance. Am J Obstet Gynecol. 1973;117:662.
18. American College of Obstetricians and Gynecologists: Hemoglobinopathies in pregnancy. Practice Bulletin No 78. January 2007.
19. Vianello A, Vencato E, Cantini M, Zanconato G, Manfrin E, Zamo A, et al. Improvement of maternal and fetal outcomes in women with sickle cell disease treated with early prophylactic erythrocytapheresis. Transfusion (Paris). 2018;58(9):2192-2201.
20. Centers for Disease control and prevention. Vaccines. [online] Available from: http://www.cdc.gov/vaccines/pubs/vis/downloads/vis mening.pdf. [Last Accessed November, 2021].
21. Vichinsky EP, Neumayr LD, Earles AN, Williams R, Lennette ET, Dea D, et al. Causes and outcomes of the acute chest syndrome in sickle cell disease. N Engl J Med. 2000;342:1855.
22. Camous J, N'da A, Etienne-Julan M, Stéphan F. Anaesthetic management of pregnant women with sickle cell disease-effect on postnatal sickling complications. Can J Anaesth. 2008;55:276.
23. Chou ST, Alsawas M, Fasano RM, Field JJ, Hendrickson JE, Howard J, et al. American Society of Hematology 2020 guidelines for sickle cell disease: transfusion support. Blood Adv. 2020;4(2):327-55.
24. Maberry MC, Mason RA, Cunningham FG, Pritchard JA. Pregnancy complicated by Hb CC and C beta-thalassemia disease. Obstet Gynecol. 1990;76:324.
25. He LN, Chen W, Yang Y, Xie YJ, Xiong ZY, Chen DY, et al. Elevated prevalence of abnormal glucose metabolism and other endocrine disorders in patients with β-thalassemia major: a meta-analysis. Biomed Res Int. 2019;2019:6573497.
26. Vichinsky E, Cohen A, Thompson AA, Giardina PJ, Lal A, Paley C, et al. Epidemiologic and clinical characteristics of nontransfusion-dependent thalassemia in the United States. Pediatr Blood Cancer. 2018;65(7):e28067.
27. Ahmadpanah M, Asadi Y, Haghighi M, Ghasemibasir H, Khanlarzadeh E, Brand S. In patients with minor beta-thalassemia, cognitive performance is related to length of education, but not to minor beta-thalassemia or hemoglobin levels. Iran J Psychiatry. 2019;14(1):47-53.

28. Leung WC, Leung KY, Lau ET, Tang MHY, Chan V. Alpha thalassemia. Semin Fetal Neonatal Med.2008;13:215-22.
29. Singha K, Taweenan W, Fucharoen G, Fucharoen S. Erythrocyte indices in a large cohort of β-thalassemia carrier: implication for population screening in an area with high prevalence and heterogeneity of thalassemia. Int J Lab Hematol. 2019; 41(4):513-8.
30. Ansari S, Rashid N, Hanifa A, Siddiqui S, Kaleem B, Naz A, et al. Laboratory diagnosis for thalassemia intermedia: are we there yet? J Clin Lab Anal. 2019;33(1):e22647.
31. Needs T, Gonzalez-Mosquera LF, Lynch DT. Beta thalassemia. StatPearls Publishing; 2020.
32. Allen A, Perera S, Perera L, Rodrigo R, Mettananda S, Matope A, et al. A "One-Stop" screening protocol for haemoglobinopathy traits and iron deficiency in Sri Lanka. Front Mol Biosci. 2019;6:66.
33. Benites BD, Cisneiros IS, Bastos SO, Lino APBL, Costa FF, Gilli SCO, et al. Echocardiografic abnormalities in patients with sickle cell/β-thalassemia do not depend on the β-thalassemia phenotype. Hematol Transfus Cell Ther. 2018;41(2):158-63.
34. Paul A, Thomson VS, Refat M, Al-Rawahi B, Taher A, Nadar SK, Cardiac involvement in beta-thalassaemia: current treatment strategies. Postgrad Med. 2019;131(4):261-7.
35. Jariwala K, Mishra K, Ghosh K. Comparative study of alloimmunization against red cell antigens in sickle cell disease & thalassemia major patients on regular red cell transfusion. Indian J Med Res. 2019;149(1):34-40.
36. Sarkar SK, Shah MS, Begum M, Yunus AM, Aziz MA, Kabir AL, et al. Red Cell alloantibodies in thalassaemia patients who received ten or more units of transfusion. Mymensingh Med J. 2019;28(2):364-9.
37. Darvishi Khezri H, Emami Zeydi A, Sharifi H, Jalali H. Is vitamin C supplementation in patients with β-thalassemia major beneficial or detrimental? Hemoglobin. 2016;40(4):293-4.
38. Kolialexi A, Vrettou C, Traeger Synodinos J. Non-invasive prenatal diagnosis of beta-thalassemia using individual fetal erythroblasts isolated from maternal blood after enrichment. Prenatal Diag. 2007;27:1228-32.
39. Manzoor I, Zakar R, Sociodemographic determinants associated with parental knowledge of screening services for thalassemia major in Lahore. Pak J Med Sci. 2019;35(2):483-8.

LONG QUESTIONS

1. Discuss the pathophysiology and inheritance of sickle cell anemia. How will you manage a pregnant woman with sickle cell anemia?
2. Describe the clinical features and complications of sickle cell anemia in a pregnant woman? How do you manage a sickling crisis?
3. Discuss the inheritance of α-thalassemia. Describe the effects of Hb Bart disease on the fetus.
4. Discuss the management of a pregnant woman with β-thalassemia major. How will you counsel her? Comment on prenatal diagnosis in this patient.

SHORT QUESTIONS

Write short notes on:
1. Pathophysiology of sickle cell disease
2. Sickle cell crisis
3. Diagnosis of sickle cell anemia
4. Pregnancy and sickle cell syndrome
5. Inheritance of α-thalassemia.

MULTIPLE CHOICE QUESTIONS

1. Which of the following is not considered effective in the management of pain from intravascular sickling?
   a. Intravenous hydration
   b. Morphine
   c. Prophylactic RBC transfusion
   d. Therapeutic RBC transfusion
2. Hb S is caused by a substitution of which of the following?
   a. Valine for glutamic acid at position 6
   b. Glutamic acid for valine at position 6
   c. Lysine for glutamic acid at position 6
   d. Glutamic acid for leucine at position 6
3. Hb C results from substitution of glutamic acid by what amino acid at position 6 of the β-chain:
   a. Valine   b. Leusine
   c. Lysine   d. Phenylalanine
4. Which of the following is not associated with Hb SC disease in pregnancy?
   a. Severe bone pain   b. Pulmonary infarction
   c. Placental abruption d. Adult chest syndrome
5. Which of the following ethnic groups is most likely to have Hb Bart?
   a. Mediterranean whites b. Asians
   c. Africans   d. Greeks
6. Which of the following characterizes β-thalassemia?
   a. Impaired production of β-globin chains
   b. Increased destruction of RBCs containing Hb F
   c. Increased production of α-globin chains
   d. Decreased production of Hb F
7. A fetus with Hb Bart can be identified at 12–13 weeks by which of the following sonographic methods?
   a. Abdominal circumference
   b. AC/BPD ratio
   c. Cardiothoracic ratio
   d. AC/FL ratio
8. Which of the following is elevated in β-thalassemia?
   a. Hb A   b. Hb A2
   c. Hb F   d. Hb H
9. Which chromosome contains the gene for α-globin chain synthesis?
   a. 6   b. 11
   c. 16   d. 21
10. Which of the following adverse pregnancy outcomes is increased in women with Hb C trait?
    a. Preterm deliveries   b. Fetal growth restriction
    c. Perinatal mortality   d. None of the above

Answers

| 1. | d | 2. | a | 3. | c | 4. | c | 5. | b | 6. | a |
| 7. | c | 8. | b | 9. | c | 10. | d | | | | |

5.7 RENAL DISEASE AND PREGNANCY

Pralhad Kushtagi

INTRODUCTION

Obstetrician needs to be prepared to provide obstetric care to women who develop renal problem during pregnancy and to those with renal disease reporting with pregnancy.

There is a paradigm change in the outlook of physicians to care of pregnancy in a woman with renal disorder. Not very long ago, renal disease was considered a contraindication to pregnancy. Improved understanding of the anatomical changes and renal physiological adaptations in pregnancy, availability and access to nephrological services, disease treatment, and pregnancy care in high-risk obstetric units have favorably changed the reproductive outcome in these women.

Women with kidney disease or systemic diseases that would put them at risk should receive preconceptional counseling. The team taking care of such women should preferably include physicians from high-risk obstetrics, maternofetal medicine, nephrology, and other concerned specialties such as rheumatology, immunology, or hematology.

The knowledge about anatomical and physiological changes in uronephrologic system is a necessity for any obstetrician to take care of pregnancy, not only the one wishing to manage renal disorders in pregnancy. The hemodynamic and cardiovascular changes that occur during pregnancy mirror in renal system. The growing expanding uterus coupled with influence of ovarian steroidal hormones ensues features mimicking obstructive uropathic changes.

I shall be excluding lower urinary tract infection (UTI) and asymptomatic bacteriuria from the purview of this chapter.

KIDNEY FUNCTION AND PREGNANCY

Anatomical Changes

The kidneys increase in size by 1–1.5 cm.[1] It may mainly be due to interstitial tissue hypertrophy and increase in renal vascular volume.[2] Pelvicalyceal system shows dilatation. The backpressure effect caused by mechanical compression of ureters at the pelvic brim could be the main reason for the dilatation. The lowered tone of the bladder and ureters along with decreased contraction pressure and decreased peristaltic activity occurring under the influence of raised maternal progesterone will add to it. The pelvicalyceal changes are more marked on the right side[3] possibly due to compression over the ureter by the dextrorotation of the growing uterus. These changes increase the overall capacity of the renal pelvis and ureter from 15 to 75 mL.

Urinary bladder undergoes marked congestion and becomes edematous in late pregnancy due to venous and lymphatic obstruction. Hypertrophy of the detrusor and elastic tissues of the bladder wall is also noticed.

Increased urinary frequency occurs in the first trimester due to changes in uterine isthmus and expanding uterus irritating the trigone. Once the uterus becomes abdominal and upright after 12 weeks of pregnancy, symptoms of frequency disappear only to reappear in late pregnancy because of pressure by presenting part. Stress urinary incontinence can be a symptom because of pressure, change in urethra-vesical angulation, and progesterone-induced changes at the meatus.

Physiological Changes

Increased cardiac output and decreased renovascular resistance is seen by mid-pregnancy, and it increases the renal perfusion by 75% with the resultant increase in glomerular filtration rate (GFR) by 50% and the increased renal clearance.[4] It may in part also be contributed by fall in oncotic pressure as a result of fall in serum albumin. Late in the third trimester of pregnancy, there will be 15–20% decrease in GFR.[5] These changes are responsible for fall in blood urea nitrogen (BUN) levels.

Circulating steroid hormones alter the salt and water metabolisms. Increased GFR, plasma clearance, and antagonism of progesterone to aldosterone increase sodium clearance. At the same time, increases in estrogen, aldosterone, and deoxycorticosterone favor sodium retention. Increased estrogen levels also predispose to increased renin, its substrate, and aldosterone. It is countered by decreased sensitivity to the pressure effect of angiotensin during pregnancy. Serum potassium usually remains in the low normal range, due to counter effects of increased excretion due to increased urine flow rate and aldosterone, and antimineralocorticoid effect of progesterone.[6]

Increased progesterone results in hyperventilation that stimulates bicarbonaturia, mild respiratory alkalosis, and to some fall in serum bicarbonate. Despite the reduction in serum bicarbonate, the anion gap is slightly reduced in normal pregnancy, may be because of an accompanying metabolic acidosis, probably of fetal origin.[7] The net result of these changes in normal pregnancy is rise in plasma pH to 7.42–7.44 and fall of arterial pCO_2 from 39 to 30 mm Hg, urinary acidification remaining normal.

There do occur some significant immunologic shifts in the function of the innate and adaptive immune systems, like a shift from T helper (T_H) cell type 1 (T_H1; cell-mediated immunity) to a T_H2 (humoral-mediated immunity) phenotype during the course of pregnancy, and increase in the number of regulatory T cells. These changes are brought about to develop tolerance to fetal antigens, aid trophoblast invasion, and assist placental formation.[8] Normal human pregnancy is associated

TABLE 1: Adaptive changes in pregnancy and clinical implications.

Adaptive changes	Clinical implications
Anatomical: • Dilatation of collecting system • ↑ Kidney size and volume	• Confusion in diagnosis of obstruction • ↑ Pyelonephritis from asymptomatic bacteriuria
Physiological: • Vasodilatation—renal and systemic • ↑ Renal plasma flow • ↑ Glomerular filtration rate • Altered tubular reabsorption—glucose, amino acids, uric acid, protein	• ↓ Blood pressure • ↓ Creatinine • Glycosuria and proteinuria

with evidence of complement activation, as determined by increased concentrations of the anaphylatoxins C3a, C4a, and C5a in the maternal circulation.[9]

Urinalysis

Protein excretion increases during pregnancy as consequence of increased GFR and increase in porosity of glomerular basement membrane, and up to 200 mg/day.[10]

Although there is normal tubular reabsorption, glucose reabsorption does not occur proportionately to the increased GFR, thus lowering the renal threshold for glucose resulting in glycosuria seen during pregnancy.[11]

Hematuria on dipstick examination is not common in pregnancy as long as urine sediment is without casts and serum creatinine is normal.[12]

Adaptive changes in pregnancy and their clinical implications are summarized in **Table 1**.

WOMAN DEVELOPING RENAL DISEASE IN PREGNANCY

The clinical consequences of the above changes are that one should consider following as reflective of impaired renal function:
- Serum creatinine above 1.2 mg/dL
- Rising urea or creatinine concentration, even within the "normal" range used outside pregnancy
- Increases in plasma sodium to those of nonpregnant women
- Increments in serum urea, particularly when accompanied by rising hemoglobin or hematocrit
- Hematuria by dipstick with active urine sediment and higher serum creatinine.

ACUTE KIDNEY INJURY

It is not very common to find acute kidney injury (AKI) developing during pregnancy. When they develop, the pregnancy-related acute kidney injury (PRAKI) episodes occur in otherwise healthy women. It is a heterogeneous syndrome with multiple etiology. It is useful to consider PRAKI as developing from (1) obstetrical complications, (2) related to pregnancy-specific disorders, and (3) miscellaneous causes. Most of these cases, nearly 75% of PRAKI occur during the late third trimester and in the early postpartum. Pregnancy-related hypertension such as severe preeclampsia (PE) and HELLP (hemolysis, elevated liver enzymes, and low platelet) syndrome is the leading cause. Other causes include antepartum hemorrhage, postpartum hemorrhage, puerperal sepsis, intrauterine death, acute fatty lever of pregnancy (AFLP), hemolytic uremic syndrome (HUS), and thrombotic microangiopathy of pregnancy. In the first half of pregnancy prerenal disease due to hyperemesis gravidarum and first trimester hemorrhages (disturbed ectopic gestation and incomplete abortion), acute tubular necrosis (ATN) from septic abortion, and those associated with viral or bacterial infection are common. Most of the other conditions can be thought of in the latter half of pregnancy or postpartum.

In these situations, the volume depletion and prerenal AKI lead to ischemic ATN if the injury is of sufficient severity and duration. Acute cortical necrosis (ACN) can also occur in the setting of severe hypotension, and it appears to occur more commonly in pregnancy mainly because of hypercoagulable state than in other conditions characterized by similar degree of hemodynamic compromise. May be because of this reason, it is also referred to as functional renal failure.

Incidence of PRAKI as noted from Canadian Database appears to be 2.68 per 10,000 deliveries, however, levels continue to be higher in India.[13] These incidence rates are low, but the trend is considered to be concerning. This could be due to several factors, including the increased use of assisted reproduction technology that allows women to become pregnant at more advanced ages, an increasing incidence of hypertensive pregnancy disorders, and increasing obesity. PRAKI requiring dialysis is less common, occurring in 1 per 10,000 pregnant women, but it is associated with increased mortality.

Criteria for the diagnosis of PRAKI are not standardized. An increase in serum creatinine level of 0.3 mg/dL, consistent with stage 1 in the AKI Network scheme, may represent a significant kidney injury since the level is typically lower in pregnancy due to hyperfiltration, as already mentioned. Smaller increases in serum creatinine levels (0.3 mg/dL) may be more sensitive for picking up early injury, and should be interpreted within the context of each clinical scenario. The working criteria for diagnosis suggested is presence of any one of the three: sudden increase in serum creatinine >1 mg/dL, oliguria/anuria, and/or need for dialysis.[14] Based on the degree of increase in serum creatinine from the baseline (to 1.5/2/3 times) and fall in urine output (from <0.5 mL/kg/h for 6 hours, 12 hours, or <0.3 mL/kg/h for 24 hours), PRAKIs are viewed in three stages.

The conditions that may develop renal injury and require detection during pregnancy are lupus nephritis, atypical HUS, and immunoglobulin nephropathy. Sometimes, it can be difficult to diagnose an acute as opposed to a chronic kidney injury, like glomerular disease that may be unmasked by the hemodynamic, inflammatory, and immunologic shifts in pregnancy.

Specific Conditions

Preeclampsia

Glomerular endotheliosis is the characteristic lesion often associated with subendothelial deposits leading to capillary luminal obstruction. Altered hemodynamic abnormalities of decreased renal plasma flow, reduction in GFR, and renal vasoconstriction make the kidney susceptible for ischemic injury in PE.[15] The impaired tubular secretion of uric acid in PE results in increased uric acid level.[16] AKI most often develops in the setting of complications of PE such as placental abruption, disseminated intravascular coagulation, postpartum hemorrhage, or intrauterine death.

HELLP (Hemolysis, Elevated Liver Enzymes, and Low Platelet) Syndrome

Cause of AKI in HELLP syndrome is not clear. Intravascular platelet activation and microvascular endothelial damage seen in HELLP syndrome can lead to intravascular microthrombosis and may cause ATN.[17]

Acute Fatty Liver of Pregnancy

Renal insufficiency is usually nonoliguric.

Intra-abdominal hemorrhage, hypovolemia, coexisting PE, coagulopathy, and hepatic failure are the different factors that may contribute to PRAKI.

Thrombotic Microangiopathy

Depending on the presentation, two clinical syndromes of thrombotic thrombocytopenic purpura (TTP) and HUS are described that can cause AKI. An acquired or constitutional deficiency of activity of Von Willebrand factor-processing protein, ADAMTS13, and pregnancy is shown to induce the onset or relapse of ADAMTS13 deficiency-related TTP. Levels of ADAMTS13 ls tend to fall during the last two trimesters of pregnancy. Pregnancy triggers episodes of HUS in women with mutation of the genes encoding complement regulatory proteins resulting in uncontrolled complement activation in them. Pregnancy-associated HUS more commonly occurs in the postpartum period.

Postrenal Acute Kidney Injury

Iatrogenic injuries to bladder and ureter in situations of cesarean deliveries, especially in late second stage of labor,[18] can result in AKI. Women with ectopic kidneys and duplication of ureters are at highest risk. Another rare cause of obstructive uropathy is compression of ureters at pelviureteric junction by gravid uterus in the third trimester. Risk factors listed are primigravida, multiple gestation, polyhydramnios, and nephrolithiasis.[19]

Causes of PRAKI are summarized in **Table 2**.

Diagnosis

In recognizing renal disease, measurement of kidney function and proteinuria are the early standard estimators of subclinical pathology. The dramatically altered changes in renal function need to be considered when assessing renal function in pregnancy and in the choice of various medications given through parturition. Renal function and filtration are also affected in PE, and recent advances have greatly expanded our understanding of the pathophysiologic mechanisms of this pregnancy-specific renal syndrome.

- *Urinalysis and microscopic examination of the sediment*: Urinalysis is usually unchanged during pregnancy, however, many variables can affect the results. Posture can affect urine concentration and specific gravity. When compared to upright position, after the lateral recumbence urine tends to be dilute.[20] The urine must be at room temperature for the dipsticks to be reliable. Dipsticks exposed to air will give false-positive results for glucose and false-negative results for blood.[21] Observational error and training also affect the sensitivity of predicting proteinuria by dipstick. The use of an automated urinalysis device for the detection of proteinuria is shown to reduce the false-positive rate. Proteinuria diagnosed on dipstick should be confirmed with a 24-hour urine.[22]
- *Proteinuria*: Quantification is done from 24-hour urine collection. It is cumbersome for the patient, is often

TABLE 2: Causes of pregnancy related acute kidney injury (AKI) according to time at manifestation.

Early pregnancy	Late pregnancy	Postpartum
• Prerenal AKI—hyperemesis gravidarum • Acute tubular necrosis—abortion hemorrhage and septic abortion • Renal cortical necrosis – postabortal sepsis, acute pyelonephritis (second trimester) • Thrombotic thrombocytopenic purpura	• Acute tubular necrosis—PE, HELLP syndrome, and placental abruption • Acute fatty liver of pregnancy • Thrombotic thrombocytopenic purpura	• Postpartum hemorrhage • Hemolytic uremic syndrome • Postrenal AKI—iatrogenic injuries to bladder and ureter in second-stage cesareans, ureteric compression in ectopic kidneys and duplication of ureters

(HELLP: hemolysis, elevated liver enzymes, and low platelet; PE: preeclampsia)

inaccurate because of under collection, and the availability of result is delayed until at least after the collection period is completed. Use of protein:creatinine ratio (uPCR) is the method of choice.
- *Serum creatinine*: Increase in the level by 0.2 mg/dL in a woman with new-onset hypertension and associated HELLP syndrome or atypical HUS is likely to indicate kidney injury.
- *Renal ultrasound*: To rule out postrenal causes of AKI; may show hydronephrosis, but this may be physiologic rather than pathologic.
- *Serum complement levels*: Increased synthesis in liver and elevated levels in pregnancy, may make the diagnosis of conditions such as lupus nephritis difficult.
- *Kidney biopsy*: It should be considered in women at <32 weeks of gestation when delivery is not a viable alternative and treatment may result in prolongation of a desired pregnancy. The potential complications of renal biopsy vary depending on the stage of pregnancy, and appear to be significantly higher in later pregnancy. The complications could be major bleeding requiring transfusion, embolization, early preterm delivery, and even fetal death. These aspects need to be considered during counseling before proceeding with a kidney biopsy.[23]

Treatment of Pregnancy-related Acute Kidney Injury

General principles to treat PRAKI are as follows:
- Identification of the underlying source of injury
- Volume resuscitation
- Prevention of further injury
- Timely initiation of renal replacement therapy (RRT)
- Prompt delivery, if necessary.

Volume repletion is central to the management of prerenal states. Rate of volume replacement requires careful monitoring, since women with either endotoxin-mediated injury or PE can easily develop pulmonary edema. Complications of AKI can be treated as in nonpregnant patients, i.e., hyperkalemia in most circumstances can be treated with cation exchange resins, metabolic acidosis with alkali therapy, volume overload with loop diuretics and anemia with blood transfusion. If these measures prove unsuccessful or if the renal injury progresses, initiation of RRT will be necessary. Specific measures to treat AKI depend on the underlying etiology of the injury.

Indications are metabolic acidosis refractory to medical management, anuria, hyperkalemia (>6.5 mEq/L), acute poisoning, volume overload not responding to diuretic therapy, and uremic organ dysfunction (pericarditis, encephalopathy, and/or neuropathy).

Steroid and immunosuppressive therapy may be warranted for biopsy-proven cases of glomerulonephritis. For the diagnoses of severe PE, HELLP syndrome, and AFLP, prompt delivery of the fetus is recommended. Treatment of the thrombotic microangiopathies (TMAs), including TTP and atypical HUS, requires plasmapheresis and administration of eculizumab (for atypical HUS). Administration of glucocorticoids is indicated should delivery of the fetus be required prior to 34 weeks of gestation in order to reduce the risk of neonatal respiratory distress syndrome.[24]

The overall incidence of AKI in pregnancy may be declining due to awareness, high index of suspicion, and availability of services, but the absolute number of deaths from AKI remain alarmingly high. Diagnosis of PRAKI is not always straightforward because of overlapping features of the encountered clinical entities (HELLP/AFLP/TMA), and can be challenging. There is a need to have disease specific diagnostic markers and prompt availability of their results to effect timely management decisions.

■ CHRONIC KIDNEY DISEASE

Chronic kidney disease (CKD) is a heterogeneous group of disorders whose manifestations are mainly dependent on underlying cause and severity of disease. The overall prevalence is estimated to be 13–14% globally with higher predilection in women. Although <5% of CKD is seen in childbearing age, the implications of it are very significant. The prevalence of CKD in pregnancy is predicted to rise due to increasing maternal age and obesity. It is characterized by alterations in the structure and functions of the kidney. Of the many causes, examples of kidney disorders in young women include glomerular disease, vascular disease, tubulointerstitial diseases, and cystic diseases. In addition, systemic diseases such as diabetes vasculitis and systemic lupus erythematosus (SLE) often involve kidneys. It significantly increases the risk of adverse maternal and perinatal outcomes.

Effect on Pregnancy of Renal Disease

Degree of renal insufficiency with the pre-existing hypertension and proteinuria are the determinants of pregnancy and perinatal outcomes. There are very few reports of prospective studies in pregnant women with CKD evaluating pregnancy outcome. However, it is generally associated with poor pregnancy outcome. Most studies have documented high rates of miscarriage, preterm delivery, PE, small for gestational age (SGA) infants, and fetal and neonatal death. Maternal acidosis may result in progressive fetal acidemia.

Even pregnant women with mild renal impairment (Cr <1.5 mg/dL) are reported to have increased rates of maternal and fetal adverse events compared to healthy individuals[25] and complications in pregnancies of women with more severe renal impairment (Cr >2.8 mg/dL) may be much higher.[26] The data on pregnancy outcome for women with significant proteinuria in early pregnancy are sparse. Women with CKD also are more likely to have higher rates of concomitant hypertension and proteinuria, which further increases the risk of adverse pregnancy outcomes.[26,27]

Maternal anemia is more common. It is due either to erythropoietin deficiency[28] or to action of circulating uremic induced inhibitors of erythropoietin.[29] Nutritional deficiency of folate, vitamin B12 deficiency due to anorexia, or washing away with dialysate compound the cause. Hypocalcemia and hyperphosphatemia could be associated with these women of advanced CKD more commonly due to secondary hyperparathyroidism.

Effect of Pregnancy on Renal Disease

The consideration a clinician has to foresee in the background of CKD on embarking the pregnancy is, does it hasten the disease progression and shorten the time to end-stage renal disease (ESRD). Absence of a uniform definition for CKD renders the counseling difficult and challenging.

Chronic kidney disease is classified as mild (stage up to 2), moderate (stages 2–3), or severe (beyond stage 3) depending on serum creatinine values (<1.4 mg/dL, >2.5 mg/dL or one in between) or based on creatinine clearance values (higher than 70%, lower than 40%, or in between; mL/min). Kidney function may decline because of pregnancy, and the severity of underlying disease determines the degree and persistence of decline.[26,30]

Most of the studies reporting effect of pregnancy have staged the disease during the pregnancy. This has the inherent problem of mis-staging due to pregnancy-related physiologic changes.

Degree or stage of kidney dysfunction is not the only variable influencing the progression, but concomitant hypertension and proteinuria also contribute to the functional decline. Even in women with moderate kidney insufficiency, inadequately treated hypertension initiate further kidney damage.[31] The greater the baseline degree of kidney function compromise with poorly controlled hypertension and proteinuria, the higher is the loss of kidney function during pregnancy.

The studies have not been consistent in recording the poor pregnancy outcome or deterioration in kidney function in women with CKD.[25,30]

Causes

The underlying disease or reason for CKD are many. These could be:

- *Glomerulonephritis*: Pregnancy is not shown to affect the course of biopsy proven primary chronic glomerulonephritis, who had normal kidney function before pregnancy.[32] Similarly, the patients who had recovered from poststreptococcal glomerulonephritis and whose kidney function had returned to normal, were not found to be at risk of fetal loss or PE.[33]
- *Mesangial immunoglobulin A (IgA) nephropathy*: Focal and segmental proliferative and hyalinosis-sclerosis changes may develop during pregnancy since they are seen more frequently in biopsies from pregnant than in nonpregnant women.[34] Occurrence of pregnancy does not appear to affect the long-term kidney function.[35,36] However, risk for pregnancy complications is high. It is advisable to discontinue angiotensin-converting enzyme (ACE) inhibitors. The pregnancy-safe alternatives to immunosuppressive agents should be prescribed. These changes should be effected preferably before conception or at the first sign of pregnancy, to minimize risk to the fetus.
- *Reflux nephropathy*: Decline in renal function, significantly high fetal loss and higher chances pf PE are noted.[37]
- *Interstitial nephritis*: Hematuria and proteinuria are not the characteristic findings in this insidious condition. Pregnancy outcome is less than optimal with higher perinatal mortality, if complicated by hypertension or PE.
- Collagen vascular diseases:
  - *SLE*: It is the most common among collagen disorders encountered in pregnancy. Effect of SLE does not depend only on disease activity. Presence of nephrotic syndrome, hypertension, and renal dysfunction are the determinants of the perinatal outcome.[38] High anticardiolipin level is considered as a sensitive predictor.[39] Neonatal lupus syndrome is described. Pregnancy per se does not appear to adversely affect SLE, but most exacerbations of lupus nephropathy noted are often the effect of hypertension or superimposed PE.[40]
  - *Scleroderma*: It is rarely encountered. Presence of extensive organ involvement or renal disease can be considered as contraindication for pregnancy.[41]
  - *Polyarteritis nodosa*: Severe hypertension, PE, and deterioration in renal function are the complications in pregnancy. Perinatal outcome is generally good.[42]
- *Diabetic nephropathy*: Most studies done in pregnancy are with small numbers. It is not clear whether diabetic nephropathy is accelerated by pregnancy. Women with diabetic nephropathy are at increased risk for adverse maternal and fetal outcome.
- *Nephrotic syndrome*: Outcome of pregnancy without deterioration in renal function depends on the cause of nephrotic syndrome. Cases with renal vein thrombosis are reported in pregnancy.
- *Hereditary renal disease*: Polycystic kidney are the common hereditary disease. It is with autosomal dominant trait and has high penetrance. Renal function status is the determinant of pregnancy outcome. Associated intracranial aneurysms pose a serious threat.
- *Tumors of the urinary tract*: Adenocarcinoma, although rare, is the common renal neoplasm occurring in pregnancy. With prompt diagnosis and treatment, it is potentially curable. In most stages, radical nephrectomy is the standard of care and should not be delayed in the first and third trimesters. If diagnosed in the second trimester, surgery can be postponed until fetal viability is attained.

Management

A high-risk obstetrician and nephrologist should evaluate women with CKD contemplating pregnancy. Counseling should involve the risks particular to their disease processes and kidney function. The CKD with well-preserved renal function and near normal blood pressure is likely to be associated with good maternal and fetal outcomes, whereas in advanced disease, there will be higher risk for pregnancy complications. Those with severe renal dysfunction may permanently lose kidney function with pregnancy. The underlying disease, such as diabetes mellitus (DM) or lupus nephritis, may impose additional disease-specific risks. Although risks such as growth restriction, preterm delivery, and SGA infants still exist, advances in neonatal care have improved the infant survival. If a histological diagnosis will change management in pregnancy, then renal biopsy can be performed in the first and early second trimester of pregnancy.

Objectives of pregnancy management in women with CKD are:
- Stabilizing disease activity in advance of pregnancy on minimized doses of pregnancy-appropriate medications
- Optimizing blood pressure control (<140/90 mm Hg) on pregnancy-appropriate medications
- Optimizing glycemic control in women with DM
- Minimizing risk of exposure to teratogenic medications
- Making a treatment plan in the event of hyperemesis or disease exacerbation or relapse during pregnancy.

Assessment of Kidney Function

- *Serum creatinine* concentrations should direct the evaluation, and not GFR or estimated GFR. Increased plasma flow and dynamic changes in filtration fraction preclude their use.
- uPCR or albumin:creatinine ratio (uACR) are used for quantification of proteinuria rather than use of dipstick[43] or 24-hour urine collection.

Diagnosis of Superimposed Preeclampsia

In a woman having chronic kidney disease (CKD) with chronic hypertension and proteinuria, the development sustained severe hypertension [>160 systolic blood pressure (SBP) and/or 110 mm Hg diastolic blood pressure (DBP)] or doubling of antihypertensive agents, and/or rising proteinuria (doubling of uPCR or uACR) should prompt assessment of superimposed PE.[44]

It should be remembered that women with CKD and more so having PE are at increased risk of developing pulmonary edema. Therefore, the fluid balance is managed throughout with the aim of maintaining normal fluid volume, avoiding dehydration, and pulmonary edema.

Management of Hypertension

Presence of hypertension increases the risk of adverse pregnancy outcomes. It is always better to optimize blood pressure before pregnancy. ACE inhibitors and angiotensin receptor blocking agents are to be changed. There is no evidence on treatment initiation thresholds or blood pressure targets. However, the blood pressure target of <140/90 mm Hg is recommended for women with CKD during pregnancy.[45] There is no need to continue hypotensive if the blood pressure consistently remains <110/70 mm Hg. Antihypertensives compatible with pregnancy include methyldopa, labetalol, nifedipine, and hydralazine.

Management of Proteinuria

Degree of proteinuria is associated with progression of underlying kidney disease and the adverse pregnancy outcomes.
- *Immunosuppression*: Pregnancy-safe options for diseases treated with immunosuppression (lupus nephritis, vasculitis, and membranous nephropathy) include prednisone, azathioprine, and the calcineurin inhibitors. Such women would require early screening and ruling out gestational diabetes. In women maintained on long-term corticosteroids, stress doses of short-acting glucocorticoids should be given during labor and delivery. If there are flares during pregnancy, pulse steroids followed by combination immunosuppression will be required.
Immunosuppressive agents to be avoided during pregnancy are mycophenolate mofetil and cyclophosphamide, since they are associated with increased risk of miscarriage. Rituximab is better avoided in pregnancy as there will be risk of neonatal B-cell depletion.
- *Severe edema*: Conservative care with compression stockings and foot end elevation will be of help; use of loop diuretic frusemide can be used judiciously, in severe cases.
- *Hypoproteinemia*: Albumin infusions will be required in severe cases for replacement.
- *Thromboprophylaxis* with low-molecular-weight-heparin will be required. Hypoalbuminemia adds to the prothrombotic state and heparin should be given throughout pregnancy and 6 months following pregnancy.

Prevention of Preeclampsia

Women with CKD are at the highest risk for PE, and importance of its prevention cannot be overemphasized. Use of micronutrient such as magnesium should be avoided since it is cleared by the kidneys.
- *Aspirin* should be started before 16 weeks of pregnancy in the recommended dose of 150 mg/day and until 34–36 weeks of pregnancy or before termination of pregnancy.[46]
- *Calcium* with *vitamin D3* have been evaluated as strategies for prevention of PE[47] and the supplementation should be continued.

Prevention and Treatment of Anemia

Prevention and treatment of anemia assumes importance since it is common in patients with CKD. Early initiation of oral or parenteral iron will be required. Intravenous administration may offer better bioavailability and tolerability.[48] In CKD, women may have insufficient capacity for gestational increase in erythropoietin. Supplementation of erythropoietin-stimulating agents can be offered. These have large molecular weight and do not cross placenta.

Other conditions that would require attention are as follows:
- *Hypocalcemia* (over and above the chemoprophylaxis against PE) and hypophosphatemia could be present in CKD due to hyperparathyroidism.
- *Hyperkalemia*: Low potassium in diet, and in severe cases, potassium-binding resins need to be initiated in time.
- *Acidosis*: Maternal acidosis will result in progressive fetal academia and may require alkalinization with sodium bicarbonate, and in severe cases, acidosis may indicate the need for dialysis.
- *UTI*: Antibiotic prophylaxis should be offered even after single episode of UTI, including asymptomatic bacteriuria.

Dialysis

Women who are already on dialysis contemplating pregnancy should receive prepregnancy counseling including the options of postponing pregnancy until transplantation (when feasible) and the need for long frequent dialysis prior to and during pregnancy. In pregnancy, risks of preterm delivery outweigh those of initiating dialysis. Dialysis needs to be considered whenever the maternal urea concentration goes beyond 100 mg/dL. The period of gestation, renal function trajectory, fluid balance, biochemical parameters, blood pressure, and uremic symptoms influence the decision-making. Women receiving hemodialysis can continue with dialysis dose prescribed accounting for residual renal function, aiming for a predialysis urea of <75 mg/dL. Those on peritoneal dialysis prior to pregnancy should convert to hemodialysis during pregnancy.

Obstetric Care

- Risk of adverse perinatal outcome is high. The antenatal care need not be any different from routine, except that frequent assessments will be required with multidisciplinary team. Antenatal assessment is done every 2 weeks until 32 weeks of pregnancy and thereafter every week.
- Women exposed to teratogenic drugs in first trimester should have assessment and counseling by fetal medicine specialist.
- The routine prenatal screening in first trimester may be less reliable. Nuchal translucency levels are unpredictable in mothers with renal compromise. Clearance by kidney of β-human chorionic gonadotropin is affected and is inversely related to creatinine clearance.[49]
- *Indications for termination of pregnancy because of the CKD are*: Severe and rapid deterioration in kidney function, symptomatic hypoalbuminemia, pulmonary edema, and refractory hypertension. In their absence, pregnancy can be carried until term.
- Indomethacin for tocolysis should be avoided because of its nephrotoxicity.
- Presence of CKD is not an indication for cesarean delivery.
- During the intrapartum, postpartum, or postoperative period, the drugs to be avoided are as follows:
  - Magnesium sulfate for care of eclampsia, when it occurs
  - Nonsteroidal anti-inflammatory drugs for analgesia
  - Gentamicin for antimicrobial cover.

SPECIAL SITUATIONS

Lupus Nephritis

Hydroxychloroquine needs to be continued during pregnancy. In women who are positive for anti-RO or anti-LA antibodies, should be evaluated with fetal echocardiography during the second trimester scan.

End-stage Renal Disease

End-stage renal disease is considered when GFR falls to <15 mL/min. Fertility rates are low in women with ESRD and those maintained on dialysis.[50] Pregnancy care in these women needs to be individualized.

Women on hemodialysis will have higher values for pregnancy-associated plasma protein A.[51] The unpredictable nuchal translucency and altered β-human chorionic gonadotropin values will necessitate looking for alternative options in chorionic villous sampling, amniocentesis, or noninvasive cell-free fetal DNA testing.

Doubled daily doses of vitamin and mineral supplements are to be prescribed because of their loss during dialysis. Protein intake should also need to be increased to 1.5–1.8 g/kg daily since significant amount of amino acids can be lost with the dialysate.[52]

Women on hemodialysis are more likely to have cervical insufficiency and in later part of pregnancy require serial assessment of cervical length.[53] Polyhydramnios is common either due to inadequate clearance of uremic toxins, increased fetal diuresis because of urea-nitrogen, or as an indicator of fluid overload.

Care during Dialysis

Objective will be to target BUN under 16 mmol/L. Dialysate concentrations used should have ≤1.5 mmol/L of potassium, calcium, and phosphate, and bicarbonate of 30 mEq/L. Intradialytic hypotension should be avoided. Volume status should be assessed every week.

If the woman is maintained on peritoneal dialysis, volume needs to be reduced as the pregnancy advances and the frequency of exchanges is increased.

With no evidence of fetal or maternal compromise, pregnancy can be carried to 37 completed weeks. Labor can be induced. Cesarean delivery will be considered only for obstetric indications. Breastfeeding is safe and is permitted.

Pregnancy after Renal Transplantation

Women with ESRD are usually encouraged to wait for at least 1 year until after the kidney transplantation to plan pregnancy. Delaying up to 2 years reduces the risks for graft rejection. Increase in GFR during pregnancy could theoretically lead to hyperfiltration and the resultant glomerulosclerosis. Pregnancy does not appear to cause excessive or irreversible problems to graft function, if the function of the transplanted kidney had been stable before the pregnancy. Pregnancy outcomes after transplantation are better when compared to the pregnancies in women dependent on dialysis. The live birth rates after transplantation are similar to that for those with the general population, but rates for PE, gestational diabetes, and preterm labor are higher.[54] These pregnancies require shared care with nephrologists. Pregnancy after transplant is a complex interplay between maternal age, comorbidities, and transplant status that requires careful, individualized counseling. The immunosuppressive regimens need to be changed to the drugs that are safe in pregnancy. Aspirin should be prescribed for PE prophylaxis. Because of being chronically under immunosuppression, UTI is most frequent and can result in pyelonephritis. Monthly surveillance is required to detect and treat promptly. If cesarean delivery is required, obstetrician should be attentive to location of transplanted kidney and ureter. Ureter is usually replanted at the dome of bladder. Review of transplant notes, ultrasonographic imaging before cesarean is necessary.

Pregnancy in Kidney Donors

Although the kidney donors are without any kidney injury or disease, they do require more careful monitoring since they are found to be at increased risk of developing PE.[55] The explanation for this amplification of risk could be the genetic predisposition in combination with a reduced GFR.

Assisted Reproduction

Reproductive capacity is affected in women with ESRD and renal transplant recipients. Renal insufficiency results in dysfunction of hypothalamic–pituitary–gonadal axis. It results in high follicle-stimulating hormone (FSH), luteinizing hormone (LH), and prolactin levels, and disruption of the normal gonadal function. In the event of laparoscopic evaluation, one has to keep in mind the changed anatomy of kidney and ureter to avoid injury to them. If she is a candidate and the attempts of induction of ovulation and intrauterine insemination have failed, the available assisted reproduction techniques can be offered as in any other patient. It is advisable to choose to transfer single embryo so as to reduce the risk of complications associated with multiple pregnancies.[56] Successful blastocyst transfer are reported. Retrieval of oocytes followed by surrogacy could be an option, especially when women have hypertension, proteinuria, graft dysfunction, and are taking potentially teratogenic drugs. Whenever assisted reproductive technologies are planned, preimplantation genetic testing (PGT) is necessary. PGT is done for diagnosis of single gene disorders, structural chromosomal abnormalities due to gains and losses, and aneuploidies.

Contraception

Safe and effective contraception should be offered postpartum and to those planning for pregnancy for optimization of disease management, avoidance of teratogenic medication, and providing awareness of an increased risk of adverse pregnancy outcomes.

- Barrier methods are relatively efficacious when correctly used and are safe.
- Long-acting reversible contraceptives such as copper and levonorgestrel releasing intrauterine devices and implants are the preferred choices.
- Surgical contraception is not contraindicated. Risks of surgery should be kept in mind.
- Progestin only options of pills (other than ones containing drospirenone), do not significantly affect blood pressure, proteinuria or increase risk of venous thromboembolism (VTE), and are safe. Drospirenone due to its anti-mineralocorticoid activity can cause hyperkalemia in at-risk women.[57]

To convert a BUN result in:	To convert serum creatinine in:
• mg/dL to mmol/L, multiply by 0.357	• mg/dL to mcmol/L, multiply by 88.42
• mmol/L to mg/dL, multiply by 6	• mcmol/L to mg/dL, multiply by 0.0113

■ KEY MESSAGES

- Preconception counseling is necessary.
- Pregnancy related acute kidney injury (PRAKI)—has numerous etiologies, diagnosis is not standardized, and treatment is targeted to the specific cause. The timing of PRAKI provides clue to underlying cause.
- Chronic kidney disease (CKD)—manifestations are dependent on underlying cause and severity of disease.
- Objectives of managing pregnancy in women with CKD is stabilizing the disease activity, optimizing blood pressure and glycemic control, minimizing risk of exposure to teratogens in addition to pregnancy care.
- Those dependent on hemodialysis before pregnancy should be continued. Those on peritoneal dialysis should be converted to hemodialysis.

- Renal disease in pregnancy imposes higher risk of miscarriage, PE, gestational diabetes, preterm labor, and having small for gestation babies.
- Presence of CKD or renal transplantation is not an indication for cesarean delivery.
- Progesterone only pills, long acting reversible contraceptives are the safe contraceptive options.

REFERENCES

1. Bailey RR, Rolleston GL. Kidney length and ureteric dilatation in the puerperium. J Obstet Gynaecol Br Commonw. 197;78(1): 55-61.
2. Roy C, Saussine C, Jahn C, Le Bras Y, Steichen G, Delepaul B, et al. Fast imaging MR assessment of ureterohydronephrosis during pregnancy. Magn Reson Imaging. 1995;13(6):767-72.
3. Rasmussen PE, Nielsen FR. Hydronephrosis during pregnancy: a literature survey. Eur J Obstet Gynecol Reprod Biol. 1988;27(3): 249-59.
4. Davidson J. Changes in renal function and other aspects of homeostasisin earily pregnancy. J Obstet Gynaecol Br Commonw. 1974;81(12):1003.
5. Davison JM, Dunlop W. Changes in renal hemodynamics and tubular function induced by normal pregnancy. Semin Nephrol. 1984;4;198-207.
6. Brown MA, Sinosich MJ, Saunders DM, Gallery EDM. Potassium regulation and progesterone aldosterone interrelationships in human pregnancy: a prospective study. Am J Obstet Gynecol. 1986;155(2):349-53.
7. Akbari A, Wilkes P, Lindheimer M, Lepage N, Filler G. Reference intervals for anion gap and strong ion difference in pregnancy: a pilot study. Hypertens Pregnancy. 2007;26(1):111-19.
8. Aluvihare VR, Kallikourdis M, Betz AG. Regulatory T cells mediate maternal tolerance to the fetus. Nat Immunol. 2004;5(3):266-271.
9. Richani K, Soto E, Romero R, Espinoza J, Chaiworapongsa T, Nien JK, et al. Normal pregnancy is characterized by systemic activation of the complement system. J Matern Fetal Neonatal Med. 2005;17(4):239-45.
10. Milne JE, Lindheimer MD, Davison JM. Glomerular heteroporous membrane modelling in third trimester and postpartum before and during amino acid infusion. Am J Physiol Renal Physiol. 2002;282(1):F170-5.
11. Christensen P. Tubular reabsorbtion of glucose during pregnancy. Scand J Clin Lab Invest. 1958;10(4):364-71.
12. Brown MA, Holt JL, Mangos GJ, Murray N, Curtis J, Homer C. Microscopic hematuria in pregnancy: Relevance to pregnancy outcome. Am J Kidney Dis. 2005; 45(4):667-73.
13. Gammill HS, Jeyabalan A. Acute renal failure in pregnancy. Crit Care Med. 2005;33 10 Suppl:S372-84.
14. Prakash J, Pant P, Prakash S, Sivasankar M, Vohra R, Doley PK, et al. Changing picture of acute kidney injury in pregnancy: Study of 259 cases over a period of 33 years. Indian J Nephrol. 2016;26(4):262-7.
15. Thornton JG, Macdonald AM. Twin mothers, pregnancy hypertension and preeclampsia. Br J Obstet Gynaecol. 1999;106(6):570-5.
16. Koopmans CM, van Pampus MG, Groen H, Aarnoudse JG, van den Berg PP, Mol BW. Accuracy of serum uric acid as a predictive test for maternal complications in pre-eclampsia: Bivariate meta-analysis and decision analysis. Eur J Obstet Gynecol Reprod Biol. 2009;146(1):8-14.
17. Abraham KA, Kennelly M, Dorman AM, Walshe JJ. Pathogenesis of acute renal failure associated with the HELLP syndrome: a case report and review of the literature. Eur J Obstet Gynecol Reprod Biol. 2003;108(1):99-102.
18. Rajasekar D, Hall M. Urinary tract injuries during obstetric intervention. Br J Obstet Gynaecol. 1997;104(6):731-4.
19. Jena M, Mitch WE. Rapidly reversible acute renal failure from ureteral obstruction in pregnancy. Am J Kidney Dis. 1996;28(3): 457-60.
20. Davison JM, Vollotton MB, Lindheimer MD. Plasma osmolality and urinal concentration and dilution during and after pregnancy: Evidence that lateral recumbency inhibits maximal urinary concentrating ability. Br J Obstet Gynaecol. 1981;88(5):472-79.
21. Lim KH, Friedman SA, Ecker JK, Kao L, Kilpatrick SJ. The clinical utility of serum uric acid measurements in hypertensive diseases of pregnancy. Am J Obstet Gynecol. 1998;178(5):1067-71.
22. Saudan PJ, Brown MA, Farrell T, Shaw L. Improved methods of assessing proteinuria hypertensive pregnancy. Br J Obstet Gynaecol. 1997;104(10):1159-64.
23. Piccoli GB, Daidola G, Attini R, Parisi S, Fassio F, Naretto C, et al. Kidney biopsy in pregnancy: evidence for counselling? A systematic narrative review. BJOG. 2013;120(4):412-27.
24. Jim B, Garovic VD. Acute kidney injury in pregnancy. Semin Nephrol. 2017;37(4): 378-85.
25. Zhang JJ, Ma XX, Hao L, Liu LJ, Lv JC, Zhang H. A systematic review and meta-analysis of outcomes of pregnancy in CKD and CKD outcomes in pregnancy. Clin J Am Soc Nephrol. 2015;10(11):1964-78.
26. Piccoli GB, Cabiddu G, Attini R, Vigotti FN, Maxia S, Lepori N, et al. Risk of adverse pregnancy outcomes in women with CKD. J Am Soc Nephrol. 2015;26(8):2011-22.
27. Piccoli GB, Fassio F, Attini R, Parisi S, Biolcati M, Ferraresi M, et al. Pregnancy in CKD: whom should we follow and why? Nephrol Dial Transpl. 2012;27(suppl 3):iii111-8.
28. Schrier RW, Besarab A, Ayyoub F. Anemia in renal disease. In: Schrier RW (eds). Diseases of the Kidney and Urinary Tract, 8th edition. Philadelphia: Lippincott Williams and Wilkins; 2007, pp. 2406-430.
29. Eschbach JW. The anemia of chronic renal failure: Pathophysiology and the effects of recombinant erythropoietin. Kidney Int. 1989;35(1):134-48.
30. Jones DC, Hayslett JP. Outcome of pregnancy in women with moderate or severe renal insufficiency. N Engl J Med. 1996; 335(4):226-32.
31. Hou SH, Grossman SD, Madias NE. Pregnancy in women with renal disease and moderate renal insufficiency. Am J Med. 1985;78(2):185-94.
32. Jungers P, Houillier P, Forget D, Labrunie M, Skhiri H, Giatras I, et al. Influence of pregnancy on the course of primary chronic glomerulonephritis. Lancet. 1995;346(8983):1122-4.
33. Kaplan AL, Smith JP, Tillman AJB. Healed acute and chronic nephritis in pregnancy. Am J Obstet Gynecol. 1962;83:1519-25.
34. Kincaid-Smith PS, Whitworth JA, Fairley KF. Mesangial IgA nephropathy in pregnancy Clin Exp Hypertens. 1980;2(5): 821-38.
35. Limardo M, Imbasciati E, Ravani P, Surian M, Torres D, Gregorini G, et al. Collaborative Group of the Italian Society of Nephrology. Pregnancy and progression of IgA nephropathy:

36. Liu Y, Ma X, Zheng J, Liu X, Yan T. A systematic review and meta-analysis of kidney and pregnancy outcomes in IgA nephropathy. Am J Nephrol. 2016;44(3):187-93.
37. Kincaid-Smith P, Fairley KF. Renal disease in pregnancy. Three controversial areas: Mesangial IgA nephropathy, focal glomerular sclerosis (focal and segmental hyalinosis and sclerosis), and reflux nephropathy. Am J Kidney Dis. 1987;9(4): 328-33.
38. Gladman DD, Tandon A, Ibanez D, Urowitz MB. The effect of lupus nephritis on pregnancy outcome and fetal and maternal complications. J Rheumatol. 2010;37(4): 754-8.
39. Lockshin MD, Druzin ML, Goei S, Qamar T, Magid MS, Jovanovic L, et al. Antibody to cardiolipin as a predictor of fetal distress or death in pregnant patients with systemic lupus erythematosus. N Engl J Med. 1985;313:152-6.
40. Hnat, M, Sibai, B. Renal disease and pregnancy. Glob Libr Women Med. 2008.
41. Zulman JI, Talal N, Hoffman GS, Epstein WV. Problems associated with the management of pregnancies in patients with systemic erythematosus. J Rheumatol. 1980;7(1):37-49.
42. Burkett G, Richards R. Periarteritis nodosa and pregnancy. Obstet Gynecol. 1982;59(2):252-4.
43. Waugh JJ, Clark TJ, Divakaran TG, Khan KS, Kilby MD. Accuracy of urinalysis dipstick techniques in predicting significant proteinuria in pregnancy. Obstet Gynecol. 2004;103(4):769-77.
44. Wiles K, Chappell L, Clark K, Elman L, Hall M, Lightstone L, et al. Clinical practice guideline on pregnancy and renal disease. BMC Nephrol. 2019;20(1):401
45. Magee LA, von Dadelszen P, Rey E, Ross S, Asztalos E, Murphy KE, et al. Less-tight versus tight control of hypertension in pregnancy. N Engl J Med. 2015;372(5):407-17.
46. Rolnik DL, Wright D, Poon LC, O'Gorman N, Syngelaki A, de Paco Matallana C, et al. Aspirin versus placebo in pregnancies at high risk for preterm preeclampsia. N Engl J Med. 2017;377(7):613-22.
47. Khaing W, Vallibhakara SA, Tantrakul V, Vallibhakara O, Rattanasiri S, McEvoy M, et al. Calcium and vitamin D supplementation for prevention of preeclampsia: a systematic review and network meta-analysis. Nutrients 2017;9(10):1141.
48. Albaramki J, Hodson EM, Craig JC, Webster AC. Parenteral versus oral iron therapy for adults and children with chronic kidney disease. Cochrane Database Syst Rev. 2012;1:CD007857.
49. Wehmann RE, Amr S, Rosa C, Nisula BC. Metabolism, distribution and excretion of purified human chorionic gonadotropin and its subunits in man. Ann Endocrinol (Paris). 1984;45(4-5):291-5.
50. Shahir AK, Briggs N, Katsoulis J, Levidiotis V. An observational outcomes study from 1966 to 2008, examining pregnancy and neonatal outcomes from dialyzed women using data from the ANZDATA registry. Nephrology (Carlton) 2013;18:276-84.
51. Wittfooth S, Tertti R, Lepäntalo M, Porela P, Qin QP, Tynjälä J, et al. Studies on the effects of heparin products on regnancyassociated plasma protein A. Clin Chim Acta 2011;412(3-4):376-81.
52. Ikizler TA, Pupim LB, Brouillette JR, Levenhagen DK, Farmer K, Hakim RM, et al. Hemodialysis stimulates muscle and whole body protein loss and alters substrate oxidation. Am J Physiol Endocrinol Metab. 2002;282(1):E107-16.
53. Hladunewich MA, Hou S, Odutayo A, Cornelis T, Pierratos A, Goldstein M, et al. Intensive hemodialysis associates with improved pregnancy outcomes: a Canadian and United States cohort comparison. J Am Soc Nephrol. 2014;25(5):1103-9.
54. Deshpande NA, James NT, Kucirka LM, Boyarsky BJ, Garonzik-Wang JM, Montgomery RA, et al. Pregnancy outcomes in kidney transplant recipients: a systematic review and meta-analysis. Am J Transplant. 2011;11(11):2388-404.
55. Garg AX, Nevis IF, McArthur E, Sontrop JM, Koval JJ, Lam NN, et al. Gestational hypertension and preeclampsia in living kidney donors. N Engl J Med. 2015;372(2):124-33.
56. Piccoli GB, Arduino S, Attini R, Parisi S, Fassio F, Biolcati M, et al. Multiple pregnancies in CKD patients: an explosive mix. Clin J Am Soc Nephrol. 2013;8(1):41-50.
57. Healthcare TFOSAR. UK medical eligibility criteria for contraceptive use; 2016.

LONG QUESTIONS

1. Pregnancy-related acute kidney injury: Discuss the definition, causes, its implications, and care of pregnancy.
2. Pregnancy in a woman with chronic kidney disease (CKD): (a) Enumerate underlying causes for CKD. (b) Discuss the effect on pregnancy and of pregnancy on kidney disease. (c) Management of pregnancy and kidney disease.
3. Discuss the effect of chronic kidney disease (CKD) on fertility, and subfertility management in women with CKD and in those after renal transplantation.

SHORT QUESTIONS

1. Chronic kidney disease with pregnancy—commonly used drugs and their hazards. Outline the alternate suggestions.
2. Chronic kidney disease—contraceptive options.
3. Obstetricians concerns in planning cesarean for women with end-stage renal disease and renal transplant.
4. Plan of antenatal care in woman with chronic kidney disease.
5. Prepregnancy counseling in woman with chronic kidney disease.

MULTIPLE CHOICE QUESTIONS

1. The condition NOT associated with chronic kidney disease is:
   a. Down syndrome   b. Fetal growth restriction
   c. Polyhydramnios   d. Preterm labor
2. The test parameter used for screening Down syndrome *unaffected* by end-stage renal disease is:
   a. β-human chorionic gonadotropin (hCG)
   b. Cell free fetal DNA
   c. Nuchal translucency
   d. Pregnancy-associated plasma protein A (PAPP-A)
3. Most common pathophysiology for pregnancy-related acute kidney injury is:
   a. Iatrogenic   b. Postrenal
   c. Prerenal   d. Renal

4. End-stage renal disease is diagnosed when glomerular filtration rate falls below:
   a. 15 mL/min
   b. 30 mL/min
   c. 40 mL/min
   d. 50 mL/min
5. In a pregnant women with end-stage renal disease receiving hemodialysis, the recommended daily intake of protein is:
   a. 0.1–0.5 g/kg
   b. 0.5–1.0 g/kg
   c. 1.0–1.5 g/kg
   d. 1.5–2.0 g/kg
6. Regarding kidney biopsy for diagnosis in pregnancy-related kidney disease, it is:
   a. Contraindicated
   b. Done after 28 weeks
   c. Done before 28 weeks
   d. Mandatory
7. In pregnant women with chronic kidney disease due to systemic lupus erythematosus:
   a. Aspirin is advised up to 34 weeks
   b. Hydroxyquinoline is continued
   c. Preeclampsia is not distinguishable from worsening nephritis
   d. Prepregnancy creatinine is an indicator of perinatal outcome
8. Most likely cause of pregnancy-related acute kidney injury diagnosed in postpartum period is:
   a. Acute fatty liver of pregnancy
   b. Hemolytic uremic syndrome
   c. Thrombotic thrombocytopenic purpura
   d. Wernicke–Korsakoff syndrome
9. Following are the indications for termination of pregnancy because of the chronic kidney disease, except:
   a. Pulmonary edema
   b. Refractory hypertension
   c. Single functioning kidney
   d. Symptomatic hypoalbuminemia
10. Following statement about use of magnesium sulfate in prescribed in pregnancy with chronic kidney disease is true:
    a. For fetal neuroprotection
    b. To inhibit preterm labor
    c. To treat eclampsia
    d. None of the above

Answers

| 1. a | 2. b | 3. c | 4. a | 5. d | 6. c |
| 7. d | 8. b | 9. c | 10. d | | |

5.8 LIVER AND GASTROINTESTINAL DISEASE: ABNORMAL PREGNANCY WITH PRE-EXISTING CONDITIONS

Sujata A Dalvi

INTRODUCTION

Gastrointestinal (GI) and liver conditions are common in women of reproductive age group. Most of them are benign and remain unaffected in case the woman becomes pregnant. There are few GI/liver conditions that can occur during pregnancy for the first time, but pregnancy per se does not alter the management and outcome of these conditions. However, select disorders such as hepatitis E can have life-threatening course during pregnancy which otherwise can have benign course in nonpregnant state.[1] The physiological changes during pregnancy can affect interpretation of diagnostic investigations and may restrict the use of some diagnostic and therapeutic procedures. There are pregnancy-related GI/liver conditions that may be challenging to physician, as they infrequently encounter them in routine practice, at the same time, it is difficult for obstetricians, as they have similar features as that of pregnancy disorders. Conditions such as gastroesophageal reflux/constipation could be troublesome, hyperemesis could be distressing and obstetric cholestasis (OC)/acute fatty liver of pregnancy (AFLP)/HELLP (hemolysis, elevated liver enzymes and low platelet counts) syndrome could be potentially fatal.[2] Select cases such as pregnancy after bariatric surgery/liver transplant need multidisciplinary tertiary care.

ANATOMY AND PHYSIOLOGY OF LIVER

A clear understanding of physiological changes in liver during pregnancy is of importance to appreciate pathological conditions.

The liver moves superior and posterior so palpable liver edge is likely to be pathological. Blood flow to liver remains unchanged, though 25% of cardiac output goes to liver for perfusion instead of 35%. There can be transient esophageal varices in up to 60% pregnant women due to increase in circulating volume, portal pressure, and diversion of venous return via azygous system due to pressure from gravid uterus on inferior vena cava (IVC). Due to peripheral vasodilatation during pregnancy—spider nevi, palmar erythema, and edema are commonly seen and should not be connected to chronic liver disease unless present before pregnancy.

Functions of Liver

- Protein synthesis, coagulation factors VII, VIII, X, and fibrinogen increases. Fibrinogen level doubles by the end of pregnancy and is probably the cause of increase in ESR. Hence, apparently normal levels may reflect abnormality in disseminated intravascular coagulation (DIC). Prolonged prothrombin time may be the first sign of coagulopathy in acute liver failure, as it has the shortest half-life. Serum albumin levels remain unchanged and up to 28 g/L is taken as normal considering hemodilution. The concentration of hormone protein binding increases due to reduced metabolism.

- Amino acids undergo oxidative deamination to produce ammonia in liver, which is converted to urea in Krebs cycle. Fall in urea level may occur in severe liver disease and should not be confused with decrease in urea level that occurs during normal pregnancy.
- Increase in cholesterol/triglyceride levels occur during normal pregnancy/liver disorders and take several months to return to normal after delivery.
- Liver is responsible for glucose storage and subsequent release during fasting. Hypoglycemia is important cause of coma in AFLP.

Liver Function Tests

Aspartate transaminase (AST), alanine transaminase (ALT), γ-glutamyl transferase (GGT), and total bilirubin levels fall during pregnancy due to hemodilution. Alkaline phosphatase rises during pregnancy reaching up to 300% in the third trimester due to heat stable placental coenzyme. The levels fall postpartum reaching nonpregnant values in 2 weeks. Transaminase levels may increase in the first 5 days of puerperium due to stress of labor and breastfeeding.

Hence, careful history and physical examination are important to identify underlying disorder such as drug-induced hepatic/biliary impairment before assuming liver dysfunction to be secondary to pregnancy.

■ LIVER DISEASE INCIDENTAL TO PREGNANCY

Jaundice (Tables 1 and 2)

Pregnancy and labor should be managed in tertiary care center with multidisciplinary consultations.[3] Avoid epidural anesthesia, if coagulopathy/thrombocytopenia is present.

TABLE 1: Jaundice can occur due to hemolysis, congenital hyperbilirubinemia and cholestasis.

Jaundice	Hemolysis	Cholestasis—intrahepatic/extrahepatic
Causes	Hereditary spherocytosis, elliptocytosis, sickle cell, thalassemia, blood group, incompatibility, drug reaction, and HELLP Syndrome	*Intrahepatic*: Viral hepatitis, drug reaction, alcohol, hyperemesis, and cirrhosis *Extrahepatic*: Gallstones, pancreatitis, bile duct, stricture, and malignancy
Laboratory investigations	Elevated unconjugated bilirubin AST, ALT, and GGT—normal	Elevated conjugated bilirubin Alkaline phosphatase Increased
Clinical features		Pale stools Dark urine

(ALT: alanine transaminase; AST: aspartate transaminase; GGT: γ-glutamyl transferase)

TABLE 2: The common cause of jaundice in pregnancy is viral hepatitis. Usually, it is hepatitis A, but occasionally, one may find B, C, or E.

Infective	Disease	Management
Hepatitis A	Unchanged	Supportive
Hepatitis B	Checked at first ANC visit—course unchanged—precaution to be taken	Vaccination/IG—newborn Antiviral to mother in PNC period depending on viral load
Hepatitis C	Checked at first ANC visit—course unchanged—increased obstetric cholestasis	Mode of delivery: Does not alter vertical transmission Precautions to be taken—avoid prolonged rupture of membranes/invasive fetal monitoring
Hepatitis E	Increased rate of infection/ fulminant hepatic failure/maternal–perinatal mortality	Supportive: Vertical transmission can cause acute hepatitis in newborn Multidisciplinary—tertiary care center approach
Herpes simplex	Increased maternal/perinatal morbidity/mortality—if present in the third trimester	Acyclovir
CMV	Congenital malformation in fetus Fetal neurological morbidity/mortality	Supportive
Inflammatory autoimmune hepatitis/primary biliary cirrhosis	Exacerbation	Immunosuppressants Assess—antibodies

(ANC: antenatal care; CMV: cytomegalovirus; Ig: immunoglobulin; PNC: postnatal care)

Budd–Chiari Syndrome

Budd–Chiari syndrome is the obstruction of large hepatic veins causing congestion and necrosis of centrilobular lobe of liver. Mainly caused by thrombosis of hepatic vein or intra/suprahepatic portion of IVC. It may be associated with antiphospholipid syndrome or factor V Leiden mutation. Patient usually has abdominal pain with hepatomegaly and ascites. Proper diagnosis with imaging and treatment with anticoagulants, thrombolytics, and diuretics is advisable. Prognosis for pregnancy is poor. Surgery like portacaval shunt/ liver transplant may be advisable.[4]

Liver Transplant Recipient

Pregnancy in liver transplant recipient is possible but clinician needs to counsel them regarding time of conception, risk of miscarriage, deterioration of mother's health, and risk of birth defects.[5] Liver plays an important role in fertility by sustaining metabolic/hormonal function and producing fetuin B protein responsible for permeability of zona pellucida. During pregnancy, immune response decreases and hence does not have effect on graft (recipient).

Contraception counseling is strictly advisable following procedure for 1–2 years for complete postoperative healing, liver functions/menstrual cycle's recovery, and stable immune modulation to avoid side effects. Women with poor liver functions have irregular menstrual cycles or amenorrhea and it is difficult for them to conceive. Menstrual cycles usually recover within 1 year of liver Transplant and have good chance of becoming pregnant.

Pregnancy can be advised in those who are on low-dose immunosuppressants with proper allograft function (stable levels of bilirubin/ALT/AST) and no failure of other organs. X-ray of chest/computed tomography (CT) of the abdomen should be included as prepregnancy investigations. Anti-HT should be changed to α-methyldopa and oral hypoglycemic agents to insulin. Assisted reproductive technology (ART) can be suggested if no spontaneous conception occurs.

Multidisciplinary approach, good nutritional advice, and regular antenatal visits are needed. Immunosuppressants such as prednisolone (<15 mg/day), azathioprine (AZA) (<2 mg/kg/day), cyclosporine A (CsA), and tacrolimus (Tac) can be used. AZA has shown to have auditory nerve agenesis in children, hence immunosuppressants based on CsA, Tac, and prednisolone are advisable. Thrombocytopenia is of concern postliver transplant and if present during pregnancy, patient needs to be hospitalized, and treated after thorough investigations.

It is advisable to give antenatal steroids for fetal lung maturity. Increased incidence of pregnancy-induced hypertension (PIH), fetal growth restriction (FGR), and preterm labor are noted. Cesarean section is indicated for obstetric reasons only. Breastfeeding is recommended by American Academy of Pediatrics.

Woman of reproductive age group following liver transplant should not be discouraged from pregnancy but only after proper counseling.

■ PREGNANCY-SPECIFIC LIVER CONDITIONS

Obstetric Cholestasis

Obstetric Cholestasis also known as intrahepatic cholestasis of pregnancy affects 1.4% women of South Asian origin. It has genetic, environment, and endocrine etiology.[6] Due to increased sensitivity of cholestatic effect of raised estrogen levels, it is commonly seen in the third trimester. Progesterone has been thought to play a role in etiology. Primary phenotype is indicative of reduced bile flow.

Generalized pruritus without rash is the classical symptom.[7] Itch may be "all over" or "on legs, palms, or soles." Rarely, pruritus in severe cases may be present in the first trimester. On inquiry, pruritus may be present for several weeks before the diagnosis is made. It tends to occur in every pregnancy so history of the same in past pregnancy may give a clue to the diagnosis. It may be associated with raised bile acids, liver transaminases, ALT, and AST. If liver function tests (LFTs) are found to be abnormal, patient should be subjected to further investigations to rule out other liver disorders.

Pruritus can be distressing symptom and if marked, can leave behind scars. It is known to recur, hence these women are advised estrogen free oral pills. Fetal risks are prematurity, fetal distress, asphyxia events, or intrauterine device (IUD). Preterm labor is thought to be due to bile acid-induced release of prostaglandins and fetal distress to its toxic effects.

Management

Active fetal surveillance and consideration of delivery after 38 weeks of gestation is recommended. Vitamin K 10 mg daily is recommended to reduce the risk of infection and postpartum hemorrhage (PPH). Antihistaminic such as chlorphenamine 4 mg every 4–6 hours provides relief for pruritus. Topical application of moisturizers will help relieve symptoms. Ursodeoxycholic acid (UDCA) 350 mg thrice a day is given to reduce bile acid levels/pruritus (stimulates bile acid release from hepatocytes—reduces symptoms). Dexamethasone 12 mg orally for 7 days followed by tapering dose results in symptomatic relief in severe cases. Postdelivery within 48 hours, pruritus practically disappears and improves within 1 week.

HELLP Syndrome

HELLP syndrome includes hypertensive disorder of pregnancy with hemolysis, elevated liver enzymes and low platelets and affects 1% of all pregnancies and 10–20% pregnancy with preeclampsia. Usually occurs in the last trimester or even postpartum. Elevated body mass index (BMI), metabolic disorders, and antiphospholipid antibody (APLA) syndrome increase risk. Patient may be asymptomatic initially but later may complain of headache, epigastric or right upper quadrant pain, and visual disturbances. The diagnosis is quite challenging as hematological and biochemical changes precede the clinical symptoms and hence, PIH profile needs to be repeated every 2–3 weekly. Mississippi classification is based on platelet count and is divided into three classes with Class 1 as most severe with high risk of morbidity and mortality.

Prompt delivery is indicated. Aggressive correction of coagulopathy and control of blood pressure is necessary. Recovery is rapid and complete. There is 25% risk of PIH in next pregnancy, though recurrence of HELLP is low.

Acute Fatty Liver of Pregnancy

Acute fatty liver of pregnancy is microvesicular fatty infiltration of hepatocytes—acute yellow atrophy/acute fatty metamorphosis. It is medical/obstetrical emergency that can be fatal for mother and child if not diagnosed and managed on time. It is rare and usually occurs in third trimester and risk factors are multiparity, underweight, multiple pregnancy, preeclampsia, and male fetus.

The clinical features are nonspecific and precede few days before presentation. The "Swansea Criteria" are usually followed to make diagnosis. They are vomiting, abdominal pain, polydipsia–polyuria, ascites, encephalopathy, elevated bilirubin, hypoglycemia, elevated urate, leukocytosis, elevated transaminase/amino acids, renal impairment, coagulopathy, and microvesicular steatosis on liver biopsy. Presence of six or more in the absence of other cause indicates AFLP. It can rapidly progress to acute liver failure with complications such as encephalopathy and coagulopathy.

Laboratory investigations show elevated transaminase, bilirubin, ammonia, uric acid, leukocyte count, and hypoglycemia. Anemia, thrombocytopenia, and altered coagulation profile may be seen. Ultrasonography (USG)/CT shows evidence of fatty infiltration.

The treatment is early recognition and delivery regardless of gestational age, as liver insult is so much in some cases that it can be life-threatening or later may require liver transplant. Differential diagnosis is HELLP but liver failure with coagulopathy, encephalopathy, hypoglycemia, and renal impairment is seen more with AFLP. There is limited data regarding recurrence in subsequent pregnancy, except in those who have β-fatty acid oxidation disorder (25% chance).

Liver Hematoma and Nontraumatic Liver Rupture

Liver hematoma is rare but its most hazardous complication is hepatic rupture. Most of these cases occur in PIH and in multipara. It is associated with high maternal and perinatal mortality. 70% have epigastric pain and 65% have hypertension. USG is helpful in diagnosis. Immediate surgical intervention is the treatment. Those who survive do not have permanent liver damage and recurrence is rare.

ANATOMY AND PHYSIOLOGY OF GASTROINTESTINAL TRACT

Nausea and vomiting during pregnancy appear to be due to combined action of estrogen, progesterone, and human chorionic gonadotropin (hCG). Gastroesophageal reflux is due to decrease in lower esophageal pressure, increase in intragastric pressure, reflux of alkaline bile, and impaired clearance of gastric acid contents. Constipation is due to progesterone-induced smooth muscle relaxation.

PREGNANCY-SPECIFIC GASTROINTESTINAL CONDITIONS

Hyperemesis Gravidarum

Hyperemesis gravidarum affects 0.5–1% pregnancies. Nausea and vomiting affect 50% pregnant women and majority maintain fluid/nutritional balance by dietary modification and medication. Apart from nausea, vomiting, and weight loss, they may complain of excessive salivation. Symptoms usually resolve by the end of first trimester. In <1%, signs of dehydration including postural hypotension—tachycardia, biochemical derangement, and nutritional deficiency may be present, if not treated. The cause is not known but is thought to result from endocrine, biochemical, and psychological factors.

The diagnosis is made by exclusion after thorough clinical examination and investigations. USG should be done to rule out multiple pregnancy/hydatidiform mole. Biochemical investigations should include electrolytes, LFTs, and thyroid function tests (hyperthyroidism).[8]

Maternal risks are hyponatremia leading to confusion, seizures, and respiratory arrest. Severe cases may develop central pontine myelinolysis. Other risks are deep vein thrombosis (DVT) due to dehydration—reduced mobility and low birth weight babies.

Management

Rehydration and vitamin supplementation should be done. Antiemetics such as dopamine antagonists (domperidone), phenothiazines (chlorpromazine), anticholinergics (dicyclomine), and antihistaminic (promethazine) can be used. Nonresponders can be given 5 hydroxytryptamine (5-HT3) receptor blocker—ondansetron—available as mouth dissolving tablets.

Admission to hospital may be needed for fluid correction and parenteral antiemetic therapy. Normal saline/Ringer's lactate (RL) should be used as dextrose-containing fluid does not have enough sodium content to correct hyponatremia. Urine output, weight, and electrolytes should be maintained.

Steroid therapy has been found to be effective in nonresponders. IV hydrocortisone 100 mg three times a day, followed by oral prednisolone 40 mg daily till relief of symptoms and then dose is tapered gradually. Inpatient should be given thromboprophylaxis. Counseling, psychological support, and consultation with a nutritionist is recommended.

GASTROINTESTINAL CONDITIONS INCIDENTAL TO PREGNANCY

Reflux Esophagitis

Most patients up to 80% experience dyspepsia/heartburn at some stage of pregnancy. It is mostly experienced in the third trimester due to combination of factors such as enlarged uterus, increase gastric pressure, reduced lower esophageal sphincter (LOS) tone, decrease gastric peristalsis/emptying time, and reduction in pyloric sphincter competence. It is seen in multiparous, elderly, with multiple pregnancy or previous history of heart burns. Estrogen and progesterone hormone may relax LOS.

Antacids are safe and mainstay of treatment. It is preferable to take it before meals and at bedtime. It is advisable to take rest with head raised and avoid late night meals. Acid suppressing agents such as H2 receptor antagonists or proton pump inhibitor (PPI) are safe and have favorable results. Metoclopramide and sucralfate are also safe.

Peptic Ulcer

Peptic ulceration is not common in pregnancy. This is due to reduced gastric acid output, increased mucus production following raised progesterone levels, healthy diet, and periodic medical supervision. Most of these are caused by *Helicobacter pylori*.

High index of suspicion helps to make the diagnosis, as symptoms of epigastric pain, dyspepsia, and nausea are commonly present during pregnancy. Smokers and nonsteroidal anti-inflammatory drug (NSAID) users are at higher risk. *H. pylori* antibodies should be measured if peptic ulcer is suspected. Gastroscopy is safe, if needed during pregnancy.

Acute GI bleeding with hematemesis, melena, and bleeding per rectum may be present. It may be associated with hypotension, tachycardia, and may result in anemia. Ulcer perforation is rare during pregnancy. If there is major maternal hemorrhage or perforation, the fetus is at risk.

Prepregnancy counseling for factors that can exaggerate peptic ulcer disease such as alcohol, smoking, or NSAIDs should be done to avoid it.

Magnesium or aluminum containing antacids are safe during pregnancy and lactation. Magnesium base is preferred over aluminum as it can cause constipation. Sodium bicarbonate containing antacids should be avoided as it may cause respiratory alkalosis and fluid overload.

Acid-suppressing drugs such as H2 receptor antagonists or PPIs and cisapride for GI reflux/pain are safe during pregnancy.

In case of *H. pylori* infection, amoxicillin, clarithromycin, and metronidazole can be given with acid-suppressing agents.

Misoprostol should not be used, as it can cause uterine contraction leading to spontaneous abortion, preterm labor, and antepartum bleeding. It is also found to be teratogenic.

Surgery is rarely needed. Upper GI endoscopy per se is not contraindicated; however, it should be done only if pregnant woman is so unwell that it could not be delayed.[9] Care should be taken regarding sedation and fetal monitoring during and after the procedure. Pregnant woman should be kept in left lateral position to reduce IVC pressure and venous return.

Constipation

Constipation is common symptom experienced by 40% of women in early phase of pregnancy. It occurs due to decreased colon motility, poor fluid intake (nausea/vomiting), and pressure on rectosigmoid due to gravid uterus. Iron supplements can cause constipation but is not dose-related.

Reassurance/dietary/fluid advice is helpful. Osmotic laxatives or bulking agents are safe/helpful and are recommended for short period.

Gastroenteritis

The incidence, investigations, and treatment remain same as in nonpregnant state. Stool examination is needed, if symptoms are not relieved with antibiotics, antidiarrheal, and antiprotozoal agents. It is advisable to consume more electrolyte fluid and avoid unhealthy food.

Inflammatory Bowel Disease

The inflammatory bowel disease includes ulcerative colitis and Crohn disease.[10] Ulcerative colitis is chronic inflammatory disease of colon and rectum. The common symptoms are diarrhea, passage of mucus, and blood. Severe cases may have fever and abdominal distention. Crohn disease is chronic granulomatous inflammatory disease of terminal ileum. Patients generally present with abdominal pain, diarrhea, anemia, weight loss, melena, and fistula. Nonintestinal symptoms such as aphthous ulcer, uveitis, and sclerosing cholangitis may be present. The causative factors for both are different though they are caused by genetic immune dysregulation in response to normal gut flora. Preconception counseling should be done to control and encourage pregnancy during quiescent phase.

Stool culture, blood for anemia, electrolyte imbalance, liver functions, and inflammatory markers such as C-reactive protein should be checked. Most patients will be diagnosed in nonpregnant state. Should the diagnosis be made during pregnancy, endoscopy (colonoscopy) and biopsy are preferable.

Reduced fertility is commonly seen. The frequency of exacerbation is same. Flares can commonly occur during first trimester. Women with colostomy or ileostomy can tolerate pregnancy well. Active disease during pregnancy may result in spontaneous abortion, low birth weight, or prematurity, hence fetal growth should be monitored. Though vaginal deliveries have been reported, caesarian section should be considered in patients with extensive perianal surgery, preferably done by experienced obstetrician. Breastfeeding is safe and should be encouraged.

5-amino salicylic acid (5-ASA) and corticosteroids are given rectally or orally. In severe attacks, intravenous therapy may be given. High doses of folic acid, diet/vitamin supplements and immunosuppressants such as AZA can be given, as it is nonteratogenic. Metronidazole and antidiarrheal agents can be used. Biological agents such as immunoglobulin G1 (IgG1) can be given and congenital anomaly have not been reported.

Celiac Disease

Celiac disease or gluten sensitive enteropathy is a disorder in which gluten containing food triggers inflammation of jejunum. It improves with consumption of gluten-free diet. Etiology is multifactorial and genetic. Gluten is present in cereals such as wheat, barley, and rye but not in oats. Histologically, villous atrophy with chronic inflammatory changes is seen in jejunum which decreases toward ileum as gluten is progressively digested.

The symptoms are variable and nonspecific, ranging from tiredness, malaise, diarrhea, steatorrhea, abdominal pain, weight loss, mouth ulcers, neurological deficiency of folate, B6 or B12, or osteoporosis.

Hemorrhoids

Hemorrhoids develop from pathological changes in anal cushion with disruption of connective tissue. Prolapse piles leads to venous stasis, erosion of epithelium leading to inflammation and bleeding. Thrombosed external hemorrhoids are common during pregnancy and postpartum.

Treatment is conservative with dietary fiber supplement, medication to relieve constipation, and local application of anesthetics—steroids. Surgery is indicated for thrombosed/higher degree of hemorrhoids with failure of conservative therapy.

■ ABDOMINAL PAIN

Abdominal pain is a common symptom during pregnancy, which may or may not be related to pregnancy. There may be delay in diagnosis, as signs and symptoms are same as pregnancy-related conditions and there is limited use of radiological or endoscopic investigations.

Appendicitis

Appendicitis is the most common gastrointestinal disorder requiring surgery during pregnancy. It accounts for 25% of surgeries for nonobstetric indication in pregnancy and incidence is 1 in 1,500–2,000 pregnancies. It occurs with equal frequency in each trimester and pregnant/nonpregnant women are at equal risk as it occurs in younger women of reproductive age group.

In the first trimester, appendix is in normal anatomical position. With advancing gestation, it displaces cephalad. By midpregnancy, it is above the right iliac crest and by late pregnancy, it is close to the gallbladder. Hence, the location of pain changes, which delays the diagnosis and makes it difficult.[11] Right lower abdominal pain, nausea, vomiting, and anorexia may be present. These symptoms are commonly present even otherwise during the first trimester. In perforated appendix, pain becomes more diffuse from localized. Retrocecal appendix may produce flank pain. Differential diagnosis of adnexal pathology should be kept in mind. Abdomen-guarding, rigidity, and rebound tenderness are usually present. Leukocytosis with high granulocyte count suggests infection. USG will be able to detect inflamed appendix or appendicular abscess. In case, appendix is not identified on USG, magnetic resonance imaging (MRI) can be used for diagnosis as it is safe during pregnancy.

Increased chances of abortion, preterm labor, and fetal loss can be seen. Maternal and fetal mortality and morbidity increase with perforation which is usually due to delayed diagnosis and its associated complications.

Surgical treatment is indicated once the diagnosis is made or following failure of conservative line of management. Open or laparoscopic approach can be used depending upon the gestation.

Gallbladder Disease

Cholecystitis is caused by cystic duct obstruction with gallstones or biliary sludge. Elevated estrogen levels during pregnancy increases lithogenicity of bile, weak contractions decrease emptying, and hence increases risk of sludge. Cholelithiasis affects 10% of pregnancies and cholecystitis 0.1% of pregnancies.

Clinical features of acute cholecystitis are nausea, vomiting, anorexia, dyspepsia, intolerance of fatty foods, midepigastric, or right upper quadrant pain. USG can detect gallstones and gallbladder wall edema with pericholecystic collection. Laboratory investigations can reveal elevated direct bilirubin and transaminase levels. In acute cholecystitis, white blood cell count and alkaline phosphatase will be increased.

Most patients are treated conservatively. Surgical intervention is done only after failure of conservative therapy. Laparoscopic approach has revolutionized treatment of biliary duct during pregnancy.

Bariatric Surgery

Bariatric surgery is one option for weight loss for those with BMI >40 kg/m$_2$ or >35 kg/m^2 with comorbidities.

Two commonly done procedures are restrictive (gastric banding) and restrictive—malabsorptive (gastric bypass).[12] Patients are advised to avoid pregnancy during the year following procedure due to significant weight loss causing serious concern about nutritional status. There is risk of malabsorption and nutritional deficiency that requires constant monitoring and correction before and during pregnancy. Due to malabsorption, contraception other than oral ones are preferred.

During antenatal period, oral drug administration should be carefully monitored due to malabsorption. Extended release preparations and oral solutions are preferable. NSAIDs are used with caution to avoid gastric ulcer. Supplementation of vitamins, minerals, and trace elements are essential to avoid deficiencies and food intake needs to be monitored by trained nutritionist. Weight gain needs to be monitored by Institute of Medicine (IOM) recommendation. Dumping syndrome can occur due to ingestion of refined sugar/high glycemic index carbohydrate. Alternative screening method such as hemo glucose test may be used for screening gestational diabetes. Differential diagnosis (D/D) of pain in the abdomen becomes wider with inclusion of band slippage, small bowel obstruction, or intussusception.[1]

Obstetric management remains unchanged and C section should be performed for obstetric indication. Breastfeeding can be done but should be monitored from mother's nutritional intake point of view.

REFERENCES

1. Frise CJ, Williamson C. Gastrointestinal and liver disease in pregnancy. Clin Med. 2013;13(3):269-74.
2. Boregowda G, Shehata HA. Gastrointestinal and liver disease in pregnancy: Best Pract Res Clin Obstet Gynecol. 2013;27(6): 835-53.
3. Geenes V, Williamson C. Gastrointestinal and liver disease in pregnancy – ScienceDirect, Obstetrics, Gynecology and Reproductive Medicine. 2017;27(3):91-8.
4. Boregowda G, Shehata HA. Gastrointestinal and liver disease in pregnancy: Best Pract Res Clin Obstet Gynaecol. 2013;27(6): 835-53.
5. Jabiry-Zieniwicz Z, Dabrowiski FA, Pietrzak B, Wyzgal J, Bomba-Opoń D, Zieniewicz K, et al. Pregnancy in the liver transplant recipient. AASLD. 2016;22(10):1408-17.
6. Kenyan AP, Girling JC. Obstetric cholestasis. Progress Obstet Gynecol. 2005;16:37-56.
7. Dixon PH, Williamson C. The molecular genetics of intrahepatic cholestasis of pregnancy. Obstet Med. 2012;4(4):141-7.
8. Williamson C, Girling J. Hepatic and gastrointestinal disease. High-risk Pregnancy, Management Options, 4th edition. Philadelphia: Saunders; 2011. pp. 839-60.
9. Gomes CF, Sousa M, Lourenço I, Martins D, Torres J. Gastrointestinal diseases during pregnancy: what does the gastroenterologist need to know? Ann Gastroenterol. 2018; 31(4):385-94.
10. Seymour CA, Chadwick VS. Liver and gastrointestinal function in pregnancy. Post Grad Med J. 1979;55(643):343-52.
11. Dietrich CS, Hill CC, Hueman M. Surgical diseases presenting in pregnancy. Surg Clin North Am. 2008;88(2):403-419.
12. ACOG Guidelines on Pregnancy after Bariatric surgery: Am Fam Physician. 2010:81(7):905-6.

LONG QUESTIONS

1. Discuss the approach to diagnosis of jaundice in pregnancy. What are the important prognostic factors in this condition?
2. What is the pathogenesis of obstetric cholestasis? Discuss the approach to a woman who presents with severe itching in pregnancy at 32 weeks gestation.
3. Discuss the management of inflammatory bowel disease in pregnancy.

SHORT QUESTIONS

1. What are the main functions of the liver and how are they affected in pregnancy?
2. What are the common causes of hepatitis in pregnancy? Rank them according to risk of maternal mortality.
3. What risks does the mother and fetus face when the mother is a liver transplant recipient?
4. What is acute fatty liver of pregnancy? State the important diagnostic criteria.
5. What is the impact of a bariatric surgery on a subsequent pregnancy?

MULTIPLE CHOICE QUESTIONS

1. In which direction does the liver move during pregnancy?
   a. Superior – Anterior
   b. Inferior – Anterior
   c. Superior – Posterior
   d. Inferior – Posterior
2. Which of the following are common findings during pregnancy?
   a. Spider nevi   b. Palmar erythema
   c. Edema   d. All of the above
3. Prolongation of which investigation is the first sign of acute liver failure?
   a. Prothrombin time
   b. Bleeding time
   c. Clotting time
   d. None of the above
4. Which of the following hormone is responsible for smooth muscle relaxation leading to constipation during pregnancy?
   a. Estrogen   b. Progesterone
   c. hCG   d. None of the above
5. What are the physiological changes of alkaline phosphatase during pregnancy?
   a. Rises   b. Falls
   c. Remains same   d. All of the above

PART 1: Obstetrics and Perinatology

6. Small amount of urobilinogen passes into liver because it is:
   a. Water soluble
   b. Fat soluble
   c. Insoluble
   d. None of the above
7. Which of following immunosuppressants used in liver transplant recipient is not safe in pregnancy?
   a. Prednisolone
   b. AZA – Azathioprine
   c. CsA – Cyclosporine A
   d. Tac – Tarcolimus
8. Classic symptom of obstetric cholestasis is generalized pruritus:
   a. With rash
   b. Without rash
   c. All of the above
   d. None of the above
9. In obstetric cholestasis, which of the following shows raised levels?
   a. Bile acids
   b. Sr Transaminase
   c. ALT and AST
   d. All of the above
10. Which of the following are fetal risks in obstetric cholestasis?
    a. Prematurity
    b. Fetal demise
    c. IUD
    d. All of the above
11. Which of the following drugs can be used to treat obstetric cholestasis?
    a. Ursodeoxycholic acid
    b. Cholestyramine
    c. Guar gum
    d. All of the above
12. Which of the following factors are responsible for hyperemesis gravidarum?
    a. Endocrine
    b. Biochemical
    c. Psychological
    d. All of the above
13. Which of the following contraception is relatively contraindicated in patients who have undergone bariatric surgery?
    a. Barrier
    b. Oral contraception
    c. Injectable
    d. IUD
14. Celiac disease is also known as:
    a. Gluten free enteropathy
    b. Gluten sensitive enteropathy
    c. Gluten allergic enteropathy
    d. None of the above
15. Appendix undergoes displacement in which direction with advancing pregnancy?
    a. Cephalad and laterally
    b. Cephalad and medially
    c. Cephalad and anterior
    d. Cephalad and posterior

Answers

1. b	2. d	3. a	4. b	5. a	6. a
7. b	8. b	9. d	10. d	11. d	12. d
13. b	14. b	15. a			

5.9 AUTOIMMUNE DISORDERS OF PREGNANCY

Vinita Salvi, Ami Surti

INTRODUCTION

The body of a normal individual recognizes its own tissues as its own. In autoimmune disorders, the body fails to recognize its own tissues as "self" and produces antibodies against itself. This results in inflammation and damage in tissues and organs. There are a great number of autoimmune disorders and while some affect particular tissues and systems such as rheumatoid arthritis (RA), others such as systemic lupus erythematosus (SLE) are more nonspecific and can cause wide-ranging effects on multiple parts of the body. The management and treatment generally consist of suppressing this immune hyperactivity.

Autoimmune disorders are more common in women, and the incidence of some of them, such as SLE, tends to peak during reproductive years. Thus, these disorders are often seen in pregnant women. Autoimmune disorders during pregnancy can have implications for both maternal and fetal/neonatal health. They may cause adverse effects due to the dysfunction they induce in various maternal organs such as the kidneys and blood vessels, which directly or indirectly affect both maternal and fetal health. On the other hand, the additional organ of consideration during a pregnancy is the placenta. Autoimmune disorders are associated with defective placentation and abruption and can affect fetal outcome in the form of miscarriage, growth restriction, oligohydramnios, fetal death, and disease-induced defects such as congenital heart block seen in neonatal lupus or adverse effects of drugs used to suppress the autoimmune dysfunction. This chapter will cover autoimmune disorders that are commonly seen in pregnancy, as well as some of the rare varieties. Type 1 diabetes will be covered in the chapter on diabetes in pregnancy.

Women with known autoimmune dysfunction are best counseled preconception with a team approach and advised to conceive when the disease is quiescent to ensure an optimum outcome. On the other hand, the obstetrician is often faced with a patient who has an undiagnosed autoimmune disease which presents for the first time during a pregnancy. The physician has to be alert to such a possibility since the management and outcome may differ. A SLE flare can mimic preeclampsia. While the first may worsen postpartum, the second generally improves after a delivery.

SYSTEMIC LUPUS ERYTHEMATOSUS

Systemic lupus erythematosus is an autoimmune disease characterized by periods of disease activity and remission. The incidence and prevalence of SLE are higher in Hispanics and Asians as compared to Caucasians, but lower than African Americans.[1] The incidence and prevalence of SLE vary with sex, age, ethnicity, and time. Women are more commonly affected than men for every age and ethnic group. Incidence peaks in middle adulthood and occurs later for males.[2] This explains the frequent occurrence of SLE-complicating pregnancy.

Women with SLE are best advised to conceive when their disease is in remission for a period of 6 months. The outcome is better if there is no active nephritis, hypertension, or thrombocytopenia. If the woman has active SLE at the time of conception, there is a higher risk of adverse pregnancy outcomes. However, even if a woman is in the active phase, the outcome will be good in almost 80% of cases (77% livebirths in the high activity patients vs. 88% in the low activity patients).[3]

The latest classification for SLE is the 2019 European League Against Rheumatism (EULAR)/American College of Rheumatology (ARA) Classification Criteria for Systemic Lupus Erythematosus **(Tables 1 and 2)**.[4]

It is based on the fact that the patient must have a positive antinuclear antibody (ANA) at least once as an obligatory entry criterion. Thereafter, there are additive weighted criteria which are grouped in seven clinical [constitutional, hematologic, neuropsychiatric, mucocutaneous **(Fig. 1)**, serosal, musculoskeletal, renal] and three immunologic [antiphospholipid antibodies (aPL), complement proteins, SLE-specific antibodies] domains and weighted from 2 to 10. Patients must accumulate 10 or more points to be diagnosed SLE. The new system has a better sensitivity (96.1%) and specificity (93.4%) as compared to earlier criteria.

EULAR/ARA Classification for Systemic Lupus Erythematosus

Entry Criteria

- ANAs at a titer of ≥1:80 on HEp-2 cells or an equivalent positive test (ever)
- If absent, do not classify as SLE
- If present, apply additive criteria.

Additive Criteria

- Do not count a criterion if there is a more likely explanation than SLE.
- Occurrence of a criterion on at least one occasion is sufficient.

TABLE 1: Systemic lupus erythematosus (SLE) diagnostic criteria—clinical.

Clinical domains and criteria	Weight
Constitutional	
Fever	2
Hematologic	
Leukopenia	3
Thrombocytopenia	4
Autoimmune hemolysis	4
Neuropsychiatric	
Delirium	2
Psychosis	3
Seizure	5
Mucocutaneous	
Nonscarring alopecia	2
Oral ulcers	2
Subacute cutaneous OR discoid lupus	4
Acute cutaneous lupus	6
Serosal	
Pleural or pericardial effusion	5
Acute pericarditis	6
Musculoskeletal	
Joint involvement	6
Renal	
Proteinuria >0.5 g/24 hours	4
Renal biopsy class II or V lupus nephritis	8
Renal biopsy class III or IV lupus nephritis	10

TABLE 2: Systemic lupus erythematosus (SLE) diagnostic criteria—immunological.

Immunology domains and criteria	Weight
Antiphospholipid antibodies Anticardiolipin IgG >40 GPL or Anti-β2GP1 antibodies IgG >40 units or Lupus anticoagulant	2
Complement proteins domain	
Low C3 or Low C4	3
Low C3 and Low C4	4
Highly specific antibodies domain	
Anti-ds DNA antibody	6
Anti-Smith antibody	6

(Ig: immunoglobulin)

- SLE classification requires at least one clinical criterion and ≥10 points.
- Criteria need not occur simultaneously.

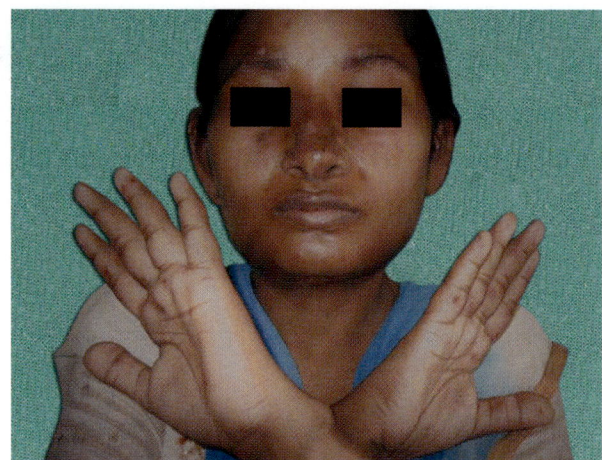

Fig. 1: Malar rash and cutaneous lupus erythematosus.

- Within each domain, only the highest weighted criterion is counted toward the total score.

Total score: Classify as SLE with a score of 10 or more if entry criterion fulfilled.

There may be antibodies to other extractable nuclear antigens (ENAs), like anti Ro/SS-A or anti La/SS-B in up to 30% patients and may be associated with neonatal lupus. Drugs commonly causing lupus erythematosus include procainamide, quinidine, and hydralazine.

It may be noted that many patients of severe preeclampsia/eclampsia satisfy the criteria for SLE, provided they test positive for antinuclear antibodies.

Planning a Pregnancy

Women with SLE should undergo preconception counseling. A team composed of a rheumatologist or experienced physician, obstetrician, and neonatologist working in collaboration with other specialists as necessary (e.g., nephrologist) would best serve the needs of the woman. The woman should be kept on medicines which are safe during pregnancy. Hydroxychloroquine sulfate (HCQS) and low-dose aspirin are relatively safe to use in pregnancy while methotrexate, cyclophosphamide, mycophenolate mofetil, and leflunomide are not. In fact, low-dose aspirin should be utilized for the prevention of preeclampsia which these women are prone to get. If the woman is on HCQS, it should be continued since it reduces the occurrence of a flare. Prednisolone should be used at the lowest possible dose necessary to prevent an activation of the disease and should preferably be maintained at 10 mg or less. Though previously, it was thought that prednisolone caused cleft lip and palate, current data does not support such an issue.[5] Nonsteroidal anti-inflammatory drugs (NSAIDs) maybe used in pregnancy. After 30 weeks of gestation, however, they may cause premature closure of the ductus arteriosus. Certain drugs are to be used after assessing the risk–benefit ratio in the given patient. Azathioprine or tacrolimus may be substituted for mycophenolate.

If a woman has hypertension, she should be converted to antihypertensives with a documented safety profile in pregnancy such as α-methyldopa, labetalol, nifedipine, or hydralazine. Angiotensin receptor blockers (ARBs) and angiotensin-converting enzyme (ACE) inhibitors are best avoided. Women with a history of nephritis should be counseled regarding the risk of a flare.

Ideally, women should attempt pregnancy only after the disease has been quiescent for 6 months. If the woman conceives during an active phase, she may need adjustment of medications.

Effect of Pregnancy on Systemic Lupus Erythematosus

With prior quiescent disease, SLE flare rate is low during pregnancy. Flares during pregnancy are mild, predominantly arthritis and cutaneous disease, and may occur at any time, including the postpartum period. Detection of lupus flares during pregnancy may be difficult due to symptom overlap between normal pregnancy and SLE flare, and between lupus nephritis and preeclampsia.

Systemic lupus erythematosus flare is a more likely diagnosis if the following features are found:
- Active disease within 6 months of conception
- Symptoms of extreme fatigue
- Skin lesions
- Arthralgia
- Lymphadenopathy
- Fever not due to infection
- Pleuritic pain
- Leukopenia with reduced complement levels
- Presence of hematuria and/or urinary casts.

Preeclampsia is more likely if serum urate levels are elevated and/or liver function tests (LFTs) are abnormal.

Effect of Systemic Lupus Erythematosus on Pregnancy

Systemic lupus erythematosus is known to be associated with adverse pregnancy outcomes. If the mother has active disease, she is more prone to preeclampsia and nephritis. There is a higher chance of abortion, preterm labor, intrauterine growth restriction and fetal death, and neonatal lupus. However, in well-controlled patients who have been in remission for over 6 months prior to conceiving and who have no additional factors such as aPL, hypertension, or lupus nephritis, the outcomes are good.

Management of a Pregnant Patient with Systemic Lupus Erythematosus

The pregnancy should be managed by a team consisting of an experienced physician, obstetrician, and neonatologist working along with other specialists such as a nephrologist, rheumatologist, or dermatologist, as required. Ideally, the woman should be counseled and evaluated prior to conceiving. A complete blood count, renal, and liver function tests should be performed periodically. Patients with renal involvement need periodic monitoring of 24 hours urinary proteins. This author evaluates the following antibodies: ANA, anti-dsDNA, lupus anticoagulant (LA), anticardiolipin (aCL), activated partial thromboplastin time, and anti-β2 glycoprotein. Anti-Ro (anti-SSA) and anti-La (anti-SSB) antibodies and complement evaluation are also a part of the evaluation profile. If the patient is positive for anti-Ro or anti-La antibodies, there is a risk of congenital heart block in the fetus. Such fetuses should be monitored by echocardiography. The neonate could also be at high risk for neonatal lupus with its hepatic, heart, and cutaneous manifestations.

Patients with SLE are often on prednisolone and low-dose aspirin. Patients on prednisolone are to be monitored for abnormal sugars and increased chance of maternal hypertension, diabetes, and infection, commonly vaginal discharge, urinary infections, and acne. In the event of being positive for anticardiolipin antibody (ACA) and/or LA and previous adverse pregnancy outcome, they are administered heparin. Besides maternal well-being, the pregnancy is also closely monitored for fetal well-being and growth. Doppler flow studies are also done serially to evaluate fetal blood supply, since SLE is associated with defective placentation and its adverse effects on pregnancy outcome.

Postpartum, there is a risk of lupus flare and steroids should never be abruptly stopped.

ANTIPHOSPHOLIPID SYNDROME

The antiphospholipid syndrome (APS) is an autoimmune disorder which is characterized by the presence of: Venous and/or arterial thrombosis and/or specific adverse pregnancy outcomes with the persistent presence of aPL.

It affects approximately 15% women with SLE, but may exist without other autoimmune disease (primary APS).

The antiphospholipid autoantibodies are:
- LA
- ACAs [immunoglobulin G (IgG) and IgM]
- Anti-β2 glycoprotein (IgG and IgM)

Antiphospholipid syndrome is defined by the Sapporo or Sydney criteria. The original Sapporo criteria were published in 1999. Since then, new clinical, laboratory, and experimental insights led to a workshop at Sydney before the Eleventh International Congress on aPL and proposed amendments to the original Sapporo criteria.[6]

Revised Classification Criteria for the Antiphospholipid Syndrome as per Sapporo/Sydney Criteria

Antiphospholipid syndrome (APS) is present if at least one of the clinical criteria and one of the laboratory criteria that follow are met.*

Clinical Criteria

- *Vascular thrombosis*: One or more clinical episodes of arterial, venous, or small vessel thrombosis, in any tissue or organ. Thrombosis must be confirmed by objective validated criteria (i.e., unequivocal findings of appropriate imaging studies or histopathology). For histopathologic confirmation, thrombosis should be present without significant evidence of inflammation in the vessel wall.
- *Pregnancy morbidity*:
  - One or more unexplained deaths of a morphologically normal fetus at or beyond the 10th week of gestation, with normal fetal morphology documented by ultrasound or by direct examination of the fetus
  - One or more premature births of a morphologically normal neonate before the 34th week of gestation because of:
    - Eclampsia or severe preeclampsia defined according to standard definitions
    - Recognized features of placental insufficiency
  - Three or more unexplained consecutive spontaneous abortions before the 10th week of gestation, with maternal anatomic or hormonal abnormalities and paternal and maternal chromosomal causes excluded.

Laboratory Criteria**

- LA present in plasma, on two or more occasions at least 12 weeks apart detected according to the guidelines of the International Society on Thrombosis and Haemostasis (Scientific Subcommittee on LAs/phospholipid-dependent antibodies)
- aCL antibody of IgG and/or IgM isotype in serum or plasma, present in medium or high titer (i.e., >40 GPL or MPL, or more than the 99th percentile), on two or more occasions, at least 12 weeks apart, measured by a standardized enzyme-linked immunosorbent assay (ELISA)
- Anti-β2 glycoprotein-I antibody of IgG and/or IgM isotype in serum or plasma (in titer >the 99th percentile), present on two or more occasions, at least 12 weeks apart, measured by a standardized ELISA, according to recommended procedures.

Generally accepted features of placental insufficiency include:
- Abnormal or non-reassuring fetal surveillance test(s), e.g., a nonreactive nonstress test, suggestive of fetal hypoxemia
- Abnormal Doppler flow velocimetry waveform analysis suggestive of fetal hypoxemia, e.g., absent end-diastolic flow in the umbilical artery
- Oligohydramnios, e.g., an amniotic fluid index of 5 cm or less
- A postnatal birth weight less than the 10th percentile for the gestational age.

---

*Classification of APS should be avoided if <12 weeks or >5 years separate the positive aPL test and the clinical manifestations.
**Investigators are strongly advised to classify APS patients in studies into one of the following categories:
- I—more than one laboratory criteria present (any combination)
- IIA—LA present alone
- IIB—aCL antibody present alone
- IIC—anti-β2 glycoprotein-I antibody present alone

It is to be noted that as per the Sapporo Sydney criteria placental insufficiency is defined even on the basis of a nonreactive nonstress test.

In 381 Indian women with two or more pregnancy losses, 176 (46.2%) patients had at least one acquired thrombophilia, while 143 (37.5%) had at least one genetic thrombophilia marker. In acquired thrombophilias, the strongest association was observed with ACA [odds ratio (OR) 32.5, 95% confidence interval (CI): 8.6–21.8, p <0.001] followed by annexin V (OR 17.1, 95% CI: 2.9–99.4, p <0.001), LA (OR 8.2, 95% CI: 1.4–47.7, p = 0.01) and anti-β2 GP1 (OR 5.8, 95% CI: 1.6–22.1, p = 0.007).[7]

Management

The hypercoagulable state of pregnancy and APS coexisting together can increase the risk of thrombosis such as a cerebrovascular accident. Pregnant women with APS who have a past history of arterial or venous thrombosis should be offered therapeutic anticoagulation with low molecular weight heparin (LMWH) and low-dose aspirin.

If there is a history of adverse pregnancy outcome in the past, women with APS are at an increased risk for miscarriage, fetal growth restriction and fetal death, preeclampsia, preterm birth, placental abruption, and thrombosis. Women with adverse pregnancy outcomes in the past but no history of arterial or venous thrombosis should be on prophylactic dose of LMWH with low-dose aspirin. Though the incidence of heparin-induced thrombocytopenia with the use of LMWH is extremely low and guidelines do not advise monitoring platelet count in obstetric patients on LMWH,[8] this author does a complete blood count 10 days after starting heparin. The safety of newer oral anticoagulants such as rivaroxaban or dabigatran during pregnancy have not been established.

The use of LMWH through a pregnancy can have considerable financial implications. Can unfractionated heparin be used instead of LMWH? Unfractionated heparin requires twice daily dosing and more intense monitoring of coagulation parameters as compared to LMWH. Though we reported[9] higher rate of successful outcomes with LMWH (9/9 patients) than unfractionated heparin (16/23 patients), the number of patients studied was very small and, we have continued to use unfractionated heparin in resource poor settings with good results.

Those women who have tested positive for aPL but have no history of an adverse pregnancy outcome or arterial or venous thrombosis, are unlikely to have an adverse pregnancy outcome and are maintained on low-dose aspirin. Women who have received anticoagulants during the antenatal period should continue to receive them in the puerperium. The choice is LMWH or warfarin. LMWH can be restarted 4–6 hours after delivery. Women on warfarin should have the international normalized ratio maintained between 2 and 3.

Women with APS who have had a history of arterial or venous thromboembolism in the past will need life-long anticoagulation, probably warfarin. Those women who have not had such a history of thromboembolism, should be counseled regarding the need for prophylactic anticoagulation, during high-risk events such as a major surgery needing immobilization (e.g., joint replacement) or a long-distance flight.

■ RHEUMATOID ARTHRITIS

Rheumatoid arthritis is a chronic inflammatory disease affecting mainly the synovial joints. It is more common in women than in men in the ratio of 3:1.

Effect of Pregnancy on Rheumatoid Arthritis

Rheumatoid arthritis commonly undergoes remission in pregnancy and especially in the second and third trimester and tends to flare postpartum. The amelioration of RA is attributed to the tolerance that develops during pregnancy of the maternal immune system to fetal antigens. Adams Waldorf and Lee[10] have postulated that during pregnancy, there is development of tolerance by the mother's immune system to fetal HLA peptides. A small quantity of apoptotic syncytiotrophoblast enters the maternal bloodstream and is engulfed by maternal immune cells which then develop a tolerance to these foreign antigens. Thus, there is a change in the recognition of maternal "self." They postulate that this decreased immunogenicity also results in an amelioration of RA during pregnancy. The greater the difference between fetal and maternal human leukocyte antigen (HLA) antigens, the greater is the amelioration in RA. Some of the other proposed theories for amelioration of RA include the decrease in cell-mediated immunity during pregnancy, elevated levels of anti-inflammatory cytokines, and the increased cortisol, estrogen, and progestin levels in pregnancy. Humoral immunity is also affected in pregnancy and neutrophil function is also altered. All these changes reverse in the postpartum period resulting in increased flares.

Effect of Rheumatoid Arthritis on Pregnancy

Rheumatoid arthritis generally does not affect the outcome of pregnancy. It is generally the drugs which are used in the management of RA, that have to be taken into consideration for their possible effects on mother and baby.

Management

Patients should be evaluated and counseled prepregnancy and made aware of the effects of DMARDs (disease-modifying anti-rheumatic drugs). Conception should be deferred till the disease is in the quiescent phase. Patients should use contraception when they are on methotrexate, cyclophosphamide, and leflunomide and for a few months after discontinuing therapy. Fertility maybe affected. Prednisone (>7.5 mg/day) and NSAIDs use may also affect fertility. Patients should be on drugs that are relatively safe during pregnancy. Corticosteroids are used commonly since they are relatively safe. Patients on steroids should be monitored for hypertension, infection, and diabetes. Osteoporosis is also a risk as well as premature rupture of membranes and small-for-gestational-age babies. Women on steroids need stress doses during labor and delivery. They should not be suddenly stopped. HCQS can be used in pregnancy. Patients on HCQS may need an ophthalmological evaluation. NSAIDs should be discontinued by 30–32 weeks gestation since they can cause oligohydramnios and premature closure of the ductus arteriosus. Nonpharmacological means of pain relief such as cold packs, splinting, paraffin baths, and decreased physical activity should be used. Cyclooxygenase 2 (COX-2) inhibitors should be avoided. Sulfasalazine may be used in pregnancy and azathioprine can be used after evaluating the risk–benefit ratio. The fetal liver is too immature to convert azathioprine to its active metabolite and thus is protected. The EULAR guidelines for the use of anti-tumor necrosis factor (TNF) medications[11] are as follows:

There is no current evidence of increased rate of congenital malformations with all of the following, except golimumab:

- *Infliximab/adalimumab*: It can be continued up to 20 weeks of gestation; if indicated, it can be used throughout pregnancy.
- *Golimumab*: Consider alternatives since there is limited evidence.
- *Etanercept*: It can be continued up to 30–32 weeks of gestation; if indicated, it can be used throughout pregnancy.
- *Certolizumab*: It can be used throughout pregnancy.

Rituximab may be used in exceptional cases in early pregnancy, since later on in pregnancy, it can cause β-cell depletion in the neonate. There is too little information on the use of other drugs such as anakinra, abatacept, and Janus kinase (JAK) inhibitors to recommend their use during pregnancy.

The range of movements at the hip joint should be evaluated before contemplating a vaginal delivery.

SCLERODERMA

Scleroderma is a progressive autoimmune connective tissue disorder that predominantly affects the skin, kidneys, lungs, heart, and blood vessels. There is excess collagen deposition in the connective tissue. The heart and lungs may get severely compromised. It affects older women and is rarely seen in pregnancy. It has exacerbations and remissions. Women with localized scleroderma which affects the skin and muscles do better during pregnancy than women with systemic scleroderma with involvement of other organ systems. Women with pulmonary hypertension are at increased risk for maternal mortality and it may be considered as a contraindication for pregnancy. Women with scleroderma may develop hypertension during pregnancy. There may be placental insufficiency affecting fetal growth. The risk to the pregnancy is highest within 4 years of the onset of the disease. As with most autoimmune disorders, it may flare postpartum.

MYASTHENIA GRAVIS

Myasthenia gravis is an autoimmune disease seen more commonly in women of childbearing age and consequently also seen in pregnancy. It occurs due to autoantibodies produced by the thymus. These autoantibodies act against the acetylcholine receptors at the neuromuscular junction. The action of acetylcholine on these receptors is prevented giving rise to muscle weakness. The antibodies are produced by a thymic neoplasm or a hyperplastic thymus. Therefore, women contemplating a pregnancy are benefited by a thymectomy before conceiving.

Myasthenia gravis behaves unpredictably in pregnancy. Some patients worsen while others improve or remain static. Due to the immunosuppression of pregnancy, patients may improve in later pregnancy and then flare postpartum. It is diagnosed by clinical evaluation and antibody levels.

Generally, myasthenia does not affect pregnancy adversely. Some neonates develop transient myasthenia due to transfer of IgG antibodies across the placenta. This manifests by day 2–4 postpartum with a weak cry, feeble sucking, ptosis, and respiratory weakness. The antibodies degrade and the baby normalizes by 3 weeks.

The mothers should be allowed normal labor since the uterus is composed of smooth muscle and therefore not affected by the antibodies. However, the second stage may need assistance with a ventouse or forceps since the pelvic floor muscles are striated and voluntary. Cesarean should be performed for obstetric indications.

Acetylcholine esterase inhibitors such as pyridostigmine and neostigmine are used in pregnancy. Prednisolone, azathioprine, cyclosporine, and rituximab are also used. The only drug to be avoided during pregnancy is mycophenolate mofetil, since there is some evidence that it may cause miscarriage and malformations.

Drugs that potentiate the effects of acetyl choline receptor antibodies are contraindicated in such patients. These include neuromuscular blocking agents such as magnesium sulfate, antiarrhythmics such as quinidine, local anesthetics, and antibiotics such as aminoglycosides, quinolones, and macrolides.

AUTOIMMUNE DISORDERS OF THE THYROID

Autoimmune disorders of the thyroid can cause either hyperthyroidism (Graves' disease) or hypothyroidism (Hashimoto thyroiditis). Postpartum thyroiditis is an autoimmune disorder which causes transient hyperthyroidism, hypothyroidism, or transient hyperthyroidism followed by hypothyroidism.

Graves' Disease

Graves' disease is an autoimmune disease of the thyroid gland which results in thyrotoxicosis. It affects women more than men and especially those who are <40 years of age. There is a genetic component. It is often associated with other autoimmune disorders such as type 1 diabetes and RA and can be aggravated by physical or mental stress and occur during pregnancy or the postpartum period. Cigarette smoking also aggravates Graves' disease. It is caused by the production of thyrotropin receptor antibodies (TRAb) which bind to the receptors on the thyroid gland and mimic the action of thyroid-stimulating hormone (TSH), resulting in overproduction of thyroid hormones. The woman suffers fatigue, anxiety, irritability, palpitations, fine tremors, heat sensitivity, diarrhea, weight loss, and sleep disturbances. Some of these may be seen even in a normal pregnancy. There may be bulging eyeballs (Graves ophthalmopathy), thyroid goiter and red thickened patches on the shin or feet (Graves' dermopathy).

During pregnancy, it may lead to preeclampsia, cardiac failure, placental abruption, and thyroid storm in the mother, while there may be a risk of miscarriage, growth restriction, prematurity, and fetal thyroid dysfunction in the fetus. If the maternal thyroid antibodies are very high and over 300% of normal, there is a risk of fetal hyperthyroidism.

Evaluation

In pregnant women, thyroid function tests and evaluation of antibodies can be done. Imaging would involve a thyroid ultrasound as radioiodine uptake studies or imaging involving radiation are not possible.

Management

Antithyroid medications are used to control the thyrotoxicosis. In the first trimester, propylthiouracil is preferred in view of the slightly increased risk of anomalies with methimazole. After the first trimester is over, the patient can take methimazole. The risk of liver dysfunction is higher with propylthiouracil as compared to methimazole. Free T_4 and TSH should be measured every 2–4 weeks at the initiation of therapy and every 4–6 weeks after stabilization.

Hashimoto Thyroiditis

These patients test positive for thyroid peroxidase antibody (anti-TPO). Many also test positive for antithyroglobulin antibodies. These pregnancies are at risk for maternal anemia, preeclampsia, cardiac dysfunction, placental abruption, and postpartum hemorrhage. There is increased risk of miscarriage, prematurity, growth restriction, and neonatal neurological development delay.

Mild cases may have only aches and pains. Lethargy and constipation may occur. Cold intolerance, stiffness, muscle cramping, dry skin and hair, and carpal tunnel syndrome may follow.

The goal of treatment is to normalize maternal TSH levels to the trimester specific range: First trimester 0.1–2.5 mIU/L, second trimester 0.2–3.0 mIU/L, third trimester 0.3–3.0 mIU/L. During pregnancy, the thyroid hormone increases by approximately 30% over prepregnancy requirements. Initially, the thyroid function tests will have to be repeated every 4 weeks till the optimum dose is reached and thereafter it may be repeated every trimester.

Postpartum Thyroiditis

This is a variant of Hashimoto thyroiditis. It may commonly occur up to 8 months after delivery. These patients have antimicrosomal antibodies. These patients are at risk for depression, permanent hypothyroidism, and recurrence of postpartum thyroiditis in subsequent pregnancies.

Vasculitis

Autoimmune vasculitis is a condition where the blood vessels get damaged due to infiltration with inflammatory cells and the blood vessel walls undergo necrosis. Vasculitis maybe primary or it may be seen as a secondary phenomenon in SLE, RA, malignancy, or infection. They are quite rare in pregnancy and may, in fact, be missed because of their rarity. As in all autoimmune disorders, vasculitis can undergo a flare or remission and patients are best advised to conceive during a remission. This condition may affect various organs and one is concerned about adverse effects such as renal damage and hypertension. These patients too are best managed with a multidisciplinary approach which should begin in the interval period. Prepregnancy evaluation and counseling are necessary. As in all autoimmune disorders, these patients too are at an increased risk of thromboembolism and may need heparin and aspirin as a part of their management scheme. Hypertension, preeclampsia, and renal function are monitored. Fetal outcome may be affected with a higher risk of adverse pregnancy outcomes, growth restriction, prematurity, stillbirths, and drug-induced teratogenicity. Nonpregnant patients are treated with immune suppressants such as prednisolone and immune modulators such as azathioprine, cyclophosphamide, methotrexate, and mycophenolate mofetil. The drugs used in pregnancy should be carefully selected with attention to their risk–benefit ratio and safety profile. Corticosteroids and azathioprine would be preferred in pregnant women. Occasionally, cytotoxic drugs such as cyclophosphamide may be necessary but they should be used only for brief periods in late pregnancy after carefully evaluating risk–benefit ratio and counseling the patient and her family. The entities are named depending on the type of vessels that are affected.

Takayasu Arteritis

Takayasu arteritis is a chronic inflammation that affects the aorta and its main branches and the pulmonary arteries. The vessels undergo fibrosis, stenosis, thrombosis, and aneurysm formation. Hypertension, stroke, valvular disease, and retinopathy are complications. It is more common in young women.

Pregnancy reduces the inflammation and erythrocyte sedimentation rate (ESR) and C-reactive protein reduce. Magnetic resonance imaging (MRI) (after first trimester) and positron emission tomography (PET) scan (nonpregnant) may be used to assess the vessels involved. Blood pressure (BP) monitoring may need a femoral cuff if the pulses in the upper arms are affected. Patients should be regularly monitored for BP, cardiac, and renal function. Corticosteroids form the mainstay of management though azathioprine is also used. If there is valvular involvement, prophylactic antibiotics should be used to prevent bacterial endocarditis during labor and delivery. During labor, BP monitoring is vital as there is a risk of an intracranial bleed.

Wegener Granulomatosis or Granulomatosis with Polyangiitis

Wegener's granulomatosis affects small blood vessels. It causes granulomatous lesions predominantly in the respiratory tract and kidneys. Cytoplasmic-staining pattern antineutrophil cytoplasmic antibody (cANCA) is a characteristic antibody seen in this condition. It is extremely rare in pregnancy since it is an unusual condition that tends to occur in older individuals. It tends to worsen in pregnancy with the possibility of a flare in those individuals who are in remission. It also has an adverse impact on the outcome of pregnancy. Cyclophosphamide is used very often to manage Wegener granulomatosis in nonpregnant individuals and this agent can have an adverse impact on ovarian function. During pregnancy, prednisolone and azathioprine are the management drugs of choice. However, occasionally, it may be necessary to introduce drugs that are toxic to the fetus and should be used for only the shortest possible time and in conjunction with joint consultation with the patient and her healthcare team.

Churg–Strauss Syndrome

This is a necrotizing vasculitis affecting medium and small arteries. Patients can present with late-onset asthma, nasal polyps, infiltrates in the lung, and eosinophilia. Typically, these patients are positive for perinuclear-staining pattern antineutrophil cytoplasmic antibody (p-ANCA). It is one more vasculitis that is encountered very rarely in pregnancy. Pregnancy may precipitate a relapse. Preconception evaluation should include echocardiography. Both cardiac and lung function should be monitored in the pregnancy. The kidneys and gut may also get affected. If the patient gets congestive cardiac failure due to myocarditis, there is a risk of mortality. Patients are managed with corticosteroids.

Polyarteritis Nodosa

Polyarteritis nodosa is a necrotizing vasculitis that affects medium vessels. It affects older individuals and is rarely seen in pregnancy. It can affect all organ systems. Arterial wall thickening and microaneurysms are seen. It is associated with hepatitis B. Renal failure with heavy proteinuria and elevated creatinine, cardiomyopathy, gastrointestinal bleeding, and neurological involvement are bad prognostic omens. Sometimes, it may be necessary to consider medical termination of pregnancy in early pregnancy. In polyarteritis nodosa, steroid monotherapy is the drug of choice but aggressive cytotoxic therapy may be necessary sometimes, late in pregnancy.

Microscopic Polyangiitis

This condition is a necrotizing vasculitis that predominantly affects small vessels of the kidneys and lungs. ANCA is positive, especially p-ANCA, which is specific for myeloperoxidase. It is an extremely rare condition and the renal and respiratory function need to be monitored both preconception and during pregnancy. Methylprednisolone, plasma exchange, and cyclophosphamide have been used in its management. It may affect the neonate as well.

INFLAMMATORY BOWEL DISEASE

Both ulcerative colitis and Crohn disease may occur during pregnancy. Ulcerative colitis tends to be more active during pregnancy while Crohn disease is not.

One-third of stable patients with inflammatory bowel disease (IBD) will relapse during pregnancy. On the other hand, two-third of those with active IBD will continue to remain active through pregnancy. With respect to fetal outcome, active disease is associated with a higher chance of adverse pregnancy outcomes including miscarriage, preterm delivery, growth restriction, stillbirth, low Apgar scores, and increased admission to neonatal intensive care unit (NICU).

Imaging of IBD during pregnancy should be by sonography, provided adequate expertise is available. Else MRI without gadolinium contrast should be utilized to evaluate the patient. If an endoscopy is absolutely necessary, it should be done after the first trimester. Flexible sigmoidoscopy can be done.

The choice of anti-inflammatory drug should be such as to be of optimal safety during pregnancy.

Antibiotics are commonly used in IBD. Amoxicillin-clavulanic acid can be safely used. Metronidazole can be used during pregnancy but preferably for short duration. Ciprofloxacin may affect growing cartilage but has not been demonstrated to have significant adverse effects as compared to controls. Sulfasalazine and 5-aminosalicylic acid (ASA) derivatives can be used during pregnancy and lactation as well as glucocorticoids. Folic acid supplementation should be routinely done. Dietary advice is necessary and iron and vitamin B12 levels should be monitored. Immunomodulatory drugs such as thiopurines (azathioprine and 6-mercaptopurine) have also been used during pregnancy with due consideration to risk–benefit ratio. Methotrexate is to be avoided since it is teratogenic. A patient on methotrexate should be advised contraception. Should she conceive during methotrexate therapy, medical termination of pregnancy should be discussed and offered. A patient should wait for 3–6 months after stopping methotrexate before attempting a pregnancy. There is insufficient data on the safety of small molecules such as tofacitinib, biological agents, and anti-TNF agents but available numbers in registries suggest no major problems.

A cesarean should be performed only for obstetric indications. However, patients with perineal involvement in Crohn disease should be delivered by a cesarean. Episiotomy should be avoided in perineal and rectal disease.

■ PSORIASIS

Psoriasis ameliorates in pregnancy in approximately half of the patients. In the remainder, it either remains static or worsens. Plaque type psoriasis generally improves while generalized pustular psoriasis or impetigo herpetiformis may worsen. Mild psoriasis generally does not impact the outcome of pregnancy. Severe cases may develop maternal preeclampsia and have an increase in perinatal morbidity and mortality. Impetigo herpetiformis can have high maternal and fetal morbidity and mortality and needs to be aggressively managed by a team approach. Impetigo herpetiformis generally occurs in late pregnancy and improves postpartum. Systemic corticosteroid is the mainstay of therapy in impetigo herpetiformis while cyclosporine A has also been used.

In mild cases of psoriasis, the doctor may reduce or stop medications. On the other hand, patients with moderate-to-severe disease should continue therapy, since otherwise the patient may deteriorate further. Moisturizer, emollient, topical mild or moderate corticosteroid application, and ultraviolet B rays are used in mild cases. PUVA (psoralens with ultraviolet B) has also been used. Systemic corticosteroids are reserved for severe cases.

Cyclosporine has been used in pregnancy. Much of the data on cyclosporine in pregnancy is derived from its use in transplant patients, where the dose used is much higher than that used in psoriasis. Though high doses have been associated with low birth weight and prematurity, there is no increase in teratogenic effect. It is not clear whether the fetal effects are due to the patient's condition or the drug.

Use of biologic agents such as infliximab and adalimumab (up to 20 weeks), etanercept (up to 30–32 weeks) is permitted as per EULAR guidelines,[11] while drugs such as ustekinumab have insufficient data for use in pregnancy. Monoclonal antibodies can cross the placenta with high concentration in the fetus. Fetal immunosuppression is a concern. However, data collected in registries suggest that they do not cause adverse effects.

■ GUILLAIN–BARRÉ SYNDROME

This autoimmune-mediated condition is extremely rare in pregnancy. The patient generally presents in the latter half of pregnancy or postpartum with pain, weakness, paralysis of the lower limbs which may progress to respiratory paralysis. In the initial stages, the pain and weakness maybe misdiagnosed as a symptom of normal pregnancy. It is often preceded 4–6 weeks prior by a bacterial or viral infection, either a flu-like illness or gastroenteritis. It is a rapidly evolving polyradiculoneuropathy. Generally, there is symmetric motor paralysis with or without sensory and autonomic involvement.

Diagnosis is confirmed by nerve conduction studies and lumbar puncture. Patients respond to intravenous Ig therapy and plasmapheresis.

Some may need ventilator support and a tracheostomy. Most patients recover.

Multiple Sclerosis

Multiple sclerosis is an autoimmune disease of the nervous system where myelin gets damaged. It maybe precipitated by a viral infection or have genetic predisposition. It affects women in the childbearing age group and therefore maybe seen during pregnancy. It may have several presentations: Fatigue, muscle weakness, muscle spasm, clonus, sensory abnormalities, paralysis, dysphagia, difficulty in talking (dysarthria), and incontinence of bladder and bowel. Some may have attention deficit, reduced concentration, and memory. The disease may remain static for a long time, while in others it may rapidly worsen leading to the patient being dependent for care. Diagnosis is by a careful neurological evaluation, MRI, and lumbar puncture. MRI may show typical plaques and scarring in the neural tissue.

Pregnancy does not generally affect multiple sclerosis. It may improve during pregnancy and flare postpartum. Urinary tract infection is more common.

Though multiple sclerosis is an incurable condition, drugs can help to delay progression. These include β-interferons, glatiramer acetate, monoclonal antibodies, dimethyl fumarate, and fingolimod. Physiotherapy, occupational therapy, cognitive therapy, speech therapy, and assistance devices such as walking sticks, walkers, and wheel chairs help. During pregnancy, the patient may find it more difficult to cope and need greater assistance than usual. If there is sensory affliction, the patient may find it difficult to appreciate the onset of labor.

■ CONCLUSION

Pregnancy has both short-term effects and long-term consequences for women. In an autoimmune disease such as RA, the disease ameliorates during pregnancy, while in others such as SLE, there may be a flare. During pregnancy, there is microtrafficking of maternal and fetal cells in both directions and this movement is responsible for the long-term effects of pregnancy.[7] This bi-directional trafficking results in persistence of fetal cells in maternal circulation and vice versa leading to a condition called microchimerism. This microchimerism persists for decades and has been implicated in some autoimmune diseases such as systemic sclerosis.[10]

In a woman with known autoimmune dysfunction, it is best to plan a pregnancy during the quiescent phase. A team approach involving experienced obstetricians, physicians, rheumatologists, endocrinologists, neonatologists, and other specialists as per the requirements of an individual patient would best serve the needs of the situation. Pregnant women are therapeutic orphans. Research on therapeutic options cannot be done easily during pregnancy because women and children are vulnerable subjects. This leads to lack of safety data on the use of most drugs during pregnancy and doctors are dependent on information collected in registries. A EULAR task force[11] found compatibility with pregnancy and lactation for the use of antimalarials, sulfasalazine, azathioprine, cyclosporine, tacrolimus, colchicine, intravenous Ig, and glucocorticoids. Methotrexate, mycophenolate mofetil, and cyclophosphamide are proven teratogens and need to be discontinued before conception. There is insufficient data on fetal safety of leflunomide, tofacitinib, abatacept, rituximab, belimumab, tocilizumab, ustekinumab, and anakinra and so they should be discontinued before a planned pregnancy. Among biologics, TNF inhibitors have been studied the most and appear to be reasonably safe for use in the first and second trimester. Thus, patients with autoimmune dysfunction can be managed reasonably with a wide variety of medications on which sufficient data is available.

REFERENCES

1. Stojan G, Petri M. Epidemiology of systemic lupus erythematosus: An update. Curr Opin Rheumatol. 2018;30(2):144-50.
2. Frances Rees, Doherty M, Grainge M, Lanyon P, Zhang W. The worldwide incidence and prevalence of systemic lupus erythematosus: a systematic review of epidemiological studies. Rheumatology. 2017;56(11):1945-61.
3. Clowse ME, Magder LS, Witter F, Petri M. The impact of increased lupus activity on obstetric outcomes. Arthritis Rheum. 2005;52(2):514-21.
4. Aringer M, Costenbader K, Daikh D, Brinks R, Mosca M, Ramsey-Goldman R, et al. 2019 European League Against Rheumatism /American College of Rheumatology Classification Criteria for Systemic Lupus Erythematosus. Arthritis Rheumatol. 2019;71(9):1400-12.
5. Bandoli G, Palmsten K, Forbess Smith CJ, Chambers CD. A review of systemic corticosteroid use in pregnancy and the risk of select pregnancy and birth outcomes. Rheum Dis Clin North Am. 2017;43(3):489-502.
6. Miyakis S, Lockshin MD, Atsumi T, Branch DW, Brey RL, Cervera R, et al. International consensus statement on an update of the classification criteria for definite antiphospholipid syndrome (APS). J Thromb Haemost. 2006;4(2):295-306.
7. Vora S, Shetty S, Salvi V, Satoskar P, Ghosh K. Thrombophilia and unexplained pregnancy loss in Indian patients. Natl Med J India. 2008;21(3):116-9.
8. Watson H, Davidson S, Keeling D. Guidelines on the diagnosis and management of heparin-induced thrombocytopenia: second edition. BJH. 2012;159(5):528-40.
9. Ghosh K, Shetty S, Vora S, Salvi V. Successful pregnancy outcome in women with bad obstetric history and recurrent fetal loss due to thrombophilia: Effect of unfractionated heparin and low—molecular weight heparin. Clin Appl Thromb Hemost. 2008;14(2):174-9.
10. Waldorf KMA, Nelson JL. Autoimmune disease during pregnancy and the microchimerism legacy of pregnancy. Immunol Invest. 2008;37(5):631-44.
11. Götestam Skorpen C, Hoeltzenbein M, Tincani A, Fischer-Betz R, Elefant E, Chambers C, et al. The EULAR points to consider for use of antirheumatic drugs before pregnancy, and during pregnancy and lactation. Ann Rheum Dis. 2016;75(5):795-810.

LONG QUESTIONS

1. A woman with SLE is planning to conceive. Discuss the plan of preconception evaluation and management.
2. Discuss the management of a pregnant patient with antiphospholipid syndrome.

SHORT QUESTIONS

1. How do you differentiate an SLE flare from preeclampsia?
2. Discuss the postpartum management of a patient with SLE.
3. What are the fetal risks due to maternal SLE?
4. Discuss Graves' disease in pregnancy.
5. Discuss the management of a pregnant lady with rheumatoid arthritis.

MULTIPLE CHOICE QUESTIONS

1. In a pregnant woman with SLE which of the following drugs cannot be used:
   a. Prednisolone   b. Methotrexate
   c. Low-dose aspirin d. HCQS
2. As per the revised Sapporo/Sydney criteria, lupus anticoagulant present in plasma should be detected on two or more occasions at least:
   a. 4 weeks apart   b. 6 weeks apart
   c. 10 weeks apart   d. 12 weeks apart
3. All of these are antiphospholipid autoantibodies, except:
   a. Lupus anticoagulant
   b. Anti-ds DNA
   c. ACL (IgG and IgM)
   d. Anti-B2 glycoprotein (IgG and IgM)
4. Autoimmune disorders that dramatically improve in pregnancy:
   a. SLE   b. Rheumatoid arthritis
   c. Myasthenia gravis d. IBD
5. If a patient with SLE is positive for Anti-Ro or Anti-La antibodies, the fetus is at risk of:
   a. Renal failure
   b. Congenital heart block
   c. Metabolic abnormalities
   d. Microcephaly
6. Bulging of eyeballs, goiter, red thickened patches on skin of feet or diarrhea are features of:
   a. Hashimoto thyroiditis b. Postpartum thyroiditis
   c. Graves' diseases   d. None of the above

Answers
1. b 2. d 3. b 4. b 5. b 6. c

5.10 RESPIRATORY CONDITIONS, THE LUNG AND PREGNANCY

Ravindra Rupwate, Sonal Kumta

INTRODUCTION

Pregnancy affects the respiratory system in profound ways. Respiratory disorders in pregnancy have some particular considerations due to the anatomical and physiological changes, symptomatology, and considerations regarding imaging and management. This chapter reviews the pregnancy-related changes, imaging modalities, and management of several respiratory disorders.

ANATOMIC CHANGES OF PREGNANCY AND IMPLICATIONS FOR PULMONARY FUNCTION TESTS

- Level of diaphragm (3–4 cm)
- Transverse diameter of the chest (2 cm)
- Subcostal angle (68–103°).

The changes in static pulmonary function tests are given in **Table 1**.[1]

PHYSIOLOGICAL AND FUNCTIONAL CHANGES IN PREGNANCY AND IMPLICATIONS FOR BLOOD GASES

- Capillary engorgement throughout the respiratory tract causes mucosal edema and hyperemia.
- Levels of progesterone, estrogen, prostaglandins, corticosteroids, and cyclic nucleotides are also higher during the course of pregnancy. The functional consequences of these changes are not very clear but higher progesterone levels are thought to be responsible for hyperventilation and rise in free cortisol levels can modify the course of steroid responsive respiratory illnesses.
- During pregnancy, minute ventilation rises markedly mainly due to increase in tidal volume. Thus, resting $PaCO_2$ decreases to 27–32 mm Hg. The pH is maintained by increased renal excretion of bicarbonates with a fall in bicarbonates level to 18–21 mEq/L. The alveolar to arterial oxygen gradient also rises due to airway closure at or near functional residual capacity (FRC) **(Table 2)**.

PHYSIOLOGICAL VARIATIONS IN RESPIRATORY PHYSIOLOGY IN PREGNANCY

Dyspnea of Pregnancy

About 60–70% of women complain of dyspnea during pregnancy; generally in the first and second trimesters. Dyspnea generally improves near term suggesting mechanical factors are not responsible for the same. Hormonal factors such as high progesterone levels play a major role. Dyspnea is probably related to increased minute ventilation. Oxygen consumption is increased during pregnancy and is 25–30% above the normal at term.

Obesity

With an increased body weight, there is increased oxygen consumption. This is related to the increase in carbohydrate utilization and increased value of respiratory quotient. In women with a normal body mass index (BMI), there is no change in oxygen saturation in pregnancy during sleep, but sleep apnea and hypopnea worsen in obese pregnant women.[3]

TABLE 1: Changes in static pulmonary function tests in pregnancy.

Decrease	Increase	No change
• Functional residual capacity (FRC) reduces by 10–25% • Mechanism—diaphragmatic elevation reduces the constituents of FRC, i.e., expiratory reserve volume (ERV) (8–40% reduced) and residual volume (RV) (7–22% reduced)	• Inspiratory capacity (IC) increases by 10% • Mechanism—increased muscle mobility of diaphragmatic and inspiratory muscles	• Vital capacity (VC) • Total lung capacity (TLC) • Flow rates • Airway resistance

TABLE 2: Arterial blood gas (ABG) changes in pregnancy (sea level).[2]

ABG parameter	Nonpregnant state	First trimester	Third trimester
PaO_2 (mm Hg)	96–100	105–106	101–106
$PaCO_2$ (mm Hg)	40 +/− 2	28–29	26–30
pH	7.40 +/− 0.02	7.42–7.46	7.43
HCO_3 (mEq/L)	22–28	18	17

Labor and Delivery

During labor, there is increase in minute ventilation and tachypnea with respiratory alkalosis. Alkalosis can reduce uterine blood flow due to vasoconstriction which can at times affect fetal oxygenation. Delivery by cesarean section (or any abdominal incision) gives rise to pain and this may cause shallow breathing with a possibility of basal, atelectasis with hypoxia. This is more commonly seen in obese patients. Physiotherapy and pain relief are useful in this situation. Lung function changes return to normal within few weeks after the delivery.

Altitude Variations

High altitude becomes physiologically relevant at altitudes >2,500 meters above the sea level. Beyond this, arterial oxygen saturation begins to fall exponentially. The following risks are increased at high altitudes.[4,5] The risks are greater when a pregnant woman moves to a high altitude in pregnancy. The risks are moderated to some extent in native highland dwellers.

- *Fetal growth restriction*: Threefold. Every 1,000 meters of elevation results in 120 g reduction in birthweights
- *Stillbirths*: Fourfold
- *Neonatal mortality*: 8–20-fold
- *Preeclampsia*: Threefold
- Higher incidence of congenital anomalies.

The effects of scuba diving on pregnancy are unclear. General recommendations are that women of childbearing age limit their dive to 60 feet and avoid strenuous dives, hypoventilation, and chilling.[6]

■ RESPIRATORY SYMPTOMS AND SIGNS

Besides dyspnea, no other symptom should be considered as physiological in pregnancy. Dyspnea should be considered physiological only if it is of static intensity (and not worsening), the onset is not acute and there is no orthopnea and paroxysmal nocturnal dyspnea. In all suspicious situations, dyspnea should be evaluated to avoid missing cardiorespiratory pathology.

Cough is usually a symptom of respiratory tract pathology. In pregnancy, there may be gastroesophageal reflux disease (GERD). This may lead to irritation of the pharynx and consequently, the woman may present with cough. This is not directly a respiratory pathology and a closer history of heartburn and retching elicits the problem.

On examination of the respiratory system, respiratory rate is increased. The baseline rate is 15–20 breaths per minute. A respiratory rate of 20–25 breaths per minute should be considered normal unless there are other features of respiratory distress. Breath sounds are generally not affected by any physiological changes in pregnancy. The presence of abnormal sounds or the absence of breath sounds should be considered as indications for further investigation.

■ DIAGNOSTIC IMAGING IN PREGNANCY

The most commonly used modality of investigation in respiratory conditions is a plain X-ray of the chest or a computed tomography (CT) scan. This poses questions in pregnancy regarding fetal radiation exposure. The scientific unit of measurement for radiation dose, commonly referred to as effective dose, is the millisievert (mSv). We are all naturally exposed to radiation and according to recent estimates, the average person receives an effective dose of about 3 mSv per year from naturally occurring radioactive materials and cosmic radiation from outer space. Radiation, is therefore, naturally occurring and not uniformly dangerous. The risk is dose-dependent. A single X-ray of the chest has very little radiation exposure, especially if the abdomen of the pregnant woman is shielded and the potential risk to the fetus is miniscule. To explain it in simple terms, we can compare the radiation exposure from one chest X-ray as equivalent to the amount of radiation exposure from our natural surroundings in 10 days. In a pregnant patient, where both the baby and mother are being imaged, other imaging modalities such as ultrasound or magnetic resonance imaging (MRI), which do not involve radiation, are sometimes used. However, when ultrasound or MRI does not give the answers, or there is a time constraint, CT may be the best imaging option.

Table 3 gives the comparison of effective radiation dose with background radiation exposure for several radiological procedures.

■ INTERVENTIONAL CHEST PROCEDURES IN PREGNANCY

In certain conditions, diagnosis and therapy of respiratory pathology will require interventional procedures. Their indications vary according to the pathology and presentation. Some considerations regarding pregnancy are mentioned here.

There are no data from well-designed prospective trials to guide recommendations for interventional pulmonary procedures in pregnancy. Clinicians who perform pulmonary interventions should have good knowledge of physiologic and mechanical changes that occur in pregnancy and the risks associated with medicines and tools used during the procedure.

Intubation

Incidence of failed intubations in obstetric patients is eight times higher and related to hormone-mediated increase in pulmonary edema.[8] Also caliber of large airways changes as lung volume decreases in later pregnancy which affects airway resistance.

Thoracentesis/Pleural Space Interventions

Use of bedside ultrasound to evaluate pleural effusions and guide thoracentesis is standard in many institutions. It is safe,

TABLE 3: Radiological imaging and radiation risk to the fetus.[7]

Procedure	Approximate effective radiation dose	Comparable natural background radiation	Additional lifetime risk of fetal cancer from radiation
Radiography—chest	0.1 mSv	10 days	Minimal
CT—chest	7 mSv	2 years	Low
CT—angiography	12 mSv	4 years	Low
X-ray of the spine	1.5 mSv	6 months	Very low
CT—spine	6 mSv	2 years	Low
X-ray of the upper GI tract	6 mSv	2 years	Low
X-ray of the lower GI tract	8 mSv	3 years	Low
CT—abdomen and pelvis	10 mSv	3 years	Low
CT—abdomen and pelvis, repeated with and without contrast	20 mSv	7 years	Moderate

(CT: computed tomography; GI: gastrointestinal)

portable, and can provide diagnosis. This does not expose the operator and the patient to radiation. When ultrasound is used in pregnancy (even for nonobstetric imaging), the rules and regulations regarding the PCPNDT (Pre-Conception and Pre-Natal Diagnostic Techniques) Act should be followed.

Placement of intercostal drains for large recurrent pleural effusions, pneumothorax can be safely performed by experienced hands.

Thoracoscopy with biopsy or pleurodesis is quiet safe in pregnancy. Pleurodesis with talc should be avoided due to concern of acute lung injury. Bleomycin and tetracycline for chemical pleurodesis are avoided in pregnancy due to fetal risk.

Bronchoscopy

It is not common to need bronchoscopy in pregnancy. Flexible fiberoptic bronchoscopy (FOB) can be safely performed in pregnancy. If possible, the procedure should be deferred to the second trimester. In case it is needed, the following principles should be followed:
- Position pregnant patient in left pelvic tilt or left lateral position to avoid inferior vena cava (IVC) or aortic compression.
- Use lowest effective dose of sedative with best safety profile.
- Maintain saturation >95% with supplemental oxygen.
- Continuous monitoring of blood pressure, pulse oximetry, and cardiac monitoring is recommended.
- Presence of fetal heart sound should be confirmed before sedation and after the procedure.
- Fluoroscopy is not recommended but when used care should be taken to minimize radiation to mother and fetus, especially during transbronchial biopsy.
- When required bipolar electrocautery is preferred over monopolar cautery. The grounding pad should be placed to minimize the flow of electrical current through the amniotic fluid.
- Obstetric support should be available in the event of pregnancy-related complication.

PREGNANCY AND TUBERCULOSIS

Pregnant women with tuberculosis (TB) poses therapeutic problem and requires good collaboration with chest physician, obstetrician, and the neonatologist. Untreated pulmonary TB in pregnancy is a definite risk for transmission of disease to the newborn. All physicians should be aware of limitations in diagnosis of TB in pregnancy, safety of anti-TB drugs, and need for prophylaxis. Today the combination of HIV (human immunodeficiency virus), resistant TB, and pregnancy is a new challenge for all.

Tuberculosis may present initially with symptoms related to normal pregnancy such as dyspnea, fatigue, and lack of energy. Pregnancy does not alter the mode of onset or presentation of initial symptoms. Cough, weight loss (absence of weight gain), fever, and hemoptysis are usual symptoms. Extrapulmonary TB is observed in approximately 20% cases and presents as lymphadenopathy or abdominal pain. Fetal growth restriction is common.

Tachycardias, anemia, raised erythrocyte sedimentation rate (ESR), and low serum albumin are seen physiologically in pregnancy and are not helpful in making a diagnosis. With history of exposure and symptoms, tuberculin skin test (TT) should be carried out. Sputum examination in suspected cases is important. A simple chest X-ray should be carried out with abdominal shield as indicated. The following diagnostic principles should be borne in mind:
- If TT is >10 mm induration, a chest X-ray should be obtained in symptomatic patient with abdominal shielding. In an asymptomatic patient, chest X-ray should be delayed until the 12th week of pregnancy.
- A chest X-ray is indicated if two sputum smears are negative and symptoms persist in spite of 2 weeks of antibiotic course.

- Suggestive radiographs with clinical symptoms and signs should be treated as sputum negative disease.

Diagnosis and treatment of extrapulmonary TB may be delayed in pregnancy. Routine hematological tests with specific investigations for the site of affected area are required for confirming the diagnosis.

The effects of TB on pregnancy are outlined here.
- TB has no adverse effect on pregnancy.
- Premature labor may occur as a consequence of general debility than TB.
- The baby is generally healthy. Congenital TB is a rare complication of maternal TB.
- Fetal infection may be hematogenous spread by the umbilical vein or more often by aerosol inhalation. Aspiration of infected amniotic fluid into lungs or ingestion into the gut also occurs.
- Prolonged labor should be avoided. The second stage of labor should be shortened by an instrumental delivery.
- Neonate should preferably be isolated from the infected mother and prophylactic isoniazid (INH) considered.
- Women with even spinal or sacroiliac TB under cover of antituberculous drugs can go through labor.

All first-line drugs except streptomycin may be safely used during pregnancy and lactation. Pyridoxine supplementation is essential in pregnant women receiving INH. Safety profile of second-line drugs has not been confirmed but they have been used with good maternal and fetal outcome. These drugs must be individualized after careful discussion of possible teratogenic effects. If the mother desires to avoid all risks related to teratogenicity and if the gestational age permits, termination of pregnancy may be considered.

Isoniazid prophylaxis is indicated for the conditions outlined in **Table 4**.

There is consensus that breastfeeding should not be discouraged. Under Revised National Tuberculosis Control Programme (RNTCP) breastfeeding is recommended, regardless of mother's disease status.[9]

Rifampicin diminishes reliability of oral contraceptives (induces P-450 enzyme), thus alternative contraception should be considered for postpartum women who require anti-TB drugs.

Coexisting HIV infection is known to augment progression of TB and worsens immunosuppression. Common infections in HIV-positive mother are *Pneumocystis jirovecii* (PCP) and *Mycobacterium tuberculosis*. Extrapulmonary TB, mediastinal/retroperitoneal adenopathy, and pleural effusions are common. Management of TB and HIV is complicated due to drug interactions, e.g., rifampicin and protease inhibitor antiretroviral drugs, and requires specialist input.

ASTHMA IN PREGNANCY

Asthma is one of the most common medical condition affecting women in the reproductive age. The course of asthma during pregnancy is variable; one-third of patients improve, one-third remain stable, and one-third worsen.[10] Exacerbations are seen most commonly between 24 and 36 weeks of gestation. Only 10% of women experience asthma exacerbation during labor and delivery. The disease severity tends to revert by 3 months' postpartum. Asthma is generally expected to follow a similar course during successive pregnancies.

A systematic review of the literature has revealed that asthma exacerbations during pregnancy which require medical intervention occur in about 20% of women, with approximately 6% of women being admitted to the hospital. These exacerbations occur primarily in the late second trimester and are either triggered by viral infection or nonadherence to inhaled corticosteroid medication. Severe exacerbations during pregnancy are a significant risk factor for a low birth weight baby and inhaled corticosteroid use may reduce the risk.[10]

Clinical features of asthma during pregnancy are the same as those in the nonpregnant patient and presents with cough, breathlessness, and wheezing with nocturnal exacerbation. Objective assessment with pulmonary function test is essential to assess the presence of airflow obstruction.

Uncontrolled asthma is associated with many maternal and fetal complications, including hyperemesis, hypertension, preeclampsia, fetal growth retardation, preterm birth, increased perinatal mortality and neonatal hypoxia, and postpartum hemorrhage.

When interpreting arterial blood gases in pregnancy, it should be remembered that the progesterone-driven increase in mechanical ventilation (MV) may lead to relative hypocapnia and a respiratory alkalosis (*see* **Table 2**).

The main aspects of long-term therapy for asthma are outlined here.[11,12]
- Avoidance and control of *asthma triggers* such as upper respiratory tract infection, sinusitis, exercise, nonsteroidal anti-inflammatory agents, irritants (e.g., tobacco smoke, chemical fumes, and humidity) and emotional disturbances. Paying close attention to asthma triggers might improve symptom control, and pregnant patients with asthma might require less medication.

TABLE 4: Indications for isoniazid (INH) prophylaxis.

Mother	Infant of mother with active tuberculosis (needs evaluation with chest X-ray, AFB in sputum/gastric lavage)
Recent tuberculin conversion	No evidence of active disease—INH for 3 months
Close contact with a household contact with active untreated TB	TT positive—INH for 6 months
Immunocompromised individual (HIV and cancer)	Mother MDR/XDR—no role of INH

(AFB: acid-fast bacilli; HIV: human immunodeficiency virus; MDR: multidrug resistance; TB: tuberculosis; XDR: extensively drug-resistant)

- Strongly encourage *smoking cessation* in patients with asthma as for any pregnant patient.
- *Gastroesophageal reflux* is commonly recognized as an asthma trigger, and approximately one-third of pregnant women have symptomatic reflux. Initial therapy might consist of small meals and raising the head of the bed by 6 inches. Some patients might require antacids or H2-receptor-blocking medications.
- *Medications* during pregnancy:[13]
  - While a natural reluctance exists to prescribe and take drug therapy in pregnancy, poorly controlled asthma is potentially more dangerous for the fetus than medication.
  - A large part of management is education of the woman and her family to take and continue medications to prevent exacerbations. Medications are added in a sequential fashion, with few differences from the nonpregnant patient. A stepped approach to asthma therapy generally is used.
  - In outpatient asthma management, β-2 agonists are used for symptomatic benefit. Inhaled corticosteroids remain the mainstay of therapy for asthma control. Initiate treatment with the lowest possible dose of inhaled steroids; the dose can be increased further as required by symptomatic and objective asthma assessment.
  - Long-acting β-2 agonists, such as salmeterol or formoterol, might be used in symptomatic patients on adequate corticosteroid therapy. The leukotriene antagonists are the newest agents available for asthma management. Their exact role in the treatment of asthma during pregnancy is unclear. No widespread experience has been gained with the use of these agents in pregnant patients. Theophylline might be used as a third-line agent after β-agonist therapy and inhaled steroids. Extensive experience has been gained with the use of theophylline during pregnancy, and it does not appear to cause developmental risk.

Managing Acute Asthma Exacerbation in Pregnancy in an Emergency

- Acute exacerbations that necessitate emergency department visits typically require a course of systemic corticosteroids. Oxygen should be used liberally, and the oxygen saturation should be maintained at or above 95% to ensure fetal well-being. A β-agonist with or without ipratropium should be given via a metered-dose inhaler with a spacer or in nebulized form. Theophylline has limited use in acute exacerbations.
- In severe cases, intravenous (IV) β-2 agonist, aminophylline, or magnesium sulfate can be tried.
- Continuous fetal monitoring is recommended for acute severe asthma.
- Pregnant women may be more difficult to intubate due to anatomical factors.
- Early referral to chest and critical care services is recommended to avoid fetal risk.

Management of Asthma during Labor

- Acute attacks of asthma are very rare in labor, perhaps due to endogenous steroid production.
- In women receiving steroid tablets, there is a theoretical risk of maternal hypothalamic–pituitary–adrenal axis suppression. Women receiving steroid tablets at a dose exceeding prednisolone 7.5 mg/day for >2 weeks prior to delivery should receive parenteral hydrocortisone 100 mg 6–8 hourly during labor.
- Women with asthma may safely use all forms of usual labor analgesia.
- In the absence of acute severe asthma, reserve cesarean section for the usual obstetric indications.
- If anesthesia is required, regional blockade is preferable to general anesthesia in women with asthma.
- Prostaglandin F2a (carboprost) used to treat postpartum hemorrhage due to uterine atony may cause bronchospasm and should be avoided.

Drug Therapy in Breastfeeding Mothers

The medicines used to treat asthma, including steroid tablets, have been shown in early studies to be safe to use in nursing mothers. <1% of the maternal dose of theophylline is excreted into breast milk. Prednisolone is secreted in breast milk, but milk concentrations of prednisolone are only 5–25% of those in serum. Encourage women with asthma for breastfeeding.

■ PNEUMONIA IN PREGNANCY

Community acquired pneumonia (CAP) is the most common cause of fatal nonobstetric infection in pregnancy.[14] The incidence varies from 0.4 to 1.47 per 1,000 pregnancies from different studies.[15,16] **Table 5** outlines the alterations in pregnancy that lead to an increased incidence of pneumonia and higher risk of severity of pneumonia in pregnancy.

Clinical findings of pneumonia are same as in nonpregnant state and include fever, cough with rusty sputum, pleuritic chest pain, chills and rigors, and breathlessness. Diagnostic investigations include chest X-ray with abdominal shield, routine blood count with biochemistry, C-reactive protein (CRP), pulse oximetry, arterial blood gas (ABG), blood culture (two sets), and sputum culture. In severe cases, serological testing for atypical pneumonia is recommended.

The bacteriology of pneumonia in pregnancy is described in **Table 6**.

Supportive treatment with hydration, antipyretic, and supplemental oxygen is important. Physiotherapy is an important tool in rehabilitation and recovery. The mainstay of

TABLE 5: Mechanisms increasing risk and severity of pneumonia in pregnancy.

Maternal physiologic changes	Coexisting conditions	Immunological
Increase in oxygen consumption	Anemia	Reduced lymphocyte proliferation response
Increase in lung water	Asthma	Diminished cell-mediated cytotoxicity
Elevation of diaphragm	Recent viral respiratory infection (influenza)	Reduced number of helper T cells
Aspiration more likely in labor and delivery especially with general anesthesia	HIV infection, diabetes, and immunosuppression	Reduced lymphokine response to alloantigens

(HIV: human immunodeficiency virus)

TABLE 6: Causative organisms for pneumonia in pregnancy.

Typical community-acquired pneumonia	Atypical community-acquired pneumonia	Viral	Hospital acquired	Immunocompromised pregnant women
Streptococcus pneumoniae 40%	Chlamydophila	Influenza A	Staphylococcus aureus (including MRSA)	Pneumocystis jirovecii
Haemophilus influenzae	Mycoplasma	COVID-19	Anaerobes, gram-negative enterococci when there has been aspiration and prolonged ventilation	Fungi: coccidioidomycosis
	Legionella	Varicella	Pseudomonas aeruginosa (with bronchiectasis and CF)	

(CF: cystic fibrosis; MRSA: methicillin-resistant Staphylococcus aureus)

the treatment is antimicrobials. The principles of antimicrobial therapy for pneumonia in pregnancy are as follows:[17]

- Antimicrobial therapy is empirical and directed for *Streptococcus pneumoniae, Haemophilus influenza*, and atypical pathogens. Penicillins, cephalosporins, and erythromycin are all safe and potentially effective for these pathogens. Fluoroquinolones are avoided during pregnancy due to fetal malformations and arthropathy. Clarithromycin and tetracyclines are not recommended in pregnancy.
- Hospitalized patients should receive IV macrolides (azithromycin/erythromycin) and ceftriaxone or cefotaxime. Patients with underlying lung disease [bronchiectasis/cystic fibrosis (CF)] should be covered with anti-pseudomonal β-lactam (imipenem, meropenem, or piperacillin-tazobactam) with aminoglycosides and a macrolide.
- MRSA should be suspected with severe CAP after influenza and vancomycin or linezolid should be used after consultation with patient.

Pneumonia-complicating HIV infection—bacterial respiratory infections are most common respiratory complication in HIV infection. Low CD4 count (<200) predisposes to bacterial pneumonia and PCP infection which can be fatal in 50% patients. Women with PCP infection should receive trimethoprim-sulfa (TMP-SMX) with steroids. Patients should be monitored for preterm labor. Due to teratogenic effect of TMP-SMX in the first trimester, pentamidine in aerosolized form is preferred due to its lack of systemic absorption.[17]

Influenza in Pregnancy

Pregnant women are at higher risk of complications due to the influenza than the general population. The risk of serious outcomes is increased by 5–7-fold. This is particularly true when the infective strain is the H1N1 virus. The usual presenting features are as for the general population. The incubation period is 8 days. Though most women will have a mild course, pregnancy is an indication to increase surveillance and consider hospitalization when influenza is detected in pregnancy. There may be superadded bacterial infection. Diagnosis is made by nasopharyngeal swab. The treatment of choice for influenza in pregnancy is oseltamivir (75 mg twice daily for 5 days) or zanamivir (25 mg inhalations twice daily for 5 days). Oseltamivir and zanamivir are both pregnancy category C drugs, but no adverse events have been reported to date among women who received these agents during pregnancy. Influenza vaccination is advocated in pregnancy.

COVID-19 in Pregnancy

The world has entered a new era with the COVID pandemic. With the emergence of new variants, knowledge on the behavior and effects of the virus in pregnant women has evolved. Pregnancy acts as comorbidity and there is an increased risk of needing critical care, death, and poor perinatal outcomes in pregnant women infected with COVID in pregnancy as compared to the general population. This is especially true if infection occurs in labor or late in pregnancy. The usual clinical features are fever, cough, breathlessness, and myalgia. Less common presentations are loss of sense of smell and taste and gastrointestinal features. Diagnosis is made by nasopharyngeal swab. There is no particular drug that has been consistently been shown to improve outcomes in COVID. Various drugs have been used at different stages of the disease including remdesivir and steroids. Their use in pregnancy should be individualized and specifically consented. COVID vaccination is advocated in pregnancy and breastfeeding.

INFILTRATIVE LUNG DISEASES IN PREGNANCY

Infiltrative lung diseases (ILDs) are a condition usually seen at an advanced age. They are not commonly associated with pregnancy. However, with the use of assisted reproduction, there has been a demographic shift in the pregnant population which makes these conditions important. Pregnancy may affect diagnosis, management, and outcome of ILD.

Some common ILDs seen in pregnancy and their important features are outlined in **Table 7**.

PREGNANCY AND PULMONARY HYPERTENSION

Pulmonary arterial hypertension (PAH) is a rare disorder that can affect women of childbearing age. Several studies have demonstrated mortality as high as 60% in women with PAH who undergo pregnancy.[21] As such, women should be advised to avoid pregnancy and there should be a consideration to terminate pregnancy. Sildenafil has been used with some success in pregnant women with PAH.

ACUTE LUNG CONDITIONS IN PREGNANCY

Pulmonary Edema in Preeclampsia

Preeclampsia is characterized by hypertension, hypoalbuminemia, edema of the peripheries, renal dysfunction, and cardiac (systolic and diastolic) dysfunction, all of which are mechanisms to induce pulmonary edema. Overzealous IV infusion and multiple blood and/or blood productions transfusion in the postpartum period can exacerbate it. Clinically tachypnea, respiratory distress with fall in saturation, crackles over lung bases, and radiological features of pulmonary edema are seen. Treatment consists of fluid restriction, oxygen, diuretics, and in severe cases, ventilatory support. Furosemide should be given in doses ranging from 40 to 120 mg as an initial bolus followed by further doses as per the clinical response. Vasopressor support is rarely needed.

Acute Respiratory Distress Syndrome in Pregnancy

Pregnancy-specific acute respiratory distress syndrome (ARDS) in our country is mostly associated with eclampsia. ARDS also results from amniotic embolism. ARDS is also seen in septic abortions or sepsis after full-term delivery. Aspiration of gastric content during labor is an important cause of aspiration pneumonia and ARDS. Clinical features are same as in nonpregnant state and management with ventilatory support is beneficial. Alkalosis during ventilator support should be avoided as it reduces placental blood flow.[22]

Tocolytic Pulmonary Edema

Premature labor occurs in approximately 7–10% deliveries. Noncardiogenic pulmonary edema has been reported with most tocolytic agents, i.e., magnesium sulfate, terbutaline, and ritodrine.[23] The incidence is higher in the presence of coexisting maternal infections, multiple gestations, hydramnios, and

TABLE 7: Infiltrative lung diseases in pregnancy.

Condition	Clinical notes	Perinatal outcomes	Therapy notes
Rheumatoid arthritis[18,19]	Improves in 70% of women in second/third trimester	Fetal risk is not increased	
Systemic lupus erythematosus (SLE)[20]	High risk of postpartum pneumonia in women with renal involvement with SLE	Fetal growth restriction is commonly seen	Wait for 6 months of stable disease to undertake pregnancy
Systemic sclerosis	Renal crisis and hypertension and high risk of maternal mortality	High risk of stillbirths and neonatal death	Pregnancy considered to be contraindicated
Sarcoidosis	Hormone-induced stability or improvement is common. Postpartum exacerbation after 3–6 months are common		Patients with advanced respiratory insufficiency, pulmonary hypertension, uncontrolled neurosarcoidosis, or myocardial sarcoidosis should be advised to avoid pregnancy
Dermatomyositis or polymyositis	Poor outcomes if there are flares in early pregnancy	Considerable fetal morbidity and mortality	Avoid general anesthesia
Pulmonary LAM (lymphangioleiomyomatosis)	Rare condition that accelerates due to hormone exposure. Pneumothorax and chylous pleural effusion are common		
Idiopathic pulmonary fibrosis	Usually, a disease of later life with high maternal mortality		Pregnancy is contraindicated
Drug-induced lung disease	Rarely diagnosed. Some common drugs (nitrofurantoin, ampicillin, and carbamazepine) can induce interstitial or eosinophilic pneumonia.		

hypertension. Steroids administered to these subjects worsen the problem further. Treatment includes cessation of tocolytic agents, antibiotics if indicated, aggressive support with diuretics and MV in select groups.

Peripartum Cardiomyopathy

Peripartum cardiomyopathy presents with dyspnea before, during, or after delivery. It is advisable to exclude pre-existing cardiac illnesses such as valvular heart disease. Tachycardia, orthopnea, dry cough, and abdominal discomforts are major symptoms. Raised jugular venous pressure (JVP), palpable tender liver, edema of the feet, crackles at lung bases, loud second heart sound, systolic murmur of functional mitral incompetence, and diastolic third heart sound at apex are the clinical findings. Chest radiograph shows enlarged heart with pulmonary edema and two-dimensional (2D) echocardiography is diagnostic. Judicial use of diuretics, low molecular weight heparin (LMWH), and inotropic support with pump dysfunction is mainstay for management. Angiotensin-converting enzyme (ACE) inhibitors are avoided in pregnancy as they cause fetal renal dysfunction. Over 50% patients gradually improve in next 6 months. Further pregnancy may cause recurrence of cardiomyopathy.

Pulmonary Thromboembolic Disease

The risk of thromboembolic disease is most often seen in postpartum period. The incidence of pregnancy-related deep vein thrombosis is 1.2% and pulmonary embolism (PE) is 0.2–0.4%, reasons being:
- Hypercoagulable state of blood
- Hormone related venous stasis in lower limbs
- Pressure effect of gravid uterus on IVC with reduced blood flow.

Diagnosis of DVT is difficult. Tests such as venography, radiolabeled fibrinogen can pose radiation risk to fetus. D-dimer may be useful but they can rise to 50% in the last trimester. Warfarin crosses placenta and can cause fetal hemorrhage and congenital abnormalities.

Low molecular weight heparin does not cross placental barrier, is effective, and does not need monitoring for clotting parameters. Women with previous history of thromboembolic disease should receive heparin prophylaxis during pregnancy.

Amniotic Fluid Embolism

Amniotic fluid embolism is a rare (1 case per 8,000–80,000 births) but potentially catastrophic complication, with a mortality rate of 10–80%.[24] This usually occurs with labor and delivery but can be associated with uterine manipulation, uterine trauma, and the early postpartum period. Amniotic fluid containing particulate cellular elements enters the vascular circulation through endocervical veins or uterine tears, obstructs the pulmonary vessels, and causes vascular spasms, resulting in pulmonary hypertension. Acute left ventricular failure might occur, probably due to humoral events mediated by cytokines. Clinical presentation usually involves a sudden onset of severe dyspnea, hypoxemia, and cardiovascular collapse. Less common presentations are hemorrhage caused by disseminated intravascular coagulation and fetal distress. The diagnosis of amniotic fluid embolism is usually based on observing the typical clinical picture. Treatment involves routine resuscitative and supportive measures with prompt attention to adequate oxygenation, ventilation, and inotropic support. No specific therapy has been shown to be effective, although corticosteroids have been suggested. Coagulation abnormalities if associated need correction.

Gestation Trophoblastic Disease

Pulmonary hypertension and pulmonary edema can complicate benign hydatidiform pregnancy due to trophoblastic PE. This commonly occurs during evacuation of the uterus, and the incidence of pulmonary complications is higher in later gestations. Molar pregnancy can also be associated with the development of choriocarcinoma, which commonly produces multiple discrete pulmonary metastases and occasional pleural effusions.

■ REFERENCES

1. Alaily AB, Caroll KB. Pulmonary ventilation in pregnancy. Br J Obstet Gynaecol. 1978;85(7):518-24.
2. Templeton A, Kelman GR. Maternal blood–gases, (PAo2-Pao2), physiological shunt and VD/VT in normal pregnancy. Br J Anaesth. 1976:48(10):1001-4.
3. Brownell LG, West P, Kryger MH. Breathing during sleep in normal pregnant women. Am Rev Respir Dis. 1986;133(1):38-41.
4. Jensen GM, Moore LG. The effect of high altitude and other risk factors on birthweight: independent or interactive effects? Am J Public Health. 1997;87(6):1003-7.
5. Palmer SK, Moore LG, Young D, Cregger B, Berman JC, Zamudio S. Altered blood pressure course during normal pregnancy and increased preeclampsia at high altitude (3100 meters) in Colorado. Am J Obstet Gynecol. 1999;180(5):1161-8.
6. Newhall JF. Scuba diving during pregnancy: a brief review. Am J Obstet Gynecol. 1981;140(8):893-4.
7. McCollough CH, Schueler BA, Atwell TD, Braun NN, Regner DM, Brown DL, et al. Radiation exposure and pregnancy: when should we be concerned? Radiographics. 2007;27(4):909-17; discussion 917-908.
8. Kuczkowski KM, Reisner LS, Benumof JL. Airway problems and new solutions for the obstetric patient. J Clin Anaesth. 2003;15(7):552-63.
9. Central TB Division Managing the Revised National Tuberculosis Control Programme in your area-A training course: Modules 1-4, New Delhi: 2001:1.
10. Madappa T, Sharma. S. (2019). Pulmonary disease and pregnancy. [online] Available from: http://emedicine.medscape.com. [Last accessed October 2021].
11. Cockcroft DW. Treatment of asthma during pregnancy. Ann Allergy Asthma Immunol. 2005;95(3):213-4.

12. Liccardi G, Cazzola M, Canonica GW, D'Amato M, D'Amato G, Passalacqua G. General strategy for the management of bronchial asthma in pregnancy. Respir Med. 2003;97(7):778-89.
13. National Asthma Education and Prevention Program. Managing asthma during pregnancy: recommendations for pharmacologic treatment. National Guideline Clearinghouse. 2005.
14. Rodrigues JM, Niederman MS. Pneumonia complicating pregnancy. Clin Chest Med 1992;13(4):679-91.
15. Benedetti TJ, Valle R, Ledger WJ. Antepartum pneumonia in pregnancy. Am J Obstet Gynecol. 1982;144(4):413-7.
16. Jin Y, Carriere KC, Marrie TJ, Predy G, Johnson DH. The effects of community acquired pneumonia during pregnancy ending in a live birth. Am J Obstet Gynecol. 2003;188(3):800-6.
17. Khan S, Niederman MS. Pneumonia in the pregnant patient. In: Rosene-Montela K, Bourjeily G, (eds). Pulmonary problems in pregnancy. New York: Humana Press; 2009. p. 177-96.
18. Nelson JL, Ostensen M. Pregnancy and rheumatoid arthritis. Rheum Dis Clin North Am. 1997;23(1):195-212.
19. Spector TD, Silman AJ. Is poor pregnancy outcome is a risk factor in rheumatoid arthritis? Ann Rheum Dis. 1990;49(1):12-4.
20. Hopkins PM. Lupus pregnancy center 1987 to 1996. Rheum Dis Clin North Am. 1997;23(1):1-13.
21. Mccaffrey R, Dunn L. Primary pulmonary hypertension in pregnancy. Obstet Gynecol Suv. 1964;19:567.
22. Bandi VD. Acute lung injury and acute respiratory distress syndrome in pregnancy. Crit Care Clin. 2004;20(4):577-607.
23. Wolff F, Fischer JH. Aspects of pathophysiology of maternal lung edema during tocolytic therapy. J Perinat Med. 1988;16(1):50-1.
24. Moore J. Amniotic fluid embolism. Crit Care Med. 2005;33(10 suppl):S279-85.

LONG QUESTIONS

1. Discuss the physiological variations in respiratory physiology in pregnancy with relation to maternal weight, altitude of stay, and labor and delivery.
2. Discuss the dilemmas in management of pregnant women with tuberculosis. What is the effect of pregnancy on tuberculosis and vice versa?
3. What are the mechanisms that increase the probability and severity of pneumonia in pregnancy? What are the usual causative agents? Discuss the principles of antimicrobial therapy for pneumonia in pregnancy.

SHORT QUESTIONS

1. What are the features of physiological dyspnea and how should it be distinguished from possible pathological conditions?
2. What is the mechanism of physiological dyspnea in pregnancy?
3. Enumerate the principles of safe bronchoscopy in pregnancy.
4. What are the main principles of medical therapy of asthma in pregnancy?
5. How should an acute exacerbation of asthma be managed in pregnancy?
6. What is tocolytic pulmonary edema? How should it be prevented and managed?

MULTIPLE CHOICE QUESTIONS

1. The following parameter of pulmonary function test is increased in pregnancy:
    a. Inspiratory capacity
    b. Functional residual capacity
    c. Expiratory reserve volume
    d. Residual volume
2. The following parameter of pulmonary function test is decreased in pregnancy:
    a. Inspiratory capacity
    b. Vital capacity
    c. Airway resistance
    d. Expiratory reserve volume
3. The following statement is true about physiological changes in pregnancy:
    a. Minute ventilation reduces
    b. Resting $PaCO_2$ decreases to 27–32 mm Hg
    c. pH is maintained by decreased renal excretion of bicarbonates
    d. Capillary perfusion is reduced
4. The following conditions are more common in high altitude dwellers in pregnancy, except:
    a. Preeclampsia   b. Fetal growth restriction
    c. Anemia   d. Congenital anomalies
5. The following are pathological findings in pregnancy, except:
    a. Respiratory rate of 23 per minute
    b. Basal rales
    c. Ronchi
    d. Absent breath sounds on the left side
6. The following is true about diagnostic imaging in pregnancy for pulmonary pathology:
    a. Ultrasound and MRI involve high doses of radiation
    b. One plain X-ray of the chest results in approximate radiation dose of 20 mSv
    c. Radiation related fetal risks are dose-dependent
    d. The fetus is most vulnerable to radiation effects in the second trimester
7. The following is true about invasive pulmonary procedures in pregnancy:
    a. Intubation is easier in obstetric patients
    b. Bleomycin and tetracycline are routinely used for chemical pleurodesis in pregnancy
    c. Fluoroscopy is recommended along with bronchoscopy
    d. Pregnant women should have bronchoscopy with the table in left pelvic tilt
8. The following is true about tuberculosis in pregnancy:
    a. Congenital tuberculosis affects 50% of neonates
    b. Streptomycin is contraindicated in pregnancy
    c. Breastfeeding is contraindicated
    d. Women should be delivered by cesarean section

9. The following are correct indications for INH prophylaxis, except:
   a. Mother—recent tuberculin conversion
   b. Mother—immunocompromised individual (HIV and cancer)
   c. Neonate of mother who is tuberculin test positive with active tuberculosis
   d. Neonate of mother with MDR/XDR TB
10. The following is true about asthma in pregnancy:
    a. Viral infection is a common trigger
    b. Asthma usually worsens in pregnancy
    c. Most women who have asthma will have an exacerbation in labor
    d. Uncontrolled asthma rarely causes fetal problems
11. The following infective agents are correctly matched for pneumonias in pregnancy, except:
    a. Typical community acquired pneumonia—S. pneumoniae
    b. Atypical community acquired pneumonia—coccidioidomycosis
    c. Hospital acquired—S. aureus
    d. Immunocompromised pregnant women—P. jirovecii

Answers
1. a 2. d 3. b 4. c 5. a 6. c
7. d 8. b 9. d 10. a 11. b

5.11 NEUROLOGICAL CONDITIONS

Jyoti Bindal

INTRODUCTION

Neurological disorders in pregnancy can be pregnancy related or can be caused by exacerbation of a pre-existing neurological condition or sometimes may even be detected for the first time during pregnancy in which it might be an incidental finding. The diagnosis and management of neurological disorders in pregnancy are always challenging tasks due to varied symptomatology and risks to fetus. The evaluation and management should be performed in stepwise fashion and requires multidisciplinary approach.

Neurological disorders in pregnancy includes:[1]
- Epilepsy and seizure disorders
- Other cerebrovascular disorders:
  - Ischemic stroke
  - Cerebral venous thrombosis
  - Subarachnoid hemorrhage
  - Hydrocephalous
  - Cerebral tumors
  - Migraine headache
  - Multiple sclerosis
  - Spinal cord disorders
  - Peripheral neuropathies
  - Disorders of cranial nerves
  - Guillain-Barré syndrome.

SEIZURE DISORDERS

The incidence of epilepsy is approximately 0.15% of all pregnancies.[2]

Definition

A seizure is defined as paroxysmal disorder of central nervous system (CNS) characterized by an abnormal neuronal discharge with or without loss of consciousness.[3]

Classification

Focal

Focal seizures have origin in one area in the brain and affect a corresponding area of neurological function. They can result from tumor, trauma, abscess, or perinatal factors.

Generalized

They involve both cerebral hemispheres and are usually preceded by an aura before an abrupt loss of consciousness. They are generalized tonic clonic in type, loss of consciousness occurs which is followed by tonic contractions of muscles and then by clonic contractions. Patient will remain confused for several hours.

Absence Seizure

They are a form of generalized epilepsy that involves a brief loss of consciousness without muscle activity. Immediate recovery of consciousness and orientation occurred.

Causes of Seizures in Pregnancy (Fig. 1)

- Pregnancy-induced causes—eclampsia and complications of general anesthesia
- Epileptic seizures
- CNS infections
- Metabolic—hypoglycemia, extreme hyperglycemia, hyponatremia, hypocalcemia, uremia, and hepatic encephalopathy
- Tumor/mass
- Antiepileptic drug (AED) withdrawal
- CNS-stimulating drugs
- Alcohol or drug withdrawal

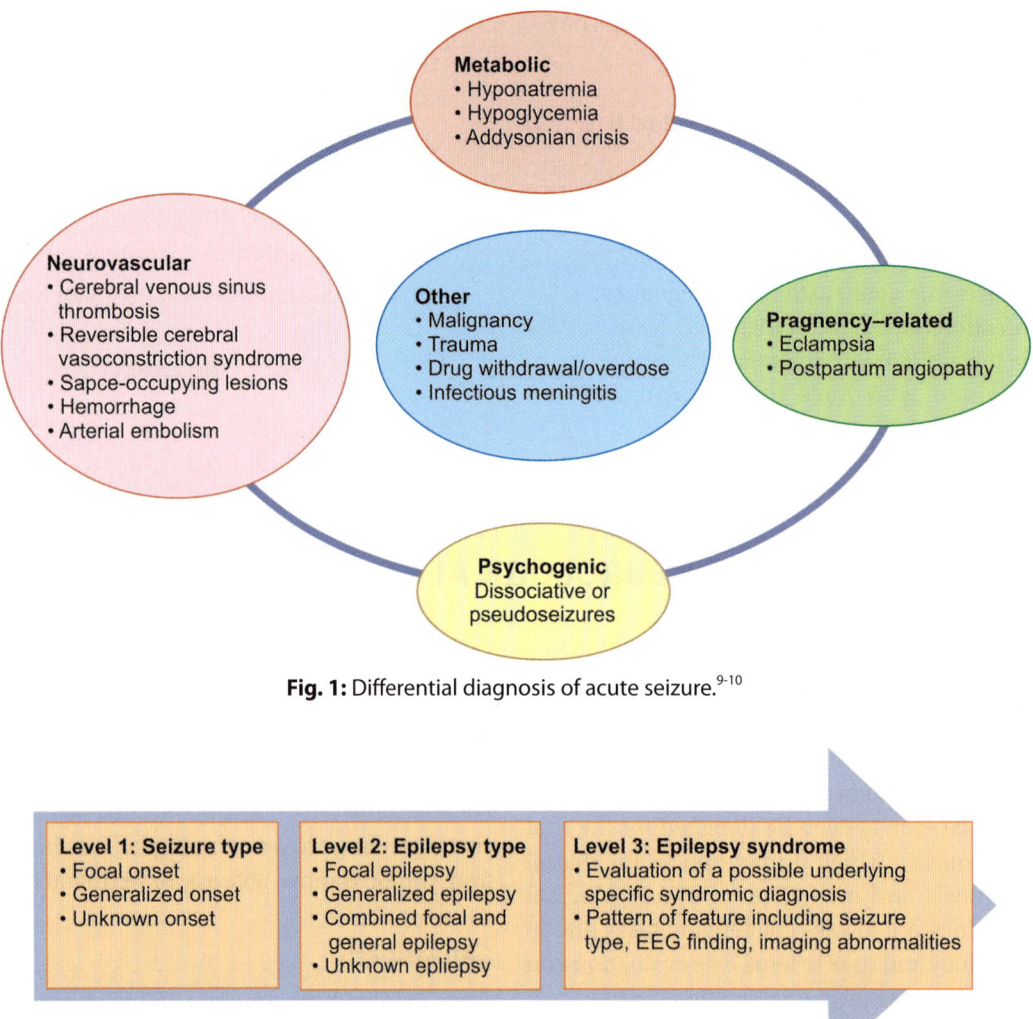

Fig. 1: Differential diagnosis of acute seizure.[9-10]

Fig. 2: The International League Aganist Epilepsy seizure classification system.[3]
(EEG: electroencephalogram)

- Trauma
- Subarachnoid or intracerebral hemorrhage
- Thromboembolism
- Psychogenic nonepileptic seizures (pseudoseizures).

Epilepsy and Seizure Disorders[4-6] (Fig. 2)

It is the most common neurological disorder to complicate pregnancy, affecting 0.5% of women of childbearing age.

Maternal implications of epilepsy in pregnancy:
- *Seizure activity*: The primary goal of treatment of epilepsy is seizure control with monotherapy. Pregnancy has a variable effect on seizure frequency. In 25% cases, frequency of fits increased during pregnancy, in 25% decreased and in 50% frequency remains unaffected. Seizures are generalized tonic clonic type. In 1–2% cases seizures occurred during labor and a further 1–2% within first 24 hours after delivery.
- Outcome of epilepsy deteriorates in pregnancy. The reasons are as follows:

- Inadequate patient information and counseling
- Poor compliance because of increased nausea and vomiting
- Poor absorption of drugs from gastrointestinal tract during labor
- Increased clearance and volume of distribution
- Hyperventilation during pregnancy
- Inadequate sleep.

Physiological changes that occur in pregnancy affect the intake, absorption, distribution, and metabolism of antiepileptic drugs. Therefore, drug dosage may need to be altered in pregnancy, not only to control seizures but also to avoid maternal and fetal toxicity.

Effect of epilepsy on pregnancy: Majority of pregnant women with controlled epilepsy have uncomplicated pregnancy and deliver healthy infants. Uncontrolled epilepsy may results in trauma, placental abruption, premature rupture of membrane, and preterm delivery.[7]

Gestational epilepsy: A seizure disorder that becomes manifest first time only during pregnancy. Most of these patients

SECTION 5: Pregnancy with Pre-existing Morbidities

TABLE 1: Antiepileptic drugs in pregananacy.[14-17]

Drug	Therapeutic level (µg/mL)	Usual nonpregnant daily dose (µg/day)	Rate of teratogenicity (%)	Maternal side effects	Fetal adverse effect
Phenytoin	10–20	300–500 in single or divided doses	0.7–7.0	Nystagmus, ataxia, hirsutism, anemia, and gum hyperplasia	Fetal hydantoin syndrome-craniofacial anomalies, fingernail hypoplasia, growth deficiency, developmental delay, cardiac anomalies, clefts, carcinogenesis, coagulopathy, and hypocalcemia
Phenobarbitone	15–40	90–180 mg in three divided doses	1 Jun	Drowsiness and ataxia	Clefts, cardiac anomalies, urinary tract malformation, coagulopathy, neonatal, depression, and withdrawal symptoms
Primidone	5–15	750–1,500 in three divided doses		Drowsiness, ataxia and nausea	Teratogenesis, coagulopathy, and neonatal depression
Carbamazepine	4–10	600–1,200 in 3–4 divided doses	2 Jun	Drowsiness, ataxia, leukopenia, and hepatotoxicity	Fetal hydantoin syndrome, spina bifida
Levetiracetam		500 twice daily	0–2	Cough; decrease appetite, diarrhea, dizziness, drowsiness, headache, and irritability	Theoretical-skeletal abnormalities, impaired growth in animals

recovered in postpartum have further seizures only during subsequent pregnancies.

Effect on fetal development **(Table 1):**
- *Hereditary effect*: An epileptic mother has a 1:30 chances of transmission of disease in to an offspring.
  - *Congenital malformations*: As compared to general population, there is two to three times increase in major malformations in children of mother exposed to AEDs in utero. The risk is highest during period of organogenesis. Risk is more in women on treatment and on polytherapy compare to women not on treatment and monotherapy exposure.

In 1976, Hanson described the *fetal hydantoin syndrome.*[8] It comprises mild-to-moderate mental retardation, growth restrictions, facial clefts, dysmorphism, finger-like thumbs, distal phalangeal and nail hypoplasia, developmental delays, and congenital heart defects.

Data from malformation birth registries suggest that:
- *Phenytoin and valproate*: Congenital heart defects
- *Phenytoin, phenobarbital, and primidone*: Orofacial clefts
- *Carbamazepine and valproate*: Neural tube defects
- *Valproate*: Skeletal defects, radial aplasia, and urogenital defects such as hypospadias
- *Carbamazepine*: Neural tube defects, cardiovascular and urinary tract anomalies (lowest risk of all monotherapy)
- *Trimethadione*: 50% risk of malformation and mental retardation (contraindicated in pregnancy)
- *Phenytoin*: Fetal hydantoin syndrome
- *Neonatal coagulopathy*: AEDs such as phenytoin, phenobarbital, primidone, and carbamazepine are enzyme-inducing drugs leads to deficiency of vitamin K-dependent clotting factors results in neonatal bleeding. However, maternal coagulation studies are normal.

Vitamin K 20 mg/day orally should be given in epileptic women from 36 weeks onward as prophylaxis for neonatal bleeding.

The American Academy of Pediatrics guidelines stipulate the need to give 1 g vitamin K at birth to all children born to mothers taking enzyme-inducing drugs.

Management

Preconceptional counseling:
- Ideally all patients should be seen prior to conception to optimize antiepileptic therapy. Seizures should be controlled preconceptionally preferably with monotherapy.
- Risk of major and minor malformations and potential longer term effects should be discussed.
- Discontinuation of therapy can be considered in women who have been seizure free for >2 years.
- Valproic acid and trimethadione should be avoided as it has increased teratogenic effect.
- Epileptic women should be advised to take supplemental folic acid 0.4 mg/day at least 1 month prior to conception and 4 mg/day, when she becomes pregnant.

Antenatal management:[9-12]
- *AEDs*: The primary goal of women with epilepsy (WWE) is seizure control with monotherapy at lowest possible dose. If patient seizures are controlled, no attempt to made change her medications.
- *Folic acid*: Folic acid 5 mg/day is recommended before conception and in first trimester in all women taking AEDs.
- *Vitamin K*: Vitamin K 20 mg/day orally should be given 36 weeks onward as prophylaxis for neonatal bleeding.
- *Antenatal screening*: All WWE should be referred for high-resolution ultrasound screening for structural anomalies. Anencephaly, neural tube defects, cleft lip and palate, and congenital cardiac defects can be detected.

Prenatal screening, using serum α-fetoprotein at 15–22 weeks combined with structural ultrasound can identify 95% fetus with open neural tube defects.

Patients should be encouraged to take her medications regularly, not deprive of her sleep. AED levels should be frequently monitored and dosage adjusted.

Intrapartum management:[13]
- Most patients are able to deliver vaginally. Cesarean sections are reserved only for obstetric indications.
- Proper administration of AEDs during labor is important, parenteral route is preferred consequent to poor absorption of drugs from gastrointestinal tract during labor.
- Lorazepam is a short-acting benzodiazepine and is the drug of choice for treating seizures acutely.
- A neonatologist must attend delivery due to possibility of malformations in the neonate.

Postpartum management:
- The baby is administered 1 mg vitamin K intramuscularly (IM) at birth.
- Breastfeeding should be encouraged as it has many beneficial effects for both mother and baby.
- Dosage of AEDs requires readjustment after delivery.
- Sleep should be adequate with the help of family.
- *Contraception*: Progesterone-only pills (POPs) are safe in lactation. Women taking enzyme-inducing AEDs require double dose of POPs.

Status epilepticus:
Definition: It is defined as ongoing seizure activity lasting for >30 minutes or recurrent seizures without full recovery of consciousness between episodes. Seizures can results in fetal hypoxia due to impaired maternal oxygenation.

Management (Flowchart 1):
- Transfer to intensive care facility
- Insert an intravenous (IV) line
- Draw blood sample for laboratory testing such as complete blood count (CBC), serum drug level, blood urea nitrogen, creatinine, glucose, serum electrolytes, calcium, and magnesium levels
- Blood for estimation of arterial blood gases
- Start administration of oxygen (8 L/min by nasal catheter/face mask)
- Document electrocardiogram
- Send urine for drug screen
- Start infusion with normal saline and not 5% dextrose. Add vitamin B complex to the infusion.
- Administer a bolus of 50 mL of 50% glucose
- Administer 100 mg thiamine injection IM
- Infuse diazepam 10 mg slows IV over 2 minutes. If seizures persist, push in an additional dose of 10 mg slowly and if seizures continue, administer a further 20 mg very slowly and if seizures continue, administer a further 20 mg very slowly (do not exceed 40 mg) to abort prolonged episodes and to prevent recurrent convulsions, whilst therapeutic brain concentrations of long-acting anticonvulsants are being achieved
- Initiate IV dilantin and infuse the loading dose of 18 mg/kg body weight administered at 50 mg/min. If hypotension develops, slow down the infusion rate
- Levetiracetam 1,000 mg IV administered followed by oral 500 mg BD may also be given
- Monitor with electrocardiogram (ECG) and watch out for atrial and ventricular conduction depression/ventricular fibrillation.

In case seizures persist:
- Initiate a phenobarbital drip and undertake endotracheal intubation and monitor vital signs. The dose of phenobarbital recommended is 20 mg/kg maximum, no faster than 100 mg/min, until seizures stop or the maximum dose has been reached.
- If seizures persist, institute general anesthesia with halothane and a neuromuscular junction blocker. If an anesthesiologist is not immediately available, administer 50–100 mg of lidocaine by IV slowly and follow it up with an IV infusion of 50–100 mg diluted in 250 mL of 5% dextrose in water at 1–2 mg/min.
- If delivery is imminent, alert the pediatrician and inform about maternal diazepam administration, as the infant will probably be born depressed. These neonates are prone to develop coagulopathy. All newborns should be administered vitamin K 1 mg after birth.
- Monitor postpartum drug levels. These changes rapidly.

CEREBROVASCULAR DISORDERS
Ischemic Stroke

Stroke in pregnancy is very uncommon. Etiology remains unknown in around 20-40% cases. Causes of strokes in pregnancy are as follows:[1]
- Antiphospholipid antibody syndrome
- Subacute bacterial endocarditis
- Paradoxical embolus
- Peripartum cardiomyopathy

Flowchart 1: Initial evaluations and intrapartum management of acute seizure.[9,10,17]

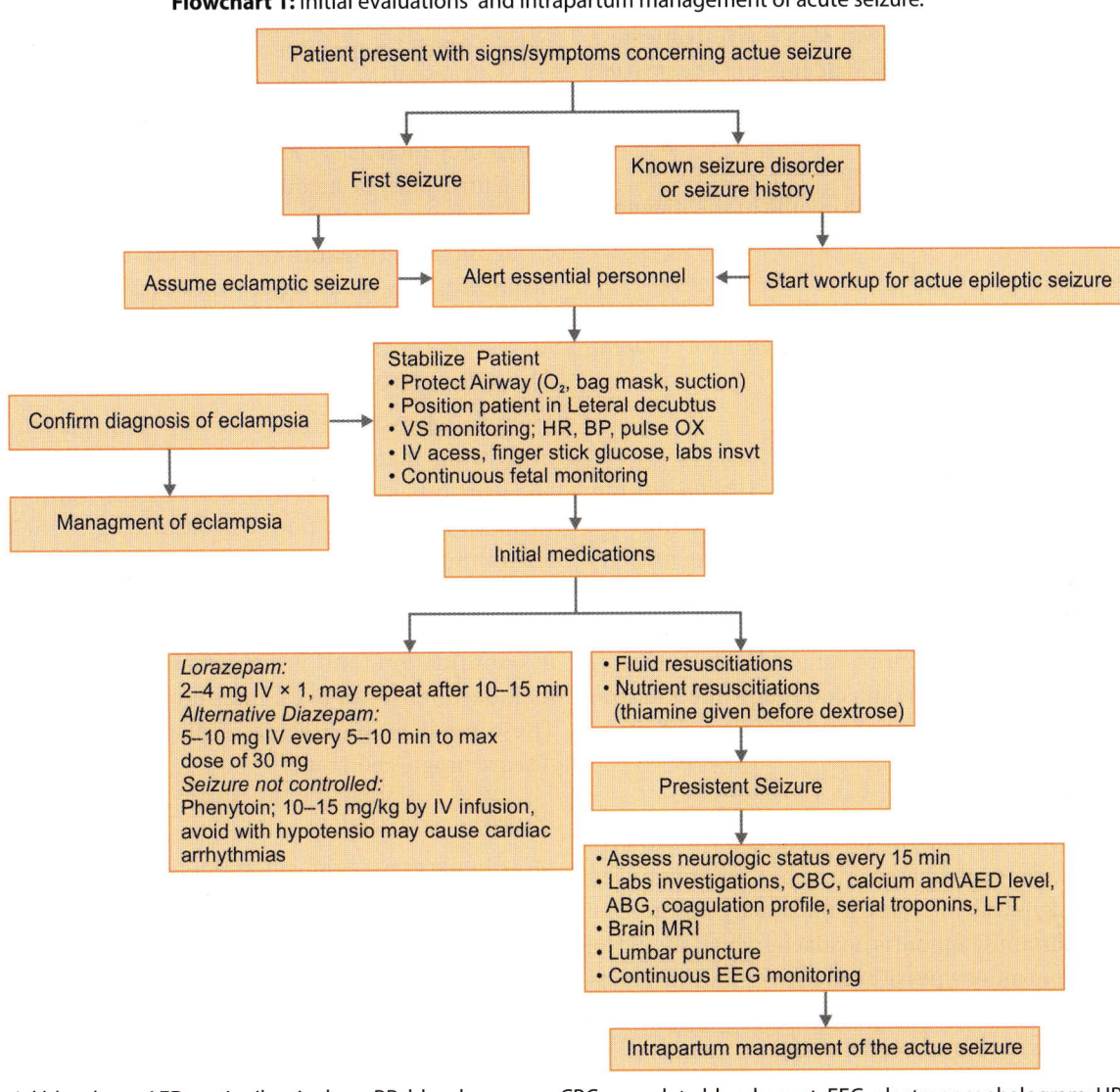

(ABG: arterial blood gas; AED: antiepileptic drug; BP: blood pressure; CBC: complete blood count; EEG: electroencephalogram; HR: heart rate; IV: intravenous; LFT: liver function test; MRI: magnetic resonance imaging)

- Pregnancy is a hypercoagulable state, prone for thrombus formation
- Most strokes associated with pregnancy occur in distribution of middle cerebral arteries. Most of the strokes in pregnancy occur in the first week of postpartum
- Magnetic resonance imaging (MRI) and computed tomography (CT) scan should be advised to confirm the diagnosis. Other investigations include CBC, coagulation profile, and echocardiography to establish the cause in pregnancy-related cerebral ischemic events
- Management includes airway patency, neurologist opinion, and to identify the cause
- Anticoagulant heparin is the drug of choice.

Cerebral Venous Thrombosis

In India, cerebral venous thrombosis is a public health problem with incidence of 40–50 per 10,000. Causes of cerebral venous thrombosis (CVT) are hypercoagulable states such as hemoglobinopathies, congenital and acquired thrombophilias, hyperviscosity syndromes, dehydration, infection, and paroxysmal nocturnal dyspnea.

Clinical features includes headache, seizures, and impaired consciousness. There may be sign of focal neurological deficit or raised intracranial tension.

Magnetic resonance imaging venography is the best modality to show venous clots and CT detects intracerebral bleeding.

Symptomatic treatment should be started. Treatment of seizures is important. Anticoagulation with heparin is required unless there is intracranial hemorrhage.

Subarachnoid Hemorrhage[1]

The main causes of subarachnoid hemorrhage are arteriovenous malformations (AVMs) and ruptured berry aneurysm. AVMs are estrogen-sensitive and therefore they dilate in pregnancy, most likely in the second trimester when the blood estrogen level reaches maximum. The risk of berry aneurysm ruptures increases with successive trimesters. Subarachnoid hemorrhage has an incidence of 1–2 per 10,000 pregnancies but causes 10% mortality. A sudden onset bursting headache is the initial symptom followed by vomiting, loss of consciousness, and sudden collapse.

Computed tomography and MRI confirm the diagnosis and site of lesion. If possible, neurosurgical excision of AVM or clipping of aneurysm should be undertaken in pregnancy. If surgical intervention is successful, then vaginal delivery is preferable. If lesion is inoperable, then elective cesarean section should be recommended.

Cerebral Tumors

Cerebral neoplasms occur primarily at extremes of life, therefore primary cancers or even metastatic tumors are uncommon during childhood period. Of the primary neoplasms, gliomas are the most common (50%), with meningiomas and pituitary adenomas accounting for 35%. Of the metastatic cerebral tumors, lung and breast tumors account for 50%. Choriocarcinoma commonly metastasizes to the cerebrum.

Clinical Features

Sign and symptoms depends on the type and the location of tumors. They are generally characterized by slow progression of neurological signs with increased intracranial pressure. One of the most important symptom is headache which should be differentiated from other types of headache. Other symptoms include pressure headache, nausea, vomiting, double vision, vertigo, seizures, and altered mental status.

Imaging Status

Magnetic resonance imaging is preferred over CT scan in pregnancy. They are of greatest assistance in revealing space-occupying lesion.

Laboratory Findings

In cerebrospinal fluid (CSF), glucose, and protein levels are normal. No evidence of infection or inflammation is present. Pleocytosis may be present, but usually it is monocytic or lymphocytic, not polymorphonucleocytes. CSF human chorionic gonadotropin (hCG) titer raises the suspicion of metastatic choriocarcinoma.

Surgery is the treatment of choice, best performed preconceptually if diagnosed prior to pregnancy, whereas in benign and low-grade malignant tumors, surgery can be deferred till after delivery, provided the patient is neurologically stable. Malignant tumors should be resected promptly. Adjuvant chemotherapy can be given after the first trimester of pregnancy. Radiation is best delayed until after delivery.

Bell's Palsy[1]

Palsy of facial nerve due to inflammation. This is strictly a motor disorder involving paralysis of muscle of facial expression on one side that are innervated by facial nerve. Pregnancy increases the frequency of this disorder. About one-fifth of palsy occur during pregnancy or shortly thereafter. Bell's palsy is usually a self-limiting illness. Treatment with corticosteroids (prednisone 40–60 mg/day) and acyclovir is helpful if given within 1 week of onset. Surgical decompression of nerve is indicated rarely.

Multiple Sclerosis[1]

Multiple sclerosis is an autoimmune demyelinating process in the white matter of CNS. It affects women as twice as men and usually has its onset between the ages of 20 and 30 years. Cause is not known, but possible etiologies include viral, environmental, and genetic. Disease has its two pattern—relapsing remitting and primary progressive. Clinical features are weakness in extremities, sensory loss, difficulty in coordination, and visual problems. Treatment option includes interferon β-1a, interferon β-1b, and glatiramer. These medications decrease relapse rates and decrease disease progression rate.

Myasthenia Gravis

Myasthenia gravis is an autoimmune disorder characterized by antibodies to acetylcholine receptors at the neuromuscular junction. It is characterized by muscle weakness, particularly with receptive movement. It is more common in females, occurs in the third decade of life. The most common symptom is easy fatigability of small muscle, usually ocular muscle, which results in double vision. Difficulty in swallowing and speech is not uncommon. The diagnosis can be confirmed by administering edrophonium (tensilon, a total of 10 mg, consisting of 2 mg followed by 8 mg 45 seconds later) to assess improvement in muscle weakness. Repetitive nerve stimulation would show decrement of >15% in a person with the condition.

One-third patients experience exacerbation during pregnancy, one-third do not experience a change in disease, and one-third experience remission during pregnancy. The disease does not affect uterine activity because uterus consists of smooth muscles. The length of labor is not affected. Exacerbations are most common during the postpartum period. Placental transfer of acetylcholine receptors antibodies can occur, so the fetus should be monitored with fetal kick counts and ultrasound. Antibodies may affect the fetal diaphragm and lead to pulmonary hypoplasia and polyhydramnios. Treatment with anticholinesterase (e.g., neostigmine) is same as in nonpregnant state, although dosage must be administered more frequently during pregnancy. Other treatment options include thymectomy, steroids, plasma exchange, and intravenous immunoglobulin (IVIg). Curare-like agents and magnesium sulfate, as well as older general anesthetics should be avoided.

Myotonic Dystrophy

Myotonic dystrophy is an inherited degenerative neuromuscular and neuroendocrine disease. The most common form is type 1 (autosomal dominant). Clinical features are progressive muscular dystrophy, muscle weakness and myotonia, cataract, cognitive impairment, cardiac conduction defects, dysphagia, and respiratory compromise.

In pregnancy, complications are miscarriage, polyhydramnios, premature labor, and postpartum hemorrhage. Myotonic dystrophy can worsen especially in the third trimester due to extra weight gain and diaphragmatic splinting from a gravid uterus. In cesarean section, general anesthesia should be avoided as drugs used in this can cause complications in these patients.

■ CONTRACEPTION

- POPs are safe in lactation. Women taking enzyme-inducing AEDs require double dose of POPs, failure rates are threefold higher.[18]
- Copper intrauterine contraceptive device (Cu-IUCD) and levonorgestrel-releasing intrauterine system (LNG-IUS)—recommended.[18]

■ KEY MESSAGES

- Neurological disorders in pregnancy can be pregnancy-related and pre-existing neurological condition.
- For neurological disorder, evaluation and management should be performed in stepwise fashion with multidisciplinary approach.
- *Gestational epilepsy*: A seizure disorder that becomes manifest first time only during pregnancy. The major congenital malformation (MCM) risk is highest during period of organogenesis.
- MCM risk is more in women on treatment with polytherapy compared to monotherapy.
- *The American Academy of Pediatrics guidelines stipulate the need to give 1 g vitamin K at birth to all children born to mothers taking enzyme-inducing drugs.*
- *Epileptic women should be advised to take supplemental folic acid 0.4 mg/day at least 1 month prior to conception and 4 mg/day, when she becomes pregnant.*
- *AEDs: The primary goal of WWE is seizure control with monotherapy at lowest possible dose.*
- *According to American College of Obstetricians and Gynecologists (ACOG) and Society of Maternal Fetal Medicine guidelines ultrasound examination at 11–14 week is recommended to confirm date and screen for neural tube defects.*
- Serum α-fetoprotein at 15–22 weeks combined with structural ultrasound can identify 95% fetus with open neural tube defects.
- *Lorazepam* is a short-acting benzodiazepine and is the drug of choice for treating seizures acutely.
- *CVT*: Pregnancy is a hypercoagulable state, prone for thrombus formation.
- Most strokes associated with pregnancy occur in distribution of middle cerebral arteries.
- Most of the strokes in pregnancy occurred in the first week of postpartum.
- The main causes of subarachnoid hemorrhage are AVMs and ruptured berry aneurysm.
- The primary neoplasms, gliomas, are the most common (50%) in pregnancy.
- Bell's palsy is usually a self-limiting illness.
- Myasthenia gravis is an autoimmune disorder. It is characterized by antibodies to acetylcholine receptors at the neuromuscular junction, most commonly occurs during the postpartum period.

■ REFERENCES

1. National Institute for Clinical Excellence. The Epilepsies. The Diagnosis and Management of the Epilepsies in Adults and Children in Primary and Secondary Care. Clinical Guideline 20. London: NICE; 2004. (www.nice.org.uk/pdf/CG20NICEguideline.pdf)
2. American College Obstetricians and Gynecologists. Seizure disorders in pregnancy. ACOG Educ Bull. 1996;231.
3. Delgado-Escueta AV, Jantz D. Consensus guidelines: preconceptional counseling, management, and care of pregnant women with epilepsy. Neurology. 1992;42(4 Suppl 5): 149-60.
4. Epilepsy in pregnancy. In: Royal College of Obstetrician & Gynaecologists Green top Guideline No. 68. 2016.
5. Gerard EE, Samuels P. Neurologic disorder in pregnancy. In: Gabbe SG, (ed). Obstetrics: Normal and Problem in Pregnancy, 7th edition. Philadelphia; Elsevier; 2017. pp. 388-95.
6. O Brien MD, Gilmour-White SK. Management of epilepsy in women. Postgrad Med J. 2005;81(955):278-85.
7. Crawford P, Appleton R, Betts T, Duncan J, Guthrie E, Morrow J. Best practice guidelines for the management of women with epilepsy. The women with epilepsy guidelines development group. Seizure. 2000;8(4):201-7.
8. Pschirrer ER. Seizure disorders in pregnancy. Obstet Gynecol Clin North Am. 2004;31(2):373-84.
9. Fisher R, vanEmde Boas W, Blume W, Elger C, Genton P, Lee P, et al. Epileptic seizures and epilepsy; definition proposed by the International League Against Epilepsy (ILAE) and the International Bureau for Epilepsy (IBE). Epilepsia. 2005;46(4):470-2.
10. Bollig KJ, Jackson DL. Seizures inPregnancy. Obstet Gynecol ClinNorth Am. 2018;45(2):349-67.
11. Kaplan PW, Norwitz ER, Menachem E, Pennwll PB, Druzin M, Robinson JR, et al. Obstetric risks for women with epilepsy during pregnancy. Epilepsy Behav. 2007;11(3):283-91.
12. LaRoche SM, Helmers SL. The new antiepileptic drugs: scientific review. JAMA. 2004;291(5):605-14.
13. Vidovic MI, Della-Marina BM. Trimestral changes of seizure frequency in pregnant epileptic women. Acta Med Croatica. 1994;48(2):85-7.

14. Morrell M. Guidelines for care of women with epilepsy. Neurology. 1998;51(5 Suppl 4):S21-7.
15. Nei M, Daly S, Liporace J. A maternal complex partial seizure in labor can effect fetal heart rate. Neurology. 1998;51(3):904-6.
16. Pennell PB. Antiepileptic drugs pharmacokinetics during pregnancy and lactation. Neurology. 2003;61(6 suppl 2):35-42.
17. Fishel Bartal M, Sibai BM. Eclampsia in the 21st century. AmJ Obstet Gynecol. 2020.
18. Nelson-Piercy C. Neurological problems. In: Nelson –Piercy C (Ed). Handbook of Obstetric Medicine, 1st edition. Taylor & Francis: Northampton; 1997. pp. 127-44.
19. Quality standards subcommittee of the American Academy of Neurology: Management issues for women with epilepsy (summary statement). Neurology. 1998;51:944.
20. Samren EB, van Duijn CM, Koch S, Hiilesmaa VK, Klepel H, Bardy AH, et al. Maternal use of antiepileptic drugs and risk of major congenital malformations: a joint European prospective study of human teratogenesis associated with maternal epilepsy. Epilepsia. 1997;38(9):981-90.
21. Yerby M, Freil PN, McCormick KB, Koerner M, Van Allen M, Leavitt AM, et al. Pharmacokinetics of anticonvulsants in pregnancy: alteration in plasma protein binding. Epilepsy Res. 1990;5(3):223-8.

LONG QUESTIONS

1. Write the definition, classification, and causes of seizures.
2. Write the antenatal, intrapartum, and postpartum management of epilepsy.
3. Write the management of status epilepticus.
4. Write the causes, clinical features, and management of stroke in pregnancy.

SHORT QUESTIONS

1. Enumerate neurological disorder in pregnancy.
2. What are the causes of seizures in pregnancy?
3. How pregnancy affects the outcome of epilepsy?
4. What are the effects of epilepsy on pregnancy?
5. What are teratogenic effects of antiepileptic drugs?
6. Write a short note on myasthenia gravis in pregnancy.
7. Write a short note on multiple sclerosis in pregnancy.

MULTIPLE CHOICE QUESTIONS

1. True statement regarding epilepsy in pregnancy:
   a. Seizure frequency decrease in majority
   b. Monotherapy is preferred to polydrug
   c. No increase in incidence of epilepsy
   d. Breastfeeding is contraindicated.
2. Which vitamin deficiency is most commonly seen in a pregnant mother who is on phenytoin therapy for epilepsy?
   a. Vitamin B6
   b. Vitamin B12
   c. Vitamin A
   d. Folic acid
3. True statement regarding the use of antiepileptic drug in pregnancy:
   a. Valproate is associated with neural tube defect
   b. Multiple drug should be given
   c. Carbamazepine is used as monotherapy
   d. Continue sodium valproate with regular monitoring of serum levels
4. What is the most common neurologic disorder in pregnancy?
   a. Seizure
   b. Headache
   c. Leg numbness
   d. Hand weakness
5. Which of the following complication is increased in women who experience Bell's palsy during pregnancy?
   a. Preterm labor
   b. Preeclampsia
   c. Premature rupture of membrane (PROM)
   d. None of the above
6. Which of the following medication is not associated with an increased risk of the congenital fetal malformation when taken in early pregnancy?
   a. Phenytoin
   b. Valproate
   c. Carbamazepine
   d. None of the above
7. Which of the following have contributed to the increase in stroke prevalence?
   a. Cocaine use
   b. Hypertension
   c. Diabetes mellitus
   d. All of the above
8. When do the pregnancy-related strokes occur?
   a. Postpartum
   b. Second trimester
   c. First trimester
   d. Third trimester
9. Which of the following organism is trigger in the development of multiple sclerosis?
   a. Herpesvirus 6
   b. Chlamydia trachomatis
   c. Influenza B
   d. All of the above
10. Antibodies are found commonly for which structure in myasthenia gravis:
    a. Acetylcholine receptor
    b. Oligodendrocyte glycoprotein
    c. Muscle-specific tyrosine kinase
    d. Nonself antigen
11. Medicine should be avoided during labor and delivery in myasthenia gravis patient:
    a. Succinylcholine
    b. Gentamicin
    c. Magnesium sulfate
    d. All of the above
12. Which of the following tumors is not commonly known to increase in pregnancy?
    a. Glioma
    b. Pituitary adenoma
    c. Meningioma
    d. Neurofibroma
13. What is the most common cause of subarachnoid hemorrhage?
    a. Trauma
    b. Cerebral venous thrombosis
    c. Ruptured saccular aneurysm
    d. Ruptured arteriovenous malformation

Answers
1. b 2. d 3. a 4. b 5. b 6. a
7. d 8. a 9. a 10. a 11. c 12. d
13. c

5.12 DERMATOLOGICAL DISORDERS IN PREGNANCY

Bharathi KR, Pooja Bhat

INTRODUCTION

Pregnancy encompasses changes in endocrine, immune, metabolic and vascular system that might have influence on skin and other organs. More than 90% of women report significant and complex skin changes during pregnancy, especially during the third trimester.[1] Although, hormones such as estrogen, progesterone, and melanocyte stimulating hormone (MSH) are attributed to these skin changes, exact etiology still remains unknown. These skin changes can be broadly categorized into physiological changes, pre-existing dermatoses affected by pregnancy, and specific dermatoses of pregnancy.[2] These dermatoses are usually benign and tend to resolve in postpartum period, some of the conditions do cause cosmetic distress, severe pruritus, few risk fetal life causing fetal distress, prematurity and still birth. Prompt, early diagnosis and treatment has significantly reduced the morbidity and mortality of the mother and improved fetal outcome.[2]

PHYSIOLOGICAL CHANGES IN PREGNANCY

Pigmentation

The most common physiological skin change observed in more than 90% of pregnant women is hyperpigmentation.[3] Although these changes tend to fade after delivery, they rarely go to their previous state. Increased estrogen, progesterone, melanocyte stimulating hormone (MSH), increased number of epidermal melanocytes and upregulation of tyrosinase by human placental lipids contribute to hyperpigmentation.

Most of these pigmentary changes are noted in third trimester and in dark skinned complexion. Linea nigra—a vertical band of pigment that usually extends from xiphisternum to pubic symphysis, is due to darkening of linea alba. Similar features of hyperpigmentation are noted in and around nipple, areola, axilla, genitalia, inner thigh, and neck. Newly formed scars, freckles might darken.

Macular pigmentation appears in centrofacial pattern on forehead, temples, cheeks, upper lip, and chin in a symmetrical fashion called mask of pregnancy or melasma. It is seen in 70% of pregnant women, out of which, epidermal type - 69.2%, dermal type - 6.2% and mixed pattern is noted in 24.6%.[4] Malar pattern involves cheeks and nose whereas the mandibular pattern involves the ramus of the mandible. Broad spectrum sunscreen and sun avoidance prevent both initial development as well as exacerbation of melisma. Topical bleaching creams, hydroquinones, retinoids, steroid treatment is done after pregnancy as these agents are potential teratogens.

Pruritus Gravidarum

Pruritus in the absence of an underlying hematological/biochemical disorder is a common complaint, occurring in 18% of pregnancies.[5] Common sites affected are scalp and abdominal skin. It may present as early as 3rd month, peak a month before delivery and resolves in the postpartum period. Recurrence rate is 50% in subsequent pregnancies. New onset persistent itch has to be considered as pruritus gravidarum if there is no rash and serum liver enzymes and bile salts are within the normal levels. Mild forms may be treated with moisturizers and topical antipruritic creams. Antihistaminics can be prescribed.

Striae Gravidarum

Striae, commonly referred to as stretch marks, are commonly seen in the lower abdomen, breasts, and thighs.[6] Incidence being 90%, it is seen during second half of pregnancy.[7] Although etiology is multifactorial, localized stretching, familial predisposition and increased estrogen, progesterone and corticosteroids are the causative factors. Rupture of collagen and elastic fires occurs in the dermis and fiber orientation shifts from perpendicular to parallel to dermoepidermal junction. They are initially seen as pink linear wrinkles and become white and atrophic with time. Several creams, emollients and oils (aloe vera, cocoa butter, olive oil) have been tried, but they do not disappear completely. Postpartum treatment includes retinoids and laser therapy.[8,9]

Vascular Changes

Nearly 50% of pregnant women develop non-pitting edema of face, eyelids, hands and feet.[10] It is commonly seen during morning and is mostly due to increased fluid retention and vascular permeability. Reassurance is done, severe cases warrants compression stockings.

Spider nevi are superficial vascular structures that branch outward from a central puncta in second trimester and regress after 3 months of delivery.[11] It occurs due to increased estrogen during pregnancy causing blood vessel dilatation and proliferation. They develop around eyes, neck, face, upper chest, arms.

Palmar erythema is seen during first trimester and resolves within 1 week after delivery. It may either present as diffuse pink mottling of whole palm or confined to the thenar and hypothenar eminences. The fingers are usually not involved.

Telangiectasia also develops under the influence of estrogen. They can involve one or more dermatomes. Gingivitis and bleeding might be noted in third trimester due to gingival hyperemia and edema. Granuloma gravidarum or pyogenic granuloma appears as soft, red or purple friable nodule that can be either sessile or pedunculated. Observation will suffice in most of the cases and if bleeding occurs, excision is done. It regresses postpartum.

Varicosities of saphenous, vulvar and hemorrhoidal veins develop due to increased venous pressure from the gravid uterus. These are seen in 40% of women, increase from 3rd month of pregnancy, and regress postpartum.[12] Treatment is elevation of legs, compression stockings and supportive garments.

Deep vein thrombosis can occur, leading to damage to the veins and death can ensue due to pulmonary embolism. Petechiae and purpura can occur due to increased hydrostatic pressure and capillary fragility. Facial flushing, pallor, hot and cold sensation and cutis marmorata can develop due to vasomotor instability.

Nearly 50% pregnant women report of non-pitting pedal edema of face, eyelids, hands and feet. It is more in the early morning and gradually subsides as day progresses. Reassurance is advocated after ruling out systemic causes of pedal edema such as cardiac, renal or preeclampsia.

Hemangiomas occur in 5% of pregnancies during second trimester and commonly seen in the hand and neck.[13]

Carpal tunnel syndrome occurs due to compression neuropathy of the median nerve when it passes beneath the flexor retinaculum. Patients present with pain, numbness, and swelling of the hand except the ring and the little finger. It regresses spontaneously post-delivery.

Appendages

Pregnancy upregulates activity of eccrine glands and downregulates apocrine gland activity, increase thyroid activity. Sebum production is increased during pregnancy due to hypertrophy and hyperactivity of sebaceous gland. Montgomery tubercles undergo hypertrophy during pregnancy.

Hair changes are marked during pregnancy. In gravid state, anagen phase increases resulting in thickening and increased scalp hair and there is slower progression of hairs from anagen to telogen stage. During postpartum, telogen phase (telogen effluvium) enters a resting phase due to which hair loss is pronounced. It begins at 4–20 weeks and recovery is usually noted by 1 year. Hair loss is less in subsequent pregnancies. No specific treatment is required apart from reassurance.

Hirsutisim may be seen on face, arms and legs. It occurs due to accentuation of ovarian and placental androgens acting on the pilosebaceous unit. It resolves postpartum but recurrence rate is high. Treatment involves reassurance and cosmetic removal.

Nail growth is accelerated during pregnancy and might become soft, brittle or dystrophic with transverse grooves (Beau's lines), subungual keratosis, or onycholysis.

Many women complain of discomfort, cracked, fissuring of nipples especially in the puerperium. This might limit suckling, and stasis, mastitis, and breast abscess ensues. Use of emollients, gentle washing are advised.

EFFECT OF PREGNANCY ON OTHER DERMATOSES

Infections

Infections tend to aggravate during pregnancy as cell-mediated immunity is suppressed. Candidiasis occurs more frequently during pregnancy and especially in gestational diabetes. 50% of neonates are reported to be positive for candidial infection, which is clinically evident in mouth and diaper area.[14] Antenatal treatment is mandatory as neonatal candidiasis can be fatal. Trichomoniasis is reported in 60% of pregnant women and is treated during second and third trimester.[14] Human papilloma virus exacerbates during pregnancy, condylomata acuminate grows rapidly and can obstruct the birth canal.[15] It can cause laryngeal papilloma in the newborn, however, prophylactic cesarean section is not recommended. Herpes simplex virus can be transmitted transplacentally in 50% of pregnant women. Recurrence rate in successive pregnancy is 5%.[16] It is sole decision of the obstetrician if elective cesarean section has to be done in such cases. Varicella zoster virus can cause viral pneumonia in 14% of affected mothers and is reported to cause neonatal death in 3%.[17] If the primary maternal infection occurs in first trimester, congenital varicella syndrome can occur in the neonate.[14]

Eczema

Atopic dermatitis develops early in childhood, commonly associated with allergies, allergic rhinitis, asthma, and environmental irritants such as soap, perfumes. Lesions are typically dry red to brownish gray, scaly and are noted in sites such as elbows, knees, hands, feet, wrist, face, neck and upper chest. Eczema is usually exacerbated during pregnancy. No adverse fetal outcome is reported however. Treatment mainly involves avoidance of allergen, reduce exposure to triggering agents such as heat, perspiration, low humidity, use of topical emollients and topical corticosteroids.

Acne Vulgaris

Acne vulgaris most commonly affects women of child bearing age group. Its effect in pregnancy is variable. Some pregnant women develop for the first time while others notice an improvement. Most of drugs used for the treatment of acne are teratogenic, therefore, withdrawal causes flare up of acne. Treatment during puerperium includes topical retinoids, benzoyl peroxide, and systemic antibiotics such as tetracycline, erythromycin or trimethoprim sulfamethoxazole.

Psoriasis

Psoriasis is typically erythematous plaques with sharp margins covered by thick silvery scale. Commonly affected sites are scalp, back, ears, nails, elbows, and knees. Psoriasis may be seen for first time during pregnancy, might aggravate or improve. Treatment in puerperium includes topical agents such as salicylic acid, steroids, ultraviolet B therapy, PUVA therapy, infliximab, cyclosporine, and methotrexate.

Impetigo herpetiformis is a rare form of psoriasis that might worsen during pregnancy. It is characterized by erythema that begins at flexures and forms superficial sterile pustules at its margins. It may be associated with fever, malaise, neutrophilia, hypocalcemia and tetany. It subsides after delivery but tends to recur in successive pregnancy. Fetal complications include still birth, neonatal death and other fetal abnormalities. Management includes fluid and electrolyte replacement, correction of hypocalcemia, assessment of fetal well-being, use of antibiotics and corticosteroids when indicated. Elective cesarean section has better outcome. Low dose methotrexate may be prescribed postpartum to prevent rebound postulation.

Leprosy

Leprosy typically manifests as hypopigmented or erythematous papules, nodules and macules. It is associated with sensory and motor loss in the areas of the lesion and also in distal extremities. Women with leprosy do well during pregnancy. Treatment includes dapsone, rifampicin, clofazimine. Dapsone is reported to cause hemolytic disease of the newborn. Type 1 and type 2 reactions are common during pregnancy. Increased incidence of twins is reported in lepromatous patients.

Collagen Vascular Diseases

Systemic lupus erythematosus (SLE) is associated with better outcome during pregnancy as per recent studies, although, pre-existing renal damage is likely to worsen leading to mortality. Neonatal lupus is reported in babies born to mothers with SLE. Pregnancy by itself, does not affect cutaneous lupus. Similarly, pregnancy does not alter the course of systemic sclerosis, dermatomyositis or polymyositis, but can deteriorate pre-existing renal damage. Ehlers-Danlos syndrome might pose problems such as excessive bleeding, wound dehiscence and uterine laceration.[14] Major gastrointestinal bleed can occur in patients with pseudoxanthoma elasticum.

Erythema Multiforme

It is an acute hypersensitivity reaction with characteristic symmetric eruption of papules, macules and vesicles – target lesion. It is preceded by nonspecific viral such as prodrome and lasts for 2–4 weeks. It is aggravated during pregnancy and tends to recur in successive pregnancy. Treatment involves avoidance of allergen and steroids in rare cases.

Neurofibromatosis

Neurofibromatosis is a neurocutaneous disorder characterized by multiple café-au-lait spots and cutaneous neurofibromas. Pregnant women with neurofibromatosis report higher incidence of first trimester abortion, still birth, IUGR, and increased cesarean rate. They present with growth of new fibroma and exacerbation of pre-existing ones. Preimplantation genetic diagnosis is new modality of diagnosing neurofibromatosis.

Melanoma

Malignant melanoma by itself is rare entity, although, if happens during pregnancy, metastasis to placenta and involvement of fetus can occur. It does not alter during pregnancy. Transplacental transmission is extremely rare but placenta of melanoma patient has to be sent for histopathology. Women with malignant melanoma are advised to delay the pregnancy by 2 years after its diagnosis. Termination of pregnancy is, however, deferred as there is no maternal benefit.

■ DERMATOSES OF PREGNANCY

Apart from the physiological changes, effect of pregnancy on other dermatoses seen earlier there are few dermatoses which are specific to pregnancy which occur due to complex interactions between profound hormonal changes seen in pregnancy along with the immune system. These are pruritic inflammatory skin disorders which may have discomfort to the mother and can be associated with fetal risks in few conditions.

Classification of Dermatoses of Pregnancy

Over the years the process of classification of Dermatoses of Pregnancy has undergone profound changes due to lack of clarity regarding etiopathogenesis and significant overlap between the clinical presentation and histopathological features. Holmes et al. in 1983 presented the first simplified classification for dematoses of pregnancy which comprised pemphigoid gestationis (PG), polymorphic eruption of pregnancy (PEP), prurigo of pregnancy (PP) and pruritic folliculitis of pregnancy (PFP).[18] Though a newer classification has been proposed by Ambros-Rudolph et al. in 2006,[19] the one which was proposed by Holmes has been accepted by most of the authors. The newer classification includes pemphigoid gestationis, polymorphic eruption of pregnancy (PEP), intrahepatic cholestasis of pregnancy and atopic eruption of pregnancy.

Pemphigoid Gestationis (Gestational Pemphigoid or Herpes Gestationis)

Pemphigoid gestationis is a rare autoimmune disease with incidence of 1 in 50,000 pregnancies.[20] It is intensely pruritic bullous eruption exclusively associated with pregnancy with autoimmune etiology. Sometimes it is seen in association with choriocarcinoma, trophoblastic disorder or hydatidiform mole. In majority of the patients the pruritic erythematous urticarial papules and plaques or vesicles begin in the periumbilical region which later spreads to trunk, thighs, breasts, palms, and soles. The face and oral mucosa is rarely involved. Bullous lesions can be seen in both inflamed and clinically normal skin which usually heals without scarring. It is mostly seen in the second half of the pregnancy although initial onset in the immediate postpartum period occurs in about 20% cases. A flare at the time of delivery precede by a period of quiescence in the late pregnancy is typically noted with spontaneous resolution of PG in the postpartum period. With each subsequent pregnancies, the severity of the disease increases.

The specific etiology is not known, but autoimmune etiology is strongly linked to PG. Histopathological examination of the PG lesions shows epidermal and papillary dermal edema with occasional foci of eosinophilic spongiosis. The bullous lesions show numerous eosinophils. Direct immunofluorescence of the perilesional skin shows linear C3 along the basement membrane zone with concomitant IgG-1 deposition. HLA-DR3, HLA-DR4 or both with its alleles are associated with PG. HLA-DR3 is an important prognostic indicator, as the absence of DR3 is associated with more mild disease in the subsequent pregnancies.[20]

Differential diagnosis for PG includes drug eruption, erythema multiforme, contact dermatitis, polymorphic eruption in pregnancy and bullous pemphigoid. Detailed history and thorough clinical examination is essential to diagnose the appropriate condition. With known autoimmune etiology, PG is associated with no maternal risks except for an increased risk of grave's disease. Vesiculobullous lesions can occur in the neonates but limited to only 10% of the cases which are mild and usually resolve spontaneously in few weeks.

Oral antihistaminics and topical steroids are used for the early urticarial lesions with good response. Topical steroids used at lower doses with or without oral steroids have good response, the dose of which is tapered 7–10 days after the achievement of the control of the disease.[20] But the dosage needs to be increased at the time of delivery to control postpartum exacerbation. As a second line of management—immunoapheresis or plasmapheresis is considered for patients who do not respond to high doses of oral steroids or when oral steroids are contraindicated.[21]

Polymorphic Eruption of Pregnancy

[Synonym: Pruritic Urticarial Papules and Plaques of Pregnancy (PUPPP)]

It is one of the most common specific dermatoses of pregnancy affecting 1 in 160–240 pregnancies. Pruritic urticarial papules and plaques of pregnancy (PUPPP) were described by Lawley and colleagues in 1979.[22] It is a self-limiting pruritic, polymorphous, urticarial eruption seen in pregnant women. It occurs predominantly in the third trimester usually after 34 weeks gestation, common in multiple pregnancies with higher order, primiparous women, and pregnancy with male fetuses. It is also seen in cases with history of rapid or excessive weight gain in pregnancy.

The exact etiology is not known but the significant stretching of the abdominal skin damages the underlying connective tissue leads to an inflammatory process causing polymorphous, urticarial and at times vesicular, purpuric, polycyclic or targetoid lesions **(Fig. 1)**. PUPPP and PG in prebullous stage have similar features clinically and not easy to differentiate. But, the lesions in the PUPPP start in the abdominal striae in majority of the cases and very characteristically show periumbilical sparing where in periumbilical onset of lesions is pathognomonic of PG. Lesions spreads over trunk and extremities usually sparing the palms and soles, also the involvement of face is unusual.

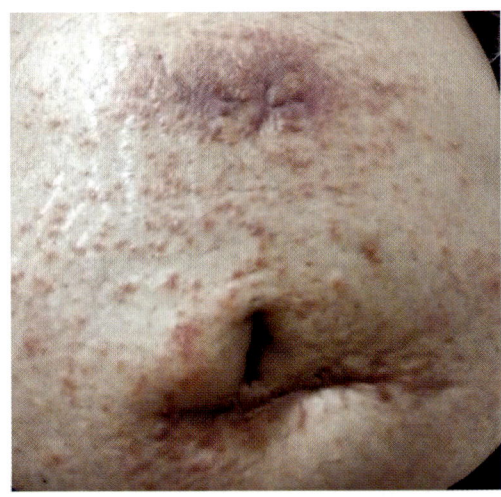

Fig. 1: Polymorphic eruptions of pregnancy or pruritic uricarial pappules and plaques of pregnancy (PUPPP).

Pruritic urticarial papules and plaques of pregnancy is predominantly a clinical diagnosis which is basically attributed to the negative results of immunofluorescence and serology results along with lack of pathognomonic histopathological features. The immunohistological studies show infiltrates predominantly of T-Helper lymphocytes which strongly suggests possibility of delayed hypersensitivity reaction to an unknown antigen. Dermatohistopathological examination reveals various epidermal spongioses with perivascular inflammatory infiltrate in the dermis. Direct immunofluorescence of the perilesional skin is negative for Linear C3 along the basement membrane zone.[12]

Mild PUPPP cases are treated symptomatically with topical corticosteroids, antipruritic medications or oral antihistaminics. If topical corticosteroids are not effective, a short course of systemic corticosteroids such as prednisolone 40–60 mg/day is effective.

Prurigo of Pregnancy (Prurigo Gestationis of Besnier)

Prurigo of pregnancy is the second most common dermatoses of pregnancy seen in the second half of the pregnancy with incidence between 1 in 300 and 450 pregnancies.[23] Usually associated with personal and family history of atopic dermatitis with atopic predisposition along with increased serum IgE, it is seen in the second half of the pregnancy with the onset between 25 and 30 weeks. Prurigo of pregnancy is the least studied dermatoses which is closely associated with obstetric cholestasis and associated conditions.

Clinically presents as itchy eruptions of the skin with grouped excoriated or crusted pruritic papules typically seen over dorsal aspect of the extremities and on the abdomen. There is no significant risk either to the mother or the fetus, but recurrence may be seen in subsequent pregnancies. Resolves following delivery but the postinflammatory hyperpigmentation develops over the lesion.

Histopathological examination is nonspecific but reveals parakeratosis, acanthosis and perivascular lymphocytic infiltrate. Immunofluorescence is negative.

Antihistaminics and topical corticosteroids form the mainstay of the treatment.

Pruritic Folliculitis of Pregnancy

Pruritic folliculitis of pregnancy is rare specific dermatoses described by Zabermann and Farmer. Because of its similarity to PUPPP and frequent misdiagnosis as PUPPP or infective folliculitis, the true prevalence of the disease is not known.

Pruritic folliculitis of pregnancy is commonly seen in 2nd trimester up to term pregnancy and resolves spontaneously at delivery or in the postpartum period. It develops as pruritic follicular erythematous papules and pustules similar to infective folliculitis. There have been no documented specific maternal or fetal risks.

The pathogenesis of the disease is not clear but histopathological examination demonstrates is typical of sterile folliculitis showing acute folliculitis with focal spongioses and exocytosis of polymorphonuclear and mononuclear cells. The cultures from the pustules rules out the most common differential diagnosis infectious folliculitis. The immunological and hormonal abnormalities seen in other dermatoses are not seen in pruritic folliculitis of pregnancy.

KEY MESSAGES

- Dermatological changes are common in pregnancy.
- Most of the changes are physiological. This should be identified and appropriate advise and reassurance should be given to the pregnant woman.
- There are some abnormal skin changes which arise as a result of pregnancy. These may have implications that are beyond dermatology.
- Conditions such as cholestasis should prompt appropriate obstetric monitoring and interventions.
- General endocrine, vascular, and immunological changes affect pre-existing dermatoses in varied manners. These should be adequately treated in pregnancy for the woman's comfort. Most drugs, especially local applications are safe in pregnancy.

REFERENCES

1. Kumari R, Jaisankar TJ, Thappa DM. A Clinical Study of Skin Changes in Pregnancy. Indian J Dermatol Venereol Leprol. 2007;73:141.
2. Warshauer E, Mercurio M. Update on dermatoses of pregnancy. Int J Dermatol. 2013;52(1):6-13.
3. Fitzpatrick TB, Eisen AZ, Wolff K. Dermatology in General Medicine. New York: McGraw Hill; 1979.
4. Muzaffar F, Hussain I, Haroon TS. Physiologic Skin Changes During Pregnancy: a study of 140 cases. Int J Dermatol. 1998;37: 429-31.
5. Black MM, Ambros-Rudolph C, Edwards L, Lynch P. Obstetric and Gynecologic Dermatology, 3rd edition. London: Mosby Elsevier; 2008.
6. Martin AG, Leal Khouri S. Physiologic skin changes associated with pregnancy. Int J Dermatol. 1992;31:375-8.
7. Kroumpouzos G, Cohen LM. Dermatoses of Pregnancy. J Am Acad Dermatol. 2001;45:1-19.
8. Kang S. Topical tretinoin therapy for management of early striae. J Am Acad Dermatol. 1998;39: S90-2.
9. McDaniel DH. Laser therapy for stretch marks. Dermatol Clin. 2002;20:67-76.
10. Dupot C. Herpes Gestationis with hydatidiform mole. Transactions of St. John's Dermatological Society. 1974;60:103.
11. Wilkin JK, Smith JG, Jr, Cullison DA. Unilateral dermatomal auperficial telangiectasia. J Am Acad Dermatol. 1983;8:468-77.
12. The Global Library of Women's Medicine. Dermatological diseases of pregnancy (Parish L, Parish J). Available from: http://www.glowm.com/section_view/heading/Dermatologic%20Diseases%20in%20Pregnancy/item/114 cited on 15.08.2014. [Last Accessed October, 2021].
13. Oumeish OY, Al-Fouzan AS. Miscellaneous diseases affected by pregnancy. Clinic Dermatolol. 2006;24:113-7.
14. Winton JB. Skin diseases aggravated by pregnancy. J Am Acad Dermatol. 1989; 20:1-13.
15. Millington GW, Graham-Brown RA. Skin and skin diseases throughout life. In: Burns T, Breathnach S, Cox N, Griffiths C (Eds). Rook's Textbook of Dermatology, 8th edition. Sussex: Wiley Blackwell; 2010. pp. 8, 9-13.
16. Torgerson RR, Marnarch ML, Bruce AJ, Rogers RS. Oral and vulvar changes in pregnancy. Clin Dermatol. 2006;24:122-32.
17. Black MM, Mayou SC. Skin diseases in pregnancy. In: de Swiet M (Ed). Medical Disorders in Obstetric Practice, 2nd edition. Oxford: Blackwell Scientific; 1989. pp. 808-29.
18. Holmes RC, Black MM. The Specific Dermatoses of Pregnancy. J Am Acad Dermatol. 1983;8:405-12.
19. Ambros-Rudolph CM, Mullegger RR, Vaughan-Jones SA, Kerl H, Balck MM. The specific dermatoses of pregnancy revisited and reclassified: result of a retrospective two centre study on 505 pregnant patients. J Am Acad Dermatol. 2005;54:395-404.
20. Engineer L, Bhol K, Ahmed AR. Pemphigoid gestationis: a review. Am J Obstet Gynecol. 2000;183:483-91.
21. Van Der Wiel A, Hart H, Flinterman J, Kerckhaert JA, Du Boeuff JA, Imhof JW. Plasma exchange in herpes gestationis. BMJ. 1980;281:1041.
22. Locksmith G, Duff P. Infection, antibiotics and preterm delivery. Semin Perinatol. 2001;25(5):295-309.
23. Nurse DS. Prurigo of late pregnancy. Austral J Dermatol. 1980;21:79-84.

LONG QUESTIONS

1. Discuss etiopathogenesis, clinical features, investigations, and management of pemphigoid gestationis.
2. Explain pruritic urticarial papules and plaques of pregnancy.
3. Describe intrahepatic cholestasis of pregnancy.

SHORT QUESTIONS

1. Write a brief note on classification of pregnancy dermatoses.
2. Physiological changes in pregnancy pertaining to skin.
3. Discuss about the effect of pregnancy on pre-existing skin disorders.
4. Immunological and hormonal changes leading to skin changes.

■ MULTIPLE CHOICE QUESTIONS

1. Common changes in skin during pregnancy includes all, except:
   a. Melasma
   b. Linea nigra
   c. Striae gravidarum
   d. Hypopigmentation
2. Main cause for skin disorders in pregnancy is:
   a. Hormonal and immunological
   b. Sunlight exposure
   c. Infections
   d. Nutritional deficiency
3. Prurigo of pregnancy is also referred as:
   a. Prurigo of Lawley
   b. Prurigo of Besnier
   c. Prurigo of Holmes
   d. Prurigo of Shronick
4. Pemphigoid gestationis is associated with deposition of:
   a. Linear C3
   b. Linear C5
   c. Linear C2
   d. Linear C8
5. A pregnant lady presents with blotchy hyperpigmentation on cheeks and nose. Diagnosis is:
   a. Senile lentigines
   b. Freckles
   c. Nevi
   d. Chloasma
6. The treatment for a pregnant diabetic patient with lakes of pus on the skin is:
   a. Cyclosporine
   b. Azathioprine
   c. Retinoids
   d. Methotrexate
7. Typical periumbilical sparing of the lesions is seen in:
   a. Pemphigoid gestationis
   b. PUPPP
   c. Prurigo of pregnancy
   d. Pruritic folliculitis of pregnancy

Answers
1. d   2. a   3. a   4. a   5. d   6. a
7. b

5.13 MENTAL HEALTH ISSUES AND SUBSTANCE USE IN PREGNANCY AND PUERPERIUM

Parul P Tank

■ INTRODUCTION

Mental health issues are one of the largest contributors to the burden of noncommunicable disease that humanity faces.[1] Women in the reproductive age group are no exception to this. Pregnancy and lactation are special situations for women with mental health issues. Women's healthcare providers should be trained to be empathetic to mental health issues, be able to acknowledge preexisting conditions, recognize new conditions that may arise and organize care in consultation with a mental health expert. They should be able to counsel women and their families on these issues. Some of the most common questions that obstetricians would face are related to the impact of mental health issues on the pregnancy or neonate, the effect of drugs used during treatment and the long-term outcomes for the mother.

■ PREVALENCE

It is difficult to have an accurate estimate of mental health problems and their subtypes in pregnancy and puerperium. Suffice it to say that these are among the most common disorders in any population. Some prevalence figures are presented below to highlight how common the problem is.[2]

- It is estimated that one in five (20%) of adults in the world have a mental health issue at some time in their lives.
- Women are more prone to anxiety and depression than men and the relative risk may be nearly two to three fold.
- About 10% of women have a preexisting mental health problem before they become pregnant. In a substantial number of women, this remains undetected and unaddressed through pregnancy.
- Approximately half of the general population has an experience with substance use that is serious enough to temporarily affect their physical or mental health. Prevalence in pregnancy may be lower due to maternal protective instincts towards a desired pregnancy.
- After childbirth, about 80% of women will experience short term mood disturbances ("blues") and about 20% of these will have postpartum depression. This has the potential to become a long term problem for women. 1% of women will have more serious mental health problems such as puerperal psychosis.

COMMON PREEXISTING MENTAL HEALTH ISSUES IN WOMEN: TYPICAL FEATURES AND RECOGNITION

The most common mental health issues that women face in the reproductive age group are mood disorders. Major depression is more common than other mood disorders such as bipolar disorder. Other mental health issues that are commonly seen are anxiety [generalized anxiety, panic, obsessive compulsive disorder (OCD), post-traumatic stress disorder (PTSD)] and substance use. Combinations of anxiety and depression are also relatively common. Psychosis, schizophrenia and related disorders, and eating disorders are also seen, but with a lower frequency.

The woman who has a preexisting mental health issue should ideally be seen in the preconception period. However, due to the prevailing stigma around mental health problems, this ideal situation may not always occur. In fact, most women would be reluctant to share the history of such a problem in the past or as an ongoing issue. The standard history taking format usually covers only physical problems (medical and surgical disease and previous obstetric history). With a small additional effort and an empathetic attitude, it is possible to draw out this history. Past mental health issues should raise a red flag for ongoing problems, flares and a higher chance of postpartum depression.

When the history of a preexisting mental health problem is not forthcoming, the healthcare provider should be alert to pick up features that should lead to a more detailed assessment with a mental health professional. Though the list given here is not exhaustive, it covers the most common symptoms.

- The woman may express typical symptoms[3]
  - *Depression:* The diagnostic criteria mentioned by the Diagnostic and Statistical Manual of Mental Disorders Version 5 (DSM-V) are elaborated in **Table 1**.
  - *Anxiety:* Disproportionate worry which stops her from functioning, panic attacks, social phobia, recurrent distressing dreams. One of the forms specific to women in pregnancy is tocophobia – an irrational and intense fear about labor, pain and vaginal birth.
  - *Obsessive compulsive disorders:* Obsessive and intrusive thoughts, repeated actions and rituals (washing hands, counting objects, pathological doubts, etc.)
  - *Schizophrenia or psychosis:* Delusions (fixed false beliefs), hallucinations, disorganized thoughts and/or behavior, catatonia, bizarre posturing or catatonia and mutism.

- Atypical symptoms which are very easy to miss or sweep away as "odd behavior" or being a difficult patient. The woman may not directly be able to or wish to express her mood. This is a cultural difference in Indian and Asian women as compared to their Western counterparts. Symptoms of the mind are expressed as somatic complaints which seem to have no organic basis on clinical evaluation and investigation. Repeated episodes of such complaints, exaggeration of symptoms and the general affect should raise the obstetrician's antennae to the possibility of a mental health issue.
- History from family members or accompanying persons is valuable. It gives an insight into the woman's behavior in her home environment, her interpersonal relationships and also gives information about the family support that she has to cope with mental and physical health problems.

NEWLY ARISING MENTAL HEALTH ISSUES IN PREGNANCY AND PUERPERIUM: FEATURES AND RECOGNITION

The postnatal period is rife with biological and sociological factors that can induce mental health problems. There are massive fluctuations in reproductive hormone levels, specifically a drop in the progesterone. Society and the mother herself expect to be happy and elated. This may run counter to the physical reality of pain, discomfort, prolonged feeding times and being responsible for the infant all the time. If there are risk factors such as undiagnosed mental health problems, poor family support, an abusive relationship, complications in childbirth and financial stressors, the probability of serious mental health problems rises.

Almost all women face some mood disturbances, which are also called postpartum blues. These disturbances of mood usually last for a few days and are mild. More significant mental health disturbances are related to depression, obsessive compulsive disorders and psychosis. The diagnosis may be missed because most units do not offer any structured screening and the team many not be sensitized to the problem. Some useful tools such as the Edinburgh Postnatal Depression scale have been specifically designed for this purpose.[4] Even if a formal assessment is not done for every woman, a bare minimum enquiry into her mood in the postnatal ward and at the postnatal visit should be mandatory. If there is a suspicion, it should be followed up with a mental health consultation. The symptoms of mood disorders have been elaborated on in **Table 1**.

SUBSTANCE USE: COMMON SUBSTANCES, RECOGNITION OF THE PROBLEM AND SCREENING

When a pregnancy is diagnosed, women who use substances may find a strong urge to stop doing so. This is a function of

TABLE 1: DSM-V criteria for major depressive disorder.

Duration	Number of symptoms and impact	Symptoms
Over the last 2 weeks Nearly every day	Five of the symptoms One symptom should be mood or interest Must cause marked distress or impairment in important areas of functioning	Depressed mood
		Markedly diminished interest or pleasure
		Insomnia or hypersomnia
		Psychomotor agitation or retardation
		Fatigue or loss of energy
		Feelings of worthlessness or guilt
		Diminished ability to concentrate
		Recurrent thoughts of death

the maternal instinct. However, substance use is a biological disorder and women may find it difficult to stop doing so. There are other sociological and environmental factors which may lead to continued use.

The most common substances used in pregnancy are nicotine and alcohol. Nicotine use may be culturally acceptable in certain populations. This is seen in the form of chewing tobacco or applying a paste of tobacco called "mishri", ostensibly to clean the gums and teeth. Cigarette smoking in young women is a rising trend in the urban population. Though a wide variety of illegal drugs and substances may be used in pregnancy, they are not as commonly seen in Indian population. Some of these are cannabis or marijuana, benzodiazepines, amphetamines, cocaine or its derivatives and stimulants such as 3,4-methylene dioxymethamphetamine (MDMA).

Enquiry about illicit substance use is a part of every history taking checklist. However, the truth may not emerge so easily. Caregivers should be alert to the circumstances that surround a particular woman and be prepared to ask more than once. Covert urine testing may be performed but may damage the fragile relationship the woman has with the healthcare provider. Screening for heavy alcohol consumption can be performed easily using the validated questionnaires which such as T-ACE, TWEAK or AUDIT **(Table 2)**. This simple method has 70% sensitivity in detecting heavy drinkers.[5] From the point of view of child care and need for child protections, patterns which involve heavy use, daily use and bingeing are the most concerning.

DOES PREGNANCY AFFECT THE COURSE OF MENTAL HEALTH PROBLEMS?

There is a complex relationship between the biological, social, psychological, behavioral and environmental forces that shape the course of mental health problems in relation to pregnancy and childbirth. It is difficult to establish linearity in this matter. Some important considerations are outlined here:

- Hormonal fluctuations, especially the withdrawal of progesterone in the postpartum period contributes to the etiology of postpartum depression. These are purely biological events over which there is no predictability or control. The same holds true for genetic predispositions.
- Social factors include marital status, status in a family hierarchy, financial status, and job continuation. These are cultural and vary significantly. The most common example of this is the status of a woman in the family depending on the child's gender. Financial status and job retention are also important for a woman's sense of self-worth and wellbeing. There are legal provisions for maternity benefits but subtle differentiations exist.
- Psychological factors such as past events, previous relationships, abuse, and the reactions to these will shape the course of mental health issues in pregnancy. The same is true for environmental factors (physical environment such as a secure dwelling, noise, crowding) and behavioral factors (substance use, nutrition, sexuality, and previous high-risk activity).

Owing to the large number of variables involved, it is not possible to accurately predict the impact that pregnancy

TABLE 2: Alcohol use screening tools.

Screening tool	Questions	Scoring	Scores requiring attention
T-ACE	T (Tolerance)—How many drinks does it take to make you feel high?	If more than 2 drinks, give 1 point	Score range is 0 to 4 Score of 2 or more requires attention
	A (Annoyance) – Have people annoyed you by criticizing your drinking?	If yes, give 1 point	
	C (Cutting Down) – Have you felt that you should cut down on drinking?	If yes, give 1 point	
	E (Eye Opener) – Have you ever had a drink first thing in the morning to steady your nerves or to get rid of a hangover?	If yes, give 1 point	
TWEAK	T (Tolerance) – How many drinks can you hold without passing out?	If more than 5 drinks, give 2 points	Score range is 0 to 7 Score of 2 or more requires attention
	W (Worried) – Have your friends or relatives expressed that they are worried about your drinking?	If yes, give 2 points	
	E (Eye Opener) - Have you ever had a drink first thing in the morning to steady your nerves or to get rid of a hangover?	If yes, give 1 point	
	A (Amnesia) - Has a friend or family member ever told you about things you said or did while you were drinking that you could not remember?	If yes, give 1 point	
	K (Cutting Down) – Have you felt that you should cut down on drinking?	If yes, give 1 point	

would have on preexisting mental health issues. The above-listed factors and their downsides are possible contributors for worsening of the condition. A multimodal and multifactorial model toward this has been proposed.[6]

IMPACT OF MENTAL HEALTH PROBLEMS ON PREGNANCY: SHORT AND LONG-TERM

All mental health problems have the potential to affect the mother and the fetus/neonate.[7] There are well-established embryological, fetal and perinatal risks with mental health problems in the mother. There is also a possibility of a much more remote impact of maternal mental health problems on the child's health in future adult life. This is a form of fetal origin of adult disease. The maternal or perinatal problems may arise from the illness, the behavioral or environmental factors one associates with the illness or from the drugs used to treat it. The behavioral or environmental factors that have been mentioned earlier are substance use, high-risk or criminal behavior, neglect of self and health care needs, violence, and abuse.

The physiological environment created by major depression adversely impacts maternal function. This is associated with poor prenatal care compliance, inadequate nutrition or obesity, substance use and suicide. There is a higher probability of preterm birth and low birth weight infants born to such women. The relationship between maternal depression and multiple childhood problems is a continuum and includes delayed milestones, lower scholastic performance, and cognitive abilities. Other sequelae include higher probabilities of infant death, abuse, neglect and accidental injuries. Children who are exposed to maternal depression in utero are four times more likely to be depressed themselves as young adults.

Women with schizophrenia are at increased risk of obstetric complications including antepartum hemorrhage, specifically placental abruption. Concurrent behavioral and socioeconomic factors also contribute to a worse perinatal outcome.

Anxiety and related disorders are associated with some adverse perinatal outcomes. However, these appear to have lesser impact as compared to depression and schizophrenia. Infants born from mothers with anxiety may have difficulties with autonomic regulation of body temperature and heart rate.

All these outcomes are not always preventable even when women are adequately treated in pregnancy and in the postpartum period. However, treated women are less likely to have such outcomes and the effect of these outcomes is blunted with adequate treatment.

IMPACT OF SUBSTANCE USE ON PREGNANCY

Acute maternal effects of substance use can include overdose, intoxication or withdrawal. This is the same as in the general population. These effects can resemble general medical conditions and obstetric disorders. Convulsions may occur with any of the three mentioned states and the differential diagnosis could be fulminant preeclampsia or eclampsia. Other acute effects affect the cardiovascular, respiratory, and neurological systems.[8]

Chronic maternal problems that are more prevalent in substance users and need attention specifically in regards to pregnancy are infections (HIV, TB, pneumonia, sexually transmitted diseases, local infections—phlebitis, abscess), anemia and malnourishment. Mental health problems such as depression and psychosis are three times more likely in substance users. Other important mental health issues are anxiety, suicidal ideation, harmful ideation or intent toward the pregnancy and unborn child. Social issues such as poverty, lack of emotional and support resources, unemployment, homelessness, physical and/or sexual abuse and criminal behaviors need to be considered in planning care.

Substance use is associated with a number of obstetric complications including: miscarriage, preterm labor, preterm rupture of membranes, placenta previa, placental abruption, preeclampsia/eclampsia, fetal growth restriction, and intrauterine fetal death. Some specific outcomes are highlighted in **Table 3**.[7-9]

MANAGEMENT STRATEGIES FOR MENTAL HEALTH PROBLEMS IN PREGNANCY AND PUERPERIUM

The general approach to managing mental health problems should include the following key elements:

- *Establishing the diagnosis:* If the diagnosis has been established from a past history or there are typical features, this is not a diagnostic challenge. However, in certain situations, one would have to proceed with a "working diagnosis" and treat accordingly. Medical and obstetric conditions which could present as mental health issues should be ruled out.
- *Assessment of risk:* The risk to the woman herself, the pregnancy in utero or the child after birth and other family members should be assessed. This depends on suicidal ideation, infanticidal thoughts, and impulses, and past history. If there is such risk, isolation of the mother from the infant is warranted. She should then be placed in an exclusive mental healthcare facility where she can be monitored and observed round the clock. These conditions justify the use of electroconvulsive therapy (ECT) in selected women.
- *Psychotherapeutics:* Medications are the mainstay of treating mental health issues today. They are discussed in the next section.
- *Non-drug treatments:* Psychotherapy is acceptable as a treatment only when the woman has mild symptoms and does not have a high risk assessment. Conditions such as mild depression, mild anxiety, PTSD and adjustment disorders are amenable to psychotherapy. A variety of

TABLE 3: Impact of substances used in pregnancy.

Substance	Embryological or Fetal effects	Perinatal effects	Comments
Nicotine	Higher risk of miscarriage. No teratogenic effects	Higher risk of preterm birth, still birth, low birth weight, placental abruption. Higher risk of sudden infant death	Risk exists with all forms of tobacco use. Smoking causes additional respiratory issues. Second hand smoke also affects outcomes
Alcohol	Alcohol is a teratogen and is responsible for Fetal Alcohol Syndrome (FAS).* Lesser degrees of affection are classified as Alcohol-related birth defects (ARBDs)	Not known	The threshold for safe alcohol consumption is not known. Therefore it is advisable for women to abstain completely
Cannabis	Higher incidence of miscarriage	Four-fold increase in low birth weight, and adverse neurodevelopment in children	
Opioids		Low birth weight, preterm birth. Neonatal abstinence syndrome (NAS)** and sudden infant deaths	
Benzodiazepines	Teratogenicity is not established but there are associations with cleft lip and cleft palate	"Floppy baby syndrome" with hypotonia, lethargy, hypothermia, breathing problems	
Illegal stimulants including cocaine, MDMA	Vascular fetal abnormalities leading to cardiac, limb and genitourinary defects	Preterm birth, hypertension, abruption	

*Fetal alcohol syndrome (FAS): The typical features are characteristic facial appearance (mid face hypoplasia, narrow palpebral fissures, thin vermillion, small philtrum, rotated low set ears and ptosis) and CNS impairment (mental retardation, small head circumference, ataxia, attention deficit disorders)
**Neonatal abstinence syndrome (NAS): Typical features are irritability, hypertonicity, tremors, exaggerated startle response, seizures, sweating, sneezing, abnormal sleep pattern, high-pitched crying, and poor sucking. As children, they have a higher risk of learning and behavior problems

treatments such as cognitive behavioral therapy (CBT), rational emotive behavior therapy (REBT) are useful in these circumstances. It should be noted that psychotherapy is not useful, and in fact the delay in treatment can be harmful when used in moderate to severe depression, obsessive compulsive disorder, and psychosis.

- *Multidisciplinary approach:* The team should include an obstetrician, psychiatrist, pediatrician, pharmacologist, internist specializing in drug use and social workers. This allows for a holistic approach to the woman's care in pregnancy and postpartum.

MANAGEMENT STRATEGIES FOR SUBSTANCE USE IN PREGNANCY

Women with serious substance use issues should be cared for by a multidisciplinary team as described earlier. Though the ideal would be to completely stop substance abuse, this may not be a practical goal. Some important aspects to consider are the levels of usage, dependence, readiness to quit, past attempts at quitting. The principle of care is minimizing harm to the mother and fetus. Initial efforts should be focused on promoting a safe and healthy lifestyle (including sexual), crime minimization, avoiding shared needles, and maintaining routine antenatal care measures. Psychosocial therapies (includes counseling, education, relapse prevention, self-help groups, formal therapies like cognitive behavior intervention) are important interventions for treatment.

- Nicotine is the most common substance used by women and the first step is to use psychosocial interventions. Nicotine replacement therapy (NRT) can have a substantial impact on the chances that a dependent smoker will be able to quit, but there is concern that its use in pregnancy may have adverse effects on the fetus. The safety and efficacy in pregnancy of pharmacotherapies such as NRT and bupropion is still debated and further research is required.
- Women abusing alcohol should be advised to minimize consumption by switching to spirits with lower alcohol content or quitting altogether.
- Women using opioids can be offered treatment with methadone maintenance. The advantages of using methadone is avoiding the high risk behavior which comes from using street drugs, effects of contaminants and the fluctuating levels of opiates. The woman may still continue using street drugs to fulfill the need for a "high". Women who are compliant may also be considered for gradual dose reduction and stopping methadone use. This should preferably be done in the second trimester. Buprenorphine is another drug which can be given for maintenance without naloxone.

PSYCHIATRIC MEDICATIONS IN PREGNANCY AND BREASTFEEDING

The range of drugs available to treat mental health disorders is vast. The principles to be followed are to use the least effective dose of the least number of medications. Polypharmacy should be avoided as far as possible. It is useful to divide the daily dose requirement in two or three portions to avoid high peak serum concentrations unless compliance is an issue. The medications used should be monitored clinically or biochemically if needed. There would be changes in the dose requirement as pregnancy advances.

Drugs are effective and have been ratified as evidence based therapy in these conditions. Medical treatment of psychiatric issues usually results in dramatic improvements in the maternal condition. The improvement is usually seen in a week and sustained improvement is seen over the next 2–3 weeks until there is a therapeutic plateau.

The use of psychoactive medications should be considered in the context of potential effects on the fetus in pregnancy and the neonate in breastfeeding women. The impact of these medications in pregnancy and breastfeeding are described in **Table 4**. The decision to use medications is based on the principle that untreated mental health problems would cause more harm to the mother or the fetus/newborn than the relatively small risk posed by the use of the medications. It is preferable to have a well-controlled mental health issue in a pregnant and breastfeeding woman rather than leaving her untreated.

Perinatal Care and Infrastructure for Women with Mental Health Issues and Substance Use

Antenatal care should focus on evaluation of the fetal anatomy to establish a normal structure. Women should be counseled that some of the abnormalities that are seen with the use of drugs are functional and not detected by ultrasound. Some abnormalities, especially nonlethal, minor ones, may be missed. The other care aspects in pregnancy should include screening for sexually transmitted infections, vaginal infections, cervical assessment for preterm birth risk stratification and growth monitoring. Routine supplements should suffice unless there are specific deficiencies. Folic acid supplement should be continued throughout pregnancy.

In labor, the short-term use of injectable medications may be considered for acute behavioral control in women who have not been treated. This can be achieved with haloperidol (2–5 mg) and promethazine (10–25 mg) administered intramuscular. This can be repeated upto three times a day. The route of delivery should be governed by obstetric factors. There are no special considerations for the use of epidural or spinal anesthesia for these women. In case a woman needs general anesthesia, it can be safely administered. Larger doses of anesthetic drug are needed for these women.

The delivery should be attended by a neonatologist. This is needed especially for women with substance use problems. Some infants of mothers who have been on psychotropic drugs may exhibit a neonatal abstinence syndrome (NAS) as outlined in **Table 3**. If resuscitation is required, naloxone is contraindicated due to the risk of severe withdrawal effects. The neonate may exhibit a metabolic and thermoregulatory imbalance and may be shifted to the special unit.

Postnatal care of the woman involves supporting her in the care of the child. Breastfeeding is encouraged for most women. Appropriate contraceptive advice and safe sex practice guidelines should be provided at discharge.

■ KEY MESSAGES

- Pregnancy and lactation are special situations for women with mental health issues.
- Women's healthcare providers should be trained to be empathetic to mental health issues.
- One in five individuals will face mental illness in their lifetimes. After childbirth, about 80% of women will experience "postpartum blues" and 20% will have postpartum depression.
- Approximately half of the general population has an experience with substance use that is serious enough to temporarily affect their physical or mental health.
- The woman who has a preexisting mental health issue should ideally be seen in the preconception period but this may not occur due to stigma.
- A bare minimum enquiry into her mood in the postnatal ward and at the postnatal visit should be mandatory.
- T-ACE, TWEAK and AUDIT are validated questionnaires for heavy substance use.
- It is not possible to accurately predict the impact that pregnancy would have on preexisting mental health issues due to complex multifactorial inputs in an individual woman.

TABLE 4: Psychotherapeutic drugs in pregnancy and breastfeeding.

No teratogenic effects demonstrated	No teratogenic effects but fertility is affected	Teratogenic effects not well established	Teratogenic
SSRI (Sertraline, Citalopram, Fluoxetine, etc.)	Typical antipsychotics (Haloperidol, Trifluoperazine) and atypical antipsychotics (Risperidone, olanzepine) Raise prolactin, may affect ovulation	Lithium and Ebstein's anomaly (<1%)	Mood stabilizers such as valproic acid and carbamazepine (1–6% risk of NTD)
Tricyclic antidepressants (amitriptyline, imipramine, etc.)		Benzodiazepines and cleft lip/palate—association is not well established.	
Lamotrigine			

- There are well-established embryological, fetal and perinatal risks with mental health problems in the mother. Treated women are less likely to have such outcomes.
- Acute maternal effects of substance use can include overdose, intoxication or withdrawal and can resemble general medical conditions and obstetric disorders.
- The principles of treating mental health issues in pregnancy and puerperium are—establishing the diagnosis, assessment of risk, use of psychotherapeutic drugs and other treatments.
- Medications are the mainstay of treating mental health issues today. Psychotherapy is acceptable as a treatment only when the woman has mild symptoms and does not have a high risk assessment.
- The decision to use medications is based on the principle that untreated mental health problems would cause more harm to the mother or the fetus/newborn than the relatively small risk posed by the use of the medications.
- In labor, acute behavioral control in women can be achieved with haloperidol (2–5 mg) and promethazine (10–25 mg) administered intramuscular. The route of delivery should be governed by obstetric factors. The delivery should be attended by a neonatologist.
- Postnatal care of the woman involves supporting her in the care of the child. Breastfeeding is encouraged for most women.

REFERENCES

1. Global, regional, and national incidence, prevalence, and years lived with disability for 354 diseases and injuries for 195 countries and territories, 1990–2017: a systematic analysis for the Global Burden of Disease Study 2017. GBD 2017 Disease and Injury Incidence and Prevalence Collaborators. Lancet. 2018;392:1789-858.
2. World Health Organization. Mental Health and Substance Use: Maternal Health. [Online] Available from: https://www.who.int/teams/mental-health-and-substance-use/maternal-mental-health. [Last Accessed October, 2021].
3. American Psychiatric Association (APA). Diagnostic and Statistical Manual of Mental Health Disorders Version 5. Washington: APA; 2013.
4. Cox JL, Holden JM, Sagovsky R. Detection of postnatal depression: Development of the 10-item Edinburgh Postnatal Depression Scale. Br J Psychiatr. 1987;150:782-6.
5. Russell M. New Assessment Tools for Risk Drinking During Pregnancy: T-ACE, TWEAK, and others. Alcohol Health Res World. 1994;18:55-61.
6. Misra DP, Guyer B, Allston A. Integrated perinatal health framework. A multiple determinants model with a lifespan approach. Am J Prev Med. 2003;25:65-75.
7. Wisner KL, Sit DKY, Bogen MA. Mental Health and Behavioral Disorders in Pregnancy. Niebyl JR, Simpson JL et al Gabbe SG (Eds). Obstetrics: Normal and Problem Pregnancies, 7th edition. New York: Elsevier; 2017. pp. 1147-72.
8. Wilson C, Peters L, Lingford-Hughes A. Substance Misuse in Pregnancy. Howard L, von Dadelszen P (Eds). The Continuous Textbook of Women's Medicine Series - Obstetrics Module Volume 7. Maternal Mental Health in Pregnancy. London: GLOWM (Global Library of Women's Medicine); 2021.
9. Royal College of Obstetricians and Gynaecologists. Alcohol in pregnancy discussed in updated patient information. [Online] Available from: https://www.rcog.org.uk/en/news/rcog-release-alcohol-in-pregnancy-discussed-in-updated-patient-information/#:~:text=The%20guidance%20states%20that%20drinking,once%20or%20twice%20a%20week. [Last Accessed October, 2021].

LONG QUESTIONS

1. Discuss the short- and long-term impact of mental health problems in pregnancy on the mother and the offspring.
2. Discuss the medical and obstetric risks that the mother faces due to substance use in pregnancy. How can these women be identified early and managed adequately?
3. Discuss the broad outline of the management strategies for mental health issues in pregnancy and breastfeeding women.

SHORT QUESTIONS

1. What are the common mental health problems that one may come across in pregnancy?
2. What are the DSM-V criteria for the diagnosis of major depression?
3. What factors contribute to depression in the postpartum period?
4. What is the Edinburgh Postnatal Depression Scale?
5. What are the questionnaires to diagnose heavy substance use?
6. What are the effects of alcohol in pregnancy?
7. Enumerate the effects of smoking in pregnancy. What is Nicotine Replacement Therapy? Can it be used in pregnancy?
8. Why is a multidisciplinary team important in managing women with mental health and substance use issues in pregnancy?

MULTIPLE CHOICE QUESTIONS

1. Approximately what proportion of women develops postpartum depression?
   a. 2%
   b. 5%
   c. 20%
   d. 80%
2. The most common mental health issue that women face in pregnancy and puerperium is:
   a. Anxiety
   b. Depression
   c. Eating disorders
   d. Schizophrenia
3. The following conditions are a part of the anxiety disorder spectrum, except:
   a. Bipolar disorder
   b. Generalize anxiety disorder
   c. Panic attacks
   d. Post-traumatic stress disorder

4. The biological factor that is contributory to the causation of postnatal depression is:
   a. Fluctuations in oxytocin and prolactin levels due to breastfeeding
   b. Withdrawal of progesterone levels
   c. Poverty
   d. Lack of partner support
5. The following are commonly used psychotherapies in pregnancy:
   a. Cognitive behavioral therapy
   b. Rational emotional behavioral therapy
   c. Hypnotherapy
   d. Electroconvulsive therapy
6. The fetal abnormality associated with Lithium use in pregnancy is:
   a. Neural tube defect
   b. Cleft lip and cleft palate
   c. Ebstein's anomaly
   d. Urogenital sinus
7. Which of the following drug is associated with a higher risk of neural tube defects:
   a. Valproic acid
   b. Lithium
   c. Benzodiazepines
   d. Imipramine
8. The following statement regarding substance use in pregnancy are true:
   a. Women who abuse drugs or alcohol usually do so in isolation and use only one substance at a time
   b. Most women using street drugs in pregnancy are careful of obtaining it in a pure form
   c. Pregnant women with substance abuse issues have a higher risk of being infected with Hepatitis C
   d. Fetal growth is not affected by recreational drugs
9. The following elements of care are essential for women abusing substance in pregnancy, except:
   a. Meeting a variety of care givers changing with every visit
   b. Multidisciplinary team approach
   c. Empathetic, nonjudgmental approach
   d. Overall assessment of socioeconomic situation
10. The following are commonly seen medical problems with women using street drugs, except:
    a. Sexually transmitted infections
    b. Thrombophlebitis
    c. Mental health problems
    d. Obesity
11. Substance use is associated with the following perinatal effects:
    a. Macrosomia
    b. Antepartum hemorrhage
    c. Postdatism
    d. Postpartum hemorrhage
12. The following is not a feature of fetal alcohol syndrome (FAS):
    a. Wide palpebral fissures
    b. Mid face hypoplasia
    c. Growth restriction
    d. Attention deficit disorder
13. The following statement regarding alcohol use in pregnancy is true:
    a. Women generally admit to alcohol use openly
    b. Fetal alcohol syndrome occurs in 50% of women with exposure to more than 6 drinks consumed in the first trimester
    c. Fetal alcohol syndrome is characterized by neural tube defects
    d. Stopping alcohol use suddenly can result in delirium tremens
14. The following is the correct drug to be used in opioid substitution therapy:
    a. Ketamine
    b. Morphine
    c. Methadone
    d. Bupropion

Answers
1. c 2. b 3. a 4. b 5. d 6. c
7. a 8. c 9. a 10. d 11. b 12. a
13. d 14. c

5.14 OBESITY

Ashis Kumar Mukhopadhyay, Maya Mukhopadhyay

INTRODUCTION

Obesity must be considered as a serious health hazard associated with several types of morbidity and consequent mortality. Obesity has now emerged as a global pandemic, marching ahead relentlessly, affecting the entire population. There is no respite from this ongoing onslaught also in sight, because with the advent of technology and our lifestyle changes, we are **"eating more and moving less!"** There is an abundant supply of cheap high calorie food around us and the young generation just loves that! This, coupled with a formidable lack of physical activities and a sedentary lifestyle, is perpetuating into a metabolic dysregulation creating an *obesity cycle!* According to World Health Organization (WHO), *worldwide obesity has nearly tripled since 1975;* 39% of adults aged 18 years and over were overweight [body mass index (BMI ≥25)] in 2016, and 13% were obese (BMI ≥30).[1]

Evidence already exists that overweight and obesity are highly prevalent among women of reproductive age, accounting for 40–60% in developed countries and 30–40% in developing countries.[2] The most modest data obtained recently was from Ethiopia where prevalence of overweight and obesity among reproductive age group women was 11.5% and 3.4% respectively in an Ethiopian demographic study.[3] In another Chinese study it was reported as 16.5%.[4] The prevalence of *overweight* and *obesity in India* is increasing faster than the world average. For instance, the prevalence of *overweight* increased from 8.4 to 15.5% among women between 1998 and 2015, and the prevalence of *obesity* increased from 2.2 to 5.1% over the same period.[5] 80% of the obese population are from urban, educated and wealthy background.

Obesity has been defined as a chronic low grade inflammatory disease. The etiopathology is multifactorial. Obesity can be primary (due to nutritional disorder) and Secondary (due to genetic, hormonal or iatrogenic factors) According to the classification based on BMI, a person is considered overweight for BMI values > 25 kg/m² and obese when BMI > 30 kg/m².

OBESITY PARADOX

World Health Organization defines obesity as a "condition in which percentage body fat (PBF) is increased to an extent at which health and well-being are impaired". Therefore, a definition based on BMI may be misleading at times, e.g., an athlete may have an increased BMI but reduced fat mass and still according to definition be called overweight. This is what is referred to as "obesity paradox".

The obese population is more prone to have comorbidities such as:
- Arterial hypertension
- Type 2 diabetes mellitus (T2DM)
- Coronary artery disease
- Cholelithiasis
- Polycystic ovary syndrome (PCOS)
- Obstructive sleep apnea
- Breast and endometrial neoplasms.

Obesity plays a significant role in the development of female specific reproductive health issues, and to understand the effects of obesity in reproduction, *we need to understand the basics first.*

Menstrual Irregularities

Due to alterations of the hypothalamic-pituitary-ovarian (HPO) axis from different reasons.

Obesity induces a hyperinsulinemic state. This reduces the level of sex hormone-binding globulin (SHBG). A large amount of free androgens are therefore released which are aromatized in the peripheral fat (already in excess) to produce large amounts of estrogens thus suppressing the gonadotropins produced by Pituitary.

Adipokines are cytokines from fat which can affect ovulation. The circulating levels of leptin are high in obese woman. These can cause suppression of HPO axis by down regulation of hypothalamic receptors.

Subfertility and Infertility

Obese women can remain subfertile even if they are ovulating regularly suggesting that the quality of oocyte is poor or below the standard.

Causes of poor quality oocytes may be some of the following:
- Obesity being a chronic inflammatory condition the levels of C-reactive proteins (CRP), adipokines and interleukin are all increased altering the follicular environment.
- The follicle contains increased levels of insulin, triglycerides, CRP and lactates which affect folliculogenesis and oocyte quality.

Pregnancy Loss and Recurrent Pregnancy Loss

Formation of a compromised zygote from fertilization of a poor quality oocyte ultimately leads to pregnancy loss which can be recurrent. The coexisting hyperinsulinemic environment causes reduction of glycodelin which is responsible for recurrent pregnancy loss (RPL). It also decreases levels of insulin-like growth factor binding protein-1 (IGFBP-1). This compromises the anchoring of the embryo to the uterine wall.

A study on the chromosomal makeup of abortus specimens from patients of RPL showed that obese women had a much higher rate of euploid pregnancy loss as compared to lean women.

Effects of Obesity on Male Reproduction

Studies are fewer in this field. But it is certain that male obesity predisposes to subfertility and infertility in a similar manner. The hypothalamic pituitary gonadal axis is disrupted in the same way as in the female by hyperinsulinemia. As a result of this, decreased Leydig cell testosterone secretion affects spermatogenesis.

The function of Sertoli cells is affected by this decreased testosterone which causes phagocytosis of mature spermatids and low sperm counts. Decrease in gonadotropins, SHBG and inhibin B—all affect Sertoli cell function leading to poor motility and morphology as well.

Male obesity can cause direct thermal damage to the testicles causing DNA fragmentation. Also, there is decreased libido, erectile and ejaculatory dysfunction due to reduced testosterone.

Obstetrical Complications in Obese Pregnant Patients (Table 1)

In simple words, obese women often suffer *early onset preeclampsia (EOPET) and gestational diabetes mellitus (GDM), apart from causing increased incidence of spontaneous abortion* (13.6% vs. 10.7%, OR: 1.31), according to the pooled data analysis of six studies which found the higher rates of miscarriage rate after spontaneous conception[6] and *RPL (three times more).*[7] Also, chromosomal analysis in these miscarriages showed that most of the miscarriages in obese women compared to their normal counterparts are euploid

TABLE 1: Risks associated and their correlation with BMI.

Condition	R/R BMI >40 versus BMI <25	Reference
Induction of labor	1.39	10
C-section	2.02	10
Emergency C-section	2.11	8
Postoperative wound healing complications	2.17	10
Complications of anesthesia and obstetric interventions	1.5	17
Severe PPH with transfusion	0.7	17
Sepsis	1.4	17
Obstetric shock	1.5	17
ICU admission	2.4	17
SAMM	1.4	17

(BMI: body mass index; ICU: intensive care unit; PPH: postpartum hemorrhage; SAMM: severe acute maternal morbidity)

in nature (58% vs. 37%), when confounding factors such as maternal age, endocrine, autoimmune and inflammatory diseases were excluded from the studies.[7]

Ovesen et al. reported a *doubling of IUFD* in obese women. A 5-min Apgar score <7 was also reported, along with fetal macrosomia (>4,500 g) in the same series.[8]

Fetal macrosomia has been extensively reviewed by a meta-analysis including 21 studies which has shown *13.4 % risk of fetal macosomia in obese women versus 7.8%* in normal weights, with a pooled *OR of 2.11*.[9]

It has been firmly established by many studies that neonates from obese mothers have a higher percentage of body fat. In another study comprising of more than 100,000 deliveries of women without any chronic diseases like DM or hypertension, it was shown that the percentage of fetal macrosomia [large for gestational age (LGA)] had shown a consistent rise in obese women, accounting for 17% compared to 8% among normal-weight mothers. Meconium aspiration syndrome, neonatal sepsis and neonatal admission at NICU were all increased twice in obese women.[10]

The pathogenesis of fetal macrosomia is complex and ill-understood. On one hand, macrosomia appears to be the consequence of increased maternal blood glucose levels, resulting from obesity-related insulin resistance[11,12] and on the other hand, however, the increase in percentage of adipose tissue in the neonate can only be attributed to the increased availability of metabolic substrates, indicating that placenta acts like a nutritive sensor.[13]

These pregnancy associated disorders increase proportionately with increasing severity of obesity during pregnancy. Even a minor 10% increase from pre-pregnancy BMI is associated with at least 10% rise in RR of HDP and GDM in the index pregnancy.[14] It has got a long-term effect (>10 years) on development of T2DM and heart disease also in future life. The effect of increased weight gain during pregnancy (>15 kg) have been associated with developing obesity later in life.[15]

Gestational diabetes mellitus shows an 11 times increase as the BMI increases from 25 to 40, whereas preeclampsia increases more than 4 times in the same BMI window of change.[16]

All forms of significant morbidities, e.g., thromboembolic diseases, CVS or CNS morbidities, respiratory morbidities or problems related to anesthesia increase 2-4 times. Risk of PPH, sepsis, obstetric shock, ICU admission and SAMM—all risks are doubled.[17]

Mechanism: Clinical and experimental evidence suggests that the metabolic alterations associated with obesity such as hyperlipidemia, hyperinsulinemia and hyperleptinemia are responsible in the pathogenesis of preeclampsia[18] and GDM. Moreover, levels of total serum cholesterol in the first and second trimester of gestation predict the onset of preeclampsia.

In obesity, there is an increased level of LDL and triglycerides and a decreased level of HDL. LDL reduces extravillous cytotrophoblastic migration and promotes trophoblast apoptosis.

Experimental studies show that hyperinsulinemia produces a shallower implantation site and altered nitric oxide (NO) synthesis which causes thickening of tunica media enhancing vasoconstriction of the arterioles and preventing relaxation. It is now accepted that optimum levels of NO production in the vascular endothelium in all tissues of the body are imperative for hemodynamic adaptation during pregnancy.

In addition to this, the low grade inflammatory state of obesity causes an increase in proinflammatory cytokines such as TNF alpha, interleukin 6 and leptin. On the other hand plasma adiponectin levels are decreased.

Adiponectin is a protein hormone which enhances insulin sensitivity by regulating fatty acid oxidation. It stimulates NO production in the endothelial cells lining the vasculature. It regulates vascular homeostasis and modulates excess inflammatory response.

Therefore there is consequent injury to the endothelial lining resulting in PET, IUGR and even IUFD.

Apart from fetal loss and RPL, there is high incidence of preterm labor both spontaneous and induced is common in obese patients. Spontaneous labor can occur as early as 32 weeks and induction of premature delivery to combat the effects of severe PET and/or GDM is often done between 35 and 36 weeks.

INCREASED INCIDENCE OF CONGENITAL ANOMALIES

As DM and abnormal glucose tolerance are common complications of obesity the incidence of congenital anomalies are expectedly on the higher side. But we have to also remember that the associated DM is not always the

TABLE 2: Malformations list and the relative risk (RR).

BMI >40 versus BMI <25	
Severe congenital malformations	1.37
CNS malformations	1.88
Spina bifida	2.24
Congenital heart disease	1.44
Cleft lip and palate	1.44
Eye malformations	1.03
GI malformations	1.54
Urinary tract malformations	1.19
Genital malformations	1.43
Limb defects	1.29
Others	1.39

causative factor; the prevalence of fetal malformations was significantly correlated with the severity of obesity **(Table 2)** and the risk increase was *independent of gestational diabetes*.[19]

Studies conducted earlier also have shown that after excluding women with DM even the risk of neonatal malformations remains high in obese pregnancies implying the possible role of other metabolic factors that are coexistent such as hyperinsulinism, hyperlipidemia and inflammation.

Apart from that, a meta-analysis comprising 18 studies reported the following obesity-associated increases in risk for specific malformations.[19]

Only the risk of gastroschisis was lower with obesity [n = 379, OR: 0.17 (0.10; 0.30)], p <0.001. However, we have to keep in mind that diagnosis is dependent on Ultrasound, which suffers from unfavorable physical scanning conditions due to excessive abdominal fat.

The adipose tissue itself acts like an endocrine organ being metabolically active producing several hormones enzymes and coenzymes. In obesity it is widely distributed in the subcutaneous and visceral tissues. The latter particularly is associated with a state of vascular malfunction. This contributes to abnormal placental metabolism which can affect organogenesis and fetal development.

The congenital anomalies in obesity are multiorgan defects but the largest organ specific risks are observed in the nervous system such as neural tube defects and cognitive impairment, viz. autism attention-deficit hyperactivity disorder (ADHD) and psychoses.

Congenital heart defects, limb defects, digestive tract defects are all increased in obese women.

PERINATAL COMPLICATIONS

Maternal obesity is associated with an elevated mortality in the 1st year of life[20] and effect was observed more in term neonates compared with the preterm ones, and this was independent of the medical and obstetric disorders such as DM and hypertension in pregnancy. This contributed to 11% of maternal deaths attributed to maternal obesity. Many other studies have confirmed this association also.

The incidence of preterm labor is higher in obese women as mentioned earlier. When induced labor may not progress desirably due to dysfunctional labor pains and in coordinate uterine contractions. Both these conditions of spontaneous and medically indicated preterm births due to pregnancy associated complications are increased in obesity and contribute significantly to the unfavorable neonatal outcome.[21]

MANAGEMENT OF OBESITY IN PREGNANCY (TABLES 3 TO 6)

We have two very recent guidelines at hand:
1. FIGO Committee guidelines for the management of prepregnancy, pregnancy and post-pregnancy obesity. First published: 07 September 2020.[22]
2. RCOG Green Top Guidelines no. 72, 21 Nov 2018, available online at https://doi.org/10.1111/1471-0528.15386.[23]

Excerpts of both these guidelines are presented here in summary.

Prepregnancy Care

All women should have their BMI calculated. Women with a BMI > or equal to 30 should be educated and advised about the effects of obesity on fertility, the risks during pregnancy and childbirth and the long-term effects of obesity on them and their offsprings.

All women with obesity should be encouraged to lose weight by diet control and adopting a healthy lifestyle which includes moderate exercise. If required, other weight management interventions may be required such as bariatric surgery. Preconception counseling, contraceptive advice or treatment of any other gynecological problem prior to pregnancy.

Assessment for sleep apnea and other comorbidities that could affect health during pregnancy have to be traced such as cardiac, pulmonary, and endocrine problems.

All women with obesity should be advised to take at least 5 mg folic acid supplementation daily for at least 1–3 months before conception.

Pregnancy Management

All women should have their height and weight checked in the first antenatal visit whereby their BMI is ascertained. Advice on required weight gain during pregnancy is stressed.

Availability of large blood pressure cuffs, appropriately sized compression stockings and pneumatic compression devices, sit-on weighing scale, large chairs without arms, large wheelchairs, ultrasound scan couches, ward and delivery beds, mattresses, theater trolleys, operating theater tables, lifting and lateral transfer equipment should be ensured at the clinic.[23]

The RCOG recommends that serial measurement of symphysis fundal height (SFH) is recommended at each antenatal appointment from 24 weeks of gestation, but women with a BMI greater than 35 kg/m^2 are more likely to have inaccurate SFH measurements and should be referred for serial assessment of fetal size using ultrasound.[23]

TABLE 3: The International Federation of Gynecology and Obstetrics (FIGO) Committee guideline for the management of prepregnancy, pregnancy, and postpartum obesity (September 2020).

Time point A: Prepregnancy

A.1	All women should have their weight and height measured and their body mass index (BMI, calculated as weight in kilograms divided by height in meters squared) calculated. Consider ethnic differences
A.2	All women with a BMI of ≥30 should be advised of the effect of obesity on fertility, the immediate risks of obesity during pregnancy and childbirth, and the subsequent long-term health effect of obesity including the higher risk of noncommunicable diseases for them and their children
A.3	All women with obesity should be encouraged to lose weight through diet and adopting a healthy lifestyle including moderate physical activity. If indicated and available, other weight management interventions might be considered, including bariatric surgery
A.4	All women with obesity should be advised to take at least 0.4 mg (400 μg) and consider up to 5 mg folic acid supplementation daily for at least 1–3 months before conception

Time point B: Pregnancy

B.1	All women should have their weight and height measured and their BMI calculated at the first antenatal visit. Consider ethnic differences. Advise on appropriate gestational weight gain
B.2	All women should receive information on diet and lifestyle appropriate to their gestation including nutrient supplements, weight management, and regular physical activity
B.3	All women with obesity should be advised of the risks of obesity and excess gestational weight gain on pregnancy, childbirth, and long-term health including risk of noncommunicable diseases for them and their children
B.4	All antenatal healthcare facilities should have well-defined multidisciplinary pathways for the clinical management of pregnant women with obesity including the identification and treatment of pregnancy-related complications

Time point C: Postpartum

C.1	All women with prepregnancy obesity should receive support on breastfeeding initiation and maintenance
C.2	All women with obesity and pregnancy complications should receive appropriate postnatal follow-up in line with local resources, care pathways, and in response to the individual health requirements of each woman and her children
C.3	All women with obesity should be encouraged to lose weight postpartum with emphasis on healthy diet, breastfeeding if possible, and regular moderate physical activity. They should be advised of the importance of long-term follow-up as they and their children are at increased risk for noncommunicable diseases
C.4	Maternal obesity should be considered when making the decision regarding the most appropriate form of postnatal contraception

TABLE 4: Good clinical practice recommendations for prepregnancy obesity (time point A).

Recommendation		Strength
A.1.1	Primary care services should support women of childbearing age with weight management before pregnancy and body mass index (BMI, calculated as weight in kilograms divided by the square of height in meters) should be measured. Advice on weight and lifestyle should be given during periodic health examinations, preconception counseling, contraceptive consultations, or other gynecologic care prior to pregnancy	Conditional
A.2.1	Women of childbearing age with obesity should receive information and advice about the effect of obesity on fertility and the risks of obesity during pregnancy and childbirth	Conditional
A.2.2	Assessment for sleep apnea and other conditions that could affect health during pregnancy, including those of the cardiac, pulmonary, renal, endocrine, and skin systems is warranted in the preconception period	Conditional
A.3.1	Weight management strategies prior to pregnancy could include dietary, exercise, medical, and surgical approaches. Diet and exercise are the cornerstones of weight management in preconception and pregnancy	Conditional
A.4.1	Women with a BMI ≥30 wishing to become pregnant should be advised to take a folic acid supplement daily, starting at least 1–3 months before conception and continuing during the first trimester of pregnancy. The dose should be at least 0.4 mg (400 μg) and consideration should be given to a higher dose (5 mg) as obesity is a risk factor for neural tube defects	Strong

TABLE 5: Good clinical practice recommendations for pregnancy obesity (time point B).

Recommendation		Strength
B.1.1	All pregnant women should have their height and weight measured at their first antenatal visit. This can be used to calculate body mass index (BMI, calculated as weight in kilograms divided by the square of height in meters). Data should be recorded in the medical records	Conditional
B.1.2	Approaches to monitor and manage gestational weight gain should be integrated into routine antenatal care practices	Strong
B.1.3	Pregnant women with a BMI ≥30 should be advised to avoid high gestational weight gain. Weight gain should be limited to 5–9 kg	Strong
B.2.1	The mainstay of weight management during pregnancy is diet and exercise. Health professionals should provide general nutrition information and advice on a healthy diet to manage weight during pregnancy. Where resources permit, individual plans for diet and exercise for weight management should be put in place	Conditional
B.2.2	Moderate intensity and appropriate exercise should be encouraged during pregnancy	Strong
B.2.3	Women with obesity should continue to take folic acid during at least the first trimester	Strong
B.2.4	Women with previous bariatric surgery require closer screening and monitoring of their nutritional status and fetal growth throughout pregnancy. They should be referred to a dietitian for advice about their nutritional needs and, where possible, have consultant-led care	Conditional
B.3.1	All pregnant women with obesity in early pregnancy should be provided with accurate and accessible information about the risks associated with obesity and how they may be minimized	Conditional
B.3.2	Women should be informed that some screening processes for chromosomal anomalies are less effective in obesity.	Strong
B.3.3	All pregnant women should be advised individually on mode of delivery, considering the risk of emergency cesarean delivery	Conditional
B.4.1	Where possible, healthcare facilities should have clearly defined pathways for the management of pregnant women with obesity. The adequacy of resources and equipment available should be considered when making decisions around care, especially for women with a BMI ≥40	Conditional
B.4.2	Women with obesity with multiple gestations require increased surveillance and may benefit from consultation with a maternal–fetal medicine consultant	Strong
B.4.3	All pregnant women with a BMI ≥30 should be screened for gestational diabetes in early pregnancy	Strong
B.4.4	Where available, an appropriately sized blood pressure cuff should be used for measurements. The cuff size used at the earliest time point should be documented in the medical records	Conditional
B.4.5	To help prevent preeclampsia, prophylactic aspirin from early pregnancy can be recommended to women with obesity who have other moderate to high risk factors	Strong
B.4.6	Clinicians should be aware that women with a BMI ≥30, before pregnancy or in early pregnancy, have a preexisting risk factor for developing venous thromboembolism during pregnancy. Risk of antenatal and postnatal venous thromboembolism should be assessed	Strong
B.4.7	If available, women with a BMI ≥35 should be referred for serial assessment of fetal size using ultrasound as they are more likely to have inaccurate symphysis–fundal height measurements	Conditional
B.4.8	Due to the elevated risk of stillbirth associated with obesity, greater fetal surveillance is recommended in the third trimester in the case of reduced fetal movements	Conditional
B.4.9	Women with a BMI ≥30 are at increased risk of mental health problems, including anxiety and depression. Healthcare professionals should offer psychological support, screen for anxiety and depression, and refer for further support where appropriate and available	Strong
B.4.10	Induction of labor is recommended at 41^{+0} weeks of gestation for women with a BMI ≥35 owing to their increased risk of intrauterine death	Strong
B.4.11	Women with a BMI ≥40 should be referred to an anesthetist for assessment in the antenatal period	Conditional
B.4.12	Electronic fetal monitoring is recommended for women in active labor with a BMI ≥35. Intrauterine pressure catheters and fetal scalp electrodes may help	Conditional
B.4.13	In the case of vaginal delivery for women with a BMI ≥40, early placement of an epidural catheter is advisable in the case of an emergency cesarean delivery	Conditional
B.4.14	Establish venous access in early labor for women with a BMI ≥40 and consider a second cannula	Conditional
B.4.15	Women with a BMI ≥30 having a cesarean delivery are at increased risk of wound infection and should receive prophylactic antibiotics at the time of surgery. Women with obesity may benefit from higher doses	Strong
B.4.16	Active management of the third stage should be recommended to reduce the risk of postpartum hemorrhage	Strong
B.4.17	Postoperative pharmacologic thromboprophylaxis should be prescribed based on maternal weight	Conditional
B.4.18	Mechanical thromboprophylaxis is recommended before and after cesarean delivery. Where available, women with a BMI ≥35 should be given graduated compression stockings, or other interventions such as sequential compression devices, after cesarean delivery until mobilization, which should be encouraged early	Conditional

TABLE 6: Good clinical practice recommendations for postpartum obesity (time point C).

Recommendation		Strength
C.1.1	Obesity is associated with low breastfeeding initiation and maintenance. Women with obesity in early pregnancy should receive specialist advice on the benefits of breastfeeding and appropriate antenatal and postnatal support for breastfeeding initiation and maintenance	Conditional
C.2.1	Women with obesity who have been diagnosed with gestational diabetes and other pregnancy complications should have appropriate postnatal follow-up	Conditional
C.2.2	Due to the increased risk associated with obesity, where available, women with obesity should be screened for postpartum mental health disorders such as depression and anxiety	Strong
C.3.1	Women should be informed that weight loss between pregnancies reduces the risk of stillbirth, hypertensive complications, and fetal macrosomia in subsequent pregnancies. Weight loss increases the chances of successful vaginal birth after cesarean delivery	Strong
C.3.2	Women with obesity should be offered further dietary and physical activity advice to support postpartum weight management	Conditional
C.4.1	Women with obesity should be counseled on the most appropriate form of postnatal contraception based on BMI	Conditional

They should be advised to use practical weight control diets not compromising on nutrition and exercise, consistent with their period of gestation. If required a dietitian may be required to map a diet chart for her.

For a woman whose BMI is 30 or more gain in weight during pregnancy should be between 5 and 9 kg, although RCOG maintains that there is a lack of consensus on optimal gestational weight gain. Until further evidence is available, a focus on a healthy diet may be more applicable than prescribed weight gain targets.[23]

Women with history of bariatric surgery need special attention toward their diet and nutrition and can be referred to a dietitian.

Obese women should be clearly informed that some tests for anomaly screening may not be foolproof in obesity such as chromosomal screening and ultrasound imaging where the gross amount of abdominal fat makes for poor viewing. RCOG recommends that all women should be offered antenatal screening for chromosomal anomalies, and consider the use of transvaginal ultrasound in women in whom it is difficult to obtain nuchal translucency measurements transabdominally.[23]

All pregnant women should be screened for gestational DM early in pregnancy. An appropriate BP cuff to measure blood pressure should be used otherwise it is only too easy to miss early onset PET.

As a means to prevent preeclampsia early tablet Aspirin can be given to those patients who have other additional risk factors. *Antiobesity or weight loss drugs are not recommended for use in pregnancy.*[23]

Patient should be made aware about the real danger of deep vein thrombosis and embolism.

In effect, obese pregnant women should undergo detailed and frequent surveillance all throughout pregnancy and particularly in the third trimester.

Mental depression and anxiety are common in most obese women.

An anesthetic checkup must be done for all women in the third trimester with close monitoring of the cardiac functions.

Labor and Delivery Issues

Electronic monitoring is always preferred during labor for these patients.

The risks associated with labor and delivery are discussed here. *The likelihood of vaginal delivery decreases with increasing obesity,*[24] as shown in **Table 1**.

Delivery by lower uterine segment cesarean section (LUCS) is found to be more common in obese mothers. We all know the reasons behind increased rates of C-section in obese mothers, especially because of the association with diabetes, hypertension and other complications, but the fat deposition that occurs in the pelvis tends to narrow down the birth passage and leads to consequent cephalopelvic disproportion (CPD). RCOG maintains that *women undergoing cesarean section who have more than 2 cm subcutaneous fat should have suturing of the subcutaneous tissue space in order to reduce the risk of wound infection and wound separation.*[23]

Where macrosomia is suspected, induction of labor may be considered. Macrosomia and cervical dystocia also predispose to surgical intervention. The decision of VBAC should be individualized.[23]

Surgical intervention itself is a complication in obesity due to high incidence of wound infection and vascular thrombosis, and they contribute to significant post-operative morbidity. Regional anesthesia is often unsuccessful and requires the services from a team of qualified anesthetists.

Active management of the third stage of labor is advised for all women, the increased risk of PPH in those with a BMI greater than 30 kg/m² makes this even more important PPH incidence is found to be increased in these cases.

Preoperative antibiotics in case LUCS is planned and prophylaxis for venous thrombosis 12 hours from after the surgery. Mechanical thromboprophylaxis such as compression stocking can be given before surgery. Early ambulation is always advocated.

POSTPARTUM MANAGEMENT

An uneventful postpartum period very much depends on the support and advice that an obese mother receives antenatally.

For instance breastfeeding initiation starts antenatally by teaching simple steps of breast and nipple care to be done regularly. Obese patients tend to suffer depression anxiety and sense of failure, the psychological support for which should come during antenatal period.

Medical disorders during pregnancy should be followed-up and referred to the appropriate specialty for review.

The importance of losing weight postpartum has to be duly emphasized to the patient with healthy diet and adequate physical exercise. The incidence of LUCS being high in such cases there is a tendency to procrastinate being active so that weight shedding postnatally becomes an issue. A high degree of motivation to loose weight comes if the patient is educated about the possibility of contracting several morbid noncommunicable diseases in later life such as T2DM, cardiac conditions, essential hypertension, etc. Also the risk of her offsprings contracting the same due to her obesity is a real risk.

Lastly an effective contraception based on her BMI to be offered to her after adequate counseling.

PREVENTION OF OBESITY: LIFESTYLE MODIFICATIONS

Easier said than done. The seeds of obesity are sown in early childhood. Breastfed infants show a less tendency to gain excess weight. They remain healthy with an excellent immune system but without the puppy fat.

In the young adulthood period, one can achieve a weight reduction to the extent of 10–15% by simple lifestyle interventions and modifications. Although you can double this weight loss by bariatric surgery, it has got many disadvantages such as fetal hypotrophy, future preterm birth, high PNMR; therefore, despite the beneficial effects of decreased incidence of GDM and fetal macrosomia, bariatric surgery is not routinely recommended.[25,26]

Similarly, weight loss during pregnancy is associated with an increased risk of neonatal hypotrophy[27,28] and weight reduction during pregnancy is not usually recommended.[29] Instead, we should recommend weight loss between two pregnancies, which has a positive effect on neonatal outcomes), although we know very well that mothers are generally poorly motivated to reduce weight once childbirth is over.[30]

There were two randomized controlled trial (RCTs) on Metformin started in pregnancy in order to effect weight loss during pregnancy. Well, weight gain was prevented but did not lower the risk of gestational diabetes and neonatal macrosomia.[31,32]

Finally, it appears that intensive and supervised physical activity started early in pregnancy (during first 3 months) can reduce maternal blood glucose levels and the rate of gestational diabetes to a clinically relevant degree.[33]

Periconceptional obesity in parents can affect the metabolic health and fertility of the offspring. Insulin resistance and obesity were transmitted to both male and female first generation offspring

Maternal obesity heightened the child's risk of CHD, stroke, T2DM and asthma.

Poor cognitive performance and increased risk of neurodevelopmental disorders, autism, attention deficit hyperactivity disorders and even cancer in later life can be a direct outcome of maternal obesity.

KEY MESSAGES

- Obesity definitely increases both maternal and fetal *morbidity* during pregnancy, and this is evidence based now. Obesity is a risk factor independent of comorbidities such as diabetes.
- An increase in prepregnancy body mass index by 10% is associated with an about 10% increase in the risk of gestational diabetes/preeclampsia.
- Excessive weight gain during pregnancy is also harmful.
- There is growing evidence that the placenta plays an important role in the regulation of fetal growth.
- In principle, weight normalization prior to getting pregnant is advantageous. Ultimately, long-term reduction of maternal and fetal morbidity can only be achieved by dietary and lifestyle changes maintained beyond pregnancy.
- The majority of studies on dietary and lifestyle interventions during pregnancy failed to show any clinically relevant maternal and fetal benefits.

REFERENCES

1. World Health Organization. (2020). Factsheet: Obesity and Overweight. [online] Available from: https://www.who.int/news-room/fact-sheets/detail/obesity-and-overweight. [Last Accessed November, 2021]
2. Black RE, Victora CG, Walker SP, Bhutta ZA, Christian P, de Onis M, et al. Maternal and child undernutrition and overweight in low-income and middle-income countries. Lancet. 2013;382(9890):427-51.
3. Kassie AM, Abate BB, Kassaw MW. Education and prevalence of overweight and obesity among reproductive age group women in Ethiopia: analysis of the 2016 Ethiopian demographic and health survey data. BMC Public Health. 2020;1189:20.
4. He Y, Pan A, Yang Y, Wang Y, Xu J, Zhang Y, et al. Prevalence of underweight, overweight, and obesity among reproductive-age women and adolescent girls in rural china. Am J Public Health. 2016;106(12):2103-10.
5. Luhar S, Timæus IM, Jones R, Cunningham S, Patel SA, Kinra S, et al. Forecasting the prevalence of overweight and obesity in India to 2040. PLoS One. 2020;15(2):e0229438.
6. Boots C, Stephenson MD. Does obesity increase the risk of miscarriage in spontaneous conception: a systematic review. Semin Reprod Med. 2011;29:507-13.
7. Boots CE, Bernardi LA, Stephenson MD. Frequency of euploid miscarriage is increased in obese women with recurrent early pregnancy loss. Fertil Steril. 2014;102:455-9.
8. Ovesen P, Rasmussen S, Kesmodel U. Effect of prepregnancy maternal overweight and obesity on pregnancy outcome. Obstet Gynecol. 2011;118:305-12.
9. Yu Z, Han S, Zhu J, Sun X, Ji C, Guo X. Prepregnancy body mass index in relation to infant birth weight and offspring overweight/obesity: a systematic review and meta-analysis. PLoS One. 2013;8:e61627.
10. Kim SS, Zhu Y, Grantz KL. Obstetric and neonatal risks among obese women without chronic disease. Obstet Gynecol. 2016;128:104-12.

11. Catalano PM, McIntyre HD, Cruickshank JK, McCance DR, Dyer AR, Metzger BE, et al. The hyperglycemia and adverse pregnancy outcome study: associations of GDM and obesity with pregnancy outcomes. Diabetes Care. 2012;35:780-6.
12. HAPO Study Cooperative Research Group, Metzger BE, Lowe LP, Dyer AR, Trimble ER, Chaovarindr U, et al. Hyperglycemia and adverse pregnancy outcomes. N Engl J Med. 2008;358:1991-2002.
13. Shapiro AL, Schmiege SJ, Brinton JT, Glueck D, Crume TL, Friedman JE, et al. Testing the fuel-mediated hypothesis: maternal insulin resistance and glucose mediate the association between maternal and neonatal adiposity, the Healthy Start study. Diabetologia. 2015;58:937-41
14. Schummers L, Hutcheon JA, Bodnar LM, Lieberman E, Himes KP. Risk of adverse pregnancy outcomes by prepregnancy body mass index: a population-based study to inform prepregnancy weight loss counseling. Obstet Gynecol. 2015;125:133-43
15. Moll U, Olsson H, Landin-Olsson M. Impact of pregestational weight and weight gain during pregnancy on long-term risk for diseases. PLoS One. 2017;12:e0168543
16. Ovesen P, Rasmussen S, Kesmodel U. Effect of prepregnancy maternal overweight and obesity on pregnancy outcome. Obstet Gynecol. 2011;118:305-12.
17. Lisonkova S, Muraca GM, Potts J, et al. Association between prepregnancy body mass index and severe maternal morbidity. JAMA. 2017;318:1777-86.
18. Hunkapiller NM, Gasperowicz M, Kapidzic M, Plaks V, Maltepe E, Kitajewski J, et al. A role for Notch signaling in trophoblast endovascular invasion and in the pathogenesis of pre-eclampsia. Development. 2011;138(14):2987-98.
19. Persson M, Cnattingius S, Villamor E. Risk of major congenital malformations in relation to maternal overweight and obesity severity: cohort study of 12 million singletons. BMJ. 2017;357:j256.
20. Johansson S, Villamor E, Altman M, Bonamy AK, Granath F, Cnattingius S. Maternal overweight and obesity in early pregnancy and risk of infant mortality: a population based cohort study in Sweden. BMJ. 2014;349:65-72.
21. Kim SS, Mendola P, Zhu Y, Hwang BS, Grantz KL. Spontaneous and indicated preterm delivery risk is increased among overweight and obese women without prepregnancy chronic disease. BJOG. 2017;124:1708-16.
22. FIGO Committee guidelines for the management of pre-pregnancy, pregnancy and post-pregnancy obesity. London: FIGO; 2020.
23. RCOG. Care of Women with Obesity in Pregnancy. Green Top Guidelines no. 72. London: RCOG; 2018.
24. Scott-Pillai R, Spence D, Cardwell CR, Hunter A, Holmes VA. The impact of body mass index on maternal and neonatal outcomes: a retrospective study in a UK obstetric population, 2004-2011. BJOG. 2013;120:932-9.
25. Legro RS. Mr Fertility Authority, tear down that weight wall! Hum Reprod. 2016;31:2662-4.
26. Johansson K, Cnattingius S, Naslund I. Outcomes of pregnancy after bariatric surgery. N Engl J Med. 2015;372:814-24.
27. Beyerlein A, Schiessl B, Lack N, von Kries R. Associations of gestational weight loss with birth-related outcome: a retrospective cohort study. BJOG. 2011;118:55-61.
28. Kapadia MZ, Park CK, Beyene J, Giglia L, Maxwell C, McDonald SD. Weight loss instead of weight gain within the guidelines in obese women during pregnancy: a systematic review and meta-analyses of maternal and infant outcomes. PLoS One. 2015;10 e0132650.
29. ACOG Practice Bulletin No 156. Obesity in pregnancy. Obstet Gynecol. 2015;126:e112-e126.
30. McBain RD, Dekker GA, Clifton VL, Mol BW, Grzeskowiak LE. Impact of inter-pregnancy BMI change on perinatal outcomes: a retrospective cohort study. Eur J Obstet Gynecol Reprod Biol. 2016;205:98-104.
31. Chiswick C, Reynolds RM, Denison F. Effect of metformin on maternal and fetal outcomes in obese pregnant women (EMPOWaR): a randomised, double-blind, placebo-controlled trial. Lancet Diabetes Endocrinol. 2015;3:778-86.
32. Syngelaki A, Nicolaides KH, Balani J. Metformin versus placebo in obese pregnant women without diabetes mellitus. N Engl J Med. 2016;374:434-43.
33. Wang C, Wei Y, Zhang X, Zhang Y, Xu Q, Sun Y, et al. A randomized clinical trial of exercise during pregnancy to prevent gestational diabetes mellitus and improve pregnancy outcome in overweight and obese pregnant women. Am J Obstet Gynecol. 2017;216:340-51.

LONG QUESTIONS
1. Discuss the etiopathogenesis of fetal anomalies in a woman with obesity. What are the barriers to detection and what are the implications of such problems?
2. What are the main interventions that should be instituted in pre-pregnancy counseling of an obese woman who is planning pregnancy?

SHORT QUESTIONS
1. Why is obesity called a state of low grade inflammation?
2. What are the common comorbidities with obesity?
3. List the common obstetric complications that are seen in a pregnancy in an obese woman.
4. What are the difficulties that should be anticipated in labor and delivery of a woman with obesity?

MULTIPLE CHOICE QUESTIONS
1. According to the WHO survey of 2016, the proportion of obesity is:
   a. 3%   b. 13%   c. 23%   d. 33%
2. The following comorbidities are commonly seen with obesity, except:
   a. Type 1 diabetes   b. PCOS
   c. Arterial hypertension c. Breast cancer
3. The following obstetric conditions are associated with obesity in pregnancy, except:
   a. Gestational diabetes   b. Intrauterine fetal death
   c. Postdates pregnancy   d. Fetal macrosomia
4. The following statement is true in the pathogenesis of obesity related obstetric complications:
   a. Hyperinsulinemia causes deep placental implantation
   b. Adiponectin levels are increased
   c. Adiponectin enhances insulin sensitivity
   d. Proinflammatory factors such as TNF-alpha levels are decreased
5. The following statement about management of the obese pregnant woman is true:
   a. There is no need for screening for gestational diabetes
   b. There is low risk for dystocia
   c. An attempt of vaginal birth after cesarean is more likely to be successful
   d. Postpartum hemorrhage is more common

Answers
1. b   2. a   3. c   4. c   5. d

5.15 CANCER IN PREGNANCY

Amita Maheshwari, Vikash K Chatrani, Sudeep Gupta

INTRODUCTION

Cancer associated with pregnancy is rare, with a reported incidence of 1/1,000–2,000 pregnancies.[1] However, as increasing number of women delaying childbearing for academic, professional and personal pursuits, along with the widespread use of assisted reproductive techniques, there has been an increase in advanced age women conceiving. Advancing age is an important risk factor for many cancers and therefore obstetricians are expected to see an upsurge in number of pregnant women with cancer. Breast cancer is the most common cancer associated with pregnancy with an incidence of 1/3,000 pregnancies; other common cancers seen during pregnancy include cervical cancer, ovarian cancer, hematological malignancies, thyroid cancer, colorectal cancer and melanoma.[1]

The management of cancer in pregnancy is complex and should involve a multidisciplinary team consists of obstetrician, oncologist, neonatologist, geneticist and psychiatrist. A careful assessment of risks and benefits to both mother and unborn child is required throughout pregnancy.

In this chapter, we will give an overview on general principles of management of cancer during pregnancy and a brief discussion on management of some important cancers seen during pregnancy.

PRINCIPLES OF MANAGEMENT OF WOMEN WITH CANCER IN PREGNANCY

In general, principles of management of cancer during pregnancy are same as for nonpregnant patient with cancer. However, certain important factors should be taken into consideration while making decision and these include—nature and stage of cancer, the expected cancer-related outcome of mother, the duration of pregnancy at diagnosis of cancer, past obstetric history, and the wishes and concerns of the family.

Diagnostic Workup during Pregnancy

The diagnostic workup should start at the earliest suspicion of malignancy and follow the general guidelines as recommended for nonpregnant patients with cancer. Blood tests, biopsy for histopathological confirmation of cancer and imaging; should be performed as indicated clinically.

Imaging during Pregnancy

Radiological imaging is often required for initial workup of cancer and also for evaluation of response to treatment. Imaging modalities without ionizing radiation such as ultrasonography and MRI, should be preferred during pregnancy over computed tomography (CT) scan. Whole-body diffusion weighted MRI can be used for characterization of primary lesion as well as for metastatic workup. Gadolinium contrast has potential to cross the placenta and should be avoided during pregnancy although no adverse effects to the neonate have been reported after gadolinium exposure.

The developing embryo and fetus are extremely sensitive to deleterious effects of ionizing radiation. The fetal toxicity depends on the gestational age at the time of exposure and includes; abortion, intrauterine growth retardation, prenatal or neonatal death, congenital malformations, mental retardation and childhood cancers and leukemia. 50 mGy has been set as margin of safety for in utero exposure to ionizing radiation however, fetal risks are low up to 100 mGy.[2] Termination of pregnancy may be considered at a cumulative radiation dose exceeding 100–150 mGy although the reported risk of gross congenital malformations is low at dose less than 200 mGy.[2] However, the general rule is that during pregnancy radiation should be avoided if possible but if inevitable, doses must be kept as low as reasonably achievable (ALARA-principle).

Generally, radiation doses with diagnostic modalities are much lower than abovementioned threshold level, e.g., chest and extremity radiographs expose fetus to a dose of <0.01 mGy and CT scan of the chest to 0.02 mGy. A chest radiograph with abdominal shield can be safely performed during pregnancy. On the other hand, CT scan of pelvis delivers a much higher dose (10–50 mGy) and therefore, should be avoided during pregnancy unless absolutely indicated.[2] Intravenous iodinated contrast material can be used if required but the thyroid function of the new born should be assessed.

18FDG-PET/CT exposes fetus to a high dose of radiation (up to 50 mGy) and therefore should not be done during pregnancy. Sentinel node procedure can be safely performed during pregnancy using lowest possible dose of radiocolloid.[3] Indocyanine green (ICG) has very limited placental transfer and seems to be safe for sentinel lymph node detection during pregnancy.[4] However, the use of blue dye should be avoided as it can rarely (in less than 0.1% cases) cause anaphylactic reaction in mother. **Table 1** summarizes recommendations for various imaging modalities during pregnancy.

Surgery during Pregnancy

Surgery is an important component of treatment for most solid cancers and the safest modality for treatment of cancer in pregnancy. It can be performed anytime during pregnancy with due precautions. However, the preferred time for surgery is beyond the stage of fetal organogenesis.

TABLE 1: Imaging modalities during pregnancy.

Imaging modality	Trimester of pregnancy		
	First	Second	Third
Ultrasonography	+	+	+
Magnetic resonance imaging (MRI)	+	+	+
Radiograph	+/−	+/−	+/−
CT scan	−/+	−/+	−/+
Sentinel lymph node biopsy for breast cancer with radiocolloid	+	+	+
Bone scintigraphy	−	−	−
PET scan	−	−	−

+: Recommended
+/−: Depending upon duration of pregnancy and location of tumor
−/+: Only if absolutely necessary
−: Not recommended

Surgery should be performed by an experienced team of surgeons and anesthesiologist. A careful monitoring of maternal hemodynamic and biochemical parameters during perioperative period is extremely important for an optimal fetal outcome. Compression of inferior vena cava should be avoided during surgery by placing patient in left lateral position. Perioperative tocolytics may be considered in the late second and third trimesters of pregnancy during abdominal surgery. Beyond the age of viability, lung maturation protocol should be offered. Laparoscopic surgery if oncologically indicated, can be performed during the first and second trimesters. However, care should be taken to limit surgical time (90–120 min) and to use low intra-abdominal pressure (10–13 mm Hg).[5] An open entry carries less risk of injury to gravid uterus and is preferred over Veress needle.

Despite taking all precautions, surgical intervention can lead to adverse fetal outcomes in the form of miscarriage, preterm delivery, IUGR and fetal distress.[5] Patient and family must be counseled regarding risks-benefits of surgical treatment during pregnancy. The incidence of adverse fetal outcomes is higher with major abdominal and pelvic procedures as compared with surgery for breast or head and neck cancer. Postoperative care of patient must include adequate pain control, hydration and thromboprophylaxis.

Systemic Therapies during Pregnancy

Chemotherapy during Pregnancy

Chemotherapy is an integral part of treatment of most malignancies and therefore many pregnant women with cancer may require chemotherapy. A number of factors should be considered prior to administration of chemotherapy during pregnancy including; gestational age, physiologic changes of pregnancy and altered pharmacokinetics of drug, placental passage of drug and fetal toxicity of drugs.

Exposure to chemotherapy drugs during the first trimester of pregnancy is associated with a 10–20% incidence of congenital malformation rates therefore chemotherapy should be started in the second trimester, after the period of organogenesis. However, accidental exposure to chemotherapy drugs in very early pregnancy (first 2 weeks after conception) generally results in "all or none" phenomena; either the pregnancy is aborted or it continues with no adverse effect.[6] Physiologic changes of pregnancy may affect efficacy of drugs by altering pharmacokinetics with regard to their distribution, metabolism, and excretion. Doses of chemotherapy drugs should be calculated based on the actual maternal weight during pregnancy. Chemotherapeutic agents cross placenta by passive diffusion, rate of which depends upon molecular size, lipid solubility, protein binding, and ionization of drug. Majority chemotherapeutic drugs have low molecular weight, not charged and are present in unbound form therefore, can easily cross the placenta and cause toxicity in fetus. Potential fetal side effects should be discussed with patient and the least toxic protocol should be used.

Chemotherapy should be discontinued 3–4 weeks prior to expected date of delivery to allow adequate time for maternal and fetal bone marrow to recover prior to delivery.

Supportive medications along with systemic therapy: Antiemetics including metoclopramide and serotonin receptor antagonists may be used during pregnancy however, safety data for neurokinin 1 inhibitors is limited. Betamethasone or dexamethasone as premedication should be avoided as these drugs freely pass to the fetus through placenta. Instead, steroids that are primarily metabolized in the placenta such as methylprednisolone, prednisolone, or hydrocortisone are preferred. Growth factors, such as granulocyte colony stimulating factors (GCSF) seem to be safe during pregnancy although data is limited.

Table 2 lists commonly used chemotherapy and supportive drugs for management of cancers during pregnancy with their mechanisms of action and potential fetal toxicities.

Targeted Therapy, Immunotherapy and Hormonal Therapy during Pregnancy

Targeted therapy acts on specific molecular pathways involved in tumorigenesis, some of which may also play a vital role in fetal growth and development. Therefore, targeted therapy increases the risk of fetal teratogenicity and morbidity and is generally not recommended during pregnancy.

Placental passage of targeted drugs depends on the class of drugs and their molecular size. Monoclonal antibodies such as trastuzumab, rituximab have large molecular size and need an active transport for transplacental passage. On the other hand, small sized molecules, e.g., tyrosine kinase inhibitors (TKIs), can freely cross the placenta throughout the pregnancy. Trastuzumab, used for treatment of HER-2 overexpressing breast cancer, may lead to severe oligohydramnios or anhydramnios and neonatal lung hypoplasia leading to respiratory failure when used in the

TABLE 2: Commonly used drugs for management of cancers during pregnancy.

Drug	Mechanism of action	Common indications	Fetal toxicity
Carboplatin	Heavy metal derived from platinum Forms DNA adduct leading to DNA damage	Ovarian cancer, breast cancer advanced stage cervical and endometrial cancers	–
Paclitaxel	Microtubule poison causing polymerization	Ovarian cancer, breast cancer, advanced stage cervical and endometrial cancers	Myelosuppression, pyloric stenosis
Cisplatin	Heavy metal derived from platinum forms DNA adduct leading to DNA damage	Cervical cancer, epithelial and nonepithelial ovarian cancer	Neutropenia, hair loss, ventriculomegaly, and hearing impairment when given within 3 weeks of delivery
Bleomycin	Inserts in the minor DNA groove causes DNA damage	Germ-cell tumors	Syndactyly
Etoposide	Podophyllotoxin derivative inhibiting topoisomerase II	Germ-cell tumors	Hearing impairment, secondary leukemias, transient pancytopenia when administered in the third trimester
Docetaxel	Microtubule poison causing polymerization	Ovarian cancer, breast cancer	–
Doxorubicin	DNA damaging agent	Breast cancer, ovarian cancer, hematological cancers	Unfavorable outcome <5% in patients with solid tumors, >20% in patients with leukemia
Fluorouracil	Pyrimidine analogue interfering with the synthesis of DNA and RNA	Cervical cancer, breast cancer	Teratogenic and abortifacient during first trimester. Possible intrauterine growth retardation
Gemcitabine	Antimetabolite of nucleotide synthesis	Ovarian cancer	Possible intrauterine growth retardation
Irinotecan	Alkaloids inhibiting topoisomerase I	Ovarian and cervical cancers	–
Topotecan	Alkaloids inhibiting topoisomerase I	Ovarian and cervical cancers	–
Vinblastine	Microtubule poison inducing depolymerization	Germ-cell tumors	Syndactyly, plagiocephaly
Vincristine	Microtubule poison inducing depolymerization	Cervical cancer	–
Supportive drugs			
Dexamethasone	Corticosteroids	Prevention of nausea	Cerebral palsy reported after repeated administration
Ondansetron	Selective serotonin receptor antagonist	Prevention of nausea	–
Promethazine	Phenothiazines	Prevention of nausea	–
Aprepitant	Substance P/neurokinin I receptor antagonist	Prevention of nausea	No reports known
Filgrastim	Cytokines	Prevention of neutropenia	No side effects recorded. May be given with caution

second or third trimester. Therefore, it is not recommended during pregnancy. Rituximab, used for the treatment of B cell malignancies, is teratogenic when given in the first trimester but may be used in the second and third trimesters with careful monitoring. Imatinib, a tyrosine kinase inhibitor used for Philadelphia chromosome positive chronic myeloid leukemia, is known to cause fetal malformations when used during the first trimester, but may be used with caution during the second and third trimesters.

Angiogenesis plays a crucial role in the normal development and growth of the fetus and placenta. As anticipated anti-angiogenesis drugs have shown to be teratogenic and can cause abortion, skeletal retardations, and fetal growth retardation in animal models. Thus, anti-vascular endothelial growth factor (anti-VEGF) and other antiangiogenic drugs are not recommended during pregnancy. Immune checkpoint inhibitors such as anti-PD1/PD-L1 have been associated with spontaneous abortions in animals and therefore, contraindicated during pregnancy.

Antiestrogenic hormonal therapy is also not recommended during pregnancy as these drugs negatively impact fetal and placental growth and development. Use of tamoxifen during the first trimester has been reported to cause birth defects in up to 25% of cases.[1] It has also been associated with vaginal bleeding, miscarriage, and fetal death.

Radiation Therapy during Pregnancy

Radiation therapy should be used with extreme caution during pregnancy and alternative treatment protocols without radiation should be offered as far as possible. The fetal exposure to ionizing radiation during radiotherapy is by a combination of internal and external scatters and radiation leakage. If radiation during pregnancy is inevitable, radiation physicist must calculate the fetal radiation dose, and modify treatment plan by changing the field size, angle, and radiation energy so that fetus receives the least possible dose. Abdominal lead shields should be used to further reduce the fetal dose. Radiotherapy to head, neck and breast may be considered during the first and second trimesters after careful evaluation and discussion with patient and her family. However, radiation to abdomen and pelvis is absolutely contraindicated during pregnancy.

■ OBSTETRIC AND PERINATAL MANAGEMENT

Obstetric Considerations

In early pregnancy, termination can be considered in patients with aggressive or advanced stage cancers or in case pregnancy is not desired. The most common obstetric complications of pregnancy with caner are intrauterine growth retardation, low birthweight and preterm delivery. Intrauterine growth retardation has been reported in up to 21%, pregnant women with cancer.[7] A number of maternal factors may contribute to fetal growth restriction including the underlying cancer, psychological stress, malnutrition, and use of chemotherapy during pregnancy. Hematologic and gastrointestinal cancers are associated with higher risk of small for gestation. Preterm birth is also common in pregnant woman with cancer. This could be either iatrogenic because of oncologic treatment scheduling or spontaneous following chemotherapy induced preterm contractions. Due to the long-term morbidities associated with prematurity, iatrogenic preterm delivery should be avoided as far as possible.[8] Intrauterine exposure to chemotherapy may cause bone marrow suppression and anemia in neonates. Fetal Doppler studies may help in detecting fetal anemia. Intrauterine fetal death may occur especially in patients with advanced malignancies and with acute hematolymphoid cancers. A combination of poor maternal health, chemotherapy and related toxicities, maternal infection, stress and poor nutrition may increase the risk of fetal demise. Maternal complications such as infections, thromboembolic events, hypertension, and blood transfusions are more common in the pregnant cancer patients compared with normal pregnancy.

It is recommended to avoid chemotherapy in the late third trimester.[9] There should be at least 3-week interval between chemotherapy cycle and delivery so as to allow both maternal and fetal bone marrow to recover from chemotoxicity. This will also provide adequate time for the placenta to metabolize and eliminate cytotoxic drugs from the fetus. Neonatal myelosuppression increases risk of bleeding, sepsis and death.

Breastfeeding

Breastfeeding is encouraged in cancer patients who are not scheduled to receive cytotoxic treatment in postpartum. However, breastfeeding is contraindicated if mother is on chemotherapy since these drugs pass into milk, and may cause toxicity in infants. Breastfeeding can be allowed few weeks after the last administered dose of chemotherapy if milk secretion can be maintained throughout chemotherapy. At least a 3-week interval between the last non-platinum chemotherapy and breastfeeding is recommended. Due to long half-life of platinum agents, a longer interval is desired for platinum containing regimens.[10] Moreover, maternal cancer and chemotherapy might have negative effect on both the quality and quantity of breast milk. Breastfeeding is also not recommended in women on endocrine therapy. In women with breast cancer, nursing may also interfere with diagnostic evaluation and therapeutic procedures.

Pediatric Outcome

Outcomes of children born to mothers treated for cancer during pregnancy are generally good although data on long term outcomes is limited. No significant differences have been reported in cognitive behavior and intelligence in children exposed to chemotherapy in utero compared to healthy controls.[11] Although the use of anthracyclines during childhood may cause short- and long-term cardiotoxicity, evaluation of children with prenatal exposure to anthracyclines has been reassuring. However, in utero exposure to cisplatin has been reported to cause hearing impairment and nephrotoxicity, therefore during pregnancy carboplatin is preferred over cisplatin. Radiotherapy, targeted therapy, or hormonal therapy are generally contraindicated during pregnancy, therefore very limited data is available on outcomes of children exposed to these treatments.

■ SPECIFIC CANCERS

Pregnancy-associated Breast Cancer

Pregnancy-associated breast cancer (PABC) is defined as breast cancer diagnosed during pregnancy or up to 1 year postpartum; some studies included breast cancer diagnosed up to 5 years postpartum as PABC.[12] Although PABC is rare, comprises only 0.2–0.4% of all breast cancers, it is the most common cancer seen in pregnancy. Early menarche and late age at first pregnancy are associated with a slight increased risk of pregnancy associated breast cancers. Pregnancy itself may temporarily increase the risk of developing breast cancer, although it has protective effect in long-term.

Clinical Presentation

The common presentation of PABC is a painless lump or thickening in the breast. Occasionally, may present as a bloody nipple discharge. A rare presentation can be unexplained refusal of a newborn to feed from a lactating breast that harbors an occult carcinoma, this is known as the "*milk rejection*" sign.

The majority of breast cancers during pregnancy are infiltrating ductal adenocarcinomas, as seen in non-pregnant women. However, PABC are often poorly differentiated and present at an advanced stage, particularly those diagnosed during lactation,[13] negative for estrogen and progesterone receptors[14] and have a higher incidence of inflammatory breast cancer.[15] Several studies and two recent meta-analyses have suggested that the survival outcome of patients who develop breast cancer during or after pregnancy is worse compared with patients who have non-pregnancy associated breast cancer.[16,17]

Diagnosis

Diagnosis of breast cancer is made by the triple test which includes clinical examination, radiological evaluation and histopathological confirmation. However, diagnostic and staging evaluations are difficult for PABC due to the engorgement and physiological hypertrophy breast during pregnancy and lactation, and the desire to limit radiation exposure to the fetus. A delay in diagnosis, both on the part of the physician and the woman, may contribute to the advanced disease at presentation. Although majority of breast masses are benign, any mass persisting for more than 2 weeks deserves detailed investigation. The differential diagnoses of a breast lump are summarized in **Box 1**.

Imaging

Sonography: Breast sonography is often the first imaging test ordered to evaluate a breast lump in a pregnant woman and is helpful in distinguishing solid from cystic mass without the risk of fetal radiation exposure. Sonography cannot differentiate benign from malignant lesions but a focal solid mass may be suggestive of gestational breast cancer.

Mammography: Mammography is not contraindicated in pregnancy as it exposes fetus to a very low dose of radiation (0.001–0.01 mGy). With abdominal shielding, which further reduces the risk, mammography is considered very safe during pregnancy. However, due to physiological changes in breast tissue during pregnancy/lactation, mammography may be associated with a high false negative rate (up to 25%).

Breast MRI: Limited data is available on the role of magnetic resonance imaging (MRI) for the evaluation of breast masses during pregnancy. Gadolinium contrast is not recommended during pregnancy and non-contrast MRI is not useful for evaluation of a breast mass.

Further imaging: Further staging evaluation will depend on the clinical assessment and may include chest radiograph (CXR) performed with maternal abdominal shielding, abdominal ultrasound, and screening non-contrast MRI of the spine to exclude bone metastases. 18-FDG-PET scan, CT scan and bone scan are not recommended during pregnancy.

Biopsy: A clinically suspicious breast mass requires biopsy for definitive diagnosis, regardless of whether or not a woman is pregnant, and despite negative mammographic or ultrasound findings. Breast biopsy (core or incisional or excisional) is the gold standard for the diagnosis of cancer and can be safely performed in pregnancy. During lactation milk suppression with bromocriptine or cabergoline before biopsy will reduce the risk of breast abscess or milk fistula.

Fine needle aspiration cytology: Fine needle aspiration cytology (FNAC) may also be used for the initial evaluation of a breast mass. It has good sensitivity but high false positive rates due to increased cellular proliferation during pregnancy and lactation. A detailed clinical information should be provided to the pathologist to avoid misdiagnosis.

Treatment

The aims of treatment of pregnancy associated breast cancer are:
- Preserve the pregnancy when possible
- Offer optimum treatment to the mother for breast cancer
- Maintain fertility and reproductive health for the future.

In general, treatment guidelines for pregnant women with breast cancer are similar to those for non-pregnant patients, with some modifications to protect the fetus. Treatment of a breast cancer should not be unnecessarily delayed because of pregnancy. **Flowcharts 1 and 2** give overview on treatment protocols for early and advanced breast cancers, respectively.

Surgery

Mastectomy: Mastectomy may be preferred during pregnancy even for stage I and II breast cancers as it may eliminate the need for adjuvant breast radiation therapy.[18] Breast reconstruction, if desired, should be delayed until after delivery.

Breast conserving surgery: The therapeutic equivalence of mastectomy and breast conserving therapy [breast conserving

---

BOX 1: Differential diagnoses of a breast lump.

- Invasive carcinoma
- Lactating adenoma
- Fibroadenoma
- Cystic disease
- Lobular hyperplasia
- Milk retention cyst (galactocele)
- Abscess
- Lipoma
- Tuberculosis
- Hamartoma

Flowchart 1: Management of early stage breast cancer in pregnancy.

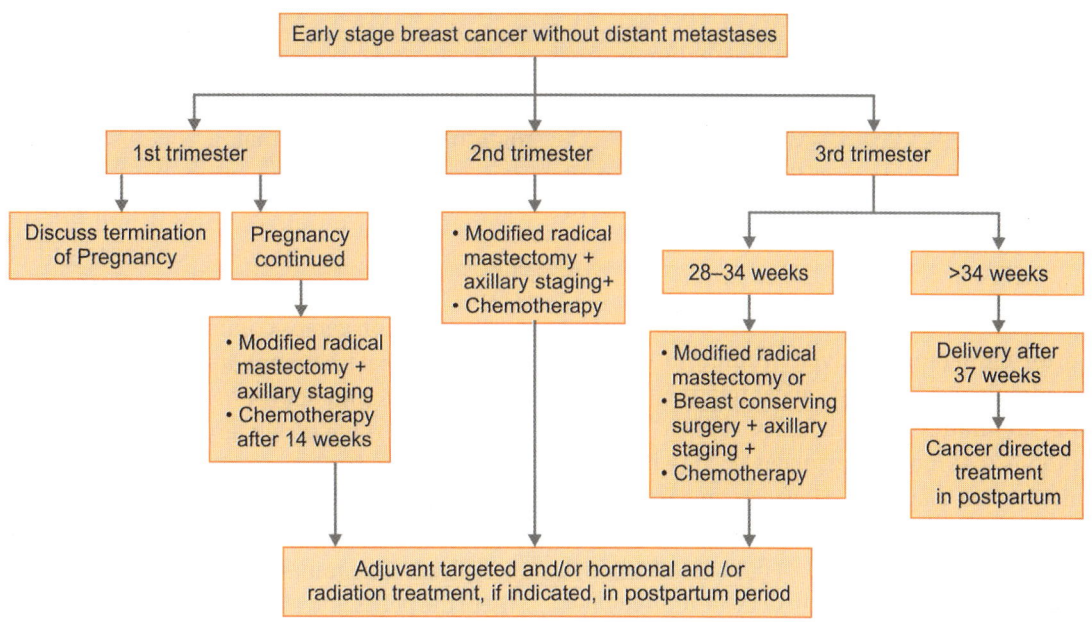

Flowchart 2: Management of late stage breast cancer in pregnancy.

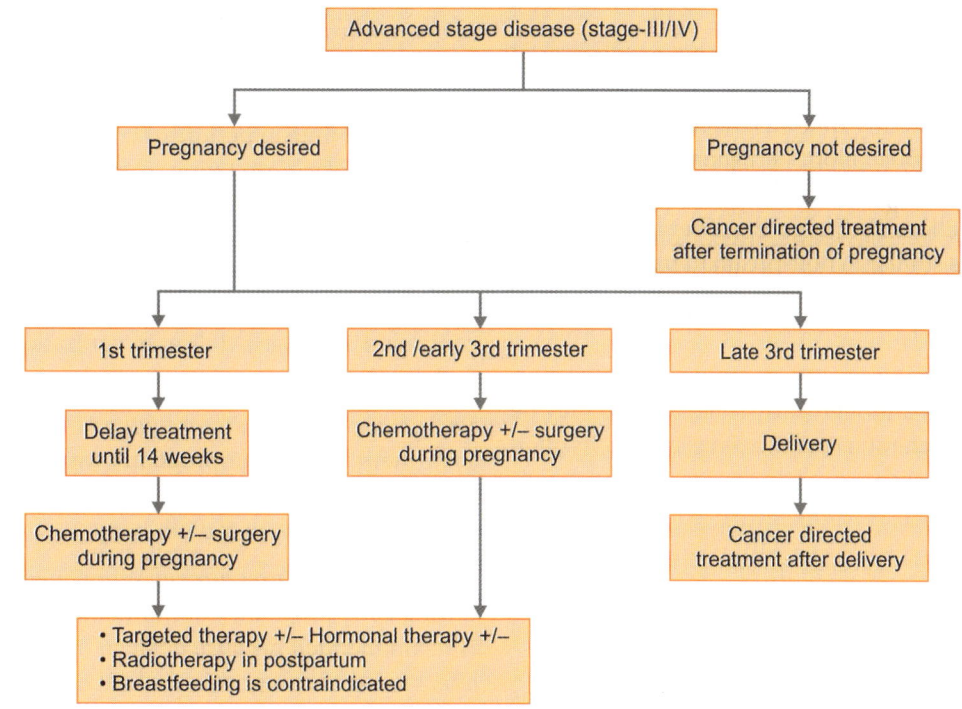

surgery (BCS) followed by radiation therapy (RT)] has been demonstrated in non-pregnant women and holds true for the pregnant patients as well. However, BCS should be offered only if adjuvant radiation therapy can be delayed until postpartum period.

Management of the axilla: Axillary staging and dissection are important components of breast cancer therapy. Assessment of nodal status provides prognostic information and is used in selecting adjuvant treatment, and axillary lymph node dissection improves local disease control.

Radiation therapy: Radiation therapy is used in the routine management of breast cancer patients who undergo BCS and also in certain high-risk cases after mastectomy. However, due to deleterious effects of therapeutic doses of radiation on fetus the use of radiation is not recommended during pregnancy.

Systemic therapy: Most women with pregnancy-associated breast cancer are candidates for systemic therapy.

Chemotherapy: Chemotherapy should be started after 14 weeks of gestation. The most commonly used regimens in pregnant women with breast cancer are doxorubicin plus cyclophosphamide (AC) or fluorouracil, doxorubicin, and cyclophosphamide (FAC).

Adjuvant targeted therapy such as trastuzumab and lapatinib and *hormonal therapy* are contraindicated during pregnancy and their use should be delayed until postpartum.

Elective termination of pregnancy: Early termination of pregnancy does not seem to improve the outcome of gestational breast cancer.

Pregnancy after Breast Cancer

It is common for clinicians to advise women to wait for 1–2 years after completion of breast cancer treatment before contemplating pregnancy. The primary reason for this recommendation is that most recurrences occur within the first 2 years after initial diagnosis. However, in case of ER/PR positive tumors, the woman should be advised selective estrogen receptor modulators (SERMs) for 5 years and advised not to get pregnant for that period, due to the risk of congenital malformations associated with tamoxifen during pregnancy.

Cervical Cancer in Pregnancy

Majority cases of cervical cancers in pregnancy are diagnosed with early disease because of regular obstetric examinations, there is also the possibility that advanced staged disease would interfere with conception.[19] Pregnancy also provides an opportunity for screening either via visual inspection or cytological examination. The prognosis of cervical cancer in pregnant patients is similar to non-pregnant patients.[20]

Clinical Presentation

Bleeding and/or discharge per vaginum are common presenting symptoms although early stage disease may be asymptomatic. Backache and constitutional symptoms often indicate advanced disease.

Diagnosis

Diagnostic evaluation of cervical carcinoma in pregnancy includes clinical assessment, colposcopy (for subclinical disease), cervical punch biopsy, and imaging.

All abnormal cervical smears should be managed as in the non-pregnant state with referral for colposcopic examination.[21] Colposcopic biopsy in pregnancy is reserved to exclude invasive disease, but when there is doubt, biopsy should not be deferred as delay in diagnosis of an early invasive and potentially curable lesion may result in progression and adverse maternal outcome. Endocervical curettage is contraindicated during pregnancy however, a gentle endocervical sample may be taken with a cytobrush if clinically indicated. Any grossly seen, suspicious cervical lesion should be biopsied. Woman with cervical cancer or pre-invasive disease should be referred to a gynecologic oncologist for further management.

Treatment

Preinvasive disease: It is preferred to manage preinvasive disease conservatively during pregnancy and defer definite treatment until the postpartum period when the fetal and maternal risks are minimal.

Invasive disease: Management of cervical cancer during pregnancy will require a careful multidisciplinary team approach and the following issues should be taken into consideration:
- Termination versus continuation of pregnancy
- Oncological treatment during pregnancy versus deferred treatment until delivery
- Time and route of delivery.

The stage of disease, duration of pregnancy and the patient's desire to continue the pregnancy or not, are the most important factors that determines management options. A good physical examination supplemented with a non-contrast MRI of the pelvis and abdomen will help in assessing the stage of disease. **Flowchart 3** gives an overview on treatment of cervical cancer during pregnancy.

Microinvasive disease
Stage IA1: Cervical conization is required to diagnose microinvasive disease and to exclude more advanced disease. The optimal time to perform a conization during pregnancy is 14–20 weeks of gestation as the risk of complications is higher in advanced pregnancy. Given the increase blood flow to the gravid uterus, cervical excisional procedures such as conization can result in substantial blood loss. There is also increased risk of abortion and preterm delivery after conization. For stage IA1 disease, conization is both diagnostic and therapeutic.

Early stage invasive disease (stage IA2, IB, non-bulky IIA): Treatment of the nonpregnant women with early stage cervical cancer is either radical hysterectomy and pelvic lymphadenectomy or radiotherapy.

Termination of pregnancy: When cancer is diagnosed during early pregnancy an immediate definitive treatment is recommended because delay in treatment may adversely affect maternal prognosis. Radical hysterectomy and pelvic lymphadenectomy can be performed either with the fetus in situ **(Figs. 1A and B)** or after elective termination of pregnancy. Alternatively, patient can be treated with definitive radiation therapy. In early pregnancy, external-beam radiation therapy can be initiated with the fetus in situ, and it usually results in fetal death. After miscarriage occurs, radiation treatment is completed with intracavitary brachytherapy.[22] However, termination of pregnancy before radiation treatment recommended for more than 20 weeks of gestation as fetal tissues is less sensitive to radiation in late second trimester.

Continuation of pregnancy: Definitive treatment may be delayed until fetal maturity in patients diagnosed after

Flowchart 3: Management of cervical cancer in pregnancy.

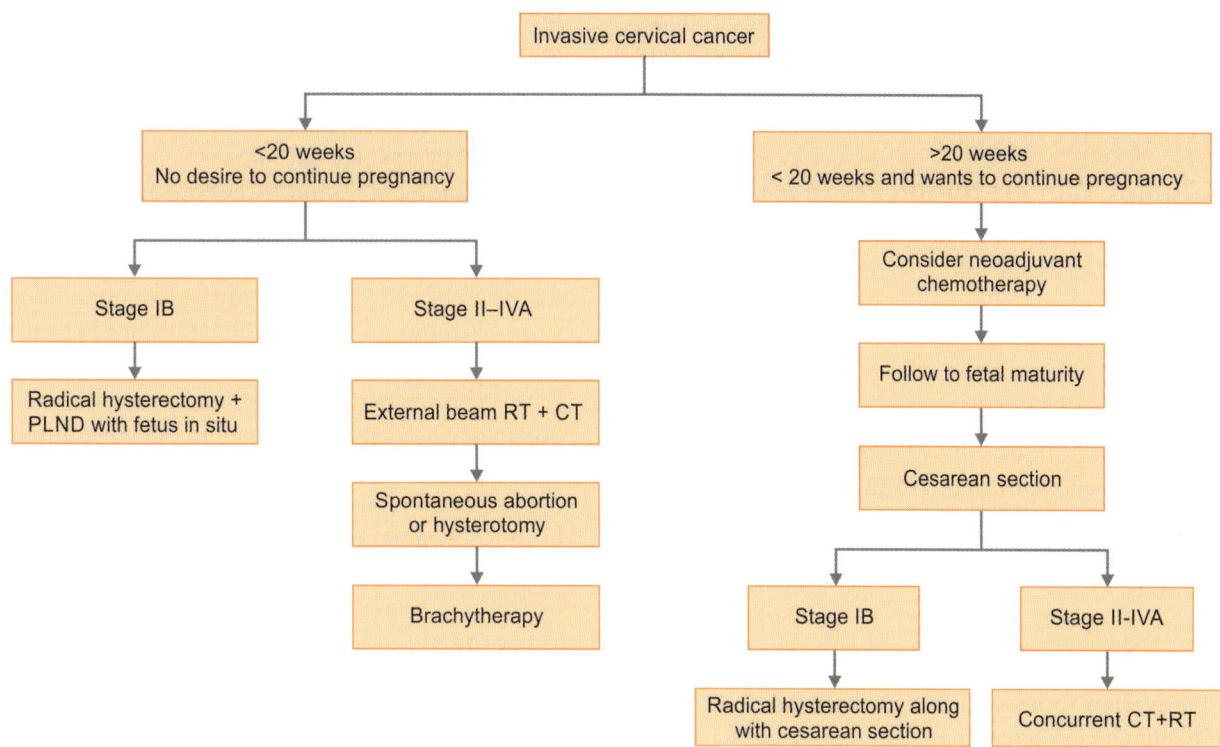

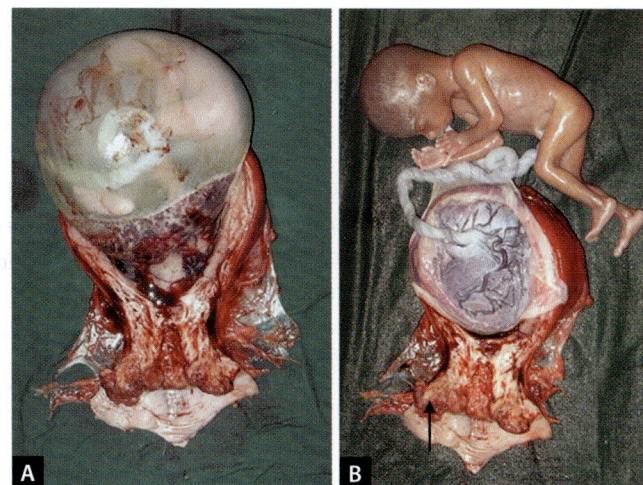

Figs. 1A and B: G4 with 20 weeks pregnancy and stage IB1 squamous cell carcinoma underwent modified radical hysterectomy with fetus in situ.

20 weeks of gestation and/or wish to continue the pregnancy. The timing of delivery should be coordinated with a multidisciplinary team including neonatologist.

Radical cesarean hysterectomy: Cesarean delivery is generally recommended for patients when gross tumor is present (stage IA2-IB-IIA disease). A radical hysterectomy and pelvic lymphadenectomy can be performed along with cesarean section. Cesarean-radical hysterectomy may be associated with greater blood loss and need for blood transfusion than radical hysterectomy in non-gravid women but the main benefit of doing radical hysterectomy at cesarean section is that it avoids further delay in cancer directed treatment.

Radical trachelectomy: Radical trachelectomy with lymphadenectomy 6–8 weeks postpartum is an alternative to radical hysterectomy for selected women with stage IA2 or small stage IB1 disease for whom fertility preservation is desired. Prior to surgery, MRI of the pelvis is a mandatory to ensure appropriateness of lesion for trachelectomy. Intraoperatively, lymph node dissection is performed initially to exclude the presence of lymph node metastasis, which would be a contraindication to fertility sparing surgery. Frozen section should be performed if a visible lesion is noted to ensure adequate resection margins. Cervical cerclage placement is recommended to avoid cervical incompetence in future pregnancy.

Advanced stage disease (stage IIB to IV disease): Chemoradiation is the standard treatment for stage IIB to IVA disease, while patients with stage IVB disease require a systemic therapy.

■ OVARIAN CANCER

The liberal use of prenatal ultrasound for evaluation of the fetus has resulted in increased detection of asymptomatic adnexal masses during pregnancy. Although the vast majority of these masses are benign, the possibility of cancer must be considered.

Clinical Presentation

Ovarian cancer during pregnancy may be an incidental diagnosis on antenatal ultrasound. In some women a palpable adnexal mass or posterior cul-de-sac nodularity identified on routine antenatal physical examination would lead to subsequent evaluation by ultrasound. Other presentations include the onset of acute abdominal pain due to torsion of the adnexa, abdominal distension, loss of weight and appetite and bladder/bowel symptoms.

Serum Tumor Markers during Pregnancy

Many ovarian cancer tumor markers including serum CA125, alpha-fetoprotein, hCG and inhibin A may be elevated during pregnancy and therefore elevated tumor makers should be interpreted with caution.

Imaging

Ultrasound examinations, followed by non-contrast MRI when the diagnosis is unclear, are the preferred imaging modalities during pregnancy **(Figs. 2A and B)**. The most common adnexal masses during pregnancy are functional or benign cysts.

Malignant Ovarian Tumors

Epithelial ovarian tumors comprise about one-half of all ovarian malignancies in pregnant women, germ cell ovarian malignancies make up about one-third, and stromal tumors and a variety of other tumor types (e.g., sarcomas, metastatic tumors) account for the remainder.

- *Epithelial ovarian tumors:* About 50% of epithelial ovarian tumors detected in pregnancy are of low malignant potential (formerly called "borderline") and the other 50% are invasive. Borderline tumors generally have an excellent prognosis and can be treated conservatively in women who wish to preserve their fertility or are pregnant at the time of diagnosis. Unilateral salpingo-oophorectomy, or, in some instances, ovarian cystectomy may be performed. Epithelial ovarian tumors of low malignant potential diagnosed in pregnancy may exhibit atypical characteristics mimicking invasive cancer. These findings include nuclear enlargement, anisocytosis, and multifocal microinvasion. For this reason, it is important that the pathologist be informed of the coexistent pregnancy and that pregnancy-associated ovarian malignancies be evaluated by a skilled pathologist.
- *Germ cell tumors:* About three-fourths of ovarian germ cell tumors occurring in pregnancy are dysgerminomas; endodermal sinus tumors, immature teratomas, and mixed germ cell tumors comprise the remainder. Most germ cell tumors are grossly limited to one adnexa except dysgerminomas which can be bilateral in 10–15% of cases.
- *Sex cord-stromal tumors:* Approximately one-half of all pregnancy-associated stromal tumors are granulosa cell tumors, one-third are Sertoli-Leydig cell tumors, and the remainders are unclassified stromal tumors. Most of these tumors are limited to one ovary at the time of diagnosis.

Management

Surgery

Surgery for an adnexal mass in pregnancy is usually indicated when the mass:

- Persists into the second trimester, or
- Is larger than 10 cm in diameter, or
- Has solid or mixed solid and cystic ultrasound characteristics highly suspicious for malignancy on imaging.

The rationale for this approach is to rule out malignancy and to prevent complications such as adnexal torsion, rupture, or obstruction of labor. The optimal time for surgery during pregnancy is the second trimester. At laparotomy, the midline incision should be adequate to minimize the need to manipulate the gravid uterus while obtaining exposure to the adnexal mass.

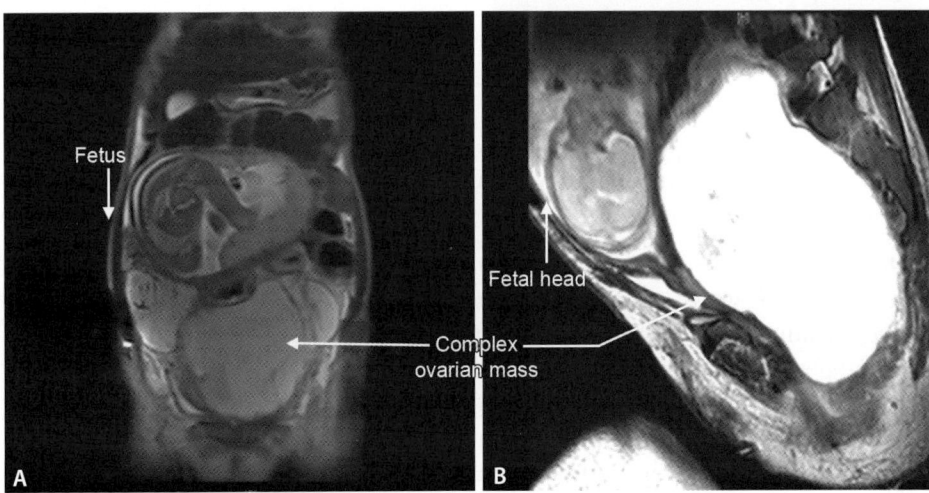

Figs. 2A and B: MRI pelvis of a 21-year-lady, G2A1 at 25 weeks of pregnancy with right complex adnexal mass. (A) Coronal view; (B) Sagittal view T2 weighted image.

Chemotherapy

Chemotherapy is recommended for all invasive epithelial ovarian cancers except stage IA/IB, well differentiated tumors. A combination of carboplatin and paclitaxel is the standard regimen. For germ cell tumors, combination chemotherapy (bleomycin, etoposide, and cisplatin) is recommended for all except stage IA dysgerminoma and stage I, grade 1 or 2 immature teratoma. Chemotherapy for ovarian epithelial and germ cell tumors can be safely given after 14 weeks of gestation.

THYROID CANCER

Considering the indolent nature of thyroid cancer, thyroidectomy is usually delayed until the postpartum period to minimize maternal and fetal complications. The patient should be monitored during pregnancy with thyroid ultrasound performed during each trimester. If by 24 weeks there is a significant increase in thyroid cancer size (50% in volume and 20% in diameter in two dimensions), surgery should be performed during the second trimester. Surgery during pregnancy is sometimes also indicated for patients with larger, more aggressive or rapidly growing cancers, or in the presence of extensive nodal or distant metastasis.

Radioactive iodine (RAI) if indicated should be started after delivery as it is absolutely contraindicated during pregnancy. RAI can negatively affect fetal brain development both directly because of its radioactive effect and indirectly by causing hypothyroidism.[23] RAI during pregnancy can lead to fetal mental retardation, malformations, as well as an increased cancer risk in the later years of its life.[24] For this reason, it is recommended to perform a pregnancy test before starting RAI treatment in a woman of reproductive age.

KEY MESSAGES

- Cancer in pregnancy is rare but its management is very challenging and requires a multidisciplinary approach; including obstetrician, oncologists, neonatologist, geneticist and psychotherapist.
- The diagnosis and treatment of cancer should not be delayed during pregnancy as it can adversely impact maternal outcome.
- Surgery can be performed throughout during pregnancy with due precautions. The optimal time for surgery is the second trimester of pregnancy.
- Majority chemotherapy drugs can be given from 14 weeks of gestation with careful monitoring of fetal wellbeing.
- Targeted therapy and hormonal therapy are generally contraindicated during pregnancy.
- Diagnostic or therapeutic modalities containing radiation should be avoided during pregnancy.
- Breastfeeding is contraindicated if the mother is receiving chemotherapy or hormonal therapy in postpartum period.
- If managed appropriately, pregnancy does not negatively impact maternal outcome.

REFERENCES

1. Silverstein J, Post A, Chien AJ, Olin R, Tsai KK, Ngo Z. Multidisciplinary management of cancer during pregnancy. JCO Oncol Pract. 2020;16:545-57.
2. Wieseler KM, Bhargava P, Kanal KM, Vaidya S, Stewart BK, Dighe MK. Imaging in pregnant patients: examination appropriateness. Radiographics. 2010;30:1215-33.
3. Han SN, Amant F, Cardonick EH, Loibl S, Peccatori FA, Gheysens O, et al. Axillary staging for breast cancer during pregnancy: feasibility and safety of sentinel lymph node biopsy. Breast Cancer Res Treat. 2018;168:551-7.
4. Rubinchik-Stern M, Shmuel M, Bar J, Eyal S, Kovo M. Maternal-fetal transfer of indocyanine green across the perfused human placenta. Reprod Toxicol. 2016;62:100-5.
5. Amant F, Berveiller P, Boere IA, Cardonick E, Fruscio R, Fumagalli M, et al. Gynecologic cancers in pregnancy: guidelines based on a third international consensus meeting. Ann Oncol. 2019;30:1601-12.
6. Cardonick E, Iacobucci A. Use of chemotherapy during human pregnancy. Lancet Oncol. 2004;5:283.
7. de Haan J, Verheecke M, Van Calsteren K, Calster BN, Shmakov RG, Gziri MM, et al. Oncological management and obstetric and neonatal outcomes for women diagnosed with cancer during pregnancy: a 20-year international cohort study of 1170 patients. Lancet Oncol. 2018;19:337-46.
8. Amant F, Van Calsteren K, Halaska MJ, Halaska MJ, Gziri MM, Hui W, et al. Long-term cognitive and cardiac outcomes after prenatal exposure to chemotherapy in children aged 18 months or older: an observational study. Lancet Oncol. 2012;13(3):256-64.
9. Weisz B, Meirow D, Schiff E, Lishner M. Impact and treatment of cancer during pregnancy. Expert Rev Anticancer Ther. 2004;4:889-902.
10. Griffin SJ, Milla M, Baker TE. Transfer of carboplatin and paclitaxel into breast milk. J Hum Lact. 2012;28:457-9.
11. Amant F, Vandenbroucke T, Verheecke M, Fumagalli M, Halaska MJ, Boere I, et al. Pediatric outcome after maternal cancer diagnosed during pregnancy. N Engl J Med. 2015;373:1824-34.
12. Lee GE, Mayer EL, Partridge A. Prognosis of pregnancy-associated breast cancer. Breast Cancer Res Treat. 2017;163:417-21.
13. Stensheim H, Møller B, van Dijk T. Cause-specific survival for women diagnosed with cancer during pregnancy or lactation: a registry-based cohort study. J Clin Oncol. 2009;27:45.
14. Ishida T, Yokoe T, Kasumi F, Sakamoto G, Makita M, Tominaga T, et al. Clinicopathologic characteristics and prognosis of breast cancer patients associated with pregnancy and lactation: analysis of case-control study in Japan. JPN J Cancer Res. 1992;83:1143-9.
15. Bonnier P, Romain S, Dilhuydy JM. Influence of pregnancy on the outcome of breast cancer: a case-control study. Societe Francaise de Senologie et de Pathologie Mammaire Study Group. Int J Cancer. 1997;72:720.
16. Woo JC, Yu T, Hurd TC. Breast cancer in pregnancy: a literature review. Arch Surg. 2003;138:91-8.

17. Hartman EK, Eslick GD. The prognosis of women diagnosed with breast cancer before, during and after pregnancy: a meta-analysis. Breast Cancer Res Treat. 2016;160:347-60.
18. Shao C, Yu Z, Xiao J, Liu L, Hong F, Zhang Y, et al. Prognosis of pregnancy-associated breast cancer: a meta-analysis. BMC Cancer. 2020;20:746.
19. Van Calsteren K, Vergote I, Amant F. Cervical neoplasia during pregnancy: diagnosis, management and prognosis. Best Pract Res Clin Obstet Gynaecol. 2005;19(4):611-30.
20. Hopkins MP, Morley GW. The prognosis and management of cervical cancer associated with pregnancy. Obstet Gynecol. 1992;80:9-13.
21. Perkins RB, Guido RS, Castle PE. 2019 ASCCP Risk-Based Management Consensus Guidelines for Abnormal Cervical Cancer Screening Tests and Cancer Precursors. J Low Genit Tract Dis. 2020;24:102-131.
22. Creasman WT. Cancer and pregnancy. Ann N Y Acad Sci. 2001;943:281-6.
23. Berg GE, Nystrom EH, Jacobsson L. Radioiodine treatment of hyperthyroidism in a pregnant women. J Nucl Med. 1998;39:357-61.
24. Hatch M, Brenner A, Bogdanova T. A screening study of thyroid cancer and other thyroid disease among individuals exposed in utero to iodine-131 from Chernobyl fallout. J Clin Endocrinol Metab. 2009;94:899-906.

LONG QUESTIONS

1. Describe principles of management of cancer in pregnancy.
2. Describe management of breast and gynecological cancers during pregnancy

SHORT QUESTIONS

1. Describe fetal toxicities of targeted therapy during pregnancy.
2. How will you manage a 30-year-old, G1 with 20 week pregnancy and 2 cm cervical lesion biopsy proven squamous cell carcinoma?
3. Describe principles of diagnostic work up for malignancy in a pregnant woman.

MULTIPLE CHOICE QUESTIONS

1. Termination of pregnancy is recommended in case of fetal exposure to ionizing radiation dose:
   a. 0.2 mGy
   b. 2 mGy
   c. 20 mGy
   d. 200 mGy
2. Which modality of radiological investigation should be avoided in cancer in pregnancy?
   a. Computed tomography of abdomen and pelvis
   b. Ultrasonography of abdomen and pelvis
   c. Magnetic resonance imaging of abdomen and pelvis
   d. Chest X-ray
3. Which of the following is not recommended for sentinel lymph node procedure during pregnancy?
   a. Methylene blue
   b. Tc 99 colloid
   c. Indocyanine green
4. Margin of safety set for in utero exposure of ionizing radiation is:
   a. 50 mGy
   b. 500 mGy
   c. 5 mGy
   d. 5,000 mGy
5. Which of the following drugs can be used in second and third trimesters of pregnancy?
   a. Trastuzumab
   b. Bevacizumab
   c. Carboplatin
   d. Tamoxifen
6. Which of the following procedures is contraindicated in evaluation of abnormal PAP smear in pregnancy?
   a. Colposcopy
   b. VIA
   c. Cervical biopsy
   d. Endocervical curettage
7. Which is the preferred surgical treatment for breast cancer in first and second trimesters of pregnancy?
   a. Breast conservative surgery
   b. Mastectomy
   c. Lumpectomy
   d. Wide local excision
8. Which of the following tumor markers is most reliable in pregnancy?
   a. AFP
   b. CA 125
   c. Beta hCG
   d. CEA
9. Which of the following is not advisable during abdominal surgery during pregnancy?
   a. Laparoscopy with intra-abdominal pressure between 10 and 13 mm Hg
   b. Laparoscopy with entry by Hasson's technique
   c. Laparoscopy with veress needle entry
   d. Laparoscopy at 16 weeks of gestation
10. Management of a 10 cm adnexal mass with solid cystic areas on USG, CA 125–500, in a 35-year-old lady with 24 weeks period of gestation
    a. Observation with no further action
    b. CE-CT abdomen and pelvis
    c. Laparotomy
    d. Laparoscopic surgery

Answers					
1. d	2. a	3. a	4. a	5. c	6. d
7. b	8. d	9. c	10. c		

5.16 HIV/AIDS AND OTHER SEXUALLY TRANSMITTED INFECTIONS

Archana Kumari, Monika Anant

BACKGROUND

Acquired immunodeficiency disease (AIDS) caused by human immunodeficiency virus (HIV) is a globally prevalent disease, but presently with no vaccine or permanent cure. HIV virus attacks the body's immune system and is spread through certain body fluids, including breast milk. There are two types of HIV—(1) type I (HIV-1) and (2) type 2 (HIV-2). The most common cause of HIV infection throughout the world is HIV-1. HIV-2 is less pathogenic than HIV-1 with slower disease progression, a much longer asymptomatic stage, slower decline in CD4 count, lower rates of vertical transmission, lower viral loads while asymptomatic and smaller gain in CD4 count in response to therapy. Mother-to-child transmission can occur during pregnancy, birth, or breastfeeding. Antiretroviral therapy (ART) has changed the outlook of HIV/AIDS from a virtual death sentence to a chronic manageable disease and also substantially reduced the risk of mother-to-child transmission (MTCT).

EPIDEMIOLOGY

India has a low HIV prevalence of 0.22%. HIV prevalence among adult males (15–49 years) was estimated at 0.24% (0.18–0.32%) and among adult females at 0.20% (0.15–0.26%). Even with this low prevalence, in terms of absolute numbers, India has third largest number of people living with HIV (PLHIV) in the world with an estimated 2.14 million people living with HIV, 87,000 estimated new infections and 69,000 AIDS-related deaths annually. Information on the epidemiology of HIV-2 and dual infection in India is limited but cases of HIV-2 infection have been reported.

The country is committed to achieving the Sustainable Development Goal (SDG) of ending AIDS as a public health threat by 2030 and is signatory to the UN strategy of 90-90-90 by 2020 which aims at ending AIDS epidemic by achieving that 90% of the estimated PLHIV know their status, of which 90% PLHIV are on ART, of which 90% PLHIV have viral suppression.

EFFECT OF PREGNANCY ON HIV AND VICE VERSA

Pregnancy does not affect disease progression. Studies from developing countries have suggested increased risk of preterm birth, stillbirth, fetal growth restriction, and perinatal mortality in HIV infected women with more risks in advanced disease. The major effect of HIV on pregnancy is risk of MTCT.

Estimated Risk and Factors Affecting Mother-to-Child Transmission

Estimated risk of perinatal transmission in the absence of any intervention and with ART intervention is mentioned in **Tables 1 and 2**. Several factors affect the rate of perinatal transmission during pregnancy, labor, and breastfeeding. The factors, which are common to all three periods are—high maternal viral load, newly acquired HIV infection and advanced disease. Specific factors operating during pregnancy, delivery and breastfeeding are mentioned in **Table 3**. The most important factor affecting the transmission is *high maternal viral load*.

TABLE 1: Risk of perinatal transmission without intervention.

Timing of transmission	Risk of transmission
During pregnancy	5–10%
During delivery	10–15%
During breastfeeding	5–20%
Overall without breastfeeding	15–25%
Overall with breastfeeding till 6 months	20–35%
Overall with breastfeeding till 18–24 months	30–45%

TABLE 2: Risk of perinatal transmission with intervention.

Short course with one antiretroviral drug (ARV); breastfeeding	15–25%
Short course with one ARV; no breastfeeding	5–15%
Short course with two ARVs; breastfeeding	5%
3 ARVs (ART) with breastfeeding	2%
3 ARVs (ART) with no breastfeeding	1%

TABLE 3: Factors that increase risk of mother to child transmission (MTCT).

Period	Factors
During pregnancy	• Viral, bacterial and parasitic infections of placenta • Maternal malnutrition • Coexisting STIs
During delivery	• Prolonged labor • Prolonged rupture of membrane • Preterm delivery • Chorioamnionitis • Invasive birth procedures • First baby of twin
During breastfeeding	• Increased duration of feeding • Mixed feeding • Oral disease in infants breast abscess, nipple fissures and mastitis
In all stages	• High viral load • Newly acquired infection • Advanced disease

Mechanisms of Mother-to-Child transmission

Antepartum: There is no mixing of maternal and fetal blood due to presence of placental barrier. In utero transmission is related to microtransfusion of virus from maternal blood to fetus due to breakdown of the integrity of the placental barrier.[1] A number of studies have shown that genital tract infections and placental inflammation, especially chorioamnionitis, can increase in utero HIV transmission.[2]

Intrapartum: Transmission during delivery occurs through contact of infant mucosal membranes with HIV virus in maternal blood and genital tract secretions. In the absence of antiretroviral treatment, membrane rupture more than four hours is associated with increased risk of transmission.[3]

Breastfeeding: HIV virus is expressed in breast milk. Transmission during breastfeeding occurs through contact of infant oral and gastrointestinal mucosa with the virus.

Factors that Decrease the Risk of Mother-to-Child Transmission

Intervention with antiretroviral (ARV) drugs containing triple drug regimen have the potential to reduce the risk of MTCT to < 5% in breastfeeding populations and < 2% in non-breastfeeding populations. The reduced risk is due to reduction of maternal viral load and loading fetus with ARVs that prevent transmitted virions from replicating. Previously used single dose Navirapine reduced the risk to 11% only. It did not cover the risk of HIV transmission during antenatal and breastfeeding periods. Further it increases the risk of drug resistance and cross resistance to efavirenz.

LABORATORY DIAGNOSIS OF HIV

In view of the low prevalence of HIV in India, it is necessary to use three different antigen-based rapid tests to confirm the diagnosis. All samples reactive in the first test should further undergo confirmatory 2nd/3rd tests based on different principles/antigens using the same serum/plasma sample as that in the 1st test. The same blood sample is utilized for performing all the tests for identifying HIV antibodies. For indeterminate results, testing should be repeated on a second sample taken after 14–28 days. Accurate diagnosis and differentiation of HIV-1 and HIV-2 is crucial for treatment, as HIV-2 is intrinsically resistant to nonnucleoside reverse-transcriptase inhibitors (NNRTI). Rapid kits that differentiate between HIV-1 and HIV-2 are being used at Integrated Counselling and Testing Centers (ICTCs). However, test results that show HIV-2 reactivity need confirmation at designated HIV-2 referral laboratory through ART centers.

ANTIRETROVIRAL DRUGS RECOMMENDED UNDER NATIONAL PROGRAM

Various ARV drugs recommended for HIV infection is shown in **Tables 4 and 5**. HIV is currently treated with combination therapy using at least three drugs from different groups—nucleoside reverse transcriptase inhibitor (NRTI) backbone (Tenofovir and Lamivudine) and one NNRTI/protease inhibitors (PIs)/integrase inhibitors. Triple drug therapy provides maximal and most durable viral suppression. Monotherapy or dual therapy should not be used due to risk of resistance. Benefits of ART other than reducing MTCT is to delay disease progression, prevent opportunistic infections (OIs), decreased rates of hospitalization, decreased transmission of HIV, increased survival and quality of life.

Dolutegravir (DTG) is a new drug under the national program that has shown to:
- Suppress viral load in a higher proportion of patients, does so faster and for longer
- Has fewer side effects
- Has a higher barrier to resistance than NNRTI
- Reduces the need to switch treatment regimen
- Adverse effects are rare and manageable.

TABLE 4: Classes of antiretroviral (ARV) drugs.

Nucleoside reverse transcriptase inhibitors (Nostril)	Non-nucleoside reverse transcriptase inhibitors (NNRTI)	Protease inhibitors (PI)
Zidovudine (AZT/ZDV)*	Nevirapine* (NVP)	Saquinavir (SQV)
Stavudine (d4T)	Efavirenz*(EFV)	Ritonavir (RTV)*
Lamivudine (3TC)*	Delavirdine (DLV)	Nelfinavir (NFV)
Abacavir (ABC)*	Rilpivirine (RPV)	Amprenavir (APV)
Didanosine (ddI)	Etravirine (ETV)	Indinavir (INV)
Zalcitabine (ddC)	*Integrase inhibitors*	Lopinavir (LPV)*
Emtricitabine (FTC)	Raltegravir (RGV)*	Fosamprenavir (FPV)
Nucleotide reverse transcriptase inhibitors (NtRTI)	Elvitegravir (EVG)	Atazanavir (ATV)*
Tenofovir (TDF)*	Dolutegravir (DTG)*	Tipranavir (TPV)
		Darunavir (DRV)*

*Drugs in National Program

TABLE 5: Antiretroviral (ARV) drugs in national program—doses and side effects.

Generic name	Dose	Side effects
Tenofovir (TDF)	300 mg daily	Nephrotoxicity, hypophosphatemia
Lamivudine (3TC)	300 mg daily	Minimal toxicity, rash (though very rare) rarely pancreatitis
Zidovudine (AZT/ZDV)	300 mg twice daily	Anemia, neutropenia, bone marrow suppression, gastrointestinal intolerance, headache, insomnia, myopathy, lactic acidosis, skin and nail hyperpigmentation
Abacavir (ABC)	300 mg twice daily or 600 mg once daily.	Hypersensitivity reaction in 3–5% (can be fatal), fever, rash, fatigue, nausea, vomiting, anorexia, respiratory symptoms (sore throat, cough, shortness of breath); rechallenging after reaction can be fatal
Efavirenz (EFV)	600 mg HS avoid taking after high fat meals	CNS symptoms (dizziness, somnolence, insomnia, confusion, hallucinations, and agitation) and personality change. Rash occurs, but less common than NVP
Lopinavir/Ritonavir (LPV/r)	400/100 mg BD	Gastrointestinal disturbance, glucose intolerance, lipodystrophy, dyslipidemia
Raltegravir (RAL)	400 mg twice daily	Rhabdomyolysis, myopathy, myalgia, diarrhea, fever, rash, Stevens-Johnson syndrome, toxic epidermal necrolysis, hepatitis
Dolutegravir (DTG)	50 mg once daily	Insomnia and headache. Dolutegravir can cause serious, life-threatening side effects. These include hypersensitivity (allergic) reactions and liver problems. People with a history of hepatitis B virus (HBV) or hepatitis C virus (HCV) infection or who have elevated results on liver function tests may have an increased risk of developing new or worsening liver problems

Key considerations about DTG for pregnant women:
- Women of childbearing age, if exposed to DTG at time of conception, there is very small potential for birth defect (neural tube defects) among infants.
- According to World Health Organization (WHO), benefits of DTG (greater viral suppression, fewer maternal deaths, fewer sexual transmissions, and less MTCT) far outweigh the risks.
- Women should be provided full information about the risks and benefits of DTG in order to make an informed choice.

When and What to Start ART in Adults and Adolescents

The current National AIDS Control Organization (NACO) guidelines (2017) is to *Treat All*, stating that all persons diagnosed with HIV infection should be initiated on ART *regardless of the CD4 count or WHO Clinical Staging or age group or population subgroups.* All patients should undergo adequate preparedness and adherence counseling before the initiation of ART. Fixed-dose combinations (FDCs) of ARVs are preferred due to ease of prescription and ease of intake and thereby improved treatment adherence. This is essential for PLHIV as *the treatment is life-long* and the chances of developing drug resistant mutants and the resultant treatment failure need to be minimized. *All PLHIV with HIV-1 infection be initiated on a first line regimen of Tenofovir (300 mg) + Lamivudine (300 mg) + Efavirenz (600 mg) (TLE) as fixed dose combination in a single pill once a day (NACO 2013 and 2017 guidelines).* A combination of clinical and laboratory monitoring is to be carried out in all PLHIV after initiation of ART. CD4 count is done at initial visit, every 6 months. Viral load is done at 6 months, 12 months, and then every 12 months. Virological suppression in context of national program means a viral load of less than 1,000 copies/mL after at least 6 months on ART.

According to recommendation of 14th meeting of Technical resource group (TRG) on ART in 2020, NACO is introducing DTG-based regime in phase wise manner.

New initiation: A fixed dose combination of Tenofovir 300 mg + Lamivudine 300 mg + DTG (50) mg (TLD) would be the preferred first line regimen for starting ART in PLHIV >10 years of age and weight >30 kg.

Transition from old regimen: Viral load test to be done before transition to DTG based regimen. Virally suppressed (<1,000 copies/mL) patients to transition to TLD, while unsuppressed patients to first undergo step-up counseling for 3 months, while continuing same regimen. The patient should have an adherence of more than 95% for conducting a second viral load test.

Prevention of Parent-to-Child Transmission and ART in Pregnant Women (Box 1 and Flowchart 1)

Under the national program, it is recommended to provide *lifelong ART for all pregnant and breastfeeding women living with HIV*, to receive a "single-pill" triple-drug ART regimen (Tenofovir, Lamivudine and Dolutegravir) -*TLD* or (Tenofovir, Lamivudine and Efavirenz -*TLE, regardless of CD4 count or clinical stage,* both for their own health and to prevent vertical HIV transmission and for additional HIV prevention benefits **(Box 2)**.

BOX 1: Goal and Objectives of Prevention of Parent to Child Transmission (PPTCT) Services in India.

Vision: Women and children, alive and free from HIV

Goal: To work toward elimination of pediatric HIV and improve maternal, new born and child health and survival in the context of HIV infection

Objectives:
- To detect more than 90% HIV infected pregnant women in India
- To provide access to comprehensive PPTCT services to more than 90% of the detected pregnant women
- To provide access to early infant diagnosis to more than 90% HIV exposed infants
- To ensure access to ARV drugs prophylaxis or ART to 100% HIV exposed infants
- To ensure more than 95% adherence with ART in HIV infected pregnant women and ARV/ART in exposed children.

PPTCT Scenarios

- *Mother diagnosed with HIV during pregnancy/ANC:* Even if the pregnant women present very late in pregnancy (including those who present after 36 weeks of gestation) the ART should be initiated promptly at ART centers only **(Table 6)**.
  - *Dose of syrup navirapine* 10 mg/mL suspension: Dose is 1.5 mL or 15 mg once daily in babies >2.5 kg, 10 mg or 1 mL once daily (Birth weight 2–2.5 kg)
  - *For HIV 2 infection- syrup zidovudine* in place of nevirapine immediately after birth till 6 weeks of age. The recommended dosages are: Birth weight > 2.5 kg: 15 mg per dose twice daily, birth weight < 2.5 kg: 10 mg per dose twice daily.

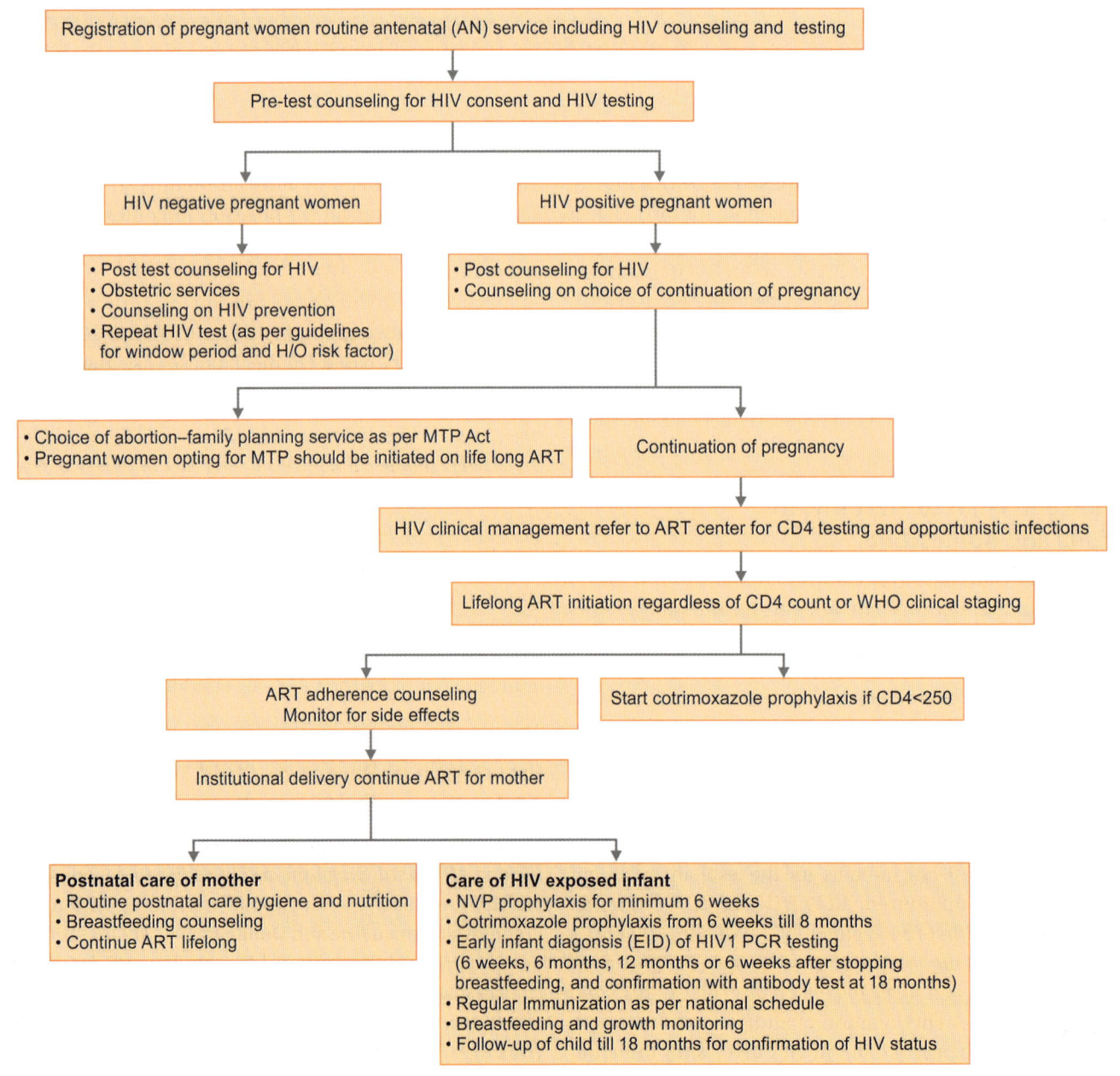

Flowchart 1: Cascade of prevention of parent to child transmission (PPTCT) services.

> **BOX 2:** Lifelong antiretroviral therapy (ART).
>
> Start lifelong ART irrespective of CD4 count and clinical stage.
> **Tenofovir (300 mg) + Lamivudine (300 mg) + Dolutegravir (50 mg) (DTG) -TLD regime to be started** (after first trimester), continue ART through pregnancy, delivery and lifelong.
> If women do want to use TLD or in first trimester:
>
> | | | |
> |---|---|---|
> | HIV type 1 | **TLE** | TDF (300 mg) + 3TC (300 mg) +EFV (600 mg) FDC to be given 2 hours after fat free meal. |
> | HIV type 2/ HIV type 1 and 2*- | **TLL** | TDF (300 mg) + 3TC (300 mg) OD FDC of LPV (200 mg)/r (50 mg) – 2 tablets BD |

*NNRTI drugs are not effective against HIV-2.

TABLE 6: ARV prophylaxis for HIV exposed infant.

Case scenario	Duration of ARV (mother)	Duration of ARV prophylaxis for infant
Mother on DTG based regime (TLD) and breast feeding	On ART for 4 weeks or more	6 weeks
Mother on DTG based regime (TLD) and breast feeding	On ART for less than 4 weeks	12 weeks
Mother on non-DTG based regime (TLE/TLL) and breast feeding	On ART for 24 weeks or more	6 weeks
Mother on non-DTG based regime and breast feeding	On ART for less than 24 weeks	12 weeks

*Extended regimen of 12 weeks applies to infants of breastfeeding women only and not those on replacement feeding.

- Pregnant women having prior exposure to NNRTI for PPTCT and ART regimen
  All HIV positive pregnant women exposed to NVP/EFV in past should be initiated on TLD regime. If in first trimester or not willing to take TLD- start her on Lopinavir/ritonavir (LPV/r) instead of Efavirenz (EFV)—**TLL regimen** as there are there are chances of HIV resistance to NNRTI. zidovudine syrup is the preferred ARV prophylaxis. If Zidovudine syrup is not available, nevirapine syrup may be used.
- HIV positive pregnant women already on ART getting pregnant
  Continue same ART regime during pregnancy, labor and delivery and lifelong. Infants (breastfeeding or replacement feeding): Daily navirapine prophylaxis for 6 weeks.
- *Women presenting directly-in-labor (unbooked cases with no HIV report)/ and is identified as new HIV positive in labor room/OR immediately postpartum*
  Labor room nurse will offer bed side counseling and HIV screening test
  - If the woman consents, screen using the "Whole Blood Finger Prick test" in delivery room or labor ward.
  - If detected HIV positive, the doctor on duty will initiate *TLD regime* and ensure immediate linkage to ART center for lifelong ART. Labor room nurse informs the ICTC counselor and lab technician for further confirmation of HIV.
  - Breastfeeding—Extended daily navirapine prophylaxis from birth for 12 weeks.
  - For replacement feeding—Daily navirapine prophylaxis for 6 weeks only.

- *Women found to be HIV positive after delivery: Women had home delivery or identified HIV positive after delivery when they bring infants to hospital*
  - *Breastfeeding:* Link to ART center for initiation of lifelong ART. If infant <6 months—navirapine prophylaxis for 12 weeks. EID testing.
  - *Replacement feeding:* Refer mother to ART center for HIV care and evaluation for treatment. Infant < 72 hours: Navirapine prophylaxis for 6 weeks.
- *Pregnant women with active tuberculosis*
  If on rifampicin based ATT regime: Along with TLD regime, additional dose of 50 mg dolutegravir to be given (12 hours after taking the regular dose) for the duration of TB treatment.

CARE OF HIV POSITIVE PREGNANT WOMEN
Care during Pregnancy

- Antiretroviral treatment for all the pregnant women irrespective of the CD4 count and WHO clinical stage
- Screening of all women for tuberculosis and treat if necessary
- *Cotrimoxazole if the CD4 count is less than 350 cells/mm^3*
- Screening for syphilis and other sexually transmitted infections
- Counseling for ART adherence, institutional delivery, exclusive breastfeeding, safe sex practice, disclosure to partner, and screening partner and other children for HIV
- Regular antenatal check-ups and follow-up
- TT, iron and folic acid, nutrition supplementation and other treatment as required.

Care during Delivery

- Follow universal work precautions
- Vaginal examinations minimized as much as possible
- Do not rupture membranes artificially. Keep membranes intact for as long as possible. Artificial rupture of membrane is reserved for cases of fetal distress or delays in the progress of labor
- Avoid invasive procedures such as fetal blood sampling and/or fetal scalp electrodes
- Avoid episiotomy as much as possible
- Avoid instrumental delivery as much as possible. Use low cavity outlet forceps instead of ventouse if there is fetal distress and maternal fatigue
- Do not milk the umbilical cord. The cord should be clamped soon after birth. Use a gloved hand to cover the cord with gauze before cutting to avoid splashing
- Suctioning the newborn with a nasogastric tube should be avoided unless the meconium is stained.

Recommendations for Cesarean Sections

HIV positive status *perse* is not an indication for cesarean sections. Cesarean is recommended only for an obstetric indication. Elective cesarean is always preferable to emergency cesarean sections.

- Ensure ARV drugs and prophylactic antibiotics before surgery.
- Follow universal work precautions and use "dry" hemostatic techniques to minimize bleeding.
- Leave the membranes intact until the head is delivered through the surgical incision.
- Use round-tip blunt needles for stitches and use forceps instead of fingers to receive and hold the needle.
- Observe good practice when transferring sharps to the surgical assistant (e.g., use a holding container/safe zones. For disposal of tissues, the placenta and other medical/infectious waste material from the delivery, standard waste disposal management guidelines should be followed.

Postpartum Care and Contraception in HIV Positive Women

- Lifelong ART for the mother with good adherence
- Follow up and treatment of mother for postpartum complications and depression
- Cu-T insertion can be done at 6 weeks, if already PPIUCD not inserted within 48 hours in addition to use of condom (Dual contraception)
- Male sterilization in father by non-scalpel vasectomy (NSV) to be encouraged between 18 months and 2 years when baby's survival has been ensured.

National Infant Feeding Guideline: The Infant and Young Child Feeding Guidelines, 2016, recommend:

- Exclusive breastfeeding in the first 6 months, irrespective of the fact that mother is on ART early or infant is provided with antiretroviral prophylaxis for 6 weeks, continue breastfeeding for 2 years of age along with complementary feeds in HIV negative babies also.
- For children who are confirmed to be HIV positive, initiate ART and continue breastfeeding until 2 years of age.
- Exclusive replacement feeding is applicable if the AFASS (affordable, feasible, acceptable, sustainable, and safe) criteria can be fulfilled or where exclusive breast feeding (EBF) cannot be done due to maternal death or severe maternal illness.
- No mixed feeding.

Management of HIV Exposed Infants

- ARV prophylaxis to be started as soon as possible
- Vaccination as per the guidelines
- *Cotrimoxazole preventive therapy (CPT):* Initiate Cotrimoxazole at 6 weeks for all HIV exposed infants, irrespective of breastfeeding or replacement feeding practice and discontinue when HIV infection has been ruled out at 18 months
- Early infant diagnosis (EID) at 6 weeks.

COVID-19, Pregnancy and HIV

People living with HIV should receive severe acute respiratory syndrome coronavirus 2 (SARS-CoV-2) vaccines regardless of CD4 count or viral load, because the potential benefits outweigh potential risks. COVID vaccination should not be withheld for pregnant women with HIV (ACOG, SMFM 2021).

Currently, there is limited data available on pregnancy and maternal outcomes in individuals with COVID-19 and HIV but pregnancy with HIV are at increased risk for severe outcomes with COVID-19 compared with people without HIV. Clinical management of pregnancy with HIV and COVID-19 coinfection remains essentially the same as SARS-CoV-2 pregnant women without HIV. Telephonic or virtual visits for routine or non-urgent care and adherence counseling should be utilized more than hospital visits. New onset or worsening dyspnea warrants an in-hospital evaluation. ART should be continued and ARV drug substitutions should be avoided. Pregnant individuals with HIV admitted for COVID-19 should continue their ARV regimen. Changes in regimens should only be done in consultation with an HIV expert if needed. The goal should be to keep pregnant women with HIV as healthy as possible during this pandemic with an uninterrupted ART supply and on a regimen which has established safety and efficacy in pregnancy. As breastfeeding is recommended for women with HIV in India, a combination of hand hygiene and a mask, and, if possible, pumping and feeding by a healthy caregiver, is recommended to provide protection from respiratory transmission of SARS-CoV-2 while mothers are still infectious.

SEXUALLY TRANSMITTED INFECTIONS IN PREGNANCY

Sexually transmitted infections (STIs) in pregnancy can change the natural course of a healthy pregnancy and fetus, can result in significant morbidity and mortality and even congenital malformation of fetus.[5] Hence, any STI diagnosed in a pregnant woman warrants early treatment. Since most STIs are asymptomatic in women, screening facilitates the identification of STIs in pregnant women **(Table 7)**. In recent times the epidemiology of STIs has changed and viral causes of STI are more common than bacterial pathogens of STI.

Syphilis

Syphilis is caused by *Treponema pallidum*, a highly transmissible spirochete. 3–10% of patients contract the disease even with a single sexual encounter. The rate of horizontal transmission is 30%. The lesions on mucous membranes or abraded skin **(Figs. 1A and B)**, blood transfusion, or transplacental from a pregnant woman to her fetus (vertical transmission) are modes of transmission. In early maternal syphilis the *maternal fetal transmission rate* can be up to 80%, whereas in late syphilis infectivity decreases **(Table 8)**.[6]

Prevalence

Globally, the estimated prevalence of maternal syphilis in 2016 was 0.69%, resulting in a global congenital syphilis rate of 473 per 100,000 live births. In India, seroprevalence of syphilis in ANC women was 0.38% (2010–11 round of HIV Sentinel Surveillance).[7] There is an increased MTCT of HIV among pregnant women coinfected with syphilis and HIV.

Diagnostic Tests

- Direct detection methods (i.e., dark-field microscopy, direct fluorescent antibody test, and nucleic acid amplification test)
- Serology (treponemal and non-treponemal tests)
- Examination of cerebrospinal fluids
  - *Non-treponemal tests:* Microscopic Venereal Diseases Research Laboratory (VDRL) test, macroscopic rapid plasma reagin (RPR) tests (qualitative or quantitative).

TABLE 7: CDC recommendations for STI screening in pregnancy.[8]

Condition	Screening recommended		Preferred test
Bacterial vaginosis*	No		—
Chlamydia	Yes	All pregnant women under 25 years of age Pregnant women, aged 25 and older if at increased risk Retest during the 3rd trimester for women under 25 years of age or at risk Pregnant women with chlamydial infection should have a test-of-cure 3–4 weeks after treatment and be retested within 3 months	NAAT
Gonorrhea	Yes	All pregnant women under 25 years of age and older women if at increased risk Retest 3 months after treatment	Women who are at risk† or living in a high-prevalence area NAAT or culture on Thayer-Martin media
Hepatitis B	Yes	Test for HBsAg at first prenatal visit of each pregnancy regardless of prior testing; retest at delivery if at high risk	HBsAg serology
Hepatitis C	Yes	Pregnant women if risk factors are present	Anti-HCV
Herpes	No	Evidence does not support routine HSV-2 serologic screening among asymptomatic pregnant women.	Culture lesions if present Culture, PCR
HIV	Yes	All pregnant women should be screened at first prenatal visit (opt-out) Retest in the third trimester if at high risk	EIA, Western blot
HPV	No		–
Syphilis	Yes	All pregnant women at the first prenatal visit Retest early in the third trimester and at delivery if at high risk	All pregnant women RPR or VDRL
Trichomoniasis	No		
Screening for vaginal infections (GOI)[9] Asymptomatic pregnant women with a history of spontaneous abortion or pre term delivery should be screened for bacterial vaginosis (BV) and trichomoniasis	Gram-stained microscopic examination of a vaginal smear Wet mount of vaginal fluid in a drop of normal saline		In the first trimester of pregnancy, treatment may be given in cases where early treatment has the best chance of preventing adverse pregnancy outcomes

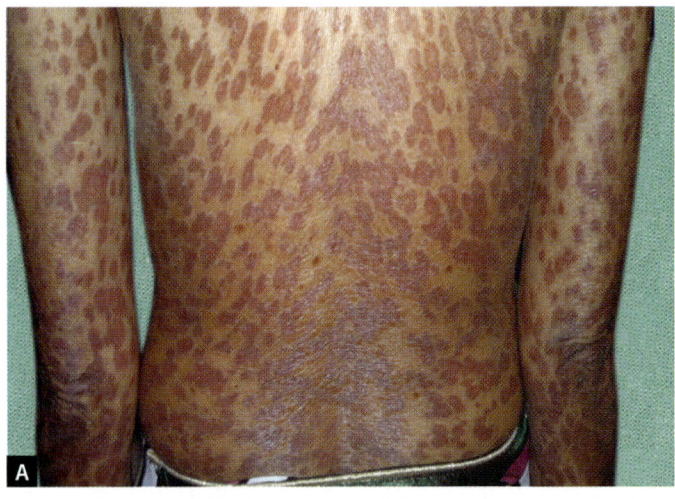
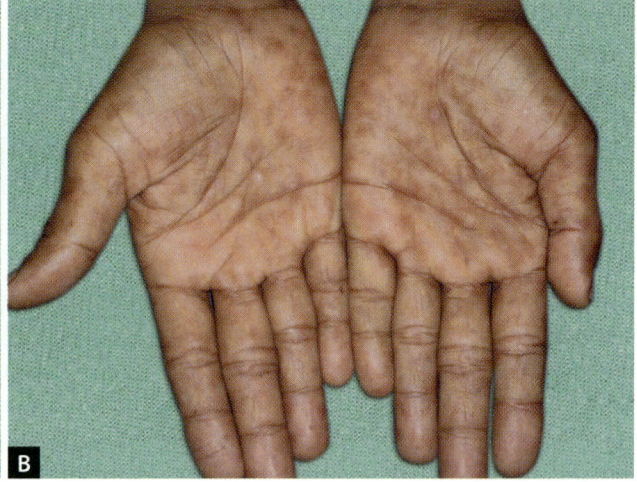

Figs. 1A and B: Secondary syphilis pappules. Generalized symmetrical coppery red maculoplaques on trunk and limbs (A) and syphilitic lesions on palms in secondary syphilis (B).

TABLE 8: Syphilis in pregnancy.

Stage	Onset of infection	Signs and symptoms	Duration of symptoms
Primary	21 days (range 10–90 days)	Painless genital ulcer	2–6 weeks
Secondary	3 weeks to 3 month	Skin rash Fever Muscle pain Latent phase: No symptoms	2–6 weeks
Tertiary	Years to decades after infection	Neurosyphilis (brain and spinal cord) Cardiosyphilis (heart) Late benign syphilis (skin)	Years

- *Treponemal tests:*
  - Treponema pallidum hemagglutination assay (TPHA)
  - Treponema pallidum particle agglutination assay (TPPA)
  - Fluorescent treponemal antibody absorption (FTA-ABS) tests.

Point-of-care test: Rapid, simple treponemal tests are immunochromatography strip (ICS)

Screening: Universal screening for syphilis in pregnancy is recommended by CDC, WHO, National guidelines because treatment of mothers can eliminate MTCT of syphilis.
- All pregnant women should be screened at the first prenatal visit
- Repeat screening at 28–32 weeks and at delivery for women with increased risk of infection
- History of stillborn >20 weeks of gestation or no history of screening in present pregnancy should be screened at delivery
- HIV testing is strongly recommended (concurrent HIV screening) in syphilis other STI, due to the high risk of coexistent disease.

Screening is performed with a blood test RPR or VDRL tests—and confirmed with FTA-ABS or TPHA. A single serologic test is insufficient because false-positives occur with other illnesses.

Complications

Maternal syphilis can cause hydramnios, spontaneous abortion, and preterm delivery. Fetal complications such as fetal syphilis, fetal hydrops, prematurity, fetal distress, and stillbirth also occur. Neonatal complications include congenital syphilis, neonatal death, and late sequelae. If syphilis is diagnosed after 20 weeks' gestation, ultrasonography should be performed to evaluate for fetal syphilis and repeated at regular interval after treatment to judge reversal of changes such as hydrops, ascites, polyhydramnios, placentomegaly and hepatomegaly caused by fetal infection. After confirming diagnosis, syphilis should be staged based on characteristic history and clinical findings. Stage will affect the treatment and risks of vertical transmission and stage is not altered by pregnant state.

Treatment: Penicillin G benzathine is the drug of choice (treatment details in **Table 9**). The fetus remains untreated with non-penicillin treatment as erythromycin and azithromycin do not cross the placental barrier completely. Hence, such infants are treated with a 10–15 day course of penicillin.

Syphilis treatment may precipitate the Jarisch–Herxheimer reaction even in pregnancy which is an acute febrile reaction with headache, myalgia, rash, and hypotension resolving only on supportive care. The reaction is seen to be more common in HIV-positive women.

Clinical response to therapy is ascertained by quantitative non-treponemal serological tests.

Successful therapy: A fourfold decline in the titer, equivalent to a change of two dilutions (e.g., from 1:16 to 1:4 or from 1:32 to 1:8).

Treatment failure: A fourfold increase in the nontreponemal titer after treatment.

Seroreversion: The loss of antibodies over time in a patient who has been treated for syphilis is considered consistent with clinical cure.

SECTION 5: Pregnancy with Pre-existing Morbidities   375

TABLE 9: Effect of sexually transmitted infections (STI) on pregnancy and pregnancy on STI, treatment summary.[9]

Interactions between STI/RTI and pregnancy	STI/RTI Effect of STI on pregnancy and neonate	Effect of pregnancy on STI	Recommended treatment
Gonorrhea	Prematurity Premature rupture of membranes	Disseminated gonococcal infection is reported to be more common	Ceftriaxone 125 mg intramuscularly in a single dose CDC recommends 500mg for weight <150 kg, 1000 mg for weight >150 kg[10] Cefixime 400 mg orally in a single dose (CDC 800 mg single dose[10]) Where Chlamydia is not excluded should receive 1 g azithromycin also
Chlamydia	Chorioamnionitis Postpartum sepsis Ophthalmia neonatorum	No effect	Azithromycin 1 g orally in a single dose or Amoxicillin 500 mg orally three times per day for 7 days
Syphilis	Abortion Prematurity Intrauterine growth retardation Stillbirth Congenital syphilis	No effect	Benzathine penicillin G 2.4 million units intramuscularly Primary Syphilis: Single dose Positive serology, no symptoms: three doses one week apart Desensitization is recommended in patients with penicillin allergy
Chancroid	No adverse effects of chancroid on pregnancy outcomes have been reported	Ulcers will increase in size and become more vascular	Azithromycin, 1 g orally as a single dose; erythromycin base, 500 mg orally 3 times daily for 7 days; or Ceftriaxone, 250 mg in a single intramuscular dose
Herpes simplex virus (HSV)	Abortion Intrauterine growth retardation Premature delivery Congenital HSV Neonatal herpes	Longer duration of symptoms Primary infection more severe dissemination may occur (DGI)	*First episode*: Acyclovir 400 mg orally three times per day or 200 mg orally five times per day for 7–10 days Valacyclovir 1 g orally two times per day for 7–10 days *Recurrent*: Acyclovir 400 mg orally three times per day for 5 days Valacyclovir 1 g orally once per day for 5 days *Suppressive therapy*: Acyclovir 400 mg orally two times per day Valacyclovir 500 mg orally once per day
Human papilloma virus (genital warts)	Laryngeal papillomatosis (rare)	Increase in size and number of warts	• Trichloroacetic acid 80–90% applied weekly. • Liquid nitrogen, electrocautery • Podofilox, imiquimod, and podophyllin are not recommended during pregnancy
Trichomoniasis	Premature rupture of membranes Preterm labor Low birth weight	No effect	Metronidazole 2 g orally in a single dose
Candidiasis	Virtually none	Increased frequency and severity of infection	Topical imidazole (clotrimazole or miconazole) vaginally for 7 days
Bacterial vaginosis	Premature rupture of membranes Chorioamnionitis Premature delivery Low birth weight Puerperal sepsis	No effect	Metronidazole 500 mg orally two times per day for 7 days

Source: National Guidelines on Prevention, Management and Control of Reproductive Tract Infections Including Sexually Transmitted Infections, Ministry Of Health And Family Welfare Government of India. New Delhi: MoHFW; 2007.

Follow-up of pregnant woman treated for syphilis and her partner is needed to know reinfection or relapse. Quantitative non-treponemal serological tests should be repeated in late pregnancy and with evidence of reinfection or relapse, retreatment is necessary. Pregnant woman and her partner should be followed up at 3, 6, 12 and 24 months after delivery. At every follow-up visit, clinical examination, qualitative and quantitative non-treponemal test (RPR) should be performed.

Congenital syphilis: T. pallidum can readily infect the developing placenta. Transplacental passage to fetus can occur as early as 9–10 weeks. Transmission usually takes place between 16 and 28 weeks of pregnancy. Increased risk of vertical transmission is seen in: mothers with untreated or inadequately treated syphilis, early stage syphilis and in mothers getting infected at later gestational age **(Box 3)**. Congenital infection has been diagnosed in 1–2% of offspring

BOX 3: Case definition of congenital syphilis.

Suspected case: "A still or live born baby of syphilis seroreactive mother"
Confirmed case: "A stillbirth, live-birth, or child aged <2 years with microbiological evidence of syphilis infection. Microbiological evidence includes anyone of the following:
- Demonstration of *T. pallidum* by dark field microscopy OR
- Fluorescent antibody detection of *T. pallidum* specific IgM in the umbilical cord or placenta, or nasal discharge or skin lesion material.
OR
A child within first 2 years of life with clinical evidence (At least 2: Swelling of joints, snuffles, bullous skin lesions, hepatosplenomegaly, jaundice, anemia, radiological changes in the long bones) of syphilis and reactive syphilis serology irrespective of the mother's serology.

TABLE 10: Recommendations on syphilis screening and treatment strategies for pregnant women (WHO 2017).[6]

Screening for maternal syphilis	Recommendation 1	*Screening all pregnant women* for syphilis during the first antenatal care visit
Screening strategies	Recommendation 2	*On-site tests* (Strategies A, B and C) rather than the standard off-site laboratory-based screening and treatment strategy
	Recommendation 3 Areas of low prevalence of syphilis (below 5%),	*A single on-site rapid syphilis test (RST)* be used to screen pregnant women (Strategy A)
	Recommendation 4 Areas of high prevalence of syphilis (5% or greater),	An on-site RST, if positive, give first dose of treatment and do a rapid plasma reagin (RPR) test If RPR test is positive, treatment modified according to duration of syphilis (Strategy C)
Treatment of Early syphilis (primary, secondary and early latent syphilis of not more than 2 years' duration)	Recommendation 5	Benzathine penicillin G 2.4 million units once intramuscularly
	Recommendation 6	Use Benzathine penicillin G 2.4 million units once intramuscularly over procaine penicillin 1.2 million units intramuscularly once daily for 10 days Alternatives: (Where Penicillin cannot be used) Erythromycin 500 mg orally four times daily for 14 days or Ceftriaxone 1 g intramuscularly once daily for 10–14 days or Azithromycin 2 g once orally
Treatment of Late syphilis (infection of more than 2 years' duration without evidence of treponemal infection)	Recommendation 7	Benzathine penicillin G 2.4 million units intramuscularly once weekly for three consecutive weeks over no treatment
	Recommendation 8	Benzathine penicillin G 2.4 million units IM once weekly for three consecutive weeks over procaine penicillin 1.2 million units IM once a day for 20 days Where penicillin cannot be used: Erythromycin 500 mg orally four times daily for 30 days
Strategy D	Standard laboratory-based screening strategy: Off-site RPR or VDRL followed (if positive) by TPPA or TPHA test and followed (if positive) by treatment	The standard screening strategy is an RPR or VDRL test, followed (if positive) by confirmation testing using TPHA or TPPA with the same blood sample; both tests are usually conducted at an off-site laboratory. Treatment is based on confirmed syphilis. Disadvantage: 1. 2–3 days to confirm 2. Two visits to the clinic for pregnant women

of women adequately treated during pregnancy compared with 70–100% of offspring of untreated mothers.

"Elimination of Parent to Child Transmission of Syphilis (e-PTCT)" is one of the new strategies launched by the STI/RTI control and prevention programme under the Department of AIDS Control (DAC) in collaboration with the Reproductive Maternal Newborn Child Health and Adolescent (RMNCH+A) programme of the National Health Mission in 2014. Its goal was to eliminate "Parent-to-Child" Transmission of Syphilis by 2017. The programmatic targets to achieve the e-PTCT goal are:
- ANC coverage (pregnant women having at least one ANC visit) of ≥95%.

- Coverage of syphilis testing of ANC attendees of ≥95%.
- Treatment of syphilis-seropositive ANC attendees of ≥95%.
- Confirmation, treatment and follow-up of 100% of suspected cases of congenital syphilis.

The other important sexually transmitted infections [Gonorrhea, Chlamydia, Chancroid, Herpes simplex virus (HSV), Human papilloma virus (genital warts), Trichomoniasis, Candidiasis, Bacterial vaginosis] in pregnancy have been outlined in **Table 10**.

REFERENCES

1. Kourtis AP, Bulterys M, Nesheim SR, Lee FK. Understanding the timing of HIV transmission from mother to infant. JAMA. 2001;285:709.
2. King CC, Ellington SR, Kourtis AP. The role of coinfections in mother-to-child transmission of HIV. Curr HIV Res. 2013;11:10-9.
3. Landesman SH, Kalish LA, Burns DN, Minkoff H, Fox HE, Zorrilla C, et al. Obstetrical factors and the transmission of human immunodeficiency virus type 1 from mother to child. The Women and Infants Transmission Study. N Engl J Med. 1996;334:1617-23.
4. James DK, Steer PJ, Weiner CP, Gonik. High Risk Pregnancy, Management options, 4th edition. Philadelphia: Saunders; 2010. pp 480-1.
5. Allstaff S, Wilson J. The management of sexually transmitted infections in pregnancy. Obstet Gynaecol. 2012;14:25-32.
6. WHO. WHO guideline on syphilis screening and treatment for pregnant women. Geneva: World Health Organization; 2017.
7. National Guidelines on Maternal Health Division Department of AIDS Control Ministry of Health and Family Welfare Government of India Prevention, Management and Control of Reproductive Tract Infections and Sexually Transmitted Infections. New Delhi: MoHFW; 2014.
8. Centers for Disease Control and Prevention. Sexually Transmitted Diseases Treatment Guidelines. Atlanta, Georgia: CDC; 2015.
9. National Guidelines on Prevention, Management and Control of Reproductive Tract Infections including Sexually Transmitted Infections Maternal Health Division Ministry of Health and Family Welfare Government of India. New Delhi: MoHFW; 2007.
10. St. Cyr S, Barbee L, Workowski KA, Bachmann LH, Pham C, Schlanger K, et al. Update to CDC's Treatment Guidelines for Gonococcal Infection, 2020. MMWR Morb Mortal Wkly Rep. 2020;69:1911-6.

LONG QUESTION

1. A 25-year-old primigravida at 28 weeks, singleton with otherwise low risk pregnancy, brings a report of positive HIV testing done at another center. How will you proceed to manage this pregnancy further?

SHORT QUESTIONS

1. What are the factors operating during pregnancy, labor and breast feeding which affect HIV transmission from mother to fetus?
2. Discuss the screening for STIs.
3. Explain the advantages and disadvantages of syndromic approach for STIs.
4. What are National Infant Feeding guidelines for HIV exposed infants?
5. Discuss the goal and objectives of PPTCT services in India.

MULTIPLE CHOICE QUESTIONS

1. Mrs A who is on ART (TLE) regimen since 2 years, visits the OPD at 18 weeks of pregnancy. Based on latest NACO guidelines, you advised her viral load test which came out to be suppressed (viral load <1,000 copies/mL). What advice you would give with regards to transition to the new TLD regimen?
   a. Transition to TLD regimen immediately
   b. Transition to TLD regimen, after providing full information about risks and benefits to make informed choice
   c. Step up counseling for 3 months, while continuing same regimen
   d. Step up counseling for 1 month, while continuing same regimen
2. What is the risk of HIV transmission from mother to child in case of HIV positive mother, who is on ART (3 ARVs) with no breastfeeding?
   a. 1%   b. 2%
   c. 3%   d. 4%
3. What is the duration of ARV prophylaxis in infants of HIV positive mother, who is taking DTG based ART regimen since 28th week of pregnancy?
   a. 6 weeks   b. 12 weeks
   c. 4 weeks   d. 24 weeks
4. Which of the following interventions should *not* be done during labor and delivery to reduce the risk of mother to child transmission in HIV positive mother?
   a. Minimize vaginal examinations
   b. Avoid prolonged labor
   c. Artificial rupture of membrane
   d. Early cord clamping, after it stops pulsating
5. Mrs D, a 24-year-old newly diagnosed HIV pregnant lady linked to the ART center. She has confirmed HIV-1 and HIV-2 coinfection. She is 4 months pregnant and her CD4 count is 700 cells/mm^3. The patient was started on TLL, as she refused TLD regimen. What ARV prophylaxis should be started to the baby after delivery?
   a. Lamivudine   b. Tenofovir
   c. Zidovudine   d. Abacavir
6. Which of the following interventions should be avoided in immediate new born care for infant born to HIV positive mother, in order to reduce the risk of mother to child transmission?
   a. Clear airway
   b. Initiate breastfeeding within 1 hour
   c. Suction using nasogastric tube, when liquor is clear
   d. ARV prophylaxis to baby as prescribed
7. What is the dose and duration of Nevirapine prophylaxis for infant of birth weight 2.2 kg born to HIV positive mother (10 mg in 1 mL suspension), who is on ART (TLE regimen) since 10th week of pregnancy?
   a. 1.5 mL once a day for 6 weeks
   b. 1.5 mL once a day for 12 weeks
   c. 1 mL once a day for 6 weeks
   d. 1 mL once a day for 12 weeks

8. Which of the following is the least toxic drug used in ART?
   a. Tenofovir
   b. Lamivudine
   c. Efavirenz
   d. Abacavir
9. Mrs L is a newly diagnosed case of PLHIV, linked to ART center. She has a 10 days old baby, who is being fed undiluted cow's milk, as mother did not want to breastfeed. Which of the following is true regarding the management of baby?
   a. Nevirapine therapy should not be started, as she has presented beyond 72 hours
   b. Nevirapine prophylaxis should be given for 12 weeks
   c. Nevirapine prophylaxis should be given for 6 weeks
   d. Zidovudine prophylaxis should be given for 6 weeks
10. Mrs A was given single dose Nevirapine prophylaxis during labor 12 years back. She has now reported to ART center, and is 4 months pregnant. Her CD4 count is 300 cells/mm^3. She is unwilling to take Dolutegravir. Which drug regimen should be started in Mrs A?
    a. Start CPT only
    b. CPT should be given first, then ART (TL+LPV/r)
    c. Start with NNRTI
    d. Continue Nevirapine
11. Treatment for external genital warts caused by HPV in pregnancy is:
    a. Acyclovir
    b. Podophyllin
    c. Local trichloroacetic acid
    d. Metronidazole
12. What characterizes "sero fast" individuals in reference to syphilis?
    a. Reduced incubation period to 1 week
    b. Response to treatment is very fast
    c. Symptoms resolve very fast
    d. Low-tire of non-treponemal test results even after successful treatment
13. Point-of-Care tests for syphilis are:
    a. Immunochromatography strip
    b. ELISA
    c. Dark field microscopy
    d. NAAT
14. CDC (2020) recommended regimen for uncomplicated gonococcal infections of the cervix, urethra, or rectum:
    a. Ceftriaxone 500 mg IM as a single dose
    b. Ceftriaxone 250 mg IM as a single dose
    c. Ceftriaxone 500 mg IV twice a day for 3 days
    d. Ceftriaxone 1000 mg IV twice a day for 3 days
15. All are objectives of PPTCT services in India, except:
    a. To detect more than 70% HIV infected pregnant women in India
    b. To provide access to comprehensive PPTCT services to more than 90% of the detected pregnant women
    c. To provide access to early infant diagnosis to more than 90% HIV exposed infants
    d. To ensure access to antiretroviral drug (ARVs) prophylaxis or antiretroviral therapy (ART) to 100% HIV exposed infants

Answers											
1.	b	2.	a	3.	a	4.	c	5.	c	6.	c
7.	c	8.	b	9.	c	10.	b	11.	c	12.	d
13.	a	14.	a	15.	a						

5.17 INFECTIONS IN PREGNANCY

Prakash K Mehta, Aparna Setia

INTRODUCTION

Infections in pregnancy are common and account for a significant proportion of maternal, fetal, and neonatal mortality and morbidity globally. Infections can be caused by viruses, bacteria, fungi, and parasites. Some infections that do not cause any problem in nonpregnant women can be dangerous in pregnancy. Other infections may not cause problems in pregnant woman, but can be harmful to the fetus and the damage may be manifested at birth or later. Maternal systemic infections like pneumonia, malaria, TB, typhoid, pyelonephritis, and worm infestations are often due to poverty, overcrowding, and malnutrition and impose health costs to the mother and risks to the fetus. The risks include spontaneous abortion, stillbirth, preterm labor and preterm birth, fetal growth restriction (FGR), and neonatal infections. Appropriate investigations and management can alleviate adverse outcomes, anxiety, and unnecessary interventions.[1]

DEFENSE MECHANISMS AGAINST INFECTION

Maternal Defenses

- *Nonspecific defenses:* These are the natural barriers to infection. Vaginal epithelium and cervix with its mucous plug are of importance in preventing ascending infection.
- *Specific defenses:* Pregnancy alters the normal immune responsiveness of the host.
  - Cellular immunity and the phagocytic defenses are altered. Pregnancy hormones, especially estriol, enhance the phagocytic activity of leukocytes and increases the metabolic activity associated with intracellular destruction of pathogens. Neutrophilia present during pregnancy could be a mechanism for added protection. Hyperglycemia inhibits leukocyte chemotaxis and thus unrecognized gestational diabetes may represent a breach in defense leading to increased infections.

- During pregnancy transferrin concentration increases and serum iron concentration declines. This results in a hostile environment for bacteria which gain access to the bloodstream and thus prevent infection.[1]
- Humoral immunity: Increased rate of IgG catabolism and transplacental transport decreases IgG levels during pregnancy. The IgA and IgM levels do not change significantly.

Fetal Defenses

- The barriers that protect the fetus from assault of microorganisms include the placenta, fetal membranes, and amniotic fluid. However, the fetal membranes are not absolutely impermeable. Bacterial contamination of the amniotic fluid can occur with intact membranes, but it appears to be minimal and gets controlled by the antibacterial factors in the amniotic fluid.[2]
- Production and maturation of T-cells and B-cells start at approximately the eighth week of gestation. The fetus is immunologically competent by 14 weeks and necessary immunologic maturity to mount an immune response is presented by the time fetus reaches maturity.[2]
- *Maternal contribution to fetal defense:* The fetal contribution to humoral immunity is minimal. Maternal antibodies cross the placenta and give immunity to the fetus. IgA and IgM do not cross the placenta, but IgG is actively transferred to the fetus.

SUSCEPTIBILITY TO INFECTION DURING PREGNANCY

Altered homeostasis during pregnancy can affect the resistance to infections. The alterations in immune and various systems and the increased immune tolerance in pregnancy to prevent the rejection of fetus can increase susceptibility. The placenta can also be colonized by pathogens, such as by *L. monocytogens* and *P. falciparum* (Table 1).

ETIOLOGY

A variety *of microbes can cause infection in pregnancy* (Tables 2 and 3).

Viral infections: Common viral infections in pregnancy are respiratory infections caused by adenovirus, corona virus, and rhinovirus. The infections are not more severe in pregnant women than in nonpregnant and cause minimal fetal effects. However, other viral infections can cause severe fetal effects (Table 4).

TABLE 1: Influence of maternal physiological changes on infection.

System	Baseline changes	Physiological impact
Cardiovascular	Decreased arterial pressure Increased heart rate (up to 30 bpm) and thus Increased cardiac output	Increased risk of hypoperfusion Masking signs of sepsis
Gastrointestinal	Decreased esophageal tone and delayed gastric emptying due to high levels of progesterone and relaxin	Risk of aspiration pneumonia
Genitourinary	Decreased vaginal pH	Increased risk of bacterial growth
Hematology	Relative anemia due increased plasma volume Increased white blood cell counts	Decreased O_2 supply to tissues Difficulty in interpreting Laboratory data
Respiratory	Increased tidal volume and minute ventilation Decreased residual volume due to elevated diaphragm	Decreased $PaCO_2$ levels A "normal" blood gas may reflect impending respiratory failure faster rate of desaturation
Renal	Ureteral dilation and increased vesicoureteral reflux Urinary stasis	Increased risk of pyelonephritis abnormal baseline may mask renal injury in sepsis

TABLE 2: Categories of infections in pregnancy.

Pregnancy-specific infections	Infections exacerbated by pregnancy	Incidental infection
Chorioamnionitis	Urinary tract infection and pyelonephritis	Lower respiratory tract infection
Endometritis (with or without retained products of conception)	Pneumonia including influenza	Tuberculosis
Lactational mastitis	Listeriosis	Viral hepatitis
Infection at site of perineal trauma	Hepatitis E	HIV
Surgical site infection, e.g., cesarean section	Herpes simplex virus	Sexually transmitted diseases
	Malaria/Varicella/Rubella	Endocarditis
	Parvovirus /cytomegalovirus	
	Toxoplasmosis	

TABLE 3: Organisms causing infection.

Virus	Bacterial	Protozoa	Fungus (Opportunistic)	Parasites
Cytomegalovirus	*Treponema pallidum*	*Toxoplasma gondii*	*Candida albicans*	Ascaris
Herpes simplex	*Mycobacterium tuberculosis*	*Plasmodium* spp	*Coccidioides immitis*	Hook worm
Parvovirus B19	*Listeria monocytogenes*	*Trypanosoma cruzi*	*Cryptococcus*	
Rubella	*Salmonella typhii*	*Trichomonas vaginalis*	*Histoplasma*	
Varicella zoster	*Chlamydia trachomatis*		*Aspergillus*	
HIV	*Borrelia burgdorferi*			
Hepatitis B	Mycoplasma	*Rickettsia*		
Hepatitis C	*Ureaplasma urealyticum*	Coxiella		
Enterovirus	*Streptococcus* species	Louse borne epidemic typhus		
H1N1	*Enterococcus*			
COVID 19	*E. coli*			
Papilloma virus	*Neisseria gonorrhoeae*			
Coxsackie virus	Group B Streptococcus			
Epstein Barr virus	*Clostridium welchii*			
	Clostridium tetani			

Bacterial infections: These can affect pregnant women from implantation to the time of delivery and even during peripartum period. Infection can also affect the fetus and newborn. Many women with these infections are asymptomatic and require a high degree of clinical awareness and adequate screening **(Table 5)**.[1]

Protozoal infections: The important protozoal infections are malaria, dengue, trichomoniasis, leishmaniasis, trypanosomiasis, and the zoonotic toxoplasmosis. They can cause problems to both mother and fetus **(Table 6)**.

Rickettsiae: They are rarely a cause of infection in pregnant women. Q fever is a zoonotic disease caused by *Coxiella burnetii* and spreads by aerosol. The clinical presentation is nonspecific. Fetal complications include abortion, FGR, fetal death, and premature delivery. Epidemic louse-borne typhus presents as chills, with high-grade fever and maculopapular rash. The specific laboratory test is OX19 agglutination test.

Fungal infections: Candidal vulvovaginitis is a common clinical problem. Common but nonspecific symptoms include thick curdy vaginal discharge, pruritus, vaginal soreness, dysuria, and inflamed vulva. Characteristic pseudohyphae are seen on KOH wet preparation. Fetal infection can occur in up to 4% cases. Treatment is by topical azole therapy for 7 days. Other fungal infections like coccidioidomycosis and aspergillosis are often opportunistic and found in immunocompromised pregnant patients.

Parasites: The soil-transmitted helminthiasis results in misery and disability in poor populations. Schistosomiasis, intestinal helminthic infections, and filariasis can impact reproductive health and cause unexplained pregnancy loss. Anemia occurs with infestation by *Necator americanus*, *Ancylostoma duodenale*, *Trichuris trichiura*, *Enterobius vermicularis*, *Strongyloides stercoralis,* and *Ascaris lumbricoides.* Thus, the Government of India program on anemia prevention, i.e., *Anaemia Mukt Bharat* follows the policy of universal deworming of pregnant women during second trimester.

Polymicrobial Infections

Urinary tract infections: The causative organisms are predominantly gram negative—*Escherichia coli, Enterobacter, Proteus, Klebsiella,* and *Pseudomonas*. Asymptomatic bacteriuria (defined as >100,000 colony-forming units in a clean-catch, midstream specimen) develops in 2–7% of pregnant women and can lead to complications such as pyelonephritis and premature labor. Empiric antibiotic therapy is started and then modified by the sensitivity of the pathogen grown in the urine culture.[22]

Pneumonia: One out of 1,000 pregnancies is complicated by pneumonia, with maximum incidence in mid-trimester, Influenza A is usually associated with epidemics and can be particularly severe in pregnancy. Causative organisms include *Streptococcus pneumonia* being most common followed by *Haemophilus influenzae*. H1N1 is a specific subtype of influenza A. Signs and symptoms include dyspnea, cough, fever, malaise, rhinitis, myalgias, headache, chills, sore throat, and pleuritic chest pain. Fine rales are heard on auscultation. Chest X-ray (CXR) with abdomen lead shield is important for diagnosis. Mortality rate is high, i.e., 12.5% for mother and 26% for fetus without antibiotics and 3.5% for mother and 17% for fetus when antibiotics cover is given.[10] Mainstay of treatment is early identification and treatment

SECTION 5: Pregnancy with Pre-existing Morbidities | 381

TABLE 4: Viral infections.[3–13]

1. Cytomegalovirus

Organism	Double-stranded DNA genome which divides in the nucleus of host cells causing cytomegalic cells, i.e., cells swollen with an enlarged nucleus, separated from the nuclear membrane by a nonstaining halo, giving cell the appearance of "owl's eyes"
Clinical features	Most common congenital infection Spreads through contact or infected blood and blood products Mild, or asymptomatic, nonspecific illness
Effect on pregnancy	*Primary infection:* 1–3% of pregnant women with fetal attack rate of 30–40% The virus remains in the body and can reactivate at various periods *Fetal effects:* Spontaneous abortion, ventriculomegaly, microcephaly, hepatosplenomegaly sensorineural hearing loss, periventricular calcifications, FGR, preterm birth, or fetal death *Infant:* Developmental delay, mental retardation, seizures
Diagnosis	*Serology:* CMV IgG and IgM, IgG/IgM paired sera IgG negative in both mother and baby rules out CMV infection. Seroconversion from negative IgG to positive IgG Identification of CMV by PCR in blood, saliva and urine Amniocentesis and PCR for diagnosis of fetal infection
Treatment	No proven or effective treatment Termination of pregnancy can be offered with high risk for fetal defects
Prevention	Routine screening is not recommended

2. Rubella

Organism	Single-stranded, linear RNA virus
Clinical features	The attack rate is 8/10,000 Infection is subclinical in up to 50% cases. Patient may present with fever, petechiae, and purpura (blueberry muffin rash)
Effect on pregnancy	Spontaneous abortion or fetal death Impact is most severe in early pregnancy. Sensorineural hearing defects, cataracts, cardiovascular, and CNS involvement with FGR and hepatosplenomegaly can occur
Diagnosis	Serology at first visit. Rubella IgM persists up to 12 weeks after infection Rubella IgG avidity distinguishes between recent and distant infections PCR for rubella RNA/viral culture Amniotic fluid rubella virus RNA PCR used for diagnosis in fetus
Treatment	No specific antiviral therapy for rubella
Prevention	Preconception or routine pregnancy testing Routine infant immunization with MMR

3. Parvovirus B19

Organism	The genome is small single-stranded, linear DNA (*parvum* in Latin means "small") and is cytotoxic to erythroid progenitor cells
Clinical features	Known as fifth disease or slapped cheek disease Spreads easily from person to person Almost 50% of child bearing women are immune Presents as fever, malaise, and myalgia
Effect on pregnancy	Transplacental transmission rises to 70% toward term Severe anemia in fetus with fetal hydrops
Diagnosis	Ultrasound and serology—specific IgM. Cordocentesis and PCR for prenatal diagnosis
Treatment	*Mother:* Symptomatic *Fetus:* Intrauterine intravascular transfusion
Prevention	No specific preventive measures

4. Herpes simplex virus

Organism	Virion is spherical with linear double-stranded DNA genome *There are 2 types:* HSV1 and HSV2
Clinical features	Affects 0.3–1% of pregnant women High index of suspicion for recognition of primary infection—may be confined to cervix Fever blister (cold sore) is a common feature of recurrent HSV-1 infection

Contd...

382 **PART 1:** Obstetrics and Perinatology

Contd...

Effect on pregnancy	Infection during later half of pregnancy and delivery—high risk of infecting fetus. With recurrent herpes risk is smaller *Fetal and neonatal effects:* Spontaneous abortion or fetal death *Prematurity, IUGR, keratoconjunctivitis, meningitis:* In newborn infection is serious and potentially life-threatening
Diagnosis	High index of clinical suspicion Clinical examination and culture at first antenatal visit *First episode: Lesion swab:* HSV1/HSV2 IgG, IgM paired sera *Recurrent:* Clinical diagnosis PCR for HSV DNA from Cx, nasopharynx, skin lesions Serology IgG/IgM
Treatment	Antiviral therapy with acyclovir and supportive care
Prevention	No vaccine is available. Safe sex including consistent and correct condom use. Elective LSCS within 4 hours of rupture of membranes
5. Hepatitis	
Organism	Infection can occur due to Hepatitis A, B, C, or E
Clinical features	Jaundice occurs in 1/3,000 pregnancies and is due to viral infection in approximately one half of the cases *Hepatitis B (HBV):* Fetal and neonatal hepatitis, low birth weight • Acute HBV infection during pregnancy usually is mild and not associated with teratogenicity or mortality • Risk in later pregnancy being higher than in early gestation • Infected newborns have a very high risk of becoming carriers of HBV and can spread the infection to others • The maternal transmission rate in untreated newborns is 10–40% in hepatitis B surface antigen (HBsAg)-positive/hepatitis B e-antigen (HBeAg)–negative mothers compared with 70–90% in HBsAg-positive/HBeAg-positive mothers • Diagnosis is by serology at first visit and focuses on HBsAg • All healthy infants should be vaccinated against HBV to give them lifelong protection. Infants born to women with evidence of ongoing HBV infection should also receive hepatitis B hyperimmune globulin as soon as possible after birth • Risk of fulminant disease and maternal mortality occurs in 20% of patients when disease presents during the third trimester • Complications include gestational hypertension, preeclampsia, and kidney disease. Premature deliveries with high infant mortality of up to 33%
Effect on pregnancy	Fetal and neonatal hepatitis (Hepatitis B), abortion or fetal death Prematurity (Hepatitis E) Transmission of less than 2% around time of birth
Diagnosis	High index of clinical suspicion Hep C antibody positive confirmed with Hep C RNA and LFT
Treatment	Supportive care Cesarean delivery should be reserved for the usual obstetrical indications. Breastfeeding is not contraindicated The course of most viral infections is not affected by pregnancy and pregnancy should not impact the management of hepatitis and vice-versa Direct-acting antivirals (DAAs), e.g., tenofovir or telbivudine in hepatitis B patients, and ribavirin for HCV
Prevention	Sanitation programs, screening of blood for transfusion, condom usage
6. Varicella zoster (VZV)	
Organism	Double-stranded DNA genome enveloped with an icosohedral capsid
Clinical features	Adults can have more severe disease along with rash including pneumonitis, hepatitis, meningoencephalitis
Effect on pregnancy	Infections in first 20 weeks may result in the congenital varicella syndrome (2%) causing microcephaly, hydrocephalus, limb deformities, fetal growth restriction, and soft tissue calcifications Spontaneous abortion or fetal death Infection in late pregnancy or labor causes neonatal varicella
Diagnosis	*Clinical:* Typical rash and lesion. Swab and PCR for VZV DNA and serology (IgM antibodies) is rarely required
Treatment	Supportive New born delivered to mothers with infection from 2 days before to 5 days after delivery should be given VZIG and if any lesion develops IV acyclovir should be given
Prevention	Immunization and avoiding contact with case
7. Human immunodeficiency virus	
Organism	Human immunodeficiency virus 1 (HIV-1) and HIV-2 virions have a diploid, linear, single-stranded RNA genome

Contd...

Contd...

Clinical features	It is sexually transmitted/blood borne or contaminated needles Primary HIV infection "mononucleosis-like" symptoms Immunodeficiency develops slowly and is less severe
Effect on Pregnancy	*Spontaneous abortion or fetal death*, FGR, preterm birth, neurodevelopmental delay Transmission is perinatal (during birth) in most cases—15–25%
Diagnosis	Serology by ELISA at first visit with pre- and post-test counseling Confirmation is by Western blot
Treatment	*Objective:* Suppress viral load Treatment every patient irrespective of viral load or CD4 count ART including 3 active drugs from 2 or more drug classes Drug classes NRTIs, NNRTIs, INSTIs, and PIs Antiretrovirals can decrease vertical transmission by two-thirds ABC/3TC 600/300 mg or ABC (600 mg) with FTC (200 mg)
Prevention	Safe sex No vaccine available C-section may reduce transmission rates
8. Dengue virus	
Organism	Single stranded RNA with four serotypes DENV-1, DENV-2, DENV-3, and DENV-4. Transmitted by female *A. egypti* mosquito
Clinical features	Undifferentiated fever, nonsevere and severe manifestation "Cytokine Tsunami" ultimately targets vascular endothelium, platelets, and various organs leading to vasculopathy and coagulopathy. Involvement of lungs and liver is also common in pregnancy
Effect on pregnancy	Vertical transmission 1.6–64%
Diagnosis	NS1 enables detection in the viremic stage
Treatment	Fever without any danger signs or complications managed symptomatically. Monitor for progression of disease
Prevention	Prevent mosquitoes bite/repellent treated mosquito nets
9. Zika virus	
Organism	Single-stranded RNA virus Transmission is from the bite of an infected mosquito *Aedes aegypti,* mother to child, sexual and blood transfusion transmissions can occur
Clinical features	Maternal symptoms are uncommon
Effect on pregnancy	Consequences of congenital infections are devastating and include pregnancy loss and birth defects Congenital Zika syndrome is characterized by microcephaly
Diagnosis	Serological diagnosis is not available RT-PCR within a week from the onset of symptoms
Treatment	There are no vaccines, preventive drugs, or specific antiviral treatments
Prevention	Prevention of insect bite, barrier method of contraception after travel
10. SARS-Conrona virus 2	
Organism	SARS-CoV-2 is a new strain of coronaviruses causing pandemic
Clinical features	Human to human transmission - Highly contagious Clinical characteristics similar to those of nonpregnant adults
Effect on pregnancy	Risk of vertical transmission of COVID-19 might be as low as that of SARS-CoV-1
Diagnosis	Throat swab RT-PCR Serology not very diagnostic
Treatment	Supportive care LSCS preferred to avoid spread
Prevention	Social distancing, hand washing, and prevention of aerosol inhalation by N 95 masks

Contd...

Contd...

11. Other viruses		
a. Rubeola Virus	*Measles:* No increase in congenital anomalies, but high perinatal mortality rate and preterm birth	Symptomatic treatment
b. Ebola and Lassa fever	Hemorrhagic fevers reported mainly from Africa but are becoming a global challenge characterized by fever, severe headache, muscle pain, abdominal pain, diarrhea, vomiting, and unexplained hemorrhage Highly transmissible Potential effect in pregnancy and the newborn	Primarily supportive Maintain plasma volume and blood pressure
c. Japanese encephalitis	Spontaneous abortion or fetal death	Supportive care
d. Mumps	Acute parotitis No increase in congenital anomalies, but elevated risk of spontaneous abortion	Symptomatic treatment
e. Enteroviruses	Diarrhea Increased risk of type 1 diabetes in childhood	Symptomatic treatment
f. Coxsackie B virus	Myocarditis no spontaneous abortion or fetal death	Symptomatic treatment

(ART: antiretroviral therapy; CMV: cytomegalovirus; CNS: central nervous system; FGR: fetal growth restriction; IUGR: intrauterine growth retardation; LFT: liver function test; LSCS: lower segment cesarean sections; MMR: Measles-mumps-rubella; PCR: polymerase chain reaction)

TABLE 5: Common bacterial infections.[14-18]

1. Syphilis	
Organism	*Treponema pallidum,* tightly coiled, unicellular, helical organisms Dark field microscopy—undulating movements of spirochete
Clinical features	*Primary syphilis:* Hard, painless red ulcer typically forms on the vulva, cervix, or vagina *Secondary syphilis:* Nonpruritic rash fever, lymphadenopathy *Latent stage:* No symptoms but fetus can get infected Tertiary syphilis results in cardiovascular or gummatous disease Neurosyphilis can occur at any stage resulting in CNS or ophthalmic presentations
Effect on pregnancy	Major cause of adverse pregnancy outcomes in developing countries Miscarriage, fetal death, stillbirth and congenital infection (mother with untreated primary infection). Transmission rate decreases with subsequent pregnancies
Diagnosis	*Serological tests:* (1) Treponemal and (2) Nontreponemal tests (used for screening—rapid plasmin reagin and VDRL) Positive results confirmed with specific antitreponemal antibody tests microhemagglutination assay–*T. pallidum* (MHA-TP) and the fluorescent treponemal antibody absorption test (FTA-ABS)
Treatment	Single dose of 2.4 million units of IM benzathine penicillin
Prevention	Safe sex including consistent, correct condom use
2. Neisseria gonorrheae	
Organism	Gram-negative Diplococcus
Clinical features	Second only to chlamydial infections among bacterial STDs-2–5% of pregnant women- Asymptomatic in 50% of patients Disseminated disease—commonly manifested as arthritis.
Effect on pregnancy	Placental transmission does not occur but vertical transmission at delivery is common *Newborn:* Ophthalmia neonatorum, sepsis, arthritis, and/or meningitis
Diagnosis	Cervical swab, Gram stain and culture, PCR (check for other STD)
Treatment	Penicillin is used for uncomplicated gonorrhea Risk of transmission decreases with treatment
Prevention	Screening by endocervical culture
3. Group B beta hemolytic streptococci	
Organism	*Streptococcus agalactiae* is a gram-positive coccus that form chains and exhibits hemolysis on blood agar

Contd...

Contd...

Clinical features	5–15% pregnant women have organisms in vagina Maternal infection is of little importance
Effect on pregnancy	*Carriers:* Asymptomatic but may develop clinical chorioamnionitis or UTI During delivery transmission causes serious neonatal sepsis
Diagnosis	History and signs and symptoms in new born
Treatment	IV penicillin G or ampicillin given during labor
Prevention	Screening-based approach and intrapartum chemoprophylaxis

4. Chlamydia trachomatis

Organism	Obligate intracellular bacterium with a biphasic life cycle
Clinical features	75% of women—asymptomatic
Effect on pregnancy	Increased risk of abortion and preterm birth *Transmission occurs in 50% infants born vaginally.* Conjunctivitis and blinding corneal injury, neonatal pneumonia, and otitis media
Diagnosis	Cervical swab, Gram stain and culture, PCR (check for other STD) Antigen test at first visit in Western countries
Treatment	Azithromycin (1 g PO as a single dose)
Prevention	Safe sex practices and early recognition

5. Mycobacterium tuberculosis

Organism	Aerobic, nonmotile with slow growth.
Clinical features	Affects 1% of obstetric population Commonly spread by respiratory droplets/patients who have smear-positive are most infective. Transmission risk is not altered by pregnancy Continuous high- or low-grade fever, fatigue, weight loss, night sweats and cough
Effect on pregnancy	Preterm birth *Congenital tuberculosis:* Very rare but usually fatal
Diagnosis	*X-ray:* Pulmonary infiltration, positive tuberculin skin test (Mantoux test) AFb in sputum and sputum culture
Treatment	INH/Rifampicin/Ethambutol and pyrazinamide for 2 months followed by INH and rifampicin for 4 months Directly observed short-term therapy strategy (DOTS)

Other bacterial infections: A. Listeriosis

Organism	Gram-positive motile rod Zoonotic disease transmitted by contaminated milk products
Clinical features	Similar to influenza with fever and muscle aches
Effect on pregnancy	The infection can be transmitted transplacentally or perinatally causing pregnancy loss, stillbirth, preterm birth, or severe infection in newborn
Diagnosis	History, microbiological findings, and culture of blood or urine
Treatment	Ampicillin
Prevention	Avoiding unpasteurized dairy products and hand washing There is no vaccine

B. Leptospirosis

Organism	*Leptospira icterohemorrhagica* transmitted by rodent excreta
Clinical features	Abrupt fever, chills, severe headache, myalgia. In severe cases, cytotoxic impact like hemorrhage and jaundice can occur
Effect on pregnancy	Transmitted transplacentally or perinatally—abortion, stillbirth, preterm or life-threatening infection of the newborn
Diagnosis	Diagnosis on suspicion in endemic area or history of contact with excreta of rodents Organisms isolated from blood/CSF. Agglutination titers develop in 7 days and last for several years
Treatment	Penicillin, cefotaxime or azithromycin
Prevention	Rodent control and protection of food from contamination

Contd...

Contd...

C. Lyme disease

Organism	*Borrelia recurrentis*—tick borne
Clinical features	*3 stages of the disease:* Early localized infection with erythema migrans, fever, malaise, fatigue, headache, myalgia, and arthralgia; early disseminated infection (occurring days to weeks later), with neurologic, musculoskeletal, or cardiovascular symptoms and multiple erythema migrans lesions; and late disseminated infection, with intermittent swelling and pain of 1 or more joints (especially knees)
Effect on pregnancy	Infection of placenta, stillbirth, congenital cardiac, and urinary tract defects. In untreated cases baby may be born with rash
Diagnosis	Clinical diagnosis
Treatment	Doxycycline or amoxicillin; erythromycin is an alternative
Prevention	Avoiding tick bite—full clothing, repellents, early shower

(CSF: cerebrospinal fluid; PCR: polymerase chain reaction; STD: sexually transmitted disease; UTI: urinary tract infection; VDRL: Venereal Diseases Research Laboratory)

TABLE 6: Protozoal infections.[19-22]

1. Toxoplasmosis

Organism	Zoonotic disease caused by intracelllular obligate parasite *Toxplasma gondii*. Cat is the primary host. Transmission by oral ingestion of the parasite through cat feces or transplacental transmission
Clinical features	Affects approximately 0.2% of pregnant women. Primary infection is generally asymptomatic. Some patients present with headache, malaise, and cervical lymphadenopathy
Effect on pregnancy	First trimester maternal toxoplasmosis causes severe fetoplacental infections leading to miscarriage or, in a few continuing pregnancies, to major fetal lesions, mainly of the central nervous system (CNS) Late maternal infection - progressively increasing incidence but decreasing severity of congenital toxoplasmosis Classic triad of congenital toxoplasmosis includes chorioretinitis, hydrocephalus, and intracranial calcifications
Diagnosis	Specific IgM antibodies. IgM levels (elevated within days and lasts for 2–3 months, but can remain positive for greater than 2 years). Seroconversion negative IgG to positive IgG. IgG appears 2 weeks after initial infection and stays lifelong A fourfold rise in IgG, paired sera indicates infection *Avidity testing:* Avidity of <30% indicated infection within past 3 months while >40% indicate infection >6 months Fetal infection - *T. gondii* PCR in amniotic fluid
Treatment	Spiramycin 1 g TID *Fetal infection:* Pyrimethamine 50 mg OD + Sulfadiazine 1 g TID + Folinic acid 5–25 mg with each dose of pyrimethamine
Prevention	Avoid eating uncooked meat and handling cat feces

2. Malaria

Organism	Intracellular protozoan parasite of the genus *Plasmodium*
Clinical features	Paroxysms of sequential chills, high fever and sweating, headache, anorexia, splenomegaly, anemia, leukopenia
Effect on pregnancy	Major cause of maternal and neonatal death Adverse effects on pregnancy (anemia) and pregnancy outcome (stillbirth, abortion, FGR, prematurity, congenital malaria) are related to the extent of placental malaria
Diagnosis	Characteristic parasites in erythrocytes, identified in thick or thin blood smears. Rapid diagnostic tests for malaria detect antigens derived from malarial parasites. PCR is accurate
Treatment	Early identification and antimalarial medication like chloroquine, artemisinin
Prevention	Insecticide treated mosquito net in endemic areas, mosquito control and chemoprophylaxis (for travellers) and intermittent chemotherapy for pregnant women

3. Trichomoniasis

Organism	*Trichomonas vaginalis* is a flagellated protozoan
Clinical features	Only about half of women are symptomatic. Symptoms and signs include excessive yellow/green vaginal discharge, vulvar itching, vaginal/vulvar erythema, vaginal odor, and occasionally a red, erythematous cervix—"strawberry cervix"
Effect on pregnancy	Preterm birth, endometritis, and an increased risk of HIV transmission
Diagnosis	Wet mount preparation for motile trichomonads

Contd...

Contd...

Treatment	Nitroimidazoles as either a stat dose or longer course. It is advisable not to use metronidazole during the first trimester in pregnancy
Prevention	Safe sex and concomitant treatment of partner
4. Chagas disease	
Organism	Zoonotic disease caused by protozoa *Trypanosoma cruizi* transmitted by insects of family Triotominae
Clinical features	Swelling, fever, and congestive heart failure
Effect on pregnancy	Spontaneous abortion or fetal death, low birth weight, preterm labor, hepatosplenomegaly, respiratory distress, anasarca, cardiac failure, meningitis/encephalitis, progression to chronic disease
Diagnosis	*Acute phase:* Thin and thick blood smear *Late phase:* Parasite-specific antibodies
Treatment	*Symptomatic:* Benznidazole and nifurtimox are contraindicated during pregnancy
Prevention	No vaccine available—vector control

(FGR: fetal growth restriction; PCR: polymerase chain reaction)

along with supportive care. Antibiotics including penicillins, cephalosporins, and macrolides can be used. Prevention is by vaccination. Hand washing, avoiding contact with respiratory droplets from diseased individuals, contact isolation, and contact prophylaxis are important for secondary prevention.

Sepsis: Septic abortion causes an estimated 5,000 maternal deaths annually.

Wound infection, endometritis, and lactation mastitis are other causes of sepsis. Generally, antibiotic like co-amoxiclav 625 mg is used every 8 hours for 7 days empirically followed by modifications according to culture reports. Endometritis presents with postpartum fever, tachycardia, and foul lochia and is causing mostly as an ascending infection. It is generally a polymicrobial infection, with two-thirds cases containing both anaerobic (Bacteroides, Clostridium, and *Peptostreptococcus* spp.) and aerobic bacteria [Group B Streptococcus (GBS), *E. coli*, and enterococcus] organisms. IV gentamicin plus clindamycin, doxycycline plus cefoxitin, or ampicillin/sulbactam are effective empirical regimes. Development of pelvic venous thrombophlebitis usually requires broad spectrum antibiotics plus anticoagulation.[23]

Chorioamnionitis: Its incidence is 20% with prelabor rupture of membranes for more than 24 hours, fetal heart rate abnormalities occur when fetus becomes infected. Bacteriological confirmation of the diagnosis before delivery is challenging.

Symptoms or signs may be subtle and nonspecific. Around 30–50% of neonatal deaths are associated with amnionitis. Co-amoxiclav 1.2 g IV every 8 hours combined with gentamicin 5 mg/kg IV per day are an empirical choice of antibiotics and started after microbiological samples have been taken.

Bacterial vaginosis: Common vaginal infections are caused by *Gardnerella vaginalis, Bacteroides*, Mobiluncus, Peptococcus, *Ureaplasma urealyticum,* and *Mycoplasma hominis*.[24] It can cause preterm labor and ascending infection leading to fetal death. A positive whiff test (i.e., a fishy odor to the vaginal discharge before or after the addition of 10% potassium hydroxide solution) is diagnostic. Oral metronidazole or clindamycin are the drugs of choice.[25]

ROUTES OF MATERNAL INFECTION

In developed countries, infections are usually transmitted by sexual, airborne, blood-borne, and skin contact while in countries with poor community hygiene waterborne transmission is also important.

- *Sexual transmission:* Transmission is through sexual contact. Common infections are syphilis, chlamydia, hepatitis B, and zika virus.
- *Airborne transmission:* Transmission through inhaling airborne droplets of the disease - a result of a cough or sneeze from an infected person and includes pneumonia and COVID-19.
- *Blood-borne transmission:* Transmission through contact with infected blood including sharing hypodermic needles, e.g., HIV, hepatitis B and C.
- *Direct skin contact:* Transmission through contact with the skin of an infected person; fungal infections, parasitic infestations.
- *Insect-borne transmission:* Transmission is through insects including mosquitoes. The insects draw blood from an infected person and later bite a healthy person transmitting the organism like malaria, dengue, and zika.
- *Foodborne transmission:* Transmission by consuming contaminated food, e.g., enteric fever, hepatitis A and E.
- *Waterborne transmission:* Transmission through contact with contaminated water, e.g., hepatitis E, cholera, typhoid.
- *Zoonotic transmission:* The transmission is through animals like cat and rodents, e.g., toxoplasmosis, leptospirosis.

EFFECT OF INFECTIONS IN PREGNANCY

Symptoms normal to pregnancy like nausea, fatigue, vague myalgia, and the physiologic leukocytosis can resemble features of infection. One of the cardinal symptoms of infections is fever.

Infections that pose significant health risks during pregnancy can be divided into three categories, based on the pathogenesis and disease outcome with some infections falling in more than one category **(Tables 7 and 8)**.[26]

Maternal Infections

Infections with increased susceptibility during pregnancy: Pneumonia and influenza to some extent appear to affect the pregnant woman more severely than the nonpregnant woman. Case fatality rate among pregnant women with hepatitis E is between 15% and 25% compared to 0.5–4% in general population. The susceptibility is higher in the third trimester. Primary herpes simplex infection, when occurring in pregnant women, particularly during the third trimester, has an increased risk of rare complications including dissemination. Recurrences of herpes genitalis are more frequent during pregnancy. Ebola infections are also more severe during pregnancy. Disseminated coccidioidomycosis occurs with increased frequency in pregnant women. Varicella occurs more frequently during pregnancy, but mortality rates are unchanged.[27]

Infections harmful to both mother and baby: Syphilis, listeriosis, hepatitis, HIV, GBS.

Placental tropism of specific pathogens (e.g., Listeria or *P. falciparum*) results in increased severity during pregnancy and poor pregnancy outcomes. The risk of severe malaria by *Plasmodium falciparum* is three times higher in pregnant women.

Fetal or Congenital Infections

These are characterized by mild or no disease in pregnant women, but vertical transmission and often severe disease in the fetus. Pathogens commonly causing intrauterine infections like toxoplasmosis, rubella, cytomegalovirus, and herpes simplex are commonly grouped under the acronym TORCH and with syphilis added the acronym is STORCH. A more comprehensive acronym, CHEAP TORCHES is also used. It includes chicken pox, hepatitis (B, C and E), enterovirus, AIDS, parvovirus, and O representing other. The "Other" infections include more and more organisms with identification of new microbes like lymphocytic choriomeningitis virus, Q fever, and increased incidence of diseases like malaria and tuberculosis. Pathogenesis of fetal infections includes:

- Disruption of placental vascular development, and
- Dysregulation of the inflammatory-angiogenic axis acting on fetal development including impaired neurodevelopment and fetal inflammatory response syndrome (FIRS).

TABLE 7: Causes of fever in pregnancy and postpartum period.

Appendicitis	Bacterial sepsis
Cholangitis	Chorioamnionitis
Mastitis	Meningitis
Pneumonia	Pyelonephritis/cystitis
Viral/Rickettsial fevers	Septic abortion
Typhoid	Malaria

TABLE 8: Susceptibility and severity of infections during pregnancy.

Infection	Increased susceptibility	Increased severity
Influenza	No	Yes
Hepatitis E	No	Yes
Herpes simplex	No	Yes
Measles	No	Yes
Dengue	No	Yes
HIV/AIDS	Yes	No
Varicella	No	Yes
Malaria	Yes	Yes
Listeriosis	Yes	No
Coccidioidomycosis	No	Yes

Neonatal and Infant Infections

Certain infections do not pose significant risk to pregnant women or fetus, but can cause severe disease in the new born, e.g., *Bordetella pertussis, Clostridium tetani,* and respiratory syncytial virus.

Many infections (e.g., Listeria, Plasmodium species, HIV, VZV, influenza viruses, Chlamydia, GBS, Treponema, and herpes viruses) may cause overlapping syndromes depending on the timing of infection during pregnancy.

RISKS TO MOTHER AND BABY

Risks to Mother

- Characterized by acute manifestations, chronic disease, and sequelae.
- Some infections mainly urinary tract infections, vaginitis, and postpartum infection pose problems primarily for the mother.
- The pregnancy-specific infections are often a result of polymicrobial infection and include chorioamnionitis, endometritis (with or without retained products of conception), perineal infections, wound infections, and lactational mastitis.
- Delayed or inappropriate treatment of these infections may lead to bacteremia or to sepsis and, subsequently, death. Maternal sepsis remains a common and potentially preventable cause of direct maternal death worldwide. Sequential organ failure assessment (SOFA) scoring

system is based on oxygenation, platelet count, bilirubin level, mean arterial blood pressure, Glasgow Coma Score, and renal assessment (creatinine and urinary output). In the high dependency unit or labor room setting, a quick SOFA (qSOFA) can be used to assess organ dysfunction. This is based on two abnormalities out of three parameters that could be assessed at the bedside, namely, altered mentation, a systolic blood pressure less than 100 mm Hg, and respiratory rate > 22/min. The qSOFA can be calculated quickly without the need for laboratory tests. This is important in resource-poor settings.

- Quite often the maternal infection cannot be confirmed microbiologically and the organism identified on culture of a high vaginal swab may not be the organism responsible for infection.[27] Growth of organisms for example in blood culture may be due to contamination rather than infection.

Risks to the Fetus[28]

- No evidence of damage
- Subclinical infection without evidence of damage
- Abortion
- Fetal death
- Stillbirth
- Death in infancy
- Fetal growth restriction
- Congenital defects
- Fetal hydrops
- Late onset of congenital disease or defects
- Preterm delivery
- Preterm premature rupture of the membranes (PPROM).

SCREENING AND DIAGNOSIS

Many infections in pregnant women are difficult or impossible to diagnose on clinical grounds. Asymptomatic or subclinical infections are commonly seen with organisms that cause congenital infection. Testing is usually done on finding sonographic markers of fetal infection during a routine ultrasound scan or when the woman is exposed to an infectious pathogen and rarely, symptomatic infection. A range of laboratory tests is available; however, interpretation of the results can be difficult. Identification of pathogens is by microbiological cultures, immunologic techniques, and polymerase chain reaction (PCR). Ultrasound plays an important role in the detection and follow-up of infection. Prenatal detection of viral infection is based on fetal sonographic findings and PCR to identify the specific infectious agent. Most affected fetuses appear sonographically normal, initially but serial scans can identify evolving defects such as FGR, ascites, hydrops, ventriculomegaly, intracranial calcifications, hydrocephaly, microcephaly, cardiac anomalies, hepatosplenomegaly, echogenic bowel, placentomegaly, and abnormal amniotic fluid volume, which though nonspecific may be indicative of fetal infection **(Table 9)**.

TABLE 9: Differential diagnosis of symptomatic infections in pregnancy.

Fever, malaise, lethargy, myalgia with or without lymphadenopathy	• Primary CMV infection • Primary toxoplasmosis • Listeriosis • Other infections including COVID 19, Dengue
Maculopapular rash ± Fever ± Arthralgia	• Rubella • Parvovirus • Enterovirus
Vesicular rash	• Varicella • Hand-foot-mouth disease (Enterovirus)
Genitourinary symptoms, Urgency/Frequency/Loin pain/Genital ulcer/Vaginal discharge	• UTI • Chlamydia • Gonorrhea • Genital Herpes
Maternal Fever near term +/- PPROM or Preterm labor	• Chorioamnionitis • UTI • GBS

(CMV: cytomegalovirus; GBS: group B *Streptococcus*; PPROM: preterm premature rupture of the membranes; UTI: urinary tract infection)

MANAGEMENT

It is mainly based on:
- Overall health and medical history
- Type of infection
- What specific medicines, procedures, or therapies are safe during pregnancy?
- Risks and benefits of treatment for the mother and unborn baby
- How long the infection is likely to last?

Antibiotics in Pregnancy

Prescribing antibiotics during pregnancy depends on:
- Whether or not the antibiotics will harm the fetus?
- Gestational age as the teratogenicity is the greatest in the first trimester.
- Altered pharmacokinetics of antibiotics during pregnancy.
- Alterations in body composition, organ functions and biological processes in both the maternal and the fetoplacental compartments may follow different trajectories over time with gestational age.
- Patient characteristics, the source of the infection, local antibiotic sensitivities, and the woman's previous and current microbiological cultures.
- Dose should be calculated based on prepregnancy weight or booking visit weight and not the weight at the time of antibiotic administration as the weight gain during pregnancy is mainly by water.[27]
- *Penicillins (category B):* Penicillin, amoxicillin, and ampicillin are the commonly used antibiotics in pregnancy because of their wide margin of safety and lack of toxicity. The increase in maternal intravascular volume and

glomerular filtration rate requires higher drug doses to achieve the same serum levels as in nonpregnant patients.
- *Cephalosporins (category B):* Generally, cephalosporins are considered safe for use in pregnancy. As they have not been well studied in the first trimester they should not be considered the first line of treatment at this stage.
- *Sulfonamides (category C):* Should be avoided in late third trimester as it can cause hyperbilirubinemia and kernicterus in the neonate. Sulfonamides may be associated with hemolysis in patients with G6PD deficiency. Combination of sulfonamides and trimethoprim in the first trimester can be associated with cardiovascular defects.
- *Tetracyclines (category D):* Tetracyclines have identifiable adverse effects in both the mother and the fetus and hence should not be used. They can cause acute fatty necrosis of the liver, pancreatitis, and renal damage in the mother and growth stunting, discoloration of teeth, and hypoplasia of dental enamel in the fetus.
- *Aminoglycosides (category D):* Aminoglycosides used in the setting of hypomagnesemia and hypocalcemia or in conjunction with calcium channel blockers may cause neuromuscular blockade. Streptomycin and kanamycin are associated with congenital deafness. No congenital abnormalities including deafness are reported with use of Gentamicin (category C).
- *Nitrofurantoin (category B):* Generally safe in pregnancy except in mothers with G6PD deficiency in whom hemolysis can occur.
- *Quinolones (category C):* Animal studies have shown arthropathies with this drug use but no human studies have been conducted and no teratogenicity has been reported.
- *Metronidazole (category B):* Controversy has surrounded the use of metronidazole during pregnancy because of mutagenicity reported in in vitro studies. However, human studies have shown no increase in congenital defects. Not using the drug in the first trimester is recommended.
- *Macrolides (category B):* These antibiotics including azithromycin have not been associated with birth defects and are considered safe for use in pregnancy.
- Clindamycin (category B) and vancomycin (category C) are not associated with birth defects based on limited data.

PREVENTION OF INFECTION IN PREGNANCY

Patient Education
- Standard precautions.
- Washing hands with soap and water.
- Avoid eating undercooked meats, such as hot dogs and deli meats.
- Avoid consumption of unpasteurized dairy products.
- Staying away from wild or pet animals and their excreta.
- Avoid sharing utensils, cups, and food with other people.
- Safe sex practices and testing for sexually transmitted infections.
- Vaccinations should be up-to-date.
- Protection during travel.
- Screening including screening for bacteriuria and serological screening.
- Surveillance of infectious morbidity.
- Isolation for contagious diseases like chicken pox or rubella to prevent both horizontal and vertical spread.

Vaccination
- Successful implementation of vaccine protocols for pregnant women requires consideration of additional challenges, such as the unplanned pregnancies and poor access to prenatal health care.
- Vaccines are made from either live, attenuated pathogen strains or from inactivated pathogens. Live, attenuated vaccines are replication-competent with the potential of becoming virulent and causing adverse effects in individuals with weakened immune systems. Due to the unknown risks to the fetus, live viruses vaccines are not recommended for use in pregnant women. Inactivated vaccines are not associated with a risk of reacquisition of virulence, but induce a weaker host–immune response.
- The goal of vaccination strategies for protecting against neonatal infections is generation of robust maternal antibody responses (IgG) during pregnancy to enhance placental transfer. Inactivated pertussis antigen in combination with tetanus and diphtheria toxoids as a single vaccine (Tdap) during third trimester is recommended for all pregnant women regardless of previous vaccine history.[29]

CONCLUSION
- Infection in pregnancy can be due to multiple overlapping etiologies with underlying obstetric complications.
- The time to provide information to mothers about these infections is preconception period.
- Strategic immunization of women, either prior to or during pregnancy, can eliminate or reduce the risk of maternal, fetal, and neonatal infection and disease.
- Screening should include rubella IgG, hepatitis B surface antigen, and serological tests for syphilis and HIV antibody either in prepregnancy period or at booking.
- If screening test is positive, confirmatory tests for maternal and, if indicated, fetal infection are essential before intervention is planned (e.g., cytomegalovirus infection).
- Appropriate investigations and management of suspected infections can reduce unnecessary intervention, prevent or decrease adverse outcomes, and relieve anxiety.

KEY MESSAGES

- Infections during pregnancy can cause maternal and fetal morbidity and mortality.
- Infections are due to viruses, bacteria, fungi, and parasites.
- Transmission of infection is by various routes.
- Maternal defense and susceptibility play an important role.
- Infection in the mother can often have trivial symptoms or even none hence diagnosis is difficult.
- Infection in the mother is not equal to fetal infection and fetal infection does not always mean the baby will be affected.
- Selection of antibiotics, preventive measures, and vaccine protocol are of paramount importance.

REFERENCES

1. Keighley CL, Skrzypek HJ, Wilson A, Bonning MA, Gilbert GL. Infections in pregnancy. Med J Aust. 2019;211(3):134-41.
2. Robbins JR, Bakardjiev AI. Pathogens and the placental fortress. Curr Opin Microbiol. 2012;15(1):36-43.
3. Kimberlin DW, Brady MT, Jackson MA, Long SS. Red Book: Report of the Committee on Infectious Diseases: Hepatitis B, 31st edition. Itasca, Illinois: American Academy of Pediatrics; 2018. pp. 401-28.
4. Naing ZW, Scott GM, Shand A, Hamilton ST, Van Zuylen WJ, Basha J, et al. Congenital cytomegalovirus infection in pregnancy: a review of prevalence, clinical features, diagnosis and prevention. Aust N Z J Obstet Gynaecol. 2016;56(1):9-18.
5. Kimberlin DW, Brady MT, Jackson MA, Long SS. Red Book: Report of the Committee on Infectious Diseases: Herpes Simplex, 31st edition. Itasca, Illinois: American Academy of Pediatrics; 2018. pp. 437-49.
6. Hollier LM, Grissom H. Human herpes viruses in pregnancy: cytomegalovirus, Epstein-Barr virus, and varicella zoster virus. Clin Perinatol. 2005;32:671-96.
7. Young NS, Brown KE. Mechanisms of disease: parvovirus B19. N Engl J Med. 2004;350:586-97.
8. Calvet GA, Santos FB, Sequeira PC. Zika virus infection: epidemiology, clinical manifestations and diagnosis. Cur Open Infect Dis. 2016;29(5):459-66.
9. Mehta N. Respiratory disease in pregnancy. Reprod Immunol. 2016;1(3):14.
10. Ghulmiyyah LM, Alame MM, Mirza FG, Zaraket H, Nassar AH. Influenza and its treatment during pregnancy: a review. J Neonatal-Perinat Med. 2015;8(4):297-306.
11. Chen H, Guo J, Wang C. Luo F, Yu X, Zhang W, et al. Clinical characteristics and intrauterine vertical transmission potential of COVID-19 infection in nine pregnant women: a retrospective review of medical records. Lancet. 2020;385:809-15.
12. Turner MJ. Bacterial Infections Specific to Pregnancy: Clinical Practice Guideline number 34. Dublin: Royal College of Physicians of Ireland; 2015.
13. Berman S. Maternal syphilis: pathophysiology and treatment. Bull WHO. 2004;82:433-8.
14. Frieden T, Sterling T, Munsiff S, Watt CJ, Dye C. Tuberculosis. Lancet. 2003;362:887-99.
15. Workowski KA, Bolan GA, Center of Disease Control and Prevention. Sexually transmitted diseases treatment guidelines. MMWR Recomm Rep. 2015;64:1-137.
16. Patel K, Williams S, Guirguis G, Williams LG, Apuzzio J. Genital tract GBS and rate of histologic chorioamnionitis in patients with preterm premature rupture of membrane. J Matern Fetal Neonatal Med. 2018;31(19):2624-27.
17. Craig AM, Dotters-Katz S, Kuller JA, Thompson JL. Listeriosis in pregnancy: a review. Obstet Gynecol Surv. 2019;74 (6):362-8.
18. Soper D. Trichomoniasis: under control or undercontrolled? Am J Obstet Gynecol. 2004;190:281-90.
19. Rogerson SJ, Desai M, Mayor A, Sicuri E, Taylor SM, Van Eijk AM. Burden, pathology, and costs of malaria in pregnancy: new developments for an old problem. Lancet Infect Dis. 2018;18(4):e107-18.
20. Wright WF, Riedel DJ, Talwani R, Gilliam BL. Diagnosis and management of Lyme disease. Am Fam Physician. 2012;85(11):1086-93.
21. Pekelharing JE, Gatluak F, Harrison T, Maldonado F, Siddiqui MR, Ritmeijer K. Outcomes of visceral leishmaniasis in pregnancy: a retrospective cohort study from South Sudan. PLoS Negl Trop Dis. 2020;14(1):1-16.
22. Nicolle LE, Gupta K, Bradley SF, Colgan R, DeMuri GP, Drekonja D, et al. Clinical Practice Guideline for the Management of Asymptomatic Bacteriuria: 2019 Update by the Infectious Diseases Society of America. Clin Infect Dis. 2019;68(10):e83.
23. Bridwell RE, Carius BM, Long B, Oliver JJ, Schmitz G. Sepsis in pregnancy: recognition and resuscitation. West J Emerg Med. 2019;20(5):822-32.
24. Murtha AP, Edwards JM. The role of Mycoplasma and Ureaplasma in adverse pregnancy outcomes. Obstet Gynecol Clin North Am. 2014;41(4):615-27.
25. Yudin MH. Bacterial vaginosis in pregnancy: diagnosis, screening, and management. Clin Perinatol. 2005;32:617-27.
26. Abduljalil K, Furness P, Johnson TN, Rostami-Hodjegan A, Soltani H. Anatomical, physiological and metabolic changes with gestational age during normal pregnancy: a database for parameters required in physiologically based pharmacokinetic modelling. Clin Pharmacokinet. 2012;51(6):365-96.
27. O'Higgins AC, Egan AF, Murphy OC, Fitzpatrick C, Sheehan SR, Turner MJ. A clinical review of maternal bacteremia. Int J Gynaecol Obstet. 2014;124(3):226-9.
28. Weckman AM, Ngai M, Wright J, McDonald CR, Kain KC. The impact of infection in pregnancy on placental vascular development and adverse birth outcomes. Front Microbiol. 2019;10:1924.
29. Vermillion MS, Klein SL. Pregnancy and infection: using disease pathogenesis to inform vaccine strategy. NPJ Vaccines. 2018;3(6).

LONG QUESTIONS

1. Discuss the various microbiological agents that cause infection during pregnancy?
2. Discuss antibiotic use during pregnancy.
3. Discuss the various causes of fever during pregnancy and their management.

SHORT QUESTIONS

1. What are the defense mechanisms against infections during pregnancy?
2. How do maternal physiological changes affect infections?

3. Write briefly about polymicrobial infections in pregnancy.
4. Describe the various routes through which infection can occur during pregnancy with examples?
5. What is the role of vaccines in preventing infections during pregnancy?

■ MULTIPLE CHOICE QUESTIONS

1. What other infection is commonly found with gonorrhea?
    a. Trichomonas
    b. Bacterial vaginosis
    c. Syphilis
    d. Chlamydia
2. What is the treatment of choice for Chlamydia in patients for whom adherence is in question?
    a. Azithromycin 1 g PO × 1
    b. Metronidazole 500 mg PO BID × 7 days
    c. Doxycycline 100 mg PO BID × 7 days
    d. Ceftriaxone 250 mg IM × 1
3. The initial symptoms of HIV infection may include:
    a. No symptoms
    b. Nonspecific flu-like symptoms
    c. Fever, headache, fatigue, and swollen glands
    d. All of the above are true
4. When is an unborn baby most at risk of developing a birth defect?
    a. First trimester
    b. Second trimester
    c. Last trimester
    d. All 9 months
5. Pregnant women should not handle cat litter to lower the risk of becoming infected with which of these?
    a. Toxoplasmosis
    b. Streptococcus
    c. *E. coli* bacteria
    d. HIV
6. Once a fetus is infected, it more susceptible to infection due to its poor immunity and lack of synthesis of which antibody?
    a. IgA
    b. IgD
    c. IgG
    d. IgM
7. *Listeria monocytogenes* is classified as a:
    a. Fungus
    b. Gram-negative rod
    c. Gram-positive cocci
    d. Gram-positive rod
8. Chorioamnionitis and maternal fever can be the result of bacterial infections due to colonization in the vagina and rectum:
    a. Group A hemolytic streptococci
    b. Group B hemolytic streptococci
    c. Candida
    d. *Staphylococcus aureus*
9. Fever with blisters is a common manifestation of:
    a. Parvovirus
    b. Recurrent HSV-1
    c. Recurrent HSV-2
    d. Varicella
10. The etiological agent most commonly associated with urinary tract infection is:
    a. *Escherichia coli*
    b. *Staphylococcus aureus*
    c. Chlamydia
    d. Mycoplasma
11. Each of the following statements regarding Toxoplasma is correct, except:
    a. Toxoplasma can cause encephalitis in immune compromised patients
    b. Toxoplasma can be transmitted across the placenta to the fetus
    c. Toxoplasma can be diagnosed by finding trophozoites in stool
    d. Toxoplasma can be transmitted by cat feces
12. Which one of the following is the most common outcome with primary herpes simplex infection?
    a. Persistent cytopathic effect in infected cells
    b. Complete eradication of virus and virus infected cells
    c. Persistent asymptomatic viremia
    d. Establishment of latent infection
13. Regarding HIV, which of the following is correct?
    a. The term viral load refers to the concentration of HIV RNA in patient plasma
    b. The antigenicity of GAG protein of HIV is highly variable, making it difficult to have a vaccine against HIV
    c. Both zidovudine and lamivudine block the HIV replication by inhibiting cleavage of precursor polypeptide by the virion protease
    d. The western blot test for HIV has more false positive results than ELISA test
14. Which of the following types of immunity to viruses would be least likely to be lifelong?
    a. Passive active immunity
    b. Passive immunity
    c. Cell-mediated immunity
    d. Active immunity
15. Which of the following are risk factors for vertical transmission of GBS?
    a. Previous history
    b. Intrapartum fever >38 degrees
    c. Current preterm labor
    d. Rupture of membranes >18 hours

Answers

1. d 2. a 3. d 4. a 5. a 6. c
7. d 8. b 9. b 10. a 11. c 12. d
13. a 14. b 15. d

5.18 COVID-19 IN PREGNANCY

Ajith S, Kasturi Donimath, Sabnam Nambiar

INTRODUCTION

Coronavirus disease 2019 (COVID-19), caused by severe acute respiratory syndrome coronavirus 2 (SARS-CoV-2) strain of corona virus and first reported from Wuhan City, China toward the end of 2019, was declared a pandemic by World Health Organization (WHO) on March 11th, 2020. The common cold, Middle East respiratory syndrome (MERS) and SARS are the other known common corona virus infections. This rapidly evolving virus has shown numerous mutations with development of various new strains, four of which – alpha, beta, gamma, and delta variants are increasingly of concern. The delta variant has been found to have a significantly higher transmission rate and resulted in a more severe disease.

The viral transmission occurs through close contact with infected person and rarely from contaminated surfaces.

Pregnancy seldom increases the chances of infection with the COVID-19 virus. In fact, various studies have shown that the affected pregnant women are rarely symptomatic and those symptomatic presenting only with mild or moderate cold/flu-like symptoms. The chief symptoms are cough, fever, sore throat, dyspnea, loss of sense of taste, anosmia, and diarrhea.[1] The impact of pregnancy, on development of prolonged symptoms or signs after acute COVID-19 infection ("long COVID" or post COVID), is rather indistinct at present.

CLINICAL STAGES OF SEVERITY

- *Mild:* No breathlessness or hypoxia, respiratory rate <24/minute, SpO_2 >94 on room air and otherwise asymptomatic
- *Moderate:* Dyspnea and/hypoxia, respiratory rate 24–29/minute, SpO_2 90–94 on room air or fever and cough
- *Severe:* Dyspnea and/hypoxia, respiratory rate > 30/minute, SpO_2 <90 on room air, pulse rate >125 with or without pneumonia
- *Critical:* Acute respiratory distress syndrome (ARDS), sepsis, or complications such as pulmonary embolism, acute coronary syndrome.

Although generally asymptomatic, the pregnant women have an increased risk of developing severe illness when compared with non-pregnant women, especially in the third trimester. The pregnant women who develop severe disease have been found to require higher rates of intensive care unit (ICU) admissions and need for ventilation.[1]

Additional risk factors for severe infection:[2]
1. *Obesity:* Body mass index (BMI) > 30 kg/m^2
2. *Pre-pregnancy comorbidity:* Diabetes, hypertension
3. Maternal age > 35 years
4. Living in areas or households of increased socioeconomic deprivation.

EFFECT OF COVID-19 ON PREGNANCY

There is no evidence of increased miscarriage rate or congenital anomalies after COVID-19 infection. There may be a 2–3 times increase in preterm deliveries in symptomatic women. According to the PregCOV-19 Living Systematic Review, risk of preterm birth is approximately 17%, most of these being iatrogenic (94%).[1] The COVID-19 infection is associated with approximately double the risk of stillbirth and a predisposition for increased incidence of small for gestational age babies.[2] The risk of vertical transmission is low, most babies tested positive are asymptomatic.

There are reports of higher rates of perinatal mental health disorders such as anxiety and depression during the pandemic. The COVID-19 infection is also associated with an increased rate of cesarean birth. The UKOSS data shows a cesarean section rate of 49% in symptomatic women compared to 29% in a historical control group in 2018.[2]

Antenatal Care during COVID Pandemic

The antenatal care is an essential service. The pregnant women should be advised to continue their antenatal visits and care although some modification of services could be advised to enable social distancing and good ventilation to reduce the risk of transmission of virus. Consideration should be given to pregnant women with comorbidities which make them susceptible to severe COVID-19. Shared waiting areas should be avoided as far as possible. There should be an area segregated to see suspected or confirmed cases.

The option of remote consultation such as video conferencing or teleconferencing should be considered if there is local lockdown. However, lack of mobile devices/computer and internet access could pose severe limitations. Lack of privacy could prevent women from disclosing personal and sensitive issues. The pandemic has caused higher levels of anxiety and other mental health problems in pregnant women than others, hence mental health should be assessed at each visit and support provided to those in need of the same.

Care of Suspected Cases

Women with symptoms suggestive of COVID-19 should undergo appropriate testing **(Fig. 1)**. They should be self-isolated and admitted to hospital if symptoms are severe, associated comorbidities are present or if near term.

Antenatal Management of Confirmed Cases

This can be divided into those of management of asymptomatic women without any comorbidities, symptomatic women, or women with comorbidities and of women with severe infection.

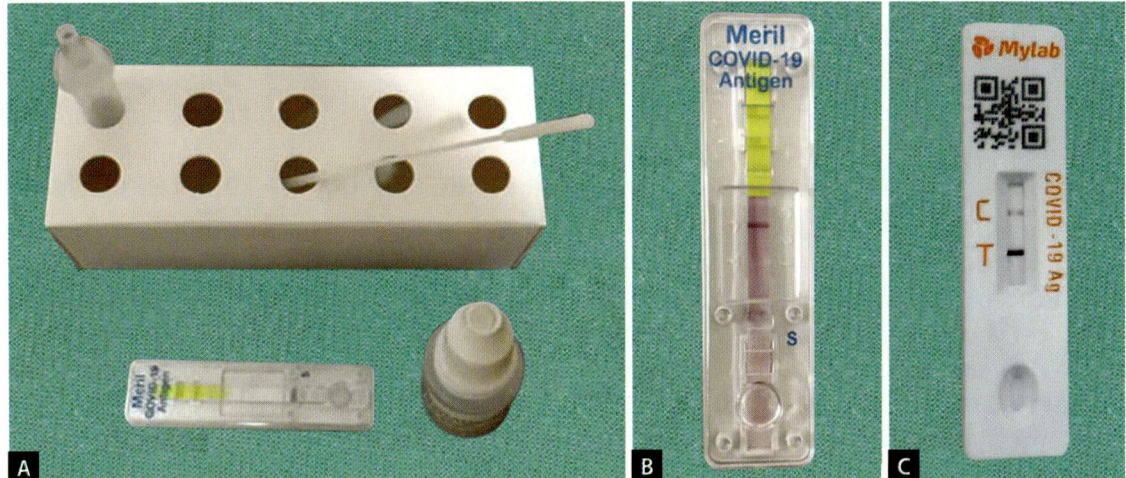

Figs. 1A to C: Rapid antigen testing for COVID-19. (A) Test set up; (B) Negative test; (C) Positive test.

Management of Asymptomatic Women without Comorbidities

They may be advised care at home especially if < 34 weeks, with advice on self isolation. They should continue iron, calcium and vitamin D supplementation and they should be advised against complete bed rest and dehydration to try and prevent venous thromboembolism. They should be informed about red flag symptoms such as breathlessness, chest pain, drowsiness, hemoptysis, cyanosis, and hypotension and should contact medical facility immediately if they are present. Severe fatigue, malaise, and persistent fever are indicative of active disease and medical advice should be taken. It is preferable to procure a pulse oximeter for personal use. They must report to the medical facility if symptomatic or if SpO_2 falls below 94%. They must be taught 6-minute walk test – where they walk for 6 minutes or take 40 steps and are told to measure the SpO_2 before and after – a fall of more than 3% from baseline is significant and they must promptly seek medical advice. Women more than 34 weeks should be assessed in a medical facility and if stable allowed home care.[3]

Management of Symptomatic Women and those with Comorbidities

They require hospital admission, investigations, and symptomatic treatment **(Table 1)**. Laboratory investigations such as complete blood count, blood sugar, liver function tests, renal function test, C–reactive protein and serum electrolytes should be sent **(Table 2)**. ECG is advised for patients with tachycardia or other heart rate abnormalities. Chest X-ray with shielding of abdomen is advised in those with persistent cough or fall in SpO_2. Additional markers such as D-dimer, serum ferritin, LDH and CPK are sent if persistent symptoms. Symptomatic treatment includes paracetamol and antitussives. Oseltamivir 75 mg twice daily for 5 days may be started if suspicion of H1N1.

TABLE 1: Laboratory investigations for hospital admitted patients.[3]

At admission	CBC, RFT, LFT, CRP, RBS, serum electrolytes, ECG, pulse oximetry
If clinically Indicated	Portable CXR, D-Dimer, ferritin, LDH, CPK, procalcitonin, blood culture, troponin T, HRCT thorax (only in case of worsening)
To repeat every 48 hours if clinically deteriorating	CBC, creatinine, AST/ALT, CRP, LDH, CPK, ferritin, D-Dimer
For immunocompromised patients, e.g., transplant recipients, HIV	Tests to rule out opportunistic infections such as *Mycobacterium tuberculosis, Pneumocystis jiroveci*, etc.

TABLE 2: Risk markers in COVID-19.

Marker	Normal value	High risk
CRP	<5	CRP >100 mg /L
D-dimer	1st trimester:169–1,202 µg/L 2nd trimester: 393–3,258 µg/L 3rd trimester: 551–3,333 µg/L	
Ferritin	<60	Ferritin >300 µg/L
LDH	<400	LDH >400 U/L
		NLR >3.13, ALC <0.8

(ALC: absolute lymphocyte count; NLR: neutrophil lymphocyte ratio)

Steroids

Steroids are generally started only after 5 days of disease onset. The appropriate dose of steroid in the right patient at the correct time can prove lifesaving. Budesonide 800 µg MDI/DPI twice a day is started when cough is persists beyond 5 days of onset of disease.

Indications of Parenteral or Oral Steroids[3]

1. Moderate to severe rise in respiratory rate or fall in SpO_2
2. 3% fall in SpO_2 with 6-minute walk test

3. Bronchopneumonia
4. Marked rise in proinflammatory markers.

Involvement of multidisciplinary team is of prime importance. The usual regime is to start with Injection dexamethasone 6 mg intramuscular 12 hourly × 4 doses, followed by Injection methylprednisolone 0.5–1 mg/kg body weight or 40 mg once daily or oral prednisolone 40 mg once daily for 10 days or until discharge whichever is earlier. Higher dose of steroids may be needed in severe cases and can be decided by the multidisciplinary team. Injection Dexamethasone can be skipped if lung maturity is not an issue. Prolonged use of dexamethasone is not recommended in pregnancy as it crosses the placenta. Methylprednisolone does not cross placenta; hence, it cannot be a substitute for dexamethasone to enhance lung maturity. Blood sugar should be monitored in patients on steroids.

Anticoagulants

Pregnancy is a hypercoagulable state. Evolving evidence suggest that patients admitted to hospital with moderate or severe COVID-19 infection are also hypercoagulable.

Women who are advised self-isolation at home should be advised regarding adequate hydration and to stay ambulant. Venous thromboembolism (VTE) risk assessment should be assessed, and appropriate anticoagulant should be advised. All pregnant admitted should be offered prophylactic low-molecular-weight heparin (LMWH), unless birth is expected within 12 hours or there is significant risk of hemorrhage. Prophylactic dose of enoxaparin is 1 mg/kg body weight, higher dose of enoxaparin may be needed in severely ill patients or those with higher D-dimer values (1 mg/kg twice daily). The LMWH should be stopped 12 hours prior to delivery or cesarean section (24 hours if taking higher dose). Thromboprophylaxis should be continued for duration of hospital stay and 10 days following hospital discharge. A longer duration thromboprophylaxis should be considered in patients with persistent morbidity. Thrombocytopenia may be associated with severe COVID-19 infection, LMWH and aspirin should be stopped if platelet count is less than 50,000.

If the woman is admitted within 6 weeks postpartum, they should be offered thromboprophylaxis during the entire period of hospital stay and for at-least 10 days following discharge. The duration may be extended to 6 weeks for those with significant ongoing morbidity.

Remdesivir

Remdesivir should only be considered in those who are not improving or who are deteriorating.[2] Though its safety in pregnancy is not established it may be offered on a compassionate basis after taking consent. It needs to be started within 10 days of onset of symptoms. The recommended dose is 200 mg IV on day 1, followed by 100 mg IV daily × 4 days. The RFT and LFT must be normal.

Tocilizumab

Tocilizumab (interleukin-6 receptor antagonist) improve outcomes, including survival, in hospitalized patients with hypoxia and evidence of systemic inflammation (CRP above 75 mg/L)[2]. The data on use of tocilizumab in pregnancy is limited, but there is no report of teratogenicity. The decision to start tocilizumab should be taken by a multidisciplinary team.

Monoclonal Antibodies

Monoclonal antibodies (casirivimab and imdevimab) may be considered in pregnant and postpartum high risk patients with COVID-19 and who are vulnerable to severe infection before progressing to hypoxia.[2]

■ CLINICAL DETERIORATION

The signs of decompensation are:[2]
1. Increasing oxygen requirements or FiO_2 above 35%
2. Increasing respiratory rate above 25 breaths/minute
3. Reduction in urine output/acute kidney injury
4. Drowsiness

Chest imaging: X-ray chest/HRCT Thorax should be performed when indicated and not to be delayed for concerns regarding radiation exposure.

A multidisciplinary team should assess the woman and a decision taken regarding need for delivery/cesarean section of a pregnant woman in third trimester to facilitate resuscitation. Oxygen should be given to maintain SpO_2 of 94–98% using nasal cannula, face mask, venturi mask, non-breather mask, noninvasive continuous positive airway pressure (CPAP), intubation and positive pressure ventilation (IPPV) and extracorporeal membrane oxygenation (ECMO) as appropriate. Care should be taken regarding fluid management, hourly input/output chart should be recorded in patients with moderate/severe symptoms and aim to maintain a neutral fluid balance. There should be suspicion of bacterial infection if white cell count is raised (lymphocytes are usually low with COVID-19) and antibiotics should be started. In patients with chest pain, worsening hypoxia or in those whose breathlessness persists or worsens after expected recovery from COVID-19, a differential diagnosis of pulmonary embolism or heart failure should be considered and additional tests such as ECG, echocardiogram, CT pulmonary angiogram and ventilation perfusion lung scan may be done.

When to Deliver?

The decision regarding timing and mode of delivery is mostly made on obstetric grounds. Sometimes decision has to be taken considering the maternal resuscitative purpose or because of concern regarding the fetal health. The decision must be taken by multidisciplinary team. It must be decided on individual basis beyond 26–28 weeks if the patient is deteriorating and not responding to noninvasive ventilation and if invasive ventilation is needed. The mode of delivery depends on the emergent nature and gestational age and will usually be through cesarean section. The mode of anesthesia also depends on general condition of patient. When iatrogenic preterm delivery is required, consider giving antepartum steroids for lung maturity and $MgSO_4$ for neuroprotection.

Intrapartum Care

Labor should be conducted in a dedicated labor room. There are reports of increased risk of fetal compromise in active labor and cesarean section in symptomatic women, hence continuous electronic fetal monitoring should be offered to symptomatic women. The number of staff members entering the room should be minimized. The hospital should have a local policy regarding companion during labor. In addition to routine parameters monitored in labor, SpO_2 also should be monitored carefully. The time taken for shifting the patient to COVID operation theater and for donning of PPE should be considered while taking decision for emergency cesarean. The option of epidural analgesia should be discussed. The Entonox (50% nitrous oxide and 50% oxygen) with single-patient microbiological filter is also safe. The delayed cord clamping and early skin to skin contact with baby in line with usual practice can be advised. The healthcare professionals should wear appropriate PPE while giving care to the woman.

Postpartum Care

The woman should be supported to take an informed decision regarding breastfeeding. The breastfeeding and rooming-in can be permitted, the risk of newborn getting infection from the mother being low especially if appropriate precautions such as wearing a mask and practicing hand hygiene are followed meticulously.[4]

Breast milk provides protection against many illnesses and is the best source of nutrition for babies. The rooming-in has the added benefit of facilitating breastfeeding and maternal-newborn bonding. The precautions recommended are washing hand with soap and water for at least 20 seconds before holding or caring the baby, keeping the baby more than 6 feet from the mother, and wearing a mask. When women are expressing breast milk in hospital a dedicated breast pump should be used and adhere to recommendations for pump cleaning after each use. The baby should be separated only if maternal critical care or additional neonatal care required.[5]

Thromboprophylaxis should be offered for at least 10 days following discharge. Proper contraception advice should be given. The family members should be given proper advice regarding self-isolation, identifying illness in newborns, and worsening of woman's symptoms and appropriate contact details if they have concerns. The institution should have proper discharge guidelines.

Follow-up of Affected Pregnancies

There should not be any change in the standard antenatal care. Those affected in first trimester or early second trimester should be offered a detailed anomaly scan. Those affected in late second trimester or in third trimester should be offered a growth scan after 2 weeks.

Vaccination

Vaccination against COVID-19 is strongly recommended in pregnancy.[2] It can be given at any time in pregnancy. The rare syndrome of vaccine-induced thrombosis and thrombocytopenia (VITT) has been reported after viral vector vaccine such as Covishield, Astra Zeneca vaccine, Johnson and Johnson vaccine, etc. It is an idiosyncratic reaction and not associated with any of the usual venous thromboembolism risk factors. The usual presentation is 5–28 days after first dose. The risk is extremely low (1:100,000). There is no evidence that pregnant and postpartum women are at higher risk of VITT. There is no known risk of VITT with Pfizer-BioNTech and Moderna vaccines. Breastfeeding is not a contraindication for COVID-19 vaccination. It does not affect fertility and vaccine can be given to those planning pregnancy and those getting fertility treatment.

■ CONCLUSION

COVID-19 is an emerging and evolving threat, more so in pregnancy. Hence, we have to prepare accordingly and adopt practical and pragmatic approaches toward containing the spread of the disease along with taking headlong the challenge of treatment and care of all those affected especially the pregnant women. The situation may continue perceptibly for some time to come, hence there has to be constant vigilance and it is not time to let down our guard, yet!

■ KEY MESSAGES

- Pregnancy seldom increase the chance of getting COVID-19 infection, most patients are asymptomatic or with mild symptoms.
- Those admitted with severe symptoms, there is more need for ICU admission and ventilatory support.
- Anticoagulant has an important role in management as both pregnancy and COVID-19 infection are hypercoagulable state.
- The right dose of right steroid in right time is life saving.
- Monoclonal antibodies may be considered in high-risk pregnant women before developing hypoxia.
- Tocilizumab may be lifesaving in patients with hypoxia.
- Delivery or cesarean section may be needed in clinically deteriorating women in third trimester to facilitate resuscitation.
- Vaccination is strongly recommended in pregnancy.

REFERENCES

1. Allotey J, Stallings E, Bonet M, Yap M, Chatterjee S, Kew T, et al. Clinical Manifestations, risk factors, and maternal and perinatal outcomes of coronavirus disease 2019 in pregnancy: living systematic review and meta-analysis. BMJ. 2020;370.
2. RCOG. Corona virus (Covid-19) infection in pregnancy. Information for healthcare professionals: Version 14. London: RCOG; 2021.
3. KFOG. GCPR on management of Covid-19 affected pregnancies. Thrissur: KFOG; 2021.
4. CDC. Information on pregnancy, Breast feeding and Caring for Newborns during the COVID-19 Pandemic. [online] Available from: https://www.cdc.gov/coronavirus/2019-ncov/if-you-are-sick/pregnancy-breastfeeding.html. [Last Accessed October, 2021].
5. Ajith C, Reshmi VP, Nambiar S, Naser S, Athulya B. Prevalence and risk factors of neonatal covid-19 infection: a single centre observational study. J Obstet Gynecol India 2021;71(3):235-8.

LONG QUESTION

1. Discuss the clinical presentation and management of COVID-19 infected pregnancies.

SHORT QUESTIONS

1. How does COVID-19 infection affect pregnancy?
2. How do you manage clinically deteriorating pregnant COVID-19 infected patients?
3. Discuss labor management of Covid-19 infected patients.
4. Discuss the post-partum management of COVID positive patients.
5. Discuss the importance of COVID vaccination in pregnancy.

MULTIPLE CHOICE QUESTIONS

1. Which COVID vaccine is associated with VITT?
    a. Covishield
    b. Moderna
    c. Pfizer-BioNTech
    d. All the above
2. Which one is true regarding postpartum care?
    a. Thromboprophylaxis is important
    b. Absolute bed rest needs to be advised
    c. Breastfeeding is contraindicated
    d. Rooming-in is not advised
3. Risk factors for severe COVID-19 infection in pregnancy are all, except:
    a. Obesity
    b. Preexisting diabetes
    c. Age >35 years
    d. Placenta previa
4. Which of the following is true?
    a. Remdesivir should be started in all symptomatic COVID positive pregnant ladies
    b. Tocilizumab is safe in pregnancy
    c. Monoclonal antibodies are option in vulnerable pregnancies before development of hypoxia
    d. Methyl prednisolone is useful in enhancing fetal lung maturity
5. Which of the following is false?
    a. Delivery should be considered in pregnant Covid positive ladies in third trimester needing intubation to help resuscitation
    b. Epidural analgesia may be used for labor analgesia
    c. Entonox is contraindicated as labor analgesia in Covid positive patients
    d. Prophylactic LMWH should be stopped 12 hours before delivery/cesarean
6. Which of the following is sign of decompensation?
    a. Acute kidney injury
    b. Drowsiness
    c. Increasing oxygen requirement FiO_2 >35
    d. All the above
7. Which of the following is true regarding management of labor in symptomatic COVID positive patients?
    a. Continuous electronic fetal monitoring is recommended
    b. Cesarean section is the best mode of delivery
    c. Early cord clamping is recommended
    d. Skin to skin contact with baby should be avoided
8. Vaccine-induced thrombosis and thrombocytopenia is:
    a. Idiosyncratic reaction
    b. More common in pregnancies compared to age matched controls
    c. More common hypertensive patients
    d. More common in patients with past history of venous thromboembolism
9. Regarding vertical transmission of COVID-19:
    a. Cesarean section is protective
    b. Vertical transmission rate low
    c. Use of antiviral medication reduce risk
    d. Early cord clamping reduce the risk
10. Upper limit of normal D-dimer value in third trimester pregnancy:
    a. 1111
    b. 2222
    c. 3333
    d. 4444

Answers
1. a 2. a 3. d 4. c 5. c 6. d 7. a 8. a 9. b 10. c

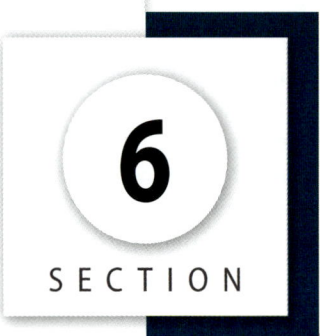

SECTION 6

Maternal Complications Arising in Pregnancy

6.1 HYPERTENSIVE DISORDERS IN PREGNANCY (GESTOSIS)

Sanjay Gupte, Arati Shah

■ INTRODUCTION

Hypertensive disorders in pregnancy (HDP) are the spectrum of disorders ranging from already existing chronic hypertension in pregnancy to complex multisystem disorder such as preeclampsia leading to complications like eclampsia, HELLP (hemolysis, elevated liver enzymes and low platelets) syndrome, pulmonary edema, stroke, and left ventricular failure (LVF).

They are responsible for a substantial burden of illness in developed as well as underdeveloped countries of the world. They are a leading cause of maternal and perinatal mortality and morbidity worldwide.

Epidemiology of Preeclampsia

Globally hypertensive disorders of pregnancy complicate approximately 5–10% of pregnancies.[1] In Africa and Asia hypertensive diseases account for 9% maternal deaths, whereas, in Latin America and the Caribbean, the figure is over 25%.[2]

Indian Statistics

Incidence of hypertensive disorders in India is found to be 10.08% as observed through the data collected by the National Eclampsia Registry (NER)[3] (11,266 out of 111,725 deliveries) with 2,554 patients out of these presenting with eclampsia. The Federation of Obstetric and Gynaecological Societies of India (FOGSI)-Indian College of Obstetricians and Gynaecologists (ICOG) NER has brought forth some revealing trends. Eclampsia prevalence among registry patients is 1.9%. This is out of the 11,725 deliveries analyzed from the cases reported by 175 reporting centers. 17% of preeclampsia patients are actually in the adolescent age group reflecting the very early age at marriage in spite of several awareness programs and legal guidelines. 76.34% of the patients were between 21 and 30 years of age thus rendering a very young population morbid and at risk of mortality. It also is a disease of the first-time pregnant woman as 81% of the patients with preeclampsia were primigravid.

CLASSIFICATION OF HDP AS PER FOGSI WORLD ORGANIZATION GESTOSIS GUIDELINES[4-6]

- *Gestational hypertension*: Blood pressure ≥ 140/90 mm Hg, detected beyond 20 weeks of gestation which returns to normal within 42nd postpartum day and is not associated with any other features of preeclampsia.
- *Chronic hypertension*: Known case of hypertension or a case of hypertension detected before 20 weeks of gestation in absence of neoplastic trophoblastic disease and multiple pregnancies.
- *Preeclampsia:* It is a multisystem inflammatory disorder beyond 20 weeks of pregnancy with significant proteinuria characterized by de novo onset of hypertension (BP ≥ 140/90 mm Hg).
- *Superimposed preeclampsia:* It is the occurrence of preeclampsia in women with chronic hypertension.
- *Eclampsia:* It is the occurrence of seizures in association with preeclampsia. It can rarely occur as atypical eclampsia without prior hypertension.

The New Definition

- The definition of preeclampsia was revised in 2014.
- Hypertension developing after 20 weeks' gestation with one or more of the following: proteinuria, maternal organ dysfunction (including renal, hepatic, hematological, or neurological complications), or fetal growth restriction. It is important to note that this definition does not require proteinuria to meet the diagnostic criteria. The inclusion

of fetal growth restriction in this definition may increase the number of women meeting the diagnostic criteria for preeclampsia and is, therefore, a significant change.

Clinical Classification of Hypertensive Disorders in Pregnancy[7,8]

Clinically, HDPs are classified as:
- *Early onset preeclampsia:* Onset of proteinuric hypertension before 34 weeks of pregnancy. The maternal complications are more severe. Low birth weight, fetal growth restriction, and iatrogenic prematurity are common.
- *Late onset preeclampsia:* Onset of proteinuric hypertension after 34 weeks of pregnancy. Here the maternal complications are less severe. Low birth weight and fetal growth restriction is less common.

Another useful way of classifying HDPs[9] is:
- *Nonsevere preeclampsia:* Blood pressure >140/90 and <160/110 mm Hg. No premonitory symptoms and normal HDP laboratory parameters.
- *Severe preeclampsia:* BP > 160/110 mm Hg with/without premonitory symptoms with/without abnormal HDP laboratory parameters. *Or* BP ≥ 140/90 mm Hg with premonitory symptoms and/or abnormal HDP laboratory parameters.

It is to be noted that nonsevere preeclampsia may get converted to severe preeclampsia in a very short time and vigilance is very important. That is why the term "mild" preeclampsia is done away with.

■ ETIOPATHOLOGY OF PREECLAMPSIA

Preeclampsia is a multisystemic disorder with profound implications for both the mother and the fetus. Abnormal interactions between fetal trophoblast and maternal decidua, including the cells of the maternal immune system, lead to inadequate placental invasion and maternal vascular remodeling. Thus the origins of preeclampsia lie in the earliest stages of pregnancy. Preeclampsia generally manifests during late pregnancy and remits after delivery attributing the critical role of its appearance to the placenta. Generally preeclampsia is considered a disorder with two components: (1) An unidentified signal from the placenta associated either with defective implantation or greater placental mass as in multifetal pregnancies or vesicular mole. (2) The aberrant maternal response to this signal which is determined by her genotype and phenotype and influenced by physiological and metabolic changes in pregnancy and also cause endothelial dysfunction with multisystemic affliction.

Two Stage Process

Etiologically preeclampsia develops in two stages **(Fig. 1)**. Asymptomatic stage involves abnormal placentation which is followed by placental elaboration of soluble factors that enter

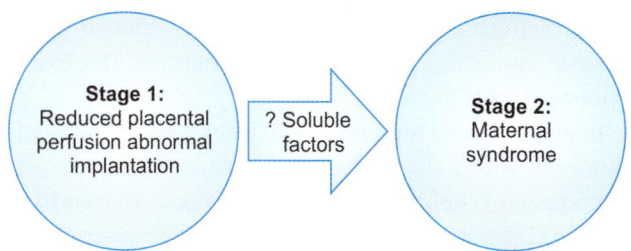

Fig. 1: The two stage model of preeclampsia.[10]

the maternal circulation and cause widespread endothelial dysfunction with signs and symptoms. This is the so-called maternal syndrome.

Stage 1: Inadequate Placental Perfusion—Failed Remodeling of Placental Vasculature

Remodeling of maternal spiral arteries leads to increased diameter of terminal vessels because of replacement of smooth muscles, thus the sphincter like action is reduced. The original conclusion was that this remodeling leads to a large increase in volume of the flow but Burton et al. (2009)[11] pointed out that flow is only increased two folds but velocity of blood is reduced from 1 m/s to 10 cm/s. So failed remodeling does not really affect the volume of the flow too much, but it keeps the speed high.

Immunology: Remodeling depends on trophoblastic invasion which depends on decidual (maternal) and trophoblast (fetal) antigen interaction.[12] This immunological interaction is intricately altered with HLA-G antigens of the trophoblast which provide protection from NK cells. To understand this we need to know the role of the highly polymorphic classical Class I molecules HLA-A, -B, -C, which are expressed on almost all somatic cells. They induce specific immune response by presenting peptide antigens to T cells. In contrast, the non-classical HLA Class I molecules HLA-G and HLA-E are thought to be involved in the induction of immune tolerance by acting as ligands for inhibitory receptors present on NK cells and macrophages. The non-classical HLA-E is also expressed ubiquitously, but HLA-G expression is characterized by a unique tissue expression mainly in the human placenta which affords specific protection to the trophoblastic cells.[13]

This is where importance of exposure to paternal antigen is intriguingly involved.

The concept of "primi paternity":[14] Robillard propagated that longer exposure to sperm antigens before pregnancy is also protective. This is now a proven fact. ICSI pregnancies and ovum donor pregnancies having more possibility of preeclampsia, also point to the importance of the immune mechanism.[14]

Effects of inadequate perfusion: Inadequate perfusion leads to many effects, like intermittent hypoxia causing oxidative stress followed by release of antiangiogenic proteins, e.g.,

SFlt and activation of inflammation. Greater velocity of blood causes fragmentation of syncytiotrophoblast, leading to more deportation of cells.

Inadequate and not reduced placental perfusion is what matters. It is not always reduced perfusion but adequacy is important. When trophoblastic mass is increased like in multiple gestations and hydropic placenta, placental perfusion is normal but still not adequate.

Stage 2: Maternal Syndrome

It is characterized by hypertension and proteinuria. Pathological examinations of organs show hemorrhage and necrosis which suggest reduced oxygen perfusion.

Also other changes seen in maternal organs are:
Vasoconstriction secondary to increased pressor sensitivity,[15] activation of the coagulation cascade with microthrombi[16] loss of fluid from the intravascular space[17] that leads to a reduction in the circulating blood volume. Interestingly, all of these are consistent with endothelial dysfunction.[18]

Important question is whether inadequate placental perfusion alone is sufficient to cause Preeclampsia? Answer is *no*. Why? Because women with FGR infants and one-third women with preterm births also showed same remodeling failure in most instances.[19]

Role of the mother: So the conclusion is effect of inadequate perfusion in PE is modified by Maternal "Constitution", i.e., maternal diseases, maternal lifestyle, genetics, environment, normal physiological changes of pregnancy (increased inflammatory response).

Implications: It implies that inadequate uterine perfusion, may not only be insufficient to cause PE, but may also not be fully necessary for PE in some cases. With a combination of maternal factors and inadequate placental perfusion together determining outcome, PE could occur with much reduced placental perfusion and almost no maternal contribution *or conversely* with minimally reduced perfusion and a profoundly abnormal maternal "Constitution". This is a crucial proposition which may help us in explaining many sub types of PE that we encounter. One such explanation was provided by Professor Redman while explaining the difference between early onset preeclampsia and late onset preeclampsia **(Fig. 2)**.

Redman[20] explained that early onset of preeclampsia is because of classical failed vascular remodeling leading to oxidative stressed placenta and syncytiotrophoblast causing antiangiogenic and inflammatory effects. For late onset of preeclampsia, he proposed a simile of pot bound placenta, which means at term some placentae overgrow the vascular supply leading to syncytiotrophoblast stress and preeclampsia.

■ DIAGNOSIS

Diagnosis of HDPs is not always conventional. In a sense, one cannot depend on the usual method of symptoms and signs. As per the NER data most of the times preeclampsia was found not to be associated with any symptoms (57%), 22% had headache and very few had vomiting, epigastric pain, giddiness, etc. Antenatal eclampsia is noted to be common (76.78%); however postpartum convulsions (13.72%) are also significant. Due to such nonspecificity of the presenting symptoms the new biomarkers are proving useful in diagnosis.

Signs and Symptoms

1. *Blood pressure:*
   - Blood pressure measurement is the most important clinical test to diagnostic HDP.
   - BP assessment is to be done with utmost care and proper technique.[21] Mercury manometer, periodically standardized; or calibrated aneroid equipment may be used.
   - The position of the pregnant mother especially after 20 weeks of gestation should be either in the sitting position or left lateral position with the zero level at

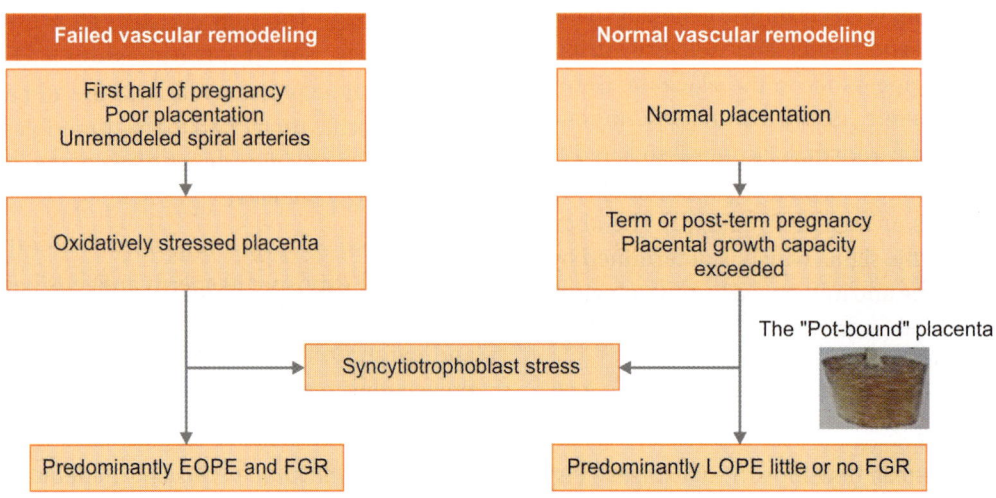

Fig. 2: Two-stage model extended.
(FGR: fetal growth restriction; EOPE: early onset preeclampsia; LOPE: late onset preeclampsia)

the level of the heart. The cuff of the appropriate size should be used.

2. *Proteinuria:*[22]
   - Significant proteinuria is urinary excretion of >300 mg protein in a 24-hour period.
   - Once significant proteinuria is established, further quantification is not required as proteinuria does not have prognostic value from management point of view.
   - However, even if proteinuria is absent, pregnant woman with hypertension still requires frequent monitoring.
   - The HDP Gestosis FOGSI scientific group recommends the following methods till further research findings are out:
     - Urinary dipstick method (Visual/by automated device)
     - *Spot urine protein:* Creatinine ratio.[23]
   - *Significant proteinuria:* Can be assessed by urinary dipstick: ≥ 2+

   Or

   Urinary protein: Creatinine ratio ≥ 30 mg/mmol.
   - Urinary dipstick method is quick and allows women with negative result to return home quickly. It also helps quick assessment of severe proteinuria.
   - The results of spot protein:creatinine also would be available within 2–4 hours.
   - It is convenient for women at risk for preeclampsia and their health professionals.
   - The gold standard of assessing proteinuria is 24-hour urine protein assessment.

3. *Laboratory investigations:* When blood pressure reading of a pregnant woman is ≥ 140/90 mm Hg (or known case of chronic hypertension visits first time to the antenatal clinic), following investigations are advisable to assess severity of the disease.
   - Baseline HDP laboratory:
     - *Urine albumin:* By dipstick method **or** urine protein: creatinine ratio
     - *Complete blood count:* Platelet count and anemia assessment
     - *Liver enzymes:* Alanine aminotransferase (ALT), aspartate transaminase (AST)
     - Lactate dehydrogenase (LDH)
     - Serum bilirubin
     - Serum creatinine
     - Serum uric acid[24,25]
   - Additional laboratory investigations:
     - Coagulation profile (when platelet count is < 100,000/mm^3)
     - Serum electrolytes (in severe disease)

4. *Ultrasonography:*
   - Maternal ultrasonography (USG abdomen and pelvis). Following things are suggested to be assessed in addition to obstetric evaluation:
     - *Liver:* Subcapsular hematoma, hepatomegaly.
     - *Kidney:* Signs of renal causes of hypertension, other changes in renal parenchyma.
     - *Ascites and pleural effusion:* As other worsening signs of preeclampsia.
   - *Fetal surveillance and placental morphology:* (Obstetric USG with Doppler):[26]
     - Fetal biometry, amniotic fluid volume (AFI), uterine artery Doppler and umbilical artery Doppler should be performed at the first diagnosis of preeclampsia.
     - In confirmed preeclampsia or in cases of fetal growth restriction, serial evaluation of fetal growth, AFI, uterine artery umbilical artery Doppler is recommended.
     - More frequent ultrasound measurements and color Doppler study are needed if there is a high resistance or absent or reversed end-diastolic flow in uterine artery with appropriate further management.
     - Placental location, morphology and any evidence of placental bed hemorrhage, abnormal adherence, and presence of sinusoids should be documented.

5. *Fundoscopy:* Fundoscopy may be required to differentiate chronic and new onset disease and to diagnose papilledema/hemorrhages as these have ominous prognosis.

6. *Additional imaging:*
   - 2D maternal ECHO: May be required in special situations where the mother is at a higher risk of developing cardiovascular complications.
   - Chest X-ray with shield: X-ray may be necessary in situations where ARDS, pulmonary edema or pulmonary embolism is suspected.
   - MRI for brain imaging may be necessary for diagnostic dilemma of eclampsia, venous sinus thrombosis, and cerebrovascular accident.

Neuroimaging is not recommended universally in all cases of eclampsia.

Maternal Alerts

Important note: PE is a dynamic and progressive process; hence continued reevaluation during pregnancy is very important. So one has to keep in mind that the following signs, symptoms, and investigations warrant urgent and prompt management.

Persistent headache, blurring of vision, difficulty in breathing, second trimester vomiting and epigastric pain, feeling of significant ill-being by the patient, uncontrolled hypertension, oliguria, brisk tendon reflexes, altered consciousness, sudden onset of massive edema, SpO$_2$ < 95%, LDH >800 u/L, S. Creatinine >1.1 mg/dL, AST/ALT >2 times the normal, platelets < 100,000/mm^3, serum uric acid >8 mg/dL.

NEED FOR UNIVERSAL SCREENING

Considering the magnitude of the mortality and morbidity associated with HDPs and especially preeclampsia there can be no two opinions regarding early and universal screening for these conditions.

HDP-Gestosis Score Provides Effective and Feasible Prediction Policy[27]

This "easy to use" score can be used for screening and prediction of preeclampsia.

Process of Risk Scoring

This score involves all the existing and emerging risk factors in the pregnant woman **(Table 1)**. Score of 1, 2 or 3 is allotted to each clinical risk factor as per its severity in development of preeclampsia. With careful history and assessment of woman a total score is obtained. When total score is ≥3, the pregnant woman should be marked as "at risk" for preeclampsia.

TABLE 1: Gestosis score.

Risk factor	Score
Age older than 35 years	1
Age younger than 19 years	1
Maternal anemia	1
Obesity (BMI > 30)	1
Primigravida	1
Short duration of paternity (cohabitation)	1
Woman born as small for gestational age	1
Polycystic ovary syndrome	1
Interpregnancy interval more than 10 years	1
Conceived with assisted reproductive (IVF/ICSI) treatment	1
Mean arterial pressure (MAP) > 85	1
Chronic vascular disease (dyslipidemia)	1
Excessive weight gain during pregnancy	1
Maternal hypothyroidism	2
Family history of preeclampsia	2
Gestational diabetes mellitus	2
Obesity (BMI > 35)	2
Multiple pregnancy	2
Hypertensive disease during previous pregnancy	2
Pregestational diabetes mellitus	3
Chronic hypertension	3
Mental disorders	3
Inherited/acquired thrombophilia	3
Maternal chronic kidney disease	3
Autoimmune disease (SLE/APLAS/RA)	3
Pregnancy with assisted reproductive (OD or surrogacy) treatment	3

This score covers all the risk factors and as per the probability and severity, the score increases.

Significance of Gestosis Score

Unlike other guidelines, which consider each factor as of equal significance, the Gestosis score gives weightage according to the severity. While completing the score sheet, it allows points to be kept blank if patient is unable to give the history. It denotes the indication for available prophylaxis (like low dose Aspirin or calcium) rather than claiming high probability of prediction.

Biomarkers in Prediction[27]

Universal screening is recommended but there is no single effective screening test. None of the tests proposed till date to predict the at-risk population for preeclampsia qualifies to be recommended for the general population screening.

The PATH Survey (2015)

Nathalie A et al., scientists from PATH international with help of Merck for Mothers recently[28] carried out the most extensive survey to date. A total of 135 unique blood and urine biomarkers and biomarker combinations associated with clinical PE presentation were identified. Of the 135 biomarkers, 118 were blood biomarkers and 17 were urine biomarkers.

Their extensive research finally has identified five practical and promising biomarkers. They are sFlt1 (*Soluble fms-like tyrosine kinase 1*), PLGF (*Placental growth factor*), CRD (*Congo Red dot test*), GlyFN (*Glycosylated fibronectin*), S. ENG (*Serum Endoglin*).

The New Predictors

Kurumachi and the team (2009)[29] found that sFlt1 concentrations are raised in established preeclampsia. The concentrations of sFlt1 are high and PLGF low in the 2nd trimester, even before the clinical onset of PE and IUGR. These changes reflect impaired placental angiogenesis and trophoblastic invasion.

sFlt1/PlGF Ratio

Increased serum levels of sFlt1 and decreased levels of PLGF, resulting in an increased sFlt1/PLGF ratio, can be detected in the second half of pregnancy in women diagnosed to have not only PE but also IUGR. Alterations are more pronounced in early-onset rather than late-onset disease and are associated with severity of the clinical disorder. The disturbances in angiogenic factors are detectable prior to the onset of clinical symptoms.

Endoglin concentrations increase well before the clinical manifestations of the disease. Furthermore, they increase most dramatically in women destined to develop early onset preeclampsia. Endoglin is a coreceptor for transforming growth factor beta-1. It prevents TGF-beta1 from binding to endothelial receptors, and thus impairs nitric-oxide synthetase-mediated vasodilatation.[30]

Using multivariate analysis, Levine et al.[31] also demonstrated that the composite ratio of (endoglin + sFlt1)/PLGF was the best predictor of both early onset and late onset preeclampsia.

Congo Red dot test[32] *and Glycosylated fibronectin*[33] are also being studied as predictive markers.

Use of Biomarkers in Diagnosis

Diagnosis of preeclampsia is based on traditional but unreliable and nonspecific clinical markers, viz. increased blood pressure and proteinuria; both are subject to observer error and poor test accuracy for identifying women at risk of adverse outcome. This clinical uncertainty leads to overuse of ancillary testing and intervention, with associated expense of antenatal monitoring and inpatient admissions. Hence biomarkers can be of value in definitive diagnosis of preeclampsia.[34]

PELICAN Study 2013[35]

This significant study concluded that in women presenting before 35 weeks' gestation with suspected preeclampsia, low PLGF has high sensitivity and negative predictive value for preeclampsia within 14 days. It is better than other currently used tests, and presents an innovative adjunct to management of such women.

This study suggested that PLGF testing presents a realistic and innovative addition to the management of women with suspected preeclampsia, especially those presenting preterm.

PREVENTION OF PREECLAMPSIA

A quote from Professor Sir Sabaratnam Arulkumaran, "the only preventive measures which seem feasible are low dose Aspirin, Calcium and $MgSO_4$ (for eclampsia)."

All "at risk" women should be started with *Aspirin 75–150 mg*.[36] Low-dose aspirin has a good maternal and fetal safety profile.[37] Aspirin for this indication should be started at or earlier than 12 weeks.[38] Defective placentation is considered the causative factor of preeclampsia. Early aspirin balances the levels of thromboxane A_2 and prostacyclin which will maintain adequate uteroplacental blood flow and improve placentation without increasing the risks of adverse maternal and perinatal outcomes. Therefore, it appears safe to use low-dose aspirin as a prophylaxis to prevent preeclampsia throughout pregnancy until 2 days prior to delivery or cesarean section.

Calcium 1–1.5 g[39] daily has been found to be useful in prevention of preeclampsia in patients with low calcium intake.

Medical Management (Flowchart 1)

FOGSI-World Organization Gestosis recommend that a systolic BP of ≥140 and/or a diastolic BP of ≥90 mm Hg warrants antihypertensive therapy.

Target range of blood pressure to be kept:[40]
- *Systolic:* ≤ 135 mm Hg
- *Diastolic:* ≤ 85 mm Hg

Antihypertensives (Mild Preeclampsia)

1. *Labetalol:*[41] *200–1200 mg/day in 2 divided doses:* It is accepted as the first line and effective medication during pregnancy. Preferred medication when baseline pulse is

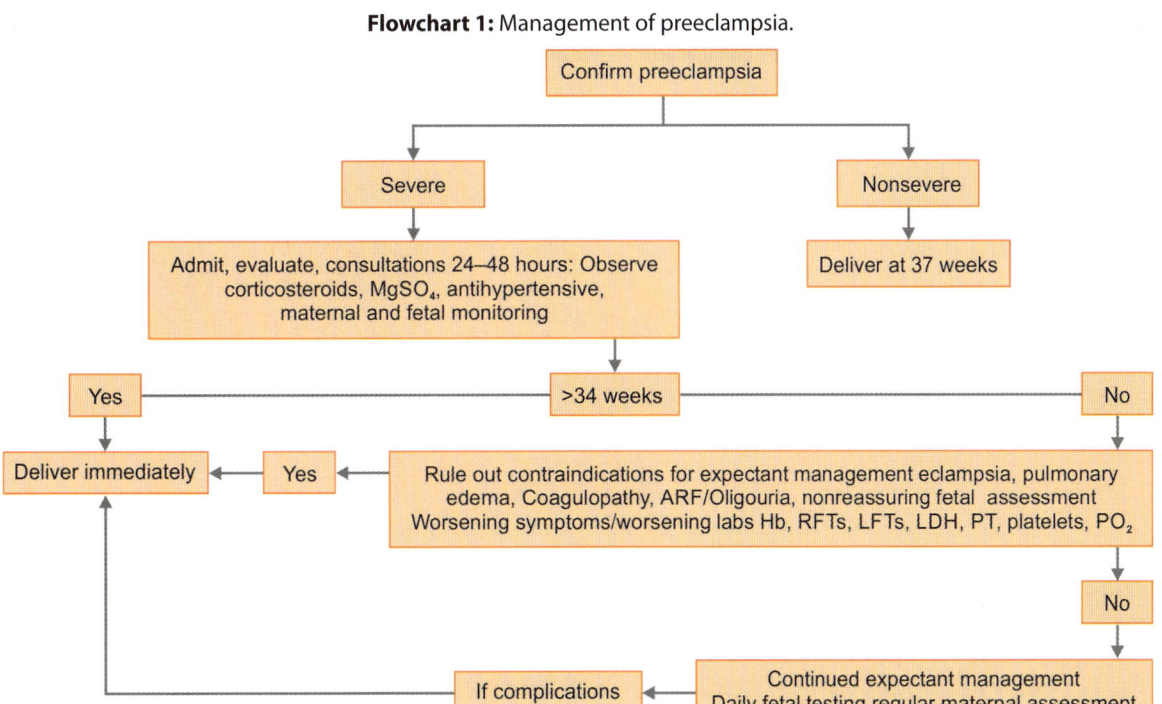

Flowchart 1: Management of preeclampsia.

(ARF: acute renal failure; Hb: hemoglobin; RFT: renal function tests; LFT: liver function tests; LDH: lactate dehydrogenase; PT: prothrombin time)

>100/min. It is contraindicated in asthma, CCF, DM and cases of bradycardia.

2. *Nifedipine:*[41] *20-120 mg/day of slow releasing preparations in 2-3 divided doses:* Preferred medication when baseline pulse is <100/min. Maternal adverse effects include tachycardia, palpitations, headaches, and facial flushing.[42] Never administer nifedipine sublingually.
3. *Methyldopa:*[43] *500-2,000 mg per day orally in 2-3 divided doses:* Methyldopa is the most time tested and safe antihypertensive. However, it is to be discontinued in the postpartum period to avoid postpartum depression.

Drugs Contraindicated in Pregnancy: ACE Inhibitors, ARBs, β-blockers and Diuretics

Antihypertensives for Rapid Control (Severe Preeclampsia)

Table 2 enumerates antihypertensives for rapid control in severe preeclampsia.

PREVENTION OF ECLAMPSIA

Loading dose of $MgSO_4$ is recommended to prevent eclampsia in all cases of severe preeclampsia.

Delivery decision:

Gestational hypertension:	Pregnancy can be continued till the term
Mild preeclampsia:	To be delivered at 37 completed weeks
Severe preeclampsia:	To be delivered after 34 completed weeks
Eclampsia:	Should be delivered once mother is stabilized after $MgSO_4$

Labor induction with appropriate method can be carried out safely.

Cesarean section is done for obstetric indications only.

Delivery decision should be carefully decided after assessing maternal and fetal risks.[46]

Timing of Delivery

Clinical convention offers women with preeclampsia delivery at 37 weeks' gestation as per NICE guidelines and the guidelines from the American College of Obstetricians and Gynecologists. Prior to 34 weeks' gestation, management is expectant with elective delivery not considered due to worse neonatal adverse outcomes (respiratory distress syndrome risk ratio 2.3, 95% CI 1.39–3.81 and necrotizing enterocolitis risk ratio 5.54, 95% CI 1.04–29.56).[47] Between 34 and 37 weeks' gestation, the optimum time to deliver to prevent morbidity for the mother and baby remained controversial. However, recently HYPITAT I (2009) and II (2015) have concluded that in both these situations, induction of labor and delivery are better options than expectant management to reduce composite of adverse maternal outcome including new-onset severe preeclampsia, HELLP syndrome, eclampsia, pulmonary edema, or placental abruption.[48]

Intrapartum Management

In addition to appropriate management of labor and delivery, the two main goals of management of women with preeclampsia during labor and delivery are: (1) prevention of seizures; and (2) control of hypertension. In the Magpie study[49] a randomized placebo-controlled trial with 10,110 participants, magnesium sulfate compared with placebo more than halved the risk of eclampsia (RR, 0.41; 95% CI, 0.29–0.58),

TABLE 2: Antihypertensives for rapid control (severe preeclampsia).

Drug	Dosage	Points to remember
Nifedipine[41]	• 10–30 mg orally (Not sublingually) • If BP is not controlled, can be repeated within 30–45 minutes • Max total dose of 120 mg is not to be exceeded • Once controlled, slow release preparations are to be started	Contraindicated in CCF and AV or SA nodal abnormalities
Labetolol[41]	Slow IV injections: • 10–20 mg IV, then 20–80 mg every 20–30 minutes • Maximum total dose of 300 mg is not to be exceeded • Alternate IV infusion regimen: • After initial loading dose, an infusion can be started at 1–2 mg/min and is titrated until desired effect • Oral tablets can be used in a conscious patient in the dose of 200 mg	Contraindicated in CCF, DM, asthma and bradycardia
Hydralazine[41]	5 mg IV or IM, then 5–10 mg every 20–40 minutes; once BP controlled repeat every 3 hours; for infusion: 0.5–10.0 mg/h; if no success with 20 mg IV or 30 mg IM, consider another drug	It has been associated with more maternal and perinatal adverse effects than intravenous labetolol or oral nifedipine such as maternal hypotension, cesarean sections, placental abruptions and oliguria[24]
Nicardipine[44,45]	• The average starting dose is 1.5 mg/h • It can be increased up to 6 mg/h for desired effect according to 0.5 μg/kg/min equation	It is 100 times more water soluble than nifedipine, so it can be administered IV making it an easily titratable IV calcium channel blocker

Target: < 140/90 mm Hg. Lower the blood pressure promptly but slowly.
(CCF: congestive cardiac failure; AV: atrioventricular; SA: sinoatrial; DM: diabetes mellitus)

reduced the risk of placental abruption (RR, 0.64;95% CI, 0.50–0.83), and reduced the risk of maternal mortality.

Mode of Delivery

It depends upon the urgency to deliver, cervical Bishop's score, gestational age, severity of FGR and Doppler study findings in the umbilical artery. It is preferable to conduct delivery in a well-equipped birthing center with the facilities of obstetrical expertise and accessible obstetric high dependency unit.

Induction of labor: It should be offered to mothers eligible for vaginal delivery. Prostaglandins (PGs) (dinoprostone gel, suppositories or tablets) can be used for induction. Misoprostol may be used in patients remote from term. Mechanical dilatation of the cervix with Foley's balloon or vaginal hygroscopic dilators may be considered. Augmentation of labor is to be done only with oxytocin.

Cesarean delivery: Severe FGR or reversed end diastolic flow (REDF) in the umbilical artery on color Doppler or any obstetric contraindication for vaginal delivery or failure of induction may make cesarean delivery a preferred choice.

Fluid Management

Inappropriate use of fluids can cause pulmonary edema and maternal death. Fluid restriction is advisable to reduce the risk of fluid overload in the intrapartum and postpartum periods. No fluid expansion should be used and total fluid restriction to 80 mL/h or 1 mL/kg/h is beneficial. Additional 700 mL can be used for nonsensical loss. Crystalloids such as Ringer's lactate or normal saline are used.

Intrapartum fetal monitoring: Close monitoring of the fetus with continuous or intermittent Doppler device or electronic fetal heart monitoring (EFM) is preferred. Laboratory investigations may be repeated when required.

Preventing Postpartum Hemorrhage

Active management of third stage of labor and prophylactic administration of oxytocics in case of cesarean delivery should be followed in all cases. It is safe to use oxytocin 5 U bolus equally diluted over 2–3 minutes or PG injections. PG can be used also as misoprostol sublingual, transrectal or transvaginal. *Methylergometrine is contraindicated.* Average blood loss of labor may not be well tolerated by these patients due to hemoconcentration. Underlying endothelial dysfunction, hypertension and use of magnesium sulfate may make the mother more susceptible to postpartum hemorrhage (PPH). The use of fluids should be judicious. Recommendation is 80 mL/h or 1 mL/kg/h as overinfusion can cause pulmonary edema in these women.

Post-delivery Management

It involves close vigilance for eclampsia, PPH, HELLP, pulmonary edema, cardiovascular, cerebrovascular events and thromboembolic complications. The National Eclampsia Registry[3] showed that in 13% of the cases, eclampsia occurred the first time after delivery. Continued postpartum surveillance has to be the norm to prevent additional morbidity as preeclampsia can develop post-delivery. During the hospital stay, blood pressure should be closely monitored for first 48 hours post-delivery. Postpartum use of NSAIDs should be avoided. Antihypertensive therapy is recommended for persistent SBP > 140 and DBP > 90 mm Hg. Persistent BP of ≥ 160 SBP and or DBP of ≥ 110 mm Hg should be treated within one hour and magnesium sulfate considered for seizure prophylaxis.

Discharge planning: After stabilization discharge can be considered with instructions for home surveillance and regular follow-up. Patients should be made aware of warning signs and symptoms and the importance of reporting to the hospital in case they are encountered.

Post discharge management: Home BP monitoring by self or a visiting HCP should be regularly practiced and OPD review must be within 3–5 days or earlier if symptoms persist or recur.

Postpartum care: Every patient of preeclampsia should be monitored closely for 3 months with advice regarding antihypertensive medicines and regular visits. They should be guided and encouraged to use contraception at least for a period of 2–3 years. The preferred method would be an IUCD. They should be counseled regarding the importance of preconceptional counseling for a subsequent pregnancy.

Long-term Surveillance

Every mother should be advised long-term surveillance as preeclampsia increases the long-term risk of chronic hypertension, ischemic heart disease (IHD), cerebrovascular disease, kidney disease, diabetes mellitus, thromboembolism, hypothyroidism and impaired memory.

THE FUTURE

It seems that enigma of gestosis will finally get solved by science of genomics. Any alteration in the gene (mutation) can lead to formation of unwanted proteins which in turn can convert health to the disease. By studying the genes and their mutations we will eventually be able to decipher the morbid process of gestosis (preeclampsia).

Emerging evidence suggests that healthy placental function requires locus-specific methylation changes in the genome at specific time points in development. Epigenetic disruptions such as maternal exposure to severe stressors, such as environmental pollutants, nutritional factors, psychosocial stress, or maternal depression during pregnancy, can increase the fetus' risk for suboptimal growth in a wide range of organ systems, and for developing a variety of disorders in adulthood.

These epigenetic regulations play a role in the pathophysiology of PE.

Interestingly, placental gene expression changes have been shown to precede PE, and candidate gene susceptibility loci where they occur are now being identified. This has wide-ranging implications in the discovery of predictive markers for

PE, which may improve the ability to provide early treatment and monitor women with high risk of PE.

A Note on Nomenclature

Eclampsia was a convulsive disorder of pregnancy known for 1,000 years. Edema, hypertension and proteinuria were noted in these cases. Even without seizures, this syndrome indicated a potentially rapidly progressive disease leading to maternal and infant morbidity and mortality. Since it generally preceded seizures, it was called preeclampsia!

Now we know that edema can be physiological in pregnancy. That is why it was discarded from definition in 1990s. Recently in 2014, proteinuria has also not been retained as the pathognomonic sign of preeclampsia. The research also shows that all preeclampsia cases (if untreated) do not proceed into eclampsia. And eclampsia can suddenly manifest without previous hypertension (preeclampsia).[50] So the time has come to change nomenclature of this condition to the original description, i.e., gestosis, meaning sterile inflammation of pregnancy which seems to be the reality.

■ REFERENCES

1. Cunningham FG, Leveno KJ, Bloom SL. Williams Obstetrics, 23rd edition. Toronto: McGraw Hill Medical; 2010. p. 34.
2. Khan KS, Wojdyla D, Say L, Gülmezoglu AM, Van Look PF. WHO analysis of causes of maternal death: a systematic review. Lancet. 2006;367(9516):1066-74.
3. Gupte S, Wagh G. Preeclampsia-eclampsia. J Obstet Gynecol India. 2014;64(1):4-13.
4. ACOG. Practice Bulletin No 202: Gestational Hypertension and Preeclampsia. Obstet Gynecol. 2019;133:e1.
5. Stella CL, Sibai BM. Preeclampsia: Diagnosis and management of the atypical presentation. J Matern Fetal Neonatal Med. 2006;19:381-6.
6. Rojas-Arias JL, Ortiz-López LD, Orduña-Aparicio WJ, Quintero-Loaiza CA, Acuña-Osorio E, Franco-Hernández A, et al. Characterization of atypical preeclampsia. Fetal Diagn Ther. 2015;38:119-25.
7. Duhig K, Vandermolen B, Shennan A. Recent advances in the diagnosis and management of pre-eclampsia. F1000 Res. 2018;7:242.
8. Tranquilli AL, Dekker G, Magee L. The classification, diagnosis and management of the hypertensive disorders of pregnancy: a revised statement from the ISSHP. Pregnancy Hypertens. 2014;4(2):97-104.
9. ACOG. Hypertension in Pregnancy. (2013b) Criteria for severe preeclampsia. Washington DC.: American College of Obstetricians and Gynecologist; 2013.
10. Roberts JM, Hubel CA. The two stage model of preeclampsia: variations on the theme. Placenta. 2009;30(Suppl A):S32-7.
11. Burton GJ, Woods AW, Jauniaux E, Kingdom JC. Rheological and physiological consequences of conversion of the maternal spiral arteries for uteroplacental blood flow during human pregnancy. Placenta. 2009;30:473-82.
12. Hiby Se, Walker JJ. Combinations of maternal KIR and fetal HLA-C genes influence the risk of preeclampsia and reproductive success. J Exp Med. 2004;200:957-65.
13. Blaschitz A, Hutter H, Dohr G. HLA class I protein expression in the human placenta. Early Pregnancy. 2001;5:67-9.
14. Robillard PY, Dekker GA, Hulsey TC. Revisiting the epidemiological standard of preeclampsia: primigravidity or primipaternity? Eur J Obstet Gynecol Reprod Biol. 1999;84(1):37-41.
15. Gant NF, Daley GL, Chand S, Whalley PJ, MacDonald PC. A study of angiotensin II pressor response throughout primigravid pregnancy. J Clin Investig. 1973;52:2682-9.
16. Kobayashi T, Tokunaga N, Sugimura M, Suzuki K, Kanayama N, Nishiguchi T, et al. Coagulation/fibrinolysis disorder in patients with severe PE. Semin Thromb Hemost. 1999,25:451-4.
17. Campbell DM, Campbell AJ. Evans blue disappearance rate in normal and pre-eclamptic pregnancy. Clinical and Experimental Hypertension. Part B. Hypertens Pregnancy. 1983;2:163-9.
18. Roberts JM, Taylor RN. Preeclampsia: an endothelial cell disorder. Am J Obstet. Gynecol. 1989;161:1200-4.
19. Brosens I, Pijnenborg R. The "Great Obstetrical Syndromes" are associated with disorders of deep placentation. Am J Obstet Gynecol. 2011;204:193-201.
20. Redman CW, Staff AC. Preeclampsia, biomarkers, syncytiotrophoblast stress, and placental capacity. Am J Obstet Gynecol. 2015;213:S9-4.
21. Bello NA, Woolley JJ, Cleary KL, Falzon L, Alpert BS, Oparil S, et al. Accuracy of Blood Pressure Measurement Devices in Pregnancy: A Systematic Review of Validation Studies. Hypertension. 2018;71:326.
22. Chappell LC, Shennan AH. Assessment of proteinuria in pregnancy. BMJ. 2008;336:968-9.
23. Wheeler TL II, Blackhurst DW, Dellinger EH, Ramsey PS. Usage of spot urine protein to creatinine ratio in the evaluation of preeclampsia. Am J Obstet Gynecol. 2007;196(5):465.el-4.
24. Bellomo G, Venanzi S, Saronio P, Verdura C, Narducci PL. Prognostic significance of serum uric acid in women with gestational hypertension. Hypertension. 2011;58:704.
25. Wu Y, Xiong X, Fraser WD, Luo ZC. Association of uric acid with progression to preeclampsia and development of adverse conditions in gestational hypertensive pregnancies. Am J Hypertens. 2012;25:711.
26. Neilson JP, Alfirevic Z. Doppler Ultrasound for fetal assessment in high risk pregnancies. Cochrane Database Syst Rev. 2000;(2):CD000073.
27. FOGSI. (2019). GCPR on Hypertensive Disorders in Pregnancy (HDP). [online] Available from: https://www.fogsi.org/fogsi-hdp-gcpr-2019/. [Last accessed November, 2019].
28. Acestor N, Goett J, Lee A, Herrick TM, Engelbrecht SM, Harner-Jay CM, et al. Towards biomarker-based tests that can facilitate decisions about prevention and management of preeclampsia in low-resource settings. Clin Chem Lab Med. 2016;54(1):17-27.
29. Steinberg G, Khankin EV, Karumanchi SA. Angiogenic factors and preeclampsia. Thromb Res. 2009;123(Suppl 2):S93-S99.
30. Levine RJ, Lam C, Qian C, Yu KF, Maynard SE, Sachs BP, et al. Soluble Endoglin and Other Circulating Antiangiogenic Factors in Preeclampsia. N Engl J Med. 2006;355:992-1005.
31. Levine RJ, Maynard SE, Qian C, Lim KH, England LJ, Yu KF, et al. Circulating angiogenic factors and the risk of preeclampsia. N Engl J Med. 2004;350:672-83.
32. Buhimschi IA, Nayeri UA, Zhao G, Shook LL, Pensalfini A, Funai EF, et al. Protein misfolding, congophilia, oligomerization, and defective amyloid processing in preeclampsia. Sci Transl Med. 2014;6:245-92.

33. Rasanen J, Quinn MJ, Laurie A, Bean E, Roberts CT Jr, Nagalla SR, et al. Maternal serum glycosylated fibronectin as a point-of care biomarker for assessment of preeclampsia. Am J Obstet Gynecol. 2015;212:82.e1-9.
34. Menzies J, Magee LA, Macnab YC, Ansermino JM, Li J, Douglas MJ, et al. Current CHS and NHBPEP criteria for severe preeclampsia do not uniformly predict adverse maternal or perinatal outcomes. Hypertens Pregnancy. 2007;26:447-62.
35. Chappell LC, Duckworth S, Seed PT, Griffin M, Myers J, Mackillop L, et al. Diagnostic accuracy of placental growth factor in women with suspected preeclampsia: a prospective multicenter study. Circulation. 2013;128:2121-31.
36. Henderson JT, Whitlock EP, O'Conner E. Low Dose Aspirin for the Prevention of Morbidity and Mortality from Preeclampsia. A Systematic Evidence Review for the U.S. Preventive Services Task force Rockville: Agency for Healthcare Research and Quality (US). 2014.
37. Atallah A, Lecarpentier E, Goffinet F, Doret-Dion M, Gaucherand P, Tsatsaris V. Aspirin for Prevention of Preeclampsia. Drugs. 2017;77:1819-31.
38. Zhu J, Huang R. A prophylactic low-dose aspirin earlier than 12 weeks until delivery should be considered to prevent preeclampsia. Med Hypotheses. 2018;121:127-30.
39. Hofmeyr G, Lawrie TA, Atallah AN, Duley L, Torloni MR. Calcium supplementation during pregnancy for preventing hypertensive disorders and related problems. Cochrane Database of Syst Rev. 2018:10.
40. Magee LA, von Dadelszen P, Singer J. Can adverse maternal and perinatal outcomes be predicted when blood pressure becomes elevated? Secondary analyses from the CHIPS (Control of Hypertension in Pregnancy Study) randomized controlled trial. Acta Obstet Gynecol Scand. 2016;95:763-76.
41. Podymow T, August P. Antihypertensive drugs in Pregnancy. Semin Nephrol. 2011;31(1):70-85.
42. Papatsonis DN, Lok CA, Bos JM, Geijn HP, Dekker GA. Calcium channel blockers in the management of preterm labour and hypertension in pregnancy. Eur J Obstet Gynecol Reprod Biol. 2001;97:122-40.
43. Magee LA, von Dadelszen P. CHIPS Randomised Contol Trial (Control of Hypertension in Pregnancy Study). Hypertension. 2016;68(5):1153-9.
44. Cornette J, Buijs EA, Duvekot JJ, Herzog E, Roos-Hesselink JW, Rizopoulos D, et al. Hemodynamic effects of intravenous nicardipine in severely pre-eclamptic women with a hypertensive crisis. Ultrasound Obstet Gynecol. 2016;47:89-95.
45. Matsuura A, Yamamoto T, Arakawa T, Suzuki Y. Management of severe hypertension by Nicardipine intravenous infusion in pregnancy induced hypertension after cesarean section. Hypertens Res Pregnan. 2015;3:28-31.
46. Broekhuijsen K, van Baaren GJ, van Pampus MG, Ganzevoort W, Sikkema JM, Woiski MD, et al. Immediate delivery versus expectant monitoring for hypertensive disorders of pregnancy between 34 and 37 weeks of gestation (HYPITAT-II): an open label, randomized controlled trial. Lancet. 2015;385:2492.
47. Churchill D, Duley L, Thornton JG. Interventionist versus expectant care for severe pre-eclampsia between 24 and 34 weeks' gestation. Cochrane Database Syst Rev. 2013;(7):CD003106.
48. Koopmans CM, Bijlenga D, Groen H, Vijgen SM, Aarnoudse JG, Bekedam DJ, et al. Induction of labour versus expectant monitoring for gestational hypertension or mild pre-eclampsia after 36 weeks' gestation (HYPITAT): a multicentre, open-label randomised controlled trial. HYPITAT study group. Lancet. 2009;374:979-88. (Level I)
49. Altman D, Carroli G, Duley L, Farrell B, Moodley J, Neilson J, et al. Do women with preeclampsia, and their babies, benefit from magnesium sulphate? The Magpie Trial: a randomised placebo-controlled trial. Lancet. 2002;359(9321):1877-90.
50. Douglas KA, Redman CW. Eclampsia in the United Kingdom. BMJ. 1994;309:1395-400.

LONG QUESTIONS

1. Describe the different classifications of HDP.
2. Describe the 2-stage model of preeclampsia.
3. Describe the methods for diagnosis of PE.
4. Describe the gestosis score of risk scoring in PE.
5. Describe the medical management of mild/moderate/severe PE.

SHORT QUESTIONS

1. What is the new definition of preeclampsia?
2. What is the maternal syndrome in the etiopathology of PE?
3. Mention the red flags in PE monitoring.
4. What are the biomarkers used for diagnosis?

MULTIPLE CHOICE QUESTIONS

1. The main age group affected by the morbidities associated with HDPs is:
   a. 21–30 years b. 31–40 years
   c. 41–50 years
2. Gestational hypertension is:
   a. Blood pressure >140/90 beyond 20 weeks of gestation, with proteinuria
   b. BP >140/90 before 20 weeks of gestation
   c. BP >140/90 after 20 weeks, returning to normal after delivery
3. The new revised definition of preeclampsia does not include proteinuria as part of its diagnostic criteria.
   a. True b. False
4. The concept of primi paternity status is based on:
   a. Sperm antigen exposure increases the risk of development of preeclampsia
   b. Longer exposure to sperm antigens is protective against preeclampsia
   c. Pregnancies achieved through egg donation have lower risk of preeclampsia
5. Inadequate perfusion leads to:
   a. Release of antiangiogenic proteins
   b. Fragmentation of syncytiotrophoblast
   c. Deportation of cells
   d. All of the above
6. Inadequate placental perfusion alone is the primary causative factor of preeclampsia:
   a. True b. False
7. Biomarkers used in preeclampsia diagnosis are:
   a. IL-6 b. sFlt
   c. TGF

8. Preventive measures for preeclampsia are:
   a. Low dose aspirin   b. Prophylactic MgSO₄
   c. Vitamin B₁₂
9. Safe antihypertensive in pregnancy is:
   a. Nifedipine   b. Labetalol
   c. Methyldopa   d. All the above
10. All cases of eclampsia should be delivered by emergency cesarean section.
    a. True   b. False
11. Nonsevere preeclampsia patients can be delivered at term.
    a. True   b. False
12. Following is the drug of choice for eclampsia:
    a. Diazepam   b. Dilantin sodium
    c. Magnesium sulfate   d. All the above

Answers
1. a   2. c   3. a   4. b   5. d   6. b
7. b   8. a   9. d   10. b   11. b   12. c

6.2 LIVER DISEASES IN PREGNANCY: (HELLP, IHCP, AFLP, HELLP AND INFECTIVE HEPATITIS)

Suyajna Joshi D, Manjula Patil

INTRODUCTION

Liver disorders during pregnancy include a spectrum of diseases seen during pregnancy and postpartum leading to abnormal liver function tests (LFT) or hepatobiliary dysfunction or both. They occur in about 3–5% of all pregnancies.[1] Pregnancy-related liver disorders contribute to significant number of maternal mortality in India but are under recognized and under reported.

Some of the unique challenges posed by liver disorders during pregnancy are:
- Few of the physiological changes of pregnancy in LFT mimic pathologic process in nonpregnancy (raised alkaline phosphate, alpha-fetoprotein, reduced serum albumin)
- Associated with the increased maternal and fetal morbidity and mortality [acute fatty liver of pregnancy (AFLP), HELLP (Hemolysis, Elevated Liver enzymes, and Low Platelet count), and pre-eclamptic liver dysfunction] and needs early diagnosis and termination of pregnancy
- Risk of vertical transmission (Hepatitis B, Hepatitis C, Hepatitis D)
- Some of the viral infections are fatal during pregnancy (Hepatitis E)
- Neonatal infection can have chronic sequelae like chronic hepatitis, cirrhosis, and hepatocellular carcinoma (HCC).

PHYSIOLOGICAL CHANGES IN THE HEPATIC SYSTEM DURING PREGNANCY

Clear understanding of the anatomical and physiological changes in the hepatobiliary system is key in managing liver disorders during pregnancy.

Anatomical changes: There is no significant change either in the size or blood flow to the liver during pregnancy and thus palpable liver during pregnancy is abnormal and needs evaluation like nonpregnant state. Palmar erythema and spider nevi are common in late gestation and may be related to increased estrogen levels.

Liver function tests: Most commonly used laboratory tests to assess the hepatobiliary system are called LFT **(Table 1)**.

TABLE 1: Physiological changes in liver function tests.

Test	Change in pregnancy
Bilirubin	No change
ALT/AST	No change
Alkaline phosphatase	↑
Alpha-fetoprotein	↑
Prothrombin time INR	No change
Hemoglobin	↓
Albumin	↓
5-Nucleotidase	No change
Gamma glutamyl transpeptidase	No change

(ALT: alanine aminotransferase; AST: aspartate aminotransferase; INR: international normalized ratio)

Abnormal LFTs are seen in 3–5% of pregnant women. Total and unconjugated bilirubin are lower in all the trimesters. Alkaline phosphatase (ALP) is increased throughout pregnancy. Bile acids synthesized from liver are mildly increased in late trimester. In general, majority of liver tests remain in the normal range in pregnancy except those produced by placenta (↑ALP, alpha-fetoprotein) and those reduced secondary to hemodilution (hemoglobin and albumin).[2]

To summarize raised bilirubin, aminotransferase, and prolonged prothrombin time needs and palpable liver need prompt evaluation during pregnancy.

CLASSIFICATION OF LIVER DISORDERS DURING PREGNANCY

Liver disorders can be those *confined* to pregnancy (conditions occur due to pregnancy status), *coincidental* to pregnancy (conditions that develop anytime and pregnancy is just a coincidence), and *chronic liver diseases* (pregnancy in pre-existing liver disease). Classification of liver disorders in pregnancy is given in **Table 2**. Early identification of pregnancy related or unrelated disorders is the corner stone of diagnosis and management since some of the pregnancy-related liver disorders need termination of pregnancy to reduce the maternal mortality.

TABLE 2: Classification of liver disease in pregnancy.

Pregnancy-related liver disease
- Hyperemesis gravidarum
- Intrahepatic cholestasis of pregnancy
- Acute fatty liver of pregnancy
- Hypertension-related liver diseases
  - Preeclampsia/eclampsia
  - HELLP syndrome

Nonpregnancy-related liver disease

Pre-existing liver disease	Coincidental with pregnancy
Chronic viral hepatitis	Acute viral hepatitis
Cirrhosis and portal hypertension	Drug-induced hepatotoxicity
Primary biliary cholangitis	Budd–Chiari syndrome
Autoimmune hepatitis	Hepatic adenoma
Wilson's disease	Hepatocellular carcinoma
Post-liver transplantation	

INTRAHEPATIC CHOLESTASIS OF PREGNANCY

Intrahepatic cholestasis of pregnancy (ICP) was first described in literature in 1883 as "recurrent jaundice in pregnancy" that resolved with delivery.[3] ICP is the most common cholestatic liver disorder seen in the late 2nd and 3rd trimester of pregnancy. It is also called "Obstetric cholestasis," "Cholestatic hepatosis," "Recurrent jaundice of pregnancy," and "Icterus gravidarum."[4] Incidence of ICP varies widely across ethnic groups and geographic regions, 0.5–1.5% in Europe,[5] 0.3% in United States among white population, and 5.6% in Latin population and in India it is 0.5–1.5%. Worldwide the highest incidence is seen in Chile of 27.6%.[6] This geographical variation may be due to differences in the environmental factors and differences in the genetic susceptibility between various ethnic groups. It is characterized by pruritus and elevation of bile acids.

Etiology

The etiology of ICP is not completely understood till date. It is a reversible type of hormonally influenced cholestasis seen in late 2nd and 3rd trimester, a period of peak estrogen level and resolves within 2–3 weeks after delivery but rarely lasts up to 6–8 weeks. Some of the risk factors are advanced maternal age, multiparous, twin gestation, past and family history of ICP, and contraceptive induced cholestasis.[3] Higher prevalence is seen in patients with hepatitis C (20 times), cholelithiasis, and nonalcoholic fatty liver.[7]

ICP has a multifactorial etiology with genetic susceptibility, environmental, and endocrinological factors playing a role. The *genetic susceptibility* is supported by the evidence of familial clustering, increased risk in first degree relatives, in certain ethnic groups and risk of recurrence of about 60–70%.[8]

Numerous mutation in the genes involved in the control of hepatocellular transportation are investigated in the recent research like the ABCB4 (adenosine triphosphate- binding cassette, subfamily B, member 4) gene encoding multidrug resistance 3 (MRD3) protein (a canalicular phospholipid translocator) is primarily involved in the subtype of *Progressive Familial Intrahepatic Cholestasis* called PFIC3,[4] genes coding for canalicular transporters or their regulators like ABCB11, ATP8B1, ABCC2, NR1H4, etc. are involved in pathogenesis.

Role of estrogen in ICP is based on the various observations like its occurrence in late 2nd and 3rd trimester with resolution following delivery, twin pregnancy, women taking oral contraceptive pills (OCPs), and early occurrence in pregnancy following ovarian hyperstimulation.

Seasonal and geographical variability indicate the *role of environmental factors* and low selenium levels in diet and low vitamin D levels due to lack of exposure to sunlight have been implicated in ICP.

Diagnosis

Clinical features: Women in late 2nd and 3rd trimester of pregnancy present with generalized pruritus with predilection for palms and soles, and of varying intensity with no skin lesions. Pruritus may be intense with excoriation due to scratching and may cause sleep disturbances. No constitutional symptoms are seen. Jaundice may be seen in 14–25% of the woman, which usually develops later,[8] thus if jaundice is seen before itching, need to evaluate for other liver disorders.[2]

Maternal and fetal risks: ICP is not associated with increased maternal morbidity or mortality except for the troublesome itching. Maternal bile acids cross the placenta and can accumulate in the fetus and amniotic fluid causing significant risk to the fetus. The adverse effects on the fetus are preterm birth, meconium staining of amniotic fluid, respiratory distress, and sudden fetal death and NICU admission, etc. These adverse perinatal outcomes are more common in higher bile acids and thus may indicate the need for delivery between 36 and 38 weeks. The pathophysiology of fetal death in ICP is poorly understood, but may be related to cardiac dysfunction,[9,10] sudden development of fetal arrhythmia or vasospasm of the placental chorionic surface vessels induced by high levels of bile acids.

Investigations

Liver function tests:
- Raised serum bile acids are hallmark of ICP. It has diagnostic as well as prognostic importance. Bile acids in normal pregnancy remain below 10 μmol/L and bile acids level more than 40 μmol/L have been shown to be associated adverse perinatal outcome[11] and levels >100 μmol/L are definitive indicators for termination of pregnancy.

- Accumulation of bile acids in the hepatocytes causes hepatotoxicity and the release of transaminases, levels are increased 2-3 times but seldom exceed 250 U/L.[4]
- Bilirubin levels are raised in about 25% of women but rarely reach 6 mg/dL, ALP is increased by 3-4 times and gamma glutamyl transferase (GGT) is increased one-third of patients.[12]
- Prothrombin time (PT) rarely prolonged and is secondary to vitamin K deficiency from fat malabsorption.
- Rule out Hepatitis C.

Ultrasound of liver and biliary tree remains normal and is done to rule out cholelithiasis and biliary obstruction.

Histopathology: Liver biopsy is not indicated for diagnosis and is rarely done in atypical cases. It shows cholestasis without inflammation with bile plug in hepatocytes and canaliculi and normal portal tracts.

ICP is disease of exclusion and thus any pregnant woman with pruritus and abnormal LFT, other most common etiologies like viral hepatitis, dermatosis of pregnancy like PUPPP (Pruritic Urticarial Papules and Plaques of Pregnancy), pre-eclampsia, HELLP, and AFLP need to be ruled out.

Management

Goals of management are:
- Relieve troublesome symptoms
- Reduce perinatal morbidity and mortality

For patients with classical clinical symptoms with normal bile acids and aminotransferase levels, antihistamines and topical emollients may give some relief from pruritus but weekly monitoring of bile acids and aminotransferase is done with definitive treatment once the levels are elevated. Ursodeoxycholic acid (UDCA) is the drug of choice, which is known to relieve pruritus, reduce bile acids, and liver enzyme levels and may reduce certain neonatal complications.[2] It is given at the dose of 10-15 mg/kg/day and with dose adjustment done weekly depending on the symptoms and continued till onset of labor. In cases refractory to UDCA and continue to have troublesome itching S-adenosyl-methionine,[13] rifampicin, and cholestyramine are used in addition to UDCA.

Antepartum fetal surveillance tests does not alter fetal prognosis, since it is not associated with uteroplacental insufficiency or fetal growth restriction (FGR) but twice weekly modified biophysical profile (BPP) can be considered. It is recommended to deliver between 36 and 37 weeks of pregnancy or at diagnosis if presented at term.[14,15] Early delivery is indicated if bile acid level increase to 100 µmol/L. Postpartum serum bile acids and aminotransferase levels are checked by 6 weeks.

Risk of recurrence is seen in about 60-70% in successive pregnancies and in women using OCPs and thus are not preferred.

ACUTE FATTY LIVER OF PREGNANCY

AFLP, also called "acute yellow atrophy" of pregnancy is a rare obstetric emergency associated with higher maternal and perinatal mortality thus require early diagnosis and termination of pregnancy. It is the result of microvesicular fatty infiltration of the liver leading to acute liver failure during pregnancy. The incidence varies from 5 per 100,000 in UK[16] to 30 per 100,000 India.

Etiopathogenesis

Acute fatty liver of pregnancy is the primary mitochondrial hepatopathy with abnormalities in mitochondrial fatty acid oxidation (FAO defect). These FAO defects can be seen in the mitochondria of the placenta, fetus, or mother. Presence of FAO defects in the fetus (homozygous or compound heterozygous) is known to increase the risk of AFLP and other pregnancy-related liver disorders by 18-fold.[17] Babies born to mothers diagnosed with AFLP need to be monitored for the manifestations of long-chain 3-hydroxyacyl-CoA dehydrogenase (LCHAD) deficiency especially hypoglycemia at birth and if found need to be screened at birth for LCHAD deficiency (testing for most common mutation *G1528C*). These defects are autosomal recessive and the most common are the mutation on the genes (*G1528C and E474Q gene on chromosome 2*) coding for long-chain-3-hydroxyacyl-CoA-dehydrogenase – known as LCHAD. Other rare mutations are for medium-chain acyl-CoA dehydrogenase – MCAD, carnitine palmitoyltransferase 1 (CPT 1) deficiency.

Late-in-gestation pregnant mother is dependent on fatty acids as a source of energy sparing glucose to fetus. Thus, defective fatty acid metabolism which will be well compensated in early pregnancy manifests and leads to accumulation of toxic intermediates like arachidonic acid in the blood which will have deleterious effect on the maternal hepatocytes causing microvascular hepatic steatosis, apoptosis, and hepatic failure.

Placenta may play a central role in the pathogenesis of AFLP as observed by the fact that preeclampsia is seen in 50% of the patients with AFLP and spontaneous recovery is seen following delivery of placenta.

Diagnosis

Clinical features: AFLP is mostly seen in late 2nd or 3rd trimester of pregnancy and may progress rapidly. The initial symptoms in mild disease are nonspecific like nausea, vomiting, abdominal pain, malaise, headache, and or anorexia. Half of the affected women will have hypertension with or without proteinuria, edema, and 20% may present with HELLP syndrome. Progression to severe disease is known with signs and symptoms of acute liver failure – jaundice, ascites, encephalopathy, disseminated intravascular coagulopathy, and hypoglycemia. Profound endothelial cell activation with capillary leakage causes hemoconcentration, acute kidney injury, ascites, and pulmonary edema and multiorgan failure.

Severe hemoconcentration leads to reduced uteroplacental perfusion and this along with maternal acidosis can cause fetal death even before women presents to hospital.

To enable rapid diagnosis of "suspected AFLP" it is important to quickly rule out the most common causes of liver failure that are endemic in the geographic area such as HEV and malaria and preeclampsia and HELLP. The Swansea criteria[18] **(Box 1)** are used in the diagnosis of AFLP. Though it has high degree of correlation with the liver biopsy, the gold standard for diagnosis of AFLP, it is more elaborate precluding rapid diagnosis. A "Simplified Criteria"[19] **(Box 2)** proposed by Goel et al. may quickly diagnose but further studies are needed to prove its diagnostic efficacy.

Investigations: Following investigations are done in suspected AFLP.

- Complete blood count (CBC) (hemoconcentration, leukocytosis, thrombocytopenia)
- LFT (bilirubin usually <10 mg/dL, serum transaminases up to maximum 1,000 U/L, reduced fibrinogen, albumin)
- Kidney function tests (raised urea, creatinine and ammonia, proteinuria)
- Coagulation profile [disseminated intravascular coagulation (DIC)]
- Hepatitis viral serology
- Peripheral smear (malarial parasite, hemolysis)
- *Imaging:* None of the imaging modalities are quite reliable in diagnosing AFLP.

Ultrasonography shows nonspecific changes like fatty infiltration with brightness.

Histology: Liver biopsy is gold standard for diagnosis of AFLP. It shows diffuse or perivenular microvesicular steatosis though it is rarely indicated either for diagnosis or for management since coagulopathy delays liver biopsy in the antenatal period and rapid resolution of these changes are observed following delivery.

Management

Early recognition and prompt delivery is the key in reducing maternal and fetal mortality and morbidity. Multidisciplinary team of obstetrician, physician, intensivist, hepatologist, transfusion medicine, nephrologist, anesthetist, and neonatologist are involved in the management early in the course of the disease. Management involves all the measures to be taken to treat patients with acute liver failure due to any other cause and is done in intensive care unit (ICU) or high dependency unit (HDU), supportive measures with fluid management, blood and blood products to correct coagulopathy, and correction of hypoglycemia. Cases presenting with fetal demise, vaginal delivery is preferred otherwise induction of labor is done keeping very low threshold for cesarean section since early delivery leads to faster recovery, in general cesarean delivery is seen in 90% of cases.

Hepatic dysfunction resolves spontaneously within a week of postpartum and recovery is complete. Two common complications in postpartum period are:
1. *Transient diabetes insipidus:* Seen in 25% and is due to increased vasopressinase concentration since reduction in its inactivating enzyme produced by liver.
2. *Acute pancreatitis:* Seen in about 20% of the women.

Maternal deaths are due to sepsis, hemorrhage, aspiration, renal failure, pancreatitis, and gastrointestinal bleeding.

PREECLAMPSIA AND ECLAMPSIA

Preeclampsia and eclampsia are spectrum of hypertensive disorders of pregnancy (HDP). HDP complicates about 6–10% of pregnancy. Hypertension and proteinuria are considered to be the classical criteria to diagnose preeclampsia but is diagnosed in the absence of proteinuria when features of other organ involvement are seen **(Box 3)**. Eclampsia is the convulsive manifestation of HDP. Eclampsia is defined by "new-onset tonic-clonic, focal, or multifocal seizures in the absence of other causative conditions such as epilepsy,

---

BOX 1: "Swansea" diagnostic criteria for acute fatty liver of pregnancy.[18]

In a patient in late pregnancy—presence of 6 of the 14 criteria in absence of alternate explanation:

Symptoms:
- Abdominal pain
- Vomiting
- Polydipsia/polyuria
- Encephalopathy

Laboratory parameters:
- Hyperbilirubinemia
- Raised aminotransferase
- Hypoglycemia (<72 mg/dL)
- Coagulopathy or PT > 14s
- Deranged renal function (AKI or creatinine >1.7 mg/dL)
- Hyperuricemia (>950 mg/dL)
- Hyperammonemia (>66 μmol/dL)
- Leukocytosis (>11 × 10^9)

Radiology and histology:
- Ascites/bright liver on ultrasound
- Diffuse/perivenular microvesicular steatosis on liver biopsy

---

BOX 2: Simplified criteria for diagnosis of acute fatty liver of pregnancy.[19]

- *Setting:* Late pregnancy (late 2nd or 3rd trimester)
- *Acute liver failure:* Jaundice with coagulopathy and/or hypoglycemia and/or encephalopathy
- No other explanation for liver failure*

Presence of all 3 criteria is required for the presumptive diagnosis of AFLP

*No history of ingestion of hepatotoxic drug, negative hepatitis viral serology, peripheral smear negative for malaria parasites.

> **BOX 3:** Diagnostic criteria for preeclampsia.[20]
>
> *Blood pressure*
> - Systolic blood pressure of 140 mm Hg or more or diastolic blood pressure of 90 mm Hg or more on two occasions at least 4 hours apart after 20 weeks of gestation in a woman with a previously normal blood pressure
> - Systolic blood pressure of 160 mm Hg or more or diastolic blood pressure of 110 mm Hg or more. [Severe hypertension can be confirmed within a short interval (minutes) to facilitate timely antihypertensive therapy], and
>
> *Proteinuria*
> - 300 mg or more per 24-hour urine collection (or this amount extrapolated from a timed collection) or
> - Protein/creatinine ratio of 0.3 mg/dL or more or
> - Dipstick reading of 2+ (used only if other quantitative methods not available)
>
> *Or in the absence of proteinuria, new-onset hypertension with the new onset of any of the following:*
> - *Thrombocytopenia:* Platelet count less than $100,000 \times 10^9$/L
> - *Renal insufficiency:* Serum creatinine concentrations greater than 1.1 mg/dL or a doubling of the serum creatinine concentration in the absence of other renal disease
> - *Impaired liver function:* Elevated blood concentrations of liver transaminases to twice normal concentration
> - Pulmonary edema
> - New-onset headache unresponsive to medication and not accounted for by alternative diagnoses or visual symptoms

> **BOX 4:** Differential diagnosis for nausea and vomiting of pregnancy.
>
> - *Gastrointestinal conditions:* Gastroenteritis, gastroparesis, achalasia cardia, biliary tract disease, hepatitis, intestinal obstruction, peptic ulcer, pancreatitis, appendicitis
> - *Genitourinary tract conditions:* Pyelonephritis, uremia, ovarian torsion, kidney stones, degenerating uterine leiomyoma
> - *Metabolic conditions:* Diabetic ketoacidosis, porphyria, Addison's disease, hyperthyroidism, hyperparathyroidism
> - *Neurological disorders:* Pseudotumor cerebri, vestibular lesions, migraine headaches, tumors of the CNS
> - *Miscellaneous conditions:* Drug toxicity or intolerance, psychologic conditions

cerebral arterial ischemia and infarction, intracranial hemorrhage, or drug use."[20] Abnormal placentation leading to placental hypoperfusion and endothelial dysfunction is the key factor involved in the etiopathogenesis of HDP.

Hepatic dysfunction is seen in up to 50% of patients with preeclampsia and portends poor prognosis. Liver involvement is described in 15–50% of preeclampsia- and eclampsia-related deaths. Liver involvement may be asymptomatic or present with epigastric and right upper quadrant pain due to stretching of Glisson's capsule secondary to hepatic edema, subcapsular hematoma, and rupture. Elevated LFTs in preeclampsia are result of vasoconstriction of hepatic blood flow secondary to endothelial damage caused by decreased prostacycline and thromboxane ratio. This in turn causes to hepatic hypoxia leading to necrosis, degeneration of hepatocytes, and elevated liver enzymes. Aspartate aminotransferase (AST) and alanine aminotransferase (ALT) can be ↑ in the range of 100–400 U/L with AST elevation more than ALT.[20] Bilirubin is increased due to hemolysis; prolonged PT is seen in only in DIC. Lactate dehydrogenase (LDH) is elevated due to hepatic damage and hemolysis **(Box 4)**.

Histology: Microvesicular fat changes, ischemic lesions, periportal and sinusoidal fibrin deposition with hemorrhagic necrosis in the surrounding parenchyma seen in liver biopsy are classical features.

Management

Control of blood pressure and termination of pregnancy are the corner stones of management of HDP. Decision to deliver is to be balanced with fetal lung maturity and control of hypertension, severity of the disease, and impending signs of eclampsia.

HELLP SYNDROME (HEMOLYSIS, ELEVATED LIVER ENZYMES, AND LOW PLATELET COUNT)

Acronym HELLP stands for Hemolysis, Elevated Liver enzymes and Low Platelet count was the term coined by *Louis Weinstein* in 1982. It is associated with severe form of preeclampsia seen in 3rd trimester or postpartum, but rarely it can be seen in normotensive and/or nonproteinuria pregnant women. Women may be asymptomatic or present with nausea, vomiting, upper abdominal pain, jaundice, or confusion. The syndrome is characterized by endothelial dysfunction, platelet aggregation and consumption, and finally hepatocellular necrosis.

Incidence: Its overall incidence is 0.1–1% of pregnancy and complicates about 4–12% of preeclampsia and eclampsia cases. Though it is most commonly found in association with hypertensive disorders of pregnancy indicating severe disease with mortality rate of 2–24%, in about 4–12% there may not be antecedent hypertension or proteinuria. It is more often seen in antenatal period with only 28% of cases seen in the postpartum period till one week of delivery with maximum cases in initial 48 hours.

Signs and Symptoms

Condition	Frequency (%)
Hypertension	85
Proteinuria	87
Right upper quadrant or epigastric pain	40–90
Nausea or vomiting	29–84
Headaches	33–60
Visual changes	10–20
Mucosal bleeding	10
Jaundice	5

Hallmarks of HELLP Syndrome

Hemolysis: Presence of microangiopathic hemolysis and diagnosis requires at least 2 of the following:
- Abnormal peripheral smear (schistocytes, spherocytes, reticulocytes, anisocytosis, and burr cells)
- Elevated serum bilirubin (≥1.2 mg/dL)
- Low serum haptoglobin
- Significant drop in hemoglobin levels, unrelated to blood loss.

Elevated liver enzymes: It signifies liver cell ischemia and/or necrosis.
- AST or ALT at least twice the upper level of normal
- LDH at least twice the upper level of normal.

Low platelets:
<100,000/mm³

Tennessee Classification

It is based on the same laboratory criteria:
- Hemolysis on peripheral smear
- AST ≥ 70 IU/L and LDH ≥600 IU/L
- Platelet count <100,000/mm³

- presence of any 2—Partial HELLP
- presence of all 3 —Full HELLP

Severity of *thrombocytopenia* is assessed using *Mississippi Classification* with platelet count <50,000 mm³ - Class I, 50,000–100,000 mm³ - Class II, and 100,000 to <15,000 mm³ as Class III.[21,22]

Treatment

There is no role of outpatient or expectant management and delivery should be expedited.

■ HYPEREMESIS GRAVIDARUM

Hyperemesis gravidarum (HG) is a severe form of nausea and vomiting of pregnancy (NVP). No single definition of HG exists. Some of the most commonly used definition includes "severe form of NVP associated with the triad of dehydration, ketosis, and weight loss of >5% of body weight."[23] "Persisting vomiting during pregnancy not related to other causes and leads to weight loss and volume depletion, resulting ketonuria and/or ketonemia."[24] NVP is very common with symptoms prevalence rates for nausea of 50–80% and for vomiting 50% and for HG 2%.

HG is the most common indication for admission in the first half of pregnancy. Symptoms usually begin from 6th to 8th week of gestation and peak by 8th to 12th week and often disappear 20th week.[25] If NVP develops for the first time beyond 9 weeks other causes need to be ruled out **(Table 3)**.[24] It is associated with abnormal liver test in 50–60% of women, mainly mild elevation in aminotransferase levels. However, if the bilirubin is >2 mg/dL and transaminases are >5 times the upper limit of normal the Indian National Association for the Study of the Liver-The Federation of Obstetric and Gynecological Societies of India (INASL-FOGSI)[12] recommends careful monitoring and look for alternative causes.

Exact etiology of HG is not known but is associated with harmonal stimulus like human chorionic gonadotropin (hCG and estrogen) and psychologic predisposition. Risk factors for HG includes HG in previous pregnancy, multiple pregnancy, hydatidiform mole, increased body mass index (BMI), overt diabetes mellitus and psychiatric illness, and fetal abnormalities (triploidy, trisomy 21, and hydrops fetalis).[2]

Severity of NVP can be assessed using pregnancy-unique quantification of emesis and nausea (PUQE) scoring[25] classified as mild, moderate, and severe. PQUE quantification is done using scores for symptoms like nausea, vomiting, hypersalivation, spitting, loss of weight, inability to tolerate food and fluids, and effect on quality of life. HG can lead to dehydration, ketosis, hypokalemia, hyponatremia, low serum urea, metabolic hypochloremic alkalosis, erythrocytosis, and renal failure and rarely vitamin deficiency in pregnancy. Most common LFT is increased serum aminotransferases

TABLE 3: Comparison of hepatitis viruses—characteristics and clinical features.

Characteristics				Clinical features		
Family	Nucleic acid	Envelope structure		Horizontal transmission	Vertical transmission	Screening and diagnostic tests
Hepatitis A	Picornaviridae	(+) RNA	No	Fecal-oral, sexual, parenteral	No	Anti-HAV IgM stool titers
Hepatitis B	Hepadnaviridae	Circular DS DNA with SS portions	Yes	Sexual, parenteral	Yes	HBsAg
Hepatitis C	Flaviviridae	(+) RNA	Yes	Sexual parenteral	Yes	Anti HCV IgM Anti HCV IgG
Hepatitis D	Deltaviridae	Circular (-)RNA	Yes	Sexual parenteral	Yes	Delta antigen Anti HDV IgM
Hepatitis E	Calciviridae	(+) RNA	No	Fecal-oral Parenteral Zoonotic	Yes	Anti HEV IgM

which usually go up to 200 U/L. Fetal complications seen with prolonged HG are FGR or small for gestational age (SGA) babies. Undernutrition in early pregnancy during fetal programming increases the risk of chronic illness in adult life of the offspring (Barkers hypothesis).

Evaluation of HG includes clinical assessment to know the degree of dehydration and weight loss and signs of ketosis. Laboratory evaluation includes CBC, serum electrolytes, renal function test (RFT), LFT, urine dipstick for quantification of ketonuria, ultrasound to demonstrate normal liver parenchyma without biliary obstruction, and obstetric ultrasound to exclude hydatiform mole and multiple gestation.

Management

Aims of management are:
- Assess severity of the condition and need for inpatient management
- Correct hypovolemia, electrolyte imbalance, and ketosis
- Provide symptomatic relief to break the cycle of vomiting
- Provide psychological support.

General principles: Early treatment of NVP is recommended to prevent progression to HG.[24] Encourage women to eat frequent small meals of whatever foods appeals to them (there is no evidence to support dietary restriction to relieve symptoms), avoid personal triggers of nausea. Best rehydrating regimen is normal saline with additional potassium chloride in each bag and guided by daily monitoring of electrolytes. Dextrose infusiones are avoided unless the serum sodium levels are normal and thiamine is administered.[23] First line antiemetics are H1 receptors antagonists and phenothiazines whereas metoclopramide due to its extrapyramidal side effects and ondansetron due to limited safety data are used as 2nd line therapy.[23,24] Combination of different drugs should be used in a women who do not respond to single antiemetic.[23]

Enteral or parenteral nutrition should be considered when all other therapies fail. Women with HG continuing in late 2nd and 3rd trimester require serial scans to monitor fetal growth.[23]

■ HEPATITIS IN PREGNANCY

Acute viral hepatitis is the most common cause of jaundice in pregnancy. Viral hepatitis can be caused by Hepatitis A, B, C, and E virus (HAV, HBV, HCV, and HEV). All these viruses have affinity for hepatocytes. The clinical presentation in all these viruses is similar, is indistinguishable, and thus requires serological testing for virus-specific diagnosis. Signs and symptoms during pregnancy are similar to general population. Women usually will have mild disease presenting with fever, nausea, vomiting, anorexia, headache, abdominal pain, and jaundice and rarely progress to severe diseases characterized by encephalopathy and coagulopathy. The viruses per se are not hepatoxic but the host–immune response secondary to infection leads to hepatic necrosis with raised ALT which is the hallmark of viral hepatitis. Others abnormal LFT include raised total and direct bilirubin (5–20 mg/dL), hypoalbuminemia, and prolonged prothrombin time.

Treatment includes supportive measures to maintain adequate hydration and good nutrition. Complete recovery occurs in majority of viral illness except Hepatitis B, D, and C, which are known to progress to chronic infections. Rarely they can be fatal like in hepatitis E and disseminated herpes simplex. Other viruses causing hepatitis are nonhepatotropic (cytomegalovirus, herpes virus, Epstein-Bar virus, and influenza virus), which are less common and infect several cell lines. In pregnant women with acute hepatitis, if serological testing for hepatotropic virus are negative, these atypical viral infections need to be tested since management varies. The characteristics of the virus and clinical features are given in **Table 3**.

Hepatitis A

This is the most common type of viral hepatitis in the developing countries and is caused by hepatitis A virus (HAV). It is transmitted by feco-oral route. Incubation period is average 30 days. The person affected with the disease will excrete maximum viral particles in the late incubation period and early prodromal phase. India is considered to be endemic for HAV and most of the individuals would have asymptomatic infection in childhood with lifelong immunity.

Diagnosis

Definitive diagnosis is by anti-HAV IgM which appears 2–5 days before the onset of infection. Anti-HAV immunoglobulin (IgG) occurs early in the course of the disease and transmitted to fetus through placenta and protects the newborn and thus congenital infection is not known.

Management

Supportive treatment with adequate fluid and maintaining good nutrition remain mainstay of treatment. There is no role of antibiotics, antivirals, and corticosteroids.

Prevention of hepatitis A: Universal vaccination of all children above the age of 12 months is recommended, two doses are given 6 months apart. Pregnant women visiting endemic area can consider both passive immunoglobulin and vaccine.[26]

Hepatitis B

Hepatitis B infection is the most common form of chronic hepatitis around the world. The prevalence of chronic hepatitis B in general population in India is 1.4–2.7%[12] and WHO estimates of 2015 shows 257 million people are living with chronic hepatitis. HBV infection is acquired by parenteral, sexual, and vertical transmission. Acute hepatitis presents similarly like other viral hepatitis. Acute infection can cause complete recovery in healthy adult in contrast to neonate where persistent infection occurs in 90–95% cases because of immature immunity. This can lead to either asymptomatic carrier state or chronic hepatitis. Around 15–40% of people with chronic infection will develop complications like cirrhosis, liver failure, or HCC.[26]

Diagnosis

Acute hepatitis B is diagnosed by detecting HBsAg and IgM core antibody. HBV core antibodies are produced secondary to infection, never vaccination **(Figs. 1A and B)**. LFT shows elevated ALT and AST levels of 500–5,000 U/L and serum bilirubin levels ≤10 mg/dL. Persistence of HBsAg after 6 months of acute infection (or diagnosis) indicates chronic infection. HBeAg indicates risk infectivity.

Diagnosis of HBV infection during pregnancy in majority of the women is during routine 1st trimester screening. Diagnosis of chronic carrier state is by presence of HBsAg and absence of HBsAb. In general, there is no effect of chronic HBV on pregnancy and vice versa except for few reported cases of preterm labor.[4] Once diagnosed with HBsAg positive, further evaluation includes assessment of viral load by HBV DNA, HBeAg, LFT, and upper abdomen ultrasound. Prevention of perinatal infection is a major intervention to reduce the HBV epidemic across the globe. Some of the measures to reduce vertical transmission are:[12,26]

- All women of childbearing age with hepatitis B infection, who plans pregnancy in near future should be treated with antiviral agents of Category B drugs preferably tenofovir.
- Universal screening of all pregnant women with HBsAg in the 1st trimester.
- Universal immunization against HBV at birth with administration of 3 doses of vaccine by 6 months of age.
- All pregnant women who are HBsAg positive and HBV DNA levels are ≥200,000 should receive antiviral prophylaxis with Tenofovir disoproxil fumarate (TDF) starting from 24–28 weeks of pregnancy and continue for up to 12 weeks postdelivery.[12]
- HBV-infected mothers who are HBeAg positive have almost 90% risk of transferring infection to neonate, but immunoprophylaxis with HBIG and vaccination within 12 hours of birth reduces the risk by 95%.[26]

Cesarean delivery is indicated for only obstetric indications. Universal precautions of infection prevention should be taken by all healthcare professionals. Breastfeeding is not risk factor for mother-to-child transmission (MTCT) even in mothers with high infectivity and thus should be encouraged. Tenofavir is not contraindicated during lactation.

Hepatitis D

It is also called as *delta hepatitis*. It is a defective RNA virus that can cause hepatitis in individuals affected by hepatitis B. It occurs as coinfection with hepatitis B or as a superinfection on chronic HBV infection. The disease transmission is similar to hepatitis B. This virus uses hepatitis B surface antigen (HBsAg) as its envelope protein essential for viral transmission. CDC 2016 estimates of the 350 million people worldwide who are chronically infected with HBV, 15–20 million of them are coinfected or superinfected with HDV. HDV infection is detected by the presence of anti-HDV and HDV DNA. Chronic coinfection with hepatitis B and D is more severe than HBV alone and up to 75% of the affected patients develop cirrhosis.

Hepatitis C

The prevalence of hepatitis C virus in India is 0.5–1.5%. Majority of acute HCV infection are asymptomatic but once infected 75–85% become chronically infected.[26] Chronic HCV may progress to cirrhosis in 20–30% and HCC. HCV is transmitted through percutaneous exposure of blood and body fluids. HCV can be transmitted to the fetus of the infected mother by intrauterine, intrapartum, and postnatal routes. Higher MTCT is seen with procedures like amniocentesis,

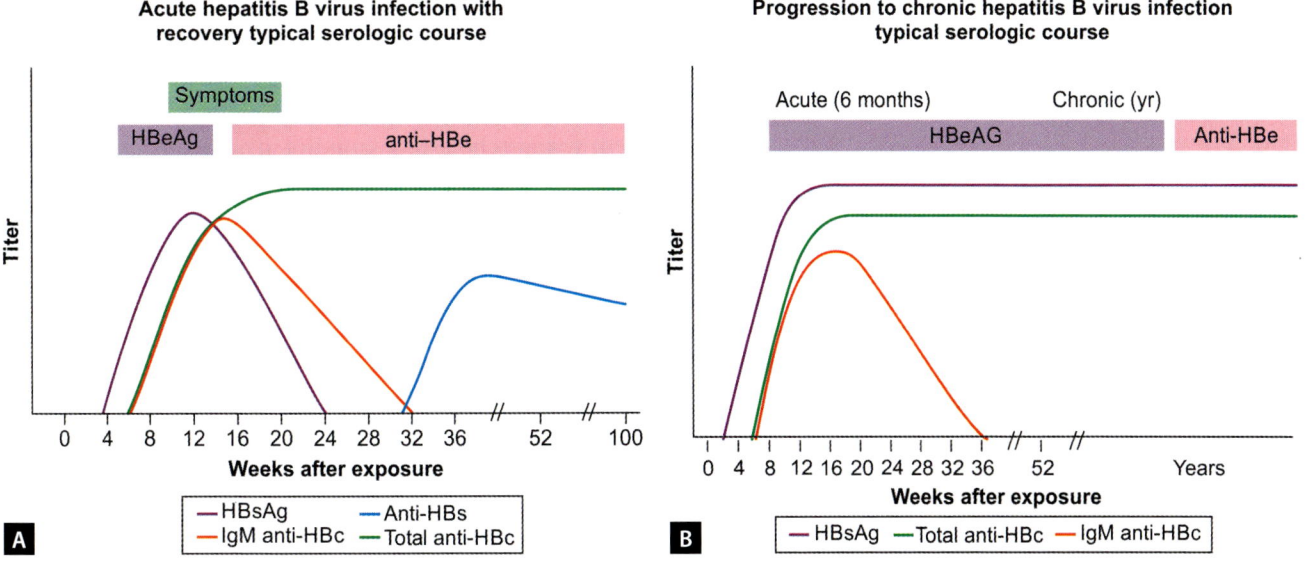

Figs. 1A and B: Immunological response in hepatitis.

invasive fetal monitoring, prolonged rupture of membranes, and high viral load and coinfection with HIV. No intervention in pregnancy is known to reduce risk of MTCT. HCV has little impact on pregnancy with minimal risk to the mother and neonate. There can be increased risk of gestational diabetes, premature rupture of membranes and preterm labor and perinatal transmission. The relative immunosuppression induced by pregnancy mirror increased viral load and ALT levels in the 2nd and 3rd trimester with diminished viral load in the postpartum period. HCV screening in pregnancy is done only for high-risk population including illicit drug users, dialysis patients, HIV infected, unexplained chronic liver disease, etc. Because of its low prevalence in general and low risk of vertical transmission ~ 5% and since no interventions are available to reduce this MTCT, presently universal screening of pregnant women is not recommended by majority of the guidelines except The American Association for the Study of Liver Disease. Vaginal delivery is not a contraindication.

Women with known HCV should be treated before planning for pregnancy to reduce the viral load. Ribavarin is teratogenic and it even causes spermatogenic abnormalities (cell toxicity, mutagenicity, and decreased epididymal sperm count) in HCV infected men and these changes revert back months after stopping treatment. Thus, INASL-FOGSI[12] recommends that if HCV therapy of the female or male partner includes ribavirin, pregnancy should be avoided for 6 months after cessation of treatment.

There is no role of treating chronic HCV during pregnancy since the safety and efficacy of directly acting antivirals (DAAs) during pregnancy is still not established and are used only as research protocol. After delivery mother should be evaluated with HCV-RNA at 9–12 months postpartum to assess for spontaneous clearance before starting therapy. Breastfeeding is not contraindicated unless cracked or bleeding nipples.

Children who have acquired HCV through vertical transmission may have spontaneous clearance (11–25%) or develop chronic asymptomatic mild disease or develop end stage liver disease.[12,26] The child should be evaluated with anti-HCV at or after 18 months and if positive HCV-RNA should be tested after 3 years of age.[12]

Hepatitis E

Hepatitis E is caused by single-stranded RNA virus. HEV is transferred by feco-oral route. Majority of the waterborne epidemic outbreaks in developing countries are due to hepatitis A or hepatitis E. Infection is usually mild-to-moderate with no chronicity and case fatality rate of 0.4–4%. Pregnant women have more severe illness with increased risk of fulminant hepatitis and mortality as high as 20%.[26] Maternal infection is associated with a high risk of fetal or neonatal mortality. The cause of increased severity in pregnancy may be due to attenuated cellular immunity. Confirmatory diagnosis is by anti-HEV IgM, the antibodies develop early in the prodromal phase, before the onset of jaundice and IgM is replaced by IgG in the convalescent period which persists for years.

The management of HEV during pregnancy requires hospitalization for supportive care because of high mortality. No role of antivirals, no pre-exposure or postexposure immunoglobulins or vaccines against HEV are available presently. Preventive measures include hygenic practice, clean drinking water, and avoid travelling to endemic areas.

PREGNANCY IN PATIENTS WITH CHRONIC LIVER DISEASES

Primary Biliary Cholangitis (Primary Biliary Cirrhosis)

PBC is a rare chronic cholestatic disease characterized by T-lymphocyte mediated destruction of the small intralobular bile ducts, leading to cirrhosis and liver failure. It is rare disease and 90% seen in women.[28] Diagnosis of PBC requires presence of two of the following three criteria:[27]

1. Biochemical evidence of cholestasis characterized by elevated ALP (>1.5 times the upper limit of normal)
2. Presence of antimitochondrial antibody (titers ≥40) and
3. Liver histology characterized by nonsuppurative cholangitis and interlobular bile duct destruction.

Women with PBC have reduced fertility. Pregnancy in women with PBC is uneventful but rarely present with intense pruritus and cholestasis. Postpartum flare up is known in 60% of women. UDCA has to be continued throughout pregnancy and found to be safe during lactation.

Primary Sclerosing Cholangitis

Primary sclerosing cholangitis (PSC) is a chronic cholestatic disease characterized by chronic inflammation, progressive fibrosis, and stricture of the medium and large sized extrahepatic and/or intrahepatic bile ducts. PSC in pregnancy may be associated with increased risk of preterm labor and cesarean delivery. There are no specific markers for PSC, but perinuclear antineutrophil cytoplasmic antibodies, antinuclear antibodies, antismooth muscle antibodies, and rheumatoid factors are found. If patients present with intense pruritus and cholestatic jaundice in pregnancy, evaluation for biliary strictures and choledocholithiasis is done using USG and magnetic resonance cholangiography. There is no specific treatment for PSC in pregnancy and postpartum.

Wilson's Disease (Hepatolenticular Degeneration)

It is an autosomal recessive disorder of copper metabolism leading to excessive copper in tissue. The disease is characterized by hepatic failure and neuropsychiatric manifestations with occasional cardiomyopathy, renal diseases. A Kayser–Fleischer ring surrounding iris is specific but seen in 50% of the affected individual.[28] The evaluation for Wilson's disease includes CBC, LFT, measurement of ceruloplasmin and copper concentration and 24-hour urinary copper excretion, ocular slit lamp examination, and molecular testing.[29,30] Treatment is mainly lifelong usage of copper chelating agents liked D-penicillamine or trientine.

Oligomenorrhea, amenorrhea, subfertility, and recurrent miscarriages are common with Wilsons disease. Pregnancy in women with Wilson's disease on anticopper therapy is safe. Continuous medical therapy throughout pregnancy and postpartum is recommended[29,30] with dose adjustments to prevent over chelation and undercoppering.[2] Since disease has autosomal inheritance, preconceptional genetic counseling is offered.

Intrapartum and postpartum periods remain uneventful with need for dose adjustment. Breast feeding is not contraindicated but may require zinc and copper supplementation.[3]

Autoimmune Hepatitis

It is progressive chronic inflammatory liver disease characterized by hypergammaglobulinemia that may progress to cirrhosis and liver failure. It usually coexists with other autoimmune diseases like autoimmune thyroid disease, Sjogren syndrome, etc. Symptoms usually are typical of acute and chronic hepatitis and 25% may remain asymptomatic. Disease is more common in childhood and adolescence. Pregnancy in a woman with autoimmune hepatitis (AIH) should be planned in remission phase of the AIH and immunosuppression should be continued throughout pregnancy and postpartum to prevent AIH flare. Both prednisolone and azathioprine used for immunosuppression are safe during pregnancy. Maternal and fetal complications in AIH especially with cirrhosis are more common and include premature birth, FGR or SGA and diabetes, and even fetal demise. Postpartum flare is seen in one-third women.[1]

Budd–Chiari Syndrome

Budd–Chiari syndrome (BCS) is a hepatic venous outflow obstruction not due to cardiac, pericardial, or veno-occlusive disease. It is caused due to thrombosis of hepatic veins or the terminal portion of inferior vena cava. BCS is associated with multiple risk factors with propensity for venous thromboembolism like pregnancy and combined oral contraceptives (COCs) use. Thrombophilia is found in up to 60% of pregnant women with BCS. BCS presents with abdominal pain, distension, ascites, nausea, vomiting, fever, and jaundice. It may present as an acute condition with obstruction of major hepatic veins or chronic with the involvement of smaller intralobular veins. In acute presentation, patient deteriorates rapidly with development of portal hypertension, variceal bleeding, and fulminant hepatic failure.[28]

Diagnosis is by Doppler ultrasound of hepatic veins and inferior vena cava, CT, or magnetic resonance imaging (MRI) imaging. LFT shows marked elevation of ALP with moderate elevation of all other tests. In addition, thrombophilia evaluation has to be done.

Treatment includes anticoagulation, diuretics, and treatment of complications of portal hypertension if present. Transjugular intrahepatic portosystemic shunting (TIPS) may be necessary to improve portal hypertension and ascites, which being noninvasive has replaced surgical shunting. Liver transplantation may be needed in severe cases.

Prevalence of pregnancy-related BCS is 6.8%. Infertility and poor pregnancy outcomes may be seen even before diagnosis of BCS. Therapeutic options like TIPS should be considered in preconception to optimize pregnancy outcome. Pregnancy may have detrimental effect on the disease due to pregnancy associated changes like hypercoagulability, volume expansion, and increased intra-abdominal pressure. Maternal complications include thrombosis, hemorrhage, and TIPS occlusion and fetal complications are increased risk of fetal loss (30%) and preterm delivery (70%). Treatment with anticoagulant low molecular weight heparin is recommended during pregnancy.

Hepatic Adenoma and Focal Nodular Hyperplasia

Hepatic adenomas are rare epithelial benign neoplasm of the liver but have 5% risk of malignant transformation and significant risk of rupture associated with hemorrhage, particularly in pregnancy.[4] They are more common in women (9:1) with strong association with oral contraceptive use, anabolic androgens, and glycogen storage disease, and less common with pregnancy.[31] Women may be asymptomatic or present with severe epigastric and right hypochondriac pain or detected during routine abdominal examination as a palpable mass, but rarely pregnant women may present in acute abdomen or shock secondary to rupture and intra-abdominal bleed. MRI or CT imaging helps to differentiate benign lesion focal nodular hyperplasia. Natural history and prognosis during pregnancy are not well established with conflicting case reports.[28]

Management includes resection or radioablation of lesion prepregnancy if it is ≥5 cm. During pregnancy large >5 cm or symptomatic adenomas should be resected in the 2nd trimester. There is no consensus managing incidentally found adenomas during pregnancy. There must be high index of suspicion to diagnose rupture and management includes resection and resuscitation.

Focal nodular hyperplasia is a benign lesion characterized by well-delineated accumulation of normal but disoriented hepatocytes that surround a central stellate scar. They remain mostly asymptomatic during pregnancy, MRI or CT scan helps to differentiate the lesion from hepatic adenoma.

Hepatocellular Carcinoma

Hepatocellular carcinoma is rare in pregnancy. Abdominal ultrasound and MRI are the first choice for evaluation of hepatic masses during pregnancy and liver biopsy is deferred due to risk of hemorrhage.[28] Accelerated growth of tumor with poor maternal and neonatal survival have been reported.

Surgical management is the primary modality of treatment. If HCC is diagnosed before the fetus is viable, pregnancy termination with definitive surgical treatment is considered. If diagnosed after fetal viability risk of expectant management must be weighed with the risk of preterm labor and synchronous cesarean delivery and liver resection can be planned.

Cirrhosis and Portal Hypertension

Cirrhosis is a late stage progressive hepatic fibrosis characterized by distortion of normal hepatic architecture and formation of regenerative nodules. Portal hypertension develops when there is resistance to portal blood flow from within liver (cirrhosis), prehepatic (portal vein thrombosis), or posthepatic (BCS). The most common causes of cirrhosis are hepatitis C, autoimmune etiologies, nonalcoholic hepatitis, and alcoholic liver disease.

Cirrhosis is associated with amenorrhea, irregular vaginal bleeding, and thus pregnancy is less likely. Pregnancy in women with cirrhosis, increases the risk of portal hypertension and massive variceal bleeding with significant maternal mortality but more recent reports show reduced mortality due to improved medical therapy and availability of timely endoscopy. Other complications during pregnancy are preeclampsia, preterm delivery, low birth weight, and fetal and neonatal death.

INASL-FOGSI recommendations[12] for management of portal hypertensive bleed in pregnancy are:
- Preconceptional screening of all cirrhosis women for gastric and esophageal varices with endoscopy, if not done, screening endoscopy has to be done at 20 weeks.
- If detected, primary prophylaxis is done with endoscopic variceal ligation (EVL) or cyanoacrylate glue.
- If patient is on β blocker, should be continued with caution on its effects on pregnancy.
- Bleeding from esophageal or gastric varices are managed like in nonpregnancy with EVL, sclerotherapy, octreotide but terlipressin is contraindicated because of teratogenic effects.

Liver Transplantation

Approximately 8% of the liver transplant recipients are women in the reproductive age. Standard recommendation[32] is to wait for at least 1 year post-transplant to ensure the acceptance of transplanted liver and time needed to stabilize immunosuppressive regimen and thus reduce pregnancy complications. Mother is at increased risk of hypertension, diabetes, preterm labor, and postpartum hemorrhage, need for cesarean delivery. Fetal complications include growth restriction and preterm delivery.

Liver transplant patients will be on lifelong immunosuppressive therapy with prednisolone, cyclosporine A and tacrolimus, and azathioprine and these are safe during pregnancy and have to be continued with the required dose adjustments. Mycophenolate mofetil (MMF) has to be discontinued 6 months before planned pregnancy. Acute cellular rejection occurs in 10–17% of patients postpartum treated with immunosuppression augmentation. Management of intrapartum and postpartum periods remains same, breastfeeding should be encouraged.

CONCLUSION

- Abnormal LFT is seen in 3–5% of all pregnancies and evaluation remains same as in general population.
- Liver disorders during pregnancy can be those confined to pregnancy such as HG, AFLP, ICP, preeclampsia, and HELLP, coincidental to pregnancy like viral hepatitis, drug-induced hepatotoxicity, BCS, hepatic adenoma, etc. or in pre-existing chronic diseases like chronic hepatitis, cirrhosis, etc.
- Evaluation of liver disorders should differentiate the pregnancy related and unrelated conditions at the earliest since some of the pregnancy-related conditions need prompt termination to reduce the maternal mortality and morbidity.
- Viral hepatitis is the most common cause of jaundice in pregnancy. Serological diagnosis is necessary to differentiate the types of virus.
- Every effort should be made to reduce the risk of vertical transmission of HBV and HCV.
- Pregnancy is well tolerated in majority of the chronic liver diseases.

REFERENCES

1. Westbrook RH, Dusheiko G, Williamson C. Pregnancy and liver disease. J Hepatol. 2016;64:933-45.
2. Tran TT, Ahn J, Reau NS. ACG clinical guideline: liver disease and pregnancy. Am J Gastroenterol. 2016;111(2):176-94.
3. Geenes V, Williamson C. Intrahepatic cholestasis of pregnancy. World J Gastroenterol. 2009;15:2049-66.
4. Cunningham FG, Leveno KJ, Bloom SL, Dashe JS, Spong CY, Hoffman BL, et al. Chapter 55: Hepatic, biliary, and pancreatic disorders. Williams Obstetrics, 25th edition. New York, NY: McGraw-Hill Education; 2018.
5. Smith DD, Rood KM. Intrahepatic cholestasis of pregnancy. Clin Obstet Gynecol. 2019;63(1):134-51.
6. Reyes H, Gonzalez MC, Ribalta J, Aburto H, Matus C, Schramm G, et al. Prevalence of intrahepatic cholestasis of pregnancy in Chile. Ann Intern Med. 1978;88:487-93.
7. Marschall HU, Shemmer EW, Ludvigsson JF. Intrahepatic cholestasis of pregnancy and associated hepatobiliary disease: a population based cohort study. Hepatology. 2013;58(4):1385.

8. Pataia V, Dixon PH, Williamson C. Pregnancy and bile acid disorders. Am J Physiol Gastrointest Liver Physiol. 2017;313:G1-G6.
9. Kondrackiene J, Kupcinskas L. Intrahepatic cholestasis of pregnancy-current achievements and unsolved problems. World J Gastroenterol. 2008;4:5781.
10. Gao H, Chen LJ, Luo QQ. Effect of cholic acid on fetal cardiac myocytes in intrahepatic cholestasis of pregnancy. J Huazhing Univ Sci Technolog Med Sci.2014;34:736.
11. Glantz A, Marschall HU, Mattsson LA. Intrahepatic cholestasis of pregnancy: relationships between bile acid levels and fatal complication rates. Hepatology. 2004;40:467-74.
12. Arora A, Kumar A, Anand AC, Puri P, Dhiman RK, Acharya AK, et al. Indian National Association for the Study of the Liver- Federation of Obstetric and Gynaecological Societies of India Position Statement on Management of Liver Diseases in Pregnancy. J. Clin. Exp. Hepatol. 2019;9(3):383-406.
13. Zhang Y, Lu L, Victor DW, Xin Y, Xuan S. Ursodeoxycholic acid and S-adenosylmethionine for the treatment for the treatment of intrahepatic cholestasis of pregnancy: a meta-analysis. Hepat Mon. 2016;16:e38558.
14. ACOG Committee Opinion No.764: Medically indicated late-preterm and early-term deliveries. Obstet Gynecol. 2019; 133:e151.
15. RCOG. Obstetric Cholestasis: Green-top guideline No. 43. London: RCOG; 2011.
16. Knight M, Nelson-Piercy C, Kurinczuk JJ, Spark P, Brocklehurst P, UK Obstetric Surveillance System. A prospective national study of acute fatty liver of pregnancy in the UK. Gut. 2008;57:83.
17. Browning MF, Levy HL, Wilkins-Haug LE, Larson C, Shih VE. Fetal fatty acid oxidation defects and maternal liver disease in pregnancy. Obstet Gynecol. 2006;107:115-20.
18. Ch'ng CL, Morgan M, Hainsworth I, Kingham JGC. Prospective study of liver dysfunction in pregnancy in Southwest Wales. Gut. 2002;51:876-80.
19. Goel A, Jamwal KD, Ramachandran A, Balasubramanian KA, Eapen CE. Pregnancy related liver disorders. J Clin Exp Hepatol. 2014;4(2):151-62.
20. ACOG. Gestational hypertension and preeclampsia. Chicago; ACOG; 2019.
21. Sibai BM. The HELLP syndrome (hemolysis, elevated liver enzymes, and low platelets): much ado about nothing? Am J Obstet Gynecol. 1990;162:311-6.
22. Martin JN Jr, Owens NY, Keiser SD, Parrish MR, Tam Tam KB, Brewer JM, et al. Standardised Mississippi protocol treatment of 190 patients with HELLP syndrome: slowing disease progression and preventing new major maternal morbidity. Hypertens Pregnancy. 2012;31:79-90.
23. RCOG. The management of nausea and vomiting of pregnancy and hyperemesis gravidarum. Green top guideline No. 69 London: RCOG; 2016.
24. ACOG. Nausea and Vomiting of Pregnancy. ACOG Practice Bulletin No. 189. Chicago: ACOG; 2018.
25. Koren G, Boskovic R, Hard M, Maltepe C, Navioz Y, Einarson A. Mother risk-PUQE (pregnancy-unique quantification of emesis) and nausea scoring system for nausea and vomiting of pregnancy. Am J Obstet Gynecol. 2002;186 suppl 2:S228-31.
26. Hamburg-Shields E, Prasad M. Infectious hepatitis in pregnancy. Clin Obstet Gynecol. 2020;63(1):175-92.
27. Lindor KD, Gershwin ME, Poupon R, Kaplan M, Bergasa NV, Heathcote JE, et al. Primary biliary cirrhosis. Hepatology. 2009;50:291-308.
28. Albright CM, Fay EE. Chronic liver disease in pregnancy. Clin Obstet Gynecol. 2020; 63(1):193-210.
29. European Association for Study of Liver (EASL) clinical practice guidelines: Wilson's disease. J Hepatol. 2012;56:671-85.
30. Roberts EA, Schilsky ML. American Association for Study of Liver Diseases (AASLD). Diagnosis and treatment of Wilson's disease: an update. Hepatology. 2018;47:2089-111.
31. Bioulac-Sage P, Sempoux C, Balabaud C. Hepatocellular adenoma: classification, variants and clinical relevance. Semin Diagn Pathol. 2017;34:112-25.
32. Lucey MR, Terrault N, Ojo L, Hay JE, Neuberger J, Blumberg E, et al. Long-term management of successful adult liver transplant: 2012 practice guideline by the American Association for the Study of Liver Diseases and the American Society of Transplantation. Liver Transpl. 2013;19:3-26.

LONG QUESTIONS

1. Classify liver disorders in pregnancy. Describe in detail etiopathogenesis, diagnosis and management of acute fatty liver of pregnancy.
2. Describe evaluation and management of jaundice in pregnancy.
3. Management of Infectious hepatitis in pregnancy.
4. Pregnancy in woman with pre-existing chronic liver disease – causes, implications, and management.

SHORT QUESTIONS

1. Define intrahepatic cholestasis of pregnancy.
2. Define HBsAg positive status in pregnancy.
3. Write in brief screening, diagnosis, and management of HCV in pregnancy.
4. Discuss pregnancy following liver transplantation.
5. Define hyperemesis gravidarum.
6. Discuss vertical transmission of HBV infection and preventive measures.

MULTIPLE CHOICE QUESTIONS

1. Increased maternal mortality is seen in following liver disorders in pregnancy, except:
   a. ICP
   b. AFLP
   c. Hepatitis E
   d. Disseminated HSV
2. High risk screening of pregnant mother is recommended in following infections:
   a. HAV
   b. HBV
   c. HCV
   d. HDV
3. Pruritus is a feature of all the conditions, except:
   a. PUPPP
   b. ICP
   c. AFLP
   d. Pemphigoid gestationis
4. Following are the physiological changes seen in LFT during pregnancy:
   a. Raised bilirubin
   b. Raised albumin
   c. Raised alkaline phosphatase
   d. Raised aminotransferases

5. Nutmeg liver is seen in following condition:
   a. Wilson's disease
   b. Budd–Chairi syndrome
   c. Hepatocellular carcinoma
   d. Primary biliary cholangitis
6. Higher prevalence of ICP is seen in all, except:
   a. HBV
   b. Cholelithiasis
   c. HCV
   d. Nonalcoholic fatty liver
7. Mutations in the genes coding for the following is seen in ICP:
   a. LCHAD
   b. ABCB4
   c. MCHAD
   d. CPT-I (carnitine palmitoyltransferase)
8. Placenta plays a key role in the pathogenesis following, except:
   a. AFLP
   b. Preeclampsia
   c. ICP
   d. HELLP
9. Indicator of risk of infectivity in HBV infection:
   a. HBeAg
   b. HBsAg
   c. HBcAg
   d. Anti HBsAg
10. Gold standard for the diagnosis of AFLP:
    a. LFT
    b. Ultrasound
    c. Liver biopsy
    d. Coagulation profile
11. Triad of Budd–Chiari syndrome includes all, except:
    a. Pain abdomen
    b. Hepatomegaly
    c. Abdominal distension
    d. Ascites
12. Post liver transplantation the following drug has to be discontinued before planning pregnancy:
    a. Prednisolone
    b. Cyclosporine A
    c. Mycophenolate mofetil
    d. Tacrolimus

Answers
1. a 2. c 3. c 4. c 5. b 6. a
7. b 8. c 9. a 10. c 11. c 12. c

6.3 GESTATIONAL DIABETES

Girija Wagh

INTRODUCTION

Gestational diabetes mellitus (GDM) is glucose intolerance developed and or detected first time in pregnancy.[1] Diabetes in pregnancy (DIP) includes women already diabetic before pregnancy, undiagnosed preexisting diabetes, as well as women with first onset hyperglycemia during pregnancy (GDM). Laboratory tests can help us differentiate between preexisting diabetes or GDM for better management and clinical approach. GDM develops in women with acquired pancreatic function insufficiency to overcome the insulin resistance associated with the pregnant state. Fetal growth in utero is ensured by abundant nutritional supply brought about by various metabolic changes in the maternal system out of which insulin resistance within the physiological limits is profound. Insulin resistance develops due to the diabetogenic hormones secreted by the placenta such as growth hormone, corticotrophin-releasing hormone, placental lactogen, and progesterone. When the insulin resistance is excessive GDM develops. GDM affects both the mother and the fetus and is associated with maternal complications such as increased risk of operative deliveries, hypertensive disorders (gestosis) and adverse fetal outcomes such as macrosomia, large for gestational age (LGA) babies, still birth, intrauterine demise, hypoglycemia and respiratory distress in the neonatal period.[2,3]

Mothers who develop GDM are at a higher risk of developing diabetes for lifetime if not diagnosed and controlled and are at risk of other metabolic and cardiovascular diseases. Likewise babies of GDM mothers are programmed to a risk of type 2 diabetes or insulin resistance disorders such as obesity and polycystic ovary syndrome (PCOS) in the female child.[4] Universal screening therefore should be offered to all pregnant women irrespective of the presence of antecedent risk factors and age.

TERMINOLOGY

Terminologies in relation to diabetes in pregnancy are defined in the **Table 1** and are suggested to be used appropriately.

INCIDENCE AND EPIDEMIOLOGY

There is a considerable rise in the occurrence of gestational diabetes (GDM) in the past decade in India and this has been attributed to the Asian ethnicity[5,6] as well as lifestyle changes and increased maternal age. The prevalence of gestational diabetes in South or East Asian women is more than in white women. Prevalence also varies because of differences in screening practices, population characteristics [e.g., average age and body mass index (BMI) of pregnant women], testing method, and diagnostic criteria. Prevalence has been increasing over time, possibly due to increase in mean maternal age and weight, particularly increasing obesity. Diabetes in pregnancy has become a global emergency needing urgent attention (**Fig. 1**) as recommended by the International Federation of Gynaecology and Obstetrics (FIGO).

Asian ethnicity and many other factors make the women from India 11 times more at risk of developing GDM as compared to women in other parts of the world.[7] Indian diversity also is reflected in the variable prevalence of GDM across the country with 3.8% in Kashmir, Western India reporting 9.5%, 6.2% in Mysore and 22% in Tamil Nadu.[8-11]

TABLE 1: Diabetes in pregnancy related terminologies.

Terminology	Description	Clinical clues
Pregestational DM	Mother who is already a diabetic may or may not be diagnosed before pregnancy	FPG is 126 mg/dL or more, glycated hemoglobin (HbA1C) is 6.5% or more, 2-hour plasma glucose level post glucose consumption of 75 g glucose is 200 mg/dL or random blood sugar level (RBSL) is 200 mg/dL or more
GDM: Gestational diabetes mellitus	Glucose intolerance first diagnosed during pregnancy or also is defined as diabetes diagnosed in the second or third trimester which is not clearly overt	First trimester if fasting plasma glucose (FPG) is 92–126 mg/dL, HbA1C is 5.7–6.4%
DGGT	Deranged gestational glucose tolerance (DGGT)	BSL between 121 and 139 2 hours after the 75 g oral glucose challenge
HIP	Hyperglycemia in pregnancy (HIP) seems to be an appropriate all-encompassing	Abnormal blood sugar levels as per all the above descriptions

(FPG: fasting plasma glucose; BSL: blood sugar level)

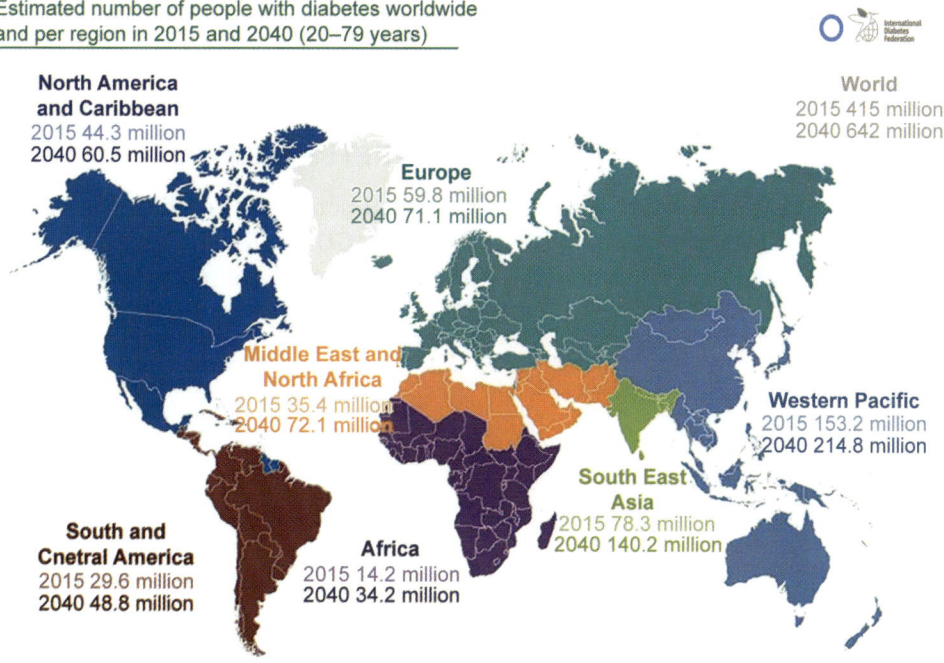

Fig. 1: Diabetes: A global emergency.

Clinical Clues for Hyperglycemia in Pregnancy

Gestational diabetes is a laboratory diagnosis and must be looked for by appropriate testing. Pregestational DM is diagnosed if FPG is 126 mg/dL or more, glycated hemoglobin (HbA1C) is 5.8% or more. GDM is diagnosed if 2-hours plasma glucose level post glucose consumption of 75 g Glucose is 140 mg/dL or more. Overt diabetes is diagnosed if random blood sugar level (RBSL) and/or 2-hours plasma glucose level post glucose consumption of 75 g Glucose is 200 mg /dl or more. Presence of classic symptoms of hyperglycemic crisis is diagnosed as diabetes.

Maternal and Fetal Metabolism in Normal Pregnancy

To understand the pathogenesis of altered insulin resistance and the occurrence of GDM the normal maternal and fetal metabolism is to be known. Each meal that the mother takes sets in motion a complex series of hormonal actions, including a rise in blood glucose and the secondary secretion of pancreatic insulin, glucagon, somatomedins, and adrenal catecholamines. This is to ensure that an ample, but not excessive, supply of glucose is available to the mother and fetus. Maternal hypoglycemia (plasma glucose mean = 65–75 mg/dL) between meals and during sleep is a common feature during pregnancy. This happens because the fetus continues to draw glucose across the placenta from the maternal bloodstream, even during periods of fasting. Maternal hypoglycemia is quite common in the first trimester itself and interprandial hypoglycemia becomes increasingly marked as pregnancy progresses and the glucose demand of the fetus increases. Insulin resistance is a result of decreased insulin action despite normal levels and is due to reasons such as defective molecular structure, receptor functioning and signal transduction pathways. To make up for these mechanisms the Langerhans's cells of pancreas secrete insulin from the finite source which eventually may completely empty. Thus, a condition which starts with GDM transits in a full blown diabetes and pregnant state has a potential of accelerating this **(Fig. 2)**. So a woman with GDM has a potential of going into overt diabetes during the index pregnancy or later on in life within the following 5 years or beyond.

Pregnancy is a Diabetogenic Condition: Why?

The placental hormones cause increased insulin inefficiency; additionally, kidney and placenta destroy insulin. Increased lipolysis is present to meet the maternal caloric needs while glucose is saved for the fetal metabolic needs. The fetus uses alanine and other amino acids preferentially and the mother is deprived of a major gluconeogenic source **(Fig. 3)**.

Fetal programming to maternal hyperglycemia: Maternal hyperglycemia is associated with large for gestational age (LGA) babies, macrosomia and fetal programming to obesity in future diabetes. Additionally, these babies also are at risk of still births due to reasons such as hypoglycemia, hypoxia, hypertension, cardiomyopathy, etc. Recurrent postprandial episodes of hyperglycemia cause episodic hyperinsulinemia leading to excessive nutrient storage. Glucose gets converted to fat and this needs energy and can consequently cause depletion of oxygen leading to FGR or intrauterine demise. The fetal hypoxia causes release of catecholamines leading to hypertension, cardiac remodeling, and hypertrophy. Stimulation of erythropoietin red cell hyperplasia in response to hypoxia causes increased hematocrit leading to polycythemia with consequent vascular sludging, poor perfusion and hyperbilirubinemia **(Fig. 4)**.

Thus, altered glucose metabolism leading to GDM is actually insulin insufficiency that becomes overpowering largely in the second half of the pregnancy but has a potential of getting into an overt diabetes. All these happens due to the mutually influencing factors and the resultant effects of diabetes on pregnancy and vice versa are enumerated in **Table 2**.

DIAGNOSIS OF GESTATIONAL DIABETES MELLITUS

Universal screening implies screening every pregnant mother for GDM and it is essential, as women of Asian origin are at a higher risk of developing GDM and subsequent

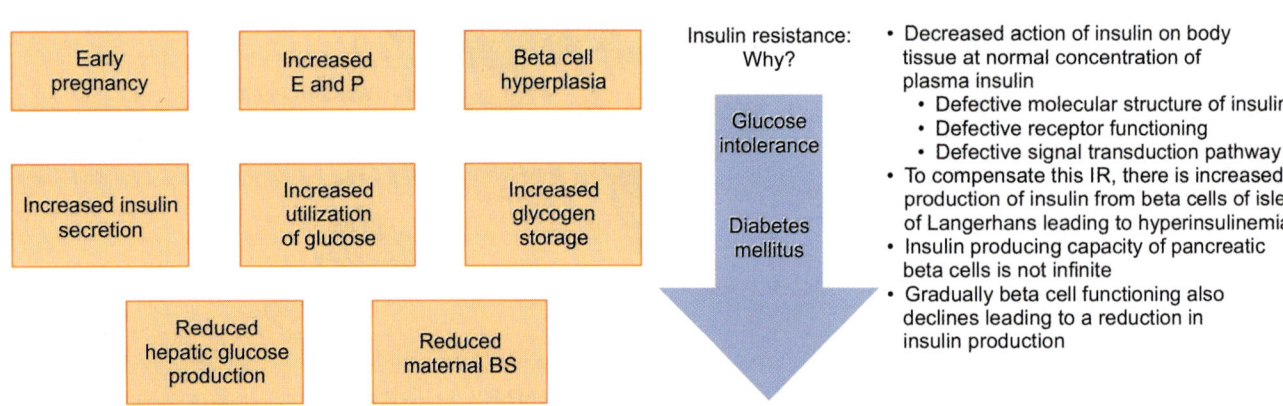

Fig. 2: Maternal and fetal glucose metabolism and insulin resistance.

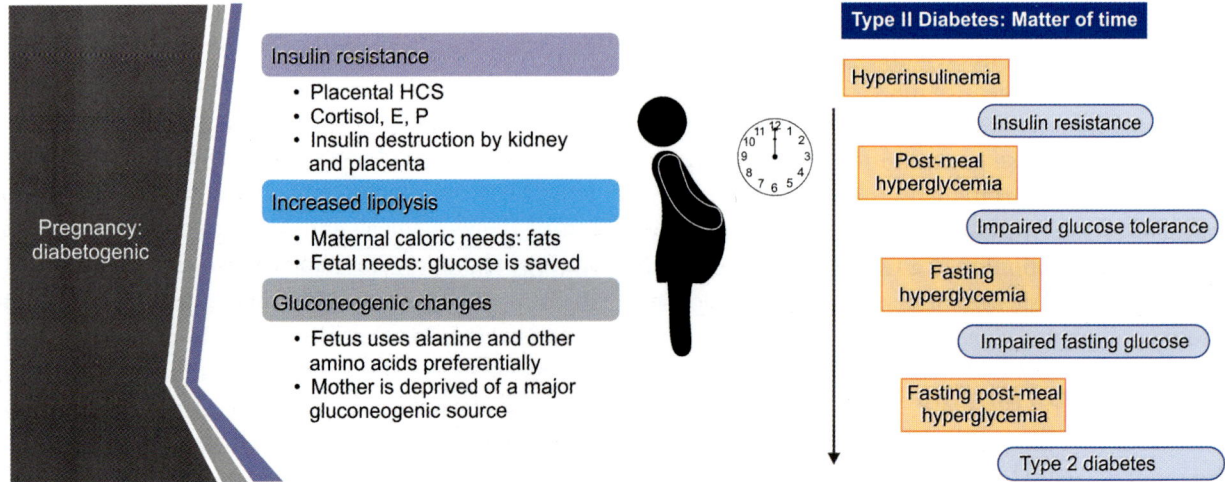

Fig. 3: The diabetogenic pregnancy and the timelines.

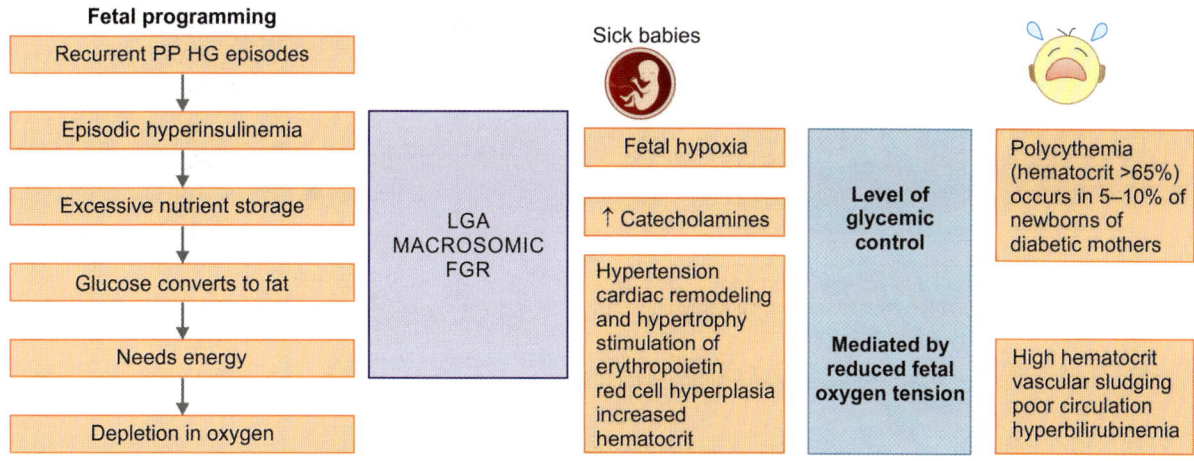

Fig. 4: Fetal programming to maternal hyperglycemia.

TABLE 2: Diabetes and pregnancy associated adverse outcomes.	
Effects of diabetes on pregnancy	*Effects of pregnancy on diabetes*
• First trimester or recurrent risk of miscarriages • Susceptibility to infections especially the genitourinary infections and chorioamnionitis and postpartum endometritis • Preeclampsia: Increased risk by 10–25% • Postpartum hemorrhage • Increased instrumentation or cesarean delivery possibilities due to macrosomia	• Increased requirement of insulin • Progression to diabetic retinopathy • Worsening of diabetic nephropathy • Increased morbidity and mortality • Increased cardiomyopathy

type 2 diabetes. Also universal screening for GDM detects more cases and improves maternal and neonatal prognosis. In order to standardize the diagnosis of GDM, the World Health Organization (WHO) recommends using a 2-hour 75 g oral glucose tolerance test (OGTT) with a threshold plasma glucose concentration of > 140 mg/dL at 2 hours, similar to that of IGT (>140 mg/dL and <199 mg/dL), outside pregnancy. Based on the WHO test a "Single-step procedure"(SSP) was developed due to the practical difficulty in performing glucose tolerance test in the fasting state, as seldom pregnant women visiting the antenatal clinic for the first time come in the fasting state and also it is unadvisable also. If they are asked to come on another day in the fasting state many of them do not return. Also the test has been validated as a screening as well as a diagnostic tool effectively in Indian pregnant mothers. It is preferable to perform the diagnostic test at the first visit itself.

Methodology (DIPSI Procedure)

In the antenatal clinic, a pregnant woman after undergoing preliminary clinical examination has to be given a 75 g oral anhydrous glucose load, irrespective of whether she is in the fasting or nonfasting state and without regard to the time of the last meal. A venous blood sample is collected at 2 hours for estimating plasma glucose by the GOD-POD method. GDM is diagnosed if 2-hour PG is ≥ 140 mg/dL (7.8 mmol/L).

Rationale: Performing this test procedure in the nonfasting state is rational, as glucose concentrations are unaffected by the time since the last meal in a normal glucose tolerant woman. On the other hand in a woman with gestational diabetes this definitely gets affected. After a meal, a normal glucose tolerant woman would be able to maintain euglycemia despite glucose challenge due to rapid and adequate insulin response, whereas, a woman with GDM who has impaired insulin secretion, her glycemic level increases with a meal and with glucose challenge, the glycemic excursion exaggerates further. This cascading effect is advantageous as this would not result in false-positive diagnosis of GDM. This single-step procedure has been approved by Ministry of Health, Government of India, DIPSI and also recommended by WHO.

Timing the tests: At the first visit ideally even if it is in the first trimester, testing will offer the chance of detecting unrecognized type 2 diabetes before pregnancy (pre-GDM). If the 2-hour PG is > 200 mg/dL in the early weeks of pregnancy, she may be a pre-GDM and HbA1C of ≥ 6.5 is confirmatory. Sometimes nausea of pregnancy may make performance of this test difficult in that case HbA1C can help to diagnose preexisting diabetes and prediabetic conditions. A pregnant woman found to have normal glucose tolerance (NGT), in the first trimester, should be tested for GDM again around 24–28th week and 32–34th week and if necessary at 36–38 weeks in presence of sudden weight gain, macrosomia or polyhydramnios or risk factors.

First trimester screening and establishment of a diabetic status or diabetogenic potential is essential. This is important as hyperglycemia has been identified as a potent teratogen **(Fig. 5)** and can cause abnormalities in the embryogenesis, organogenesis and placentation and mother's health can also be challenged if she is already a diabetic. Pregnant women with overt diabetes and suboptimal blood glucose control

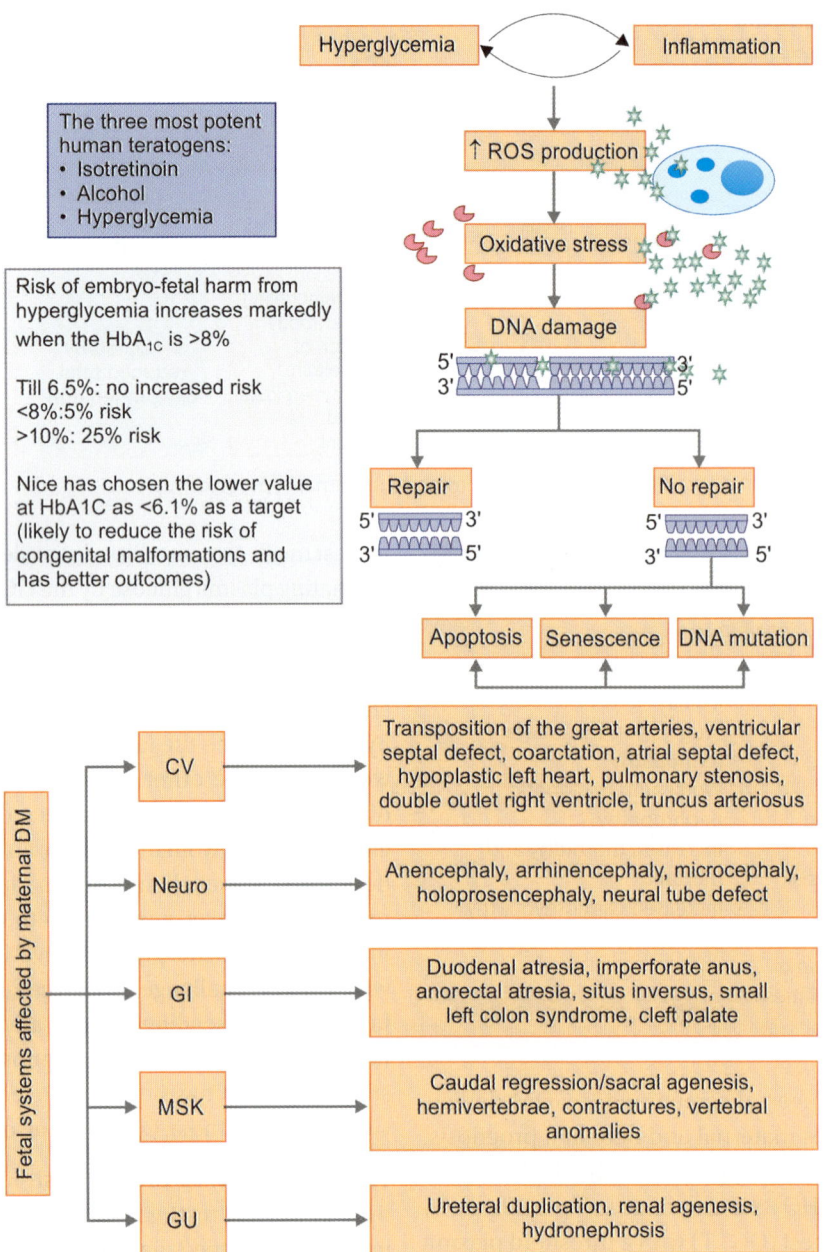

Fig. 5: Maternal and fetal risks due to teratogens.
(CV: cardiovascular; GI: gastrointestinal; GU: genitourinary; MSK: musculoskeletal)

in early pregnancy are at increased risk of having a fetus with congenital anomalies **(Fig. 5)** and are also at increased personal risk of worsening of diabetic retinopathy and nephropathy.

Early diagnosis of previously undiscovered overt diabetes in a pregnant woman helps in optimizing outcomes. Early effective screening for GDM can be achieved based on maternal characteristics and history.

MANAGEMENT OF GESTATIONAL DIABETES MELLITUS

Approach to GDM includes nutritional modification and structured physical activity as supportive measures but the mainstay is pharmacotherapy either with insulin or oral antihyperglycemic agents.

Strict control of sugars, throughout pregnancy, is imperative to decrease the incidence of ketoacidosis in mother, congenital anomalies and macrosomia in the fetus, and neonatal morbidity. A Cochrane review of four studies involving 612 women with GDM treated with primary dietary therapy or no specific treatment found no differences in birthweight greater than 4,000 g (OR 0.78, 95% CI 0.45–1.35) or cesarean deliveries (OR 0.97, 95% CI 0.65–1.44) suggesting that macrosomia cannot be prevented by dietary therapy alone. This is possibly due the fetal programming for macrosomia being around 16 weeks during which time such a dietary modification may not have been practiced. There is insufficient evidence to support the use of myoinositol supplementation for treatment of GDM but it seems to have promise in reducing the dosages of metformin, occurrence of overt diabetes and need of insulin therapy. When medical nutritional therapy (MNT) fails to achieve sugar control one has to start pharmacologic therapy.

Medical Nutritional Therapy

Medical nutrition therapy should be offered to all women with GDM. The meal pattern should provide adequate calories [sourced form complex carbohydrates (low glycemic index), proteins and healthy fats in moderations], and nutrients (sourced from soluble and nonsoluble fibers) to meet the needs of pregnancy. The expected weight gain during pregnancy is 300–400 g per week and total weight gain is 10–12 kg by term. After 2 weeks of initial treatment with MNT if the targeted control of FPG ~90 mg/dL and/or postmeal glucose ~120 mg/dL, is not achieved then insulin may be initiated.

Antenatal Exercises

Physical activity such as walking and stretching exercises have been identified to reduce the insulin resistance and are to be advised in a structured manner and are mentioned in the GOI guidelines on GDM.

Maternal Surveillance in GDM

Regular antenatal care with meticulous weight, blood pressure and hyperglycemia surveillance should be undertaken. Regular check for genitourinary infections through history and /or clinical examination can be done. Along with normal laboratory tests, glycosylated hemoglobin, blood urea, serum creatinine, thyroid-stimulating hormone, spot urine protein-to-creatinine ratio can be undertaken. Daily self-sugar surveillance can be individualized. In a mother with preexisting DM, cardiac health evaluation, fundoscopy can be undertaken.

Fetal Surveillance in GDM

Antenatal Pharmacologic Therapy

Optimum threshold for initiating pharmacologic therapy has not been established, usually any of the following ACOG and ADA and ACOG recommended cut offs are considered:
- Fasting blood glucose concentration >95 mg/dL (5.3 mmol/L)
- 1-hour postprandial blood glucose concentration >140 mg/dL (7.8 mmol/L)
- 2-hour postprandial glucose concentration >120 mg/dL (6.7 mmol/L)
- Some still use old criteria of fasting >105 mg/dL and any value >200 mg/dL.

There are two pharmacologic options in pregnant patients:
1. Insulin
2. Selected oral antidiabetic agents

Conventionally, insulin therapy has been the mainstay of management because of its efficacy in achieving strict sugar control and it does not cross the placenta. But it is an invasive and expensive treatment hence patient compliance is poor. Since GDM and type 2 diabetes are characterized by insulin resistance and relatively decreased insulin secretion, it is only logical to use insulin sensitizers. Moreover, they are oral and inexpensive. Off late, more and more obstetricians are preferring oral antidiabetic agents as their first choice. As per 2013 ACOG guidelines insulin and oral antidiabetic agents are equal in efficacy and either can be used as first-line therapy.

Metformin Therapy

Metformin in doses of 500 mg once or twice a day may be enough in mild elevations of sugar, especially in lean or moderately overweight women developing GDM late in pregnancy. Metformin may especially be used in women who had used it before conception as a part of infertility treatment. The advantages of metformin are:
- Evidence suggests that it prevents abortion in post PCOS pregnancies, if continued in first trimester
- It is used in the prepregnancy control of sugars
- Placental crossing is minimal
- It does not cause severe hypoglycemia
- It does not stimulate the fetal pancreas
- Lesser incidence of macrosomia
- Minimal secretion in breast milk.

Metformin does not have serious adverse side effects except for mild gastrointestinal discomfort. However, it has limited long-term follow-up information. Hospitalization is not necessary and monitoring can be done on outpatient basis.

Insulin Therapy

Premix insulin 30/70 of any brand is preferred with a starting dose: 4 units before breakfast. Every 4th day increase 2 units till 10 units. If FPG remains >90 mg/dL advise 6 units before breakfast and 4 units before dinner. Review with blood sugar test and adjust dose further. Total daily insulin dose can be divided as two-thirds in the morning and one-third in the evening. Initially if post-breakfast plasma glucose is high then start Premix 50/50. If GDM is diagnosed in the third trimester; MNT is advised for a week. Insulin is initiated if MNT fails. If 2-hour PG > 200 mg/dL at diagnosis, a starting dose of 8 units of premixed insulin could be administered straightaway before breakfast and the dose has to be titrated on follow-up. Along with insulin therapy, MNT is also advised. The target for glycemic control is maintaining a mean plasma glucose (MPG) level ~105–110 mg/ dL. This is possible if FPG and 2-hour postprandial peaks are ~90 mg/dL and ~120 mg/dL, respectively, and ensures good fetal outcome.

One-third of women using metformin may need supplemental insulin to achieve glycemic targets. Hospitalization is better to titrate the dosage and teach the technique of insulin injections and self-monitoring of blood glucose.

Strict glucose monitoring is important once the insulin is started. It has been shown that postprandial monitoring was associated with better glycemic control, lower incidence of macrosomia and lower cesarean rates as compared to preprandial monitoring.

There is no fixed dose or ideal regimen of insulin therapy. There are several methods and each center may have their own. Moreover, dose of insulin varies in different individuals based on presence of obesity, degree of hyperglycemia, and other demographic criteria.

General consensus is that the total insulin dose ranges from 0.7 to 2 units per kg (present pregnant weight) through the different trimesters to achieve glucose control. The dose and type of insulin used is calculated based upon the specific abnormality of blood glucose noted during monitoring.

Glyburide Therapy

Glyburide has been used commonly for the treatment of GDM. As with insulin therapy, glyburide must be carefully balanced with meals and snacks to prevent maternal hypoglycemia. Starting doses of 2.5–5 mg once daily are commonly used, and the dose is increased as needed to a maximum of 20 mg/day. Twice daily dosing is often necessary to maintain euglycemia. When glyburide was compared with metformin in a 2017 systematic review, there were no statistical differences in important outcomes such as perinatal mortality, macrosomia, or neonatal hypoglycemia.

Tolbutamide and Chlorpropamide

Tolbutamide or chlorpropamide (older sulfonylureas) therapy is not recommended in women with GDM because these drugs cross the placenta and can cause fetal hyperinsulinemia, which can lead to macrosomia and prolonged neonatal hypoglycemia.

Other

Acarbose, an alpha glucosidase inhibitor, acts in the gastrointestinal tract. Since a small proportion of this drug may be absorbed systemically, potential transplacental passage and fetal effects should be studied.

Use of thiazolidinediones, meglitinides (repaglinide and nateglinide), DPP-4 inhibitors, amylin mimetics, and GLP-1 inhibitors during pregnancy is considered experimental.

Other supportive measures: Correction of anemia, screening for preeclampsia and UTI regularly. Screening for dyslipidemia and renal function with serum creatinine in overt diabetes should be done. Regular exercise regimen and self-glucose monitoring with counseling about complications need to be done.

Fetal Surveillance

Fetal surveillance should include every trimester biometry, 22 weeks uterine artery Doppler for prediction of preeclampsia and NST weekly 34 weeks onwards can be undertaken.

Delivery before full term is not indicated unless there is evidence of macrosomia, polyhydramnios, poor metabolic control or other obstetric indications (e.g., preeclampsia or intrauterine growth retardation). A few obstetricians prefer to deliver around 38 gestational weeks to avoid stillbirth.

Delivery: During labor, it is essential to maintain good glycemic control, while avoiding hypoglycemia. Lower insulin requirements are common during labor (often no insulin is necessary). Maternal blood glucose level should be monitored after delivery, 24 hours postpartum and if found to be high, checked again on follow-up. Cesarean delivery is considered for obstetric indication. A neonatologist's presence at the time of delivery is ideal.

Prepartum and Intrapartum Management

Insulin management on the day of planned cesarean section or induction of labor:
- Skip morning dose of insulin
- Perform blood glucose levels and urine ketones for every 4 hour
- 5% dextrose is infused with neutralizing dose (6–8 units of actrapid) of insulin
- Add one additional unit to the drip for every rise of 10 mg/dL after 180 mg/dL
- Inject 10 U SC if urine ketones are present.

If the patient comes in labor after taking morning dose of insulin, then the regular schedule is suspended from that point and aforementioned regimen is followed.

Postnatal Management

One must keep in mind that insulin requirement comes down drastically after the delivery. Good practice would be to perform sugar profile after 24–48 hours and titrate the insulin accordingly.

Insulin-diabetic Ketoacidosis

- Insulin infusion of 40 U in 40 mL of normal saline
- Rate decided by blood glues levels done for every 2 hours
- Hydration with 0.9% NS through a parallel line
- Serum potassium, urine ketones and arterial blood gas (ABG) are done at every 4 hour.

Contraception: IUCD or barriers are recommended. Oral contraceptive pills especially progesterone only pills and injectable progesterone are avoided as they interfere with carbohydrate metabolism and may increase sugar levels. Either copper IUCD or conventional methods may be used.

Long-term follow-up: Gestational diabetic women require follow-up. An OGTT with 75 g oral glucose, using WHO criteria for the nonpregnant population should be performed at 6–8 weeks postpartum. If found normal, glucose tolerance test is repeated after 6 months and every year to determine whether the glucose tolerance has returned to normal or progressed. A considerable proportion of gestational diabetic women may continue to have glucose intolerance. It is important that women with GDM be counseled with regard to their increased risk of developing overt diabetes and possible cardiovascular disorders. Life style changes and regular surveillance lifelong are recommended.

CONCLUSION

Hyperglycemia has important implications for the mother and fetus. The screening for gestational diabetes should be universally instituted in our country. Simple and feasible tests such as the WHO 75 gram 2 hour test or DIPSI test should be used. The early management of blood sugar levels gives an opportunity to reduce maternal and perinatal complications. Blood sugar control may be achieved by nutritional therapy, oral hypoglycemic agents or insulin. Fetal surveillance should be started at 32–34 weeks of pregnancy and the timing and route of delivery should be optimized. Women who develop gestational diabetes will require long-term follow-up to detect the onset of type 2 diabetes in later life.

REFERENCES

1. Yogev Y, Ben-Haroush A, Hod M. Pathogenesis of gestational diabetes mellitus. In: Hod M, Jovanovic L, Di Renzo GC, de Leiva A, Langer O (Eds). Textbook of Diabetes and Pregnancy, 1st edition. London: Martin Dunitz, Taylor and Francis Group PLC; 2003. pp. 46.
2. American Diabetes Association. Standards of medical care in diabetes–2017. Diabetes Care. 2017;40:S1-135.
3. Mithal A, Bansal B, Kalra S. Gestational diabetes in India: science and society. Indian J Endocrinol Metab. 2015;19:701-4.
4. Plows JF, Stanley JL, Baker PN, Reynolds CM, Vickers MH. The pathophysiology of gestational diabetes mellitus. Int J Mol Sci. 2018;19(11):3342.
5. Savitz DA, Janevic TM, Engel SM, Kaufman JS, Herring AH. Ethnicity and gestational diabetes in New York City, 1995-2003. BJOG. 2008;115:969-78.
6. Chu SY, Abe K, Hall LR, Kim SY, Njoroge T, Qin C. Gestational diabetes mellitus: all Asians are not alike. Prev Med. 2009;49:265-8.
7. Kayal A, Mohan V, Malanda B, Anjana RM, Bhavadharini B, Mahalakshmi MM, et al. Women in India with Gestational Diabetes Mellitus Strategy (WINGS): Methodology and development of model of care for gestational diabetes mellitus (WINGS 4). Indian J Endocrinol Metab. 2016;20(5):707-15.
8. Raja MW, Baba TA, Hanga AJ, Bilquees S, Rasheed, Haq IU, et al. A study to estimate the prevalence of gestational diabetes mellitus in an urban block of Kashmir valley (North India). Int J Med Sci Public Health. 2014;3:191-5.
9. Bhatt AA, Dhore PB, Purandare VB, Sayyad MG, Mandal MK, Unnikrishnan AG. Gestational diabetes mellitus in rural population of Western India-Results of a community survey. Indian J Endocrinol Metab. 2015;19:507-10.
10. Swami SR, Mehetre R, Shivane V, Bandgar TR, Menon PS, Shah NS. Prevalence of carbohydrate intolerance of varying degrees in pregnant females in western India (Maharashtra) – a hospital-based study. J Indian Med Assoc. 2008;106:712-4, 735.
11. Seshiah V, Balaji V, Balaji MS, Sanjeevi CB, Green A. Gestational diabetes mellitus in India. J Assoc Physicians India. 2004;52:707-11.

LONG QUESTIONS

1. Describe carbohydrate metabolism in pregnancy. Add a note on GDM screening and diagnosis. What are its complications?
2. Define pregestational diabetes. Write a note on maternal and fetal impacts of pregestational diabetes.
3. Describe the management of diabetes mellitus during pregnancy.

SHORT QUESTIONS

1. What is deranged gestational glucose tolerance?
2. Why pregnancy is a diabetogenic condition?
3. What is the DIPSI procedure?
4. What is medical nutritional therapy (MNT) for gestational diabetes?
5. What is the ideal postnatal management for a woman who had been diagnosed with GDM?

MULTIPLE CHOICE QUESTIONS

1. The best time for GDM screening is at:
   a. 14 weeks of gestation
   b. 18 weeks of gestation
   c. 22 weeks of gestation
   d. 28 weeks of gestation
   e. 32 weeks of gestation
2. Endocrinopathies associated with diabetes:
   a. Cushing Syndrome
   b. Pheochromocytoma
   c. Hypothyroidism
   d. a + b
   e. a + b + c
3. What are the cut-off values in 2-hour oral glucose tolerance test for fasting and at 1 hour and 2 hours after meals respectively?
   a. 92, 182, 155
   b. 92, 180, 153
   c. 95, 180, 155
   d. 92,180, 155
4. Complications of diabetes in pregnancy include all, except:
   a. Macrosomia
   b. Shoulder dystocia
   c. Hyperglycemia in new-born
   d. Hypocalcemia
5. Most sensitive screening test in diabetic mothers for congenital malformation is:
   a. AFP
   b. Blood glucose
   c. Amniotic fluid AFP
   d. HbA1C
   e. Urine glucose
6. In a known diabetic fundoscopy is recommended at:
   a. When visual symptoms appear
   b. At 1st antenatal visit
   c. At 28 weeks
   d. 34 weeks
   e. Not done

Answers
1. a 2. e 3. c 4. c 5. d 6. a

6.4 THE SURGICAL ABDOMEN IN PREGNANCY

Shashank Parulekar

◼ INTRODUCTION

"Surgical abdomen" is a clinical term that means a condition that is of a short duration, painful, and for which an urgent surgical intervention would be required.[1] Surgical disorders can affect a pregnant woman just like they affect a nonpregnant woman. The differential diagnosis of an acute abdomen is sometimes quite difficult in nonpregnant state, because there are a number of organs in the abdomen, a number of structures in the retroperitoneum, and the number of conditions affecting them is truly large. In a pregnant woman, there are the added difficulties of occurrence of acute conditions of obstetric origin, and the alteration in anatomy and function due to pregnancy. The Pandora's box becomes much more complex due to pregnancy. A management of an acute abdomen of surgical origin is based on a correct diagnosis, which needs to be reached early so as to reduce morbidity and mortality.[2] It is more important in pregnancy because there is the fetus whose well-being also needs to be taken into consideration.

An acute abdominal pain lasts for a few hours to a few days. A chronic abdominal pain lasts for a few months to a few years. The duration of a subacute pain is between that of an acute and chronic pain.[3] A patient with a subacute or chronic pain may present with an acute exacerbation of the condition. Acute abdominal pain is the cause for 5–10% of all visits of women of reproductive age to the emergency room of a hospital. It is also one of the most common conditions necessitating hospital admission.

◼ ETIOLOGY

The causes of an acute abdomen in pregnancy can be obstetric, gynecological or other, as discussed here.[3,4] Medical causes have been listed as well, because they need to be ruled out in differential diagnosis of the acute abdomen.[5]

Obstetric Causes

- First half of pregnancy:
  - Abortion
  - Ectopic pregnancy
- Second half of pregnancy:
  - Abortion
  - Placental abruption
  - Preeclampsia and its complications.
  - HELLP syndrome
  - Uterine rupture
  - Stretching of the round ligament(s)
  - Acute fatty liver
  - Torsion of uterus
  - Intraperitoneal hemorrhage from a placenta percreta.

Gynaecological Causes

- Acute pelvic infection
- Torsion of an ovarian cyst or tumor
- Bleeding into an ovarian cyst
- *Acute degeneration of a leiomyoma:* Cystic, red
- Torsion of normal adnexa
- Rupture of an endometriosis
- Torsion of subserous pedunculated leiomyoma
- Rupture of a corpus luteum hematoma.

Surgical Causes

Various surgical causes of acute abdomen in pregnancy are as follows:[3,6-9]

- Acute appendicitis
- *Perforated ulcer:* Gastric, duodenal
- Bowel obstruction
- Perforative peritonitis
- Cholelithiasis
- Cholecystitis
- Acute pancreatitis
- Hepatic rupture
- Rupture of a visceral artery aneurysm
- Dissecting aneurysm of abdominal aorta
- Inflammatory bowel disease
- Diverticulitis
- Rectus sheath hematoma
- Adrenal hemorrhage
- Nephrolithiasis
- Mesenteric venous thrombosis
- Abdominal wall hernia
- Spontaneous rupture of the urinary tract.

Medical Causes

These conditions do not require surgical treatment. Hence, making their diagnosis is important when evaluating the cause an acute abdomen.[6,7,10]

- Gastrointestinal:
  - Gastroenteritis
  - Acute hepatitis
  - Constipation
- Endocrine and metabolic disorders:[6]
  - Diabetic crisis
  - Uremia
  - Addisonian crisis
  - Acute hyperlipoproteinemia
  - Acute intermittent porphyria
- Infections and inflammatory conditions:[6]
  - Abdominal malaria
  - Dengue

- Herpes zoster
- Tabes dorsalis
- Henoch-Schönlein purpura
- Acute rheumatic fever
- Polyarteritis nodosa
- Systemic lupus erythematosus
- Hematologic disorders:
  - Sickle cell abdominal crisis
  - Acute leukemia
- Thoracic referred pain:
  - Myocardial infarction
  - Pulmonary embolus
  - Pneumonia
  - Pleurisy
  - Acute pericarditis
  - Pneumothorax
- Miscellaneous:
  - Lead poisoning
  - Other heavy metal poisoning
  - Hereditary angioedema
  - Narcotic withdrawal.

■ CLINICAL EVALUATION

Differential diagnosis of causes of acute abdomen in pregnancy is difficult, because it is anyway difficult even in the nonpregnant state, and there are additional causes to be considered related to pregnancy. It is made more difficult by the presence of a large uterus, which may mask some signs and alter the presentation of others.[11] It is important to reach a diagnosis early and accurately, because urgent management is important in some cases to save the life of the gravida and the fetus and reduce their morbidity too.

Standard method of history taking and examination is followed. Points of importance are as follows:

History

Details of pain such as site, radiation, severity, quality, chronology, aggravating and relieving factors must be taken. The site of abdominal pain often indicates the underlying cause, as shown in **Figure 1**.

Sometimes the pain radiates from the site of origin or is felt at a distant site, which suggests the underlying cause.[3,12] A loin to groin pain is seen with ureteric colic. Pain of pancreatitis is experienced in the back. Pain in the left shoulder may be due to conditions affecting the caudal pancreas, spleen, heart, or left hemidiaphragm. Pain in the right shoulder may be due to conditions affecting the liver, bile duct, or right hemidiaphragm. Hepatobiliary pain sometimes radiates from the right hypochondrium to the back.

The quality of the pain changes depending on the cause.[3,12] Burning or gnawing pain is seen in gastroesophageal reflux disease and peptic ulcer disease. Colicky pain is due to gastroenteritis, intestinal obstruction, cholelithiasis and ureteric colic. Intermittent, crescendo-decrescendo pain is typical of labor pain. A sharp and continuous pain is due to inflammation of the parietal peritoneum. Agonizing and continuous pain is due to ischemia of bowel. Throbbing pain is due to an abscess, as with appendiceal abscess or hepatic amebic abscess. Burning or boring pain is suggestive of peptic ulcer or acute pancreatitis. Pain of sudden onset is due to perforation of peptic ulcer or biliary tract. Central abdominal colicky pain followed by sharp and continuous pain in the right iliac fossa, followed by agonizing and continuous pain is indicative of gangrene of the appendix.

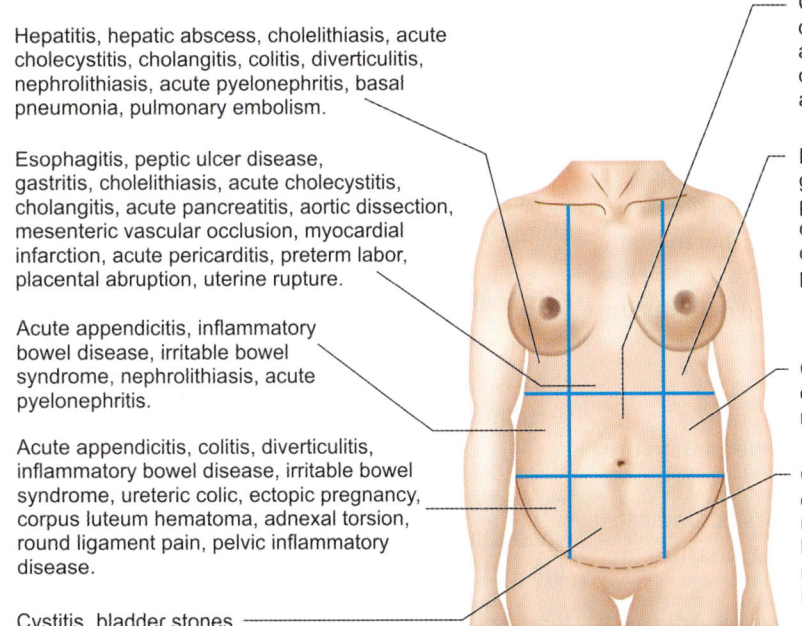

Fig. 1: Causes of acute abdominal pain, based on the site of the pain.

The precipitating, aggravating, and relieving factors also help differentiate the causes of acute pain in abdomen in pregnancy.[3,12] The pain due to gastritis and gastric ulcer starts after food and is relieved a few hours after eating. The pain of duodenal ulcer starts several hours after eating and is relieved by food. Pain due to mesenteric ischemia starts in 1 hour of eating. Pain due to acute pancreatitis is relieved by sitting up and leaning forward. Pain due to peritonitis is aggravated by movements.

Some symptoms associated with the pain help pinpoint the cause with reasonable certainty.[7,12] Nausea, vomiting, diarrhea, constipation, alternating diarrhea and constipation, rectal bleeding, melena are due to conditions affecting the gastrointestinal system. Jaundice, nausea, vomiting, high color of urine and clay colored stool are due to conditions affecting the hepatobiliary system. Dysuria, frequency, urgency, hematuria, and retention of urine suggest the presence of conditions affecting the genitourinary system. The presence of fever is most often due to infection. This may be due to perforation of a typhoid ulcer or tuberculous ulcer of the intestine, abdominal malaria, dengue, acute pyelonephritis or basal pneumonia.

If the woman has a single episode of vomiting at the beginning, it may be due to most of the causes of an acute abdomen. But if vomiting started before the abdominal pain, it is mostly due to obstruction of the bowel.[7,12] Frequent and profuse vomiting is due to small bowel obstruction. It is infrequent with colonic obstruction. Severe persistent vomiting is indicative of small bowel obstruction or acute pancreatitis. Vomiting at the height of a pain is associated with intestinal or renal colic. A combination of vomiting with fever and acidosis is due to diabetes mellitus. The content of the vomited material also helps in making a diagnosis.[7,12] Stomach contents and bile are seen with acute gastritis. Greenish jejunal content is seen with colic. Feculent matter is seen with late stages of small bowel obstruction. Frequent retching with little vomitus is suggestive of torsion of a viscus.

The past history may be very important in suggesting the likely diagnosis. Past abdominopelvic surgery, tuberculosis, peritonitis or endometriosis may suggest the presence of intraperitoneal adhesions, causing intestinal obstruction.[12] A history of gallstones or urinary stones indicates that the pain is due to the stones or their complications. A case of sickle cell disease may present with acute abdominal pain due to sickle cell crisis.

Examination

A general examination is done, with special attention to the following.

A poor general condition and unstable vital signs indicate a need for emergency measures, including possibly an exploratory laparotomy.

Severe degree of pallor, associated with tachycardia and hypotension, is due to a severe hemorrhage. Intraperitoneal hemorrhage may be due to injury to a viscus such as liver or spleen, or a vascular accident such as dissection of abdominal aorta or rupture of an aneurysm of a vessel. It must be kept in mind that some degree of anemia is almost universal in pregnancy, and tachycardia is seen as a physiological change of pregnancy. Presence of fever is indicative of an underlying infection. A shallow, occasionally grunting respiration is seen in peritonitis. Rapid and shallow respiration is characteristic of shock. Localized splinting of abdominal respiratory movements is seen when there is an inflammation under that part of the abdominal wall. Respiratory rate almost twice the normal rate is seen with pneumonia. If the patient is in shock, it may be hemorrhagic or septic. Septic shock may be seen as a complication of peritonitis, acute pyelonephritis and septicemia.

The patient's face is said to be gray in cases of perforation of peptic ulcer, acute pancreatitis, and strangulation of bowel. It is deathly pale with massive intraperitoneal hemorrhage. The eyes are sunken and mouth dry with dehydration.

The patient's attitude in bed is important.[12] A patient with severe colic or hemorrhage is restless in bed. She is constantly moving about with ureteral colic. She is straight at one moment and doubled up next in case of intestinal or biliary colic. She lies still in case of perforated gastric ulcer and peritonitis, as movement aggravates her pain. Her right hip and knee are flexed in case of appendiceal or right psoas abscess. The left hip and knee are flexed in case of left psoas abscess.

Abdominal tenderness indicates an acute inflammation of the underlying structure. The site of tenderness indicates possible diagnosis, as shown in **Table 1**.

Tenderness is never encountered in a normal pregnancy without a surgical cause.[10] Guarding and rigidity indicate widespread intraperitoneal inflammation such as peritonitis. Rebound tenderness is also looked for. It is seen in case of peritonitis. But its value is considered to be less in modern times.

An abdominal lump is felt in case of an appendiceal lump, pyonephrosis, and amebic liver abscess. A pulsatile abdominal lump is due to aortic dissection.

A rectal examination may show blood or mucus on the examining finger. Pelvic tenderness can also be appreciated.[13]

Clinical Tests

Cough pain test: The patient is asked to cough and asked to show where maximal pain is experienced. It is positive in peritonitis, but not in case of colic.[12]

Murphy's sign: The patient is asked to take a deep breath. Her inspiration is arrested abruptly by pain in acute cholecystitis, when the gallbladder fundus touches the examining fingers due to the descent of the diaphragm and liver.[14]

Iliopsoas test: The patient is made to lie down, turned to the side opposite to the side of pain. The thigh on the affected side

TABLE 1: Site of tenderness.

Site of tenderness	Possible diagnosis
Epigastrium	Gastritis, peptic ulcer disease
Right hypochondrium	Hepatitis, hepatic abscess, acute cholecystitis
Right costal border anteriorly	Cholecystitis
McBurney's point	Appendicitis in early pregnancy
Uterus	Acute degeneration of a leiomyoma, placental abruption, threatened rupture of uterus
Lateral vaginal fornix	Ectopic pregnancy, corpus luteum hematoma, adnexal torsion, pelvic inflammatory disease
Posterior fornix	Pelvic abscess, pelvic inflammatory disease
Anterior fornix	Cystitis
Hypogastrium	Cystitis, abortion, threatened rupture of scar of previous cesarean section
Right iliac fossa	Appendicitis, typhlitis, ectopic pregnancy
Left iliac fossa	Colitis, ectopic pregnancy
Rebound tenderness	Peritonitis
All over abdomen	Peritonitis
Costovertebral angle	Acute pyelonephritis

is extended to the fullest extent. If that causes pain, the test is positive. It is positive in cases of iliac abscess, pyomyositis of iliacus, and appendiceal abscess on the right side.[15] It is done only if the patient is moderately sick and does not have generalized peritonitis.

Obturator test: The patient is made to lie down in supine position and her flexed thigh of the affected side is rotated internally. If it causes pain, the test is positive, as seen in cases of pus or hematocele in contact with the obturator internus.[16]

Fist percussion test: Gentle percussion is done with a closed fist over the lower chest wall. It is said to be positive if it causes pain. It is positive on the right side in case of a lesion of the liver or diaphragm, and on the left side with a lesion of the spleen, stomach or diaphragm.[12]

Carnett's sign: The patient is made to lie down in supine position. The point of maximal tenderness on the abdominal wall is identified. Then the patient is asked to raise her head and extend lower limbs. The test is said to be positive if the pain increases, as in case of abdominal wall pain caused by intercostal neuralgia, nerve entrapment syndrome, herniation of thoracic intervertebral disc, hernias, myofascial pain, rectus sheath hematoma, and costoiliac impingement syndrome. The test is said to be negative, if the pain decreases on tensing the abdominal wall, as with intra-abdominal painful conditions.[17]

Lateral position test: The patient is made to lie down in supine position and the point of tenderness is determined. She is asked to turn on her side opposite to the side of pain, while the examining hand is kept at the site of tenderness. If there is tenderness at that site while the uterus has moved away from the palpating hand, the tenderness is over a structure outside the uterus. But if the tenderness has moved along with the uterus, it is due to a painful lesion of the uterus, like a red degeneration off a leiomyoma.[3]

Auscultation

Peristaltic sounds are reduced or absent in peritonitis and ileus. Loud rushes are heard in gastroenteritis. A rub is heard over the spleen in a case of splenic infarct. A rush of high pitched tinkling coinciding with worsening of pain is characteristic of bowel obstruction. Crackles and bronchial breath sounds are heard over the chest in pneumonia.

DIFFICULTIES IN DIAGNOSIS DUE TO PREGNANCY

The diagnosis of the cause of an acute abdominal pain is made difficult in pregnancy by a number of factors.[18]

1. Nausea and vomiting of pregnancy may mask vomiting due to bowel obstruction.
2. The point of tenderness may be shifted by the gravid uterus, if it pushes the inflamed structure away from its normal position. This is seen in acute appendicitis, when the appendix gets gradually pushed upward toward the liver as the pregnancy advances. The point of tenderness shifts upward accordingly.
3. Diagnosis of free fluid in the peritoneal cavity like blood or ascites is more difficult to identify because the abdomen is filled significantly by the gravid uterus in the second half of pregnancy.
4. Palpation of abdominal masses is difficult due to space occupied by the gravid uterus.
5. Presence of the gravid uterus makes palpation of intra-abdominal structures difficult.
6. Accumulation of fat in the abdominal wall makes palpation of intra-abdominal structures difficult.

A comparison of different features of common and important causes of an acute abdomen is given in **Table 2**.

INVESTIGATIONS

Specific investigations are done to confirm specific diagnosis **(Table 3)**.

White blood cell count increases to a 10,000–14,000/mm^3 during pregnancy,[18] It may increase to 20,000–30,000/mm^3 in labor.[19] Thus it cannot be used very reliably to diagnose an infection in pregnancy. But appearance of band forms definitely indicates an infective process.

Imaging Studies

- Ultrasonography is the first diagnostic imaging modality for evaluation of an acute abdomen in pregnancy.[20] It easily

TABLE 2: Comparison of common causes of acute abdomen.

Pain	Perforated peptic ulcer	Appendicitis	Cholecystitis	Pancreatitis	Bowel obstruction	Diverticulitis	Mesenteric vascular obstruction	Gastroenteritis	Rupture of aortic aneurysm
Onset	Sudden	Gradual	Sudden	Sudden	Gradual	Gradual	Sudden	Gradual	Sudden
Site	Epigastrium	Periumbilical, later RLQ	RUQ	Epigastrium, back	Periumbilical	LLQ	Periumbilical	Periumbilical	Abdomen, back, side
Radiation	Nil	Nil	Scapula	Back	Nil	Nil	Nil	Nil	Nil
Nature	Initially localized, diffuse later	Initially diffuse, localized later	Localized	Localized	Diffuse	Localized	Diffuse	Diffuse	Diffuse
Quality	Burning	Ache	Gripping	Ache	Cramp	Ache	Sharp	Spasm	Sharp
Severity	+++	++	++	++/+++	++	++	+++	+/++	+++

(RLQ: right lower quadrant, RUQ: right upper quadrant; LLQ: left lower quadrant)

available in most places, economical, and noninvasive. It is useful in evaluating upper abdominal pain (other than ulcer pain or bowel obstruction) and abdominal masses. Its diagnostic sensitivity is 80% for acute appendicitis. Color Doppler study helps diagnose avascular cysts, torsion of adnexal masses and inflective masses. When it does not yield the information required, magnetic resonance imaging (MRI) without using gadolinium and computerized tomography (CT) (as a last resort, since it causes maternal and fetal irradiation) can be used.

- *Plain chest radiograph:* It is done if one suspects lower lobe pneumonia or pleural effusion due to subphrenic inflammatory lesions.[21,22]
- *Plain abdominal radiograph:* It may be done in pregnancy only if absolutely required. Usually the diagnosis of perforative peritonitis and intestinal obstruction, for which this test is usually done, can be made by other means.[21,22]
- *CT scan:* It is useful to detect small quantity of free gas under the diaphragm, site of inflammation, and masses. It helps decide which cases require a laparotomy (e.g., perforative peritonitis) and which do not (e.g., diverticulitis and pancreatitis). It should not be done indiscriminately, but can be done in pregnancy when required. The threshold dose for abortion at preimplantation stage is more than 10 rads, for causing organ malformation is more than 5 rads, and for causing growth retardation or mental impairment is more than 10 rads.[21,22] Fetal dose with an abdominal CT scan is 2.6 rads. Thus it appears to be safe.
- *Therapeutic endoscopic retrograde cholangiopancreatography:* It has been reported to be safe in pregnancy, provided additional intraprocedure safety measures are taken.
- *Radionuclide scans:* Hepatobiliary iminodiacetic acid (HIDA) scans, liver-spleen scans and gallium scans are not required in pregnancy, as a CT scan is usually adequate and safer.

Endoscopy

Proctosigmoidoscopy may be done when large bowel obstruction is suspected or there is gross blood in stools. Colonoscopy helps reduce a sigmoid volvulus and may also locate the site of bleeding from lower gastrointestinal tract. Laparoscopy is better avoided in the second half of pregnancy.

Abdominal Paracentesis

It is done under ultrasonic scan. If the aspirate is blood, bile, or bowel contents, an urgent laparotomy is warranted.

MANAGEMENT

Indications for an urgent exploratory laparotomy are as follows:
- Clinical:
  - Increasing or severe localized tenderness
  - Guarding or rigidity
  - Progressive or tense distention of abdomen
  - Septicemia
  - Failure of conservative treatment
  - Tender abdominal or pelvic mass
  - Shock
- Investigational:
  - Pneumoperitoneum on imaging
  - Mesenteric occlusion
  - Blood, pus, bowel contents, bile or urine on abdominal paracentesis.

Management of all the conditions that present as an acute abdomen is beyond the scope of this article. Interested readers are referred to textbooks of surgery and scientific articles. It should be borne in mind that though surgical treatment takes priority in the management of these patients, the well-being of the mother and the fetus should be kept in mind. Thus hypoxia should be avoided during anesthesia and surgery,

SECTION 6: Maternal Complications Arising in Pregnancy   433

TABLE 3: Interpretation of investigations.

Test	Importance
Hemogram	• Low hemoglobin with intraperitoneal hemorrhage • Leukocytosis with infection, bowel ischemia, perforated peptic ulcer • For fitness for anesthesia and surgery
Urinalysis	• Urinary tract infections • Hepatic dysfunction • Urinary calculi • Diabetes mellitus
Stool • Occult blood • Warm stool smears • Culture	• A mucosal lesion obstructing the colon or unsuspected carcinoma • Bacteria, ova, and amebic trophozoites • Gastroenteritis, cholera or dysentery
C-reactive protein	Infection
Plasma sugar	Diabetes mellitus
Liver function tests	Hepatic dysfunction
Renal function tests	Renal dysfunction
Electrolytes	• Electrolyte abnormalities • Diabetic ketoacidosis • Metabolic acidosis
Lipase and/or amylase	• Pancreatitis • Bowel obstruction • Bowel perforation • Mesenteric ischemia
Abdominal and pelvic USG	• All structural diseases and their complications • Doppler studies for vascular disease
Abdominal radiography	Gas under diaphragm with bowel perforation
MRI	All structural diseases and their complications
CT	All structural diseases and their complications
Laparoscopy	Diagnostic and operative
ECG	Angina, myocardial infarction
Pulse oximetry	• Pneumonia • Pulmonary embolism
Chest radiograph	• Pneumonia • Gas under diaphragm with bowel perforation
Viral markers	Hepatitis

hypotension should be managed well, acid-base balance and fluid electrolyte balance should be maintained. Drugs harmful to the fetus should be avoided unless required from surgical point of view and alternatives are not available.[3]

KEY MESSAGES

Surgical abdomen is an acute condition that could be due to large number of conditions. The cause needs to be diagnosed early, so that the management will minimize maternal and fetal morbidity and prevent their mortality. The symptoms, signs, and laboratory and imaging results can be influenced by the pregnancy, which make the diagnostic process difficult. Investigations which cause fetal irradiation have to be used with caution, so as to prevent fetal teratogenic effects and toxic effects. Fetotoxic drugs should be avoided unless they are essential in maternal interest. Surgery should not be deferred in view of pregnancy.

REFERENCES

1. Siewert B, Raptopoulos V. CT of the acute abdomen: findings and impact on diagnosis and treatment. Am J Roentgenol. 1994;163(6):1317-24.
2. Firstenberg MS, Malangoni MA. Gastrointestinal surgery during pregnancy. Gastroenterol Clin North Am, 1998;27:73.
3. Parulekar SV. Surgical disorders in pregnancy, 1st edition. Mumbai: Project Gutenberg; 2019. pp. 102-111.
4. Stone K. Acute abdominal emergencies associated with pregnancy. Clin Obstet Gynecol. 2002;45:553.
5. Squires R, Postier RG. Acute Abdomen. In: Townsend C, Beauchamp RD, Evers BM, Mattrox K (Eds). Sabiston Textbook of Surgery, 19th edition. New York: Saunders Elsevier; 2012.
6. Augustin G, Majerovic M. Non-obstetrical acute abdomen during pregnancy. Eur J Obstet Gynecol Reprod Biol. 2007;131(1):4-12.
7. Martin RF, Rossi RL. The acute abdomen. Surg Clin North Am. 1997;77(6):1227-43.
8. Dietrich CS, Hill CC, Hueman M. Surgical diseases presenting in pregnancy. Surg Clin North Am. 2008;88(2):403-19.
9. Cormier CM, Canzoneri BJ, Lewis DF. Urolithiasis in pregnancy: current diagnosis, treatment, and pregnancy complications. Obstet Gynecol Surv. 2006;61:733.
10. Parangi S, Levine D, Henry A, Isakovich N, Pories S. Surgical gastrointestinal disorders during pregnancy. Am J Surg. 2007;193:223.
11. Kilpatrick CC, Monga M. Approach to the acute abdomen in pregnancy. Obstet Gynecol Clin North Am. 2007;34:389.
12. King M, Bewes PC, Cairns J, Thornton J. Primary Surgery: Non-trauma. Oxford: Oxford University Press; 1990. pp. 142-8.
13. Elhardello OA, MacFie J. Digital rectal examination in patients with acute abdominal pain. Emerg Med J. 2018;35(9):579-80.
14. Musana KA, Yale SH. Murphy's Sign. Clin Med Res. 2005;3(3):132.
15. Nelson DB, Manders DB, Shivvers SA. Primary iliopsoas abscess and pregnancy. Obstet Gynecol. 2010;116(Suppl 2):479.
16. Rastogi V, Singh D, Tekiner H, Ye F, Mazza JJ, Yale SH. Abdominal Physical signs and medical eponyms: movements and compression. Clin Med Res. 2018;16(3-4):76-82.
17. Rastogi V, Singh D, Tekiner H, Ye F, Mazza JJ, Yale SH. Abdominal Physical Signs and Medical Eponyms: Part III. Physical Examination of Palpation, 1926-1976. Clin Med Res. 2019;17(3-4):107-14.
18. Tan EK, Tan EL. Alterations in physiology and anatomy during pregnancy. Best Pract Res Clin Obstet Gynaecol. 2013;27(6):791-802.
19. Acker DB, Johnson MP, Sachs BP, Friedman EA. The leukocyte count in labor. Am J Obstet Gynecol. 1985;153:737.

20. Scoutt LM, Sawyers SR, Bokhari J, Hamper UM. Ultrasound evaluation of the acute abdomen. Ultrasound Clin. 2007;2(3):493-523.
21. Masselli G, Brunelli R, Monti R, Guida M, Laghi F, Casciani E, et al. Imaging for acute pelvic pain in pregnancy. Insights Imaging. 2014;5(2):165-81.
22. Woodfield CA, Lazarus E, Chen KC, Mayo-Smith WW. Abdominal pain in pregnancy: diagnoses and imaging unique to pregnancy—review. Am J Roentgenol. 2010;194:WS14.

LONG QUESTIONS

1. What are the difficulties in making a diagnosis of the causes of acute abdomen in pregnancy?
2. How will you differentiate the causes of acute abdomen depending on the site of abdominal pain?
3. How will you differentiate the causes of acute abdomen depending on the nature of abdominal pain?
4. How will you differentiate the causes of acute abdomen depending on the type of vomiting?

SHORT QUESTIONS

1. What are the obstetric causes of acute abdomen?
2. What are the gynecological causes of acute abdomen?
3. What are the surgical causes of acute abdomen?
4. What are the medical causes of acute abdomen?

MULTIPLE CHOICE QUESTIONS

1. The duration of pain in acute abdomen is _____.
   a. Few minutes to few hours
   b. Few hours to few days
   c. Few days to few weeks
   d. Few weeks to few months
2. The cause of an acute abdomen cannot be _____.
   a. Medical   b. Orthopedic
   c. Cardiovascular   d. Urogenital
3. Acute pain in right iliac fossa may be due to _____.
   a. Tubal ectopic pregnancy
   b. Acute appendicitis
   c. Torsion of right ovarian cyst
   d. All of the above
4. Acute pain in the epigastrium may be due to _____.
   a. Esophagitis   b. Myocardial infarction
   c. Aortic dissection   d. All of the above
5. Acute pain in the right hypochondrium may be due to _____.
   a. Basal pneumonia   b. Pulmonary embolism
   c. Neither a nor b   d. Both a and b
6. Acute pain in the left hypochondrium may be due to _____.
   a. Acute gastritis   b. Acute pyelonephritis
   c. Myocardial infarction d. All of the above
7. Acute pain in the left iliac fossa may be due to _____.
   a. Diverticulitis
   b. Left tubal ectopic pregnancy
   c. Left ureteric colic
   d. All of the above
8. Acute pain in the hypogastrium cannot be due to _____.
   a. Cystitis   b. Bladder calculus
   c. Aortic dissection   d. All of the above
9. Acute pain in the right lumbar region may be due to _____.
   a. Acute appendicitis
   b. Inflammatory bowel disease
   c. Nephrolithiasis
   d. All of the above
10. Acute pain in the left lumbar region may be due to _____.
    a. Gastroenteritis
    b. Inflammatory bowel disease
    c. Nephrolithiasis
    d. All of the above
11. Pain of a thoracic condition can be referred to abdomen in _____.
    a. Myocardial infarction   b. Pulmonary embolus
    c. Pneumonia   d. All of the above
12. Acute abdominal pain can be due to _____.
    a. Lead poisoning   b. Hereditary angioedema
    c. Narcotic withdrawal d. Any of the above

Answers

| 1. b | 2. b | 3. d | 4. d | 5. d | 6. d |
| 7. d | 8. c | 9. d | 10. d | 11. d | 12. d |

6.5 TRAUMA IN PREGNANCY

Alok Sharma, Aanya Sharma

INTRODUCTION

Over the past centuries, trauma has presented as unique challenge during pregnancy. From the early 1600s, from the first report of Ambrose Pare gunshot wound to the uterus till date, diagnosis, management, prognosis and outcome still remains a dilemma for both mother and attending obstetrician. The basal precept of trauma evaluation, and prompt aggressive resuscitation is the keystone for management of the expectant mother. The addition of fetus, as smaller patient is highlighted as anxiety in evaluating prognosis and outcome of traumatic pregnant patient. Hence, trauma to an obstetric patient is trauma with a double magnitude.

Trauma today, is one of the leading causes among the non-obstetric causes of maternal morbidity and mortality, around one in twelve pregnancies.[1,2] The diverse causes of trauma could be attributed to wide spectra, either minor or major. Around 60-70% fetal losses in the pregnancies are experienced during minor trauma during their antepartum period. With advancing gestational age, incidence of trauma further increases.[3] More than over half of trauma, occurs in third trimester. The prevalence of different subtypes of trauma as per a systemic review account for 8,307/100,000 live birth for domestic abuse and around 207/100,000 live birth for motor vehicle crash.[4]

Several adverse outcomes including placental abruption, preterm delivery, uterine rupture, and pelvic fracture, are to be anticipated during same. An alignment of policies, within each system optimizes triage, and integration of care. The successful maternal therapy is the key to fetal survival.[5] The multidisciplinary focused approach is essential component in management of trauma in pregnancy. It is useful to determine the type of trauma, better clinical judgments, outlining early diagnosis and identifying measures toward efficient action in both emergency room and delivery room. The successful maternal therapy is the key to fetal survival.[5]

CONSIDERATION OF ANATOMICAL AND PHYSIOLOGICAL CHANGES DURING TRAUMA IN PREGNANCY[6,7]

Understanding and integration of key anatomical and physiology changes in pregnancy, are key when evaluating a pregnant trauma patient. The major systems affected during trauma, are described understated.

Physiological Considerations during Pregnancy

Hematological and Cardiovascular Changes

The hemodynamic physiological changes in pregnancy include increase in plasma volume by 50% leading to dilution anemia, and reduced oxygen capacity, further signs of shock could be recognized late, due to blood loss, in case of moderate to severe trauma. There is increase in heart rate by 15-20 beats/minutes and in cardiac output by 50%, both these demands, increase the efforts put in cardiopulmonary resuscitation in case of trauma. Simultaneously, any return of blood pressure to normal levels, so be treated as a caution to a sign of hypovolemia. It is suggested that maternal blood pressure tends to fall as in nonpregnant trauma patient, by the time mother experiences almost 30% of blood loss.

The redistribution of blood flow, as increase in uterine blood flow, is a response as a protective feature to the uterus and fetus, it does impend toward potential rapid massive hemorrhage during any trauma.[4] There is evident sequestration of blood during trauma, attributable to decreased systemic vascular resistance.

The liver becomes hypermetabolic state during the pregnancy. The concentration of clotting factors increases, during the pregnancy, these activated coagulated cascade leads to increased risk of deep vein thrombosis and disseminated intravascular coagulation. DIC should be evaluated with utmost caution during any event of trauma in a pregnant woman. At term pregnancy, there are elevated fibrinogen levels, as a normal physiological adaptation of pregnancy, therefore a keen eye should be kept, even in case of normal or elevated fibrinogen levels. The constellation of symptoms resulting from compression of inferior vena cava, in pregnancy leads to high venous return, leading increase difficulty cardiopulmonary resuscitation.

Respiratory Changes

Similarly increased respiratory rate, increased oxygen consumption by 20%, decreased arterial partial carbon dioxide leads to decreased buffering capacity, acidosis and hypoxia develops quickly.[8] Pregnancy also presents as a state of chronically compensated respiratory alkalosis. Therefore during the evaluation of blood gases always this must be taken into account.

Decreased residual capacity and even laryngeal edema hint towards more chances of hypoxemia, acidosis and difficult intubation when required. Mucosal congestion leads to more airway bleeding. Due to increased upper airway blood flow, there is evidence of friable mucosa leading to increased bleeding and difficult intubation. The diaphragm is elevated 2-3 cm in pregnancy. In an event of trauma, the thoracotomy thus needs to be performed in upper intercostal spaces in midaxillary line, unlike in a nonpregnant patient, to avoid trauma to liver and spleen.[9]

Abdominal Changes

The relaxed lower esophageal sphincter, and decreased gastric mobility, increase the risk of aspiration. Because of these risk factors, there is increased risk of aspiration.[7] There is peritoneal irritation, more commonly seen in third trimester, due to over stretching of peritoneum. The superior displacement of bowel, leads to chances of massive injury to it, during a trauma.

Anatomical Consideration during Pregnancy

The main anatomical changes during pregnancy, which include elevated diaphragm, progressive uterine growth and changes in different trimester which impact the response to fetal trauma. During the first trimester, the uterus is a pelvic organ thick walled and is protected by the pelvic girdle.[10] In the second trimester, uterus is enlarged beyond the pelvis with abundant amniotic fluid, protecting the growing fetus and providing cushioning effect.

During the third trimester, uterus becomes a prominent abdominal organ, larger in size with thinned out walls, more exposed to abdominal trauma and sudden compression shearing forces.[11] The vertex presentation being the most common, the pelvic factures are related to more fetal skull fractures and trauma. With the advancement of the period of gestation, the placenta being inelastic, is prone to the shearing forces of trauma. Both placenta and fetus are extremely sensitive to catecholamine stimulation too. Placental abruption remains an unavoidable squeal in pregnancy in many cases of trauma.[12]

Implications of enlarged gravid uterus and inelastic placenta are as follows:[8]
- Aortocaval compression leads to increased supine hypotension, reduced venous return
- Lack of autoregulation
- Increased sensitivity to maternal blood pressure changes
- Diaphragmatic splinting decreases the residual capacity, leading to difficult ventilation
- Every 10 minutes the entire blood volume passes through the uterus, leading to massive hemorrhage in case of any trauma
- Heart rotation to left axis seen, normal in ECG especially in third trimester.

CAUSES OF TRAUMA IN PREGNANCY

The most common causes of trauma in pregnancy are as follows:

Intentional: Assaults, intimate partner violence, domestic violence, homicide, gunshots, suicides

Unintentional: Motor vehicle crashes, electrical injuries, falls, poisoning and burns.

Other classification includes:

Minor trauma: Does not involve abdominal, rapid compression, deceleration or shearing forces. Patient remains largely asymptomatic. Example: Minor blunt trauma, motor vehicle crashes.

Major trauma: It involves sudden abdominal trauma, rapid compression or shearing forces and associated with vaginal bleeding, abdominal pain, fluid loss or even loss/absent fetal movements.

Nine out of ten trauma patients, experience minor trauma during the event. The more common minor traumas such as motor vehicle crashes are mostly associated with 60–70% of fetal losses.[13]

ASSESSMENT AND MANAGEMENT OF TRAUMA IN PREGNANCY

Advanced trauma life support remains the underlying baseline for management and treatment of trauma, in a pregnant woman similar to a nonpregnant woman. Understanding and interpretation with clinical assessment, due to anatomical and physiological changes should guide an obstetrician led team to formulate the protocols for same.

The best and early treatment for the fetus is early stabilization of mother.

The extent of maternal and fetal involvement depends upon the type of trauma experienced, clinical assessment helps for identifying the same. The prompt response should remain same both in minor as well as major trauma. Fetal monitoring evaluation, should be dealt with equal importance irrespective of nature or insignificant trauma inflicted.

The survey should be streamlined as two major categories (**Table 1**).

Primary Survey

First and foremost, consideration is to evaluate airways, breathing and circulation in trauma during pregnancy.

Airway needs to be secured and maintained.

The intubation in a pregnant woman is to be considered difficult and should be done by experienced health provider.

Laryngeal mask airway can be used in difficult intubation.

Ensuring early gastric decompression is important as there is delayed gastric emptying in pregnancy.

The various reasons stated for difficult intubation include decreased respiratory system compliance, decreased residual capacity, increased hyperemia, friable mucosal congestion and increased oxygen requirements.[14]

Breathing should be kept patent in evaluation of trauma, providing oxygen supplementation to maintain oxygen saturation > 95% to ensure adequate fetal oxygenation. There is increased risk of sudden desaturation, thus active watch on saturation is very important.

Due to raised elevated diaphragm, if a chest tube is indicated, insert one to two intercostals spaces higher to avoid abdominal injury during same.[9]

Circulation: An attempt to control obvious external hemorrhage is needed, to maintain hemodynamic *circulation*. The patient should be tilted to 15–30 degree to avoid uterine compression. As there is uterocaval compression, avoid femoral lines to establish circulation.[8]

Maternal vital signs are established late and less sensitive. Maternal hypovolemia is a sign of impending redistribution and shunting of blood in reverse direction from fetus to mother.

TABLE 1: Two major categories of survey.

Primary survey	Secondary survey
Follow basic principles of trauma: – Airway – Breathing – Circulation	Obstetric and non-obstetric causes Fetal well-being

Even with the release of vasopressors and catecholamines as a response to stress and trauma, both in maternal and placenta system, does pose a threat to fetus. Hence, a prompt step should be taken to deal with maternal hypotension and immediate resuscitation is indicated.

If severely injured establish two bore cannula and assess response, maintaining an awareness of pregnancy related physiological parameters. There is low oncotic pressure in pregnancy, and chances of pulmonary edema is very high, hence avoid excessive crystalloid overload. Keep fluid therapy < 1 liter.

If patient is hemodynamically unstable, a focused abdominal sonography for trauma (FAST) should be done to identify free fluid intra-abdominal and intrapleural cavity. In cases of spinal injury, we can proceed with magnetic resonance imaging.

Cardiopulmonary Resuscitation

Three basic principles to be followed during the cardiopulmonary resuscitation include:
1. *Maternal abdominal tilt:* Around 25–30 degree, leads to decreases uterocaval compression.
2. *Manual uterine displacement:* Avoids complete maternal tilt and may provide better and adequate chest compressions.
3. *Medications and advanced cardiac support:* Remains similar in all kinds of inflicted trauma and comparable to nonpregnant patient, but with more caution with both maternal and fetal monitoring.
4. *In case of cardiac arrest:* While receiving a patient in emergency, the preparedness of cardiac arrest as a possibility should be kept in mind. The standard guidelines of advanced cardiac life support should be followed.

Mother resuscitation becomes the priority, and consider these four main points. At this moment, do not focus on fetal monitoring.[8] Remove all internal and external fetal monitoring devices.
- Prevent circulatory collapse
- Secure safe and patent airway
- Chest decompression
- Plan for perimortem cesarean as indicated.

First priority, start with chest compressions with similar hand placements like in a nonpregnant patient. Proceed with resuscitative hysterotomy as soon as possible. All the resuscitation drugs can be administered in similar way as in nonpregnant patient.[14,15] In case of defibrillation, defibrillate same as a nonpregnant patient, no evidence explains transfer of shock to the fetus. Initially always ventilate with 100% oxygen.[16]

Evidence states that perimortem cesarean delivery in case of an acute emergency improves both neonatal and maternal outcome and is not harmful.

Disability: Assess Glasgow coma scale and look for any neurological deficit.

Expose the patient to look for all signs of trauma, but keep a check on hypothermia.

The primary survey can be remembered as TILT ABCDE:
- Tilt the patient
- Airway, Breathing, Circulation
- Disability assessment
- Expose and examine

Points to remember in initial evaluation:[17]
- In the reproductive age group, every female with trauma, should be considered pregnant unless and until proven.
- Adequate oxygenation saturation should be maintained >95%, to ensure adequate fetal circulation.
- Two wide bore intravenous lines to be established as a resuscitation precaution.
- A nasogastric tube can be used in semiconscious and unconscious women.
- If needed thoracotomy tube should be inserted, 1–2 intercostal spaces above the routine procedure.
- A left lateral tilt should be given to prevent supine hypotension, but spine cord injury should not be over ruled.
- In cases of major trauma, to evaluate the feotmaternal hemorrhage, the Kleihauer–Betke test should be done in all pregnant patients with trauma, irrespective of the Rh status.
- Anti-D immunoglobulin should be given to all rhesus D-negative pregnant trauma patients. If blood transfusion is needed, always transfuse for O negative packed red cell blood, if blood group not known.
- Injection tetanus, should be given to the patient, if they did not receive same during routine antenatal care.
- Intimate partner violence should be evaluated as a complete protocol, as it remains an important perspective. Detailed history for mental health and depression should be elicited.
- Appropriate timely referral to a higher center after primary stabilization of the pregnant patient should be done.

Secondary Assessment

Once primary life threats are excluded, secondary assessment is carried out. This includes two aspects: Maternal monitoring and fetal monitoring.

Maternal Assessment

- *Detailed history:* Reevaluate the history, with an intent to evaluate any mental, domestic or sexual assault. The symptoms such as diminished self-image, suicidal attempts, frequent physician visits, unexplained change in behavior, self-harm, any substance abuse, unwanted fondling should be documented **(Box 1)**. Any patient reporting with inconsistent history again and again to the obstetrician should be eyed with suspicion of intimate partner violence.

> **BOX 1:** Signs and symptoms of trauma.[18]
> - Fear, anxiety, depression
> - Agitation
> - Irritability and emotional outbursts
> - Mood swings and self-harm
> - Self-shame and self-blame
> - Unexplained behavioral changes
> - Retraumatization: Repetitive similar hurtful experiences
> - Palpitations and sweating episodes
> - Difficulty in trusting peer and lack of concentration

- *Detailed clinical examination:* It is utmost to establish the extent of injury. Per abdomen examination is done to look for ecchymosis, any seat belt marks, marked bruising. Look for any abdominal markers for blows, kicks or any other injury. Placental abruption, due to the shearing forces on the uterus is one of the causes for fetal demise and an eye for the same is must. Per abdomen needs assessment of uterine contractions, tone, tenderness, fetal parts is needed. Fundal height corresponds to gestational age, and should be noted.

Per speculum and vaginal examination should be done according to gestational age, to evaluate ruptured membranes, vaginal bleeding, cervical dilation, and effacement. Preferably avoid per vaginal examination unless placenta previa is excluded. Per rectal examination is equally important especially in case of any spinal injury. Look for anal reflex and anal tone.

Fetal Assessment

After the detailed primary survey and stabilizing the maternal status, a fetal assessment is important. When the gestational age greater than 20 weeks for a woman, fetal monitoring needs to be initiated as soon as she is stabilized. Detailed obstetric history including number of fetus, lie, presentation, and placental location should be evaluated.[17]

The fetal monitoring should be done at least minimum 4 hours with tocodynamometry after the trauma inflicted. There is 100% chance of placental abruption, if uterine contractions greater than eight contractions/minute are observed. Estimation of gestational age and fundal height should be done. Detailed ultrasound scan for determining the fetal status, biophysical profile should be carried out, and the need of delivery should be anticipated.

The continuous fetal heart rate monitoring is crucial in a case of pregnant trauma patient. A blood loss of around 1,500 mL, is easily tolerated by a women in late gestation but fetal heart rate is sensitive indicator of maternal blood volume, as it reflects the maternal vascular filling, as compensation of hypovolemia inflicted during trauma. The compensation of maternal hypovolemia is very well picked by continuous cardiotocography (CTG) changes. Hence, monitoring via fetal heart rate via CTG for minimum 4 hours is essential in all pregnant trauma patients, with gestation > 20 weeks.

Diagnostic Evaluation

Radiographic studies indicated for maternal evaluation including chest X-ray and abdominal computed tomography should not be deferred or delayed due to concerns regarding fetal exposure to radiation.

Ultrasonography has poor sensitivity (24%) for detection of placental abruption however, it is very specific (96%).[11] Focused abdominal sonography for trauma should be considered for free fluid in intra-abdominal and intraperitoneal cavity.

In case of spinal cord injury, magnetic resonance imaging is preferred with any risk radiation exposure to the fetus.

The American College of Obstetricians and Gynecologists (ACOG) recommendation states always and always counsel and inform the patient and attendant regarding the risk of exposure.[19]

Explain that the risk of early diagnosis of trauma management outweighs the risk of fetal exposure and hence should be proceeded with prompt evaluation with these diagnostic tools.

Concerns regarding the side effects of high ionizing radiation should be addressed and should be used in medically indicated patients. Magnetic resonance imaging and ultrasound should be used in whichever possible cases.

For dosimetry calculation, an expert should be consulted for the same, especially in cases of multiple exposures.

Special Circumstances pertaining to Management of Trauma[8]

Hemorrhage

Trauma in a pregnant female, is often associated with concealed and massive hemorrhage. Due to limitation of changes in clinical features and concealing of hemorrhage symptoms, form the challenge in identification. Always keep in mind that clinical signs may not become apparent, unless or until there is loss of around 1,500–2,000 mL of blood loss. Principles for the management protocol remain same as a nonpregnant woman.

Identify the cause of bleeding: Both internal and external. In case of any limb injury, proceed as required with specialized trauma teams. Initiate massive hemorrhage protocol according to department guidelines. Arrange for blood products and aim for balanced transfusion as needed. Avoid excessive fluid resuscitation.

Perimortem Cesarean Section or Resuscitative Hysterotomy

A cesarean section done for fetus which is initiated after cardiopulmonary resuscitation is known as resuscitative hysterotomy. The main aim is to stabilize the mother. Golden period for resuscitative hysterotomy is 4–5 minutes and is associated with potentially better maternal and fetal outcome. For a gestational age greater than 20 weeks, it is preferred.[20]

It is preferred to perform the same, as soon resuscitation is started with no later than 4–5 minutes. Do not delay the procedure for a proper operation area or assessing fetal viability. Vertical incision is preferred for easy and early technique. Quick in and out response is needed, with continuation of cardiopulmonary resuscitation throughout and after the procedure.

Placental Abruption

It is the most common sequelae in a case of trauma. Identification of signs and symptoms very important which includes vaginal bleeding, uterine contractions, abdominal pain, loss of fetal movements, fetal distress. A keen eye to identify is important. Management is similar to abruption in any other pregnant women. In case of stable patient with reassuring fetal status, go for conservative management and administer corticosteroids. In case of nonreassuring fetal status, plan for emergency cesarean section.

MECHANISMS AND CAUSES OF TRAUMA IN PREGNANCY (FLOWCHART 1)[8]

Blunt Trauma

It is most common trauma in pregnancy (80–85%).
The most common etiology is motor vehicle collision.[12]

Motor vehicle collision: Most common type. Other causes are fall and direct assault

Mechanism of injury: Direct impact on the uterus.
During pregnancy wearing a seat belt in a motor vehicle is effective in reducing risk of adverse outcomes.

Outcome is related to:
- Placental abruption as a result of shearing forces and abrupt changes
- Mechanism of collision and acceleration-deceleration velocities
- Use of protective devices such as seat belts and air bags
- Positioning of motor vehicle seat belts while pregnant

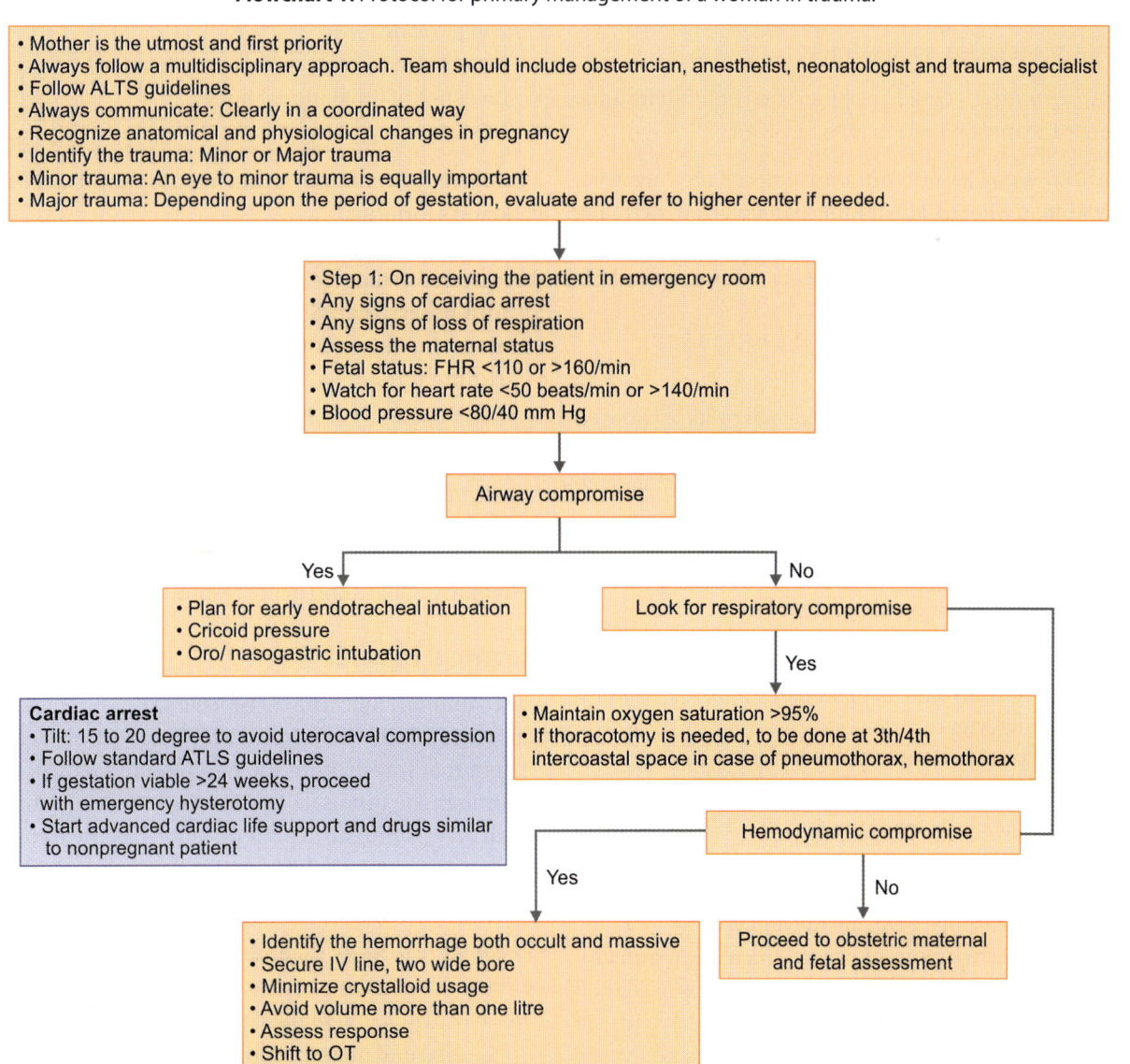

Flowchart 1: Protocol for primary management of a woman in trauma.[8]

Consequences include:
- Direct injury to fetus: Intracranial injury
- Fetomaternal hemorrhage
- Abruption
- Preterm labor
- More chances of postpartum hemorrhage.

Correct positioning of seat belt during pregnancy: Sash between breast and above uterus and lap belt below uterus above hips.[8]

Domestic Violence and Abuse

The domestic violence and abuse is also termed as intimate partner violence.

The incidence of domestic abuse and violence is increased in both in developed and developing nations especially in lower socioeconomic strata.

It is more commonly seen in third trimester.

ACOG recommends screening for intimate partner violence privately in cases of trauma in all reproductive age group.[21] Try establishing and maintaining relationships with community resources in such women.

Mechanism of injury: It could be penetrating or blunt trauma. Abdomen is the most common area involved.

Outcomes are related: Severity of traumatic force, area involved.

Every woman who sustains trauma particularly penetrating trauma, should be evaluated in detail for any domestic injury. Careful, detailed, and contemporaneous documentation is essential.

Penetrating Trauma

Penetrating injuries in pregnant trauma patients are managed in essentially the same way as in non-pregnant patients.[22] By the end of second trimester, bowel is most likely to be affected due to its protection to gravid uterus.

It includes stab wounds and gunshot wounds.

Stab wounds are clean wounds and easily manageable in comparison to gunshot wounds.

Mechanism of injury: Uterus and fetus are both susceptible to injury. Fetus is more involved in penetrating injuries. Complex bowel injuries are even common.

Outcomes are related to the level of the injury. The impact of maternal and fetal outcomes depends majorly on the gestational age of the fetus. In cases of upper abdominal injury, more damage to visceral organs.

Consequences include—fetal death, preterm labor, maternal shock, uteroplacental insufficiency.

Surgery is the treatment of choice in cases of gunshot wounds, during trauma in pregnancy.[3] It is recommended that if the patient is hemodynamically stable, with no hematochezia or hematemesis and the bullet is below the fundus, the bullet is radiologically anterior to the posterior uterine walls, and the fetus is dead, can be delivered later not an emergency. If the fetus is salvageable, requires immediate abdominal laparotomy.[23]

Factors that can influence the decision to proceed with cesarean section are gestational age, extent and severity of fetal injury, degree of uteroplacental compromise, parameters of fetal well-being, and the need for hysterectomy with extensive uterine injury.[6] Emergency cesarean is associated with 45% fetal survival.

Thermal Injury

Maternal and fetal outcomes are both dependent on the total body surface area involved in the burns.

Mechanism of injury: Due to extreme dehydration after the burns and pregnancy itself, there is a fluid shift to the interstitial and difficult resuscitation. Fetal injury is not direct but dependent on the maternal state. If the total body surface area is more than 50%, more chances of fetal death.

Outcomes related to:
- Extent of total body surface area involved
- Presence of inhalational injury
- Gestational age and fetal monitoring in viable pregnancies.

Management includes: Fluid resuscitation according to Parkland's formula.[8]

If the total body surface area involved is greater than 55%, there is need of emergency cesarean delivery, if fetus is viable.

And in less than 55%, administer corticosteroids with expectant management.

Thromboprophylaxis is recommended in some centers, though the risk of increased thrombosis is attributable to immobilization more than burns.[24]

Consequences: Preterm birth, puerperal sepsis, maternal shock, fetal death. Increased vascular permeability throughout the microcirculation may contribute to the development of pulmonary edema and acute respiratory distress syndrome.

Electrical Injuries

Most common clinical impact is feeling of transient unpleasant sensation felt by the mother and no effect on her fetus. A current that travels from the hand to the foot will probably go through the uterus, stimulating myometrial contractions, which may culminate in preterm labor. Electrical current that traverses the amniotic fluid (an excellent conductor) may lead to spontaneous abortion, fetal demise, or fetal burns.[25]

Outcomes related to: Magnitude of the current, duration of contact, maternal body weight, blunt trauma following the electrical insult, and being wet.

The fetal and maternal outcomes are not well established in electric injuries.[26]

Musculoskeletal Injuries

For spinal cord injuries: Always consider multidisciplinary approach. Immobilization of the spine adequately is important. Right lateral tilt is important for avoiding uterocaval compression.

Consider early and prompt delivery in case of late gestation.

For pelvic fractures: Multidisciplinary approach is very important. Immobilize the pelvis. Fetal head injury is the most common injury inflicted in these patients. Cesarean delivery is indicated in case of disruption of pelvic anatomy or unstable book fracture of pelvis. Vaginal delivery is not absolutely contraindicated.[27]

Thromboprophylaxis is considered beneficial in long-term immobilization and lower limb fractures.

Minor Injuries

All the minor injuries should also be attended with caution and prompt response, as fetal response at times could be unpredictable.

Always prefer continuous fetal monitoring for such patients. Admission is considered a safer option for both maternal and fetus outcomes.

Consider discharge if:
- Normal CTG for minimum 4 hours
- No vaginal bleeding
- No uterine contractions
- No maternal distress
- Normal laboratory parameters
- Counsel the mother, to report to hospital in case of vaginal bleeding, contractions, signs of preterm labor, and change in fetal movements.

■ COMPLICATIONS OF TRAUMA IN A PREGNANT WOMAN

- Vaginal bleeding
- Placental abruption around 1.6% in minor trauma and 37.5% in major accidents
- Preterm labor
- Maternal pelvis fractures, musculoskeletal injury
- Intracranial hemorrhage
- Fetal fractures especially skull, clavicles, long bones
- Fetomaternal hemorrhage (rare and severe): RBC isoimmunization
- Uterine rupture
- Amniotic fluid embolism
- Disseminated intravascular coagulation.

■ REFERENCES

1. Mirza FG, Devine PC, Gaddipati S. Trauma in pregnancy: a systematic approach. Am J Perinatol. 2010;27(7):579-86.
2. El Kady D. Perinatal outcomes of traumatic injuries during pregnancy. Clin Obstet Gynecol. 2007;50(3):582-91.
3. Barraco RD, Chiu WC, Clancy TV, Como JJ, Ebert JB, Hess LW, et al. Practice Management Guidelines for the Diagnosis and Management of Injury in the Pregnant Patient: The EAST Practice Management Guidelines Work Group. J Trauma. 2010;69(1).
4. Mendez-Figueroa H, Dahlke JD, Vrees RA, Rouse DJ. Trauma in pregnancy: an updated systematic review. Am J Obstet Gynecol. 2013;209(1):1-10.
5. Lavery JP, Staten-McCormick M. Management of moderate to severe trauma in pregnancy. Obstet Gynecol Clin North Am. 1995;22(1):69-90.
6. Houseman B, Semien G. Florida Domestic Violence [Internet]. StatPearls Publishing; Treasure Island (FL): 2021.
7. Huls CK, Detlefs C. Trauma in pregnancy. Semin Perinatol. 2018;42(1):13-20.
8. Queensland Clinical Guidelines. Trauma in pregnancy. Guideline No. MN19.31-V2-R24. [Internet]. Queensland: Queensland Health; 2019.
9. Krywko DM, Toy FK, Mahan ME. Pregnancy Trauma. In: StatPearls [Internet]. Treasure Island (FL): StatPearls Publishing; 202.
10. McAuley DJ. Trauma in pregnancy: anatomical and physiological considerations. Trauma 2004;6(4):293-300.
11. Brown S, Mozurkewich E. Trauma during pregnancy. Obstet Gynecol Clin North Am. 2013;40(1):47-57.
12. Royal College of Obstetricians and Gynaecologists. Antepartum haemorrhage. Green-top Guideline No. 63. London: RCOG; 2011.
13. El-Kady D, Gilbert WM, Anderson J, Danielsen B, Towner D, Smith LH. Trauma during pregnancy: an analysis of maternal and fetal outcomes in a large population. Am J Obstet Gynecol. 2004;190(6):1661-8.
14. Jeejeebhoy FM, Zelop CM, Windrim R, Carvalho JC, Dorian P, Morrison LJ. Management of cardiac arrest in pregnancy: a systematic review. Resuscitation. 2011;82(7):801-9.
15. Jones R, Baird SM, Thurman S, Gaskin IM. Maternal cardiac arrest: an overview. J Perinat Neonatal Nurs 2012;26(2):117-25.
16. Vanden Hoek TL, Morrison LJ, Shuster M, Donnino M, Sinz E, Lavonas EJ, et al. Part 12: cardiac arrest in special situations: 2010 American Heart Association guidelines for cardiopulmonary resuscitation and emergency cardiovascular care [published corrections appear in Circulation. 2011;123(6):e239, and Circulation. 2011;124(15):e405]. Circulation. 2010;122(18 Suppl 3): S829-61.
17. Jain V, Chari R, Maslovitz S, Farine D, Bujold E. Guidelines f or the management of a pregnant trauma patient. J Obstet Gynaecol Can. 2015;37(6):553-74.
18. Substance Abuse and Mental Health Services Administration. SAMHSA's Concept of Trauma and Guidance for a Trauma-Informed Approach. HHS Publication No. (SMA) 14-4884. Rockville: SAMHSA; 2014.
19. Guidelines for diagnostic imaging during pregnancy and lactation. Committee Opinion No. 723. American College of Obstetricians and Gynecologists. Obstet Gynecol. 2017;130:e210-6.
20. Rose CH, Faksh A, Tray nor KD, Cabrera D, Arendt KW, Brost BC. Challenging the 4- to 5-minute rule: from perimortem cesarean to resuscitative hysterotomy. Am J Obstet Gynecol. 2015;213(5):653-6.e1.

21. ACOG Committee Opinion No. 518: Intimate partner violence. Obstet Gynecol. 2012;119(2 Pt 1):412-7.
22. Mattox KL, Goetzl L. Trauma in pregnancy. Crit Care Med. 2005;33(Suppl):S385-9.
23. Molina GA, Aguayo WG, Cevallos JM, Gálvez PF, Calispa JF, Arroyo KA, et al. Prenatal gunshot wound, a rare cause of maternal and fetus trauma, a case report. Int J Surg Case Rep. 2019;59:201-4.
24. Parikh P, Sunesara I, Lutz E, Kolb J, Sawardecker S, Martin JN Jr. Burns during pregnancy: implications for maternal-perinatal providers and guidelines for practice. Obstet Gynecol Surv. 2015;70(10):633-43.
25. Deshpande NA, Kucirka LM, Smith RN, Oxford CM. Pregnant trauma victims experience nearly 2-fold higher mortality compared to their nonpregnant counterparts. Am J Obstet Gynecol. 2017;217(5):590.e1-e9.
26. Reddy SV, Shaik NA, Gunakala K. Trauma during pregnancy. J Obstet Anaesth Crit Care. 2012;2:3-9.
27. McGoldrick NP, Green C, Burke N, Quinlan C, McCormack D. Pregnancy and the orthopaedic patient. Orthopaed Trauma. 2012;26(3):212-9.
28. American College of Surgeons. Advanced trauma life support: Student course manual, 9th edition. Chicago: ACS; 2013.

LONG QUESTIONS

1. Enumerate the causes for trauma in pregnancy. Enumerate the steps for initial evaluation of a trauma and for individual causes in a pregnant woman.
2. A 24-year-old pregnant woman was involved in a motor vehicle accident and her period of gestation is 32 weeks. On examination in the emergency room, her pulse rate is 84/minutes, blood pressure is 120/80 mm Hg, with respiratory rate 20/min, with SpO$_2$ 100% with Glasgow coma scale of 12/15. Enumerate the scheme of management for this patient.
3. Enumerate the different causes and mechanism of action of individual kinds of trauma.
4. Formulate the plan for management of a feeble pulse, hypotensive pregnant patient with limb fracture at period of gestation at 25 weeks and 5 days.

SHORT QUESTIONS

1. What are the complications of trauma during pregnancy?
2. What are the anatomical and physiological considerations of a trauma patient during pregnancy?

MULTIPLE CHOICE QUESTIONS

1. Kleihauer–Betke test is performed to patient:
   a. Presence of fetal cells in maternal circulation
   b. Mothers Rh status
   c. Presence of disseminated intravascular coagulation
   d. Fetal maturity
2. The cardiovascular changes in pregnancy include which of the following:
   a. Decreased systemic vascular resistance, increased blood volume, increased cardiac output
   b. Increased systolic blood pressure, decreased cardiac output, decreased hematocrit
   c. Decreased cardiac output, increase blood volume, increased colloidal pressure
   d. Increased blood pressure, decreased hematocrit, and decreased heart rate decrease in systemic vascular resistance (SVR)
3. Which of the following is not a complication of trauma in pregnancy?
   a. Rupture of amniotic membrane
   b. Preeclampsia
   c. Placental abruption
   d. Uterine rupture

Answers

1. a   2. a   3. b

6.6 POISONING IN PREGNANCY

Sujata Sharma, Amarjeet Kaur

INTRODUCTION

Poisons: These are the substances which are injurious or deleterious to the body leading to disease, deformity or death or illness, infirmity or death.

Poisoning: It is defined as any substance exposure which may be unintentional or intentional or any drug overdose that is injurious to health or interferes with normal body functioning or cause death.[1] Poisoning may be acute or chronic, local or systemic, suicidal or homicidal or accidental or stupefying. Poisoning can resemble other illnesses, thus resulting in difficulty in diagnosis. The correct diagnosis can be established by history, physical examination, routine and toxicological investigations and characteristic clinical course of poison.[2,3]

The poisons can be corrosives, irritants, neurotics, cardiac, asphyxiants and miscellaneous. Poisons can be administered through following routes, e.g., enteral, parenteral, inhalational, external application on broken skin, sublingual or introduction to natural orifices.

Among the injury-related hospital admissions in pregnancy, poisoning is the third leading cause; first and second being traffic accidents and falls respectively. It accounts for 0.6% of all exposures recorded in Toxic registry.[1-4] Toxicological exposure not only harms the mother but also affects fetus leading to various fetal complications like fetal distress, intrauterine growth restriction (IUGR), teratogenicity or even fetal demise. Majority of the cases in pregnancy are accidental but one-fifth may be intentional.

As reported in a study, 32% of poisonings occurred in the first trimester, 37.6% in the second trimester and 30.5% in the third trimester.[5] Self-poisoning attempts are highest in first trimester and decreases with advancing age. As per the American Association of Poison Control Centers (AAPCC) National Poison Data System (NPDS); in USA, approximately 7,500–8,000 cases of poisoning in pregnancy are reported each year to the center of poison control.[1] There is limited evidence based data to manage the poisoning in pregnancy and the efficacy and safety profile of antidotes.

The common poisonings during pregnancy are: acetaminophen, non-steroidal anti-inflammatory drugs (NSAIDs), selective serotonin reuptake inhibitors (SSRIs) and iron excluding the abuse drugs. Most common drug class poisoning in pregnancy is of non-opioid analgesics; among this class, acetaminophen (APAP) poisoning is present in 81.2% of all cases and 25.2% in all the poisoning cases in pregnancy. The second most commonly involved drug category is sedatives and hypnotics or muscle relaxants (18.4%); third being the opioids. As per the APPCC in 2012, analgesics were the most commonly involved in exposure during pregnancy followed by cleansing substances and pesticides.[1-4]

Poisoning and Physiological Changes in Pregnancy

Due to physiological and psychological changes in pregnancy; absorption, metabolism and distribution of various poisons get altered. Certain clinical features of different types of poisoning may resemble pregnancy related complications, thus making the diagnosis difficult.

Poisoning in Pregnancy: Risk Factors

Poisoning is more common in the presence of following high risk factors as shown in **Table 1**.

EFFECTS OF POISONING ON FETUS AND MOTHER

Acute poisoning in pregnancy can be challenging to the clinicians due to potential immediate life-threatening risk to mother and fetus and lifelong complications to two lives. The fetal complications depend on the gestational age at the time of exposure. Certain poisons are teratogenic, their exposure in first trimester leads to teratogenicity in fetus. Exposure to some of the chemicals in pregnancy leads to adverse birth outcomes such as pregnancy loss, preterm birth, low birth weight, congenital anomalies, cognitive dysfunction, impaired immune system development, adult disease and mortality. Poisoning affects the maternal health, thus leading to various maternal complications and indirectly the fetal complications. Chronic exposure to chemicals in pregnancy can also lead to adverse maternal health, LBW, IUGR, teratogenicity, etc. Poisoning in pregnancy should be thoroughly investigated due to potential self-harm, psychiatric consideration and social implications.

DIAGNOSIS OF POISONING IN PREGNANCY

It can be made by history, examination, investigations including both toxicology and routine investigations and poison specific clinical picture. Proper history must include time of exposure, route of exposure, duration since exposure, name and amount of poison consumed, circumstances leading to poisoning in woman, intention of poisoning and location of poisoning. Medical and psychiatric history should be taken. Sudden unexplained illness in a healthy woman or a group, any history of domestic violence, recent changes in health, any psychiatric disorder, pregnancy in the unmarried girl and history of drug abuse are some of the suspicious conditions pointing to the diagnosis.[6,7]

The relevant information should be obtained from family, friends, police, etc., as most of the time, patient is not able to provide history due to confused or comatose condition. Ingredients can be identified by labels on the poison and poison can be identified by referring to available text or computerized information of the poison along with history of exposure. Proper obstetric history should be taken. Past, personal and family history should be taken.

Physical Examination

It includes measuring the vital signs, general physical examination, the cardiopulmonary system, and neurologic status and obstetrics examination. The final step is to identify the particular agent involved by looking for relatively poison specific signs and symptoms and investigations.

Laboratory Assessment

Routine investigations, serum electrolytes, arterial blood gas (ABG), prothrombin time (PT) and international normalized ratio (INR), liver function tests, renal function tests, urine analysis and toxicological examination should be done. ECG and shielded chest X-ray should be done.

Toxicologic analysis: Toxicologic analysis of urine, blood, gastric lavage/aspirate and samples of chemicals can be done for confirming or ruling out poisoning.

Rapid qualitative urine tests are the screening tests for drugs of abuse. Confirmatory tests with gas chromatography/

TABLE 1: High risk factors for poisoning in pregnancy.

• Young age (18–20 years) • Primigravidity • Lower socioeconomic status • Psychiatric disturbances and illnesses • Drug addiction • Domestic violence • Unplanned pregnancy	Psychosocial factors leading to poisoning in pregnancy: • Lifestyle • Suppression of women in society • Women's lower authority in the family • Lack of economic independence and lack of family planning knowledge

mass spectrometry can be done. Ultrasonography for fetal evaluation and Doppler studies should be done. USG to rule out anomalies should be done in case of chronic poisoning. Response to antidotes can be used as a diagnostic purpose. For example, normalization of vitals and altered mental status after intravenous administration of naloxone or flumazenil is diagnostic of opioid or benzodiazepine poisoning respectively.

MANAGEMENT

Management of poisoning in pregnancy is similar to the non-pregnant patient, but fetal health should be kept in mind. Approach to acute poisoning in pregnancy is different because of physiological changes in pregnancy and the potential risk to both mother and fetus. Mother's life should be the priority. Any intervention that can harm the fetus in utero should be avoided unless the mother's life is in danger.[8]

It should be managed in collaboration with intensivist, physician, forensic expert, toxicologist, psychiatrist, and sociologist. Mild to moderate cases can be managed in emergency or high dependency unit (HDU). Severe cases should be managed in ICU. The main goal of treatment is to maintain the vitals, decontamination, preventing further absorption of poison, enhancing the elimination of poison, administration of antidotes and preventing re-exposure to poison. Specific treatment depends on the identification of poison, route of administration, amount of poison exposure and severity of poisoning. Pharmacokinetics and pharmacodynamics of the poison must be known.[5] Patient should be kept warm and comfortable. Good nursing care should be given especially for unconscious patient.

Principles of treatment of poisoning in pregnancy are:
- By treating mother, fetus gets treated
- Maternal stabilization is priority with immediate evaluation of ventilatory, hemodynamics and mental status
- In mental status change, suspect hypoglycemia or narcotic overdose first and treat accordingly (dextrose and/or naloxone)
- Withholding or delaying the required treatment to mother can cause more harm and damage
- General toxicologic and decontamination principles are same as in non-pregnant state.

MEDICOLEGAL ASPECTS OF POISONING

The medicolegal aspects of poisoning in pregnancy are as given in **Box 1**.

Decontamination is most valuable prior to the onset of poisoning during the pretoxic phase. Gastric lavage should be done. Gastric lavage is contraindicated in corrosive or petroleum poisoning, in patients at risk of hemorrhage/perforation in gastric or esophageal pathology, in combative patients and patients with unprotected airway. Both activated charcoal and gastric lavage are safe for the fetus.

> **BOX 1:** Medicolegal aspects of poisoning.
> - All cases should be informed to the police whether suicidal, homicidal or accidental
> - The doctor must notify the public health authorities at once
> - He/she should take every precaution to prevent the possibility of further administration of the poison
> - The records of the case should be kept in meticulous details
> - Stomach washings, sample of vomit and urine passed in his/her presence and blood should be preserved in separate containers and sent to forensic science laboratory
> - Any suspicious objects such as bottles, linen soiled with vomit, stools, etc., should be preserved

In the toxic phase, i.e., the interval between the onset of poisoning and peak effect of poison, management depends mainly on the clinical findings and investigations. Resuscitation and stabilization are the priority. The measures that enhance the elimination of poison may shorten the severity and duration of the toxic phase. The diagnosis of the type of poison is required to choose the correct agent to enhance elimination. Urinary alkalinization can enhance salicylates elimination and of few other poisons. Investigations to check acid base balance and serum electrolytes should be monitored carefully.[9] Chelation therapy can enhance the elimination of metals.

Antidotes are the remedies which neutralize or counteract the effect of poison without causing significant harm to the patient. Their safe use requires the correct identification of the poison. For example, demulcents, bulky food, and activated charcoal, diazepam for strychnine, naloxone for morphine, N-acetylcysteine (NAC) for acetaminophen and certain chelating agents act as specific antidote for heavy metals.[10]

In the resolution phase of poisoning, supportive care must be continued until the clinical features, ECG and laboratory parameters return to the normal. Strict fetal monitoring should be continued. In case of fetal distress or IUD, the termination of pregnancy can be considered after stabilization of maternal condition. In case of abortion, termination should be planned if the maternal condition permits.

Obstetric management: It depends on the gestational age and condition of the mother and the fetus.

SPECIAL POISONING SYNDROMES

Some common poisoning syndromes in pregnancy are described here.

Acetaminophen Poisoning

Besides drug of abuse, it is the most common type of poisoning in pregnancy.

Pathophysiology

Most of the APAP metabolism occurs in the liver after conjugation with glucuronide or sulfate leading to the formation of non-toxic metabolites. These non-toxic metabolites are then excreted in the urine. Around 7% of the APAP metabolism in the liver and kidney occurs by chytochrome P450 enzyme leading to the formation of toxic compound NAPQI (N acetyl-p-benzoquinone imine). This molecule (NAPQI) forms a covalent bond with a macromolecule resulting in cell injury and death. NAPQI detoxification occurs by combining with glutathione. This leads to formation of mercapturic acid metabolite which is a nontoxic compound and gets excreted in the urine. In APAP poisoning, NAPQI is formed in more amount leading to the depletion of glutathione stores resulting in NAPQI induced cell toxicity. It mainly affects the liver; kidney is also affected but to a lesser extent.[11-13] The pathophysiology is shown in **Figure 1**.

Symptoms can be described under three stages that include: Gastrointestinal, latent, hepatic failure.

1. *Gastrointestinal:* The symptoms are mild. Vomiting is seldom severe or accompanied by other symptoms and patient remains fully conscious.
2. *Latent:* After 24 hours, though the liver undergoes damage, patient is relatively pain free. Anorexia, epigastric pain, malaise occur due to hepatic damage.
3. *Hepatic failure:* This stage is seen after about 3–5 days. It is characterized by liver failure, gastrointestinal hemorrhage, cerebral edema, renal tubular necrosis and cardiomyopathy. In cases where patient survives the 3rd stage, complete resolution of the liver injury occurs.

Fetal Effects of Poisoning

Acetaminophen crosses the placental barrier and metabolism occurs in liver of the fetus leading to generation of NAPQI. Cases of fetal hepatic necrosis had been reported if there was delay in the treatment; but at a lower rate than in adults. This is due to the immaturity of the fetal cytochrome P450 enzymes.

Treatment

Patient should be hospitalized immediately as the history and clinical state of the patient may mislead the diagnosis. A patient who is apparently well 12 hours after taking the overdose of APAP can die due to acute hepatic failure 5 days later. Gastric lavage must be done within 4 hours of poisoning. Adequate hydration should be maintained in protracted poisoning. Fluid retention can occur in APAP poisoning, therefore IV fluids should be restricted to 2.5L in that cases.

Severe hepatic necrosis in APAP leads to complications such as metabolic acidosis, hypoglycemia and bleeding tendencies. These complications should be treated with supportive therapy such as bicarbonate infusion, dextrose, vitamin K injection and whole blood or plasma therapy. N-acetyl cysteine is the antidote. It is the most commonly used antidote. It should be given in 16–24 hours of poisoning, thus preventing hepatic damage. Initially, 140 mg/kg of NAC should be given followed by infusion of 50 mg/kg over 4 hours, then 100 mg/kg over 16 hours. It crosses the placental barrier and also provides protection to fetus. It is not teratogenic in therapeutic doses, so its administration should not be delayed.

Salicylate Poisoning in Pregnancy

Salicylates cross the placenta leading to the accumulation in the fetal blood stream. Severe acute toxicity can lead to intrauterine fetal demise. Due to immature fetal glucuronidation and renal excretion pathways, fetal salicylate elimination occurs slowly; thus concentrating in fetal brain due to less intracellular/intravascular pH gradient in fetus. This leads to increased risk of intracerebral hemorrhage. This intracerebral salicylate accumulation is the major cause of fetal morbidity and mortality.

Signs and symptoms in pregnant patient include hematemesis, tinnitus, agitation, tachypnea, and tachycardia.

Investigations

Serum salicylate levels, bicarbonate levels, ABG, ultrasound for fetal well-being, electrolyte levels. Urine toxicology screen should be sent.

Treatment

Soda bicarbonate and glucose drip and intravenous fluids should be given. Bicarbonate drip should be continued for urinary alkalinization. In salicylate poisoning, maternal hemodialysis is not of much benefit to the fetus. In pregnant

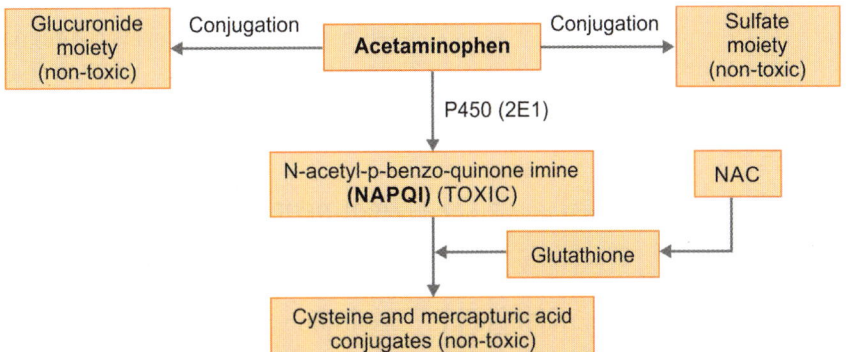

Fig. 1: The pathophysiology and the formation of toxic compounds. (NAPQI: N acetyl-p-benzoquinone imine; NAC: N-acetylcysteine)

patient, no reports of dialysis use for any toxic overdose have been found. Delivery should be delayed until the maternal status is optimized. Fetus acidosis persists despite the patients' alkalosis due to bicarbonate therapy leading to fetal distress. Emergent delivery is the treatment for the fetus exposed to in utero salicylate poisoning at or near term.

Acute Iron Intoxication in Pregnancy

Intentional poisoning is more common in females and is associated with higher mortality.[13] Consequences depend on the ingested amount of elemental iron. Symptoms are absent if dose is below 20 mg/kg, between doses of 20 and 40 mg/kg, severe toxicity can occur. Death is reported with doses from 60 to 300 mg/kg.[14]

Iron poisoning or intoxication occurs in five stages. This includes gastrointestinal stage, latent stage, shock and metabolic acidosis, hepatotoxicity and bowel obstruction. Gastrointestinal stage results from the mucosal damage which occurs in 30 minutes to 6 hours after the ingestion. Signs and symptoms include vomiting, diarrhea, abdominal pain, lethargy, malena, hematemesis, metabolic acidosis and shock. Latent stage may not be apparent in all cases and it is a period of stability that can leads to recovery or can be the anticipation of clinical deterioration. Metabolic acidosis and shock usually occur 6 to 72 hours after ingestion. Signs and symptoms of gastrointestinal bleed, perforation of bowel, pulmonary dysfunction, hypoglycemia or hyperglycemia, renal and neurologic dysfunction, iron induced coagulopathy develop in this stage. Hepatotoxicity usually occurs in 2 days of poisoning. It can also develop 12–96 hours after tablets ingestion. Bowel obstruction occurs in consequence to bowel mucosal injury and scarring. It usually occurs 2–8 weeks after the acute event. Vomiting is the main symptom of bowel obstruction.

Risk to Fetus

In pregnancy, the fetus is protected from the effects of iron as the placental absorption of iron is saturable process. Fetus is at risk only when the mother is clinically decompensated as in hypotension, liver failure or pulmonary failure. Maternal organ failure leads to increased risk of spontaneous abortion, preterm delivery and intrauterine death.

Investigations

Peak serum iron concentration is the investigation of choice.

Treatment

Gastric lavage should be done. In severe iron intoxication, treatment of choice is desferrioxamine.

Following are the indications of desferrioxamine: severe signs and symptoms, peak serum iron concentration more than 500 µg/dL, metabolic acidosis or a significant number of pills in the X-ray.

It is contraindicated in anuria and severe chronic renal disease. Adverse effects include urticaria, rash, hypotension and acute respiratory syndrome. Acute respiratory syndrome is reported for longer perfusions of more than 32 hours.

Criteria to stop desferrioxamine:
- Improvement in patient's condition.
- Return to normal color of urine. During chelation therapy, "vinrose" discoloration of urine occurs due to chelation production.
- Modification of serum or urine iron concentration by desferrioxamine use.

Tranquilizer Poisoning

These drugs relieve anxiety and mental tension without producing sedation or sleep. They are also used in anesthesia for their muscle-relaxant properties. Common examples are diazepam and razepam. Signs and symptoms of tranquilizer poisoning include restlessness, tremor, diplopia, hallucinations, drowsiness, weakness, incoordination followed by cyanosis, respiratory depression, coma and collapse.[15,16]

Treatment

Stomach wash, emetics and symptomatic treatment. Flumazenil orally or IV injection 0.3 to 1 mg is the antidote. It is classified as a pregnancy category C drug by FDA. It should be used only if benefits outweigh the risk.

Lead Poisoning

Lead poisoning is of two types: (1) acute or (2) chronic. Chronic poisoning is more common than the acute. The toxic effects are due to the fixation of lead in brain or peripheral nervous tissue. Lead is stored in the bones. As the calcium is released from the bones and delivered to the fetus, lead is also released into the blood stream. This results in very high lead levels in the fetus, both before and after the birth of the baby. Neonates and infants need aggressive management to lower the lead levels as early as possible.

Signs and symptoms of acute lead poisoning are metallic astringent taste, dry throat, thirst, nausea and vomiting with abdominal pain, headache, drowsiness, constipation, offensive and black feces, limb paralysis, collapse and death. Elevated lead levels in pregnancy are associated with spontaneous abortion, IUGR, impaired neurodevelopment of fetus and risk of gestational hypertension. Acute cases may survive and develop the symptoms of chronic poisoning.[17]

Treatment

Stomach should be washed. A diet rich in calcium and vitamin D and administration of calcium salts are helpful as calcium favors disposition of lead in the skeleton. Calcium versenate (EDTA) and penicillamine are useful antidotes. Chelation therapy should be considered for pregnant women with confirmed blood lead level (BLL) > 45 μg/dL in consultation with expert in toxicology. The rest of the treatment is symptomatic.[17]

Chronic Lead Poisoning

Chronic lead poisoning is more common as compared to acute lead poisoning. It occurs in chronic occupational exposure to lead. Chronic poisoning may occur from the mobilization of lead which is already stored in the body tissues like bones, e.g., in acidosis. Therefore, symptoms of chronic or acute poisoning can develop years after the originally absorbed lead.

Signs and symptoms of chronic poisoning are pallor, anemia with punctuate basophilia, colic and constipation, lead line, encephalopathy, paralysis, endovascular manifestation, reproductive system manifestations and general symptoms.

Investigations
Blood lead levels should be tested.

Treatment
Treatment includes removal of source of exposure and enhancing the excretion of the stored lead. EDTA combines with lead, thus promoting its mobilization and urinary excretion in an inactive form, resulting in the rapid clearance of signs and symptoms of poisoning. Nutritional status makes a woman more susceptible to lead exposure. Appropriate dietary intake of certain nutrients such as iron, calcium, vitamin C, D and E and zinc decreases the lead absorption. In pregnant with BLL > 5 μg/dL with history of lead exposure, a dietary calcium intake of 2,000 mg daily should be maintained.

Food Poisoning

Pregnant women are more at risk of food poisoning because of the metabolic and circulatory changes and due to alteration in immune system. It is often characterized by nausea, vomiting and diarrhea, headache, fever, abdominal pain or discomfort, dehydration, bloody stools. Common types of food poisoning are *E. coli, Salmonella spp., Listeria spp.*

Complications during Pregnancy
Excessive vomiting and diarrhea can lead to dehydration in short time span. Listeria can lead to long term neurological developments problems in fetus. *E. coli* leads to damage to blood vessel lining or kidney failure indicated by bloody stools. *Salmonella* can cause dehydration, meningitis, reactive arthritis (Reiter's syndrome) and bacteremia. Patients on antacids, inflammatory bowel disease (IBD), recently used antibiotics, immunocompromised states like HIV are high risk factors.

Fetal complications: Miscarriage, stillbirth, preterm birth.

Treatment
Fluid loss should be replenished. Severe dehydration might require hospitalization or IV fluids. Antibiotics should be added. Both maternal and fetal monitoring should be done.

■ POISONING OF DRUGS OF ABUSE

It can be in the form of chronic addiction (chronic poisoning) or overdose (acute poisoning).

Substance Abuse

Substance abuse is increasing in young women, and this produces significant maternal and fetal morbidity during pregnancy. The associated social problems of poor hygiene, nutrition, and social deprivation are responsible for much of the risk, rather than abuse itself. Substance exposed pregnancies are high risk pregnancies. Therefore, proper and adequate antenatal care should be provided to these patients including tackling her social and medical problems.

Alcohol Poisoning in Pregnancy

As per the data from a global cohort study, it was found that 34% of first time mothers had history of binge alcohol drinking in the 3 months before pregnancy, out of which 23% of these mothers continued binge alcohol drinking during the first 15 weeks of pregnancy.[18] Binge drinking, i.e., taking more than five units at a time can be more harmful than taking same quantity in divided doses. Alcohol related damage can occur throughout the pregnancy. Only complete abstinence during pregnancy is considered safe.

Acute Alcohol Poisoning
Ethyl alcohol depresses the CNS, irregularly in the descending order from cortex to medulla. It first depresses the higher centers which control judgment and behavior (stage of excitement), then motor centers (stage of incoordination) and finally the vital centers in the medulla (stage of narcosis). Alcohol can be lethal at relatively lower blood levels when combined with other central nervous system depressants such as barbiturates, carbon monoxide, and morphine.

Treatment: Stomach lavage should be done with care. Isotonic saline with 5% glucose should be given to treat symptoms of hypoglycemia. Artificial respiration should be given if there is respiratory depression.

Chronic Alcohol Abuse and Pregnancy
Heavy drinking during pregnancy can cause fetal alcohol syndrome (FAS) and other birth defects. Higher miscarriage rates have been associated with consumption of more than 6 units in a day for many days.

Drinking heavily during pregnancy can result in:
- Increase miscarriage
- Fetal growth restriction and low birth weight
- Risk of stillbirth
- Congenital malformations
- Preterm labor
- *Fetal alcohol spectrum disorder (FASD) or FAS:* It includes microcephaly, fetal growth restriction, nervous system dysfunction (learning disability, ataxia, impaired intellect,

and attention deficits) and characteristic facial appearances (narrow palpebral fissures, mid-face hypoplasia, ptosis, underdeveloped philtrum and rotated low-set ears). FAS is a relatively rare disorder with an incidence of less than 1 in 1,000 live births, increasing to 4.3% among heavy drinkers. FASD is less severe than FAS. Children with FASD can have learning disabilities, physical disability, behavior problems and emotional and psychiatric problems that last for lifelong.

Stopping drinking alcohol at any point during pregnancy can be beneficial. Fetus can start growing at a normal rate. Maternal alcohol intake of more than 20 g/day is associated with an increase in preterm delivery and neonatal jaundice. Moderate intake of alcohol during pregnancy of less than 12 to 14 units/week has no apparent detrimental effect on fetal growth. Liver function tests should be checked.

Treatment

Planned detoxification should be considered. Detoxification is normally undertaken with benzodiazepines, with the addition of phenobarbitone to manage convulsions. Benzodiazepines given in the first trimester may be associated with cleft palate abnormalities. If delivery is likely within next few days, benzodiazepines should be given with care because neonatal sedation and "floppy baby syndrome" can occur. Disulfiram should not be used because it is considered a potential teratogen, although the incidence is conflicting.

Opium Poisoning

Opium is easily available in India. For suicidal purposes, it is a poison of choice. It can be chronic addiction or acute poisoning. As the pregnancy progresses, rate of overdose events decreases and again increases after delivery. Signs and symptoms usually appear within half an hour to 1 hour after ingestion and within about 3–5 minutes after injection. It acts on the central nervous system, first leading to stimulation and later to depression followed by narcosis.

Treatment

Stomach wash should be done with tepid water. Intestines should be cleared out by enema. Nalorphine and naloxone are the antidotes. Rest of the treatment given is symptomatic as per the condition of the patient.

Naloxone

Naloxone should be used cautiously in opioid dependent pregnant females. This can lead to adverse effects such as hypertensive crisis, preterm labor, fetal distress and precipitation of withdrawal symptoms. It should be used in pregnancy only if clearly required to save maternal life.

Chronic Opioid Poisoning or Opioid use Disorder

As per the recent estimate, opioid use disorder (OUD) ranges from 0.4 to 0.8% during pregnancy.[5] Pregnant women with OUD have an increased risk of fetal growth restriction, preterm labor, placental abruption, preeclampsia and stillbirth.

Risk of overdose increases in patients with OUD. Temporary withdrawal symptoms can occur after delivery if patient does not get enough drug. Neonate of patient with OUD can develop temporary withdrawal symptoms. This is called neonatal abstinence syndrome (NAS).[9,19] The behavioral therapy and drug replacement therapy with buprenorphine or methadone improves the obstetrical and infant outcomes in patients with OUD.[19] It has been found that opioid replacement medication does not cause birth defects. Breastfeeding can be continued in patients taking methadone or buprenorphine. Naloxone can cause fetal distress when given in pregnancy but its use should not be delayed to save the maternal life.

CONCLUSION

Poisoning in pregnancy is a challenging situation and difficult to manage due to the limited data available. Poisoning affected pregnancies are high risk pregnancies and should be managed in tertiary care center in collaboration with experts of other specialties also to provide best possible maternal care. Aim is to save both the mother and the fetus.

REFERENCES

1. Zelner I, Matlow J, Hutson JR, Wax P, Koren G, Brent J, et al. Acute Poisoning During Pregnancy: Observations from the Toxicology Investigators Consortium. J Med Toxicol. 2015;11(3):301-8.
2. Bronstein AC, Spyker DA, Cantilena LR, Green JL, Rumack BH, Dart RC. 2010 Annual Report of the American Association of Poison Control Centers' National Poison Data System (NPDS): 28th Annual Report. Clin Toxicol. 2011;49(10):910-41.
3. Bronstein AC, Spyker DA, Cantilena LR, Green JL, Rumack BH, Dart RC. 2011 Annual report of the American Association of Poison Control Centers' National Poison Data System (NPDS): 29th Annual Report. Clin Toxicol. 2012;50:911-1164.
4. Mowry JB, Spyker DA, Cantilena LR, Bailey JE, Ford M. 2012 Annual Report of the American Association of Poison Control Centers' National Poison Data System (NPDS): 30th Annual Report. Clin Toxicol. 2013;51(10):949-1229.
5. Watson WA, Litovitz TL, Rodgers GC, Jr, Klein-Schwartz W, Reid N, Youniss J, et al. 2004 annual report of the American association of poison control centers toxic exposure surveillance system. Am J Emerg Med. 2005;23:589-666.
6. Ann Howland M, Lewin NA, Nelson LS, Goldfrank LR. Goldfrank's Toxicologic Emergencies, 10th edition. New York: McGraw-Hill; 2015.
7. Thompson TM, Theobald J, Lu J, Erickson TB. The general approach to the poisoned patient. Dis Mon. 2004;60:509.
8. Gei AF, Suarez VR, Van Hook JW. Overdose, Poisoning, and Envenomation during Pregnancy. In: Phelan JP, Pacheco LD, Foley MR, Saade GR, Dildy GA, Belfort MA (Eds). Critical Care Obstetrics. London: Wiley-Blackwell; 2020.
9. ACOG Committee on Health Care for Underserved Women, American Society of Addiction Medicine ACOG Committee Opinion No. 524: opioid abuse, dependence, and addiction in pregnancy. Obstet Gynecol. 2012;119:1070-6.

10. Dart RC, Borron SW, Caravati EM, Cobaugh DJ, Curry SC, Falk JL, et al. Expert consensus guidelines for stocking of antidotes in hospitals that provide emergency care. Ann Emerg Med. 2009;54:386.
11. McElhatton PR, Sullivan FM, Volans GN, Fitzpatrick R. Paracetamol poisoning in pregnancy: an analysis of the outcomes of cases referred to the Teratology Information Service of the National Poisons Information Service. Hum Exp Toxicol. 1990;9(3):147-53.
12. McElhatton PR, Sullivan FM, Volans GN. Paracetamol overdose in pregnancy analysis of the outcomes of 300 cases referred to the Teratology Information Service. Reprod Toxicol. 1997;11(1):85-94.
13. Riggs BS, Bronstein AC, Kulig K, Archer PG, Rumack BH. Acute acetaminophen overdose during pregnancy. Obstet Gynecol. 1989;74(2):247-53.
14. Tran T, Wax JR, Philput C, Steinfeld JD, Ingardia CJ. Intentional iron overdose in pregnancy—management and outcome. J Emerg Med. 2000;18(2):225-8.
15. Stahl MM, Saldeen P, Vinge E. Reversal of fetal benzodiazepine intoxication using flumazenil. BJOG. 1993;100(2):185-8.
16. Dolovich LR, Addis A, Vaillancourt JM, Power JD, Koren G, Einarson TR. Benzodiazepine use in pregnancy and major malformations or oral cleft: meta-analysis of cohort and case control studies. BMJ. 1998;317:839-43.
17. Shannon M. Severe lead poisoning in pregnancy. Ambul Pediatr. 2003;3(1):37-9.
18. McCarthy FP, O'Keffee LM, Khashan AS. Association between maternal alcohol consumption in early pregnancy and pregnancy outcomes. Obstet Gynecol. 2013;122:830-7.
19. Binder T, Vavrinkova B. Prospective randomized comparative study of the effect of buprenorphine, methadone and heroin on the course of pregnancy, birthweight of newborns, early postpartum adaptation and course of the neonatal abstinence syndrome (NAS) in women followed up in the outpatient department. Neuroendocrinol Lett. 2008;29:80-6.

LONG QUESTIONS

1. What is the incidence and risk factors of poisoning in pregnancy? How will you proceed to diagnose poisoning in pregnancy?
2. Describe in detail the general principles and line of management of poisoning in pregnancy.
3. Describe acetaminophen poisoning in pregnancy, its pathophysiology and management.
4. Describe lead poisoning in pregnancy. How it can be prevented and what is the treatment?
5. Describe the iron intoxication in pregnancy. How will you diagnose and manage the case of iron intoxication in pregnancy?

SHORT QUESTIONS

1. Define the poison and poisoning. Classify the poisons.
2. What are the risk factors for poisoning in pregnancy?
3. What are the effects of poisoning on mother and fetus?
4. What are the medicolegal aspects of poisoning in pregnancy?
5. What is FAS or FSAD?

MULTIPLE CHOICE QUESTIONS

1. Which is the most common poisoning in pregnancy?
   a. Non-opioid analgesics
   b. SSRIs (selective Serotonin reuptake inhibitors)
   c. Lead poisoning
   d. OPC poisoning
2. Which is not the risk factor for poisoning in pregnancy?
   a. Lower socioeconomic status
   b. Domestic violence
   c. Psychiatric disorder
   d. Multigravida
3. What should be done in cases of poisoning in pregnancy?
   a. Inform the police
   b. Records should be kept in meticulous details
   c. Any suspicious objects should be preserved
   d. All the above
4. Which is the active metabolite in acetaminophen poisoning?
   a. N-acetyl cysteine (NAC)
   b. Acetaminophen
   c. NAPQI (N acetyl-p-benzoquinone imine)
   d. None of the above
5. Which is not the effect of poisoning in pregnancy?
   a. Preterm birth   b. Low birth weight
   c. Teratogenicity   d. Big baby
6. What is the antidote of acetaminophen poisoning?
   a. NAC(N-acetyl cysteine)   b. Soda bicarbonate
   c. Flumazenil   d. None of the above
7. What is the FDA category of flumazenil?
   a. A   b. B
   c. C   d. X
8. Which is the typical feature of listeria food poisoning?
   a. Neurological development problems in fetus
   b. Dehydration
   c. Reiter's syndrome
   d. Vomiting
9. Which of the following is the feature of fetal alcohol spectrum disorder (FASD) or fetal alcohol syndrome (FAS)?
   a. Microcephaly   b. Ptosis
   c. Learning disability d. All the above
10. What is the antidote for opium poisoning?
    a. Flumazenil   b. Naloxone
    c. NaHCO$_3$ d. None of the above
11. Which of the following is the adverse effect of opioid use disorder (OUD) in pregnancy?
    a. Abruptio placentae   b. Stillbirth
    c. Preeclampsia   d. Al the above

Answers

1. a   2. d   3. d   4. c   5. d   6. a
7. c   8. a   9. d   10. b   11. d

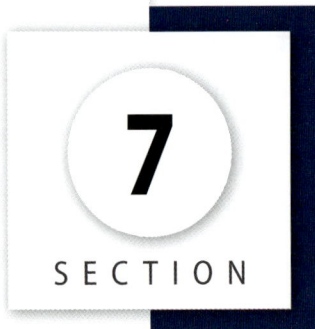

SECTION 7

Fetal Complications

7.1 FETAL INFECTIONS

Geetha Balsarkar

■ CASE SCENARIO

A 35-year-old primigravida patient visits the antenatal clinic for registration of pregnancy. She has been known to be HIV positive on antiretroviral prophylaxis. Extensive one to one counseling is given to the patient regarding percentage of vertical transmission of HIV to the fetus with antiretroviral therapy and without therapy. It is advised to her that she continue antiretroviral therapy during the pregnancy also to decrease the vertical transmission rate. She is very concerned about the congenital malformations possible after retroviral therapy. After discussing these options with her husband and family, the patient chooses not to take the antiretroviral and opts for a vaginal delivery. About 25–30% is the approximate risk of vertical transmission from the mother to the fetus for this patient.

■ INTRODUCTION

Although the immune system changes that occur during pregnancy are not well understood by us till date, a shift from cell-mediated immunity as primary defense to humoral immunity is believed to occur. These immunologic changes may alter susceptibility to and severity of infectious diseases in pregnant women, which affects the fetus too inside the uterus. For example, pregnancy may increase susceptibility to toxoplasmosis and malaria, may increase severity of these illness and increase mortality rates from influenza and varicella. Pregnant women's altered response to infectious diseases also plays a role in severity of these infections and which infections are transmitted to the fetus in utero and in what severity.[1]

Maternal infections during pregnancy and fetal infections have been a major cause of worry since many centuries. The pregnant mother and her developing fetus during organogenesis are susceptible to several infectious diseases, epidemics and pandemics and complications that normally do not occur in healthy adults or children. Hence, fetal infection as a cause of reproductive wastage, obstetric mishaps and neonatal morbidities were often overlooked generally or were investigated after other causes are ruled out. This is not true any longer. "What the mind does not know, the eye does not see," hence suspicion is the prime requirement for diagnosing fetal infections.[2,3]

Fetal infections should be suspected in the following cases:
- History of fetal infection in previous pregnancy or baby after birth
- Early repeated abortions
- Unexplained stillbirths, sometimes repeatedly
- Presence of malformations such as hydrocephalus, microcephaly, cataracts, cardiac anomalies in mid trimester scans or after birth
- Mental retardation and deafness in small children
- Multiple neurological deficits with symptoms such as convulsions.

While inside the uterus, the fetus is protected by layers of chorion and amnion, the placenta and amniotic fluid which in itself have antibacterial factors. Organisms causing the fetal infection can reach the fetus in many ways. "Vertical transmission" is a term that refers to the spread of infections from mother to the baby. These infections may occur:
- While the fetus is still in the uterus ("in utero")
- During the process of labor and delivery
- Handling of baby after delivery (such as while breastfeeding).

Important points about fetal infections:
1. The appropriate time to provide knowledge to the mothers about these infections is in the pre pregnancy period, 3–6 months before because this is the best time for intervention and preventive measures if any to be taken.
2. The first trimester of pregnancy is usually the most dangerous time for the mother to acquire these infections, as organogenesis occurs during this period and hence there is a greater risk of the fetus getting affected.

3. Infection in the mother can often be accompanied by no symptoms or very trivial symptoms, so the condition is not usually diagnosed as there are no complaints.
4. Infection in the mother does not always mean that the baby will always be affected. For many infections, the baby is more at risk at particular stages of pregnancy (for example, first trimester for Rubella, at delivery for HSV).
5. Some infections can be avoided by the mother through simple measures, such as immunization (Rubella, VZV) during childhood and before pregnancy. Some infections are treatable (e.g., syphilis is treated effectively with penicillin).
6. Fetal adaptive immune responses are common in neonates who have been exposed to maternal infection during pregnancy but not infected themselves. Such responses could affect the development of immunity to the homologous pathogens and their control during the first few years of life. Fetal innate and regulatory responses might also affect immunity to unrelated pathogens and responses to vaccines. Strategies to improve child health should integrate the possible clinical implications of in-utero exposure to chronic maternal infections.[4]

CLASSIFICATION OF ETIOLOGIC AGENTS

- Bacterial infections
- *Viral infections:* HIV, hepatitis infection
- TORCH infections
- Protozoal infections
- Syphilis infection
- Listeriosis.

The more common organisms causing congenital infections include **(Table 1)**: CMV, HSV, Erythrovirus (Parvovirus) B19, Rubella, Hepatitis B virus, HIV, VZV, *Treponema pallidum, Toxoplasma gondii*.

BACTERIAL INFECTIONS

Among the important maternal bacterial infections, causing neonatal infection are the group B *Streptococcus* (GBS) and *E. coli*, both of which account for about 70% of all systemic bacterial infection. The pathogenesis of these infections may relate to lack of type specific antibodies to these organisms in the neonate. A specific polysaccharide, sialic acid, found on the outer capsules of both GBS and *E. coli* prevents activation of alternate complement pathway and hence destruction of bacilli by the host immune system.

Following maternal infection, the organisms enter blood stream. If the maternal infection increases, it would lead to placentitis or if the infection is contained within, then the neonate is not infected. Even with placentitis seen on histopathology, there may or may not be fetal infection. Fetal infection affects either fetal viability or growth. In the varying stages of infection, there may be embryonic death or

TABLE 1: Effect of infection on the fetus.

Organism or disease	Prematurity	In utero growth retardation and low birth weight	Developmental anomalies	Congenital disease	Persistent postnatal infection
Viruses					
Rubella	−	+	+	+	+
CMV	+	+	+	+	+
HSV	+	−	−	+	+
VZV	−	(+)	+	+	+
Enteroviruses	−	−	(+)	+	−
Hepatitis B	+	−	−	+	+
HIV	(+)	(+)	(+)	+	+
Erythrovirus B19 (Parvovirus B19)	−	−	−	+	−
Bacteria					
Treponema pallidum	+	−	−	+	+
Mycobacterium tuberculosis	+	−	−	+	+
Listeria monocytogenes	+	−	−	+	−
Campylobacter fetus	+	−	−	+	−
Salmonella typhosa	+	−	−	+	−
B. burgdorferi	−	−	−	+	−
Parasites					
Toxoplasma gondii	+	+	−	+	+
Plasmodium spp.	(+)	+	−	+	+
Trypanosoma cruzi	+	+	−	+	−

resorption, abortion, still birth, low birth weight, prematurity, developmental anomalies, congenital disease and persistent postnatal infection.

Maternal conditions predisposing to neonatal sepsis include premature rupture of the membranes, prolonged rupture of membranes, urinary tract infection and chorioamnionitis. Suspicious labor characteristics include preterm labor and fetal tachycardia without maternal fever, blood loss, hypotension or tachycardia inducing medication. Sepsis should be considered in all of these situations as well as in the setting of unexplained fetal distress or birth asphyxia. Predisposing factors for early onset neonatal sepsis include male sex.

TORCH INFECTIONS

Rubella

From the year 1941, when Gregg started associating rubella with fetal congenital anomalies to the year 1969, when rubella vaccine was developed, a lot of congenital anomalies were reported. In the prevaccination era, 80% of women of childbearing age were already infected atleast once due to the existing custom of kitty parties. The clinical features of Rubella are maculopapular rash, fever, lymphadenopathy and arthropathy. The risks of rubella infection during pregnancy can be classified according to weeks of gestation.

- *Preconception:* Minimal risk
- *0 to 12 weeks:* 100% fetus infected congenitally. Very high risk of abortio
- *13 to 16 weeks:* Spontaneous abortion in 20%, deafness and retinopathy in 15%
- *>16 weeks:* Normal development, slight risk of deafness and retinopath.

With the availability of vaccine, these anomalies have reduced.[5] Congenital rubella syndrome requires termination.

Toxoplasmosis

Toxoplasma is an obligatory intracellular parasite infecting a wide range of birds and small mammals. The human being is not normally a vector. However, the humans can acquire the parasite by contamination with cat feces or by ingestion of uncooked meat following which the organism infects the mother and later on the fetus by transplacental infection. In India, 80–85% of women are infected by the age of 20, compared to the rates of 20% in the UK and USA. Although most cases of maternal toxoplasmosis are asymptomatic, when infection is evident, the most common form of presentation is a glandular fever like illness.

Toxoplasmosis appears to be harmful to the fetus by way of fetal infection if the primary infection occurs during pregnancy. The earlier the infection in pregnancy, the more severe is its effect on the fetus. Because most mothers will not give a history of infection, a high index of suspicion is needed for diagnosing congenital toxoplasmosis. On ultrasonography, hydrocephalus, unilateral or bilateral, calcification in the cranial region should give a high index of suspicion of fetal toxoplasmosis. Neonatal manifestations include chorioretinitis, hydrocephalus, microcephaly, hepatosplenomegaly, anemia and a maculopapular rash. The diagnosis is made from maternal and neonatal serology, but more recent techniques include direct culture and use of reverse transcriptase polymerase chain reaction. Umbilical cord blood sampling can also be used for serology in fetal infections suspected on ultrasonography when other causes need to be ruled out.[3]

There is a significant role of maternal treatment with spiramycin during pregnancy to prevent fetal infection. Recent evidence suggests that the outcome improves with early recognition and treatment of congenital infection.

However, even with treatment, these infants are at considerable risk of cerebral palsy, mental retardation and visual disturbance. If the infection is identified in an infant, the treatment protocol includes spiramycin alternating with sulfadiazine or clindamycin and pyrimethamine.

Cytomegalovirus Infection

Cytomegalovirus (CMV) is the most common cause of congenital infection, complicating 0.4–2.4% of all births. About 50–85% of women of child bearing age are seropositive. Primary infection in pregnancy is often acquired from other young children or from sexual partners. About 30–40% of infants born to mothers sustaining their primary CMV infection during pregnancy will have congenital infection, of which 10% are asymptomatic. Features suggestive of congenital CMV include growth retardation, hepatosplenomegaly, jaundice, petechiae, microcephaly, hydrocephalus, periventricular calcification and chorioretinitis. However, the most common manifestation of congenital CMV is sensorineural hearing loss that occurs in 15% of symptomatic and 5% of asymptomatic infants. The diagnosis is best made by culturing the virus from neonatal urine or saliva. Demonstrable seroconversion during pregnancy may be helpful, but paired sera are not usually available. At present, there is no effective antiviral therapy for congenital CMV, although there are a number of ongoing multicenter trials regarding the use of ganciclovir. Common long-term complications, even among asymptomatic infant include deafness and learning disabilities.[3]

Herpes Simplex

Neonatal herpes simplex virus infections are rare. Infections usually results from the perinatal acquisition of HSV, usually type 2, from the maternal genital tract in about 85% of cases. The recurrence rate of genital herpes appears to be higher in pregnant than in non-pregnant women, with the likelihood of recurrence increasing as the patient reaches term. Maternal HSV antibodies are protective, particularly if type specific. Infants at highest risk are of those delivered vaginally to mothers who have acquired the primary infection late in pregnancy, as they may be still shedding the virus from the genital tract without having the opportunity to produce protective antibodies. Neonatal infection usually presents toward the end of the first week of life. Neonatal HSV may be localized to the eye, skin or mouth, or be generalized, or cause isolated pneumonitis or meningoencephalitis. Only localized external disease has a good prognosis. Without antiviral treatment, 70% of localized external cases of neonatal HSV will become disseminated. Therefore, prompt recognition of neonatal herpes using direct immunofluorescence techniques, electron microscopy or PCR is important in improving outcome. Acyclovir will decrease the likelihood of disseminated disease in the neonate. Although acyclovir therapy decreases infant mortality associated with perinatal HSV transmission, development of permanent neurological disabilities is not uncommon. Mother-to-neonate HSV transmission is most efficient when maternal genital tract HSV infection is acquired proximate to the time of delivery, signifying that neonatal herpes prevention strategies need to focus on decreasing the incidence of maternal infection during pregnancy and more precisely identifying infants most likely to benefit from prophylactic antiviral therapy.[6]

A mother with primary genital HSV in labor should be delivered by cesarean section if the membranes have not been ruptured for more than 24 hours. The management of asymptomatic recurrences in labor is less clear. When the infant is delivered vaginally to primary genital HSV, swabs are sent from the infant's nasopharynx and conjunctiva, and if positive, treated with acyclovir to prevent fulminant infection.

Current ACOG guidelines do not recommend routine antepartum genital HSV cultures in asymptomatic patients with recurrent disease, nor they recommend routine screening of pregnant women for HSV. Suppressive antiviral therapy with acyclovir should be given to pregnant women who have a primary episode or active recurrent genital HSV at or beyond 36 weeks of gestation. It should also be given to women with an active genital herpes infection, primary or secondary, near term or at the time of delivery. A recent statement by ACOG supports the use of antiviral therapy in pregnant women with outbreaks of genital herpes. Acyclovir therapy started at 36 weeks of gestation may decrease viral shedding, prevent neonatal herpes, reduce the need for cesarean delivery and decrease clinical recurrences of herpes simplex virus infection. Valacyclovir is a promising substitute of acyclovir with similar efficacy, as well as the increased bioavailability of valacyclovir and famciclovir results in their less frequent dosing to achieve the same therapeutic benefits as acyclovir. All these three drugs, acyclovir, famciclovir and valacyclovir have been labeled as category B drugs. Valacyclovir is prodrug of acyclovir, which is rapidly converted to acyclovir, hence safety profile quite similar to the second one.[7]

CONGENITAL SYPHILIS

Congenital syphilis is the oldest recognized congenital infection with severe, disabling infection often with grave consequences seen in infants. This long forgotten disease continues to affect pregnant women resulting in perinatal morbidity and mortality. The continuing prevalence of this disease reveals the failure of control measures established for its prevention. WHO's recommendation is that all pregnant women should be screened for syphilis in the first antenatal visit in the first trimester and again in the late pregnancy.[8]

The transmission to the infant is by the transplacental passage of *Treponema pallidum* from an infected mother to her fetus. The newborn can also be infected by contact with an active genital lesion at the time of delivery. The highest risk to the fetus is in untreated primary syphilis or in the early stages of secondary syphilis. Early recognition and treatment of the mother will prevent 98% of cases of neonatal infection. Penicillin is the antibiotic of choice. Treatment with erythromycin causes treatment failures as high as 30%.

The clinical signs and symptoms of congenital syphilis are nonspecific and similar to those with other intrauterine infections such as CMV and toxoplasmosis. Serum testing for nontreponemal titers or VDRL titers is diagnostic. If in doubt, it is best to treat the infant with aqueous crystalline penicillin or procaine penicillin for 10-14 days. Treated infants should be followed up for at least 12 months with repeated serological testing.

HEPATITIS B

Hepatitis B is acquired following contact with blood or genital secretions. The disease course in pregnancy is similar to that seen in the general population. Acute HBV infection does not have any teratogenic effects. However, a higher incidence of low birth weight and prematurity has been reported.

About 10-20% of women seropositive for HBsAg transmit the virus to their neonates in the absence of immunoprophylaxis. In women, who are seropositive for both HBsAg and HBeAg, vertical transmission is approximately 90%. In patients with acute hepatitis B, vertical transmission occurs in up to 10% of neonates when infection occurs in the first trimester and in 80-90% of neonates when acute infection occurs in the third trimester. Risk for HBV transmission at delivery is mainly due to exposure to cervical secretions and maternal blood. Minority of infections are not prevented by prompt neonatal immunization, hence a lot of transplacental transmission is also presumed. Risk factors for transplacental transmission of HBV include maternal HBeAg positivity, high HBsAg titer and HBV DNA level. HBV infection during pregnancy does not alter the natural course of the disease; however, chronic infection occurs in about 90% of infected infants. Though routine prenatal screening of all pregnant women for HBsAg is the need of the hour, especially until hepatitis B vaccine is included in the scheme of compulsory vaccination of all newborns it is not practiced routinely currently.[9]

Pregnancy is not a contraindication for HBV vaccination, and pregnant females can receive three doses of the vaccine at 0, 1 and 6 months. If the female is exposed to a person with acute hepatitis B as a result of sexual contact, then a course of HBV vaccine into the deltoid along with a dose of hepatitis B immunoglobulin (HBIg) 0.06 mL/kg IM into the contralateral arm should be given within 14 days after the most recent sexual contact. However, in cases with exposure to chronic carriers hepatitis B vaccine alone is recommended. Neonatal vaccination prevents newborn infection in about 80–95% of cases. Interferon, lamivudine, adefovir and entecavir are classified by the Food and Drug Administration as Class C, and telbivudine and tenofovir as Class B. In most cases, this is because there are insufficient data in humans to demonstrate teratogenic or embryotoxic effects. For these reasons, in most instances, it is reasonable to defer therapy until after delivery, to avoid fetal exposure to the therapeutic agents.[10]

HUMAN IMMUNODEFICIENCY VIRUS

Around the world, about 50% of all adults living with human immunodeficiency virus (HIV) are women and the prevalence of HIV positive children is 2.5 million. In 2001, the United Nations General Assembly Special Session on HIV/AIDS committed countries to reduce the proportion of infants infected with HIV by 20% by 2005 and by 50% by 2010. Twenty seven million new pregnancies occur per year in India of which 97,000 pregnancies occur in HIV +ve mothers (prevalence 0.36%). There are 30,000 HIV-infected babies (25–30% transmission rate) born every year. Still, significant number of pregnant women needs to be covered under the umbrella of HIV testing and preventive medicine.[11,12]

Human immunodeficiency virus transmission from an HIV-positive mother to her child can occur during pregnancy, labor, delivery or breastfeeding. Without treatment, around 15–30% of babies born to HIV positive women become infected with HIV during pregnancy and delivery. A further 5–20% become infected through breastfeeding.

The risks associated with perinatal transmission of HIV-1 are multifactorial. Known risk factors include high maternal plasma viremia, advanced clinical HIV-1 disease, reduced maternal immunocompetence, vaginal delivery and a lengthy interval between rupture of the amniotic membrane and delivery. In addition, direct exposure to maternal blood, presence of ulcerative genital infection in the maternal vaginal tract at the time of delivery, illicit drug use during pregnancy, prematurity, and low birth weight have all been associated with increased mother-to-child transmission.[12]

Human immunodeficiency virus transmission to the fetus can occur as early as the 15th week of pregnancy. Prenatal infection may cause a HIV-specific embryopathy in the majority of infected children. It is characterized by a small forehead, short flat nose, pronounced philtrum, microcephaly, thick lips and hypertelorism. There is evidence suggesting that pregnancy also favors the progression of the HIV disease in the mother. The most important determinant is the virus load present in the mother.[11]

Current policies with respect to breastfeeding by mothers who are infected with HIV are guided by observational evidence that exclusive breastfeeding for the first 4–6 months of life reduces the risk of transmission of HIV as compared with mixed breastfeeding (i.e., feeding both breast milk and formula) and may have survival benefits at 18–24 months that are similar to those for exclusive formula feeding. Other measures that may minimize risk of transmission through breast milk are:

- Good lactation management so that breastfeeding problems such as cracked nipples, engorgement and mastitis are prevented.
- Where the mother does develop mastitis or abscesses, she must express milk from the affected side frequently, discard it and continue feeding from the unaffected side.
- Condoms must be used throughout the lactation period.
- If the infant has oral thrush, it must be treated promptly.

World Health Organization (WHO) recommends that "where replacement feeding is acceptable, feasible, affordable, sustainable and safe HIV-infected women should avoid breast-feeding". Although peripartum prophylaxis with a single dose or a short course of antiretroviral agents effectively reduces intrapartum HIV transmission, its effect does not extend much beyond 4–6 weeks in breastfeeding populations.[13]

World Health Organization also recommends that infants born to HIV-infected women receiving ART for their own health should receive:

- *Breastfeeding infants:* Daily NVP from birth until 6 weeks of age
- *Non-breastfeeding infants:* Daily AZT or NVP from birth until 6 weeks of age.

In case of breastfeeding infants of HIV-infected pregnant women who are not in need of ART for their own health, maternal ARV prophylaxis should be coupled with daily administration of NVP to the infant from birth until 1 week after all exposure to breast milk has ended. In non-breastfeeding infants, maternal ARV prophylaxis should be coupled with daily administration of AZT or NVP from birth until 6 weeks of age.

An elective cesarean section substantially reduces vertical transmission among untreated or highly active ART (HAART) treated pregnant women. However, CS has higher postpartum morbidity than vaginal delivery especially in HIV-infected women, compared with their non-HIV-infected counterparts. ACOG thus recommends, "the decision regarding mode of delivery must be individualized". In the HAART era, vaginal delivery should be considered if woman is treated with HAART and has a viral load before labor of below 1,000 copies/mL. A meta-analysis of 15 prospective cohort studies also suggested that elective CS reduces vertical transmission of HIV-1 independent of zidovudine therapy. Although not recommended in the United States, elective CS is routinely recommended in some European countries for HIV-1-infected pregnant women after 36 weeks of gestation.[12]

CHALLENGES

Emerging infectious diseases, defined as infectious diseases whose incidence in humans has increased during the past 2 decades or threatens to increase in the near future, are increasingly recognized by physicians as an important threat to pregnant women. Emerging infectious diseases include novel pathogens that have newly emerged, such as severe acute respiratory syndrome (SARS), H1N1 as well as pathogens that could potentially be used as biologic weapons.

The coronavirus disease 2019 (COVID-19) has spread from isolated cases of pneumonia in Wuhan, Hubei province, China, to become a worldwide pandemic as declared by the WHO on March 11, 2020.

Coronaviruses are single-stranded RNA viruses. Although there are many coronaviruses, the particular coronavirus that is responsible for this pandemic is the severe acute respiratory syndrome coronavirus 2 (SARS-CoV-2). After 2–7 days of incubation, most symptomatic patients typically experience fever, cough, or loss of taste or smell, with some cases developing into life-threatening pneumonia and acute respiratory distress syndrome.

Pregnant women are not at an increased risk of spontaneous abortion or spontaneous preterm birth but have higher rates of cesarean delivery.

Vertical transmission of severe acute respiratory syndrome coronavirus 2 is possible and seems to occur in a minority of cases of maternal coronavirus disease 2019 infection in the third trimester. The rates of infection are similar to those of other pathogens that cause congenital infections. However, given the paucity of early trimester data, no assessment can yet be made regarding the rates of vertical transmission in early pregnancy and potential risk for consequent fetal morbidity and mortality.[14]

In conclusion, there is currently no concrete evidence of intrauterine vertical transmission of SARS-CoV-2, but further high-quality research is needed.[15]

Pregnant patients should follow the same general precautions as nonpregnant persons for avoiding exposure to the virus in community transmission like physical distancing [at least 6 feet (2 m)], wearing a three layer cloth face mask or nonmedical disposable mask when contact with anyone not from the same household, avoiding indoor crowded spaces such as theaters and restaurants and crowded places, washing or sanitizing hands frequently, disinfecting frequently touched surfaces, avoiding close contact with ill individuals. Face masks should also be used when a household member is infected or has had recent potential COVID-19 exposure. Those who contact with a confirmed or suspected case of COVID-19 should be monitored.

CONCLUSION

Changes in immune function during pregnancy alter a pregnant woman's susceptibility to and severity of certain infectious diseases. These alterations are particularly problematic because physicians may hesitate to provide prophylaxis or aggressive treatment to pregnant women because of concerns about effects on the fetus. Compared with what is known about conventional disease threats, knowledge about currently recognized emerging infectious diseases is quite limited. Soon we will likely be faced with novel pathogens about which little or nothing is known. Because the effects of emerging infections in pregnant women might differ from those in the general population, pregnancy must be considered a potential risk factor for disease susceptibility as well as for illness and death. Unfortunately, pregnancy issues are often not well addressed in outbreak investigations, ongoing prospective studies, or emergency preparedness planning. Future scientific inquiry and medical investigations must include pregnancy-related issues as a vital component

REFERENCES

1. Szekeres-Bartho J. Immunological relationship between the mother and the fetus. Int Rev Immunol. 2002;21:471-95.
2. Menezes EV, Yakoob MV, Soomro T, Haws RA, Darmstadt GL, Bhutta ZA. Reducing stillbirths: prevention and management of medical disorders and infections in pregnancy. BMC Pregnancy Childbirth. 2009;9(Suppl 1):S4.
3. Yamamoto R, Ishii K, Shimada M, Hayashi S, Hidaka N, Nakayama M, et al. Significance of maternal screening for Toxoplasmosis, rubella cytomegalovirus and herpes simplex infection in cases of fetal growth restriction. J Obstet Gynaecol Res. 2013;39(3):653-7.
4. Dauby N, Goetghebuer T, Kollmann TR, Levy J, Marchant A. Uninfected but not unaffected: chronic maternal infections during pregnancy, fetal immunity, and susceptibility to postnatal infections. Lancet Infect Dis. 2012;12(4):330-40.
5. Reef SE, Chu SY, Cochi SL, Kezaala R, Kezaala R, van den Ent M, et al. Reducing the global burden of congenital rubella syndrome. Lancet. 2012;380(9848):1145-6.
6. Cherpes TL, Matthews DB, Maryak SA. Neonatal herpes virus infection. Clin Obstet Gynecol. 2012;55(4):938-44.
7. American College of Obstetricians and Gynecologists (ACOG). Management of herpes in pregnancy. Washington (DC): American College of Obstetricians and Gynecologists (ACOG); 2007.
8. Murali MV, Nirmala C, Rao JV. Symptomatic early congenital syphilis: a common but forgotten disease. Case rep Pediatr 2012;2012:934634.
9. American College of Obstetricians and Gynecologists. ACOG Practice Bulletin No. 86: Viral hepatitis in pregnancy. Obstet Gynecol. 2007;110:941-56.
10. Velu PP, Gravett CA, Roberts JK, Wagner TA, Zhang JS, Rubens CE, et al. Epidemiology and etiology of maternal bacterial and viral infections in low- and middle-income countries. J Glob Health. 2011;1(2):171-88.
11. WHO. RAPID ADVICE—Use of antiretroviral drugs for treating pregnant women and preventing HIV infection in infants. [online] Available from: http://www.who.int/hiv/pub/mtct/rapid_advice_mtct.pdf. [Last Accessed October, 2021].
12. Singhal P, Naswa S, Marfatia YS. Pregnancy and sexually transmitted viral infections Indian J Sex Transm Dis. 2009;30(2): 71-8.

13. Ishaque S, Yakoob MY, Imdad A, Goldenberg RL, Eisele TP, Bhutta ZA. Effectiveness of interventions to screen and manage infections during pregnancy on reducing stillbirths: a review. BMC Public Health. 2011;11(Suppl 3):S3.
14. Kotlyar AM, Grechukhina O, Chen A, Popkhadze S, Grimshaw A, Tal O, et al. Vertical transmission of coronavirus disease 2019: a systematic review and meta-analysis. Am J Obstet Gynecol. 2020.
15. Wang C, Zhou YH, Yang HX, Poon LC. Intrauterine vertical transmission of SARS-CoV-2: what we know so far. Ultrasound Obstet Gynecol. 2020;55(6):724-5.

LONG QUESTIONS

1. Review current concepts in perinatal infections.
2. Review major perinatal pathogens and clinical problems.
3. Discuss examples of successful practices in prevention.
4. Discuss areas of possible intervention in settings with limited resources.

SHORT QUESTIONS

1. Describe the major causes of congenital and perinatal infections.
2. Describe the common means of transmission of the perinatal infections.
3. Describe the major manifestations of congenital and perinatal infections.
4. Describe how you diagnose and prevent these infections.
5. Describe the "important points to remember concerning congenital infections".

MULTIPLE CHOICE QUESTIONS

1. Which of the following condition is most common cause of perinatal morbidity and mortality?
   a. Congenital malformation
   b. Preterm delivery
   c. IUGR
   d. Infection
   e. Abnormal karyotype

2. A 22 year-old female patient 28 weeks gestation comes because of an increased vaginal discharge. She developed this symptom 2 days ago. She also complains of dysuria. She is sexually active with one partner and uses condoms intermittently. Examination reveals some erythema of the cervix but is otherwise unremarkable. A urine culture is sent which comes back negative. Sexually transmitted disease testing is performed and the patient is found to have gonorrhea. While treating this patient's gonorrhea infection, treatment must also be given for which of the following to prevent preterm labor?
   a. Bacterial vaginosis   b. Chlamydia
   c. Herpes   d. Syphilis
   e. Trichomoniasis

3. A 31-year-old primigravid woman comes for a prenatal visit. She is known to be HIV positive. Extensive counseling is given to the patient regarding vertical transmission of HIV to the fetus. It is recommended to her that she might take antiretroviral therapy during the pregnancy to decrease the vertical transmission rate. It is also recommended to her that she have a scheduled cesarean delivery. After consideration of these options, the patient chooses not to take the antiretrovirals and opts for a vaginal delivery. Which of the following represents the approximate risk of vertical transmission (from the mother to the fetus) for this patient?
   a. 2%   b. 8%
   c. 25%   d. 50%
   e. 100%

4. A 22-year-old woman, gravida 4, para 3, at 38 weeks' gestation comes to the labor and delivery ward with a gush of fluid. Sterile speculum examination reveals a pool of fluid that is nitrazine positive and forms ferns when viewed under the microscope. The fetal heart rate is in the 150 s and reactive. An ultrasound demonstrates that the fetus is in the breech position. A cesarean delivery is performed. During the operation, the physician, who has received no recent immunizations, is stuck with a needle that had been used on the patient. Which of the following is this physician at greatest risk of contracting?
   a. HIV   b. Hepatitis B
   c. Hepatitis C   d. Scabies
   e. Syphilis

5. A 39-year-old woman, gravida 4, para 3, comes for a prenatal visit. Her last menstrual period was 8 weeks ago. She has had no abdominal pain or vaginal bleeding. She has no medical problems. Examination is unremarkable except for an 8-week sized, nontender uterus. Among investigations sent VDRL came positive. Which of the following is the most appropriate pharmacotherapy?
   a. Erythromycin   b. Levofloxacin
   c. Metronidazole   d. Penicillin
   e. Tetracycline

6. All of the following statements are true about congenital rubella, except:
   a. It is diagnosed when the infant has IgM antibodies at birth
   b. It is diagnosed when IgG antibodies persist from more than 6 months
   c. Most common congenital defects are deafness, cardiac malformations and cataract
   d. Infection after 16 weeks of gestation results in major congenital defects
   e. Fetal Infection does not occur in immunized mother

7. The following marker is useful to prognosticate transmission from mother to fetus in hepatitis B infection:
   a. HbeAg   b. Anti-HBc IgG
   c. Anti-HBc IgM d. HBV-DNA
   e. HbsAg

8. WHO EPI schedule for developing countries for women of reproductive age:
   a. Tetanus
   b. Hepatitis B
   c. Rubella
   d. Typhoid
   e. Influenza
9. In cases of premature rupture of the membranes, chorioamnionitis should be suspected if:
   a. The maternal platelet count rises
   b. A leaking of fluid occurs per vaginum
   c. Maternal sweating occurs
   d. Fetal movements increases
   e. The fetal heart becomes tachycardic
10. The most common of all infections in pregnancy:
    a. Dental infections
    b. Fungal infections of skin
    c. Vaginal Candida infection
    d. Urinary tract infection
    e. Amebic infection
11. Indication for cesarean section in pregnant woman affected with HPV is:
    a. Presence of genital warts
    b. Giant warts obstructing the introitus
    c. To prevent JORRP
    d. H/O HPV in previous pregnancy
    e. HPV not vaccinated women

Answers

1. d 2. b 3. c 4. b 5. d 6. d
7. a 8. a 9. e 10. c 11. a

7.2 MULTIPLE PREGNANCY

Sanjay Singh, Parag Biniwale

INTRODUCTION

Pregnancy with more than one fetus is called multiple pregnancy that may result from the fertilization of two or more than two ovum or from the fertilization of a single ovum with the subsequent division of the zygote, or from the combination of the two. Multifetal pregnancy, on a rise largely because of infertility therapy, is a high risk pregnancy, even today. It poses a risk to the fetus in form of prematurity and its consequences, fetal anomalies and increased perinatal mortality and morbidity. The mother too faces very high risk of preeclampsia, postpartum hemorrhage, peripartum hysterectomy and maternal death. More the number of fetuses, higher are the rate of these complications. Hence, for optimization of the maternal as well as neonatal outcome, early diagnosis and a regular and evidence based antenatal care is of paramount importance.

INCIDENCE

The incidence of the multiple births rose significantly till 1998 in USA and all along the world.[1] However, it has declined to 1.43/1,000 total births since then, because of the evolving infertility management. The incidence of twin pregnancy rose steeply from 1980 to 2004, but has stabilized after that. Presently, the global incidence of twin pregnancy is 32.6/1,000 live births, i.e., 3.26%.[2]

The frequency of twin pregnancies varies among different countries and populations mostly due to the variation in dizygotic twinning. It is highest in Nigeria (1 in 20) and lowest in eastern countries (1 in 200 pregnancies). In India the incidence is about 1 in 80.

Hellin's law, also called *Hellin-Zeleny's law (1895)*, is used to guess the approximate rate of multiple births (dizygotic), which is one in 80^{n-1}, where n stands for number of fetuses: twin births occur about once per 80 singleton births, triplets about once per $80,^2$ quadruplets about once per $80,^3$ and so on.

Rate of monozygotic twining however is relatively constant (3.5–4 per 1,000 births/1 in 250) and its etiology has not yet been well understood. In contrast to dizygotic twins, it has got no ethnic variations.

MECHANISM OF MULTIFETAL GESTATIONS

Twin pregnancy in approximately 70% cases occurs as a result of fertilization of two ova with two sperm during a single ovarian cycle. This is known as dizygotic (DZ) twins/fraternal twins/binovular twins. In approximately 30% cases it results from fertilization of a single ovum that subsequently divides into two. This is called monozygotic (MZ) twins/uniovular twins/identical twins. Either or both processes may be involved in the formation of triplet/quadruplets or further higher number of pregnancies.

Superfecundation refers to fertilization of two different ova that has been released in the same menstrual cycle, by separate acts of coitus, in a short span of time. Since this may occur following assisted reproductive technology (ART), the woman should be advised not to have intercourse following transfer of the embryo. *Superfetation* on the other hand refers to fertilization of two ova released in different menstrual cycle. The implantation of the embryo and the development of one fetus over another is theoretically possible (known to occur in mares), till 12 weeks, when there is obliteration of the uterine cavity by fusion of decidua capsularis to the decidua parietalis.

Zygosity: Dizygotic versus Monozygotic Twinning

By zygosity we mean genetic makeup of the twin pregnancy. Since, dizygotic twins acquire genetic material from different ova and sperm; they are not considered true twins. They may resemble or differ like any of their sibling. Monozygotic twins since they share same genetic material are also called identical twins. However, as rule they may not be considered always identical. For example, after division of a single zygote into two, both may not carry the similar genetic material. Moreover, after division the post zygotic mutation may not be the same in both.

The ART procedure has significantly increased the incidence of dizygotic twins but has got only marginal effect (2-5 fold increase) on incidence of monozygotic twins. The inciting factor resulting in division of the zygote in monozygotics may be any of the following: specimen handling, growth media, sperm DNA microinjection. It may also arise from intrinsic abnormalities related to infertility.

Unlike dizygotic twins, monozygotic twins do not show ethnic variations. The monozygotic twins are associated with increased adverse perinatal outcome comparing dizygotic twins.

The timing of division of the zygote, in monozygotic twins, decides the outcome of monozygotic twinning, though it has not been proven in humans **(Table 1)**.[3]

Determining Zygosity

As the organ transplant is much in vogue now a day, determination of zygosity in twins is important. Zygosity may be predicted by fetal gender, type of placenta and genetic testing. DNA finger printing however is definitive method for confirmation of zygosity. **Table 2** gives the summary of determination of zygosity.

TABLE 1: Outcome of monozygotic twinning based on the timing of division of the zygote.

Timing of division of the zygote	Result	Frequency
Within first 72 hours	Two embryos, two amnions, two chorions, diamniotic dichorionic (DADC) twin. The placenta may be two or single in case it is fused	25–30%
Between 4th and 7th day	Two embryos, two amnions, one chorion, diamniotic and monochorionic (DAMC) twin pregnancy	70–75%
Between 8th and 12th day (the chorion and amnion already differentiated)	Two embryos in same amniotic sac, monochorionic monoamniotic (MCMA) twin pregnancy	1–2%
Between 13 and 16 day	Conjoint twins	Rare (1 in 200,000)

Chorionicity: Determination

Chorionicity implies the number of chorionic (outer) membranes that surround babies in a multiple pregnancy. Amnionicity on the other hand implies the number of amnions (inner membranes) that surround babies in a multiple pregnancy. Chorionicity is the main determinant of the perinatal outcome in twin pregnancies: perinatal mortality and morbidity are significantly higher in monochorionic than dichorionic twins. The chorionicity is best determined by USG **(Table 3)**. **Figure 1** shows a monochorionic twin.

The ideal time to determine chorionicity is the first trimester. First trimester transvaginal ultrasonography is highly reliable with a sensitivity rate of approximately 95–100%.

First Trimester USG

By using transvaginal sonography, as early as 4–5 weeks postmenstrual weeks, when gestational sac appear, by simply counting the chorionic sacs it is possible to establish whether the pregnancy will be monochorionic, dichorionic, trichorionic and so on **(Fig. 2)**. However at this period of gestation (POG) if only one sac is visualized, it does not exclude the possibility of a monochorionic twin. Hence, by 6th week when yolk sac

TABLE 2: Determination of zygosity.

Feature	Monozygotic	Dizygotic
Phenotype	Identical	Nonidentical
Genotype	Identical	Nonidentical
Gender	Same	Same or different
Placenta	One	Two (often fused)
Communicating vessels	Present	Absent
Intervening membranes	2 (amnions)	4 (2 amnions, 2 chorions)
DNA finger printing	Same	Differ
Skin grafting (Reciprocal)	Accept	Reject

TABLE 3: Determination of chorionicity by sonography.

Features	Dichorionic	Monochorionic
First trimester USG		
Gestational Sac	Two	One
Twin peak sign	Present	Absent
T-sign	Absent	Present
Second and third trimester		
Fetal gender	Identical	Identical/may differ
Placenta	Two	One
Dividing membrane	Three or four layers	Two layers
Thickness of dividing membrane	Thin (<2 mm)	Thick (>2 mm)

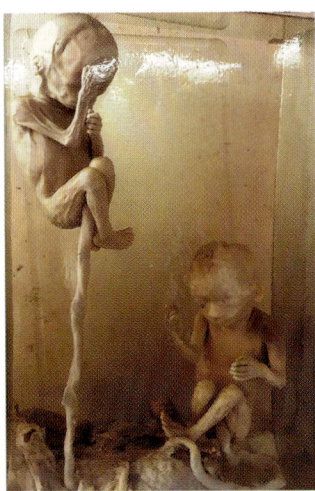

Fig. 1: Monochorionic twins.

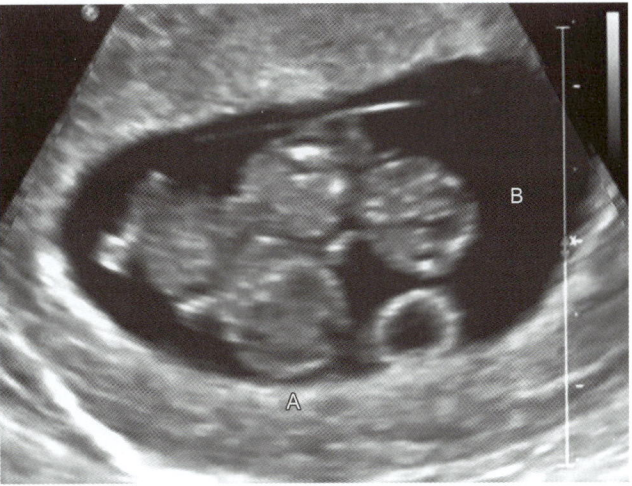

Fig. 3: Monoamniotic twins: Ultrasonography shows two fetuses in same gestational sac without any intervening membrane.

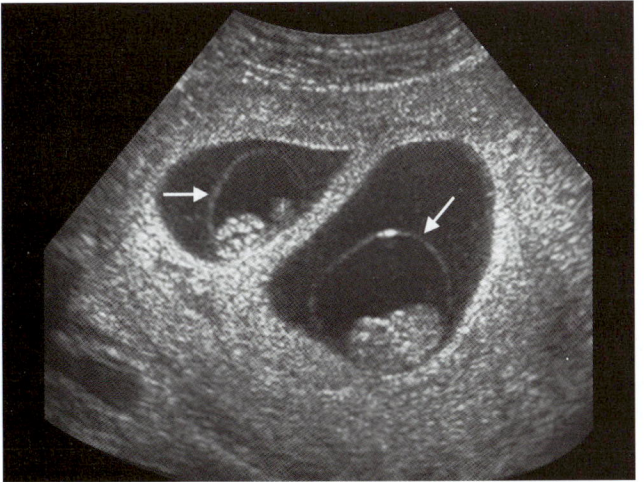

Fig. 2: Dichorionic twins. Ultrasonography at 7 weeks gestation showing two fetuses with thick intervening membrane.

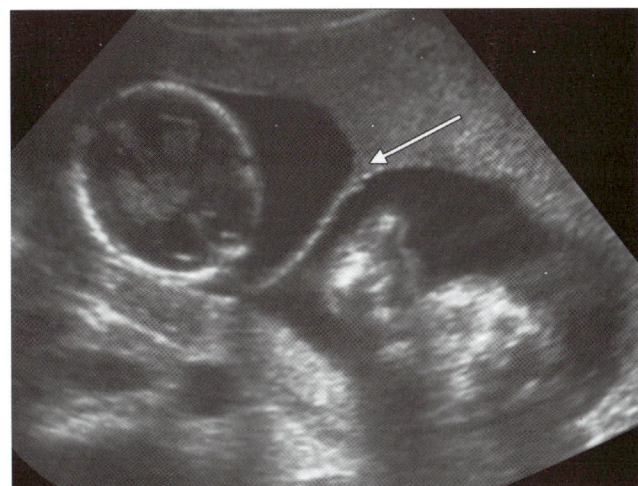

Fig. 4: A triangular projection of placenta is seen between two amnion layers near placental surface. This is *twin peak sign or lambda sign* present only in DC twins.

and the embryo can be seen inside the chorionic sac, the definitive diagnosis of a single pregnancy or monochorionic twin pregnancy can be done. That means, single chorionic sac containing two yolk sacs and two embryonic poles, will suggest monochorionic twin.

Because the amnion is still too close to the embryo, determination of amnionicity is difficult until 8 weeks of gestation. So even after 8 weeks, if the amniotic membrane is not visualized the diagnosis of monochorionic monoamniotic twins is confirmed **(Fig. 3)**. In this, depending on the time of cell division, the number of yolk sac seen may be one or two.

After 10 weeks of gestation, chorionicity is determined by the evaluation of the number of the placental masses and, in case of a single placental mass, by the characteristics of the membrane dividing the amniotic sacs. In DC twins with fused placentas, one may find a triangular projection of placenta between two amnion layers near placental surface. This is twin peak sign or lambda sign present only in DC twins **(Fig. 4)**. In MC twins, however, there is no such projection and both the layers of amnions are attached perpendicularly to placental surface, known as T sign **(Fig. 5)**. The sensitivity of these two tests have been reported ranging from 89.8 to 100%; the specificity ranging from 97.4 to 99.8%.[4] Evaluation of the number of layers of the intertwin membrane by TVS, (two layers in monochorionic and four layers in dichorionic), though mainly used in second and third trimester, has also been used to assess chorionicity in the first trimester. Second trimester assessment of chorionicity in the second and third trimester is problematic and the diagnostic accuracy is also lower than in the first trimester. The diagnosis relies on the evaluation of fetal gender, number of the placental masses and characteristics of the intertwin membrane.[5] Whereas, separate placental sites are an indicator of dichorionic twins, a single placental mass may be indication of both monochorionic and dichorionic twins with fused placentas. Hence, if single placenta has been seen, one must rely on other sonographic marker of chorionicity.

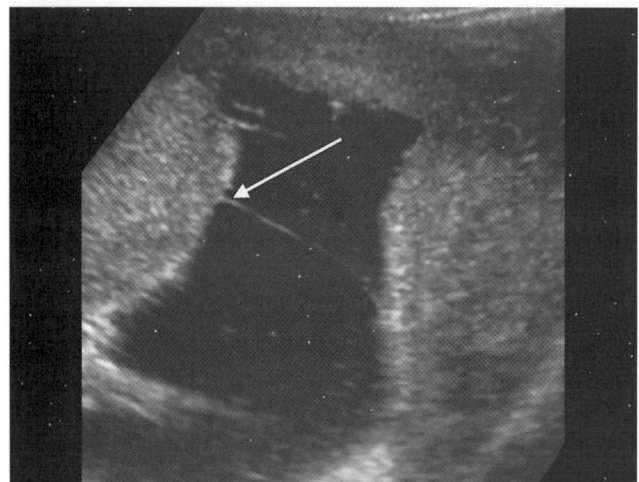

Fig. 5: T sign: In monochorionic twins there is no such projection and both the layers of amnions are attached perpendicularly to placental surface, known as *T sign*.

In the second and third trimester, the lambda sign and T sign has a limited diagnostic value as compared to the first trimester. Both the signs may be obscured by the fetus especially in third trimester and posteriorly attached placenta. Furthermore, as the pregnancy progresses the lambda sign may disappear as a result of the progressive regression of the chorion frondosum to form chorion leave. Thus, it may be concluded that presence of lambda sign suggests dichorionicity but its absence does not exclude the possibility.

The intertwin membrane thickness measured with high resolution ultrasound, is used to assess chorionicity. The DC membrane with four layers is thicker than MC membrane with two layers only. A cut off of 2 mm has been used for the differentiation. As the diagnostic sensitivity of membrane thickness reduces as gestation prolongs and as it is technically challenging, it has got limited value in determining chorionicity in the second and third trimesters.

Using high resolution equipment and magnified images, it is possible to recognize the layers. Counting more than two layers helps diagnose dichorionicity. As there is tinning of the membrane with progressing gestational age, the technique is more accurate in the second rather than the third trimester. As this technique is time consuming, technically difficult and operator dependent, counting of the layers in the inter-twin membrane is not commonly used in the clinical practice.

After delivery on examination of placenta, unlike MC twins where only two intervening layers of amnion is present, in DC twins one may note two amnions and two chorions (four layers) or two amnions and one fused chorion (three layers).

ETIOLOGY/FACTORS AFFECTING TWINNING

The etiology of the monozygotic twinning is not clearly known with an exception that its rate is marginally increased following ART. Unlike DZ twinning, its frequency is fairly constant (1 in 250 births) throughout the globe.

Dizygotic twinning is the more common variety and its incidence is influenced by maternal age, parity, nutrition, race, heredity and treatment for infertility.

Age: The chance of dizygotic twinning increases fourfold between the ages of 15 and 37 years.

Parity: In Nigerian population there is 8 fold rise in multifetal pregnancy with a parity of ≤4 and a 20-fold rise with a parity of ≥5.

Nutrition: It has been found that taller and heavier woman had 25–30% higher chance of having dizygotic twins than short and nutritionally deprived woman.

Race: The frequency is highest in Nigerians (1 in 20 births). Hispanic, Asian and Native American women have relatively lower rates than white woman.

Heredity: The risk of twinning is more if there is a family history of the mother than that of the father.

Use of oral contraceptive pills (OCPs): The risk of dizygotic twins increases in women who conceive within one month after stopping OCPs.

The increased level of FSH has been attributed as the causative factor, for high risk of dizygotic twins linked with age, parity, nutrition, race, heredity and use of OCPs.

Assisted reproductive techniques: Ovulation induction with FSH and hCG or clomiphene citrate has increased the chance of DZ twinning. During IVF procedures more the number of embryos transferred higher is the risk of DZ twinning. Recently, guidelines have been developed regarding the number of embryos to be transferred, in order to reduce the frequency of higher order pregnancy, which has fetched positive results.[6]

MATERNAL PHYSIOLOGICAL ADAPTATIONS/CHANGES

To accommodate more than one fetus, physiological changes during pregnancy gets multiplied, that increases the likelihood of maternal complications. Because of higher beta-hCG level in the first trimester the mother gets more nausea and vomiting comparing singleton pregnancy. In third trimester, because of substantial uterine growth, the mother may face cardiorespiratory embarrassment and the resultant iliac vein/venacaval compression predisposes her to develop swelling of legs, varicose veins and hemorrhoids. Over this, development of hydramnios predisposes her to obstructive uropathy. In view of relatively more expansion of blood volume (50–60%) comparing singleton pregnancy (40–50%), the stroke volume and cardiac output increases. This hypervolemia is very much needed to counter double the blood loss following vaginal delivery in twin than singleton pregnancy. Proportionately lesser rises in RBC count coupled with increased requirement of iron and folic acid, the mother develops anemia. In twin pregnancy, the diastolic blood pressure has been noted to be lower than singleton as early as by 8 weeks gestation. However, it rises to a greater degree at term. Throughout pregnancy the vascular resistance in twin gestation remains significantly low than singleton ones.

DIAGNOSIS OF MULTIFETAL GESTATION

To optimize the outcome of twin pregnancy, its detection at earliest possible opportunity, is important. Based only on clinical criteria however, the diagnosis of multifetal gestation is not reliable.[7] Twin pregnancy should be suspected on history and clinical examination and confirmed by USG.

History

History containing risk factors for twinning as mentioned earlier (advance maternal age, high parity, obesity, belonging to a specific race, conception in the first month of stopping OCP, maternal history of twins, and history of ovulation induction or ART) may suggest possibility of twin pregnancy. The mother having twin gestation may be found symptomatic with increased nausea and vomiting in first trimester, may have pressure symptoms because of over distended uterus in form of swelling of legs, bleeding hemorrhoids, varicose veins, breathlessness, GI symptoms and backache. She may also perceive excessive fetal movements.

Examination

On general examination, she may have pallor, pedal edema, abnormal weight gain and evidence of preeclampsia. On obstetric examination the abdomen is unduly enlarged and the fundal height is approximately 4–5 cm more than expected for that period of gestation for a singleton pregnancy. Palpation of multiple body parts, diagnostic of twin, may be obscured by obesity, polyhydramnios and one fetus overlying other. In lean and thin patient though, all the 4 poles (two cephalic and two podalic) may be palpable, palpation of only two heads or three poles are considered adequate for the diagnosis of twin pregnancy. Simultaneous auscultation of two fetal hearts, heard by two examiners with a difference of 10 beats, is considered diagnostic.

Sonography

Sonography can detect almost all types of multiorder pregnancy. Apart from detecting twin at a very early gestation, it is used to estimate fetal number, gestational age, chorionicity and amnionicity. Later, ideally two fetal heads or two abdomens should be visualized in the same image plane, in order to prevent identifying the same fetus twice and presuming it to be a twin gestation.

Ultrasonography also plays a crucial role in detection of fetal anomalies, assessment of fetal growth and wellbeing, measurement of cervical length, diagnosis of malpresentation and assisting certain obstetric procedures e.g. selective termination or selective fetal reduction, amniocentesis, amnioreduction and septostomy.

Radiography and Magnetic Resonance Imaging

As the fetal skeletal system are not adequately radiopaque before 18 weeks and as fetuses may move at the time of radiography, radiographs by and large has very limited utility in diagnosing twin. MRI is generally not used to diagnose twin pregnancy; however, it is a useful tool for detection of various complications in monochorionic twin.

Biochemical Tests

In twin pregnancy, the maternal serum beta-hCG, α-fetoprotein and unconjugated estriol are generally higher than that of a singleton pregnancy, however these biological markers do not reliably diagnose twin pregnancy.

PREGNANCY COMPLICATIONS

Maternal Complications

Maternal complications may occur during antenatal, intrapartum and postpartum period.

Antenatal Complications

Excessive nausea and vomiting: Because of higher beta-hCG level in the first trimester the mother gets more nausea and vomiting comparing singleton pregnancy.

Spontaneous abortion: The rate of spontaneous abortion in twin pregnancy is 7.3% per live birth, which is higher than singleton pregnancy (0.9%). 1 in 8 pregnancies though begin with twin, but are spontaneously reduced. Monochorionic twins and twins conceived post IVF, have higher rate of spontaneous abortion. It must be noted that the spontaneous abortion of one of the twin may alter prenatal diagnostic tests including cell free dNA (cfdna), by altering levels of several serum analytes used for the test. Curnow KJ et al. suggest that single-nucleotide polymorphism-based noninvasive prenatal testing (NIPT) is useful to identify triploid, unrecognized twin, and vanishing twin pregnancies.[8]

Anemia: Proportionately less rise in RBC mass comparing plasma volume and increased requirement of folic acid and iron, leads to development of anemia, usually dimorphic in nature.

Pregnancy related hypertension: With an incidence of around 20%, development of preeclampsia is three times more in twin pregnancy than singleton gestation. Fetal number and placental mass are in the root of genesis of preeclampsia. The hypertension develops at early gestation and tends to be more severe in nature with multiple pregnancies.

Hydramnios: Occurs in around 5% of twin pregnancies. They are more common in monozygotic twins, having abnormal placental vascular communication leading to twin to twin transfusion syndrome. The twin that gets more blood produces more urine. Development of acute polyhydramnios may occur at or around 28 weeks of gestation.

Antepartum hemorrhage (APH): Slightly increased incidence of placenta previa and abruptio placenta increases the risk of APH in twin pregnancy. The bigger placental mass because of fused placentas or because of overcrowding one of the placentas may be attached to lower uterine segment, giving rise to placenta previa in twin. The increased incidence of abruptio is mainly because of increased incidence of preeclampsia in twin pregnancy. However, deficiency of folic acid, sudden decompression of uterus after rupture of membrane in polyhydramnios cases, premature separation of placenta following delivery of first twin, may also increase the risk of abruptio in twin.

Pressure symptoms: In third trimester, because of substantial uterine growth, the mother may face cardiorespiratory embarrassment and the resultant iliac veins/vena caval compression predisposes her to develop swelling of legs, varicose veins, and hemorrhoids. The exaggerated lordosis gives rise to backache. Dyspepsia and early satiety is because of displacement and pressure on gastrointestinal (GI) tract.

Malpresentation: More so in the second fetus, is quite common in twins than singleton pregnancies.

Preterm Birth

The duration of gestation reduces as the fetal number increases. The mean gestational age for the delivery of twin is 36 weeks. Almost 40–70% of the twins are delivered preterm out of which 50% are indicated and induced birth, 30% are the result of spontaneous labor and 10% birth occur because of premature rupture of membranes.[9] The risk is higher in MC pregnancies. Around one-third of the twin pregnancy cases result from intra-amniotic infection. Since preterm birth is most important cause of perinatal mortality its prediction and prevention is important, to improve perinatal outcome.

Prediction

Cervical (Cx) length measurement has been considered as a good predictor of preterm labor in singleton and twin pregnancy. Conde-Augudelo et al., in their review have found out that a Cx length of 20 mm at 20–24 weeks' gestation is most accurate parameter for predicting preterm labor before 34 weeks with a specificity of 97%.[10] Melamed et al. have concluded that serial cervical measurement (every 2–3 weeks between 14–18 weeks and 28–32 weeks of gestation) is more useful than single measurement for predicting preterm labor in asymptomatic women.[11] Some suggest that addition of maternal serum fetal fibronectin with cervical length improves the predictability of preterm. McMahon et al. based on their study opined that at 24 weeks of gestation, a normal digital examination (closed internal os) is equally effective predictor of delivery at >32 weeks of gestation in twin, as a negative fetal fibronectin level, a normal cervical length on sonographic scan, or the combination of a negative fetal fibronectin level and a normal cervical length. However, Gordon et al. suggest that routine second-trimester transvaginal ultrasound assessment of cervical length is not associated with improved outcomes.[12]

Prevention

A number of strategies have been proposed to prevent preterm deliveries: Hospitalization, bed rest, tocolytics, home uterine activity monitoring, cerclage, and most recently, progesterone. Unfortunately, none have been proved to be effective.

Crowther et al. in their meta-analysis opine that there is currently not enough evidence to support a policy of routine hospitalization for bed rest in multiple pregnancies and it does not reduce the risk of preterm birth or perinatal death.[13] However, patients with twin pregnancy may require admission for specific reasons such as preeclampsia and threatened preterm labor. Little evidence suggest that limited physical activity, frequent ante natal visits and serial sonography examinations, may have some role in prevention of preterm birth in twin pregnancy.

Evidences are lacking to support the view that long-term prophylactic tocolysis may prevent preterm birth. In fact injudicious use of beta-sympathomimetic in twin pregnancy may lead to iatrogenic pulmonary edema in the pregnant mother, hence it is condemned. Short time use of tocolytic during preterm labor, for giving the benefit to corticosteroid for lung maturity to act, may have some role.

Adequately powered studies suggest that weekly injection of intramuscular 17 alpha-hydroxyprogesterone caproate (17-OHP-C) is not effective in preventing preterm labor in cases of twin pregnancy even to those with short cervix.[14]

Vaginal insertion of micronized progesterone in order to prevent preterm delivery in twin has got conflicting report. Whereas few of the studies have found this practice (vaginal insertion of 100 or 200 mg of micronized progesterone) useful,[15] several other studies have failed to demonstrate this beneficial effect.[16] Prophylactic cervical cerclage in unindicted cases as well as cases with sonographically proven short cervix has been found to be of no benefit.[17] However, few of the studies suggest a role of rescue cerclage in second trimester twin pregnancy with dilated cervix.[18]

Though few of the studies talk about beneficial role of vaginal pessary in prevention of preterm labor by encircling and compressing the cervix;[19] ACOG (2016) does not recommend this to be used for prevention of preterm in twin.[7]

Treatment of Preterm Labor

Like singleton pregnancy, corticosteroid for acceleration of lung maturity is indicated in women with twin pregnancy in preterm labor. Short-term tocolytics in established preterm labor may prolong pregnancy, so that corticosteroid given for the lung maturity may work. Limited physical activity, light work, regular antenatal visits and serial sonography evaluation may have some role.

Intrapartum and Postpartum Complications

Because of high incidence of malpresentation there is increased risk of pre labor rupture of membrane (PROM), cord prolapse (five times more than singleton), increased operative vaginal delivery and cesarean section. Labor may get prolonged because of over distension of the uterus, needing labor augmentation. Premature separation of placenta following delivery of first twin may lead to APH. Inadequate uterine contractions, because of overdistended uterus, may cause atonic PPH and retained placenta. There is increased risk of postpartum infection because of increased operative interference, preexisting anemia, and larger raw area in the decidua underneath larger placenta. Risk of subinovulation of the uterus because of its overdistension during antenatal period, lactational difficulties and thromboembolism is more in twins than singleton pregnancies.

Fetal Complications

Fetal complications are relatively more in twins that result in high perinatal mortality and morbidity. Fetal complications occur both in monozygotic as well as dizygotic twin pregnancy, however certain unique complications occur only in monozygotic twin.

Common Fetal Complications (Mono- and Dizygotic Twins)

Congenital anomalies: The congenital malformation rate in twins has been reported as 4.06% comparing 2.38% in singleton pregnancy. It is two times more in monozygotic than dizygotic twins. The rate of anomalies in dizygotic twins has also risen over a period of time because of increased availability of ART and it is now well-known that infants conceived after ART had a higher prevalence of certain birth defects.[20]

Fetal growth restriction: More the number of fetuses more are the risk of growth restriction. Ideally parameters of growth of multiorder pregnancies and not singleton pregnancy are to be taken in account to identify these fetuses. Twins grow like their singleton counterpart till 28–30 weeks, thereafter their growth start lagging. Monozygotics have more growth lag because of unequal distribution of blastomere, abnormal vascular anastomosis within placenta with unequal nutrient supply and structural anomaly in one fetus. In dizygotic twins on the other hand growth discordancy may occur because of unequal placental mass, different genetic growth potential of the fetuses, umbilical cord abnormalities, e.g., vasa previa, velamentous insertion or marginal insertion, fetal malformations or infections. Prematurity as discussed above, prematurity rate is quite high in twin pregnancy and is an important cause perinatal mortality and morbidity.

Asphyxia and stillbirth: Because of increased incidence of preeclampsia, malpresentation, abruption placentae, malpresentation and increased operative interference the risk of asphyxia and stillbirth is more common among twins, especially monochorionic twins.

Long-term fetal consequences: Normal birth weight twin fetuses like their single counterpart have similar cognitive outcomes. However, it has been noticed that the cerebral palsy rate is higher in twins and other higher order gestation than singleton pregnancy, among normal birth weight neonates.[21] This high risk is probably because of fetal growth lag, congenital anomalies, TTTS or fetal demise of a cotwin.

COMPLICATIONS UNIQUE TO MONOZYGOTIC TWINS

As has been emphasized most of the fetal complications in twins occur in cases of monozygotic twins. Few of the unique complications related to MZ twins are discussed here.

Monoamniotic Twins

Its incidence is approximately 1% of all monozygotic twins. The risk of fetal death is as high as 70% that occurs because of spontaneous abortions, fetal anomalies, cord entanglement, preterm birth or twin–twin transfusion syndrome (TTTS). In monoamniotic twins congenital anomaly rate is 18–20% with very high risk of cardiac anomalies for which fetal echocardiogram is recommended. Only one-fourth of these twins may have similar anomalies, highlighting the fact that absence of anomaly in one fetus does not deny the presence in other. Since both twins are genetically identical, both or none of the fetuses may have similar chromosomal abnormalities. Screening for the Down syndrome is similar to that of singleton pregnancy.

Comparing MCDA, MCMA twins have fewer incidences of TTTS, probably because of almost universal presence of arterioarterial anastomoses, which are considered protective.

Umbilical cord entanglement is quite frequent **(Fig. 6)**. If cord entanglement occurs early, the morbidity and mortality of the fetuses are high. However, if pregnancy successfully crosses 30–32 weeks the risk is reduced. The perinatal mortality rate in monoamniotic twins is 17%. Color flow Doppler sonography can detect it. Women with MCMA pregnancy may be admitted at 26–28 weeks or may be called on OPD basis for 1 hour daily fetal heart rate monitoring. Injection corticosteroid exhibition is to be done for fetal lung maturity. These patients need elective cesarean at 32–34 weeks.[7]

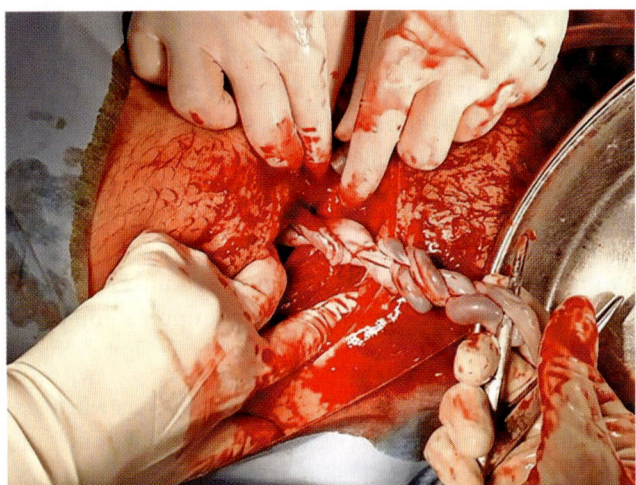

Fig. 6: Cord entanglement in a case of monoamniotic twin.

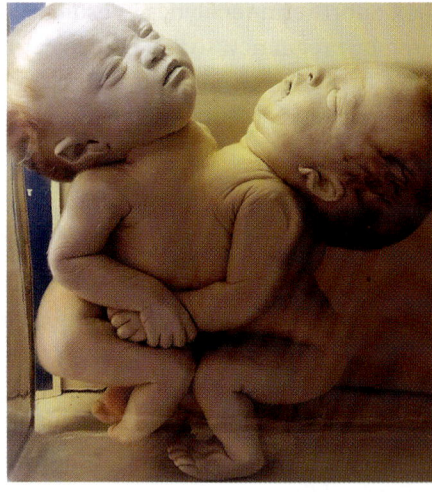

Fig. 7: Conjoint twin: Conjoint twins are joined at the level of thorax.

Aberrant Twinning

This implies incomplete splitting of an embryo into two separate twins or early secondary fusion of two separate embryos. These separate embryos are either symmetrical or asymmetrical whereas symmetrical monozygotic twins may be separate or conjoint, asymmetrical monozygotic twins may be external acardiac, external parasitic or internal fetus in fetu.

Conjoined Twins

The incidence of conjoint twin also called Siamese twins-after Chang and Bunker of Siam, located in Thailand, is a rare entity (1 in 60,000) with very high mortality. The twins may be connected at any level and it is named after which body parts are joint or shared. Thoracophagus is the most common variety **(Fig. 7)**. It may be identified by USG at mid pregnancy. Identification during first trimester is also possible. MRI is more sensitive especially in later trimester when liquor is less and there is crowding of fetal parts. It also clearly demonstrates the sharing organs. Surgical separation after birth is possible provided vital organs are not shared. Viable conjoint twins or mature fetuses are delivered by cesarean. In cases of premature conjoint twins vaginal delivery may be possible as union is most often pliable.

External Parasitic Twin

Grossly defective fetus or merely fetal parts (supernumerary limbs with some viscera) are attached externally to a relatively normal twin. Typically, however, brain and heart are absent. Parasite results from its demise with its surviving tissue attached to and is vascularized by normal twin. It accounts for 4% of all conjoint twins and more in male fetuses.

Fetus in Fetu

This occurs when early in development one of the fetuses is enfolded within its twin. However, they cannot normally grow and their normal development gets arrested in first trimester. Classically vertebral and axial bones are found without any heart or brain. These masses are supported by their host by large parasitic vessels.

Twin Reversed Arterial Perfusion Sequence/ Acardiac twin

The incidence of twin reversed arterial perfusion sequence (TRAP) is 1 in 35,000. It is a complication of monochorionic multifetal gestation wherein single placenta is shared. It occurs between a well-formed donor twin that develops heart failure and recipient twin that lacks a heart and other structure. It is caused by large artery to artery and also vein to vein shunt. Arterial perfusion pressure in donor twin is more than recipient twin, who thus receives reverse blood flow of deoxygenated arterial blood from its co twin. This "used" arterial blood reaches the recipient twin through its umbilical arteries and preferentially goes to its iliac vessels thus only lower body is perfused, leading to disrupted growth of upper body. Failure of growth of head is called acardius acephalus. Partially developed head is known as acardius myelacephalus and failure of any recognizable structure is recognized as acardius amorphous. Donor twin pumps blood for self and cotwin, resulting in cardiomegaly and high output failure. The risk of fetal demise was more than 50% in the past. Risk appears to be directly related to the size of acardiac twin. Treatment of choice is radio frequency ablation, done at around 20 weeks of gestation. The outcome of TRAP sequence occurring in monoamniotic pregnancy is poorer than that in MCDA pregnancy.

Monochorionic Twins with Vascular Anastomosis

All monochorionic placentas share some vascular anastomosis **(Fig. 8)**, whose number (median number of anastomosis being 8), size and direction varies considerably.[22] Artery to artery anastomosis located at chorionic surface of monochorionic

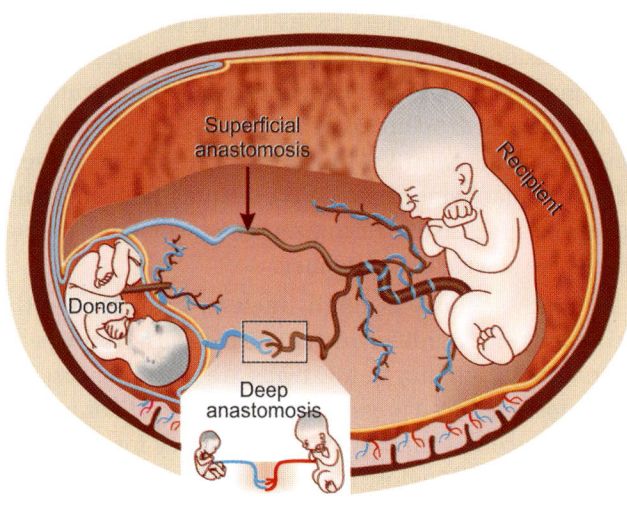

Fig. 8: Twin to twin transfusion syndrome. Showing anastomoses between donor and recipient twin.

twin placenta, are most common (75% cases). Artery to vein and vein to vein anastomosis each is found in 50%. One vessel may have several communications-at times to artery as well as to vein. Apart from these superficial connections over the surface of chorion, deep artery to vein communications may also exist in 50% of the cases. This deep communication creates a common villous compartment also known as third circulation. Harmful effect of these anastomoses to the fetus depends on degree to which they are hemodynamically balanced. Those with significant pressure gradient may develop a shunt between two fetuses. This chronic transfusion may result in several clinical problems; twin–twin transfusion syndrome (TTTS), twin anemia polycythemia syndrome (TAPS), TRAP/acardiac twinning.

Twin–Twin Transfusion Syndrome

The prevalence of TTTS is around 1–3/10,000 births.[23] In this syndrome the donor twin pumps blood to the recipient twin as a consequence of which the donor twin becomes anemic and growth restricted whereas the recipient twin becomes polycythemic and develops circulatory overload, heart failure, and fetal hydrops.

The donor and the donor side placenta become pale and the recipient and the recipient side placenta become plethoric. Recipient neonate after birth shows features of circulatory overload, heart failure, polycythemia, hyperviscosity, hyperbilirubinemia and kernicterus.

The pathogenesis of TTTS is not yet been clearly understood and is more complex. The problem is presumed to result from unidirectional flow through deep arteriovenous anastomosis. If this unidirectional flow is not compensated through superficial arterioarterial anastomosis—this unidirectional flow leads to imbalance in blood volume between both fetuses. This syndrome typically manifests in mid pregnancy. The donor because of hypovolemia becomes oliguric leading to oligohydramnios which prevents movement of the fetus giving it a name; stuck twin. This fetus becomes growth restricted and oligohydramnios may result in contracture and pulmonary hypoplasia. Recipient twin on the other hand, because of development of hypervolemia may develop heart failure. It produces more urine resulting in polyhydramnios that puts this fetus under the risk of PROM too. Because of disparity in amniotic fluid level, this syndrome is also called polyhydramnios oligohydramnios syndrome.

Fetal brain damage such as cerebral palsy, microcephaly, multicystic encephalomalacia is associated with vascular anastomosis. However the exact cause is not known. The likely cause is ischemic necrosis leading to cavitary brain lesions. Donor-ischemia results from hypotension, anemia or both. Recipient ischemia results from-blood pressure instability and episodes of severe hypotension. If one twin dies, cerebral pathology in survivor results from acute hypotension, as a result of acute transfusion of blood from high pressure vessels of living fetus to low resistance vessels of the dead fetus. Emboli originating from dead fetus appear to be the less likely cause. The risk of neurodevelopmental problem following single fetal demise is more in monochorionic twins (26%) than 2% dichorionic twins.[24] This morbidity is also related to gestational age of one of the twins at the time of death. Death occurring at an earlier POG (28–33 Weeks) has a higher risk of neurodevelopmental problem than that occurring (>34 weeks). The onset of hypotension following death of one twin with TTTS may be so quick that successful intervention for survivor becomes impossible. The clinical implication is that in absence of another indication, immediate delivery of live twin is not beneficial. Previous criteria for diagnosing and classifying TTS by taking in account the weight and Hb difference has been discarded as these are considered late manifestations of the problem. As per Society for Maternal Fetal Med (SMFM) 2013, two sonographic criteria are considered for this purpose: first one is diagnosis of MCDA twins and second one is the diagnosis of polyhydramnios (largest vertical pocket >8 cm) or oligohydramnios (largest vertical pocket <2 cm).[23] So that the problem is detected earlier, it is recommended that ultrasonography (USG) in high risk group should be done first at 16 weeks and then every 2 weeks.[7,23] Once identified TTTS is staged as per Quintero staging system as described in **Table 4**.[25]

The prognosis depends on Quintero stage and gestational age of the twins. In Stage 1, more than three-fourths remain stable and regress without intervention. However, Stage 3–5 has worse prognosis with a perinatal loss of 70–100% without intervention.

Several therapies such as serial amnioreduction, laser ablation of vascular anastomoses and selective feticide have been recommended as treatment for TTTS. Septostomy is no more practiced now a day. For Stage 1, the optimal treatment is controversial and for Stage 2–4, laser ablation is preferred modality with surveillance.

TABLE 4: Quintero staging: Staging of severity of TTTS based on sonographic and Doppler findings.

Stage	USG feature
Stage 1	Discordant amniotic fluid volume but urine still visible sonographically in bladder of the donor twin
Stage 2	Criteria of Stage 1, but no urine in bladder
Stage 3	Criteria of Stage 2 and abnormal Doppler studies of umbilical artery, ductus venosus, or umbilical vein
Stage 4	Ascites or frank hydrops in either twin
Stage 5	Demise of either fetus

Selective reduction is done in case severe oligohydramnios and IUGR develops before 20 weeks of gestation. Since use of drug to kill one fetus may harm other also because of shared circulation, several other methods instead are used to occlude circulation. These include umbilical vein or umbilical cord occlusion by radiofrequency ablation, fetoscopic ligation/laser ablation and mono or bipolar cauterization. Even after these procedures, risk to remaining fetus is still high.

Twin Anemia Polycythemia Sequence

It implies significant Hb difference between donor and recipient twins without discrepancies in amniotic fluid volume typical of TTTS. It is diagnosed when middle cerebral artery (MCA) peak systolic velocity (PSV) is >1.5 MoM in recipient twin.[23] It has got two verities–(1) spontaneous (develops after 26 weeks) and (2) iatrogenic that develops after laser photocoagulation (within 5 weeks of procedure). Further studies required to guess its natural history and management.

HYDATIDIFORM MOLE WITH COEXISTING NORMAL FETUS/TWIN MOLAR PREGNANCY

The prevalence of one twin with complete molar pregnancy coexisting with a normal cotwin is 1 in 22,000 to 1 in 100,000 pregnancies. This case needs to be distinguished from a single partial molar pregnancy (usually triploid) with its abnormal associated fetus. There also exists a possibility of having a normal fetus in one sac and a partial molar pregnancy in another. The optimal management of this problem is not known. If the diagnosis is made in first half of pregnancy, it may be terminated. For karyotypically normal and nonanomalous fetus, declining beta-hCG level and no early preeclampsia, pregnancy continuation is recommended. However, preterm delivery is frequently required in view of development of severe preeclampsia or APH. Risk of development of placental site trophoblastic tumor (PSTT) is same as singleton.

DISCORDANT GROWTH OF TWIN FETUSES

Fifteen percent twins may have discordant growth, resulting in abnormal growth restriction in one of the twins. As the weight difference between two twins increase, perinatal mortality rate increases proportionately. Since single placenta is not equally shared in MC twins, these twins have greater discordant growth outside of TTTS than DC twins. Restricted growth in one twin develops late in the second or early third trimester. Discordant growth before 20 weeks carries higher risk of fetal demise in smaller twin (20%). Incidence of respiratory distress, intraventricular hemorrhage (IVH), seizures, periventricular leukomalacia, sepsis and necrotizing enterocololitis increases with degree of weight discordancy.

Etiopathogenesis is often unclear. Etiology for the discordancy in MC is different than DC twins. The responsible factors for discordancy in MC twins are placental vascular anastomosis, reduced pressure and perfusion of donor twin, unequal placental sharing and discordancy for structural anomalies. In DC twins, discordancy in growth may be because of different genetic growth potential, suboptimal of one placenta, uterine crowding and histological placental abnormality. Discordancy in weight is calculated by sonography. Some diagnose selective fetal growth restriction if abdominal circumference that reflects fetal nutrition differs by >20 mm or if effective fetal weight difference is 20% or more. Percent discordancy helps in prediction of adverse perinatal outcome which is calculated as weight of larger twin minus the weight of smaller twin divided by weight of larger twin. A weight discordancy of >25–30% is associated with adverse perinatal outcome. The relative risk of fetal death is 5.6 if percent discordancy is >30% and 18.9 if it is >40%.

Since growth restricted fetus is at a risk of fetal demise, sonographic monitoring of growth is crucial in the management. Presence of oligohydramnios helps gauging fetal risk. MC twins are monitored more frequently as risk of death (3.6% vs. 1.1%) and neurological damage is more than DC twins. Though there is no uniformity in thought process, some recommend serial USG evaluation at every 2 weeks in both monochorionic,[23] and DC twins.[26] However, ACOG guidelines 2016 recommends that the indications for antenatal fetal wellbeing assessment for the twin fetuses remains the same as is there for singleton pregnancy. Based on degree of discordancy and period of gestation, frequency of fetal surveillance may be increased. Nonstress tests (NST), biophysical profile (BPP), umbilical artery Doppler all have been suggested to assess fetal wellbeing. Optimal time of delivery has not yet been established for these twins and delivery is not prompted by size discordancy alone.

FETAL DEMISE

One or both may die either simultaneously or sequentially. Causes and incidence of fetal demise are related to zygosity, chorionicity and growth concordance.

Death of One Fetus

Prognosis of live cotwin depends on time of demise of another twin, chorionicity, time between demise and delivery.

Death in early pregnancy results in vanishing twin. Death in slightly advanced gestation, i.e., after 1st trimester results in fetus compressus or fetus papyraceous (conspicuously flat due to desiccation: **Figure 9**). Risk of still birth is higher before 32 weeks. The risk of fetal demise is much higher for MC than DC twins. After demise of one twin the odds of cotwin demise is five times higher in MC than DC twins. With demise of vanishing twin the risk of death is not increased for survivor. Cotwin demise rate remains unaffected regardless of gestational age at time of death of other twin.[24] However, odds of preterm birth (spontaneous/iatrogenic) for the remaining twin are increased. It is more for MC twin if death has occurred between 28 and 32 weeks and same for both (MC and DC) for death beyond 34 weeks. Neurological prognosis for a surviving twin depends almost exclusively on chorionicity (18% MC vs. 1% DC). For a fetal demise before 34 weeks, there is fivefold increased risk of neurological developmental morbidity in MC twin. After 34 weeks it is same for both (MC and DC). Coagulopathy is rare after single fetal demise.

Management is based on gestational age, cause of death and risk to surviving fetus. Vanishing twin is harmless to survivor (**Fig. 10**). In cases of loss after 1st trimester, the risk of death or damage is to MC twins. Morbidity in MC twin survivor is almost always due to vascular anastomosis which often causes demise of one twin followed by sudden hypotension in other. If one MC twin dies before age of viability termination of pregnancy can be considered. If death of one DC twin has occurred due to discordant anomaly, pregnancy can be continued. In case of single fetal demise after late 2nd or early 3rd trimester, risk of subsequent death or neurological damage is more for MC twins. Risk of preterm birth is equally increased for both (DC and MC). Delivery generally occurs within 3 weeks. Corticosteroid for fetal lung maturity is to be exhibited and pregnancy is to be continued unless intrauterine environment becomes hostile. Timing of delivery after conservative management of a late 2nd and early 3rd trimester single fetal demise is a matter of debate. DC twins can be safely delivered at term whereas MC twins should be delivered by 34–37 weeks gestation.[27] In case of death at term delivery can be expedited.

KEY MESSAGES

- Multifetal pregnancy, especially dizygotic twin, on a rise largely because of infertility therapy, is a high risk pregnancy.
- It poses a risk to the fetus in form of prematurity and its consequences, fetal anomalies and increased perinatal mortality and morbidities.
- The mother too faces very high risk of preeclampsia, postpartum hemorrhage, peripartum hysterectomy and maternal death.
- Dizygotic twinning is the more common variety and its incidence unlike monozygotic twin is influenced

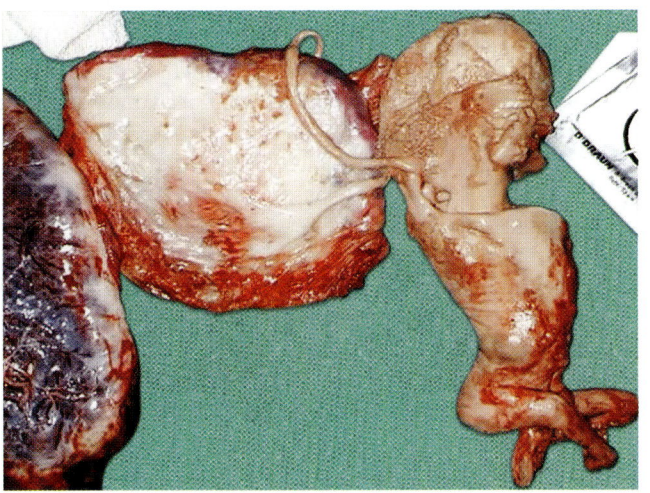

Fig. 9: Fetus papyraceous.

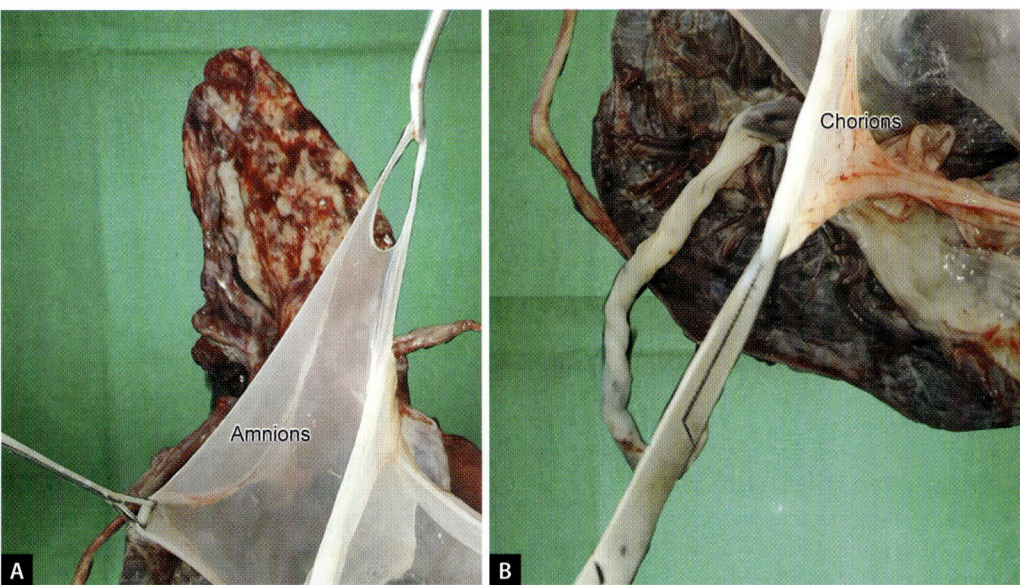

Figs. 10A and B: Dichorionic diamniotic placenta showing two amnions and two chorions.

- by maternal age, parity, nutrition, race, heredity and treatment for infertility.
- Zygosity can be convincingly ascertained by DNA finger printing.
- Diagnosis of chorionicity, done in first and or second trimester by USG, is essential, to predict maternal and perinatal outcome and planning management. Monochorionic twins have more complications.
- To accommodate more than one fetus, physiological changes during pregnancy gets multiplied, that increases the likelihood of maternal complications.
- Diagnosis of twin pregnancy is based on history, obstetric examination and sonography.
- Most of the fetal complications in twins occur in cases of monozygotic twins. Few of the unique complications related to MZ twins are: monoamniotic twins, aberrant twinning mechanism (conjoint twins, external acardiac twin-Reversed Arterial Perfusion Sequence, external parasitic twin, internal fetus in fetus), monochorionic twins with vascular anastomosis (twin to twin transfusion syndrome, twin anemia polycythemia syndrome, acardiac twinning).
- The risk of fetal death in monoamniotic twin is as high as 70% that occurs because of spontaneous abortions, fetal anomalies, cord entanglement, preterm birth or TTTS. They should be frequently monitored and delivered at 32–34 weeks by elective cesarean section.
- TTTS is presumed to result from uncompensated unidirectional flow through deep placental arteriovenous anastomosis. The donor twin becomes growth restricted and develops oligohydramnios. Laser ablation of the communicating vessels is useful.
- Early diagnosis of discordant growth is important in order to optimize the management of growth restricted fetus.
- In case of single fetal demise prognosis of live cotwin depends on time of demise of another twin, chorionicity and time between demise and delivery.

REFERENCES

1. ACOG Practice Bulletin No. 144: Multifetal gestations: twin, triplet, and higher-order multifetal pregnancies. Obstet Gynecol. 2014;123(5):1118-32.
2. Martin JA, Hamilton BE, Osterman MJK. Births in the United States, 2018. NCHS Data Brief. 2019:1-8.
3. Blikstein I, Keith LG. On the possible cause of monozygotic twinning: lessons from the 9-banded armadillo and from assisted reproduction. Twins Res Hum Genet. 2007;10:394-9.
4. Dias T, Arcangeli T, Bhide A, Napolitano R, Mahsud-Dornan S, Thilaganathan B. First-trimester ultrasound determination of chorionicity in twin pregnancy. Ultrasound Obstet Gynecol, 2011;38:530-2.
5. Monteagudo A, Timor-Tritsch IE. Second- and third-trimester ultrasound evaluation of chorionicity and amnionicity in twin pregnancy. A simple algorithm. J Reprod Med. 2000;45:476-80.
6. American Society for Reproductive Medicine, Society for Assisted Reproductive Technology: Guidance on the limits to the number of embryos to transfer: a committee opinion. Fertil Steril. 2017;107(4):901-3.
7. American College of Obstetricians and Gynecologists. Multifetal Gestations: Twin, Triplet, and Higher-Order Multifetal Pregnancies. Practice Bulletin No. 169, Washington DC: ACOG; 2016.
8. Curnow KJ, Wilkins-Haug L, Ryan A. Detection of triploid, molar, and vanishing twin pregnancies by a single-nucleotide polymorphism-based noninvasive prenatal test. Am J Obstet Gynecol. 2015;212(1):79.e1-9.
9. Chauhan SP, Scardo JA, Hayes E, Abuhamad AZ, Berghella V. Twins: prevalence, problems, and preterm births. Am J Obstet Gynecol. 2010;203(4):305-15.
10. Conde-Agudelo A, Romero R, Hassan SS, Yeo L. Transvaginal sonographic cervical length for the prediction of spontaneous preterm birth in twin pregnancies: a systematic review and meta-analysis. Am J Obstet Gynecol. 2010;203(2):128.
11. Melamed N, Pittini A, Hiersch L, Yogev Y, Korzeniewski SJ, Romero R, et al. Do serial measurements of cervical length improve the prediction of preterm birth in asymptomatic women with twin gestations? Am J Obstet Gynecol. 2016;215(5):616.e1-616.
12. Gordon MC, McKenna DS, Stewart TL, Howard BC, Foster KF, Higby K, et al. Transvaginal cervical length scans to prevent prematurity in twins: a randomized controlled trial. Am J Obstet Gynecol. 2016;214(2):277.e1-277.
13. Crowther CA, Han S. Hospitalisation and bed rest for multiple pregnancy. Cochrane Database Syst Rev. 2010;(7).
14. Senat MV, Porcher R, Winer N, Vayssière C. Prevention of preterm delivery by 17 alpha-hydroxyprogesterone caproate in asymptomatic twin pregnancies with a short cervix: a randomized controlled trial. Am J Obstet Gynecol. 2013;208(3):194.
15. Romero R, Conde-Agudelo A, El-Refaie W. Vaginal progesterone decreases preterm birth and neonatal morbidity and mortality in women with a twin gestation and a short cervix: an updated meta-analysis of individual patient data. Ultrasound Obstet Gynecol. 2017;49(3):303-14.
16. Rode L, Klein K, Nicolaides KH, et al: Prevention of preterm delivery in twin gestations (PREDICT): a multicenter, randomized, placebo-controlled trial on the effect of vaginal micronized progesterone. Ultrasound Obstet Gynecol. 2011;38:272.
17. Houlihan C, Poon LC, Ciarlo M, Kim E, Krampl-Bettelheim E, Tabor A; PREDICT Group. Cervical cerclage for preterm birth prevention in twin gestation with short cervix: a retrospective cohort study. Ultrasound Obstet Gynecol. 2016;48(6):752-6.
18. Roman A, Rochelson B, Martinelli P, Saccone G, Harris K, Zork N, et al. Cerclage in twin pregnancy with dilated cervix between 16 to 24 weeks of gestation: retrospective cohort study. Am J Obstet Gynecol. 2016;215(1):98.e1-98.e11.
19. Goya M, de la Calle M, Pratcorona L. Cervical pessary to prevent preterm birth in women with twin gestation and sonographic short cervix: a multicenter randomized controlled trial (PECEP-Twins). Am J Obstet Gynecol. 2016;214(2):145-52.
20. Boulet SL, Kirby RS, Reefhuis J, Zhang Y, Zhang Y, Sunderam S, Cohen B, et al. Assisted Reproductive Technology and Birth Defects Among Liveborn Infants in Florida, Massachusetts, and Michigan, 2000-2010. JAMA Pediatr. 2016;170(6):e154934.
21. Giuffre M, Piro E, Corsello G. Prematurity and twinning. J Matern Fetal Neonatal Med. 2012;25(53):6.

22. Zhao DP, de Villiers SF, Slaghekke F, Walther FJ, Middeldorp JM, Oepkes D, et al. Prevalence, size, number and localization of vascular anastomoses in monochorionic placentas. Placenta. 2013;34:589
23. Society for Maternal-Fetal Medicine, Simpson LL. Twin-twin transfusion syndrome. Am J Obstet Gynecol. 2013;208(1):3.
24. Hillman SC, Morris RK, Kilby MD. Co-twin prognosis after single fetal death. A systematic review and meta-analysis. Obstet Gynecol. 2011;118(4):928.
25. Quintero RA, Morales WJ, Allen MH. Staging of twin-twin transfusion syndrome. J Perinatol. 1999;19:550.
26. Corcoran S, Breathnach F, Burke G. Dichorionic twin ultrasound surveillance: sonography every 4 weeks significantly underperforms sonography every 2 weeks: results of the Prospective Multicenter ESPRiT Study. Am J Obstet Gynecol. 2015;213(4):551.e1-5.
27. Blickstein I, Perlman S. Single fetal death in twin gestations. J Perinat Med. 2013;41:65.

LONG QUESTIONS

1. Discuss the mechanism of twinning. Enumerate the maternofetal complications of twin pregnancy. How will you manage a case of single fetal demise in twin pregnancy?
2. Define and enumerate the causes of discordant growth in twins. How will you diagnose discordant growth? Discuss the management of a case of twin pregnancy at 30 weeks with discordant growth.
3. Enumerate unique fetal complications of monozygotic twins. How do you diagnose twin to twin transfusion syndrome? How will you manage a case of twin to twin transfusion syndrome at 30 weeks?

SHORT QUESTIONS

1. What are different physiological changes during twin pregnancy?
2. Determination of chorionicity.
3. Explain maternal and fetal complications of twin pregnancy.
4. Define conjoint twins.
5. What is twin-to-twin transfusion syndrome?
6. Define Quintero staging.
7. What is selective fetal reduction?

MULTIPLE CHOICE QUESTIONS

1. Which of the following increases the risk of monozygotic twinning?
    a. Increased parity
    b. Increased maternal age
    c. Heredity
    d. None of the above
2. After how many days of fertilization, division of the zygote results in formation of a conjoint twin?
    a. 0–3 days
    b. 4–7 days
    c. 8–12 days
    d. More than 13 days
3. Which statement is true regarding chorionicity in multifetal pregnancy?
    a. Chorionicity can be diagnosed by sonographically measuring the thickness of the dividing membrane during first trimester
    b. Dichorionic pregnancies are always dizygotic
    c. Monochorionic pregnancies are always monozygotic
    d. Monochorionic membrane should have four layers
4. Comparing singleton pregnancy which of the following is lower in twin pregnancy?
    a. Blood volume expansion
    b. Blood pressure at term
    c. Systemic vascular resistance
    d. Blood loss at delivery
5. Which complication may be seen in dichorionic pregnancy?
    a. Complete mole with coexisting normal twin
    b. Fetus in fetu
    c. Twin-twin transfusion syndrome
    d. Acardiac twins
6. What is the most common cause of increased neonatal morbidity rates in twins?
    a. Congenital malformation
    b. Preterm birth
    c. Abnormal growth pattern
    d. Twin–twin transfusion syndrome
7. Which are the most common vascular communications seen in monochorionic placenta?
    a. Deep artery-vein   b. Deep vein-vein
    c. Superficial artery-artery d. Superficial artery-vein
8. What percentage of Quintero stage 1 remains stable without intervention?
    a. 25%   b. 50%
    c. 75%   d. 100%
9. Which is the most important predictor of neurological outcome of the survivor after death of a cotwin?
    a. Gestational age at time of demise
    b. Malformations present in the deceased twin
    c. Length of time between demise and delivery of second twin
    d. Chorionicity
10. Which of the following interventions has shown to reduce the preterm birth rate in twins?
    a. Cervical encirclage
    b. β-sympathomimetics
    c. 17 hydroxyprogesterone caproate
    d. None of the above
11. The most common presentation of twins in labor is:
    a. Vertex/vertex   b. Vertex/breech
    c. Breech/vertex   d. Vertex/transverse

Answers

| 1. | d | 2. | d | 3. | a | 4. | c | 5. | a | 6. | b |
| 7. | c | 8. | c | 9. | d | 10. | d | 11. | a | | |

7.3 ABNORMALITIES OF AMNIOTIC FLUID VOLUME

Sasikala Kola, Vidya M Ranga Rao

INTRODUCTION

Amniotic fluid is the liquid, which surrounds the fetus, it progressively increases from 8 weeks of gestation, peaks at 34 weeks, declines thereafter, markedly after 40 weeks.

- It provides the necessary fluid, space and growth factors to permit normal development of the fetal lungs and musculoskeletal and gastrointestinal systems.
- It helps to protect fetus from trauma to the maternal abdomen.
- It cushions the umbilical cord from compression between the fetus and uterus.
- It has antibacterial properties that protect from infection.
- It serves as reservoir of fluid and nutrients.

Abnormalities of amniotic fluid volume (AFV) are associated with increased maternal morbidity, perinatal morbidity, and perinatal mortality. Although clinical assessment is done, it often is too late to diagnose oligohydramnios (less amniotic fluid) or polyhydramnios (more amniotic fluid).

Ultrasonography (USG) is the best tool for early diagnosis, prognosis, and management of the pregnancy with abnormal amniotic fluid volume. USG is a noninvasive, integral and essential component of any obstetric ultrasound evaluation.

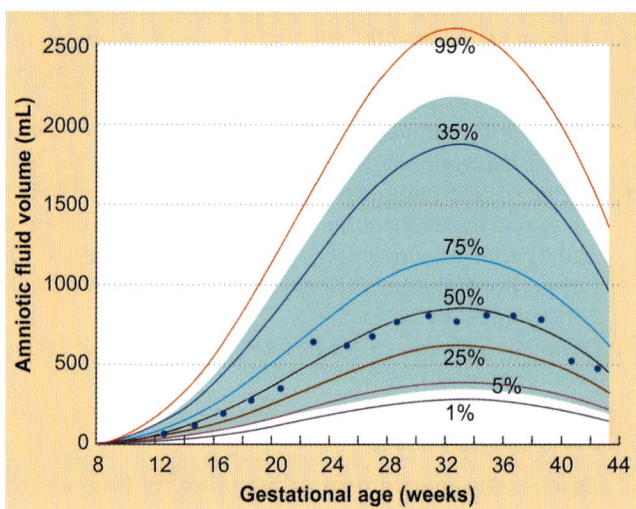

Fig. 1: Amniotic fluid volume as a parameter of gestational age.

AMNIOTIC FLUID: PHYSIOLOGY AND REGULATION

The maintenance of amniotic fluid is a dynamic process throughout pregnancy but with differing origins as the gestational age advances. Amniotic fluid is not a static collection of fluid, it is rather a circulatory process with fetal urine and lung fluid production being balanced by fetal swallowing and intramembranous absorption across amnion and vessels into fetal circulation **(Fig. 1)**.

DYNAMICS OF AMNIOTIC FLUID VOLUME (FIGS. 2 AND 3)

Production

First trimester: Amniotic fluid arises as a transudate of plasma through the non-keratinized fetal skin, uterine decidua and placental surface.[1] Amniotic fluid at this time is isotonic with maternal plasma,[2] has low oxygen tension and increased sugar alcohols suggesting anaerobic metabolism.[3]

Second trimester: In the second trimester the production of dilute urine is well noted, which is a major component of amniotic fluid. Osmolality decreases by 20–30 mOsm/Kg, while amniotic fluid urea, creatinine and uric acid increase.[4] Fetal urine is excreted at the rate of 110 mL/kg/24 hour at 25 weeks to 200 mL/kg/24 hours at term.[5] Fetal urine production

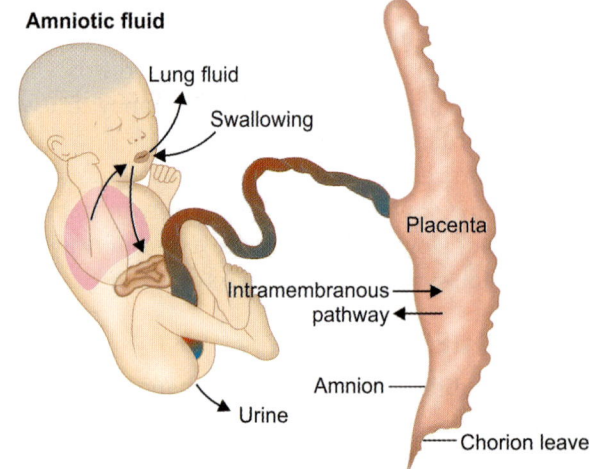

Fig. 2: Circulation of amniotic fluid water to and from the fetus.
Source: Modified from Seeds AE. Current concepts of amniotic fluid dynamics. Am J Obstet Gynecol. 1980;138:575.

is ranges from 300 to 600 mL/kg/day, that is 25% of estimated fetal weight per 24 hours.[6] Fetal lung fluid is secreted at a rate of 100 mL/kg/24 hours. Transudation across umbilical cord and skin water is produced as a byproduct of fetal metabolism. Fetal skin keratinizes the beginning of third trimester (approximately at 25 weeks age).

Resorption of Amniotic Fluid

Fetal swallowing occurs at a rate of 190–760 mL/day, which is less than the volume produced per day. Intramembranous flow across amnion to fetal vessels possibly helps to normalize amniotic fluid volume.[7] Aquaporins are cell membrane water channel proteins present in the chorioamniotic membrane and placenta play a key role.[8]

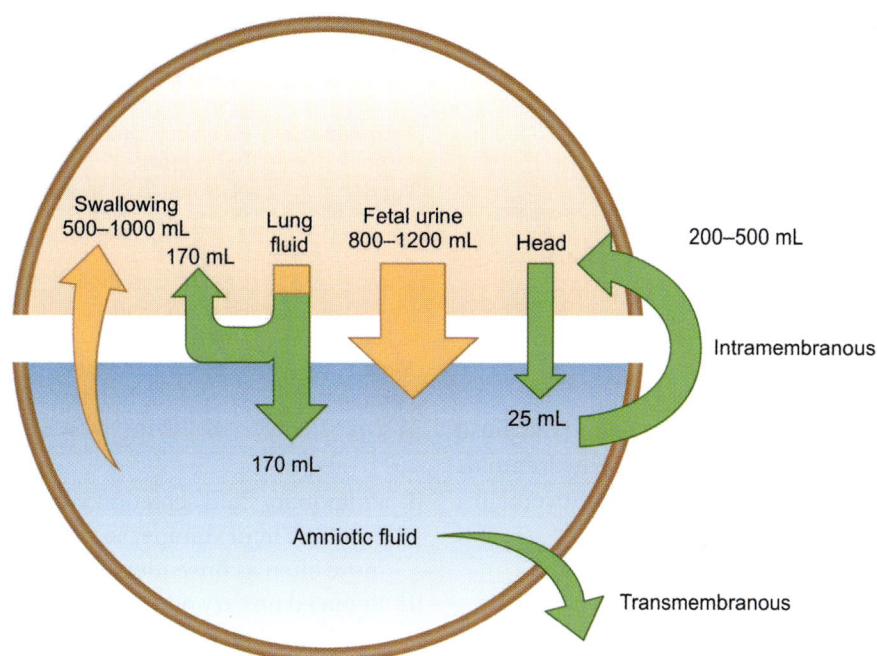

Fig. 3: Summary of water flows into and out of amniotic space in late gestation (arrow size proportional to flow).
Source: Gilbert WM, Brace RA. Amniotic fluid volume and normal flows to and from the amniotic cavity. Semin Perinatol. 1993;17:150-7.

Alterations in maternal hydration can result in changes in transplacental flow.

In oligoamnios aquaporin 1 and 3 are increased and in polyhydramnios 3 and 8 are increased. In human's orexin-A, a stimulator of fetal swallowing was increased in umbilical cord blood in idiopathic polyhydramnios.

The approximate normal volumes at different gestational ages are given in **Table 1**.[9]

Assessment of Amniotic Fluid Volume

In current practice, ultrasound is the best available semiquantitative method to assess AFV, fetal development and well-being.

Two methods of measuring the amniotic fluid are:
1. *SDP/DVP:* Single deepest pocket/Deepest (maximal) vertical pocket (Chamberlain)[10]
2. *AFI:* Amniotic fluid index (Phelan)[11]

The uterine cavity is divided into four quadrants, using imaginary lines drawn through the maternal sagittal plane, with the midline vertically and a transverse line midway between the symphysis pubis and the upper edge of uterine fundus **(Fig. 4)**. The transducer should be perpendicular to the floor and parallel to maternal sagittal plane. The measurements in centimeters of the deepest pocket, free of cord or fetal parts in each quadrant are added to get AFI. Doppler is used to identify and exclude umbilical cord be used whenever necessary.

Normal ranges 5–95th centile and its almost similar to fixed cut-offs for **(Table 2)**:
- SDP: 2–8 cm
- AFI: 5–24 cm (5–18 cm in Asians)

TABLE 1: Approximate normal volumes at different gestational ages.[9]

Weeks (of gestational age)	Normal volumes
10 weeks	25 mL
20–22 weeks	400–630 mL
24–37 weeks	770–800 mL (30 weeks maximum 800 mL)
36–38 weeks	Unchanged
40 weeks	<600 mL
41 weeks	500 mL
>41 weeks	33% decline per week (60–70 mL fall after 40 weeks)

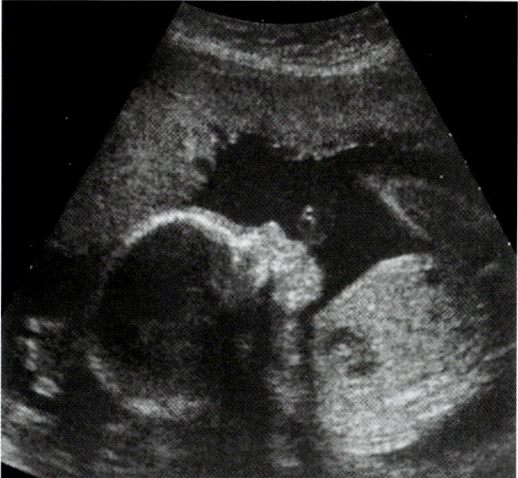

Fig. 4: Amniotic fluid pocket with normal volume in 2nd trimester.

- SDP over diagnoses polyhydramnios and AFI over diagnoses oligoamnios

Khadilkar et al. reported 95 percentile value for Indian women as 18.2 cm.[12] So AFI should be 12.9 ± 4.6 cm on average.

TABLE 2: Abnormal levels of amniotic fluid.

Mild oligohydramnios	Moderate oligohydramnios	Severe oligohydramnios
SDP <3 cm	<2 cm	<1 cm
AFI <8 cm	5–8 cm	<5 cm
Mild polyhydramnios	**Moderate polyhydramnios**	**Severe polyhydramnios**
SDP >3	>5	>8 cm
AFI 8–11	12–16	>16 cm

TABLE 3: Etiology of oligohydramnios.

Maternal	Maternal dehydration, hypertension, autoimmune disorders, medications
Fetomaternal	Prelabor rupture of membranes (PROM), Postdatism
Fetal	Placental insufficiency
	Urinary tract abnormalities: Structural and/or functional
	Genetic conditions
	Gastrointestinal
	Miscellaneous
Most common:	• PROM 25% cases • Placental insufficiency (IUGR) • Post-term pregnancies

Though accuracy of ultrasound indices is good to diagnose normal liquor, sensitivity for both oligo- and polyhydramnios is poor, the limitations being 2D imaging, fetal movements, and loops of cord.

Pitfalls (Fok et al.)[13]

1. Central lying fetus leads to higher AFI calculation higher.
2. Excess maternal abdominal pressure.
3. Umbilical cord filled quadrant should not be used (if measured color Doppler is to be used).
4. Fat: Obesity produces artifactual echoes, vernix.
5. SDP on static image not a representative of amniotic fluid volume, always real time imaging is better.
6. AFI is strongly dependent on weight of the baby.

Amniotic fluid index is the best semiquantitative method to predict poly- and oligohydramnios but it is isolated use is likely to lead to increased obstetric intervention without improvement in perinatal outcome.[14]

■ OLIGOHYDRAMNIOS

By definition it is less than 300–500 mL amniotic fluid after mid trimester. Manning et al.[15] defined oligohydramnios as <2 cm SDP and Phelan et al.[11] defined it as AFI <5 cm.

Pregnancies complicated by oligohydramnios have an increased risk of labor induction, non-reassuring FHR patterns, cesarean deliveries, NICU admissions, meconium aspiration, still birth and neonatal death.[16]

Incidence

0.5–5% (11% in postdated pregnancy).

Etiology

The etiology of oligohydramnios is described in **Table 3**.

Pathogenesis

Reduction in amniotic fluid production in IInd and IIIrd trimester.

Causes

I. Reduced/absent urinary output
II. Pulmonary fluid secretion contributes very little to total amniotic fluid volume, so pulmonary hypoplasia itself is more often a consequence of reduced amniotic fluid.
III. Reduced urinary output may be due to
   a. Altered renal function (more common)
   b. Abnormality in fetal urinary tract.

Placental insufficiency (IUGR): Results in reduced amniotic fluid volume mediated through reduced fetal urinary output. These changes are mediated through a variety of mechanisms including chemo- and baroreceptors, influence of renin angiotensin system and release of vasopressin.

Hypoxia leads to redistribution of blood flow leading to increased cerebral perfusion at the expense of perfusion to viscera including renal perfusion changes detected by Doppler. This is seen as low resistance resistance in MCA and high in renal arteries.

Abnormalities in fetal renal tract: Only one functioning kidney is required to maintain adequate fetal urine production.

Oligohydramnios sequence: Potter facies, limb deformities, growth retardation, pulmonary hypoplasia.[17]

Bilateral renal agenesis (BRA): Amniotic fluid volume is normal until 20 weeks then decreases resulting oligo-and anhydramnios which is diagnosed by inability to visualize bladder, kidneys, expansion of adrenals and fetal renal arteries on Doppler. Diagnostic amnioinfusion is suggested in these cases **(Fig. 5)**.

- Bilateral renal dysplasia, polycystic kidney disease (PCKD, autosomal recessive, autosomal dominant), bilateral multicystic dysplastic kidney (MCDK): All these cause renal tubular dysgenesis resulting in interstitial renal dysfunction and oligohydramnios/ anhydramnios before <26 weeks, severe oligohydramnios affects the canalicular phase of fetal lung development resulting in severe pulmonary hypoplasia incompatible with life resulting in IUFD or still birth.
- Congenital urinary tract obstruction affecting drainage of urine from both kidneys leads to oligohydramnios.

Urethral obstruction: Posterior urethral valves, ureteroceles, urogenital septum, mal formations and bilateral uretero vesical or pelvi ureteric junction obstruction.

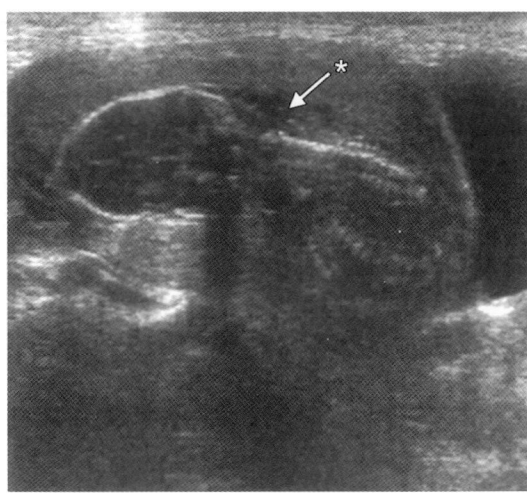

Fig. 5: Sonogram of fetus with renal agenesis.

Lower urinary tract obstruction (LUTO)
- Bladder overdistension (megacystis)
- Back pressure on kidneys (kidney damage)
- Bladder rupture (prune belly syndrome).

Genetic conditions associated with renal anomalies:
- *Smith-Lemli-Opitz syndrome:* Hypoplastic kidney, small cortical cysts, ectopic kidney, hydronephrosis, hydroureter.[18]
- *Meckel Gruber syndrome:* Autosomal recessive, lethal anomalies of CNS (encephalocele), enlarged kidneys cystic dysplasia, malformations of hands and feet.

Gastrointestinal conditions and miscellaneous conditions:
- Gastroschisis
- Megacystis microcolon
- Genetic syndromes
- Metabolic conditions, e.g., hypothyroidism
- Indomethacin, nimesulide use.

Maternal Hydration

Acute maternal hypovolemnia leads to decrease in amniotic fluid volume which is restored back to normal after appropriate hydration.[19]

In the screening arm of RADIUS trial low risk women had routine USG at 15–22 weeks then 31–35 weeks, 0.8% had oligohyramnios of which 50% had isolated oligohydramnios. Perinatal outcomes were similar to those with normal amniotic fluid volume.[20]

Post-term Pregnancies

The risk of adverse perinatal outcome was increased even in low-risk pregnancies when oligohydranios was diagnosed after 40 weeks.[21]

Prognosis

- *1st trimester (up to 12 weeks):* If the difference between the gestational sac and crown rump length (CRL) is < 5 mm poor outcome in the form of 94% fetal loss is noted.
- *2nd trimester (13–24 weeks):* Fetal anomaly 51% (65% aneuploidies), PPROM 34%, FGR 5%, Unknown 4% poor outcome.
- *3rd trimester (after 24 weeks):* Uteroplacental Insufficiency, preeclampsia, maternal vascular disease, FGR, idiopathic, post-term.

Evaluation

- *Maternal history, clinical examination:* Small for dates uterus, easily felt fetal parts; irritability
- *Sonography:* Exclusion of structural anomalies—renal, cardiac and limb anomalies
- *Doppler velocimetry:* Helps identify fetuses at risk—80% fetuses had adverse fetal outcome when S/D ratio is increased
- *Amnioinfusion and MRI* for complex anomalies
- *Genetic testing* if anomalous fetus
- *TORCH* testing when history suggests.

Other parameters of biophysical profile (BPP) should be taken into consideration along with Doppler to avoid unnecessary intervention as it would lead to morbidity due to prematurity.

In a high risk patient < 41 weeks and AFI ≥ 8 cm the risk of oligohydramnios occurring in the next 4 days is 1.7%, in next 7 days is 2.2%, so assessment is to be done weekly. If AFI ≤ 5 cm, assess biweekly and if >41 weeks, irrespective of prior value biweekly.

Management

Remote from term:
Lethal anomalies → termination

Nonlethal → endeavor to prolong pregnancy with close fetal monitoring

Near term: IUGR or preeclampsia – termination

If Doppler abnormalities seen
BPP + antenatal steroids to be given and terminate after 34 weeks.

Continuous intrapartum fetal monitoring and maternal hydration when necessary

In idiopathic oligohydramnios termination has been advised is between 37 and 37[+6] days, as there is no benefit of waiting till term.[22]

Strategies to increase AFV, when indicated however no treatment has been proven to be effective long term.

I. Amnioinfusion (AI)[23]
1. To improve the detection rate of fetal anomalies. If done in the 2nd trimester using 200 mL NS the visualization of fetal structure improves from 51 to 77% after AI.

2. To facilitate ECV.
3. To prevent fetal sequelae of oligohydramnios.

II. Maternal hydration: In isolated oligohydramnios where delivery is not indicated, oral hydration with 2 liters of water may be useful. Hypotonic saline is more effective than isotonic saline.[24]

Experimental Therapies (Only in Research Situations)

- *Hydration and DDAVP:* Combined use of oral water ingestion and desmopressin (DDAVP) increases AFI and maternal hydration causes anti diuresis.
- *Tissue sealants in PPROM:* Fibrin glue, gelatin sponge, and amniopatch have shown some success but safety and effectivity not known
- *Hydration and sildenafil citrate*: If oligohydramnios is diagnosed > 30 weeks, sildenafil 25 mg TID and 1 L IV fluids followed by oral hydration if used,[25] has shown to result in a lower rate of LSCS and NICU admissions. However, a Dutch trial (STRIDER) was stopped early because of higher rate of lung disease and deaths in neonates,[26] so sildenafil use has been stopped till further research.
- *Vesicoamniotic shunt*: To be attempted in LUTO to limit renal, lung and orthopaedic sequelae.
- Open fetal surgery, fetal cystoscopy, electrocautery of PUV, puncture/septostomy and renal transplant in surviving infant might become necessary.[27]

■ POLYHYDRAMNIOS

Definition

Polyhydramnios is defined as when the amniotic fluid is more than 1,500–2,000 mL.

AFI: 24–29.9 cm (mild), 30–34.9 cm (moderate), >35 cm (severe)

DVP/SDP: 8–11 cm (mild), 12–15 cm (moderate), > 16 cm (severe

Incidence

About 1–3.5%, out of which in 5% it is severe. It is independent of race, ethnicity, but more common in multigravidae.[28]

Polyhydramnios causes distress to mother in the form of an unmanageable girth, shortness of breath, digestive discomfort, edema, varicose veins, hyperemesis and preterm labor/PROM. Distress to fetus is due to malpresentations, SGA and macrosomia which increases perinatal morbidity.

Acute polyhydramnios can be catastrophic and resembles abruptio placentae. Idiopathic polyhydramnios are mild in 80% cases.

Etiology

I. *Maternal:* Diabetes
II. *Fetal:* Abnormalities, multiple gestations

In mild to moderate polyhydramnios, 80% are idiopathic.
In severe polyhydramnios, 80% are due to an underlying abnormality.

Fetal abnormality incidence in polyhydramnios is as follows:[29]
- Mild polyhydramnios: 1%
- Moderate polyhydramnios: 2%
- Severe polyhydramnios: 11%

Pathogenesis of Polyhydramnios

Abnormal or interrupted turnover of amniotic fluid which may be due to inability to swallow and absorb fluid that interrupts normal turnover of amniotic fluid resulting in net accumulation.

Fetal Causes

1. **Structural abnormalities of upper GI (intrinsic/extrinsic) (Figs. 6 and 7)**
   a. *Esophageal atresia:* In only 40% of cases with esophageal atresia polyhydramnios seen. There is failure to visualize stomach on USG. Amniotic fluid

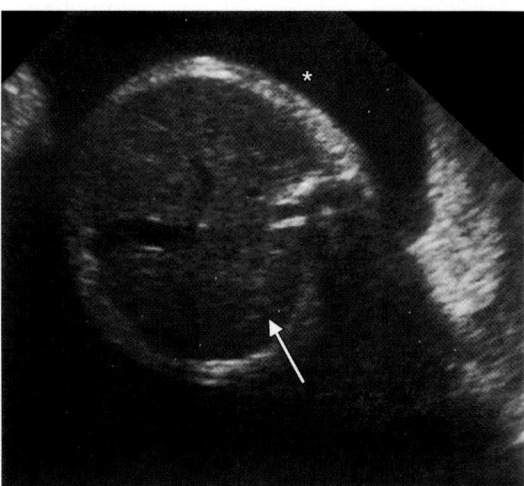

Fig. 6: Sonogram of a patient with esophageal atresia.

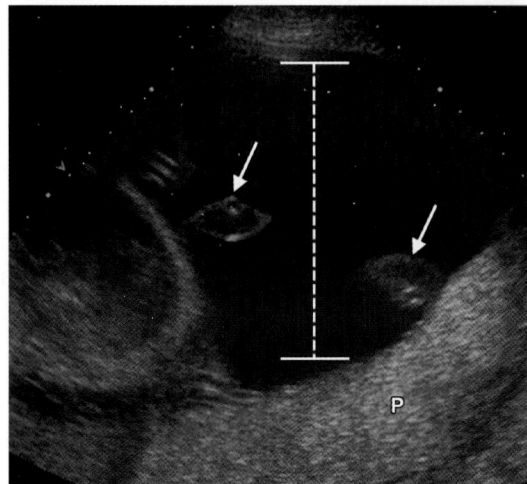

Fig. 7: Sonogram of a patient with duodenal atresia.

cannot progress beyond upper GI and refluxes back into the amniotic cavity.
  b. Pyloric stenosis.
  c. Duodenal atresia (double bubble sign).
  d. *Large head and neck masses:* Physical obstruction of oropharynx and upper esophagus is noted.
  e. *Congenital high airway obstruction syndrome (CHAOS):* Lung secretions are tapped within pulmonary tree and the resulting distension and mediastinal venous and cardiac compression may give rise to both ascites and polyhydramnios.
  f. *Intrathoracic masses:* Upper GI compression, e.g., diaphragmatic hernia, congenital adenomatoid malformation of lung, bronchogenic cysts, bronchopulmonary sequestration, e.g., skeletal dysplasia.
2. *Neurological conditions* which interfere with swallowing process. Neurological disruption of swallowing is noted in myotonic dystrophy, anencephaly and progressive fetal paralysis in arthrogryposis. Also in genetic conditions such as Beckwith – Wiedemann syndrome there is macroglossia which interferes with the swallowing process.
3. *Fetal hydrops* (high output cardiac failure) **(Figs. 8 and 9)**
  a. Immune
  b. Nonimmune: AV anastomosis
4. *Multiple gestations:* In multichorionic gestations the causes of polyhydramnios and oligohydramnios are similar to single gestation. However in a monochorionic twin gestation, fetofetal transfusion might occur.[30]

Maternal Causes

Diabetes Mellitus and Insipidus

Suboptimal glycemic control → fetal hyperglycemia.

Fetal hyperinsulinemia → osmotic action → Polyuria → Fetal macrosomia → Polyhydramnios.

Gestational diabetes with polyhydramnios → no ↑ in perinatal morbidity.[31]

Lithium to Mother

Maternal lithium consumption may cause polyhydramnios.

Placental Abnormalities

Chorioangioma is associated with polyhydramnios in 30% cases. Laser photo coagulation is suggested as therapy.

Clinical Evaluation

- Malpresentations
- Difficult to feel fetal parts and "large for dates" uterus (other causes to be ruled out like multiple pregnancy, wrong dates, hydrops fetalis, hydatidiform mole, full bladder, pregnancy with ovarian cyst/fibroid and obesity)
- Maternal diabetes.

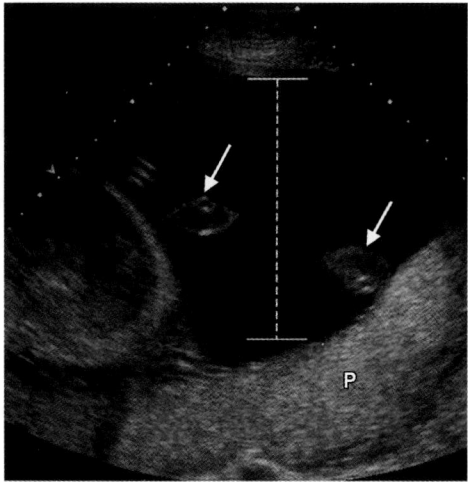

Fig. 8: Pocket of amniotic fluid in a patient with hydrops fetalis and polyhydramnios.

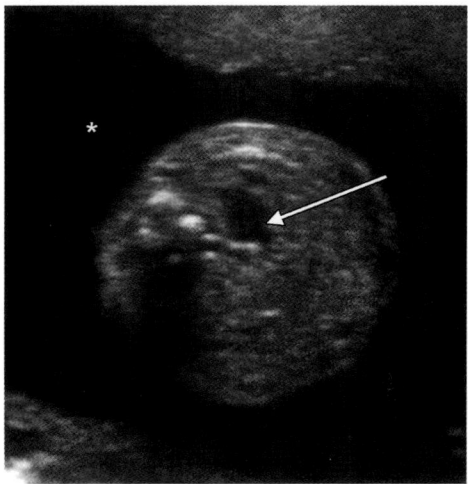

Fig. 9: Polyhydramnios in a patient with unilateral ureteropelvic junction obstruction.

In Fetal Hydrops

- Antibody screen: D, C, Kell, Duffy to exclude alloimmunization
- CMV, toxoplasmosis, parvovirus: IgA, IgM
- Alpha thalassemia to be looked for by Hb electrophoresis

Ultrasonography

Ultrasonography is best for correct diagnosis. Concerns are excess fluid makes it difficult to visualize an organ or structure. If the fetus is beyond range of transducer ask the patient to turn to one side. Placenta appears thin even though it is thick because of abnormal expansion.

Heart may be abnormally enlarged but it appears normal because of elongation and compression by over distended lungs. Congenital infection usually presents with additional sonographic findings such as nonimmune hydrops, hepatosplenomegaly and splenomegaly.

Imaging

Detailed examination of fetal brain, upper GI, head and neck and chest/long bones and thorax to be done.

To look for congenital cardiac disease a detailed echocardiography of fetus is necessary.

Fetal movements, tone, examinations of knee, wrist and elbow should be evaluated, as all these are key to diagnosis of neuromuscular abnormalities such as arthrogryposis.

To diagnose aneuploidies which may be seen in about 5–20% of cases, karyotyping and FISH with amniocentesis is recommended

Cervical length must for be measured along with funneling assessment.

Cordocentesis in hydrops to determine fetal Hb and subsequent intrauterine transfusion (IUT).

Earlier CNS anomalies were more commonly diagnosed, however now GI anomalies more common because of early detection and greater termination of CNS anomalies.

In mild polyhydramnios only 1% anomalies noted while in in severe polyhydramnios 10% anomalies detected postnatally in spite of imaging. Hence it is important to counsel the patient.

Management

1. *Rest/Conservative:* If respiratory distress, amnioreduction indicated in only in severe maternal discomfort and dyspnea or both
2. *Amnioreduction:* To be done under local anesthesia with 10 mL 1–2% Xylocaine using a 20–22 G needle under USG control along with a 3-way stop cock and 50 mL syringe. 5–10 liters can be removed with low complication rate of 1.5%. Complications include PPROM, Placental abruption, chorioamnionitis, membrane detachment, and perforation of amniotic septum in MCDC twins. In serial amnioreduction a perinatal survival rate of 66% has been reported.
3. *Prostaglandin inhibitors:*
   - *Indomethacin:* 1.4–3 mg/kg daily (25 mg 4–6 hourly to 75 mg 12 hourly)
     - Prostaglandins inhibitors stimulate ADH and affect vasopressin leading water resorption from the tubules and decrease urine output in fetus
     - AFI is done twice weekly during treatment
     - Majority fluid reduction occurs in the first week
     - When two-thirds of pretreatment level is achieved it is advised to stop indomethacin
     - Fetal echo important to detect ductus closure. So restrict usage <32–34 weeks.
     - Necrotizing enterocolitis, intestinal perforation, IVH and LBW are other complications.[32]
   - Sulindac (prostaglandin inhibitor) 250 mg 12 hourly has been used. It has milder effect on ductus and greater effect in reducing AFV[32]
   - *Nimesulide:* PG inhibitor has also been tried.

Intrapartum Care

During labor complications often encountered may be malpresentation, cord prolapse, and PPH. In cases of idiopathic mild polyhydramnios, there is no need of increased antenatal surveillance and patient should be allowed to go into spontaneous labor. Mode of delivery depends on obstetric indications.[33]

Uncommonly done procedures for relief of polyhydramnios in certain fetal anomalies are:
- *Cyst adenoid malformation of fetal lungs:* Needle puncture and drainage of cystic lesions
- *Congenital diaphragmatic hernia:* Fetal endotracheal balloon occlusion
- *Twin-twin transfusion syndrome:* Fetoscopic photo-coagulation of vascular anastomosis identified on placental surface, serial amnioreduction or amnion septostomy

■ CONCLUSION

Aberrant amniotic fluid volume complicates up to 7% pregnancies. In many instances the alteration is mild and idiopathic and occurs in third trimester and does not produce any adverse sequelae. In contrast severe oligohydramnios or polyhydramnios in mid trimester is associated with substantial perinatal morbidity and mortality. It is observed that as weight of fetus increases amniotic fluid volume increases. USG and Doppler are extremely useful aids in diagnosis and management

■ REFERENCES

1. Gillibrand PN. Changes in the electrolytes, urea and osmolality of the amniotic fluid with advancing pregnancy. J Obstet Gynaec Brit Cwlth. 1969;76:898-905.
2. Campbell J, Walter N, Macintosh M, Cass P, Chard T, Mainwaring Burton R. Biochemical composition of amniotic fluid and extraembryonic coelomic fluid in first trimester. BJOG. 1992;99:563-5.
3. Jauniaux E, Hempstock J, Teng C, et al. Polyol Concentrations in the Fluid Compartments of the Human Conceptus during the First Trimester of Pregnancy: Maintenance of Redox Potential in a Low Oxygen Environment. J Chin Endocrinology Metabolism. 2005;90:1171-5.
4. Faber JJ, Gault CF, Green JJ. Chloride and generators of AF in early embryo. J Exp. 2001;183:343-52.
5. Lotgering FK, Wallenburg HC, Halperin JL, Fuster V. Mechanism of Action and Pharmacology of Unfractionated Heparin. Sepin Perinatol 1986;10:94-102.
6. Rabinonitz R, Peters MT, Vyas S, Camp bell S, Nicolaides KH. Measurement of fetal urine production in normal pregnancy by real-time ultrasonography. Am J Obstet Gynecol. 1989;161:1264-6.
7. Adams EA, Choi HM, Cheung CY, Brace RA. Comparison of Amniotic and Intramembranous permeability in late gestation. Am J Obstet Gynecol. 2005;193:247-55.
8. Wang S, Kallichanda N, Song W, Ramirez BA, Ross MG. Expression of aquaporin-8 in human placenta and

chorioamniotic membranes: evidence of molecular mechanism for intramembranous amniotic fluid resorption. AJOG. 2001;185:1226-31.
9. Brace RA. Physiology of amniotic fluid volume regulation. Clin Obstet Gynecol. 1997;40:280-9.
10. Chambulern PF, Manning FA, Morrison. USG evaluation of AFV. AJOJ. 1984;150:245-9.
11. Phelan JP, Smith CV, Bronssard P, Small M. AF volume assessment at 36-42 weeks. J Reprod Med. 1987;32:540-2.
12. Khadilkar SS, Desai, Tayade, Purandare CN. AFI in normal pregnancy (Indian). J Obstet Gyn. 2003;131:136-41.
13. Fok WY, Chan LY, Tau TK. The influence of fetal position on amniotic fluid index and single deepest pocket. Ultrasound Obstet Gynecol. 2006;28:162.
14. Morns JM, Thampson K, Smithey J, et al. The usefulness of ultrasound assessment of amniotic fluid in predicting adverse outcome in prolonged pregnancy: a prospective blinded observational study. BJOG. 2003;110(11):989-94..
15. Manning FA, Hill LM, Platt LD. Qualitative AFV determination and detection of IUGR. Am J Obstet Gynecol. 1981:139:254-8.
16. Jeng CJ, Lee JF, Wang KG, Yang YC, Lan CL. Decreased AFI in term pregnancy - clinical significance. J Reprod. 1992;37(9):789-92.
17. Potter EL. Facial characteristics of infants with bilateral renal agenesis. Am J Obstet Gynecol. 1946;51:885-8.
18. Lowry RB, Opitz JM, Variability in Smith-Lemli opitz syndrome - A J Med Genetics 2005, 14:429-433
19. Sherer DM, Cullen JBH, Thampson HO, Woods JR. Transient oligohydramnios in severe hypovolemic gravid women at 35 weeks. Am J Obstet Gynecol. 1990;162 (3):770-1.
20. Zhang J, Troendle J, Meikle S, Klebanoff MA, Rayburn WF. Isolated oligohydramnios. BJOG. 2004:111(3)220-5.
21. Locatelhi A, Zagarelle A. Serial assessment AFI in uncomplicated term pregnancy. J Mat Fetal Neonatal Med. 2004;15(4): 233-6.
22. Bannerman CG, Chauhan SP. Oligohydramnios at 34-36 weeks: observe or deliver. AJOG. 2011:205:163.
23. Pryde PG, Hallak M, Lauria MR, Littman L, Bottoms SF, Johnson MP, et al. Severe oligohydramnios with intact membranes: an indication for diagnostic amnioinfusion. Fetal Diagn Ther. 2000;15;46.
24. Gizzo S, Noventa M, Vitagliano A, et al. An update on maternal hydration. PLoS One 2015; 10:e 0144334
25. Maher MA, Sayyed TM, Ekhouly N. Sildenafil citrate therapy for oligohydramnios: a randomized controlled trial. Obstet Gynecol. 2017;129;615-20.
26. Hawkes N. Trial of Viagra for FGR halted after baby deaths. BMJ. 2018;362;K3247.
27. Holmes N, Harrison MR, Baskin LS. Fetal surgery for posterior urethral valves: long-term postnatal outcomes. Pediatrics. 2001:108:E7.
28. Moise KJ Jr. Polyhydramnios. Clin Obstet Gynecol. 1997;40(2):266-79.
29. Dashe JS, MC Intire DD, Ramus RM, Santos-Ramos Rx Twickler DM. Hydramnios—anomaly prevalence and sonographic detection. Obstet Gynecol. 2002:100:134-9.
30. Denbon ML, Fisk NM. The consequences of monochorionic placentation. Baillieres Clin Obstet Gynecol. 1998;12:37-51.
31. Vink JY, Poggi SH, Glindini A, Spong CY. Amniotic fluid index and birth weight: is there a relationship in diabetics with poor glycemic control? Am J Obstet Gynecol. 2006;195:845-50.
32. Amin SB, Sinkin RA, Glantz JC. Indomethacin on neonatal outcomes. AJOG. 2007;197;486e1-10.
33. Luo QQ, Zou L, Gao H, Zheng YF, Zhao Y, Zhang WY. Idiopathic polyhydramnios at term and pregnancy outcomes, multicenter observational study. J Matern Fetal Neonatal Med. 2017:30;1755-9.

LONG QUESTIONS

1. Write a description of amniotic fluid regulation and illustrate it with an appropriate diagram.
2. How do you counsel a woman with oligoamnios? What other specialists do you have to involve?

SHORT QUESTIONS

1. What contributes maximum to AF volume? Explain briefly why an aberration can occur?
2. How does ultrasound contribute to diagnosis of abnormal AFV and mention a few pitfalls?
3. How important is US Doppler in managing FGR ± PIH with oligohydramnios?
4. How does BPP complement Doppler in management of a pregnancy with oligohydramnios and uteroplacental insufficiency?
5. Write a short note on maternal diabetes and polyhydramnios.

MULTIPLE CHOICE QUESTIONS

1. Amniotic fluid helps in normal development of:
    a. Muscles   b. Lungs
    c. Intestines   d. Bones
    e. All of the above
2. The volume of AF is maximum at:
    a. 28 weeks   b. 30 weeks
    c. 34 weeks   d. 40 weeks
3. The fetal urine output is.........mL/kg wt/24 hours at term.
    a. 100 mL   b. 200 mL
    c. 150 mL   d. 110 mL
4. After 40 weeks rate of decline per week in AFV is:
    a. 25%   b. 15%
    c. 21%   d. 33%
5. Keratinization of fetal skin occurs around:
    a. 12 weeks   b. 15 weeks
    c. 22 weeks   d. 25 weeks
6. In Indian women, average AFI is:
    a. 20 ± 5 cm   b. 10 ± 3 cm
    c. 24 ± 6 cm   d. 12.9 ± 4.6 cm
7. AFI forms a part of................
    a. BPP   b. BPT
    c. NST   d. NTT
8. The most common cause of oligoamnios:
    a. PROM   b. Postdates
    c. Placental insufficiency   d. Fetal renal anomalies
9. Oligoamnios before........is lethal.
    a. 15 weeks   b. 20 weeks
    c. 30 weeks   d. 26 weeks

10. Amnioinfusion can be recommended in MSAF in labor in............settings.
    a. Resource poor
    b. Where all facilities available
    c. Developing countries
    d. a and c
11. Vesicoamniotic shunt is done in LUTO to limit.......... damage.
    a. Lung   b. Renal
    c. Gastrointestinal   d. CNS
12. Polyhydramnios is defined as:
    a. More than 1,500–2,000 mL
    b. SDP >3 cm
    c. AFI >18 cm
    d. All of the above
13. At what percentage, polyhydramnios is severe—
    a. 2%   b. 6%
    c. 10%   d. 5%
14. Fetal malformations associated with polyhydramnios are:
    a. GIT   b. Neck
    c. Viral infections d. All of the above
15. What is the DD of PH?
    a. Hydatidiform mole b. Ovarian cyst
    c. Full bladder   d. Fibroid
    e. All of the above
16. Dosage of Indomethacin in PH:
    a. 1.4–3 mg/kg daily b. 0.5–1 mg/kg
    c. 20 mg/kg   d. 12 mg/kg
17. Adverse effects of indomethacin:
    a. Premature closure of DA
    b. LBW
    c. Necrotizing enterocolitis
    d. IVH
    e. All of the above
18. Evaluation of placenta important in PH to rule out:
    a. Low implantation b. Thickness
    c. Chorioangioma   d. None
19. Evaluation of fetal movements, swallowing, knee and elbow movements is important to rule out:
    a. Structural defects b. Neurological defects
    c. Genetic conditions d. None
20. Lifesaving invasive procedure in hydrops is:
    a. Photocoagulation   b. Intrauterine transfusion
    c. Cordocentesis   d. Vesicoamniotic shunts

Answers
1. b   2. c   3. d   4. d   5. d   6. d
7. a   8. a   9. a   10. a 11. b 12. a
13. d 14. d 15. e 16. a 17. e 18. c
19. a 20. b

7.4 ABNORMALITIES OF THE PLACENTA AND CORD

Tamkin Khan, Ayesha Ahmad

■ INTRODUCTION[1]

Placenta is a fetomaternal organ derived from trophoblast of the blastocyst, with contributions from both fetus (chorion frondosum) and mother (decidua basalis). Its functional component is formed by chorionic villi which provide a surface for gaseous and substrate exchange. They start as primary villi containing only trophoblast to secondary villi containing both trophoblast and mesoderm and finally, tertiary villi containing trophoblast, mesoderm and blood vessels. There is fibrinoid deposition in placenta, starting as early as 4th month. It occurs within the chorionic plate (Subchorial Langhans' layer), beneath the stem villi in basal plate (Rohr's layer) and in Nitabuch's layer within decidua basalis in the basal plate.

A normal placenta is round or oval shaped with a mean diameter of 22 cm and a central thickness of 2–2.5cm. It weighs about one-sixth of the fetal birth weight. The surface overlying uterine wall is called basal plate, which is divided by clefts into cotyledons. The fetal surface or the chorionic plate has umbilical cord inserted in its center. The chorionic plate and umbilical vessels are covered by a thin amnion. Fetal membranes refer to structures derived from blastocyst that do not contribute to the embryo. They consist of amnion, chorion, yolk sac, and allantois.

On ultrasonographic examination, the placenta has a homogeneous consistency, with a retroplacental hypoechoic area separating basal plate from myometrium. Its functions include nutrition, excretion, immunologic and endocrine function. **Table 1** lists different placental abnormalities. Evaluation of placenta, cord and membranes is essential as abnormalities can be associated with adverse pregnancy outcome.

■ ABNORMALITIES OF PLACENTAL SHAPE[2]

The usual round or oval outline of the placenta may be replaced by a wide spectrum of shapes which are largely innocuous variants. Occasionally, they may assume clinical significance and be associated with fetal complications. We will be discussing some common placental shape abnormalities of clinical relevance.

Bilobate Placenta

Morphologically, the placenta is separated into two roughly equal sized lobes, separated by membranes. It is called a

	TABLE 1: Common placental abnormalities.
A	**Abnormalities of placental shape and size**
	Bilobate
	Multilobate
	Annular
	Membranous
	Extrachorial Circumvallate Placenta marginata
	Large placenta
B	**Abnormalities of placental implantation**
	Placenta previa
	Morbid adherence of placenta
C	**Abnormalities of placental circulation**
	Infarction
	Calcification
D	**Inflammation of placenta**
	Chorioamnionitis
E	**Tumors of placenta**
	Gestational trophoblastic disease
	Gestational trophoblastic neoplasia
	Chorioangioma
	Metastatic tumors
F	**Miscellaneous**
	Degenerative lesions
	Hypertrophic lesions of chorionic plate

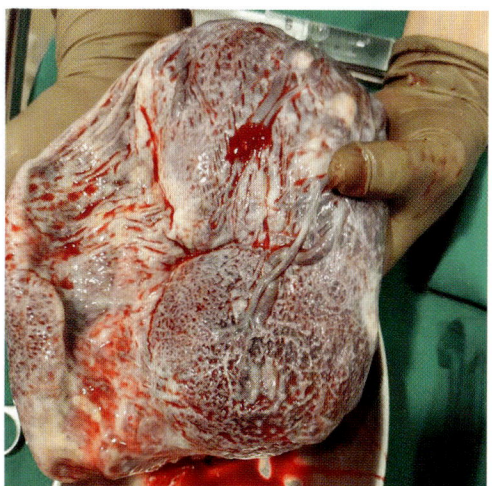

Fig. 1: Succenturiate placenta.

multilobate placenta when there are more than two lobes. This variant of placenta is found to have an incidence of 2–8%.

Diagnosis

The diagnosis is made on ultrasound when two separate placental disks of nearly equal sizes are noted.

Clinical Implication

It has been found to be associated with first trimester bleeding, velamentous insertion of cord, vasa previa, polyhydramnios, abruption and retained placenta.

Succenturiate Placenta (Fig. 1)

It is a morphological abnormality in which one or more accessory lobes of the placenta develop in the membranes away from the main placenta. The accessory lobe is connected to the main placenta by communicating blood vessels present in the membranes. If there are no vascular connections in the placental membranes, it is called placenta spuria. Development of the accessory lobe is attributed to activation of chorion laeve, which normally disappear during embryogenesis. The incidence is found to be increased with advanced maternal age and assisted reproductive technology.

Diagnosis

The separate lobes may be identified on ultrasound: the main portion to which the umbilical cord is attached and the succenturiate lobe. Occasionally, a myometrial contraction may simulate an accessory lobe, but there will be no defining boundary between the lobe and myometrium. A repeat scan would confirm the diagnosis.

Clinical Implication

- Retention of placental lobe during third stage of labor:
  - Primary postpartum hemorrhage
  - Sub-involution of uterus, puerperal sepsis and secondary postpartum hemorrhage
- Development of placental polyp.

Circumvallate Placenta

It is an annular placenta with basal plate is larger than the chorion frondosum **(Figs. 2A and B)**. As a result, the placental edges are raised and rolled back to form a ring, leaving a rim of uncovered placental tissue (extrachorial portion). The fetal surface has a central depressed zone, surrounded by a thick gray white ring. The ring is composed of a double fold of chorion, amnion, degenerated decidua and fibrin deposits. Branching vessels radiate from the cord insertion upto the ring only. The area outside the ring is thicker, elevated and rounded. The incidence of this variant is around 0.5–18%.

Diagnosis

The prenatal diagnosis can be suspected when the peripheral rim of chorionic tissue appears echo dense.

Clinical Implication

It has a high association with single umbilical artery (SUA) and placental insufficiency. There is an increased risk of miscarriage, fetal congenital malformations, fetal growth restriction, antepartum hemorrhage and preterm labor.

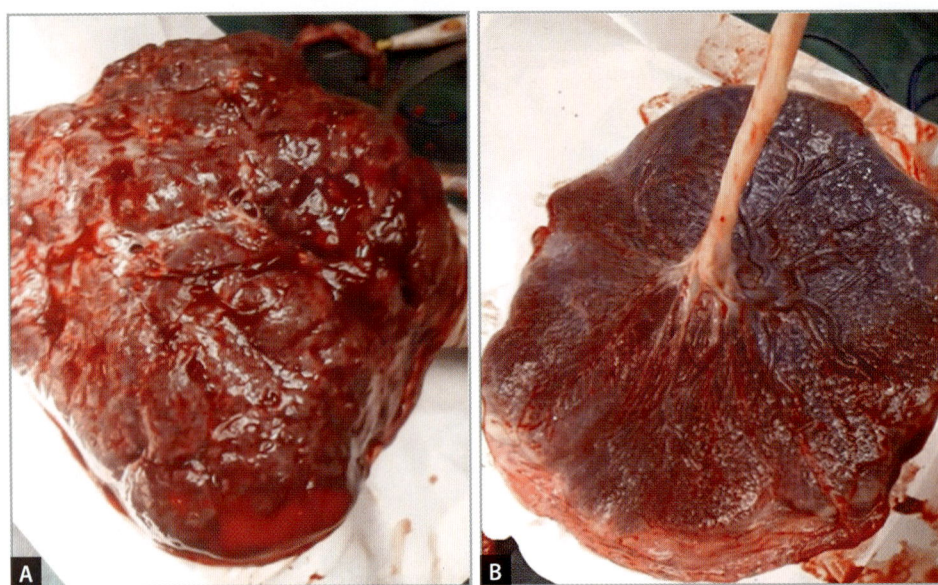

Figs. 2A and B: Gross examination of placenta. (A) Maternal surface: Develops from decidua basalis. Rough, shaggy, fleshy and dull red in appearance; (B) Fetal surface: Develops from chorion frondosum and chorionic plate. Smooth in appearance. The umbilical cord is attached centrally.

Membranous Placenta (Placenta Diffusa)

It is a rare condition in which the entire chorion is covered by functioning villi.

Diagnosis

Placenta appears as a thin, membranous structure.

Clinical Implication

Placental tissue may be adherent and difficult to remove resulting in postpartum hemorrhage.

ABNORMALITIES OF PLACENTAL SIZE

Placentomegaly is associated with multiple pregnancies, diabetes mellitus, syphilis, macrosomia, and hydrops fetalis. Small placentae are seen in fetal growth restriction, placental infarcts and postdated pregnancies.

Morbidly Adherent Placenta[3]

The term is used for a placenta firmly adherent to the uterine wall due to partial or total absence of decidua basalis and the fibrinoid layer (Nitabuch layer). Pathologically, there is abnormal attachment of the chorionic villi to myometrium (accreta), invasion beyond myometrium (increta) or into the serosa (percreta). Risk factors for morbidly adherent placenta (MAP) are previous uterine surgeries such as cesarean section, dilatation and curettage, myomectomy, uterine adhesiolysis, etc., placenta previa, previous manual removal of placenta and grand multiparity.

Diagnosis

Morbidly adherent placenta can be diagnosed on antenatal ultrasound. In case of doubtful diagnosis, magnetic resonance imaging (MRI) may be done. The ultrasonographic diagnostic features of MAP are:

- *Swiss cheese appearance:* Multiple vascular lacunae within the placenta. Color Doppler shows a turbulent flow within the lacunae with a peak systolic velocity of more than 15 cm/s
- Loss of normal retroplacental hypoechogenic zone
- Retroplacental myometrial thickness of less than 1 mm
- Increased blood flow at the uterine placental margin and myometrial bladder interface. Occasionally, exophytic masses can be seen invading the urinary bladder.

Clinical Implications

Morbidly adherent placenta is associated with severe postpartum hemorrhage. Its incidence is increasing due to rise in risk factors. MAP is one of the most common causes of obstetric hysterectomy. Maternal mortality can be as high as 5–10%, with a morbidity as high as 75%. An early diagnosis is imperative to plan the course of management and reduce complications of MAP.

Placental Tumors

Chorioangioma

These are common benign placental tumors with an incidence of around 1%. They are hamartomas of primitive chorionic mesenchyme. Small tumors are usually asymptomatic. Large tumors may cause fetal anemia and thrombocytopenia—due to sequestration of red blood cells and platelets, leading to fetal hydrops and cardiac failure. Placentomegaly is a usual feature, attributed to a hyperdynamic circulation as a result of arteriovenous shunting. Hydramnios, preterm delivery, fetal growth restriction, and intrauterine death are other sequelae. They may be associated with maternal mirror syndrome in which mother may also present with similar features (e.g., cardiac failure). Symptomatic chorioangiomas may be associated with a perinatal mortality of up to 40%.

Diagnosis: On ultrasonography, chorioangioma appears as a well circumscribed mass (hypo- or hyperechoic) usually located underneath the chorionic plate, close to the insertion of umbilical cord. Large vascular channels are visualized around and within the tumor on color Doppler imaging.

Clinical implication: Once the diagnosis of chorioangioma is made, a detailed ultrasound examination should be done including fetal echocardiography for assessment of cardiac function. Fetal middle cerebral artery peak systolic velocity is measured for diagnosis for fetal anemia. Follow-up scans are usually done every 2–3 weeks to monitor growth of tumor, cardiac function and fetal anemia. Intrauterine procedures such as ultrasound guided laser coagulation of tumor vessels, amniodrainage and intrauterine transfusions may be done in advanced centers.

Metastatic Tumors

Placenta is an unusual site of metastasis of maternal malignant tumors, melanomas, leukemia, lymphomas and breast cancer are the common ones that metastasize. The tumor cells usually remain confined to the intervillous space due to which metastasis to fetus is uncommon.

Umbilical Cord[4]

It is a helical and tubular blood conduit connecting fetus to placenta. By 4th week of intrauterine life, the rudimentary umbilical cord starts forming and achieves its final form by 12th week of gestation. Blood flow is established by 5th week of gestation. The umbilical arteries start as continuation of the primitive dorsal aortae but finally arise from the internal iliac arteries. After birth, the proximal portion of intra-abdominal umbilical arteries persists as the internal iliac and superior vesicle arteries and the distal portions are obliterated and form the medial umbilical ligaments. The right umbilical vein disappears by the end of 6th week of gestation leaving the left umbilical vein behind. This obliterates at birth and the remnant persists as ligamentum teres.

Contents of umbilical cord: It contains two arteries, one vein, and remnants of allantois, protected by a gelatinous substance known as Wharton's jelly and surrounded by a single layer of amnion **(Fig. 3)**. The two arteries are smaller in diameter than the vein. When fixed in their normally distended sate, the umbilical arteries exhibit transverse intimal folds of Hoboken across their lumen. The folding and tortuosity of the vessels within the cord itself creates false knots, which are essentially varices. The umbilical cord is assessed by different parameters as length, coiling, vessel number, etc. **Table 2** lists some common abnormalities of umbilical cord.

Length: The mean length of an umbilical cord is 50–60 cm but it can range from 30 to 100 cm. A short cord (<30 cm)

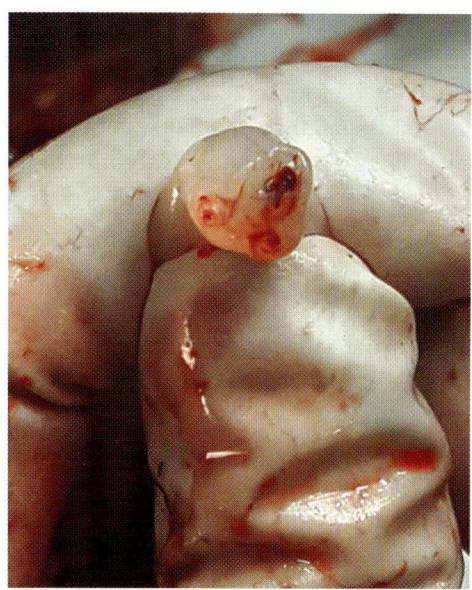

Fig. 3: Umbilical cord. The cut surface shows two umbilical arteries and one umbilical vein.

TABLE 2: Abnormalities of umbilical cord.	
A	**Length abnormalities**
	Absent cord
	Long cord
	Short cord
B	**Coiling abnormalities**
	Hypocoiled
	Hypercoiled
C	**Cord insertion abnormalities**
	Battledore placenta
	Velamentous insertion
D	**Knots**
	True knot
	False knot
E	**Vascular abnormalities**
	Single umbilical artery
	Four vessel cord
	Hypoplastic umbilical artery
	Persistent right umbilical vein
F	**Miscellaneous**

may be associated with congenital abnormalities, fetal growth restriction, premature separation of placenta (abruption), fetal distress, intrauterine death and inversion of uterus. A long cord (> 100 cm) may be associated with looping of cord around baby's neck, cord entanglement, fetal distress, cord prolapse and intra uterine death.

Diagnosis: Antenatal determination of cord length on ultrasound is limited, so cord diameter has been investigated as a predictive marker for fetal outcomes. Although studies have found an association of adverse fetal outcome with lean as well as large diameter umbilical cords, the data is still sketchy.

Coiling

The two umbilical arteries form a cylindrical helix around the umbilical vein, which are dextral in 90% of cases and sinistral in the remaining. The normal cord has one coil per 5 cm of cord length. The cord may develop upto 40 spirals and there may be straight portions in different segments. The factors responsible for spiraling are helical muscle layers in walls of umbilical arteries, rotational movements of the fetus, asymmetry in sizes and growth rate of umbilical arteries and uterine contractions. Both hypocoiled and hypercoiled variants of umbilical cord have been associated with suboptimal pregnancy outcomes. Hypocoiled cords are associated with a higher incidence of fetal distress, abnormal cord blood pH and chances of operative delivery. Hypercoiled cords have been associated with preterm labor, fetal growth restriction, fetal distress during labor and increased chances of cesarean section.

Diagnosis: Ultrasound can be used to determine umbilical cord coiling. Umbilical coiling index (UCI) is defined as number of complete coils per centimeter of cord length. The normal UCI is approximately 0.2, with <10th centile termed as hypo coiled and >90th centile as hypercoiled umbilical cord.

Vessel Number

Embryos start with four vessels in umbilical cord - two arteries and two veins. In the first trimester, the right umbilical vein atrophies resulting in a three vessel umbilical cord. The most common aberration is the presence of single umbilical artery resulting in a two vessel cord. Rarely, a four vessel cord may be seen.

Single Umbilical Artery[5-7]

The absence of one of the umbilical arteries is a common ultrasonographic finding with an incidence of 0.7–0.8% in singletons and higher in twin pregnancies 5%. The pathogenesis is attributed to either primary agenesis of umbilical artery or secondary atresia of a normally developed artery. Persistence of the original allantoic artery of the body stalk is another theory. SUA is often a normal variant found in healthy fetuses. However, it has been associated with a higher incidence of chromosomal abnormalities (5%) mainly trisomy 13, 18 triploidy, structural abnormalities (20%) most commonly genitourinary and cardiac abnormalities, fetal growth restriction (10%), preterm birth and perinatal mortality. It is more common in diabetic pregnancies, eclampsia, epilepsy, and abnormalities of liquor (oligohydramnios, polyhydramnios).

Diagnosis: Single umbilical artery is diagnosed on color Doppler (with settings on low pulse repetition frequency and high color gain) when only one artery is seen around fetal bladder.

Clinical implication: The presence of SUA warrants a detailed ultrasound to exclude abnormalities, fetal echocardiography and consideration for chromosomal analysis of fetus (karyotyping, chromosomal micro array). Serial scans are recommended at 28, 32 and 36 weeks' gestation to assess fetal growth and well-being. The pediatrician should be informed about the existence of SUA, so that a more detailed examination of the baby is carried out after birth.

Hypoplastic Umbilical Artery

An artery to artery diameter difference of more than 50% is abnormal and is considered to represent a milder form of SUA. It is found to be associated with fetal anomalies, growth restriction, placental infarction, cord hematoma and still birth.

Persistent Right Umbilical Vein

Unusual persistence of right umbilical vein instead of the left umbilical vein is associated with congenital anomalies such as cardiac, genitourinary, and skeletal anomalies, situs inversus, etc. The diagnosis is made on ultrasound when umbilical vein is seen connected with the right portal vein instead of the left and fetal gallbladder is seen between umbilical vein and stomach.

Four Vessel Umbilical Cord

The persistence of distal portion of right umbilical vein along with left umbilical vein, leading to the appearance of four vessel umbilical cord is found rarely. It is associated with major congenital malformations.

CORD INSERTION ABNORMALITIES[8]

Battledore Placenta

The umbilical cord is attached to the placental margin instead of having a central attachment. It usually has no clinical significance.

Velamentous Cord Insertion

This condition is seen in 1% of all pregnancies and is characterized by cord insertion into the chorioamniotic membranes instead of the placental mass. The vessels are surrounded by fetal membranes only, without the cushioning support of Wharton's jelly. The incidence increases in multiple pregnancies and placenta previa and vasa previa.

Clinical Implication

It has found to be associated with congenital malformation, growth restriction, preterm labor, fetal distress, intrauterine death and retained placenta.

Vasa Previa

This condition is characterized by coursing of vessels within the membranes and overlying cervical os. They can be compressed by the fetal part or rupture with cervical dilation or membrane rupture. Vasa previa is uncommon with an estimated prevalence of around 1 in 3,000 pregnancies. Vasa previa is classified as type 1, in which vessels are part of velamentous cord insertion and type 2, in which vessels span between portions of a bilobate or succenturiate placenta. The incidence of vasa previa is increased in multiple pregnancy, placenta previa, IVF conceptions (1 in 300). A detailed ultrasound with color Doppler is used for diagnosis. On ultrasound, the umbilical vessels are seen traversing lower segment above the cervix, unsupported by umbilical cord or placenta. If diagnosed antenatally, it is managed by elective cesarean section.

True Knot[9]

It is a rare finding with an incidence of 0.3–2%. True knots are found more commonly in long umbilical cords, polyhydramnios, small fetuses, male gender, gestational diabetes mellitus, monoamniotic twins, and multiparous women. The clinical significance of true knot is debatable with majority of cases having satisfactory obstetric outcome. Rarely, there may be an association with intrauterine fetal death when it results in obstructing blood circulation to the fetus.

Diagnosis

Ultrasound shows a typical "cloverleaf pattern" on gray scale.[10] In monoamniotic twins, when the true knot is purposely sought for, the sensitivity of ultrasonographic diagnosis increases.[11]

Umbilical Cord Cyst

Found in 1% of pregnancies, the cysts are divided into true cysts and pseudocysts. Pseudocysts are more frequently seen and can be found anywhere along the cord. They represent localized edema and liquefaction of Wharton's jelly and do not have an epithelial lining. True cysts are embryological remnants of allantois or omphalomesenteric duct and are usually located toward fetal insertion of the cord. Single cysts are usually innocuous and transient. The presence of multiple umbilical cord cysts is associated with an increased risk of miscarriage, chromosomal anomalies, structural abnormalities, and fetal growth restriction. A detailed ultrasound examination is recommended, with consideration to fetal karyotyping in nonisolated cases.

PLACENTAL EVALUATION IN ADVERSE PERINATAL OUTCOME[12]

Placental evaluation is considered essential in cases of stillbirth, late miscarriage, neonatal unit admission, prematurity, severe fetal growth restriction, fetal hydrops and maternal pyrexia (>38°C).[13] It is considered desirable in abruption, fetal congenital malformation, rhesus isoimmunization, morbidly adherent placenta, multiple pregnancy, abnormal placental shape, two vessel cord, prolonged rupture of membranes (>36 hours), gestational diabetes, maternal group B *Streptococcus* infection, preeclampsia, maternal coagulopathy and substance abuse. The placental examination should be undertaken by a perinatal pathologist. It involves naked eye examination **(Table 3)**, karyotyping, microbial culture and histopathology **(Box 1)**. The most viable tissues for karyotyping include placenta, umbilical cord close to placenta, cartilage from costochondral junction, patella and amniotic fluid.[14] Common histopathological findings are discussed here.[15]

Maternal Vascular Malperfusion

Maternal vascular malperfusion (MVM) occurs due to abnormal spiral artery blood flow and is characterized by agglutinated villi, increased syncytial knots, distal villous hypoplasia (affecting >30% of distal villi) and infarcts. It is associated with preeclampsia, fetal growth restriction and altered Doppler indices.

Massive Perivillous Fibrin Deposition

It is a rare placental condition associated with increased perinatal morbidity and mortality. It is also known as maternal

TABLE 3: Naked eye examination of placenta, cord and membranes.

Placenta	
	Weight
	Calcifications
	Diameter
	Retroplacental clots
Umbilical cord	
	Insertion
	Length
	Coiling
	Diameter
	Entanglement
	Knots: True or false
	Stricture
	Aneurysm
	Pseudocyst
	Ulcer
Membranes	
	Insertion
	Color
	Thickness
	Intact/not intact
	Surface characteristics

> **BOX 1:** Sample collection and processing of placenta.
>
> - Placenta should be stored in a sealed, correctly labeled container
> - Sample should be stored at 4°C
> - It should be submitted to laboratory in a fresh state
> - In case refrigerated storage is not available or if delay is anticipated in sending to laboratory, placenta can be formalin fixed. Primary formalin fixation has the advantage of rendering placentae less infectious, easier to section and better assessment of infarction. However, it renders placenta unsuitable for bacteriologic examination and tissue culture. The container should be adequately sized and formalin (10%) volume should be ample to minimize distortion
> - Relevant clinical details should be sent along with the placenta
> - Prior to grossing, a photographic record is useful which may be referred to later
> - Hematoxylin and Eosin (H & E) stain is used for histopathological examination
> - Other special assays such as chromosome analysis, mRNA, chromosomal microarray, etc., are done by a perinatal pathologist. They require special collection and sampling procedures

floor infarction which is a misnomer as there are no signs of infarction. There is excessive fibrin deposition in at least 30% of distal villi. It is associated with recurrent miscarriage, fetal growth restriction, stillbirth, preterm birth and neonatal neurological morbidity. The high recurrence rate of massive perivillous fibrin deposition (MPVFD) makes it clinically significant.

Fetal Thrombotic Vasculopathy

It can occur as a result of placental or umbilical pathology such as hypercoiling of cord, stricture, cord entanglement, and long cord. Characteristic pathological changes include intimal fibrin cushion, fibromuscular sclerosis, and hemorrhagic endovasculopathy. Fetal thrombotic vasculopathy (FTV) has association with oligohydramnios, fetal growth restriction, maternal or fetal thrombophilia, severe chorioamnionitis and fetal distress in labor.

Villitis of Unknown Etiology

It is a common finding in 5–15% of near term placentas and belongs to the group of placental inflammatory immune processes. It is characterized by chronic inflammation, destructive changes, and T cell infiltration into the chorionic villi. Villitis of unknown etiology (VUE) may be suspected when higher levels of human chorionic gonadotropin or alpha-fetoprotein levels are found in antenatal screening. It is found to be associated with fetal growth restriction, perinatal asphyxia, preeclampsia, prematurity and twin discordance.

Villous Dysmaturity

It is associated with maternal diabetes. The characteristic features include enlarged terminal villi, increase in number of capillaries and macrophages, with fluid within villous structure. These changes decrease the exchange of nutrients and oxygen between mother and fetus, and confirm presence of chronic fetal hypoxemia.

Chorioamnionitis

It is defined as an inflammation of amnion and chorion. It is classified according to the intensity of inflammation into two grades: Grade 1 (mild to moderate) and Grade 2 (severe). Microbial invasion of the amniotic cavity may occur either as an ascending infection from the lower genital tract or via hematogenous spread. While rupture of membranes is a risk factor, bacteria have been found to invade the amniotic cavity, even with intact membranes.

■ REFERENCES

1. Ugwumadu A. General Embryology. In: Basic Sciences for Obstetrics and Gynaecology, 1st edition. Oxford, United Kingdom: Oxford University Press; 2014. pp. 1-18.
2. Cunningham FG, Leveno K, Bloom S, Dashe J, Hoffman B, Casey B, et al. Placental Abnormalities. In: Williams Obstetrics, 25th edition. New York: McGraw Hill; 2018. pp. 111-23.
3. Fetal Medicine Foundation. (2020). Morbid Adherent Placenta. Fetal Abnormalities. [online] Available from: https://fetalmedicine.org/education/fetal-abnormalities/placenta-umbilical-cord/morbid-adherent-placenta. [Last Accessed October, 2021].
4. Predanic M. Sonographic assessment of the umbilical cord. Donald Sch J Ultrasound Obstet Gynaecol. 2009;3(2):48-57.
5. Hua M, Odibo AO, MacOnes GA, Roehl KA, Crane JP, Cahill AG. Single umbilical artery and its associated findings. Obstet Gynecol. 2010;115(5):930-4.
6. Geipel A, Germer U, Welp T, Schwinger E, Gembruch U. Prenatal diagnosis of single umbilical artery: determination of the absent side, associated anomalies. Doppler findings and perinatal outcome. Ultrasound Obstet Gynecol. 2000;15(2):114-7.
7. Gornall AS, Kurinczuk JJ, Konje JC. Antenatal detection of a single umbilical artery: does it matter? Prenat Diagn. 2003;23(2):117-23.
8. Sharma JB. Abnormalities of Placenta, Cord, Amniotic Fluid and Membranes. In: Textbook of Obstetrics, 1st edition. New Delhi: Avichal Publishing Company; 2014. pp. 324-33.
9. Ikechebelu J, Eleje G, Ofojebe C. True umbilical cord knot leading to fetal demise. Ann Med Health Sci Res. 2014;4(Suppl 2):S155-S158.
10. Ramón Y Cajal CL, Martínez RO. Four-dimensional ultrasonography of a true knot of the umbilical cord. Am J Obstet Gynecol. 2006;195(4):896-8.
11. Deutsch AB, Miller E, Spellacy WN, Mabry RT. Ultrasound to identify cord knotting in monoamniotic monochorionic twins. Res Hum Genet. 2007;10(1):216-8.
12. Yetter JF. Examination of the Placenta. Am Fam Physician. 1998;1;57(5):1045-54.
13. Cox P, Evans C. Tissue pathway for histopathological examination of the placenta. London: Royal College of Pathologists; 2017.
14. Jaiman S. Gross Examination of the Placenta and Its Importance in Evaluating: an Unexplained Intrauterine Fetal demise. J Fetal Med. 2015;2:113-20.
15. Thirumalaikumar L, Ramalingam K, Marton T. Placental histopathological abnormalities and poor perinatal outcomes. Obstet Gynaecol. 2019;21:135-42.

LONG QUESTIONS

1. What are the ultrasonographic features in morbid adhesion of placenta?
2. Write a note on the work up of placental evaluation in adverse perinatal outcome.

SHORT QUESTIONS

1. Write short notes on the following:
   a. Succenturiate placenta
   b. Single umbilical artery
   c. Contents of umbilical cord

MULTIPLE CHOICE QUESTIONS

1. The normal umbilical coiling index is:
   a. 0.2
   b. 0.1
   c. 0.4
   d. 0.5
2. A normal umbilical cord has ___ vessels:
   a. 1
   b. 2
   c. 3
   d. 4
3. The finding of a single umbilical artery on examination of the umbilical cord after delivery is:
   a. Insignificant
   b. Occurs in 10% of newborns
   c. An indicator of considerably increased incidence of major malformation of the fetus
   d. Equally common in newborn of diabetic and nondiabetic mothers
4. Fetal blood loss in abnormal cord insertion is seen in:
   a. Vasa previa
   b. Decidua basalis
   c. Battledore placenta
   d. Succenturiate placenta
5. Placenta succenturiata may have all, except:
   a. Preterm delivery
   b. Postpartum hemorrhage
   c. Missing lobe
   d. Sepsis and sub-involution
6. Human placenta is best described as:
   a. Discoidal
   b. Hemochorial
   c. Deciduate
   d. All of the above

Answers
1. a 2. c 3. c 4. a 5. a 6. d

7.5 FETAL GROWTH RESTRICTION

Pratik Tambe, Sarita Bhalerao, Usha Krishna

INTRODUCTION

There are several determinants of fetal birth weight including hereditary, familial, ethnic predisposition, genetics, adequate maternal nutrition, an uneventful antenatal course and a normally functioning placenta which forms the link between the mother and the baby. Various etiologies have been implicated in fetal growth restriction which may be of maternal, fetal and placental origin. Common conditions include maternal disease, hypertensive disorders of pregnancy (HDP) and other pathologies which involve compromised uteroplacental blood flow and circulation. Of particular importance are diseases which involve an inadequate second wave of trophoblastic invasion, e.g., HDP as noted earlier.

ETIOLOGY

Fetal Origin

- Commonly associated aneuplodies such as trisomy 13, 18, 21, Turner syndrome, aberrations such as deletions
- Multiple pregnancies.

Placental Factors

Various conditions including placenta previa, circumvallate placenta, chorioangiomata, multiple placental infarcts, infections such as syphilis and malaria can cause FGR. According to a review by Burton G, placental origin FGR arises from a lack of conversion of the spiral arteries into a capacitance system in early pregnancy. This leads to fibrin deposition and infarction and are seen in HDP. The consequent reduction in placental size leads to reduced surface area and the gas exchange therefore suffers.[1]

Maternal Conditions

- Nutritional deficiency specifically Vitamins C and E
- Chronic infections such as tuberculosis, malaria, toxoplasmosis, HIV, rubella, CMV, herpes, varicella in first trimester
- Chronic hypertension or pregnancy induced hypertension can cause reduced uteroplacental blood flow
- Smoking, tobacco use
- Endocrine disorders such as diabetes mellitus and thyroid disorders
- Anemia
- Cardiorespiratory diseases such as COPD and valvular heart disease
- Antiphospholipid antibody (APLA) syndrome
  This syndrome is associated with multiple/recurrent miscarriages, second and third trimester intrauterine fetal deaths (IUFD), HDP and FGR. Immune complexes are formed along with complement activation and vascular endothelial damage. Micro and macrothromboses lead to placental infarcts, fetal compromise, and occasionally IUFD.

- Renal diseases like chronic glomerulonephritis can also cause FGR.
  Oxidative stress is an important cause of FGR. Karowics-Bilinska et al. found elevated levels of malondialdehyde and 4-hydroxyalkenals and decreased alpha-1 antitrypsin which point to lowered antioxidant capacity when compared with a healthy pregnancy. Treatment with 3 g of L-arginine and 75 mg of acetylsalicylic acid daily for 3 weeks resulted in a decrease lipid peroxidation and improvement in alpha 1 antitrypsin activity.[2]
- Postmaturity: The word "postmature" refers to a clinical syndrome of uteroplacental insufficiency resulting in oligohydramnios, meconium passage, fetal hypoxia and fetal death. Changes in the placenta are meconium staining of cord and placenta, calcium deposition, infarcts at placental borders. Placental infarcts are seen in 10–25% of term pregnancies and 60–89% of post-term placentae.
- Congenital abnormalities of the uterus.

DIAGNOSIS

The first step is to estimate the gestational age as per a dating scan, typically from the first trimester if available. While this is typically calculated from the last menstrual period, it may be fallacious in women with irregular cycles.

Worldwide, irrespective of racial and ethnic differences, there is a positive correlation between maternal weight gain during pregnancy and the fetal birth weight. Absence of weight gain <4.3 kg prior to 24 weeks is considered an independent predictor of FGR.

Serial fundal height estimation is commonly used in antenatal clinics as a marker for identifying adequate growth of the baby. This method utilizes a tape measure from the fundus till the pubic symphysis, ideally with its marking side face down to avoid errors/bias on the part of the obstetrician.

BIOCHEMICAL MARKERS

Coyle and Brown (1963) reported significantly lower urinary estriol levels in pregnancies with small babies. With advancement in laboratory methods, there was a shift from urinary to blood estriol level estimation. However, there is significant diurnal and day to day variation in plasma as well as urinary estriol levels. Hence, this cannot be reliably used as a predictor for FGR.

Human placental lactogen (hPL) was widely studied in the late 1960s. Plasma hPL concentrations <4 μg/mL beyond 30 weeks gestation are considered abnormally low and indicative high risk of FGR. However, a significant number of IUFDs could also occur when hPL levels were normal, so this is no longer considered a reliable predictor for FGR.[3]

ULTRASONOGRAPHIC BIOMETRY

Ultrasound has emerged as the gold standard in assessment of fetal growth over the past few decades. The standard measurement of the biparietal diameter (BPD), head circumference (HC), abdominal circumference (AC) and femur length (FL) performed by the radiologist/sonographer are compared with the 50th centile in population charts via the integrated software. When below the 10th centile, these are considered highly suspicious of FGR. Any measurement below the 3rd centile is labeled as unequivocal evidence of FGR.

Ponderal index

This is calculated by the formula estimated fetal weight (EFW)/FL^3 and when less than the 10th centile, is considered significant. Based on the Ponderal index two types of FGR have traditionally been described:

1. Symmetric FGR: The Ponderal index is normal, HC is less and weight and length are both lower than the normal population. This is owing to early onset growth restriction.
2. Asymmetric FGR: The Ponderal index is low and the fetal weight is restricted more than the length, presumably from late onset growth restriction.

Amniotic Fluid Index

The fetus is surrounded by amniotic fluid which includes the fetal urine, GI and respiratory tract secretions. As a consequence of FGR, there is reduced renal blood flow, lower glomerular filtration rate, diversion of blood to the fetal brain and therefore, less liquor is seen. The amniotic fluid index (AFI) consists of the vertical depth of vertical measurements of amniotic fluid in each of the four uterine quadrants. An AFI of ≥5 cm and/ or any single vertical pocket >2 cm is considered as normal. Placental aging as reflected by placental calcium deposits is also another clue to a compromised circulation and FGR. The presence of a Grade 3 placenta before 36 weeks is considered as corroborative evidence of FGR.[4]

SCREENING FOR FETAL GROWTH RESTRICTION

Effective screening for FGR has the potential to reduce the mortality and morbidity due to FGR. The new maternal biomarker placental growth factor offers much potential in this context. Society of Obstetricians and Gynaecologists of Canada (SOGC) recommend that all women should be screened for clinical risk factors. Screening tests using biomarkers of placental function and ultrasound have been evaluated.

Sotiriadis et al. in a retrospective study of women in antenatal care who were subjected to antenatal ultrasound surveillance identified a combination of factors which may be used to predict FGR. Their first trimester screening model which included factors on history such as the type of conception, maternal smoking, mother's height and investigations including pregnancy associated plasma protein-A (PAPP-A) and uterine artery pulsatility index (UtAPI) could predict 50.0% of the antenatally diagnosed and 36.7% of the late FGR with a 10% false positive rate.

Furthermore, a model which included both first and second trimester screening parameters (type of conception, maternal smoking, s PAPP-A levels, second trimester EFW, HC/AC ratio and UtAPI) could predict 78.6% of the antenatally detected and 59.6% of the late FGR with a 10% FPR [area under the curve 0.901 (95% CI, 0.856–0.947) and 0.855 (95% CI, 0.818–0.891), respectively]. Unfortunately, the prediction of FGR was less than ideal for both first trimester and combined screening.[5]

■ MANAGEMENT PRINCIPLES

A practice bulletin on FGR issued by the ACOG notes that intrauterine growth retardation (IUGR) is a common complication during pregnancy and is associated with a variety of adverse perinatal outcomes. There is confusion surrounding the exact terminology, varying etiology and appropriate diagnostic criteria for fetal growth restriction. There is also uncertainty regarding the preferred management and correct gestational age to deliver in such cases. Other conditions such as genetically or constitutionally small babies can present as a small fetus further confusing the issue.[6]

■ EVALUATION

As noted earlier, inadequacy in growth is associated with poor fetal and neonatal outcomes. Clinical evidence suggests that there are broadly two groups: (1) FGR and (2) constitutional SGA. The former are more prone to in utero compromise, stillbirth, and worse perinatal outcomes when compared with AGA fetuses. Doppler findings in FGR suggest a hemodynamic redistribution owing to fetal adaptation to undernutrition and in utero hypoxia. These findings are classically absent in constitutional SGA fetuses.

Figueras F et al. note that this is an important distinction owing to the impact on perinatal outcomes. Most international authorities recommend delivery in FGR fetuses when lung maturation is achieved. It may be hastened if there is deterioration during monitoring. This is in contradistinction to SGA fetuses where active intervention is often unwarranted. In clinical practice, differentiating between these two may be difficult and relies on Doppler identification of various fetal changes consequent to placental insufficiency **(Fig. 1)**.[7]

Fallacy of Umbilical Artery Doppler

A large number of studies have demonstrated that abnormal UA Doppler correlated with poor outcomes in FGR babies. Hence, for nearly two decades, Doppler evaluation of the umbilical artery has now been widely accepted as the gold standard for diagnosis, evaluation and treatment follow-up in FGR. However, small fetuses with normal UA Doppler have been missed due to this approach which considers them as constitutional SGA. UA Doppler observations are correct when there is severe FGR consequent to severe placental compromise. Unfortunately, it may not identify mild placental insufficiency which is seen in some early onset FGR and almost all cases of delayed onset FGR. Hence, UA Doppler should not be used as a single criterion for the diagnosis of FGR.[8]

Doppler Cerebroplacental Ratio

The Doppler cerebroplacental ratio (CPR) is an important index of fetal well-being and is obtained by dividing the middle cerebral artery (MCA) PI by the UA Doppler PI. This is probably a better indicator of FGR when compared with routine Doppler evaluation. It has been postulated to reflect mild increases in placental resistance and with compensatory mild reductions in fetal cerebrovascular resistance. Alterations in the CPR are more frequently encountered when there is hypoxia than either MCA PI and/or UA PI and correlates better with poor perinatal morbidity and mortality.

In fetuses below the 10th centile, those with an EFW < 3rd centile have a greater risk of adverse perinatal outcome no matter what may be the CPR and UtA Doppler indices. When either CPR or uterine artery PI are abnormal or EFW is < 3rd centile, the risk of adverse perinatal outcome is increased. Hence, it has been proposed that a modern definition of FGR should ideally include all of these three parameters.

Early versus Late Onset FGR[8]

Early onset FGR in up to 50% of cases and is consequent to HDP, severe placental insufficiency and chronic fetal hypoxia **(Table 1; Figs. 2 and 3)**. Long duration of compromise results in hypoxia and acidosis, abnormal UA PI and raised PI in the ductus venosus (DV). These changes on Doppler monitoring help assessing the progression of fetal deterioration and allow us to plan elective delivery.

On the other hand, late onset FGR may show normal UA Doppler values but there will still be abnormalities in CPR values as noted above. Advanced brain vasodilation which is seen in chronic hypoxia is reflected by an MCA PI <p5 and may occur in 25% of late FGR. Signs of fetal compromise including changes in DV are virtually never seen in late FGR. There is a high risk of severe deterioration, intrapartum fetal distress, and late pregnancy mortality.

While treatment is easily instituted in late onset FGR, the challenge remains to diagnose it in time before complications have ensued. Management in early onset FGR requires achieving a balance between the risks of continuing the pregnancy against the risk of prematurity and NICU admission.

■ MONITORING AND PATHOPHYSIOLOGICAL PROGRESSION

Role of Cardiotocography

Conventional cardiotocography (CTG) has been shown to have 50% false positive rate for prediction of fetal outcomes

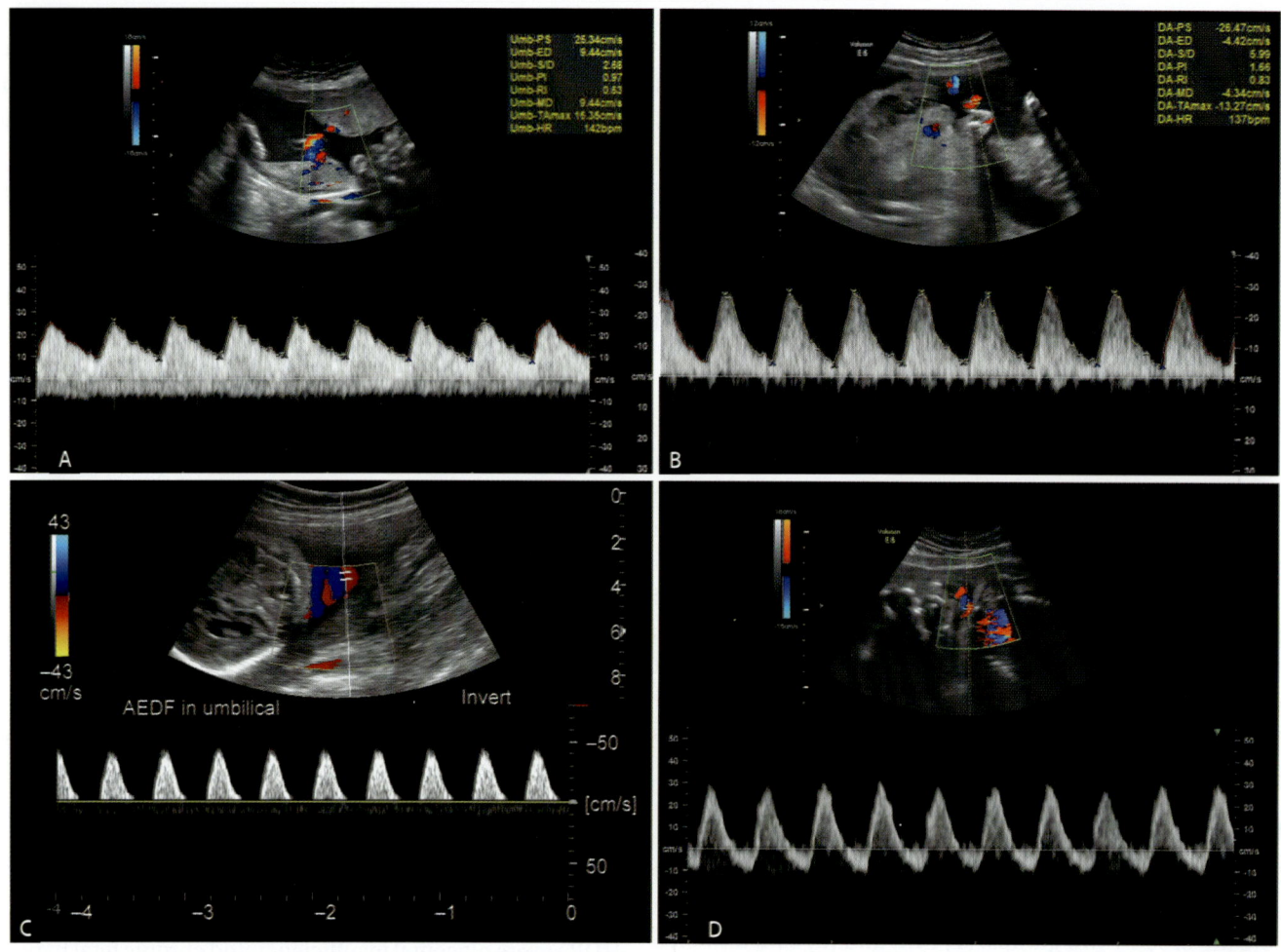

Figs. 1A to D: Umbilical artery Doppler waveforms. (A) Normal umbilical artery Doppler; (B) High resistance umbilical artery Doppler; (C) Absent diastolic flow umbilical artery Doppler; (D) Reversed diastolic flow umbilical artery Doppler (AEDF: absent end-diastolic flow).

TABLE 1: Early onset and late onset FGR.	
Early-onset FGR (1–2%)	*Late-onset FGR (3–5%)*
Problem: Management	*Problem:* Diagnosis
Placental disease: Severe (UA Doppler abnormal, high association with preeclampsia)	*Place ntal disease:* Mild (UA Doppler normal, low association with preeclampsia)
Hypoxia++: Systemic cardiovascular adaptation	*Hypoxia +/–:* Central cardiovascular adaptation
Immature fetus = higher tolerance to hypoxia = natural history	Mature fetus = lower tolerance to hypoxia = no (or very short) natural history
High mortality and morbidity; lower prevalence	Lower mortality (but common cause of late stillbirth); poor long-term outcome; affects large fraction of pregnancies

and has been proven in meta-analysis to be ineffective in reducing perinatal mortality. However, computerized CTG with analysis of the short term variation (STV) of FHR is non-subjective and better associated with prediction of advanced fetal deterioration. STV closely correlates with fetal acidosis and severe hypoxia.[9,10]

Biophysical Profile and Amniotic Fluid Index

The biophysical profile (BPP) has a high false positive rate similar to CTG while low amniotic fluid index (AFI) is considered a chronic marker of fetal compromise. In current practice, the preference is for color Doppler evaluation over the BPP or AFI to diagnose and predict complications including timing of delivery.

Bed Rest

Bed rest as a methodology of treatment is commonly prescribed, whether in hospital or at home. This enables close monitoring and supervision but the benefits of bed rest must be balanced with the risk of thrombosis. Scientific

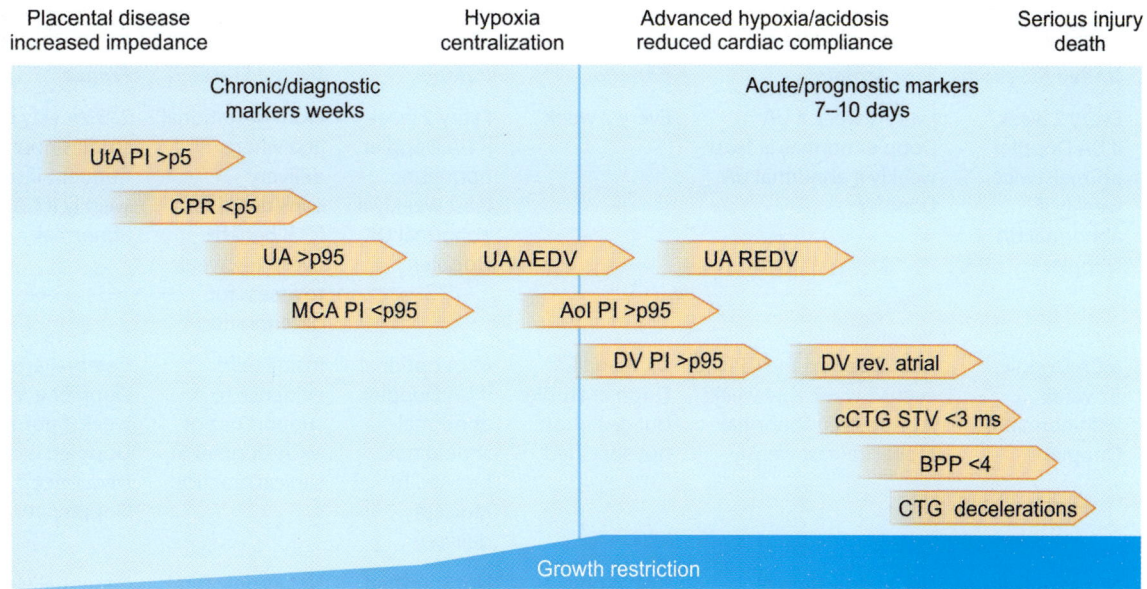

Fig. 2: Early onset FGR.[8]

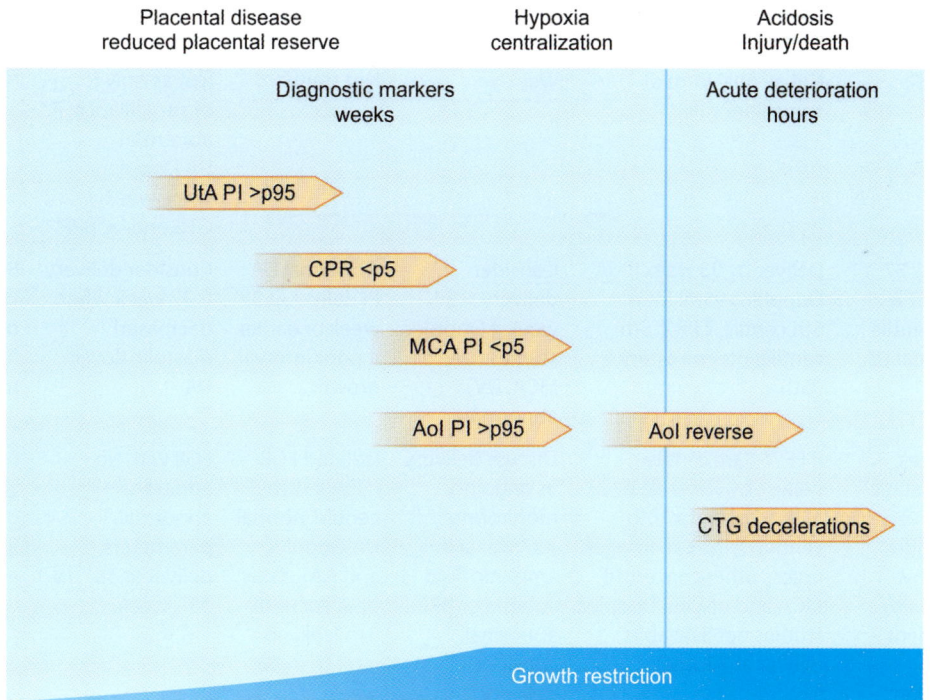

Fig. 3: Late onset FGR.[8]

studies, which compare bed rest with ambulatory treatment have shown minor differences in birth weights but this is not statistically significant.

Maternal Dietary Supplementation

Implementing general dietary supplementation vis-a-vis specific protein supplementation has a small and variable effect on fetal growth to the extent of an increase. When there is a low dietary intake of DHA, such antenatal DHA supplementation may result in increased neonatal weight.

■ SURVEILLANCE AND TIMING OF BIRTH

McCowan et al. performed a systematic review of evidence based national guidelines for the management of FGR. These included those from the UK, USA, France, Canada, New Zealand, and Ireland. A summary of their findings is highlighted in the **Table 2**.[11]

There is consensus in recommending fundal height measurement in the third trimester and three guidelines specify the use of a customized growth chart. Routine scanning is not recommended and should be restricted to women who

TABLE 2: Monitoring and timing of birth for late onset FGR.

Country	United Kingdom	New Zealand	Canada	Ireland	United States	France
UA Doppler frequency	Every 2 week if UA Doppler normal, twice weekly if abnormal UA Doppler	Every 2 week if UA Doppler normal, at least weekly if abnormal UA Doppler	Every 2 week	Every 2 week if UA Doppler normal, at least weekly if abnormal UA Doppler	From gestational age where delivery considered for fetal benefit every 1–2 week to assess for deterioration[b]	2–3 Weekly if Doppler studies normal, more frequent if severe FGR; weekly if UA Doppler abnormal
Cerebral Doppler studies	MCA Doppler > 32 week with normal UA Doppler	MCA Doppler and CPR every 2 week ≥ 34 week; if Doppler(s) abnormal repeat at least weekly	MCA and DV Doppler studies but gestation not specified	MCA optional if UA Doppler abnormal—should not be used to indicate delivery	Insufficient evidence to support use of MCA Doppler in clinical practice	Cerebral artery Doppler every 2–3 week if normal UA Doppler; increase frequency if UA Doppler abnormal
CTG	Not as only form of surveillance	Not as only form of surveillance; at least weekly if abnormal UA, MCA, CPR, uterine artery Doppler or EFW <3rd centile	Not as only form of surveillance, consider if BPP abnormal	Not specified	Not as only form of surveillance; if abnormal UA Doppler, twice-weekly CTG and/or BPP[b]	"Essential element in assessment of SGA fetus," frequency not specified
BPP	Do not use	Not as only form of surveillance	Weekly	Not standard	Not as only form of surveillance; if abnormal UA Doppler, twice weekly CTG and/or BPP[b]	Not discussed
Timing of birth abnormal Doppler[a]	Deliver by 37 week if MCA PI <5th centile or abnormal UA Doppler	Deliver by 38 week if UA Doppler >95th, MCA < 5th centile, CPR < 5th centile, uterine artery > 95th	Consider delivery > 34 week if Doppler studies (UA, MCA, DV) abnormal	Abnormal UA PI deliver at 37 week or earlier if poor interval growth	Consider delivery > 37 week when decreased diastolic flow in UA	Birth from ≥37 week depending on EFW, amniotic fluid, and Doppler measurements
Timing of birth normal Doppler	If >34 week deliver if static growth over 3 week; offer delivery by 37 week with involvement of senior obstetrician	If EFW <3rd centile deliver by 38 week; if EFW >3rd and <10th centile deliver at 40 week unless other concern; if MCA and uterine Doppler studies not available, deliver at 38 week	Discuss delivery vs ongoing monitoring >37 week; if amniotic fluid volume or BPP abnormal, consider delivery	Isolated FGR (EFW <10th centile, normal UA Doppler, and AA), delay delivery until 37 week, no later than 40 week	FGR with no additional abnormal parameters, deliver at 38^{+0} to 39^{+6} week	Birth from ≥37 week depending on EFW, amniotic fluid, and Doppler measurements
Mode of birth	If UA end-diastolic flow present, induction of labor with continuous CTG recommended	Individualize care; high risk of CS with abnormal CPR, MCA, or UA Doppler—continuous fetal monitoring from onset of labor	Not specified	Individualize care; consider CS <34 week	FGR alone not indication for CS	Routine CS for FGR not recommended; CS recommended for very preterm FGR or severe UA Doppler abnormalities; continuous fetal monitoring in labor

(AFI: amniotic fluid index; BPP: biophysical profile; CPR: cerebroplacental ratio; CS: cesarean delivery; CTG: cardiotocography; DV: ductus venosus; EFW: estimated fetal weight; FGR: fetal growth restriction; MCA: middle cerebral artery; PI: pulsatility index; SGA: small for gestational age; UA: umbilical artery
[a]Pregnancies with absent or reversed end-diastolic volume are considered in Table 5; [b]Society of maternal-fetal medicine guideline.
McCowan evidence-based national guidelines for management os suspected fetal growth restriction. Am J Obstet Gynecol 2018.

have major risk factors and should be recommended serial scanning in the third trimester. UA Doppler is universally advised but the recommended frequency varies (2–4 weekly). In late-onset FGR >32 weeks, the consensus fetal cerebral Doppler studies should be utilized to plan the time of delivery. Fetal surveillance using CTG is recommended but timing of delivery recommended is not consistent.[11]

Low Dose Aspirin

Low dose aspirin is recommended for women risk of HDP. There is a marked reduction in risk of early onset HDP in women identified as exhibiting high risk during first trimester screening. These parameters include maternal history, uterine artery Doppler, blood pressure, serum pregnancy associated plasma protein (PAPP)-A and placental growth factor who were treated with low-dose aspirin 150 mg. A reduction in FGR has been demonstrated and a systematic review concluded that aspirin was more effective in preventing HDP and FGR when started at or before 16 weeks and in a dose of 100 mg.[12-15]

Low Molecular Weight Heparin

Based on an earlier meta-analysis, the Canadian guideline recommends that heparin should be offered in selected women. However, the Enoxaparin for Prevention of Preeclampsia and Intrauterine Growth Restriction trial has demonstrated that enoxaparin is not effective in preventing FGR in women with previous severe or early onset FGR and is not recommended.[16,17]

FOLLOW-UP AND MONITORING PROTOCOLS (TABLE 3)

Several authorities have proposed monitoring and follow-up protocols and one such algorithm is reproduced in **Figure 4**.

Timing of Delivery in Late Onset FGR

In FGR where color Doppler studies are abnormal or EFW <3rd centile, international guidelines suggest that delivery should be planned at 37–38 weeks. When color Doppler findings are normal and the EFW not <3rd centile, a more conservative approach may be prudent.

The Disproportionate Intrauterine Growth Intervention Trial at Term study included 650 women with suspected FGR >36 weeks. They were randomized to 2 groups: induction of labor or expectant management with twice weekly surveillance. The women who were expectantly managed had double the incidence of HDP (7.9% vs. 3.7%, p <.05) and were more likely to have fetal birth weight <3rd centile (30% vs. 13%, p <.001). Additional data on outcomes in the children showed that there was no difference in neonatal morbidity between induction of labor and expectant management groups. However, induction of labor at <38 weeks was associated with increased NICU admissions. The study concluded that planning delivery at 38 weeks in FGR fetuses may be ideal.[18-23]

Timing of Delivery in Early Onset FGR

The Trial of Randomized Umbilical and Fetal Flow in Europe (TRUFFLE) of management of preterm FGR between 26 and 32 weeks was an important and landmark trial as far as management strategies is concerned. This trial was a study on early onset FGR where mothers were allocated to 1 of 3 monitoring strategies to indicate timing of delivery: reduced fetal heart rate short-term variability on CTG, early changes in fetal ductus venosus (DV) waveform or late changes in fetal DV waveform. The TRUFFLE trial has shown that waiting until late changes occur in the DV Doppler or abnormal CTG correlates with improved outcomes at 2 years of age.[24]

Management Protocols for Early Onset FGR[6]

Monitoring and timing of birth for early onset FGR in different countries are given in **Table 4**.

RECENT ADVANCES

As elucidated earlier, if the risk of hypoxia, fetal acidosis and intrauterine death is severe, the only solution is the maternal

TABLE 3: Classification of FGR and prognostication based on Doppler indices.				
Stage	**Pathophysiological correlate**	**Criteria (any of)**	**Monitoring**	**GA/mode of delivery**
I	Severe smallness or mild placental insufficiency	EFW <3rd centile EPR <p5 UA IP >p95 MCA PI <p5 UtA PI >p95	Weekly	37 weeks
II	Severe placental insufficiency	UAAEDV Reverse AoI	Biweekly	34 weeks CS
III	Low-suspicion fetal acidosis	UA REDV DV-PI >3 ms FHR decelerations	1–2 days	30 weeks CS
IV	High-suspicion fetal acidosis	DV reverse a flow cCTG <3 ms FHR decelerations	12h	26 weeks CS

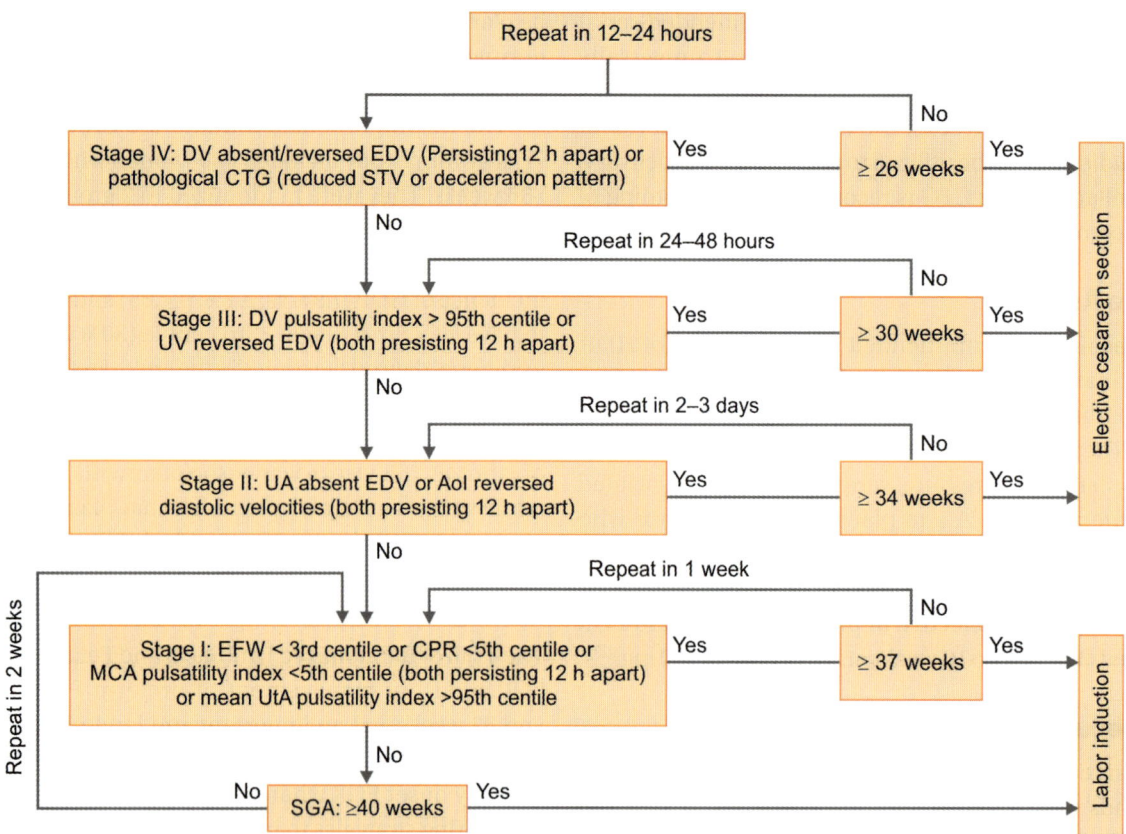

Fig. 4: Surveillance algorithm.

TABLE 4: Monitoring and timing of birth for early onset FGR.						
Country	*United Kingdom*	*New Zealand*	*Canada*	*Ireland*	*United States*	*France*
Corticosteroids	Up to 35^{+6} week	Up to 34^{+0} week	Up to 34^{+0} week	Up to 34^{+0} week	Up to 34^{+0} week	Up to 34^{+0} week
Magnesium sulfate	Not specified	<30 week[b]	Not specified	32 week	<32 week	<32–33 week
Recommended timing of delivery with AEDV and REDV	AEDV by 32 week; REDV by 32 week	AEDV by 34 week; REDV by 32 week	AEDV not specified; REDV not specified; "Requires intervention and possibly delivery	AEDV no later than 34 week; REDV no later than 30 week	AEDV ≥ 34 week[a]; REDV ≥ 32 week	AEDV ≥34 week; REDV ≥34 week
Indication for delivery	Abnormal computerized CTG or DV Doppler	Not applicable—NZMFMN guideline for SGA ≥34 week	Abnormal BPP, CTG or DV Doppler	Abnormal computerized CTG	Abnormal fetal surveillance (CTG, amniotic fluid, or BPP)	Abnormal computerized CTG or DV Doppler
Mode of delivery	CS for AEDV and REDV	CS for AEDV and REDV	Not specified	CS for AEDV and REDV	FGR alone not indication for CS	CS for AEDV and REDV

Include survaillance for AEDV as this usually occur <32 week gestation, and >32 week gestation delivery is usual practice.
AEDV: absent end-diastolic volume; BPP: biophysical profile; CS: cesarean section; CTG: cardiotocography; DV: ductus venosus; FGR: fetal growth restriction; NZMFMN: New Zealand Maternal Fetal Medicine Network; REDV: revereesed end diastolic volume; SGA: small for gestational age
[a]Society for Maternal-fetal medicine Doppler guideline; [b]New Zealand magnesium sulfate guidelines.
McCowan evidence-based national guidelines for management os suspected fetal growth restriction. Am J Obstet Gynecol 2018.

administration of magnesium sulfate for fetal neuroprotection and administering corticosteroids to achieve fetal lung maturity followed by delivery and transfer to an NICU.

Several promising approaches in recent years utilize varying approaches and strategies aiming to increase fetal growth by improving uterine blood flow and enhancing the placental circulation. Phosphodiesterase type 5 inhibitors that which act by increasing nitric oxide availability (e.g., sildenafil citrate) have been extensively studied. The results from the Sildenafil TheRapy In Dismal Prognosis Early onset intrauterine growth Restriction (STRIDER) randomized controlled clinical trials are as yet awaited.[25]

Maternal vascular endothelial growth factor (VEGF) gene therapy is one such avenue which is being explored. Other approaches include nanoparticles and microRNA to deliver drugs to the uterine arterial endothelium or trophoblast. Research into melatonin, creatine and N-acetyl cysteine suggests they may have potential as neuro- and cardioprotective agents in fetal growth restriction.[26]

CONCLUSION

The management of FGR is a subject for eternal debate. While early onset FGR is easily detected, the optimal route and timing of delivery is a subject for much discussion. Late onset FGR is often missed with devastating consequences and there is much scope for improvement of surveillance protocols for timely identification of this condition. Therapeutic options are limited in that they need to be initiated at an appropriate duration of pregnancy and the advantages that they offer may be minimal necessitating close surveillance and pose a dilemma regarding how to proceed with a view to optimizing the fetal outcome.

KEY MESSAGES

Fetal growth restriction (FGR) is a pathological condition associated with a decrease in the rate of fetal growth. FGR may occur secondary to uteroplacental compromise leading to an inadequate supply of nutrients and oxygen to the growing fetus. This is commonly classified as symmetrical and asymmetrical depending on ultrasonographic biometry. In symmetrical FGR, fetal chromosomal anomalies, structural abnormalities, and intrauterine infections should be excluded. Owing to absence of uteroplacental vascular remodeling during the second wave of trophoblastic invasion in conditions such as hypertensive disorders of pregnancy, there is an increase in placental bed vascular resistance and lowered oxygen delivery to the growing fetus. This underperfusion of the placenta also causes villous damage, the total tertiary villous capillary bed surface area is reduced further enhancing the detrimental effects of increased placental resistance. These changes can be diagnosed by color Doppler and with changes seen in the uterine, umbilical, fetal middle cerebral arteries and ductus venosus vessels and their indices. In severe cases, careful surveillance, planning the delivery of the fetus balancing the risks and advantages is essential to achieve a good perinatal outcome.

REFERENCES

1. Burton GJ. Pathophysiology of placental-derived fetal growth restriction. Am J Obstet Gynecol. 2018;218(2):S745-61.
2. Karowicz-Bilinska A, Kedziora-Kornatowska K, Bartosz G. Indices of oxidative stress in pregnancy with fetal growth restriction. Informa Healthcare (London). 2007.41,870-873.
3. John F. Biochemical prediction of the low birth weight growth restricted baby. In: Tambyraja RL, Mongelli M (Eds). The Low Birth Weight Baby. Obstetrics and Gynecology in Perspective. Hyderabad: Orient Longman Private Limited; 2003.
4. Suhas O, Coyaji K. Fetal growth restriction. In: Krishna U, Shah D, Salvi V, Sheriar N, Damania K (Eds). Pregnancy at Risk, 5th edition. New Delhi: Jaypee Brothers Medical Publishers (P) Ltd.; 2010.
5. Sotiriadis A, Figueras F, Eleftheriades M, Papaioannou GK, Chorozoglou G, Dinas K, et al. Ultrasound Obstet Gynecol. 2019;53(1):55-61.
6. ACOG Practice Bulletin No. 204. Fetal Growth Restriction. Obstet Gynecol. 2019;133(2):e97-e109.
7. Figueras F, Gratacós E. Update on the Diagnosis and Classification of Fetal Growth Restriction and Proposal of a Stage-Based Management Protocol. Fetal Diagn Ther. 2014;36:86-98.
8. Oros D. Longitudinal changes in uterine, umbilical and fetal cerebral Doppler indices in late-onset small-for-gestational age fetuses. Ultrasound Obstet Gynecol. 2011;37:191-5.
9. Pattison N, McCowan L. Cardiotocography for antepartum fetal assessment. Cochrane Database Syst Rev. 2000:CD001068.
10. Grivell RM. Antenatal cardiotocography for fetal assessment. Cochrane Database Syst Rev. 2010:CD007863.
11. McCowan LM, Figueras F, Anderson NH. Evidence-based national guidelines for the management of suspected fetal growth restriction: comparison, consensus, and controversy. Am J Obstet Gynecol. 2018;218(2S):S855-S868.
12. Alfirevic Z, Stampalija T, Dowswell T. Fetal and umbilical Doppler ultrasound in high-risk pregnancies. Cochrane Database Syst Rev. 2017;6:CD007529.
13. World Health Organization. WHO recommendations for prevention and treatment of preeclampsia and eclampsia. Geneva: World Health Organization; 2011.
14. Rolnik DL, Wright D, Poon LCY. ASPRE trial: performance of screening for preterm pre-eclampsia. Ultrasound Obstet Gynecol. 2017;50:492-5.
15. Roberge S, Nicolaides K, Demers S, Hyett J, Chaillet N, Bujold E. The role of aspirin dose on the prevention of preeclampsia and fetal growth restriction: systematic review and meta-analysis. Am J Obstet Gynecol. 2017;216:110-20.e116.
16. Rodger MA, Gris JC, de Vries JIP. Low molecular weight heparin and recurrent placenta mediated pregnancy complications: a meta-analysis of individual patient data from randomized controlled trials. Lancet. 2016;388:2629-41.
17. Groom KM, McCowan LM, Mackay LK. Enoxaparin for the prevention of preeclampsia and intrauterine growth restriction in women with a history: a randomized trial. Am J Obstet Gynecol. 2017;216:296.e1-14.
18. Boers KE, Vijgen SM, Bijlenga D. Induction versus expectant monitoring for intrauterine growth restriction at term: randomized equivalence trial (DIGITAT). BMJ. 2010;341:c7087.
19. Royal College of Obstetricians and Gynecologists. The investigation and management of the small-for-gestational-age fetus. Green-top guideline no. 31. London: RCOG; 2013.
20. Lausman A, Kingdom J. Intrauterine growth restriction: screening, diagnosis and management. SOGC clinical practice guideline no. 295. J Obstet Gynaecol Can. 2013;35:741-8.

21. New Zealand Maternal Fetal Medicine Network. Guideline for the management of suspected small for gestational age singleton pregnancies and infants after 34 wk' gestation. New Zealand Maternal Fetal Medicine Network. 2014.
22. Institute of Obstetricians and Gynecologists Royal College of Physicians of Ireland. Fetal growth restriction-recognition, diagnosis management. Clinical practice guideline no. 28. 2017. Version 1.1. Updated March 2017.
23. Vayssiere C, Sentilhes L, Ego A. Fetal growth restriction and intra-uterine growth restriction: guidelines for clinical practice from the French College of Gynecologists and Obstetricians. Eur J Obstet Gynecol Reprod Biol. 2015;193:10-8.
24. Lees CC, Marlow N, van Wassenaer-Leemhuis A, Arabin B, Bilardo CM, Brezinka C, et al. 2 year Neurodevelopmental and intermediate perinatal outcomes in infants with very preterm fetal growth restriction (TRUFFLE): a randomized trial. Lancet. 2015;385:2162-72.
25. Pels A, Kenny LC, Alfirevic Z, Baker PN, von Dadelszen P, Gluud C, et al. STRIDER (Sildenafil TheRapy in dismal prognosis early onset fetal growth restriction): an international consortium of randomised placebo-controlled trials. BMC Pregnancy Childbirth. 2017;17(1):440.
26. Groom KM, David AL. The role of aspirin, heparin, and other interventions in the prevention and treatment of fetal growth restriction. Am J Obstet Gynecol. 2018;218(2S):S829-S840.

LONG QUESTIONS

1. Discuss uteroplacental circulations and its importance?
2. Discuss different drugs used for the treatment of FGR?

SHORT QUESTIONS

1. What are the fetal causes of FGR?
2. What are the color Doppler changes seen in FGR?
3. What are neonatal complications of FGR?

MULTIPLE CHOICE QUESTIONS

1. Fetal birth weight is determined by:
    a. Genetic growth potential
    b. Intrauterine nutrition
    c. Uteroplacental blood flow
    d. Maternal height and weight
    e. All of the above
2. Placental growth involves:
    a. Trophoblast invasion in 1st trimester
    b. Trophoblast invasion in 2nd trimester
    c. Conversion of rigid vessels into capacitance vessels
    d. Decreased vascular resistance
    e. All of the above
3. Fetal growth restriction is not seen in:
    a. Trisomy 13   b. Trisomy 21
    c. Turner syndrome   d. Klinefelter syndrome
    e. Chromosomal deletions
4. Factors not responsible for FGR include:
    a. Vitamin C deficiency   b. Malaria
    c. Hepatitis B   d. Varicella
    e. COPD
5. Markers not indicative of FGR include:
    a. Serial fundal height estimation
    b. Inadequate maternal weight gain
    c. Serum estriol levels
    d. Inadequate increase in maternal AG
    e. Serum hPL levels
6. Ultrasound findings indicative of FGR:
    a. BPD less than 50th centile
    b. HC less than 50th centile
    c. FL less than 10th centile
    d. AC less than 3rd centile
    e. AC less than 10th centile
7. Physiological changes which do not occur in pregnancy:
    a. Trophoblast invasion into spiral arteries
    b. Uterine blood flow increases 10–15 fold
    c. Decreased end diastolic flow
    d. 50% increase in maternal blood volume
    e. Low resistance flow in uteroplacental circulation
8. Abnormal flow on Doppler is not seen in FGR in:
    a. Umbilical artery   b. Spiral arteries
    c. Uterine artery   d. Middle cerebral artery
    e. Ductus venosus
9. The following are early findings associated with FGR:
    a. Absent uterine artery end diastolic flow
    b. Pulsatile pattern in ductus venosus
    c. Reversed uterine artery end diastolic flow
    d. Absent flow in ductus venosus
    e. Abnormal pulsatility in fetal MCA
10. Evidence based management of FGR does not include:
    a. DHA supplementation
    b. L-arginine
    c. Bed rest
    d. Low dose aspirin
    e. Low molecular weight heparin
11. Indications for delivery of the FGR fetus include:
    a. Absent variability on NST
    b. Absent end diastolic flow on Doppler
    c. BPP score 6
    d. Absent DV flow during atrial systole
    e. All of the above
12. The most sensitive method to detect intrapartum fetal acidemia is:
    a. FHR auscultation
    b. Electronic fetal monitoring
    c. Scalp blood pH
    d. Fetal pulse oximetry
    e. Arterial blood gases

Answers

| 1. | e | 2. | e | 3. | d | 4. | c | 5. | d | 6. | d |
| 7. | c | 8. | b | 9. | c | 10. | c | 11. | e | 12. | c |

7.6 FETAL HYDROPS

Muralidhar V Pai, Krishnendu Gupta

INTRODUCTION

Abnormal (excessive) collection of serous fluid in at least two places (fetal skin edema, ascites, pleural effusions, or pericardial effusions) or one effusion plus anasarca, is called *fetal hydrops* (**Fig. 1**). It is usually accompanied by big placenta and polyhydramnios. In the past the diagnosis was made only after the delivery of a massively edematous dead fetus. With the advent of ultrasound it can be diagnosed prenatally.

There were two types:
1. Immune fetal hydrops (IFH) which is due to alloimmunization as occurs in RhD alloimmunization
2. Nonimmune fetal hydrops (NIFH) which may be due to causes such as multiple fetal anatomic and functional disorders.

This chapter discusses causes, investigation, and management of both the types.

IMMUNE FETAL HYDROPS

The incidence of IFH has drastically come down due to better understanding of alloimmunization, use of anti-D immune globulin and improved diagnosis, monitoring as well as therapeutic interventions with intrauterine transfusion in fetal medicine units.

Immune fetal hydrops is a part of advanced stage of hemolytic disease of the fetus and new-born and is due to the destruction of fetal red cells by RhD antibodies that are developed by mother to the RhD positive antigen of the fetus. These antibodies are transferred antenatally through the placenta. Fetal hydrops occurs when the fetal hemoglobin deficit is at least 7 g/dL below the mean for gestational age (consistent with a hematocrit less than approximately 15% or hemoglobin <5 g/dL).[1] It is usually associated with thrombocytopenia and neutropenia and the risk of both increases with severity of anemia.[2] However, platelet transfusion is generally not required during intrauterine transfusion.

Diagnosis and Management

Steps toward diagnosis of fetal hydrops in RhD negative pregnant woman:
1. Husband's/partner's blood group and RhD type to be determined
2. If positive, his zygosity should be determined
3. If homozygous, all offspring would be positive hence fetal RhD typing is not necessary
4. If heterozygous, if facilities are available and affordable, then fetal RhD typing is determined by cell-free DNA (cfDNA) testing on maternal plasma
5. If cfDNA testing is not available, fetal *RhD* gene status may be determined by PCR on uncultured amniocytes obtained by amniocentesis after 15 weeks of gestation[3]
6. If both cfDNA or PCR tests are not possible then fetus is presumed to be RhD positive and indirect Coombs test (ICT) is performed
7. If ICT is negative it should be repeated every 4 weeks to check if it becomes positive later in pregnancy
8. If ICT is positive, then alloimmunization and hence the risk of fetal hydrops exists. Therefore, ICT titer is repeated monthly as long as it remains stable; rising titers should be repeated every 2 weeks until the titer reaches the "critical" level (16–32). A threshold value of 15 IU/mL is the critical value.[4]
9. Since titers are only screening tests and not diagnostic of severe anemia, they are discontinued once a critical titer is reached.
10. Doppler velocimetry of the middle cerebral arterial-peak systolic velocity (MCA-PSV) is performed to identify fetuses that are likely to be severely anemic. Doppler assessment of the fetal MCA-PSV is based on the principle that the fetal hemoglobin level determines blood flow in the MCA: MCA-PSV increases as fetal hemoglobin level falls.[5]

Middle cerebral arterial-peak systolic velocity is performed, when clinically indicated, after 20 weeks of gestation and repeated every 2 weeks. The frequency is increased if multiples of the median (MoMs) approach 1.5. An MCA-PSV ≤1.5 MoMs for gestational age is unlikely to have moderate to severe anemia. However, MoMs >1.5 for gestational age, indicate cordocentesis for determining fetal hemoglobin and if it shows severe anemia, then intrauterine

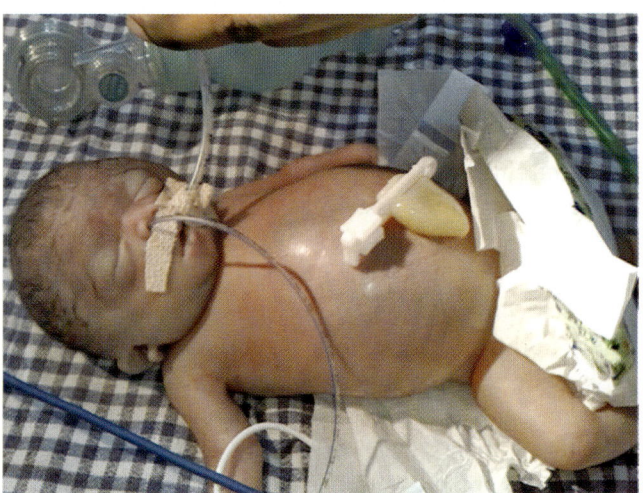

Fig. 1: Neonate with hydrops.

fetal transfusion (IUT) is indicated, especially if hematocrit is less than 30% to avoid fetal hydrops.[6] Though IUT may be repeated at intervals of 2–3 weeks many prefer early delivery and exchange transfusion post-delivery. Same is preferred if there is established hydrops as seen by ultrasound (vide infra). Obstetric principles of management of preterm delivery (steroid and $MgSO_4$ prophylaxis, cesarean delivery of very and extreme preterm babies and delayed cord clamping) should be followed.

NONIMMUNE FETAL HYDROPS

When first described, NIFH constituted 20% of all cases, but with decrease in immune fetal hydrops, NIFH constitutes 90% cases of fetal hydrops.[7] The prevalence of NIFH ranges from 1/1,500 to 1/4,000 births.[8]

Etiology

The main reason for NIFH is transfer of fluid from vascular to interstitial spaces and this can happen because of any or all of the following:[7]

- Obstructed lymphatic drainage in the thoracic and abdominal cavities
- Increased capillary permeability
- Increased central venous pressure
- Decreased osmotic pressure.

The above may happen in fetuses with any of the following disorders:[7]

- Cardiovascular (22%)
  - Structural defects
    - Ebstein anomaly, Fallot's tetralogy with absent pulmonary valve, hypoplastic left or right heart, premature closure of ductus arteriosus, arteriovenous malformation (vein of Galen aneurysm)
  - Cardiomyopathies
  - Tachyarrhythmias, bradycardia, as may occur in heterotaxy syndrome with endocardial cushion defect or in maternal SLE with anti-Ro/La antibodies
- Chromosomal (13%)
  - Turner syndrome (45,X), triploidy, trisomies 21, 18, and 13
- Hematological (10%)
  - Hemoglobinopathies, such as α4-thalassemia
  - Erythrocyte enzyme and membrane disorders
  - Erythrocyte aplasia/dyserythropoiesis
  - Decreased erythrocyte production (myeloproliferative disorders)
  - Fetomaternal hemorrhage
- Infections (7%)
  - Parvovirus B19, syphilis, cytomegalovirus, toxoplasmosis, rubella, enterovirus, varicella, herpes simplex, coxsackievirus, listeriosis, leptospirosis, Chagas disease, Lyme disease
- Thoracic abnormalities (6%)
  - Cystic adenomatoid malformation
  - Pulmonary sequestration
  - Diaphragmatic hernia
  - Hydro/chylothorax
  - Congenital high airway obstruction sequence
  - Mediastinal tumors
  - Skeletal dysplasia with very small thorax
- Lymphatic abnormalities (6%)
  - Cystic hygroma, systemic lymphangiectasis, pulmonary lymphangiectasis[6]
- Placental, twin, and cord abnormalities (6%)
  - Placental chorioangioma, twin-twin transfusion syndrome, twin reversed arterial perfusion sequence, twin anemia polycythemia sequence, cord vessel thrombosis
- Kidney and urinary tract (2%)
  - Kidney malformations
  - Bladder outlet obstructions
  - Congenital (Finnish) nephrosis, Bartter syndrome, mesoblastic nephroma
- Syndromic (4%)
  - Arthrogryposis multiplex congenita, lethal multiple pterygium, congenital lymphedema, myotonic dystrophy type I, Neu-Laxova, Noonan, and Pena-Shokeir syndromes
- Other rare disorders (6%)
  - *Inborn errors of metabolism:* Gaucher disease, galactosialidosis, GM1 gangliosidosis, sialidosis, mucopolysaccharidoses, mucolipidoses
  - *Tumors:* Sacrococcygeal teratoma, hemangioendothelioma with Kasabach Merritt syndrome
- Idiopathic (18%).

Diagnosis

On abdominal examination the uterine height may be bigger than period of gestation and there will be evidence of polyhydramnios. However, fetal hydrops is diagnosed prenatally by ultrasound when two or more of the following is seen:

- Fetal ascites—if ascitic fluid is large, the bowel may appear compressed
- Pleural effusions—may be unilateral or bilateral, and may compress the lung tissue
- Pericardial effusions—may be difficult to visualize with standard two-dimensional images. It is important not to mistake physiologic pericardial fluid or the hypoechoic myocardium for an abnormal effusion
- Skin edema—late sign of fetal hydrops. Pathologic skin edema has been defined as subcutaneous tissue thickness on the chest or scalp greater than 5 mm
- Polyhydramnios—amniotic fluid index (AFI) > 25/single vertical pocket > 8 cm.

Placental thickening ≥4 cm in the second trimester and ≥6 cm in the third trimester is considered abnormal and should prompt further investigation. However, massive polyhydramnios can cause the placenta to appear thinned or compressed.

An attempt should be made to find out the etiology of the hydrops as several of them can be confirmed or excluded by ultrasound (e.g., fetal echo can rule out cardiac anomalies and arrhythmias).

Management

General principles are:
- Identification of in utero treatable causes
- Delivering the fetus if continuation of pregnancy has risk of fetal demise.

If fetal echo and targeted anomaly scan does not reveal any abnormalities then Doppler assessment of the fetal MCA-PSV should be performed to diagnose moderate to severe fetal anemia of any etiology (i.e., immune or nonimmune).[9] Attempts should be made to diagnose the cause of anemia (e.g., parvovirus infection, fetomaternal bleeding, hemoglobinopathy). Irrespective of the etiology, fetal anemia is treated with IUT as in case of an immune hydrops and an early delivery should be contemplated.

Fetal tachyarrhythmias can often be treated by maternal administration of rate controlling agents.

Maternal treatment with propylthiouracil or methimazole is an effective transplacental treatment of affected fetuses due to maternal Graves' disease.

The prognosis is poor for fetuses with aneuploidy. In nonlethal aneuploidies, early delivery is indicated.

Prognosis of hydropic fetuses with congenital pulmonary lesions depends on the gestational age at the time of development of the lesion, earlier the development poorer the prognosis due to poor lung growth and function. Therapeutic options include:
- Needle aspiration if shunting is planned[10]
- Placement of a pleuroamniotic shunt[11]
- Open fetal surgery.

In twin gestation, if hydrops is due to twin-to-twin transfusion syndrome, treatment involves an in utero ablation procedure. Selective feticide of a hydropic twin can also reverse the maternal disorder, thereby allowing prolongation of the pregnancy.[12]

Nonimmune fetal hydrops is associated with an overall perinatal mortality rate of 50–98%.[13] Among the live born infants, mortality was 43%.[14]

Pregnancy counseling and management are guided by the etiology and severity of NIFH and whether it can be treated successfully.

When the etiology is not known or untreatable, options include fetal monitoring with active intervention or pregnancy termination.

Fetal hydrops may be associated with maternal preeclampsia (Mirror syndrome). Delivery is indicated if maternal condition deteriorates. Maternal symptoms disappear in few days.

All said and done usually early delivery is common in 66% of pregnancies.[15] Mode of delivery is decided by the gestational age, fetal condition, and chances of neonatal survival.

The risk of recurrent NIFH depends upon the underlying etiology; therefore, every effort should be made to determine the cause.

■ REFERENCES

1. Nicolaides KH, Thilaganathan B, Rodeck CH, Mibashan RS, Erythroblastosis and reticulocytosis in anemic fetuses. Am J Obstet Gynecol. 1988;159(5):1063.
2. van den Akker ES, de Haan TR, Lopriore E, Brand A, Kanhai HH, Oepkes D. Severe fetal thrombocytopenia in Rhesus D alloimmunized pregnancies. Am J Obstet Gynecol. 2008;199(4):387.e1.
3. Goebel JC, Soergel P, Pruggmayer M, Mühlhaus K, Stuhrmann M, Scharf A. Prenatal diagnosis of the Rhesus D fetal blood type on amniotic fluid in daily practice. Arch Gynecol Obstet. 2008;277(2):155-60.
4. Nicolaides KH, Rodeck CH. Maternal serum anti-D antibody concentration and assessment of rhesus isoimmunisation. BMJ. 1992;304(6835):1155.
5. Picklesimer AH, Oepkes D, Moise KJ Jr, Kush ML, Weiner CP, Harman CR, et al. Determinants of the middle cerebral artery peak systolic velocity in the human fetus. Am J Obstet Gynecol. 2007;197(5):526.e1.
6. Moise KJ Jr. Management of rhesus alloimmunization in pregnancy. Obstet Gynecol. 2008;112(1):164.
7. Bellini C, Hennekam RC, Fulcheri E, Rutigliani M, Morcaldi G, Boccardo F, et al. Etiology of nonimmune hydrops fetalis: a systematic review. Am J Med Genet A. 2009;149A(5):844-51.
8. Steurer MA, Peyvandi S, Baer RJ, MacKenzie T, Li BC, Norton ME, et al. Epidemiology of Live Born Infants with Nonimmune Hydrops Fetalis-Insights from a Population-Based Dataset. J Pediatr. 2017;187:182-3.
9. Borna S, Mirzaie F, Hanthoush-Zadeh S, Khazardoost S, Rahimi-Sharbaf F. Middle cerebral artery peak systolic velocity and ductus venosus velocity in the investigation of nonimmune hydrops. J Clin Ultrasound. 2009;37:385.
10. Deurloo KL, Devlieger R, Lopriore E, lumper FJ, Oepkes D. Isolated fetal hydrothorax with hydrops: a systematic review of prenatal treatment options. Prenat Diagn. 2007;27:893.
11. Pellegrinelli JM, Kohler A, Kohler M, Weingertner AS, Favre R. Prenatal management and thoracoamniotic shunting in primary fetal pleural effusions: a single centre experience. Prenat Diagn. 2012;32:467.
12. Okby R, Mazor M, Erez O, Beer-Weizel R, Hershkovitz R. Reversal of mirror syndrome after selective feticide of a hydropic fetus in a dichorionic diamniotic twin pregnancy. J Ultrasound Med. 2015;34:351.
13. Santo S, Mansour S, Thilaganathan B, Homfray T, Papageorghiou A, Calvert S, et al. Prenatal diagnosis of non-immune hydrops fetalis: what do we tell the parents? Prenat Diagn. 2011;31:186.
14. Steurer MA, Peyvandi S, Baer RJ, MacKenzie T, Li BC, Norton ME, et al. Epidemiology of Live Born Infants with Nonimmune Hydrops Fetalis-Insights from a Population-Based Dataset. J Pediatr. 2017;187:182.

15. Mascaretti RS, Falcão MC, Silva AM, Vaz FA, Leone CR. Characterization of newborns with nonimmune hydrops fetalis admitted to a neonatal intensive care unit. Rev Hosp Clin Fac Med Sao Paulo. 2003;58:125.

LONG QUESTION

1. Define fetal hydrops. What are the types? What are the etiological factors of fetal hydrops? Describe the diagnosis and management of fetal hydrops.

SHORT QUESTIONS

1. Ultrasound diagnosis of fetal hydrops.
2. Diagnostic approach of Immune fetal hydrops.
3. Intrauterine transfusion.
4. Management of congenital pulmonary lesions leading to hydrops.
5. Etiology of nonimmune hydrops.

MULTIPLE CHOICE QUESTIONS

1. Fetal hydrops is excessive collection of serous fluid in:
   a. Plural cavity
   b. Pericardial cavity
   c. Peritoneal cavity
   d. Two places
2. Fetal hydrops is accompanied with:
   a. Big placenta
   b. Oligohydramnios
   c. Macrosomia
   d. Small placenta
3. The incidence of immune fetal hydrops (IFH) has:
   a. Drastically come down
   b. Gone up
   c. Remained same
   d. Been fluctuating
4. Immune fetal hydrops is due to:
   a. Cardiac anomaly
   b. Destruction of fetal RBC
   c. Intrauterine infection
   d. Trisomy 21
5. Fetal hydrops occurs when fetal Hb deficit is below following mean for gestational age:
   a. 3 g/dL
   b. 5 g/dL
   c. 7 g/dL
   d. 9 g/dL
6. With regards to steps toward diagnosis of fetal hydrops following statement is not correct:
   a. If homozygous, all offsprings would be positive hence fetal RhD typing is necessary
   b. If heterozygous fetal RhD typing is determined by cell-free DNA (cfDNA) testing on maternal plasma
   c. If cfDNA testing is not available, fetal RhD gene status may be determined by PCR on uncultured amniocytes
   d. If both cfDNA or PCR tests are not possible then fetus is presumed to be RhD positive and indirect Coomb's Test (ICT) is performed
7. Critical ICT value is:
   a. 4
   b. 8
   c. 12
   d. 16
8. Severe fetal anemia is suspected when MCA-PSV is:
   a. ≤0.5 MoMs for gestational age
   b. 0.5–1.0 MoMs for gestational age
   c. 1.0–1.5 MoM for gestational age
   d. >1.5 MoM for gestational age
9. In nonimmune fetal hydrops transfer of fluid happens because of the following, except:
   a. Increased capillary permeability
   b. Increased central venous permeability
   c. Open lymphatic drainage in the thoracic and abdominal cavities
   d. Decreased osmotic pressure
10. Following can cause nonimmune fetal hydrops, except:
    a. Fallot Tetralogy
    b. Trisomy 21
    c. Parvovirus B1
    d. Rh D

Answers

1. d 2. a 3. a 4. b 5. c 6. a
7. d 8. d 9. c 10. d

SECTION 8

Late Pregnancy Complications

8.1 ANTENATAL CARE: MALPRESENTATIONS

N Palaniappan

INTRODUCTION

One of the objectives of antenatal care is to identify high risk pregnancies, recognize the deviation from normal, and refer such cases for specialized management. Out of all the malpresentations breech presentation and transverse lie need recognition and management in third trimester. These malpresentations may lead to increased fetal morbidity and mortality (3–5 times more than vertex) and higher maternal morbidity and mortality due to increased need of operative deliveries. In one of the studies, cesarean rate in breech was 43.4% as compared to overall rate of 16% for all cases. Maternal morbidity was higher, 10.3% with cesarean section (C-section) versus 5.8% for vaginal delivery. Before 28 weeks if the patient goes in labor with these malpresentations, can deliver mostly spontaneously due to small size of the fetus.

Cephalic malpresentations such as face and brow can be suspected sometimes in the antenatal period due to more prominent occipital pole and by detecting sulcus between neck and back, are to be observed carefully in early labor as these can get corrected spontaneously. However, all the persistent malpresentations will lead to abnormal labor.

MALPRESENTATIONS

Pointers to the malpresentations can be:
- Grand multipara
- Short stature.
- Contracted pelvis
  The malpresentations are 4–5 times more common in the above three conditions.
- Uterine obliquity and pendulous belly – 10 times increase in transverse lie
- Prematurity – incidence of breech is 20% at 28 weeks as compared to 3.7% at term[1]
- Placenta previa and cornu fundal attachment of placenta can lead to breech presentation
- Tumors in the lower segment and pelvis such as fibroids or ovarian
- Polyhydramnios and oligohydramnios
- Congenital anomalies of the fetus such as hydrocephalous and anencephaly
- Congenital anomalies of the uterus such as bicornuate, subseptate, arcuate
- Intrauterine death (IUD)
- Cord around the neck, dolichocephalic fetal head (face presentation). Recurrent breech and transverse lie can be associated with contracted pelvis and congenital anomalies of the uterus
- Abnormalities of the bony pelvis
- Poliomyelitis and traumatic injuries of the pelvis.

Management

In third trimester, besides routine antenatal examination, abdominal examination should be done to diagnose lie and presentation.

Diagnosis

Diagnosis of breech and transverse lie in antenatal period is described in **Table 1**.

Differential Diagnosis

It is blunder to diagnose shoulder as breech. Breech sometimes can be wrongly diagnosed as cephalic presentation. Whenever malpresentations are suspected or diagnosis is in doubt, ultrasound should be done to confirm the diagnosis. Patient with transverse lie if allowed to go in labor can have life-threatening complications such as hand prolapse, obstructed labor and ruptured uterus and in neglected cases baby too can be lost **(Box 1)**.

TABLE 1: Diagnosis of breech and transverse lie in antenatal period.

Examination abdominal	Breech	Transverse lie
Fundal height	Corresponds to period of amenorrhea and shape of abdomen is similar to cephalic presentation	Smaller than period of amenorrhea, abdomen looks broader from side to side
Fundal grip	Head is felt as a well-defined hard globular ballotable mass. In extended breech it may not be defined well due to extended legs obscuring the head and feet may be felt as small parts	Empty
Lateral grip	Back on one side and limbs on the other side	Head on one side felt as hard ballotable well defined and buttocks on the other side felt as soft irregular non-ballotable
Pelvic grip	Soft irregular non-ballotable, sometimes in extended breech sacrum feels hard and can be mistaken for vertex	Empty
Lie	Longitudinal	Transverse
Fetal heart sound (FHS)	Near umbilicus or at a higher level in spinoumbilical line	FHS can be below umbilicus in dorsoanterior position and at a higher level in dorsoposterior position
Vaginal examination (rule out placenta previa by ultrasound before examination)	Soft irregular part felt higher at pelvic brim	Presenting part higher up, neither breech nor vertex is felt. Sometimes shoulder of good sized baby can be wrongly diagnosed as breech

BOX 1: Complications of transverse lie.

Transverse lie in labor can have life-threatening complications like hand prolapse, obstructed labor and ruptured uterus and in neglected cases baby too can be lost.

BOX 2: Role of ultrasonography in malpresentations.

Ultrasound is done in these patients to confirm diagnosis, maturity, type of breech, attitude of head such as hyperextended, locate placenta, amount of liquor detection of congenital anomalies of fetus and uterus, IUGR, estimated fetal weight and fetal number.

Investigations

Routine investigations are carried out. Ultrasonography is necessary in these patients:

- To confirm the diagnosis and know the number of fetuses
- To know the maturity
- To know the type of breech, attitude, such as hyperextended star gazing appearance of the fetus
- To locate placenta
- To know the amount of liquor
- For detection of congenital anomalies of fetus such as hydrocephalus, spina bifida or anencephaly
- To detect IUGR, estimated fetal weight and fetal well-being
- To identify uterine anomaly or fibroid **(Box 2)**.

Once the diagnosis is confirmed, the patient should be counseled about malpresentation and note should be made in the records of the patient. As the fetus keeps on moving the malpresentation can get corrected on its own. If the patient goes in preterm labor then this information may help the obstetricians in managing the case properly. Patient should be offered external cephalic version (ECV) from 36 weeks onwards if there are no contraindications. Before 36 weeks, the chances of spontaneous version are high. As the pregnancy grows beyond 36 weeks, the amount of liquor is reduced and chances of spontaneous version are less. If complications at the time of version happen then baby can be salvaged by C-section as enough maturity of baby is achieved by that time.

She can be examined at 2-weekly interval upto 36 weeks and after version at weekly interval to confirm that breech or transverse lie has not recurred. In case of failure of version and contraindications to version, decision regarding mode of delivery is made as follows: Vaginal delivery is planned in breech cases if there is no fetopelvic disproportion, no maternal complicating factors such as heart disease, severe preeclampsia, precious pregnancy and antepartum hemorrhage (APH), estimated fetal weight of <3.5 kg, congenital malformation of the fetus incompatible with life or IUD, favorable breech attitude such as frank breech with no hyperextension of fetal head and availability of experienced obstetrician and pediatrician. The decision is tilted in favor of C-section[2] if fetal weight is >3.5 kg, suspected fetopelvic disproportion, precious pregnancy, bad obstetric history (BOH), associated maternal complications such as severe pregnancy-induced hypertension (PIH), hyperextended fetal head, footling presentation, abnormal cardiotocography (CTG) and dysfunctional labor **(Box 3)**.

Patient with persistent transverse lie with salvageable baby will require C-Section at term. She is counseled for the same and investigations and preanesthesia checkup is done for the same. A multigravida should be counseled regarding family planning methods also such as tubectomy, etc.

> **BOX 3:** Fetal complications of breech presentations.
> - Inherent to the fetus
>   – Prematurity
>   – Congenital anomalies
>   – Chromosomal anomalies
>   – Neuromuscular disorders
> - Inherent to breech delivery
>   – Cord accidents
>   – Birth asphyxia
>   – Entrapment of after coming head
>   – Birth trauma

External Cephalic Version

It is manipulation of fetus through maternal abdomen so that breech or oblique or transverse lie is converted to cephalic presentation. It can be done from 36 weeks onwards and even in early labor with intact membranes. Spontaneous version is common before 36 weeks if liquor is adequate but after 36 weeks it happens in 8% cases only.[3] Success rate of external cephalic version can be 35–86% with average being 58%.[4]

Success rate for external cephalic version for transverse lie can be 90%.[5] It was 37.5% in a study done at MAMC and Lok Nayak Hospital[1] when nifedipine is used for tocolysis. Success rates are more in multigravida with breech not engaged and uterus well relaxed. Tocolysis increases the success rate of ECV (Evidence level A)[6,7] if ritodrine, salbutamol and terbutaline are used as tocolytic agents but not with glycerol trinitrate (GTN) or nifedipine. However, there is two-fold increase in C-Section rate in ECV corrected presentations. Immediate C-Section may be required in 0.5% cases.[8,9]

In our country there is higher rate of unsupervised deliveries (scar rupture can take place in previous C-Section cases) and high perinatal mortality; ECV should be offered to all low risk cases of breech and transverse lie from 36 weeks to early labor with intact membranes. ECV is contraindicated in 4% cases.[10] Contraindications for ECV are as follows:
- Abnormal CTG
- High risk cases such as elderly primi, BOH, PIH and diabetes mellitus
- Contracted pelvis
- APH
- Multiple pregnancy
- Uterine anomalies
- Oligohydramnios, ruptured membranes
- Nuchal cord
- Scarred uterus
- Fetal growth restriction
- Fetal macrosomia.

Essential steps before ECV: Exclude contraindications, do ultrasound to exclude placenta previa and do pelvic assessment to exclude fetopelvic disproportion. CTG should be reactive, counsel the patient regarding risks and procedure, take consent, give anti-D immunoprophylaxis to Rh (-ve) non-immunized mother. Patient is asked to empty bladder, she lies in dorsal position with head and shoulders slightly raised and thighs semiflexed so that the abdominal muscles are relaxed. In engaged breech cases, Trendelenburg position can be used to disengage the breech.

Procedure: It can be done on OPD basis but preferably under ultrasound guidance. Doctor stands on rights side of the mother, breech is held with right hand and is placed toward one iliac fossa and then carried to lumbar region. Simultaneously the head is held with left hand and is pushed toward the lumbar region of the mother keeping the flexed attitude of the fetus. Thus the lie is made transverse first. Fetal heart sound is heard if the procedure is not being done under ultrasound. The procedure should be done gently avoiding too much force causing pain to the patient. Hands of the obstetrician are changed now. The right hand holds the head of the baby and left hand holds the podalic pole and head is pushed toward the pelvis of the mother and breech toward the fundus. This step is same for transverse lie. In case of failure tocolysis can be used if it has not been used earlier. Terbutaline 250 µm subcutaneously or intravenously at the rate of 5–8 drops per minute for 15 minutes can be used before procedure.

The maternal pulse and FHS should be continuously monitored. The procedure should be stopped if the patient complaints of pain. The patient should be taken for C-section in case she has bleeding or leaking PV or if there is fetal distress.

What is done after version?[11]
- Listen to FHS. Sometimes bradycardia can be there which settles down in 5–10 minutes time. If it does not settle, emergency C-Section may be needed.
- Observe the patient for 20 minutes for any bleeding or leaking per vagina or for onset of labor.
  These complications will require admission and further management.
- Call the patient after 1 week for checking presentation. Version can be repeated in case of recurrence. In case of unstable lie per se or after correction of abnormal presentation induction of labor and oxytocin stabilizing drip can be carried out at 37–38 weeks.

Causes of failure of version can be:
- Tight abdominal muscles and failure of patient to relax
- Breech with extended legs
- Oligohydramnios
- Undiagnosed congenital malformations of uterus
- Undiagnosed twins
- Short cord.

Complications of external version: Complications such as premature labor, preterm premature rupture of membranes, accidental hemorrhage, ruptured uterus, fetomaternal hemorrhage, fetal distress, and fetal death can occur. Fetal loss was seen in 1.7% cases[12] **(Box 4)**.

Indications for elective C-section in breech presentation:
- Estimated fetal weight more than 4 kg
- Footling breech
- Knee presentation

PART 1: Obstetrics and Perinatology

> **BOX 4:** Complications of external cephalic version (ECV).
> - Premature labor
> - Preterm premature rupture of membranes
> - Accidental hemorrhage
> - Ruptured uterus
> - Fetomaternal hemorrhage
> - Fetal distress
> - Fetal death

- Hyper extended fetal head
- Nuchal arms
- Placenta previa
- Contracted pelvis.

Transverse Lie

In case of failure of version or contraindications to version, patient needs C-section and so investigations and preanesthesia checkup is done accordingly. If baby is dead or congenitally malformed then further management such as destructive operation or internal podalic version is decided in labor, but in modern day obstetrics, cesarean section is considered much safer unless the baby is very small and/or preterm.

Patients with breech and shoulder presentation (transverse lie) should preferably be kept admitted during the last 2 weeks of pregnancy even when elective cesarean section is planned, as they can go in labor or have PROM before their surgery. In case of breech presentation, even if vaginal delivery is contemplated, patient should be admitted in ward close by to labor room to prevent intrapartum complications.

CONCLUSION

Malpresentations become relevant to clinical management in the later part of the third trimester. There is an increase in perinatal morbidity and mortality, operative interventions and maternal complications in pregnancies where the fetus is in a malpresentation. The clinical diagnosis of a malpresentation should be confirmed by ultrasound before an intervention is performed. An attempt should also be made to look for the underlying etiology and possible problems that may occur with malpresentations. External cephalic version is an evidence based approach to reducing the cesarean section rate in this group of women. It should be used with a view on the contraindications and with due counseling and preparation.

REFERENCES

1. Rohini R, Rathore AM, Manaktala U. Evidence of external cephalic version in the management of breech pregnancies ≥ 34 weeks period of gestation. Thesis, Doctor of Medicine, Obstetrics and Gynaecology. Delhi: MAMC/LNH/Delhi University; 2006.
2. Hannah ME, Hannah WJ, Hewson SA, Hodnett ED, Saigal S, Willian AR. Planned caesarean section versus planned vaginal birth for breech presentation at term: a randomized multicentre trial. Term Breech Trial Collaborative Group. Lancet. 2000;356:1375-83.
3. Westgren M, Edvall H, Nordstrom L, Svalenius E, ranstam J. Spontaneous cephalic version of breech presentation in the last trimester.Br J Obstet Gynaecol. 1985;92:19-22.
4. American College of Obstetrics and Gynecology. External cephalic version: Practice Bulletin no.13. Washington, DC: ACOG; 2000.
5. Newman RD, Peacock BS, Van Dorsten JB. Predicting Success of External cephalic version. Am J Obstet Gynecol. 1993;169:245.
6. Royal College of Obstetricians and Gynaecologists. Guideline No. 20a. London: RCOG; 2010.
7. Hofmeyr GJ. Interventions to help external cephalic version for breech presentation at term. Cochrane Database Syst Rev. 2004;(1):CD 000184.
8. Impey L, Lissoni D. Outcome of external cephalic version after 36 weeks gestation without tocolysis. J Matern Fetal Med. 1999;8:203-7.
9. Collins S, Ellaway P, Harrington D, Pandit M, Impey LW. The complications of External Cephalic Version; Results from 805 consecutive attempts. Br J Obstet Gynaecol. 2007;114(5):636.
10. Impey L, Pandit M. Tocolysis for repeat external cephalic version after a failed version for breech presentation at term: randomized double blind placebo control trial. BJOG. 2005;112:627-31.
11. Prasad S, Mala YM, Batra S. Common Viva discussion in Obstetrics and Gynaecology. New Delhi: Jaypee Brothers Medical Publishers (P) Ltd.; 2003. p. 96.
12. Van Dorsten JP, Sehifrin BS, Wallace RL. Randomized Control trial of external cephalic version with tocolysis in late pregnancy. Am J Obstet Gynecol. 1981;141:417.

LONG QUESTIONS

1. Discuss the antenatal diagnosis and management of transverse lie in third trimester.
2. Discuss the management of a second gravida, previous normal vaginal delivery, at 38 weeks of gestation with an extended breech presentation.
3. Debate the merits versus demerits of an assisted breech delivery versus elective C-section for a breech presentation in a primigravida at term gestation.

SHORT QUESTIONS

1. What are the common associations or etiologies for malpresentations?
2. Enumerate the contraindications for ECV.
3. What are the immediate measures that one can take in case of a cord or hand prolapse with malpresentation?
4. What are the complications of a transverse lie?
5. What are the advantages of a USG in a breech presentation at term?

MULTIPLE CHOICE QUESTIONS

1. Following are the contraindications for external cephalic version, except:
   a. Severe preeclampsia   b. Previous cesarean
   c. Twins   d. Contracted pelvis
   e. Transverse lie at term
2. External cephalic version is done at all gestations, except one:
   a. 34 weeks   b. 36 weeks
   c. 37 weeks   d. 38 weeks
   e. 39 weeks

3. The most common cause for breech presentation is:
   a. Prematurity
   b. Twins
   c. Hydrocephalous
   d. Placenta previa
   e. Contracted pelvis
4. Antenatal diagnosis for the following malpresentation is a must to reduce maternal morbidity and mortality in:
   a. Face presentation
   b. Occipitoposterior position
   c. Brow presentation
   d. Breech presentation
   e. Transverse lie
5. Tick true (T) or false (F):
   a. X-ray is safer than ultrasound to confirm diagnosis of breech. (T/F)
   b. MRI and CT are frequently done to assess pelvis. (T/F)
   c. Rule out placenta previa before doing pelvic examination in transverse lie. (T/F)
   d. Spontaneous version takes place in 2% cases of breech after 36 weeks. (T/F)
   e. Fundal and pelvic grip is empty in transverse lie. (T/F)

Answers
1. e 2. a 3. a 4. e
5. a (F), b (F), c (T), d (F), e (T)

8.2 PRETERM LABOR

MB Bellad, Bhawna Garg

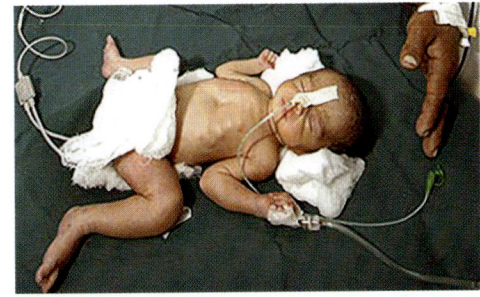

INTRODUCTION

Preterm labor (PTL) is one of the leading causes of perinatal morbidity and mortality. It is one of the major public health problems, especially with reference to mortality, disability and healthcare expenses.[1] This problem in developing countries (such as India) has different magnitude, as the cost involved in caring for these preterm babies is enormous, that is not within the reach of the poor.

In spite of the great scientific advances in the last half century, there is no change or little change in the incidence of PTL. Effective preventive and therapeutic measures are still not available because of the persistence of uncertainties of measures to either prevent or treat PTL. Effective strategy for both prevention and management will reduce morbidity and mortality associated with preterm births.

MAGNITUDE OF THE PROBLEM

The overall incidence of PTL is around 10–15% (6–15% range).[2] Out of all PTL, 50% occur spontaneously, 25% following preterm premature rupture of membranes (PPROM) and remaining 25% iatrogenic (induced due to maternal and/or fetal risks—hypertension, antepartum hemorrhage and others). Fortunately, most of the preterm births (71%) occur between 34 and 36 weeks, 13%, 10% and 6% at 32–33 weeks, 28–31 weeks and <28 weeks respectively.[3] It is the leading cause of neonatal death and disability (both short term and long term) especially, cerebral palsy, deafness, blindness and chronic lung disease.

Viability

Since the survival of extremely premature baby, 22–24 weeks, is lower without morbidity every aspect of the prognosis must be discussed with woman and the concerned before taking decisions. Some of the institutes do not offer cesarean section for fetuses with estimated fetal weight of< 750 g. The care of the preterm neonates is highly expensive and not within the reach of the poor, this is one of the main reasons for increased mortality in developing countries.

DEFINITION

Preterm labor is defined as occurrence of regular uterine contractions (four or more in 20 minutes or eight or more in 1 hour) and associated cervical changes (effacement equal to or greater than 80% and dilatation equal to or greater than 1 cm) in women with intact fetal membranes with gestational age more than 20 weeks and less than 37 weeks.[4] Uterine contractions are better noted by tocodynamometer.

RISK FACTORS

Previous history of PTL is one of the important risk factors as it is estimated that the recurrence of PTL in subsequent pregnancies is 14.3% after one preterm birth and it is almost double after two preterm births (28%).[5] Other risk factors include multiple pregnancies, uterine over distension (polyhydramnios, macrosomia and fibroids), uterine anomalies, cervical incompetence, bacterial vaginosis, bleeding in early pregnancy, poor socioeconomic status, elderly and adolescent age and tobacco use (smoking and smokeless). However, these risk factors have variable sensitivities and predictive values.

DIAGNOSIS OF PRETERM LABOR

The diagnosis of PTL is based on following:

Regular uterine contractions (four or more in 20 minutes or eight or more in 1 hour) associated with cervical changes (effacement equal to or greater than 80% and dilatation equal to or greater than 1 cm). Though difficult to correlate effacement is used in percentage and not in length.

In conditions where the uterine contractions are noted or other symptoms (lower abdominal pain, heaviness in pelvis and back ache etc.) without the cervical changes, the transvaginal sonography assists in the diagnosis. If cervical length of ≤ 2.5 cm, the condition is called threatened PTL. If the cervical length is more than ≥ 2.5 cm then PTL is ruled out.[4]

PREDICTORS

Fetal fibronectin (fFN): This is the glycoprotein produced in 20 different forms by a different cell types, e.g., hepatocytes, fibroblasts, endothelial cells and fetal amnion. It is present in high concentration in maternal blood and in amniotic fluid, it is thought to play a mole in intercellular adhesion during implantation and in the maintenance of placental adhesion to deciduas.[6]

It is also described as the basement membrane protein, acts as an adhesion binder (facilitates the attachment of the placental membranes to the uterine deciduas). The fetal fibronectin is normally detectable in cervical secretions up to 20 weeks. Presence or detection of fFN in cervical secretions after 24 weeks of pregnancy is an indication of disruption of membranes due to inflammation that usually precedes the onset of PTL. fFN has high negative predictive value, nearly >95% (absent fFN correlates with very less chance of PTL).[7] This is very useful especially when there are symptoms suggestive of PTL without evidences. The positive fFN test, however, has lower specificity indicating that women may or may not go into PTL.

Cervical length: Transvaginal assessment of the length of the cervix has been extensively evaluated. The mean cervical length of 35 mm in women at 24 weeks did not experience PTL and progressively shorter cervices experienced more PTL.[8] In high risk women short cervical length was increasingly associated with PTL.[9] Funneling of membranes into endocervical canal with short cervix and previous preterm birth were good predictors of PTL.[10] Cervical length and fFN in combination are also useful in prediction of PTL **(Fig. 1)**.[11]

Amniotic fluid sludge: Presence of amniotic fluid sludge above the internal os, observed as dense hyperechogenic matter in the amniotic fluid is an additional predictor of preterm birth.[12]

Home uterine activity monitoring (HUAM): HUAM device was designed to monitor uterine contractions at home for women at the risk of PTL.

However, it has a limited role as it does not decrease the rate of preterm birth.[13]

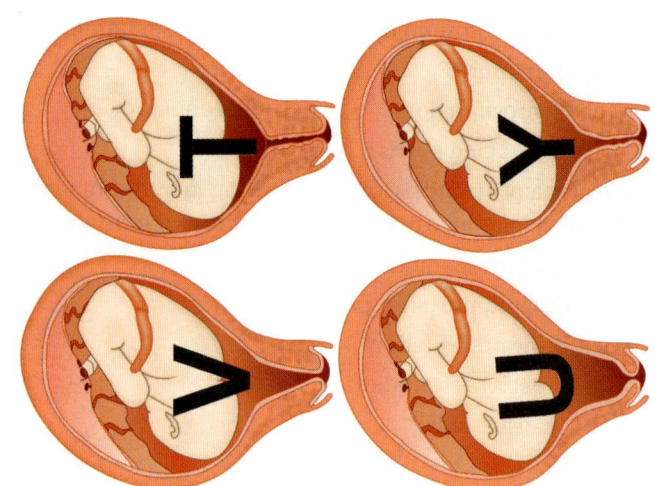

Fig. 1: Funneling of the cervix with the changes in forms T, Y, V, U (correlation between the length of the cervix and the changes in the cervical internal os).
Source: Zilianti M, Azuaga A, Calderon F, Pagés G, Mendoza G. Monitoring the effacement of the uterine cervix by transperineal sonography: a new perspective. J Ultrasound Med. 1995;14(10):719-24.

Salivary estriol: Detection of salivary estriol surge maybe helpful in prediction of PTL. However, the evidence is limited therefore it is not used in routine screening.

Cytokines: Proinflammatory cytokines including interleukin (IL)-6, IL-8, IL-16 have been found to have diagnostic and predictive role in PTL.[14]

Phosphorylated insulin-like growth factor binding protein-1/ Actim® Partus Test Kit **(Fig. 2):** Highly phosphorylated IGFBP is found in decidua, whereas amniotic fluid contains non-phosphorylated forms. Initiation of labor disrupts the choriodecidual interface thus releasing PIGFBP. It is a one-step dipstick test for detecting PIGFBP-1 in cervical secretions to assess the risk of imminent preterm delivery.[15]

Infection: Intrauterine infection has emerged as a frequent and important mechanism of disease in PTL.[16-20] It is the only pathological process for which a firm causal link with PTL has been established for which a defined molecular pathophysiology is known **(Fig. 3)**.[16-20] The two common microorganisms associated with PTL are *Ureaplasma urealyticum* and *Mycoplasma hominis*.[21]

Bacterial vaginosis (BV): It is not an infection per se but maldistribution of vaginal flora. Most of the lactobacilli are replaced with anaerobic bacteria such as *Gardnerella vaginalis, Mobiluncus* and *Bacteroides* species. There is an association between BV and PTL. However, the treatment does not reduce the PTL and routine screening for BV is not recommended.[22]

Human placental alpha microglobulin-1 (PAMG-1): This test is available as ParstoSure™ kits **(Fig. 4)**.[23] This is based on immunochromatographic assay of monoclonal antibodies which are sensitive to detect 4 pg/dL of PAMG-1 in cervicovaginal discharge. Significant correlation has been

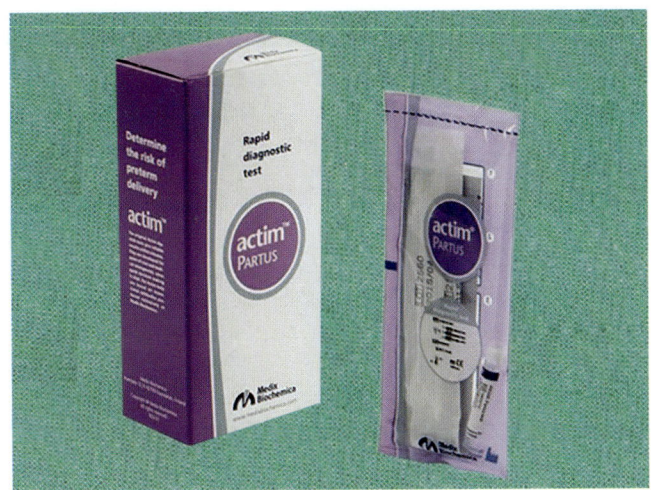

Fig. 2: Actim® Partus kit.

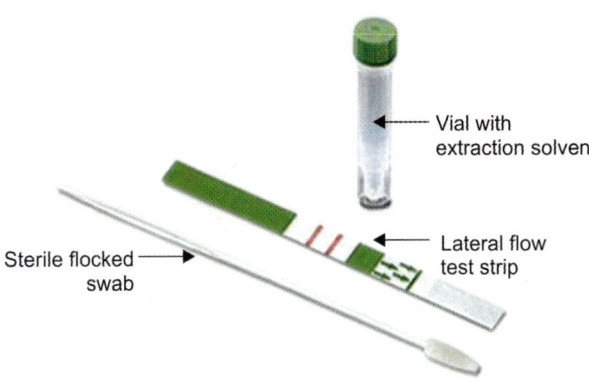

Fig. 4: PartoSure™ Kits- rapidly assess the risk of preterm delivery in ≤7 or ≤14 days from the time of cervicovaginal sample collection in pregnant women with signs and symptoms of early preterm labor.
Source: FDA Summary of Safety and Effectiveness Data. Available from: https://www.accessdata.fda.gov/cdrh_docs/pdf16/P160052B.pdf.

Cerclage: Cerclage prevent PTL if used in the following:
- Women with recurrent second trimester losses.
- Diagnosed as having incompetent cervix.
- TVS demonstrates short cervix.
- Emergency cerclage (rescue cerclage) in threatened PTL.
Cervical cerclage prevents PTL in subset of women with previous history of PTL.[24]

Antibiotics: Though infection is more commonly associated with PTL, the use of antibiotics was not associated with reduction of PTL. Although antibiotics such as erythromycin, azithromycin, metronidazole, vaginal clindamycin either alone or in combination were not associated with reduction of PTL. However, oral clindamycin 300 mg twice daily versus placebo early pregnancy (early second trimester in women with abnormal flora was associated with reduction in PTL).[31]

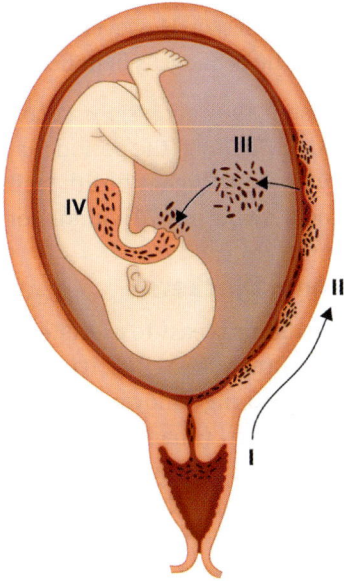

Fig. 3: Stages of Intrauterine infections leading to preterm labor: (I) Vaginal infection, (II) Inflammation of fetal membranes, (III) Microbial infection of amniotic cavity, (IV) Fetal inflammation.
Source: Goncalves LF, Chaiworapongsa T, Romero R. Intrauterine infection and prematurity. Ment Retard Dev Disabil Res Rev. 2002:8:3-13.

found between positive PAMG-1 test and imminent preterm delivery.

■ PREVENTION OF PRETERM LABOR

Progesterone: Progesterone is associated with uterine quiescence and prevents the labor initiation as reported by Csapo in 1956.[24] Use of 17-hydroxy progesterone caproate weekly from 16 to 36 weeks reduced significantly PTL compared to placebo.[25] Use of progesterone suppositories 100 mg or 200 mg were associated with significant reduction of preterm birth compared to placebo.[26,27] However, progesterone gel in the dose of 90 mg versus placebo was not associated with reduction in PTB.[28] Use of 17-hydroxy progesterone caproate was not associated with improvement in twins or triplets.[29,30] There is a need for further studies on dose, preparation and route of administration progesterone.

■ MANAGEMENT (TABLE 1)

The main stay of the management of PTL with intact membranes is to ensure the pregnancy to continue at least up to 34 weeks.

In spite of evidences supporting the intra-amniotic infections, amniocentesis as a part of management to demonstrate is not recommended in PTL and PPROM.

Bed Rest

Earlier studies neither supported, nor refuted the role of bed rest in the treatment of PTL.[32,33] The later studies have clearly not only refuted the role of bed rest in the management but also warned about thromboembolic and bone loss risks associated with bed rest.[32-37]

Corticosteroids

The effectiveness of glucocorticoids in fetal lung maturity and its impact on neonatal survival was evaluated with proven benefit, if delivery or birth is delayed by at least 24 hours after the initiation of steroids (Betamethasone or Dexamethasone).[38]

TABLE 1: Drugs used in management of preterm labor.

Drug	Dose	Contraindication	Side effects (Maternal)	Side effect (Fetal)
Nifedipine	*Oral:* 20 mg stat followed by 10–20 mg every 6–8 hourly for 48 hours	Cardiac disease, diabetes mellitus (uncontrolled), deranged liver function and concurrent use of other tocolytics	Tachycardia, hypotension, headache, hot flushes, nausea and vomiting	Tachycardia
Atosiban	Initial bolus dose of 6.75 mg over 1 minute IV slowly followed by infusion of 18 mg per hour for 3 hours and then 6 mg per hour for 45 hours (Total 48 hours)	Deranged hepatic and renal function	Nausea, allergic reaction, headache, chest pain and dyspnea	Not known

Currently one course of glucocorticoids (betamethasone two doses of 12 mg each 12/24 hours apart or Dexamethasone 6 mg 6 hourly for 4 doses or 12 mg 12 hourly, 2 doses) is recommended to all PTL even when there is insufficient data to assess its effectiveness (hypertension, diabetes, multiple pregnancy, fetal growth restriction and fetal hydrops and in threatened PTL).

The American College of Obstetricians and Gynecologists (ACOG) recommends a single dose of corticosteroids for women between 24[+0] and 33[+6] weeks of gestation who are in preterm labor when delivery is likely within next 7 days.[39,40]

However National Institute for Health and Care Excellence (NICE) guidelines recommend administration of steroids after 26 weeks of gestation.

ACOG and NICE, both recommend a single dose of antenatal steroids of women in labor between 34 + 0 and 36 + 6 weeks of gestation when delivery is likely within 7 days.

At present the rescue steroid therapy (administration of repeat dose of steroid when pregnancy is prolonged more than 7 days after first course) is not recommended due to conflicting observations and without added perinatal benefits.[41,42]

However, it has been seen that the repeated doses of antenatal corticosteroids is associated with higher incidence of cerebral palsy.[43]

Which Corticosteroid to use?

The two corticosteroids (Betamethasone and Dexamethasone) are comparable in its effectiveness in PTL.

It has been seen that there is decrease incidence of intraventricular hemorrhage when dexamethasone was given.[44,45] Whereas another study reported better neurological outcome when betamethasone was given.

Betamethasone is available in two forms: (1) Betamethasone acetate and (2) Betamethasone sodium phosphate.

Betamethasone sodium phosphate has comparatively lesser half-life (36–72 hours). However both the formulations cross the placental barrier, thus ensuring the adequacy of surfactant.[44]

Role of antimicrobials: Their use is not recommended as these do not arrest PTL nor improve the neonatal outcome. Currently there is no role of antimicrobials with intact membranes with PTL.[46]

Emergency Cerclage (Rescue Cerclage)

Cerclage that is performed after established PTL or with bulging membranes is called emergency (rescue) cerclage. In cases with bulging membranes the success of rescue/emergency cerclage is lesser. However if only cervical length is ≤ 15 mm on TVS the cerclage is beneficial.

Tocolysis: At present the tocolysis is recommended for a maximum period of 72 hours (the period that allows steroids to act and shift women to higher health facility). Long-term (maintenance) tocolysis beyond 72 hours is not recommended.

Calcium Channel Blockers

Currently oral nifedipine is easy to use, effective in temporary arrest of uterine contractions in PTL. It is effective with initial loading dose of 20–30 mg followed by maintenance dose 10–20 mg every 6 hours. (Loading dose of 30mg followed by 20mg every 6 hours is effective).[4] The observed side effects are headache and tachycardia, rarely hypotension. Combination with other tocolysis is not recommended. These are economical in comparison to Atosiban. Currently these are first choice drugs.[4]

Magnesium sulfate: This is used with the loading dose of intravenous 4 g followed by 1 g/h for 24 hours is recommended with close monitoring.[47] Because of its neuroprotective effects (as noted in adults to stabilize intracranial tone, reduce fluctuations in cerebral blood flow, reduce reperfusion injury and block calcium medicated cell damage and minimize inflammation.[48-53] It is recommended for use in very early PTL up to 32 weeks.

Proposed mechanisms of action of MgSO$_4$:
- Calcium channel antagonist thereby blocks entry of calcium in N-methyl-D-aspartic acid (NDMA) receptors on oligodendrocytes. This prevents white matter injury.
- Stabilizes neuronal membranes
- Blocks excitatory transmitters
- Protects against oxidative injury
- Anti-inflammatory effects.

Prostaglandin inhibitors: Indomethacin either orally or rectally (more rapidly absorbed) is recommended in the dose

50–100 mg every 8 hourly with a maximum of 200 mg in 24 hours. The duration of use of indomethacin is restricted to 24–48 hours due to its effect on amniotic fluid (oligoamnios). There is increased incidence of necrotizing enterocolitis, intraventricular hemorrhage and patent ductus arteriosus in indomethacin group.[54] Other investigators have challenged these side effects and risks.[55] Now it is found that there is no association with these effects with indomethacin.[55,56] Use of indomethacin in infants helps to reduce/prevent pulmonary hypertension and patent ductus arteriosus.

Beta-adrenergic receptors agonists: Ritodrine, terbutaline are used in PTL. Current evidences suggest they should not be used as first-line drugs due to the life-threatening risks such as pulmonary edema, tachycardia, hyperglycemia, hypotension, cardiac failure, myocardial ischemia and death. Both intravenous and oral preparations are not recommended as their efficacy is inferior to calcium channel blocker.

Atosiban: It is commonly used in Europe and now available in India. It is an oxytocin receptor antagonist. It is less effective compared to calcium channel blockers but has lesser side effects. Though commonly used in Europe, the FDA has not approved its use due to its concern on its efficacy and fetal/newborn safety.[57,58]

Nitric oxide donors: These are potent smooth muscle relaxants specially affecting gastrointestinal tract, vessels, and uterus. These have not been found to be superior to other tocolytics (nitroglycerine) when administered orally, transdermally or intravenously. Use of these nitric oxide donors is usually associated with hypotension.[59]

INTRAPARTUM MANAGEMENT

Lesser the gestational age at labor greater the risks of labor birth.
- Labor weather induced/spontaneous, CTG is a must.
- Tachycardia suggests infection in PPROM – prevention of acidemia is important.
- Antibiotic prophylaxis to prevent infection in newborn.
- Episiotomy to be given to deliver the soft preterm baby in rigid/nonrelaxed perineum.
- Preparedness for neonatal resuscitation with neonatologist.
- No prophylactic forceps.
- Delivery by cesarean section in preterm to prevent intracranial hemorrhage has conflicting evidences.
- Close monitoring of the neonate in neonatal intensive care unit and outside for early evidences of complications and for prevention and treatment of same.

COMPLICATIONS

Preterm labor poses risks to fetus during labor for
- Intracranial hemorrhage
- Birth asphyxia
- Sepsis
- Stillbirth.

NEONATAL RISKS

Neonate is at risk for short term and long term problems.[60]

Short-term Problems

- *Pulmonary:* Respiratory distress syndrome, air leak, bronchopulmonary dysplasia, apnea of prematurity.
- *Gastrointestinal:* Hyperbilirubinemia, feeding intolerance, necrotizing enterocolitis, growth failure.
- *Immunological:* Hospital acquired infection, immune deficiency, perinatal infection.
- *Central nervous system:* Intraventricular hemorrhage, periventricular leukomalacia, hydrocephalus.
- *Ophthalmological:* Retinopathy of prematurity.
- *Cardiovascular:* Hypotension, patent ductus arteriosus, pulmonary hypertension.
- *Renal:* Water and electrolyte imbalance, acid base disturbances.
- *Hematological:* Iatrogenic anemia, need for frequent transfusions, anemia of prematurity.
- *Endocrinological:* Hypoglycemia, transiently low thyroxin levels, cortisol deficiency.

Long-term Complications

- *Pulmonary:* Bronchopulmonary dysplasia, reactive airway disease, asthma.
- *Gastrointestinal:* Failure to thrive, short bowel syndrome, cholestasis.
- *Immunological:* Respiratory syncytial virus infection, bronchiolitis.
- *Central nervous system:* Cerebral palsy, hydrocephalus, cerebral atrophy, neurodevelopmental delay, hearing loss.
- *Ophthalmological:* Blindness, retinal detachment, myopia, strabismus.
- *Cardiovascular:* Pulmonary hypertension, hypertension in adult.
- *Renal:* Hypertension in adulthood.
- *Endocrinological:* Impaired glucose regulation, increased insulin resistance.

NEWER ASPECTS IN MANAGEMENT OF PRETERM LABOR

- *Silk based injectable biomaterial*
  - Silk polyethylene glycol (PEG), restores the natural properties of cervical tissue and hence the cervical function.
  - It stiffens the tissue of cervix thus providing better support to the weakened tissue **(Figs. 5A to C)**.[61,62]
- *Arabin cervical pessary* **(Fig. 6)**[63]
  - It is a pessary available in different sizes.
  - It encircles the cervix completely and supports it.
  - It can be continued till term.
  - Removal is done in case of PPROM, IUD, and labor.[64-66]

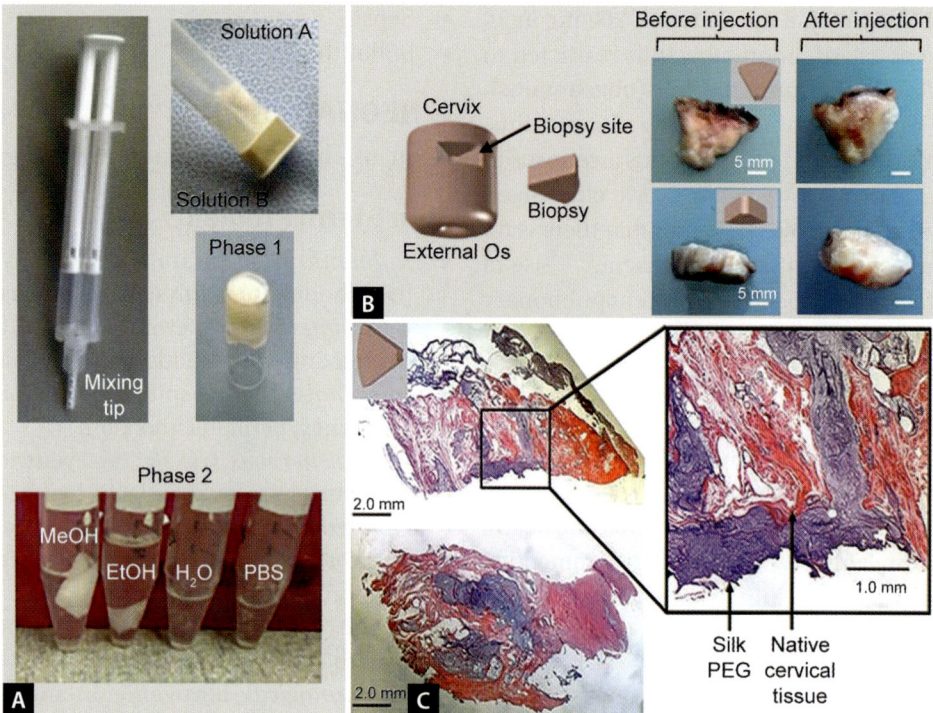

Figs. 5A to C: Biomaterial formation, gross morphology, and histology. (A) The 2-step gelation process is shown. Mixing of the 2 solutions results in a chemically cross-linked gel due to the reaction between the thiol and the maleimide functional groups. Further stabilization arises due to β-sheet formation in silk, which occurs when the silk–polyethylene glycol (PEG) is exposed to methanol or ethanol (white color) but not to water or phosphate-buffered saline (PBS); (B) After injection, the cervical tissue appears larger due to the increase in mass. The silk–polyethylene glycol appears as a translucent, white material on the tissue; (C) Hematoxylin and eosin histology of cervical tissue after injection shows integration of the silk–polyethylene glycol biomaterial (purple) into the tissue. For reference to color, please see online version.
Source: Brown JE, Partlow BP, Berman AM, House MD, Kaplan DL. Injectable Silk-based biomaterials for cervical tissue augmentation: an in vitro study. Am J Obstet Gynecol. 2016;214(1):118.e1-9.

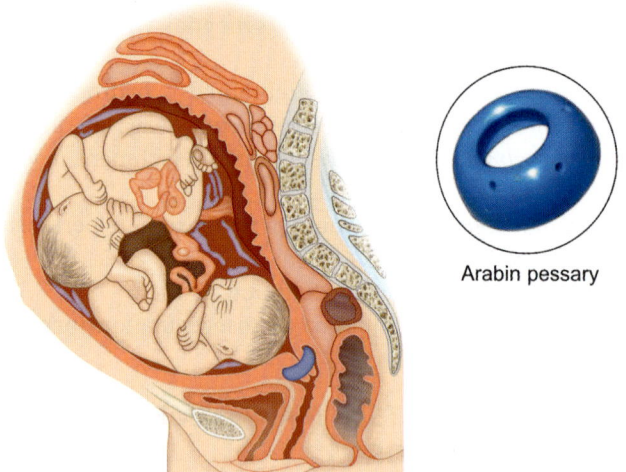

Fig. 6: Use of Arabin cervical pessary.
Source: https://elht.nhs.uk/application/files/1316/2125/8529/W37_Arabin_Leafet_Jan_2021.pdf

- *QUiPP app (Quantitative instrument in prediction of preterm births)*
  - Helps in clinical decision making during managing a case of preterm labor.
  - It is based on previous pregnancy outcomes, last miscarriage, symptoms, quantitative fFN and cervical length.[67]

- Decreases inappropriate admissions and transfers to higher center.

Antenatal corticosteroids: The use of antenatal corticosteroids must be on the basis of prediction of preterm birth within 7 days of its administration. Use of corticosteroids and continuation of pregnancy to term was associated with increased perinatal morbidity and mortality.[68,69]

The research is underway to find out the correct dose and time interval of administration of corticosteroids.

■ KEY MESSAGES

- Preterm labor and birth is one of the leading causes of neonatal and perinatal morbidity and mortality.
- Diagnosis of PTL is assisted by tocodynamometer and cervical length by transvaginal sonography.
- For pregnancies ≤ 34 weeks, prolongation till corticosteroids to act must be considered.
- Nifedipine is the first line tocolytic agent. In pregnancies between 24 and 28 weeks, magnesium sulfate is the tocolytic of choice.
- Proper counseling is essential with respect to prognosis, course, cost and complications by obstetricians and neonatologist.

- In developing countries, it is better to use steroids up to 36 weeks.
- Antibiotics in PTL mainly help to prevent neonatal infections.
- Intranatal close monitoring is essential with necessary pre-requisites.
- Routine use of forceps is not recommended.
- Correct resuscitation of newborn by neonatologist is the key issue.
- Specialized neonatal care both in neonatal intensive care unit and outside is essential.
- Woman must be educated with reference to care of such neonates.
- Regular follow-up is the key to ensure proper growth and development of the preterm infant.

REFERENCES

1. Chandraharan E, Arulkumaran S. Recent advances in management of preterm labor. J Obstet Gynecol India. 2005;55(2):118-24.
2. Slattery MM, Morrison JJ. Preterm Delivery. Lancet. 2002;360:1489-97.
3. Martin JA, Hamilton BE, Sutton PD. Births: Final data for 2004. National vital statistics reports, Vol 55, No1. Hyattsville, MD: National Centre for Health Statistics; 2006.
4. Arias F, Daftary SN, Bhide AG. Textbook of practical guide to high-risk pregnancy and delivery, A South-Asian Perspective, 3rd edition. Gurugram: Elsevier (A Division of Reed Elsevier India Pvt. Ltd.); 2008. pp. 194-261.
5. Bakketeig LS, Hoffman HJ, Harley EE. The tendency to repeat gestational age and birth weight in successive births. BMJ. 1979;135:1086-103.
6. Leeson SC, Maresh MJA, Martindale EA. Detection of fetal fibronectin as a predictor of preterm delivery in high risk symptomatic pregnancy. Br J Obstet Gynaecol. 1996;103:48.
7. Leitich H, Kaider A. Fetal fibronectin – how useful is it in the prediction of preterm birth? BJOG. 2003;10(Suppl 20):66-70.
8. Oakeshott P, Kerry S, Hay S. Bacterial vaginosis and preterm birth: a prospective community based cohort study. Br J Gen Pract. 2004;54:119-22.
9. Owen J, Iams JD, Hauth JC. Vaginal sonographic and cervical incompetence. Am J Obstet Gynecol. 2003;188:586.
10. De Carvalho MH, Bittar RE, Brizot Mde L. Prediction of preterm delivery in the second trimester. Obstet Gynecol. 2005;105:532.
11. SonoWorld. Cervical incompetence. [online] Available from: https://sonoworld.com/fetus/page.aspx?id=274. [Last Accessed October, 2021].
12. Kusanovic JP, Espinoza J, Romero R, Gonçalves LF, Nien JK, Soto E, et al. Clinical significance of the presence of amniotic fluid 'sludge' in asymptomatic patients at high risk for spontaneous preterm delivery. Ultrasound Obstet Gynecol. 2007;30(5):706-14.
13. Reichmann JP. Home Uterine activity monitoring: the role of medical evidence. Obstet Gynecol. 2008;112(2 Part1):325-7.
14. Van Vliet EO, Askie LA, Mol BW. Antiplatelet agents and the prevention os spontaneous preterm birth; a systemic review and meta-analysis. Obstet Gynecol. 2017;29(2):327-36.
15. Lee MS, Romero R, Park JW. The clinical significance of a positive Amniosure test in women with preterm labor. J Matern-fetal Neonatal Med. 2012;25(9):1690-8.
16. Minkoff H. Prematurity: infection as an etiologic factor. Obstet Gynecol. 1983:62:137-44.
17. Romero R, Mazor M Wu, Sirtori M, Oyarzun E, Mitchell MD, Hobbins JC. Infection in the pathogenesis of preterm labor. Semin Perinatol. 1988:12:262-79.
18. Romero R, Sirtori M, Oyarzun E, Avila C, Mazor M, Callahan R, et al. Infection and labor. Prevalence, microbiology, and clinical significance of intra-amniotic infection in women with preterm labor and intact membranes. Am J Obstet Gynecol. 1989:161:817-24.
19. Goncalves LF, Chaiworapongsa T, Romero R. Intrauterine infection and prematurity. Ment Retard Dev Disabil Res Rev. 2002:8:3-13.
20. Romero R, Espinoza J, Kusanovic JP, Gotsch F, Hassan S, Erez O, et al. The preterm parturition syndrome. BJOG. 2006:195:17-42.
21. Goldenberg RL, Andrews WW, Goepfert AR, Faye-Petersen O, Cliver SP, Carlo WA, et al. The Alabama preterm birth study: umbilical cord blood *Ureaplasma urealyticum* and *Mycoplasma hominis* cultures in very preterm newborn infants. Am J Obstet Gynecol. 2008a;198:43.
22. American College of Obstetricians and Gynecologists. Assessment of risk factors for preterm birth. Practice Bulletin No. 31. Washingto, DC.: ACOG; 2001.
23. FDA. PartoSure Test (p160052). [online] Available from: https://www.fda.gov/medical-devices/recently-approved-devices/partosure-test-p160052. [Last Accessed October, 2021].
24. Cunningham FG, Leveno KJ, Bloom SL, Hauth JC, Rouse DJ, Spong CY. Textbook of William's Obstetrics. 23rd edition. New York: The McGraw-Hill Companies Inc.; 2012. Pp. 804-31.
25. Meis PJ, Klebanoff M, Thom E. Prevention of recurrent preterm delivery by 17 alpha-hydroxyprogesterone caproate. National Institute of Child Health and Human Development Maternal-Fetal Medicine Units Network. N Engl J Med. 2003;348:2379.
26. da Fonseca EB, Bittar RE, de Carvalho MH. Prophylactic administration of progesterone by vaginal suppository to reduce the incidence of spontaneous preterm birth in women at increased risk: A randomized placebo-controlled double-blind study. Am J Obstet Gynecol. 2003;188:419.
27. da Fonseca EB, Celik E, Parra M. Progesterone and the risk of preterm birth among women with a short cervix. N Engl J Med. 2007;357:462.
28. O'Brien JM, Adair CD, Lewis DF, Hall DR, Defranco EA, Fusey S, et al. Progesterone vaginal gel for the reduction of recurrent preterm birth: Primary results from a randomized, double-blind, placebo-controlled trial. Ultrasound Obstet Gynecol. 2007;30:687.
29. Caritis SN, Rouse DJ, Peaceman AM, Varner MW, Sorokin Y, Hirtz DG, et al. Prevention of preterm birth in triplets using 17 alpha-hydroxyprogesterone caproate. Obstet Gynecol. 2009;113:285.
30. Rouse DJ, Caritis SN, Peaceman AM, Sciscione A, Thom EA, Spong CY, et al. A trial of 17 alpha-hydroxyprogesterone caproate to prevent prematurity in twins. National Institute of Child Health and Human Development Maternal-Fetal Medicine Units Network. N Engl J Med. 2007;357:454.
31. Ugwumadu A, Manyonda I, Reid F, Hay P. Effect of early oral clindamycin on late miscarriage and preterm delivery in

asymptomatic women with abnormal vaginal flora and bacterial vaginosis: a randomized controlled trial. Lancet. 2003;361:983-8.
32. Sosa C, Althabe F, Belizan J, Bergel E. Bed rest in singleton pregnancies for preventing preterm birth. Cochrane Database Syst Rev. 2004;1:CD003581.
33. Goldenberg RL, Cliver SP, Bronstein J. Bed rest in pregnancy. Obstet Gynecol. 1994;84:131.
34. Goulet C, Gevry H, Lemay M, et al: A randomized clinical trial of care for women with preterm labour: Home management versus hospital management. CMAJ 164:985, 2001.
35. Kovacevich GJ, Gaich SA, Lavin JP, Hopkins MP, Crane SS, Stewart J, et al. The prevalence of thromboembolic events among women with extended bed rest prescribed as part of the treatment for premature labor or preterm premature rupture of membranes. Am J Obstet Gynecol. 2000;182:1089.
36. Promislow JH, Hertz-Picciotto I, Schramm M, Watt-Morse M, Anderson JJ. Bed rest and other determinants of bone loss during pregnancy. Am J Obstet Gynecol. 2004;191:1077.
37. Yost NP, Bloom SL, McIntire DD, Lenevo KJ. Hospitalization for women with arrested preterm labor: a randomized trial. Obstet Gynecol. 2005;106:14.
38. Liggins GC, Howie RN. A controlled trial of antepartum glucocorticoid treatment for prevention of the respiratory distress syndrome in premature infants. Pediatrics. 1972;50:515.
39. ACOG. Antenatal corticosteroid therapy for fetal lung maturation. ACOG committee opinion. 2017;130(2).
40. NICE. Preterm Labor and birth. NICE Guideline. London: NICE; 2015.
41. Peltoniemi OM, Kari MA, Tammela O. Randomized trial of a single repeat dose of prenatal betamethasone treatment in imminent preterm birth. Pediatrics. 2007;119:290.
42. Kurtzman J, Garite T, Clark R, MAurel K. Impact of a "rescue course" of antenatal corticosteroids (ACS): a multicenter randomized placebo controlled trial. Am J Obstet Gynecol. 2010;202(6):544.
43. Wapner RJ, Sorokin Y, Mele L, Johnson F, Dudley DJ, Spong CY, et al. Long-term outcomes after repeat doses of antenatal corticosteroids. National Institute of Child Health and Human Development Maternal-fetal medicine units network. N Engl J Med. 2007;357(12):1190-8.
44. Katzung BG. Basic and clinical Pharmacology. New York: McGraw Hill; 2004. pp. 641-60.
45. Brownfoot FC, Crowther CA, Middleton P. Different corticosteroids and regimens for accelerating fetal lung maturation for women at risk of preterm birth. Cochrane Database Syst Rev. 2015;(4):CD006764.
46. Kenyon SL, Taylor DJ, Tarnow-Mordi W. Broad Spectrum antibiotics for spontaneous preterm labor: the ORACLE II randomized trial. ORACLE collaborative group. Lancet. 2008;372(9646):1319-27.
47. Crowther CA, Hiller JE, Doyle LW, Haslam RR, Australasian Collaborative Trial of Magnesium Sulphate (ACTO-Mg SO4) Collaborative Group. Effect of magnesium sulfate given for neuroprotection before preterm birth: a randomized controlled trial. JAMA. 2003;290(20):2669-76.
48. Grether JK, Hoogstrate J, Walsh-Greene E. Magnesium sulfate for tocolysis and risk of spastic cerebral palsy in premature children born to women without preeclampsia. Am J Obstet Gynecol. 2000;183:717.
49. Nelson KB, Grether JK. Can magnesium sulfate reduce the risk of cerebral palsy in very-low-birthweight infants? Pediatrics. 1995;95:263.
50. Nelson KB, Grether JK. More on prenatal magnesium sulfate and risk of cerebral palsy. JAMA. 1997;278(18):1493.
51. Aslanyan S, Weir CJ, Muir KW. Magnesium for treatment of acute lacunar stroke syndromes: Further analysis of the IMAGES trial. Stroke. 2007;38(4):1269.
52. Marret S, Gressens P, Gadisseux JF. Prevention by magnesium of excitotoxic neuronal death in the developing brain: an animal model for clinical intervention studies. Dev Med Child Neurol 1995;37(6):473.
53. Norton ME, Merrill J, Cooper BA, et al. Neonatal complications after the administration of indomethacin for preterm labor. N Engl J Med. 1993;329:1602.
54. Muench V, Harman CR, Baschat AA, Alger LS, Weiner CP. Early fetal exposure to long term indomethacin therapy to prevent preterm delivery: neonatal outcome. Am J Obstet Gynecol. 2001;185:S149.
55. Abbasi S, Gerdes JS, Sehdev HM, Samimi SS, Ludmir J. Neonatal outcomes after exposure to indomethacin in utero: A retrospective case cohort study. Am J Obstet Gynecol. 2003;189:782.
56. Gardner MO, Owen J, Skelly S. Preterm delivery after indomethacin: a risk factor for neonatal complications? J Reprod Med. 1996;41:903.
57. Romero R, Sibai BM, Sanchez-Ramos L. An oxytocin receptor antagonist (atosiban) in the treatment of preterm labor: a randomized, double-blind, placebo-controlled trial with tocolytic rescue. Am J Obstet Gynecol. 2000;182:1173.
58. Fullerton GM, Black M, Shetty A, Bhattacharya S. Atosiban in the Management of Preterm Labour. Clinical Medicine Insights: Women's Health. 2011;4:1-8.
59. Bisits A, Madsen G, Knox M. The randomized nitric oxide tocolysis trial (RNOTT) for the treatment of preterm labor. Am J Obstet Gynecol. 2004;191:683.
60. Eichenwald EC, Stark AR. Management and outcomes of very low birth weight. N Engl J Med. 2008;358:1700.
61. Heard AJ, Socrate S, Burke K.A. Silk-Based Injectable Biomaterial as an Alternative to Cervical Cerclage: An In Vitro Study. Reprod Sci. 2013;20:929-36.
62. Brown JE, Partlow BP, Berman AM. Injectable Silk-based biomaterials for cervical tissue augmentation: an in vitro study. Am J Obstet Gynecol. 2016;214(1):118.e1-9.
63. Mathews Open Access Publishers. Pregnancy Outcomes upon Using Arabin Pessary in Cases of Premature Cervical Shortening. [online] Available from: http://mathewsopenaccesspublishers.blogspot.com/2017/03/hi_13.html?m=0. [Last Accessed October, 2021].
64. Liem S, Schuit E, Hegeman M, Bais J, de Boer K, Bloemenkamp K, et al. Cervical pessaries for prevention of preterm birth in women with a multiple pregnancy (ProTWIN): a multicentre, open-label randomised controlled trial. Lancet. 2013;382(9901):1341-9.
65. Nicolaids KH, Syngelaki A, Poon LC. A randomized Trial of a cervical pessary to prevent preterm singleton birth. N Eng J Med. 2016;374(11):1044-52.
66. Goya M, Pratcorona L, Merced C. Cervical pessary in pregnant women with a short cervix (PECEP): an open label randomized controlled trial. Lancet. 2012;379:1800-6.

67. Watson HA, Carlisle N, Kuhrt K, Tribe RM, Carter J, Seed P, et al. EQUIPTT: The Evaluation of the QUiPP app for Triage and Transfer protocol for a cluster randomised trial to evaluate the impact of the QUiPP app on inappropriate management for threatened preterm labour. BMC Pregnancy Childbirth. 2019;19(1):68.
68. Melamed N, Shah J, Soraisham A, Yoon EW, Lee SK, Shah PS, et al. Association between antenatal corticosteroid administration-to-birth interval and outcomes of preterm neonates. Obstet Gynecol. 2015;125(6):1377-84.
69. Wilms FF, Vis JY, Pattinaja DA, Kuin RA, Stam MC, Reuvers JM, et al. Relationship between the time interval from antenatal corticosteroid administration until preterm birth and the occurrence of respiratory morbidity. Am J Obstet Gynecol. 2011;205(1):49.e1-7.

LONG QUESTIONS

1. What are the prediction and prevention strategies for preterm labor in modern obstetric practice?
2. Discuss critically the role of cervical cerclage based on current evidence in the prevention of preterm birth.
3. Evaluate the currently available tocolytic agents and summarize the current state of therapy with these agents.

SHORT QUESTIONS

1. Discuss modifiable risk factors and preterm birth risk.
2. Iatrogenic preterm birth is on the rise. Give possible reasons.
3. Explain Role of assisted reproduction in preterm birth.
4. Comment on antenatal corticosteroids in terms of drug of choice, regimen and repeat doses.
5. What is in utero transfer? When should it be practiced?

MULTIPLE CHOICE QUESTIONS

1. The preferred tocolytic in very early PTL of 24–28 weeks is:
    a. Nifedipine
    b. Magnesium sulfate
    c. Terbutaline
    d. Ritodrine
2. In preterm labor contractions will be:
    a. Contractions at least 4 in 20 minutes
    b. Contractions of at least 3 in 20 minutes
    c. Contractions of at least 6 in 1 hour
    d. Contractions of at least 4 in 1 hour
3. Risk of preterm labor with prior history of one preterm birth is present is:
    a. 04.3%
    b. 14.3%
    c. 24.3%
    d. 34.3%
4. The mean cervical length in second trimester for which preterm labor is less likely:
    a. 15 mm
    b. 25 mm
    c. 35 mm
    d. 45 mm
5. Only pathological process for which a defined molecular pathophysiology is known:
    a. Infection
    b. Cervical length
    c. Fetal fibronectin
    d. Overdistension
6. Steroids has beneficial effect brought by production substance that brings the change in:
    a. Fetal lung
    b. Fetal kidney
    c. Fetal liver
    d. Fetal skin
7. Beta adrenergic receptor agonists cause:
    a. Tachycardia
    b. Hypotension
    c. Hyperglycemia
    d. All of the above
8. Magnesium sulfate has neuroprotective mechanism as:
    a. Stabilize intracranial blood flow
    b. Reduce reperfusion flow
    c. Minimize inflammation
    d. All above
9. Atosiban acts as:
    a. Calcium channel blocker
    b. Oxytocin receptor agonist
    c. Oxytocin receptor antagonist
    d. Nitric oxide donor
10. Common complication of preterm baby are following, except:
    a. RDS
    b. Congenital dislocation of Hip
    c. Sepsis
    d. Hypothermia
11. Newer modalities for prediction of preterm labor:
    a. Arabin pessary
    b. Silk based injectable biomaterial
    c. QUiPP app
    d. All the above
12. Repeated dose of corticosteroids lead to:
    a. Cerebral palsy
    b. Immunosuppression in mother
    c. Asthma
    d. Hypothyroidism
13. What are the presenting features of chorioamnionitis?
    a. Maternal tachycardia
    b. Fetal tachycardia
    c. Elevated total leukocyte count
    d. All the above

Answers

1. b 2. a 3. b 4. c 5. a 6. a
7. d 8. d 9. c 10. b 11. d 12. a
13. d

8.3 PRETERM PREMATURE RUPTURE OF MEMBRANES

Shyam V Desai, Gaurav S Desai

■ INTRODUCTION

The rupture of fetal bag of waters during pregnancy prior to 37 weeks before the onset of labor is known as preterm premature rupture of membranes (PPROM). It occurs in 3% of pregnancies and results in approximately one-third of preterm deliveries. Meis JP et al. in 1987 stated that PROM and PPROM complicate one-quarter to one-third of preterm births.[1]

Although it can occur in all strata of society, it is seen much more commonly in the patients of the lower socioeconomic strata. It can lead to significant perinatal morbidity, including respiratory distress syndrome, neonatal sepsis, umbilical cord prolapse, placental abruption, and fetal death. It can lead to a number of other perinatal and neonatal complications, including a 1–2% risk of fetal death.

As the period of viability is decreasing over the years with improving neonatal support babies of 23 weeks' gestation or over can be expected to survive. Therefore, some other definitions are also relevant and worth considering, e.g.,

- *Previable PROM*, i.e., ROM which occurs prior to viability, i.e., at 23 weeks.
- *Preterm PROM remote from term* which occurs from viability, i.e., 23 weeks till 32 weeks gestation.
- *Preterm PROM near term*, which occurs from 32 weeks till 36 weeks gestation.

It is important to identify each of these entities and manage according to the period of gestation as each subset has an optimal methodology of management to obtain the best results.

It is important for obstetricians to correctly identify patients at risk for PPROM and thereby prevent the occurrence of, and if not correctly diagnose and manage PPROM. These steps eventually lead to an improved outcome in these patients.

■ ETIOLOGY

- Choriodecidual infections and sexually transmitted diseases (STDs)
- Obstetric factors such as incompetent os, and over distension of the uterus.
- Lower socioeconomic status
- Malnutrition and low body mass index (BMI)
- Smoking
- Lack of education
- Coitus in the third trimester.

A number of factors lead to an elevated risk of PPROM. These include African-American descent.[2] Additionally, being from the lower socioeconomic strata of society, a history of sexually transferred infections, smoking addiction, a past occurrence of vaginal bleeding, or preterm delivery can lead to PPROM. Uterine distension due to hydramnios or from multifetal gestation may also increase the risk.[3] Choriodecidual infection or inflammation may cause preterm PROM.

Cerclage and amniocentesis can also increase the risk of PPROM. Multifactorial reasons for PPROM is seen in many patients.[4] PPROM can result from a reduction in the quantity of collagen in bag of waters.[5] Even though many of the cases would have one or more of the above factors responsible in a fairly large number of cases none of the above factors may be noted.

■ INFECTIONS

Intrauterine and choriodecidual infections are an important causative factor leading to PPROM. Infection either intrauterine or cervical results in an innate immune system response followed by release of inflammatory chemokine and cytokines such as interleukin 1B and tumor necrosis factor (TNF). Degradation of the extracellular matrix in the fetal membranes predisposes them to rupture prematurely. 33% of patients with PPROM shows a positive microbial culture from the amniotic fluid which could be as a result of ascending infection from the vagina. Several studies show that a positive PCR for *Ureaplasma urealyticum* is noted even though the culture is negative. The earlier gestation that PPROM occurs the higher is the rate of intrauterine infection.[6]

Ascending infection from the vagina is the most common cause of infection and a variety of organisms have been implicated. Mycoplasma, chlamydia, yeast, *Neisseria gonorrhoeae*, Group B *Streptococcus* and bacterial vaginosis all cause production of phospholipase and result in PROM. Bacterial vaginosis is associated with a 2-fold increase in the incidence of PPROM as are infections such as *Trichomoniasis* and *Mycoplasma hominis* colonization. Urinary tract infections are also notorious in causing PPROM in as many as 5–10% of cases.

Obstetric Factors

Over distension of the uterus due to polyhydramnios and multiple gestation cause an increase in intrauterine pressure and this can result in underperfusion of the membranes resulting in rupture. Polyhydramnios could be as a result of fetal anomalies and gestational diabetes and further investigations may be warranted. As a result of an increase in assisted reproductive technology (ART) pregnancies the incidence of multiple gestations is on the increase and with a precious pregnancy the event could be disastrous. Incompetence of the cervix is known to be associated with PPROM as the membranes lie unsupported in the cervical region. The incidence of the cervical factor may be seen in 1 in 54 to 1 in 2,000 deliveries. Several reasons are listed for a cervical incompetence and it is well documented that a cervix <2.5 cm on transvaginal sonography (TVS) is associated with PPROM in multigravidae as well as primigravidae.

Other Factors

Women who are non-Whites, women of extremes of age, i.e., below 20 years and above 34 years with low body weight, malnourished and smokers are known to be at a higher risk for early rupture of membranes. The exact mechanism is not very clear but it could be assumed that these women are more likely to suffer from infectious morbidity; their overall resistance being on the lower side.

In the USA, in a study carried out over a 3-year period 22,657 women delivered at term and 2,030 delivered prematurely. Women of African origin had a rate of almost twice that of the white women. The effect of education, good nutrition, and employment are all very significant in avoidance of this complication.

■ PREDICTION OF PPROM

As the consequences and complications of PPROM are profound; there is always a benefit if we are able to identify those patients or situations which are likely to result in this problem and rectify them in time.

In women who have compromised general health, the incidence of PPROM is on the higher side and it would be well to advise such patients to improve their nutrition and treat any infection: urinary, vaginal, or systemic in good time.

Infections such as bacterial, vaginosis, and STDs are easily identified and treated.

Physical work in pregnancy could be curtailed.

Obstetric complications such as a short cervix and incompetent os can be identified and treated. The presence of a cervix of <2.5 cm is known to predispose to PPROM in primigravidae as well as multigravidae.

The fibronectin test can serve as a valuable means of identifying the risk of PPROM in nulliparas with a positive cervical fetal fibronectin (FFN) test and a short cervix had a 16.7% of having PPROM.

Multigravidae with a prior history of PPROM, a short cervix and positive FFN had a 25% risk of PPROM. However, the larger picture shows that the cost of screening all patients for the parameters would be impractical, inconvenient, and also exorbitant and hence we prefer to treat PPROM after it has occurred rather than concentrating on the preventive aspect.

■ COMPLICATIONS

Preterm delivery is arguably the most feared complication. Studies have shown that the period of rupture of membranes to delivery is inversely proportional to the gestational age.[7,8] As a consequence of PPROM, surviving neonates have a possibility to have malpresentations, compression of the umbilical cord, and resultant oligohydramnios. Additionally pitfalls of PPROM include respiratory distress syndrome, necrotizing enterocolitis, impairment of the fetal nervous system, and intraventricular hemorrhage.[9,10]

■ DIAGNOSING PRETERM PROM

The diagnosis of PPROM is based upon the patient's history, physical examination as well as laboratory tests. A sudden gush of fluid with continued leakage per vaginum especially at rest raises possibility of PPROM. One must elicit history of uterine contractions, recent sexual activity or vaginal bleeding or even a febrile illness. Accurate documentation of patients, last normal menstrual period, and due date are of paramount importance.

A speculum examination is the preferred method of assessment of the cervix rather than digital cervical examination which increases morbidity.[11,12] It has been shown that digital cervical examinations shorten latency thereby increasing morbidity due to infections.[13] Obstetricians may be concerned that not doing digital examinations may lead to an incorrect diagnosis however this has not been proven.[14]

Sigs of ruptured membranes is evident from the presence of fluid in the vagina which gushes after fundal pressure and evidenced by outflow of fluid from the cervix on speculum examination. Presence of ferning is an evidence of amniotic fluid presence.[15] The amniotic fluid is more alkaline (pH of 7.1–7.3) leading to nitrazine paper turning blue **(Figs. 1A to C)**. However, contaminants like blood semen can also cause this false positive result.

Presence of ferrying pattern also indicates presence of amniotic fluid. False positive result can be abstained because of cervical mucus and blood. A DNA probe or culture should be performed for chlamydia and gonorrhea as this is a strong possibility in PPROM.[16] Vaginal or perianal swab for group B streptococci should also be obtained.

Ultrasound is useful in showing low amniotic fluid volume. Amniocentesis with instillation of 1 mL of indigo carmine dye mixed in sterile saline can show ROM in ambiguous cases (no presence of fluid in vagina but nitrate test positive). If the membranes are ruptured, the blue dye should pass onto a vaginal tampon within 30 minutes of instillation.[17]

■ MANAGEMENT OF PPROM

Management of PPROM depends on the gestational age at which it occurs, the maternal and fetal status. Medications that can be safely administered and must be considered are given here.

Medications

Corticosteroids

Liggins and Howie from New Zealand carried out a randomized controlled trial (RCT) between 1969 and 1970 and demonstrated that antepartum glucocorticoid treatment could reduce the idiopathic respiratory distress syndrome (RDS) in preterm infants delivered between 26 and 32 weeks gestation.

The risk of RDS is between 15 and 30% at 32–36 weeks and rises sharply in gestations between 24 and 28 weeks

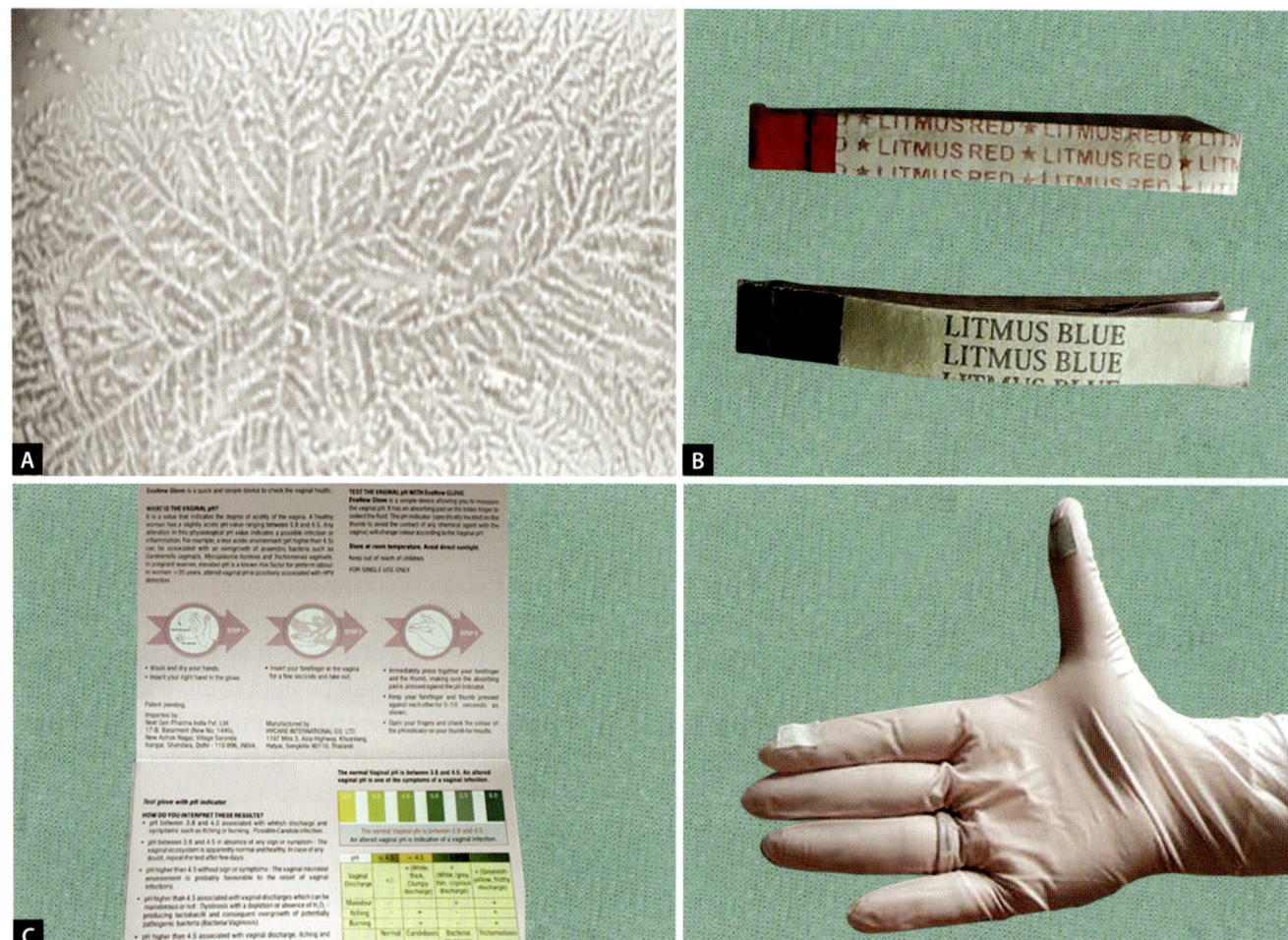

Figs. 1A to C: Tests to detect amniotic fluid. (A) Ferning pattern of dried amniotic fluid on microscopy; (B) Litmus paper (red turns blue indicates alkaline content such as amniotic fluid); (C) Nitrazine paper loaded gloves.

Corticosteroids decrease perinatal morbidity and mortality after preterm PROM.[18] A recent meta-analysis[18] found that corticosteroid administration after preterm PROM versus no administration, reduced the risk of respiratory distress syndrome (20% vs. 35.4%), intraventricular hemorrhage (7.5% vs. 15.9%), and necrotizing enterocolitis (0.8% vs. 4.6%) without an increase in the risk of maternal or neonatal infection.

Because corticosteroids are effective at decreasing perinatal morbidity and mortality, all physicians caring for pregnant women should understand the dosing and indications for corticosteroid administration during pregnancy.

The most widely used and recommended regimens include intramuscular betamethasone 12 mg every 24 hours for 2 days, or intramuscular dexamethasone 6 mg every 12 hours for 2 days.[19]

Administration of dexamethasone is cheaper and hence more useful in low income situations. The administration of antenatal corticosteroids has greatly helped reduce the perinatal mortality of the preterm babies. Administration of corticosteroids also reduces neonatal deaths less than 24 hours before delivery and has been shown to enhance the benefits of surfactant therapy.

The National Institutes of Health recommends administration of corticosteroids before 30–32 weeks' gestation, assuming fetal viability and no evidence of intra-amniotic infection. Use of corticosteroids between 32 and 34 weeks is controversial. Administration of corticosteroids after 34 weeks' gestation is not recommended unless there is evidence of fetal lung immaturity by amniocentesis.

Multiple courses are not recommended because studies have shown that two or more courses can result in decreased infant birth weight, decreased head circumference, and body length as well as neurological development delay as well as placental infarction and neonatal sepsis.[20]

Antibiotics

A large proportion of cases of PPROM are as a result of infectious etiology. Giving antibiotics to patients with preterm PROM can reduce neonatal infections and prolong the latent period. A meta-analysis[6] showed that patients receiving antibiotics after preterm PROM, compared with those not receiving antibiotics experienced reduced postpartum endometritis, chorioamnionitis, neonatal sepsis, neonatal pneumonia, and intraventricular hemorrhage. Another meta-analysis[21] found a decrease in neonatal intraventricular hemorrhage and sepsis.

Antibiotics can improve outcomes in two ways one they delay the progression to labor by controlling the infectious status and modulating the subsequent inflammatory process and second by reducing fetal infection (FIRS, fetal inflammatory response syndrome) can directly improve neonatal outcome.

A number of antibiotic regimens are advocated for use after preterm PROM. Most of the recommendations are for a duration of 3-7 days period. The regimen studied by the National Institute of Child Health and Human Development trial[22] uses an intravenous combination of 2 g of ampicillin and 250 mg of erythromycin every 6 hours for 48 hours, followed by 250 mg of amoxicillin and 333 mg of erythromycin every 8 hours for 5 days. Women given this combination were more likely to stay undelivered for 3 weeks despite discontinuation of the antibiotics after 7 days.

It is advisable to administer appropriate antibiotics for intrapartum group B *Streptococcus* prophylaxis to women who are carriers, even if these patients have previously received a course of antibiotics after preterm PROM.

The ACOG recommends a 7-day course of parenteral and oral therapy with ampicillin or amoxicillin and erythromycin during expectant management. Ampicillin with clavulanic acid should be avoided in view of the risk of necrotizing enterocolitis. Prophylaxis to B *Streptococcus* is required during labor.[23]

Tocolytic Therapy

Evidence is lacking on use of tocolytics and more is desired. Combination of tocolysis with antibiotics and steroid use required further investigation.

Short-term tocolysis helps to extend steroid use but does not help in neonatal outcomes.[24] Giving tocolysis allows for initiation of antibiotics, corticosteroid administration, and maternal transport.[25] Long-term tocolytic therapy in patients with PROM is not advisable.

Magnesium Sulfate

Cerebral palsy is a dreaded complication of preterm births the incidence being 2 of 1,000 births. There is evidence that magnesium sulfate given to patients prior to 34 weeks' gestation reduces risk of cerebral palsy. The first article on the use of magnesium sulfate was published by Karen Nelson and Judith Grether and they stated that babies with cerebral palsy were much less exposed to magnesium sulfate. Magnesium sulfate reduces vascular instability, lessens hypoxic damage, and protects against cytokine or excitatory amino acid damage which are all associated with damage to the venerable preterm brain.

Magnesium sulfate is to be administered to the mother in preterm labor as a bolus of 4 g IV over 20 minutes followed by a maintenance infusion of 1g per hour over 24 hours. The time honored antidote for magnesium toxicity 1 g calcium gluconate should always be kept available. Common problems with magnesium infusion include flushing and pain at injection site.

Randomized controlled trials with placebo control trials were held in 3 countries France, USA, and UK and all three trials showed that the risk of cerebral palsy was reduced with no increase in fetal/neonatal mortality. The cord blood concentration was inversely correlated with fetal demise, i.e., higher the concentration the lower the risk. No significant risk of major maternal complications, adverse neonatal outcomes was noted. The cost effectiveness remains extremely high. The benefit of magnesium therapy is best prior to 32 weeks.

Flowchart 1 is a useful guide in outlining the plan of action in a patient with PPROM.

Management Based on Gestational Age

34 to 36 Weeks

It is wise not to prolong pregnancy in cases of PPROM occurring after 34 weeks of gestation. Expectant treatment between 34 and 36 weeks results in an increased risk of chorioamnionitis and lower than average umbilical cord pH.[26] There is also evidence to suggest that the neonatal condition does not necessarily improve significantly after 34 weeks.[27] Preterm PROM is not a contraindication to vaginal delivery. Steroids use in this subset of the patients is not needed however the use of antibiotics but be considered especially if the pregnant woman is being transferred to higher center.[28-30]

32 to 33 Weeks

In cases where the fetal lungs are mature the woman should be transferred to an equipped hospital with NICU backup and the goal is to deliver the baby. Chances of maternal and fetal infection increase if the pregnancy is unnecessarily prolonged.

Patients in whom PPROM has occurred but lack of pulmonary maturity are more tricky to handle. The obstetrician must weigh the pros and cons of delivering in this situation. On one hand prolonging delivery to wait for lung maturity will increase risk of chorioamnionitis and sepsis. On the other hand, lies the risk of respiratory distress if delivered too early.

Administration of steroids and antibiotics must be done in those patients without lung maturity in fetuses and try to prolong as much as possible without compromising on risk of infection. Antibiotics must cover both gram positive and negative organisms in addition to anaerobes.

24 to 31 Weeks

The goal of treatment is to try to prolong the pregnancy till fetal maturity or 34 weeks at least in the absence of evidence of infection. However, most deliver before this time.[8] Any evidence of fetal or maternal compromise necessitates early delivery and admission of baby to NICU. Corticosteroid and antibiotics should be given.

Fetal and maternal monitoring to rule out complications like cord compression and amnionitis is paramount in this gestation age. Signs of amnionitis include fetal or maternal tachycardia, febrile temperature, and raised C reactive proteins.

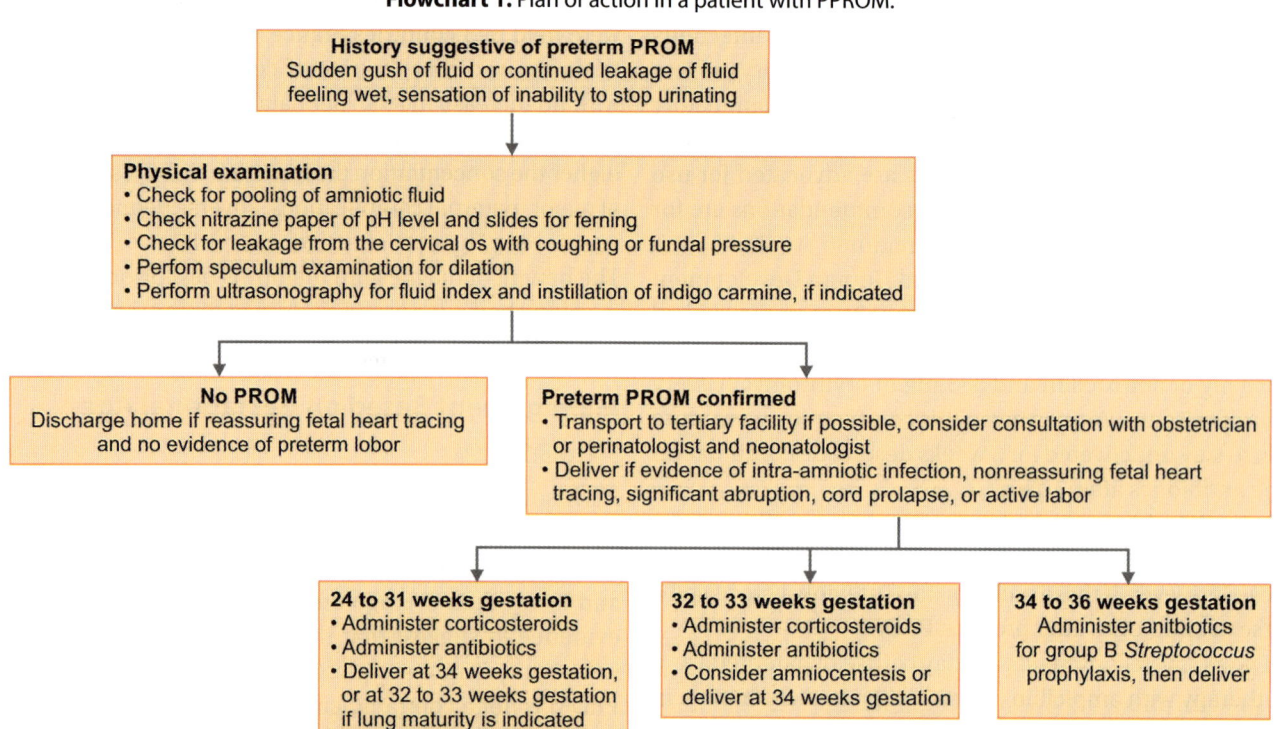

Flowchart 1: Plan of action in a patient with PPROM.

Increasing the latency of pregnancy PPROM leads to the increase risk of amnionitis and infection.[31] Any evidence of this must entail delivery. Decreased glucose level or a positive Gram stain and differential count can signify amnionitis.[28] For those, that are fortunate to progress to 34 weeks assessment of fetal lung maturity and maternal status must be done. If lungs are mature, delivery should be attempted.

Before 24 Weeks

Preterm premature rupture of membranes before 24 weeks usually does not continue for long.[12] Parents must be consoled as to the severe morbidity of these preterm babies including extended hospital NICU stay and cerebral palsy not to mention the higher chance of lung injury and infection. Potters syndrome is another problem faced.

This is more common at earlier gestations and is a result of absence of the fluid cushion resulting in crushing of limbs.[32] Best place to deliver these extreme PPROM is at a well-equipped tertiary care institution with NICU backup. Home management and bed rest are controversial ideas. Close monitoring of the mother and the fetus is important in these patients.[33]

KEY MESSAGES

- Administration of antibiotics to patients with PPROM improves maternal and fetal outcome.
- Administration of corticosteroids in cases of PPROM between 24 and 32 weeks of gestation prevents and reduces complications associated with PPROM, e.g., IVH and RDS.
- Per vaginal examination during PPROM should be deferred and speculum examination is preferred in PPROM.
- Short-term tocolysis helps in shifting the mother and fetus in utero along with action of steroid. However, long-term tocolysis has no place in PPROM.
- Corticosteroid use after 34 weeks does not add any beneficial value.

REFERENCES

1. Meis PJ, Ernest JM, Moore ML. Causes of low birth weight births in public and private patients. Am J Obstet Gynecol. 1987;156:1165-8.
2. Savitz DA, Blackmore CA, Thorp JM. Epidemiologic characteristics of preterm delivery: etiologic heterogeneity. Am J Obstet Gynecol. 1991;164:467-71.
3. American College of Obstetricians and Gynecologists. Premature rupture of membranes. Clinical management guidelines for obstetrician-gynecologists. ACOG practice bulletin no. 1. Int J Gynaecol Obstet. 1998;63:75-84.
4. Bendon RW, Faye-Petersen O, Pavlova Z, Qureshi F, Mercer B, Miodovnik M, et al. Fetal membrane histology in preterm premature rupture of membranes: comparison to controls, and between antibiotic and placebo treatment. Pediatr Dev Pathol. 1999;2:552-8.
5. Stuart EL, Evans GS, Lin YS, Powers HJ. Reduced collagen and ascorbic acid concentrations and increased proteolytic susceptibility with prelabor fetal membrane rupture in women. Biol Reprod. 2005;72:230-5.
6. Mercer BM, Arheart KL. Antimicrobial therapy in expectant management of preterm premature rupture of the membranes. Lancet. 1995;346:1271-9.

7. Hannah ME, Ohlsson A, Farine D, Hewson SA, Hodnett ED, Myhr TL, et al. Induction of labor compared with expectant management for prelabor rupture of the membranes at term. N Engl J Med. 1996;334:1005-10.
8. Schucker JL, Mercer BM. Midtrimester premature rupture of the membranes. Semin Perinatol. 1996;20:389-400.
9. Ananth CV, Savitz DA, Williams MA. Placental abruption and its association with hypertension and prolonged rupture of membranes: a methodologic review and meta-analysis. Obstet Gynecol. 1996;88:309-18.
10. Gonen R, Hannah ME, Milligan JE. Does prolonged preterm premature rupture of the membranes predispose to abruptio placentae?. Obstet Gynecol. 1989;74(3 pt 1):347-50.
11. Alexander JM, Mercer BM, Miodovnik M, Thurnau GR, Goldenburg RL, Das AF, et al. The impact of digital cervical examination on expectantly managed preterm rupture of membranes. Am J Obstet Gynecol. 2000;183:1003-7.
12. Schutte MF, Treffers PE, Kloosterman GJ, Soepatmi S. Management of premature rupture of membranes: the risk of vaginal examination to the infant. Am J Obstet Gynecol. 1983;146:395-400.
13. Lewis DF, Major CA, Towers CV, Asrat T, Harding JA, Garite TJ. Effects of digital vaginal examinations on latency period in preterm premature rupture of membranes. Obstet Gynecol. 1992;80:630-4.
14. Munson LA, Graham A, Koos BJ, Valenzuela GJ. Is there a need for digital examination in patients with spontaneous rupture of the membranes?. Am J Obstet Gynecol. 1985;153:562-3.
15. Davidson KM. Detection of premature rupture of the membranes. Clin Obstet Gynecol. 1991;34:715-22.
16. Ekwo EE, Gosselink CA, Woolson R, Moawad A. Risks for premature rupture of amniotic membranes. Int J Epidemiol. 1993;22:495-503.
17. Naylor CS, Gregory K, Hobel C. Premature rupture of the membranes: an evidence-based approach to clinical care. Am J Perinatol. 2001;18:397-413.
18. Harding JE, Pang J, Knight DB, Liggins GC. Do antenatal corticosteroids help in the setting of preterm rupture of membranes? Am J Obstet Gynecol. 2001;184:131-9.
19. Effect of corticosteroids for fetal maturation on perinatal outcomes. NIH Consens Statement. 1994;12:1-24.
20. Vidaeff AC, Doyle NM, Gilstrap LC III. Antenatal corticosteroids for fetal maturation in women at risk for preterm delivery. Clin Perinatol. 2003;30:825-40,vii.
21. Egarter C, Leitich H, Karas H, Wieser F, Husslein P, Kaider A, et al. Antibiotic treatment in preterm premature rupture of membranes and neonatal morbidity: a meta-analysis. Am J Obstet Gynecol. 1996;174:589-97.
22. Mercer BM, Miodovnik M, Thurnau GR, Goldenburg RL, Das AF, Ramsey RD, et al. Antibiotic therapy for reduction of infant morbidity after preterm premature rupture of the membranes. A randomized controlled trial. JAMA. 1997;278:989-95.
23. Ehernberg HM, Mercer BM. Antibiotics and the management of preterm premature rupture of the fetal membranes. Clin Perinatol. 2001;28:807-18.
24. Weiner CP, Renk K, Klugman M. The therapeutic efficacy and cost-effectiveness of aggressive tocolysis for premature labor associated with premature rupture of the membranes [published correction appears in Am J Obstet Gynecol 1991;165:785]. Am J Obstet Gynecol. 1988;159:216-22.
25. Fontenot T, Lewis DF. Tocolytic therapy with preterm premature rupture of membranes. Clin Perinatol. 2001;28:787-96,vi.
26. Naef RW III, Allbert JR, Ross EL, Weber BM, Martin RW, Morrison JC. Premature rupture of membranes at 34 to 37 weeks' gestation: aggressive versus conservative management. Am J Obstet Gynecol. 1998;178(1 pt 1):126-30.
27. Lieman JM, Brumfield CG, Carlo W, Ramsey PS. Preterm premature rupture of membranes: is there an optimal gestational age for delivery?. Obstet Gynecol. 2005;105:12-7.
28. Mercer BM. Preterm premature rupture of the membranes. Obstet Gynecol. 2003;101:178-93.
29. Smith CV, Greenspoon J, Phelan JP, Platt LD. Clinical utility of the nonstress test in the conservative management of women with preterm spontaneous premature rupture of the membranes. J Reprod Med. 1987;32:1-4.
30. Cox SM, Leveno KJ. Intentional delivery versus expectant management with preterm ruptured membranes at 30–34 weeks' gestation. Obstet Gynecol. 1995;86:875-9.
31. Gopalani S, Krohn M, Meyn L, Hitti J, Crombleholma WR. Contemporary management of preterm premature rupture of membranes: determinants of latency and neonatal outcome. Obstet Gynecol. 2005;60:16-7.
32. Rotschild A, Ling EW, Puterman ML, Farquharson D. Neonatal outcome after prolonged preterm rupture of the membranes. Am J Obstet Gynecol. 1990;162:46-52.
33. Carlan SJ, O'Brien WF, Parsons MT, Lense JJ. Preterm premature rupture of membranes: a randomized study of home versus hospital management. Obstet Gynecol. 1993;81:61-4.

■ LONG QUESTIONS

1. Define PPROM. Describe the causes and management in a primigravida at 31 weeks' gestation.
2. Discuss the rationale and use of corticosteroids and magnesium sulfate in PPROM.
3. Enumerate the complications of PPROM. Describe the antibiotic use in PPROM.
4. What is previable PPROM? Discuss the management of a multigravida with PPROM at 24 weeks' gestation.
5. Discuss the protocols in management of early and late PPROM.

■ SHORT QUESTIONS

1. Define fetal fibronectin.
2. Define Corticosteroids in PPROM.
3. Define diagnosis of PPROM.
4. Discuss magnesium sulfate in PPROM.
5. Discuss complications of PPROM.

■ MULTIPLE CHOICE QUESTIONS

1. Magnesium sulfate is used for neuroprotection in preterm delivery. Its antidote is:
   a. Strontium   b. Calcium
   c. Manganese   d. Copper
2. Antibiotics given in a case of PPROM reduce the incidence of:
   a. Endometritis   b. Neonatal sepsis
   c. IVH   d. All of the above

3. Corticosteroids are given to PPROM patients to reduce the incidence of all, except:
   a. IVH
   b. Necrotizingenterocolitis
   c. Diabetes mellitus
   d. RDS
4. All are risk factors for PPROM, except:
   a. Diabetes mellitus
   b. Polyhydramnios
   c. Multiple gestation
   d. Oligohydramnios
5. Fetal fibronectin test is used in:
   a. Oligohydramnios
   b. GDM
   c. FGR
   d. PPROM
6. Previable ROM occur before:
   a. 23 weeks
   b. 25 weeks
   c. 27 weeks
   d. 28 weeks
7. Primigravida at 31 weeks' gestation has PPROM. She falls in the category:
   a. Previable
   b. Preterm PROM remote from term
   c. PROM near term
   d. None of the above
8. Prophylaxis to which of the following organism is recommended in PPROM?
   a. Chlamydia
   b. Group B streptococci
   c. Staphyloocci
   d. Acinetobacter
9. PPROM occurs before:
   a. 38 weeks
   b. 37 weeks
   c. 26 weeks
   d. 34 weeks
10. A G2 P1L1 at 31^{+2} weeks' gestation with diabetes mellitus and multiple gestation comes to the ER complaining of leaking per vaginum. On examination liquor is demonstrated per speculum. She will require which of the following in her management?
    a. Antibiotic
    b. Corticosteroids
    c. Magnesium sulfate
    d. All of the above

Answers
1. b 2. d 3. c 4. a 5. d 6. a
7. b 8. b 9. b 10. d

8.4 ANTEPARTUM HEMORRHAGE

Madhuri Chandra

DEFINITION

Antepartum hemorrhage (APH) is defined as bleeding from or in to the genital tract, occurring from the period of viability (24^{+0} weeks of pregnancy) and prior to the birth of the baby.[1] It complicates about 3–5% of all pregnancies.[1] APH remains a major cause of maternal and perinatal mortality and morbidity in the developing world.

CAUSES OF ANTEPARTUM HEMORRHAGE (BLEEDING IN SECOND HALF OF PREGNANCY)

The most important causes of APH are placenta previa and placental abruption. Abruptio placenta is twice as frequent as placenta previa, the incidences being roughly abruptio placenta 40%, placenta previa 20%, undetermined APH 35% and the remaining 5% are due to pregnancy unrelated and local genital tract disorders **(Table 1)**.

In this chapter we will discuss the main causes of placental site bleeding:
- Placenta previa
- Abruptio placenta
- Vasa previa.

PLACENTA PREVIA/UNAVOIDABLE HEMORRHAGE

Definition

Placenta previa is defined as a placenta that occupies part or whole of the lower uterine segment.[1] The placenta instead of becoming implanted at the usual site in upper uterine segment,

TABLE 1: Causes of antepartum hemorrhage (APH).

Pregnancy related	Local causes/other than due to pregnancy
Excessive show	Cervical polyp
Placenta previa	Cancer cervix or cervical dysplasia
Abruptio placenta	Cervicitis
Vasa previa	Vaginal varicosities
Rupture uterus	Vaginal lacerations/trauma
DIC/coagulation defects	Vaginal infections

(DIC: disseminated intravascular coagulation)

implants over or very near the internal os. The incidence of placenta previa is 1/200 pregnancies.[2-4] The incidence increases with age, parity and number of cesarean deliveries.

Etiology

The fertilized ovum implants in lower segment and the decidua basalis forms in lower uterine segment, this is seen in scarred uterus and in ART pregnancies. The placenta may be large and thin, and spread to lower segment as in multiple pregnancy, infections, and Rh incompatibility. In routine 2nd trimester scan, placenta is frequently seen in lower segment but at term the incidence of placenta previa is much lower. This is due to differential growth of uterus and placenta, initially placenta occupies about one-half to one-third of uterine wall and may occupy the lower segment, however the change in ratio permits a degree of apparent placental movement (placental migration). In the first 7 months of pregnancy it is the upper segment that grows and in the last 2 months there is formation of lower segment. With the cervical effacement and dilatation the placenta is sheared of the lower segment resulting in bleeding.

Risk Factors[1,2,4,6-8]

- *Previous placenta previa:* Increases the risk by 12 fold
- *Previous cesarean sections:* The risk increases linearly with the number of cesarean sections
- Previous termination of pregnancy
- Multiparity (5 or more deliveries)
- Advanced maternal age > 40 years
- Pregnancy following assisted reproductive technology
- *Multiple pregnancy:* More likely with dichorionic twin pregnancy
- *Smoking:* Heavier, thinner placentas with larger surface areas
- *Deficient endometrium due to presence or history of:* Uterine scar, endometritis, manual removal of placenta, curettage and submucous fibroids.

Classification

Clinical[3,6]

- *Type 1:* Lateral placenta previa. The greater part of placenta is in the upper segment but its lower edge dips into the lower segment.
- *Type 2:* Marginal placenta previa, the edge of the placenta touches the margin of the internal os.
- *Type 3:* Partial placenta previa, the cervical os is partly covered by the placenta.
- *Type 4:* Total placenta previa, the cervical os is completely covered by the placenta, even when fully dilated. This classification is now obsolete.[2]

Transabdominal Sonography/Transvaginal Sonography (Fig. 1)

With the advent of real time sonography, most women will have placental localization with their routine 2nd trimester sonography. The modified classification based on sonography >16 weeks is (AIUM):[5]

- *Placenta previa:* When the placenta lies directly over the internal os
- *Low lying placenta:* In pregnancies >16 weeks of gestation, the placenta is reported as "low lying" when the placental edge is less than 20 mm from the internal os
- *Normal:* In pregnancies >16 weeks of gestation, when the placental edge is 20 mm or more from the internal os on transabdominal sonography/scan (TAS) or transvaginal sonography/scan (TVS).

A TAS should be advised in any woman presenting with vaginal bleeding in second half of pregnancy. There are

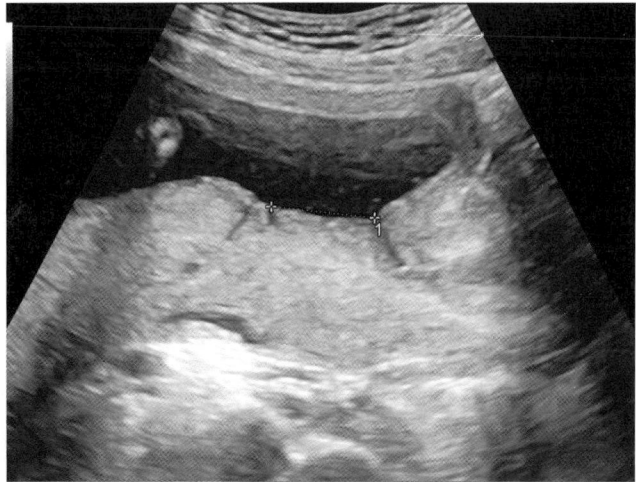

Fig. 1: Measurement of the distance between the placental edge and internal os for diagnosis of placenta previa.

difficulties in diagnosis and a false positive rate of 25% with TAS, as in cases of over distention of the maternal urinary bladder, focal low-lying myometrial contractions, low-lying leiomyomas and hematomas. A posterior placenta previa is more difficult to visualize on TAS and in case of doubt a TVS is recommended.[3,5] There are concerns that a TVS may provoke more bleeding in a patient of APH but the vaginal probe is inserted under direct ultrasonic visualization and avoids any direct contact with the cervix. There is about 2–3 cm distance between the tip of the vaginal probe and the cervix. Thus low lying placenta must be confirmed and followed up by a transvaginal scan.

The incidence of placenta previa at 16–18 weeks is 2–6%.[8,9] But not all low-lying placenta or placenta previa diagnosed by sonography in midtrimester scan, would remain previa by term.[9] Apparent placental "migration" following the development of the lower uterine segment during the third trimester of pregnancy results in the resolution of the low-lying placenta in 90% of the cases before term.[6,9] Thus scan must be repeated at 32 weeks gestation and if required at term. Placental migration is less likely if placenta is posterior, thick and lower edge is <2cm from internal os or there is history of previous section. Color Doppler will aid in ruling out abnormal placental attachment [placenta accreta spectrum disorders (PASD)] and vasa previa.[6]

A TAS or TVS is adequate for diagnosis of APH and magnetic resonance imaging (MRI) is not required, though MRI do have potentially better tissue differentiation and an ability to highlight blood and may be advised if invasive placenta or PASD is suspected. Here MRI is better able to delineate the depth of invasion and lateral extension of myometrial invasion.[6] Placenta accreta is characterized by a thin, incompletely developed or absent decidua basalis and the villi invade the uterine wall to different degrees. Though placenta accreta is rare and occurs in about 1 in 1,600 pregnancies, its incidence is increased in pregnancies with placenta previa. Placenta accreta must be kept in mind in all anterior placenta previa and in presence of a prior uterine scar.[6] Placenta accreta may be total, partial or focal, depending on surface area of placenta adherent.

Placenta accreta is classified according to the degree of myometrial invasion.
- *Placenta accreta:* The abnormally adherent placental villi are attached directly into the myometrium, but do not invade it.
- *Placenta increta:* The villi invade the myometrium.
- *Placenta percreta:* The placental villi penetrate through the myometrium, reaching the serosal surface of the uterus.

The placenta accreta spectrum disorders are covered in the next chapter.

Clinical Picture

With the advent of routine midtrimester sonography, most low-lying placenta and placenta previa will be picked up at second trimester scan. The presenting symptoms are painless, causeless, recurrent and revealed vaginal bleeding. The initial bleeding may be slight and is called "warning hemorrhage". The bleeding is due to disruption of the placental attachment to the lower uterine segment and may be provoked by sexual intercourse or vaginal examination. The amount of bleeding is usually proportional to the degree of placenta previa and tends to occur at an earlier gestation in major degree of placenta previa.

About one-third of women have initial bleeding before 30 weeks of gestation, these are at higher risk of preterm births, preterm premature rupture of membranes, severe bleeding, and may require emergent cesarean section and blood transfusions.

The initial bleeding subsides to be followed by brisker hemorrhage but this is not the rule and the woman may present with sudden profuse bleeding and collapse at the first episode. On examination in contrast to abruptio there is an absence of abdominal discomfort and usually a normal fetal heart tracing. About 10–20% may present with both bleeding and uterine contractions. The uterus tends to be soft, relaxed, nontender and fetal parts can be palpated. The lower segment of uterus is empty and presenting part lies high up. There is fetal malpresentation or malposition in 30% cases. An increased risk of congenital malformations and intrauterine growth restriction has been reported in pregnancies complicated by placenta previa.[6]

There is no role of vaginal examination in patients with diagnosed placenta previa. However we may still have women presenting with vaginal bleeding and no prior sonography. If on examination the uterus is contracting, the presenting part is engaged or nearly so, facilities of sonography not available, an examination in "double set up", a gentle palpation through the fornices followed by examination of cervical os may be done, to determine the cause of antepartum hemorrhage and progress of labor. By double setup is implied, patient is shifted to operation theater, one person does the internal examination, while team is ready to proceed with cesarean section if placenta is encountered or there is torrential hemorrhage.

Management

Placenta previa must be suspected in any woman who presents with vaginal bleeding beyond 20 weeks of pregnancy and an ultrasonography for placental localization is mandatory before any digital examination. Women with APH must be managed in tertiary care center with facilities of blood transfusion, skilled anesthetist and 24/7 facility for operative deliveries.

Asymptomatic Women Diagnosed with Placenta Previa at Mid-trimester Scan

Women diagnosed with low lying or placenta previa on second trimester scan must have a repeat scan at 32 weeks.[6] About 90% placenta previa resolve by that time.[6,9] If at 32 weeks, the placental edge is >2 cm from internal os, the placental position is reported as normal and she may be scheduled for vaginal delivery if there is no other contraindication. If the placental edge still covers the os or is <2 cm from os, a repeat scan at 36 weeks is advisable. Color Doppler is useful to confirm the position of placental edge, exclude vasa previa, and exclude any placenta accreta spectrum disorders. If the placental edge covers the internal os at 36 weeks, cesarean delivery is advised. If the placental edge does not cover but is <2 cm from the internal os, the woman is counseled on risks and benefits of a trial of labor.

Women Presenting with Vaginal Bleeding at <34 Weeks

Management will depend on clinical presentation, severity of bleeding (**Table 2**), degree of placenta previa and hemodynamic condition of woman.

A thorough history taking to establish duration of pregnancy, any pain, review of previous records including sonographies, an assessment of the extent of vaginal bleeding, the cardiovascular condition of the mother, and an assessment of fetal wellbeing.

All women with diagnosed placenta previa, must be counseled about the need to report any vaginal bleeding however mild. Written informed consent about risk of preterm

TABLE 2: Assessment of amount of bleeding.[1]

Spotting	Staining, streaking or blood spotting noted on underwear or sanitary protection
Minor hemorrhage	Blood loss < 50 mL that has settled
Major hemorrhage	Blood loss of 50–1,000 mL, with no signs of clinical shock
Massive hemorrhage	Blood loss > 1,000 mL and/or signs of clinical shock[1]

birth, cord complications, need for blood transfusion and operative delivery and if required hysterectomy must be recorded. There is a need to avoid heavy work and sexual intercourse. Any anemia should be corrected with iron and folic acid supplementations. She must be hospitalized if any bleeding or uterine contractions are present.

The time and route of delivery would depend on gestational age, sonographic findings (placental localization, relation of placental edge to internal os and fetal head) and severity of hemorrhage.

Expectant Management

Women who presented with spotting and are no longer bleeding, where placenta praevia has been excluded with a reassuring initial clinical assessment, can go home 48 hours after all bleeding ceases.[1]

All women with APH heavier than spotting and women with ongoing bleeding should remain in hospital at least until the bleeding has stopped.[1] Such women should follow-up in OPD after discharge and the above instructions are relevant to them. Any anemia must be corrected by supplements and/or blood transfusion. Regular monitoring of fetal growth is done. About 50% of pregnancies with initial bleeding but who are not in labor, who are hemodynamically stable with normal fetal heart rate, respond to supportive therapy and prolong pregnancy by 2-4 weeks. This expectant management with aim to further fetal growth and maturation was first suggested by Macafee,[7] with high fetal salvage.

Women who are Rh negative must receive anti-D immunoglobulin (Ig) at time of bleed in order to prevent RhD alloimmunization. Repeat dose is not necessary if delivery occurs within 3 weeks of administration.

In women who present with vaginal bleeding in early third trimester (<34 weeks), and are hemodynamically stable, short term tocolysis (for 48 hours) in order to gain time for corticosteroid prophylaxis for fetal lung maturity may be done with Injection magnesium sulfate.[6] This additionally has a neuroprotective effect on the fetus. Otherwise tocolytic drugs are to be avoided. If bleeding is controlled, woman is stable, fetal status is reassuring, expectant management can be continued as described earlier.

Immediate Cesarean Section

For women with major bleeding, the mother's life should take priority. She should be resuscitated and stabilized before any decision is made regarding delivery of the baby.[1] Major degrees of placenta previa with brisk hemorrhage will require immediate operative delivery to save the mother's life.

A short cervical length on TVS before 34 weeks of gestation increases the risk of preterm emergency delivery and massive hemorrhage at cesarean section.[1] However, there is no role of cervical cerclage, which may provoke bleeding.

Emergency cesarean section is advisable for any woman with placenta previa in active labor, with vaginal bleeding and fetal distress, severe persistent vaginal bleeding or significant bleeding in pregnancy at >34 weeks.

Women Presenting with Vaginal Bleeding at 34 or >34 Weeks

All women with major degrees of placenta previa must be hospitalized at 34 weeks. In cases of complete placenta previa, if patients remain otherwise stable, documentation of fetal lung maturity and elective cesarean delivery are usually advocated at 34–36 weeks' gestation under regional anesthesia.[8,10] With uncomplicated placenta previa, the cesarean delivery can be planned at 36–37 weeks.[8,10]

While in those with low-lying placenta, the route of delivery would depend on the distance between placental edge and internal os and fetal head position relative to leading edge of placenta. In most cases, when the placental edge is less than 2 cm from the cervical os, it is considered preferable to proceed with elective cesarean to prevent massive hemorrhage and its complications. When the placental edge is at least 2 cm from the cervical edge, patient is asymptomatic and the fetus is in vertex presentation, it is usually safe to allow the patient a trial of vaginal labor **(Table 3)**.

Cesarean Section

The cesarean section should be planned with presence of senior obstetrician and anesthetist.[6] Preoperative ultrasonography should exclude placenta accreta spectrum disorders and vasa previa. Ample blood must be cross matched and ready. Regional anesthesia is preferred for the hemodynamically stable woman, this avoids risk of atonic postpartum hemorrhage associated with general anesthesia.

In preterm placenta previa with transverse lie or unformed lower segment a low vertical uterine incision may be used. Consider using preoperative and/or intraoperative ultrasonography to precisely determine placental location and the optimal place for uterine incision.[6] If anterior placenta previa, all efforts should be made to avoid transecting the

TABLE 3: Management guidelines (TVS preformed within 28 days of term).[3]

Placenta previa/overlap of internal os	Cesarean delivery only
Placental edge 0–10 mm from internal os	Higher likelihood of bleeding and need for cesarean section delivery
Placental edge 11–20 mm from the internal cervical os	Lower likelihood of bleeding and need for CS, if trail of labor is decided upon, facility must have ability to perform emergency cesarean section 24/7
Placenta edge is ≥ 20 mm from the internal cervical os	Trial of labor is appropriate

placenta and fingers must find edge of placenta to deliver the baby. Clamp cord early to avoid fetal blood loss.

Active management of third stage of labor using oxytocics: Oxytocin and methylergonovine are advised. Tranexamic acid injection may be used to control postpartum hemorrhage **(Table 4)**. If pharmacological measures fail to control hemorrhage, initiate intrauterine balloon tamponade and/or surgical hemostatic techniques (Affronti hemostatic square sutures, B Lynch compression suture, gel foam at bleeding site, stepwise devascularization of uterus) sooner rather than later. Early recourse to hysterectomy is recommended if conservative medical and surgical interventions prove ineffective.[6]

Facilities with interventional ultrasonography, may consider uterine artery embolization to control hemorrhage, however this is more helpful in placenta previa with placenta accreta spectrum disorders in which the catheter may be placed preoperative and embolization done if required intra or postoperative.

Complications

Woman with placenta previa are at risk is of preterm labor and hemorrhage. Assessment of the cervical length at sonography will guide toward the risk of both. Anterior placenta previa in previous cesarean section or scarred uterus is risk of placenta accreta with resultant massive hemorrhage, emergency hysterectomy, massive blood transfusion, disseminated intravascular coagulation (DIC) and acute respiratory distress syndrome.

Postpartum complications include postpartum hemorrhage, amniotic fluid embolism, postpartum collapse, and venous thromboembolism.

There is increased neonatal mortality and morbidity due to preterm labor, intrauterine growth restriction (IUGR), congenital malformation, malpresentation, and fetal anemia and cord complications. During labor there is increased incidence of fetal bradycardia and late decelerations in posterior marginal placenta previa.

ABRUPTIO PLACENTAE/ ACCIDENTAL HEMORRHAGE

Definition

Placental abruption is the premature separation of a normally situated placenta from the uterine wall, resulting in hemorrhage before the delivery of the fetus.[2,4] It is variously known as abruptio placentae, ablation placentae, and accidental hemorrhage. Women with abruptio placenta typically present with bleeding, uterine contractions, and fetal heart rate abnormalities.

Incidence

Placental abruption of some degree is seen in 1 in 80–100 deliveries.[11] The risk of abruption recurring in a subsequent pregnancy is increased by 10-fold.

Pathophysiology

In normal pregnancy, the second wave of trophoblastic invasion occurs at 15–16 weeks, transforming the spiral arteries into large low resistance vessels relatively unresponsive to vasoactive substances. In patients with placental abruption, there is absence of this physiological transformation[12] with decreased placental blood flow and abnormal endothelial response to vasoactive substances.

Although the exact cause is not clear, the rupture of an uteroplacental blood vessel leads to bleeding into the decidua basalis with formation of a hematoma. This hematoma dissects the decidua basalis causing placental separation with resultant fetal hypoxia. The bleeding extends in to myometrium, with disruption of the myometrial muscle fibers with blood dissecting into the broad ligaments and under the pelvic peritoneum. Blood may trickle to the serosal surface of

TABLE 4: Drugs to control postpartum hemorrhage.

Drug	Dosage	Side effects	Contraindications
Oxytocin	• 10 units IM • 20 units/500 mL IV infusion	• Nausea • Water intoxication	Known hypersensitivity
Methylergonovine	0.25 mg IM, repeat every 15 mins to maximum 5 doses	• Peripheral vasospasm • Hypertension • Nausea, vomiting	• Hypertension • Peripheral vascular disease • Known hypersensitivity
Carboprost tromethamine	0.25 mg IM, repeat every 15 mins to maximum 8 doses	• Bronchospasm • Flushing • Diarrhea, vomiting	• Bronchial asthma • Acute renal or liver disease hypersensitivity
Misoprostol	600 µg oral or rectal	Flushing, diarrhea, vomiting	Known hypersensitivity
Tranexamic acid	1 g (10 mL in 100 mL saline) IV, over 10–20 min. May be repeated if bleeding persists after 30 min	Anaphylaxis, nausea, vomiting, DVT, pulmonary embolism	History of stroke, subarachnoid hemorrhage, convulsions, color blindness, and renal dysfunction

(DVT: deep vein thrombosis)

the uterus and produce the typical boggy, purple ecchymosis of the Couvelaire uterus. These uteri are prone to atonic postpartum hemorrhage (PPH).

The hematoma may remain small, with insignificant placental separation and normal fetal heart. Or it may expand completely separating the basal plate from the decidua until complete placental detachment results. There will be signs of maternal acute blood loss, fetal distress, and fetal death. The rupture of spiral arterioles causes a "high pressure" bleed in central area of placenta with near complete placental separation.[4] It is associated with hypertension and vascular diseases.[4] With >50% placental separation, fetal death and DIC ensues.[11] While tears in marginal veins of placenta, cause "low pressure venous bleed" with small placental separation. It is associated with cigarette smoking.[4]

The retroplacental bleeding extends to placental edge between the chorion and decidua parietalis to present at the os and vagina as revealed hemorrhage, or it may break through the amniotic membranes and enter the amniotic fluid (blood stained liquor). At other times the bleeding remains retroplacental, separating the center of placenta, while the margins remain adherent to uterine wall, thus bleeding is completely retained inside the uterus and is termed concealed hemorrhage. Revealed hemorrhage is seen in 80% cases and concealed hemorrhage in 20% and often the hemorrhage is mixed.

Compression from the hematoma obliterates the overlying intervillous space with further damage of placental vessels. Decidual bleeding and hypoxia leads to release of tissue factor (thromboplastin) from the decidual cells. Thrombin generation would lead to uterine contractions, uterine hypertonus,[11] enhanced expression of matrix metalloproteinases, apoptosis, and induced expression of inflammatory cytokines leading to tissue necrosis and degradation of extracellular matrix resulting in further vascular disruption, initiation of labor and premature rupture of membranes.

The tissue thromboplastin release into maternal circulation, activates coagulation cascade with consumption of coagulation factors.[11] The maternal fibrinolytic system is then activated with critical depletion of platelets, fibrinogen and other clotting factors and consequent DIC. Hemorrhage associated with DIC leads to further consumption of coagulation factors, setting off a vicious circle.[11] Large amounts of fibrinogen and other clotting factors are lost in the large retroplacental clot.

Risk Factors[1,2,4,11,13]

- *Hypertension:* Increased fragility of vessels, vascular malformations, or abnormalities in placentation. Placental abruption is seen more often in gestational hypertensive disease
- *Previous placental abruption:* A prior placental abruption is associated with 10-fold higher risk in subsequent pregnancy
- Low body mass index (BMI), poor nourishment, low socioeconomic class
- Pregnancy following assisted reproductive techniques
- First trimester bleeding in current pregnancy
- Advanced maternal age
- Parity >4
- *Multiple gestations, polyhydramnios, and short cord:* Rapid uterine decompression as occurs after delivery of first twin or after rupture of membranes in polyhydramnios may cause placental bleed and separation
- Chorioamnionitis, intrauterine infection, premature rupture of membranes and prolonged rupture of membranes
- *Trauma:* Blunt injury to abdomen, road side accident
- Uterine malformations, submucous fibroids
- *Thrombophilias:* Activated protein C resistance, deficiencies of protein C, protein S, and antithrombin III), hyperhomocystinemia and rarely congenital hypofibrinogenemia
- *Maternal cocaine, smoking and tobacco use:* Vasoactive substances in tobacco cause placental hypoperfusion, decidual ischemia and hemorrhage
- *Abnormal maternal serum biochemical markers:* Elevated maternal serum alpha-fetoprotein (MSAFP) and human chorionic gonadotropins, decreased PAPP A, inhibin A levels in the second trimester.

Clinical Picture

Placental abruption presents classically with triad of abrupt vaginal bleeding, abdominal pain and tenderness, and uterine contractions. Placental separation causes fetal hypoxia and fetal heart rate abnormalities.

There may be high risk factors such as hypertension, previous abruptio, overdistended uterus or a history of blunt injury to abdomen.

On clinical examination, the uterus is irritable, with increased baseline tone. It is firm to rigid in consistency, and tender to touch. The fetal parts may be difficult to palpate and there is evidence of fetal distress. In posterior placenta, backache may be the presenting complains. In concealed hemorrhage, the uterine size is greater than period of gestation, there is an increasing fundal height and abdominal girth. On internal examination, the patient is usually in labor with cervical effacement and dilatation. The presenting part is felt and may be engaged in contrast to the empty lower segment and high presenting part seen in placenta previa.

Vaginal bleeding may be mild and clinically insignificant to severe and life threatening. The clinical signs of blood loss are out of proportion to the amount of vaginal bleeding.[2,11]

With mild cases, there may be only abdominal pain, uterine irritability, and scant vaginal bleeding. The diagnosis is confirmed on examination of placenta postdelivery, which reveals intervillious hemorrhage, a clot and/or depression in the maternal surface.

In severe acute blood loss, the woman may present with signs of shock, a low or rapidly falling blood pressure, a rapid and weak pulse, generalized pallor with cold and clammy extremities, tachypnea, and mental cloudiness. In severe cases, the entire uterus develops a board-like rigidity, so that palpation of fetal parts and auscultation of fetal heart sounds are difficult. The severity of fetal distress correlates with the degree of placental separation. In severe abruption with placental separation >50%, there is high risk of fetal death and DIC.[11] A fibrinogen level <200 mg%, best correlates with severity of bleeding, postpartum hemorrhage, DIC and need for multiple blood transfusions.

Some women may present as chronic abruption with light, chronic, intermittent bleeding in late second to third trimester of pregnancy. This is marginal venous bleeding and is associated with features of placental insufficiency such as oligohydramnios, IUGR, preeclampsia, preterm labor and preterm premature rupture of membranes.

Ultrasonography (Fig. 2): Abruptio placenta is a clinical diagnosis and sonography may be negative in presence of abruption. If sonographic evidences of placental abruption are present, it is associated with worst maternal and perinatal outcomes.[11] The classic picture is of a retroplacental hematoma, which is initially hyperechoic. It becomes hypoechoic after a week and sonolucent after 2 weeks. Other findings are subchorionic collection of fluid, echogenic debris in amniotic fluid, thickened placenta which shimmers with maternal movement (Jello sign).[11]

Complications

Table 5 lists the maternal and fetal complications of abruptio placenta.

Classification[2,4]

Placental abruption is graded in three degrees of severity.
- *Grade 1 (40% of cases):* Mild vaginal bleeding, slightly tender uterus, normal maternal blood pressure and heart rate, no coagulopathy and no fetal distress. It is diagnosed after delivery of placenta by the presence of a retroplacental clot.
- *Grade 2 (45% of cases):* The classical signs of abruption are present but the fetus is still alive. There is mild to moderate vaginal bleeding, uterine tenderness with possible tetanic contractions, and maternal tachycardia with postural hypotension and fetal distress. Hypofibrinogenemia (150–250 mg/dL) may be present.
- *Grade 3 (15% of cases):* Bleeding is moderate to severe, but may be concealed. Painful tetanic uterus, maternal shock, hypofibrinogenemia (< 150 mg/dL), coagulopathy, and fetal death.

Ananth[14] has defined placental abruption, taking into consideration maternal, fetal and neonatal complications. "Severe abruption" should include at least one of maternal (disseminated intravascular coagulation, hypovolemic shock, blood transfusion, hysterectomy, renal failure, or in-hospital death), fetal (nonreassuring fetal status, intrauterine growth restriction, or fetal death), or neonatal (neonatal death, preterm delivery, or small for gestational age) complications. All other cases are termed mild abruption.

Management

Any women presenting with vaginal bleeding in late pregnancy must be assessed for coexisting symptoms such as pain, backache, uterine contractions, extent of vaginal bleeding, and the maternal and fetal status.

A per speculum examination is permissible to identify cervical dilatation or visualize a lower genital tract cause for the APH. However digital vaginal examination, to assess chance of vaginal delivery should not be performed until an ultrasound has excluded placenta previa.

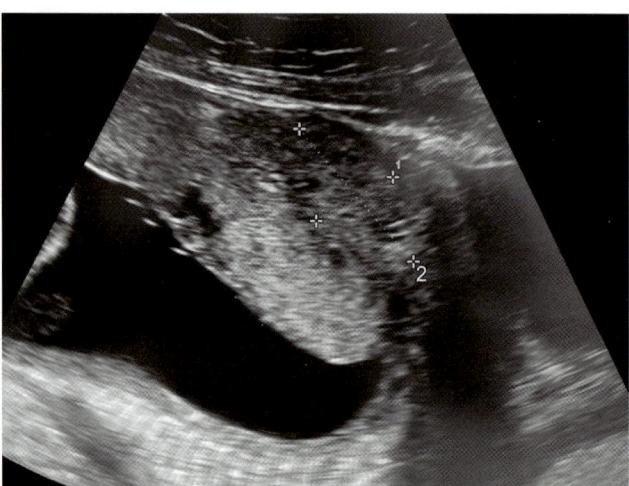

Fig. 2: Abruptio placenta – Retroplacental hematoma on ultrasound. It should be noted that this is not always visualized and abruptio is a clinical diagnosis.

TABLE 5: Maternal and fetal complications of abruptio placenta.

Maternal (severity of placental separation)	Fetal (severity of placental separation + gestation)
Hemorrhage, hypovolemic shock	Preterm birth, preterm PROM
DIC	Hypoxia, asphyxia
Renal failure, bilateral cortical necrosis in concealed hemorrhage and acute tubular necrosis as a result of shock	IUGR
ARDS	Fetal anemia hyperbilirubinemia
Multiple blood transfusion	RDS
Operative delivery, peripartum hysterectomy	Stillbirths, 10-fold increase
Couvelaire uterus, postpartum hemorrhage	

(ARDS: acute respiratory distress syndrome; DIC: disseminated intravascular coagulation; IUGR: intrauterine growth restriction; PROM: prolonged rupture of membranes)

Initial Assessment and Resuscitation in Woman with Vaginal Bleeding (Suspected Abruptio)

Rapid assessment of maternal and fetal condition is done. Rule out preeclampsia, HELLP syndrome and trauma to abdomen.

Secure intravenous assess with wide bore cannula. Send blood for laboratory investigations: Complete blood picture, platelet count, blood group and type, coagulation profile (fibrinogen level, prothrombin time, and activated partial thromboplastin time), liver function test and renal profile. Urine examination should be done for protein and sugar. When DIC is suspected, estimate fibrin degradation products by D dimer assay.

Bedside clot observation test: Take 5 mL of woman's blood in a test tube. Do not shake. A clot should form within 6–8 minutes. If it does not or if it forms and lyses within 30 minutes to 2 hours, a significant coagulopathy and low fibrinogen level is present.

Administer crystalloids to maintain urine output at 30 mL/hour. In dwelling Foley's catheter is placed and urine output must be monitored closely.

Monitor hemodynamic condition of mother. Pulse, blood pressure, pO_2, urine output, vaginal bleeding, uterine contractions, increase in fundal height and abdominal girth.

Initiate continuous fetal heart rate monitoring. Fetal tachycardia/bradycardia, loss of variability, sinusoidal pattern, and late decelerations signify fetal compromise.

Replace blood and blood products: Target hematocrit >25%, platelets >75,000/uL, fibrinogen >300 mg/dL and PT, PTT at <1.5 times control.

Tocolysis should not be used to delay delivery in a woman presenting with a major APH, or who is hemodynamically unstable, or if there is evidence of fetal compromise. Tocolytic therapy is contraindicated in placental abruption and is relatively contraindicated in "mild hemorrhage" due to placenta previa.

Administer antenatal corticosteroids for pregnancies < 34 weeks, some advise up to 36 weeks.

Neuroprotective dose of magnesium sulfate for pregnancies <32 weeks is advisable.

Anti-D Ig 500 IU should be given to all non-sensitized Rh D-negative women after any presentation with APH. A Kleihauer Betke test is advised in Rh negative mothers to check amount of fetomaternal hemorrhage.[4]

Subsequent Management

Further management would depend on gestational age, maternal and fetal condition. The maternal and fetal condition reflects the severity of abruption.

Term pregnancies and pregnancies complicated by severe abruption (DIC, hypovolemic shock, need for blood transfusion, impending renal failure, IUGR, fetal distress or fetal death) must be delivered.

The route of delivery would depend on hemodynamic condition of mother, fetal status, and progress of labor.

Immediate delivery: If patient in labor, she is hemodynamically stable, uterus is contracting and cervical dilatation has progressed, or vaginal delivery is imminent, a spontaneous or assisted vaginal delivery is preferred. Practice active management of third stage of labor (AMTSL) and watch out for postpartum hemorrhage.

If the mother is hemodynamic unstable, there is evidence of continuous hemorrhage or significant coagulopathy, and vaginal delivery is not imminent, irrespective of fetal condition a cesarean delivery is the best option.[11] Blood and blood products must be used to correct hypovolemia and coagulopathy prior to cesarean section **(Table 6)**.

TABLE 6: Blood and blood products.

Blood product	Component	Indication/Comment
Fresh whole blood 350 mL	↑ fibrinogen by 12.5 mg% and adds 10,000–15,000 platelets/mm³	• Hemorrhage • Usually unavailable because of screening procedure
Whole blood 350 mL	RBC, plasma, 600 mg fibrinogen, no platelets	• *Hemorrhage:* ↑ Hct 3–4% per unit • Only whole blood stored for < 24 hours at 20–24°C is the source of viable platelets and labile coagulation factors V and VIII
Packed red cells 200–250 mL	Hematocrit (Hct: 55–80%, contents RBCs only, increases Hct 3–4% per unit	• Severe anemia and acute blood loss • Improves oxygen carrying capacity
Fresh frozen plasma 150 mL	All coagulation factors	Severe bleeding, DIC, liver disease 1 pack/15 kg body weight/24 hours
Cryoprecipitate	200 mg fibrinogen plus other clotting factors	• Fibrinogen deficiency, acute DIC or massive transfusion • About 3,000–4,000 mg is needed to restore maternal fibrinogen to > 150 mg%
Platelets 50 mL	1 bag: 5.5×10^{10} platelets	Massive transfusion when the platelet count is $<50 \times 10^9$/L; or in the management of DIC when the platelet count is $<100 \times 10^9$L 6–10 units usually transfused, each increases platelets by 5,000/mL

(DIC: disseminated intravascular coagulation)

Expectant Management

Expectant management of suspected placental abruption is the exception and not the rule.[4] The goal is to prolong pregnancy with the hope of improving fetal maturity and survival.[2]

If mother is hemodynamically stable and fetal status is reassuring (normal CTG) and gestational age is <34 weeks, administer antenatal corticosteroids. Monitor mother daily, ask her to report any further bleeding, contractions, pain, or decrease in fetal movement. Assess fetus by sonography for fetal growth, biophysical profile, nonstress test and target delivery at 36–37 weeks.

Women who present at 34–36 weeks with acute abruption should be delivered as there is risk of progressive or recurrent abruption and neonatal morbidity is low at this gestation. Vaginal delivery is the least morbid route of delivery for mother and provided there is no indication of cesarean section (CPD, malpresentation), an artificial rupture of membranes (ARM) and oxytocin infusion is advisable. The uterus is frequently contracting, ARM stops further bleeding, stimulates uterine contractions, and stops entry of thromboplastins into maternal circulation, oxytocin infusion will augment the contractions with rapid vaginal birth.

In a patient with Couvelaire uterus and uncontrollable blood loss, a hysterectomy may be indicated. A bruised Couvelaire uterus by itself not a reason for hysterectomy as in most cases, the uterus will still be able to contract sufficiently in response to oxytocics given to prevent postpartum hemorrhage **(Figs. 3A and B)**.[4]

The risk of placental abruptio in subsequent pregnancy is increased tenfold. Maternal hypertension should be controlled, smoking, tobacco and cocaine should be avoided before considering next pregnancy. Though folic acid supplementation is advised in early pregnancy, its ability to prevent abruptio is uncertain. Also uncertain role for antithrombotic therapy (low dose aspirin ± low molecular weight heparin) in the prevention of abruption in women with thrombophilia.[1] Serial growth scans every 4 weeks are advised in third trimester and in women with >2 prior abruptions, documentation of fetal lung maturity and delivery at about 37 weeks gestation seems reasonable.[11]

■ VASA PREVIA

Definition

Vasa previa is the presence of fetal vessels (unsupported by umbilical or placental tissue) below the fetal presenting part. The fetal vessels run through the free placental membranes overlying the cervical os. Vasa previa may rupture in active labor or when amniotomy is performed to induce or augment labor and should be suspected whenever bleeding occurs after rupture of membranes and is associated with falling fetal heart rate.

Incidence

It is rare, prevalence ranging between 1 in 1,200 and 1 in 5,000 pregnancies.[15] More common with twin gestation, low-lying placenta, velamentous insertion of cord and succenturiate placental lobe.

Classification

- *Type I:* When the vessel is connected to a velamentous umbilical cord
- *Type II:* When it connects the placenta with a succenturiate or accessory lobe.

Clinical Presentation

The woman presents in labor with painless vaginal bleeding (Benckiser's hemorrhage). The vessels may be felt pulsating through the intact membrane. As the cervix dilates and is effaced and the membranes rupture spontaneously and bleeding from the torn vessel starts. Given the total fetal blood volume at term is approximately 80–100 mL/kg, the loss of small amount of blood can cause fetal exsanguination and fetal death.[15]

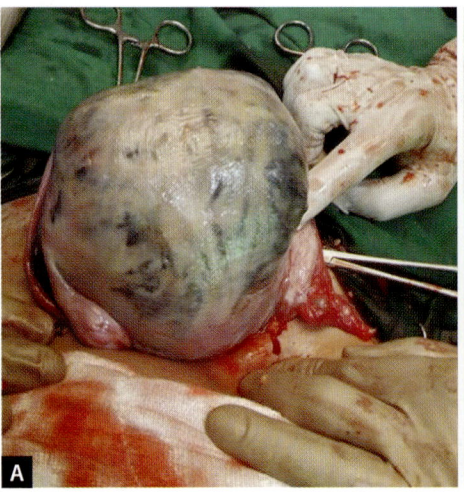
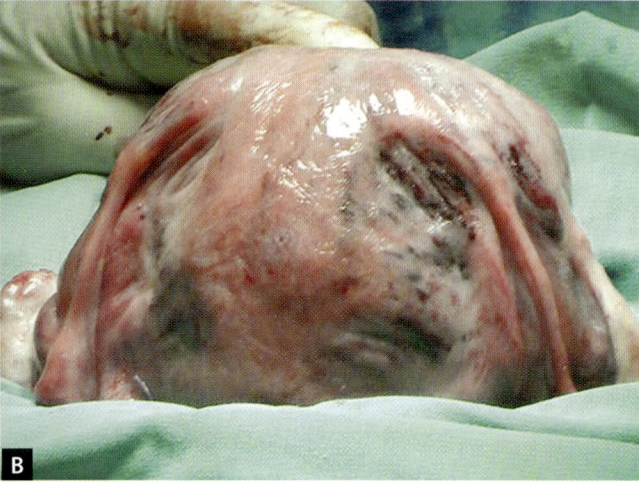

Figs. 3A and B: Couvelaire uterus in abruptio placenta.

Diagnosis

On ultrasonography with color Doppler: Vasa praevia has been defined as a vessel running in the free placental membranes within 2 cm of the cervix in mid trimester scan, its needs to be confirmed in third trimester (32 weeks).[15]

Management

High risk women with diagnosed vasa previa, preterm labor, any bleeding or multiple gestations must be admitted at 30–32 weeks of gestation. Administration of corticosteroids for fetal lung maturity is recommended.

Delivery should be planned by elective cesarean section after fetal pulmonary maturity (34–36 weeks) is established and prior to the onset of labor, in women with confirmed vasa previa.

Emergency cesarean delivery and neonatal resuscitation are essential in the management of ruptured vasa previa diagnosed during labor, fetal mortality rate in this situation is at least 60%.

UNEXPLAINED ANTEPARTUM HEMORRHAGE

In about half the cases with vaginal bleeding in second half of pregnancy, the cause of bleeding remains uncertain.[4] Most cases of unexplained APH would go into labor within 2 weeks. Unexplained APH is associated with an increased risk of oligohydramnios, fetal growth restriction, and preterm labor, premature rupture of membranes, stillbirth, fetal anomalies, and cesarean delivery.

REFERENCES

1. RCOG. Antepartum Hemorrhage: Green-top Guideline No. 63. London: RCOG; 2011.
2. Giordano R, Cacciatore A, Cignini A, Vigna R, Romano M. Antepartum Hemorrhage. J Prenat Med. 2010;4(1):12-6.
3. Oppenheimer LW. A new classification of placenta previa: measuring progress in obstetrics. Am J Obstet Gynecol. 2009:226-9.
4. FOGSI Focus. Antepartum Hemorrhage. Mumbai: FOGSI; 2010.
5. AIUM Practice Parameter for the Performance of Limited Obstetric Ultrasound Examinations by Advanced Clinical Providers. J Ultrasound Med. 2018;37:1587-96.
6. RCOG. Placenta Praevia and Placenta Accreta: Diagnosis and Management. Green-top Guideline No. 27a. London: RCOG; 2018.
7. MacAfee CHG. Placenta previa: a study of 174 cases. J Obstet Gynecol Br Commonwealth. 1945;52:313-7.
8. Oppenheimer L, Society of Obstetricians and Gynaecologists of Canada. Diagnosis and management of placenta previa. J Obstet Gynaecol Can. 2007;29:261.
9. Rizos N, Doran TA, Miskin M, Benzie RJ, Ford JA. Natural history of placenta previa ascertained by diagnostic ultrasound. Am J Obstet Gynecol. 1979;133(3):287-91.
10. Vergani P, Ornaghi S, Pozzi I. Placenta previa: distance to internal os and mode of delivery. Am J Obstet Gynecol. 2009;201:266.
11. Oyelese Y, Ananth CV. Placental abruption. Obstet Gynecol. 2006;108(4):1005-16.
12. Dommisse J, Tiltman AJ. Placental bed biopsies in placental abruption. Br J Obstet Gynaecol. 1992;99(8):651-4.
13. Williams MA, Lieberman E, Mittendorf R, Monson RR, Schoenbaum SC. Risk factors for abruptio placentae Am J Epidemiol. 1991;134(9):965-72.
14. Ananth CV, Lavery JA, Vintzileos AM, Skupski DW, Varner M, Saade G, et al. Severe placental abruption: clinical definition and associations with maternal complications. Am J Obstet Gynecol. 2016;214:272.
15. RCOG. Vasa Praevia: Diagnosis and Management. Green-top Guideline No. 27b. London: RCOG; 2018.

LONG QUESTIONS

1. A 26-year-old primigravida is under your care, her scan at 18 weeks shows placenta covering the os. What is the chance of her having placenta previa at term? How will you manage her during the antenatal period?
    a. Her 32 week scan shows low-lying placenta. She has had no episode of vaginal bleeding. What will be your further management?
    b. How do you plan her delivery?
2. A 34-year-old para 3, live 3, no abortions, unbooked patient reports to emergency with about 7 months gestation, abdominal pain and bleeding per vaginum since past 2 hours. She had one previous antenatal checkup, where her BP is recorded as 140/90 mm Hg. On examination, her pulse is 110/min, BP 150/94 mm Hg, uterus is irritable, FHS audible.
    a. What will be your management?
    b. What is her risk of developing coagulopathy? What investigations are advisable?

SHORT QUESTIONS

1. Write short note on placental localization by ultrasonography.
2. Explain principles of expectant management in placenta previa.
3. What is abruptio placenta? How do you grade placental abruption?
4. Enumerate maternal and fetal complications following placental abruption.
5. What are vasa previa? What risk do they pose to mother and fetus?

MULTIPLE CHOICE QUESTIONS

1. Common placental causes of APH are all but:
    a. Placenta previa   b. Vasa previa
    c. Abruptio placenta   d. Rupture uterus
2. Regarding placenta previa, which is correct?
    a. It complicates 2% pregnancies
    b. Majority of low lying placenta diagnosed at 20 weeks remain so at term
    c. It presents as painless, causeless, recurrent hemorrhage
    d. If placenta previa is diagnosed by sonography, patient must be admitted in hospital

3. Risk factors for placenta previa are all, except:
   a. Previous placenta previa
   b. Previous cesarean section
   c. Pregnancy following artificial reproductive technology (ART)
   d. Hypothyroidism in mother
4. On USG, "low-lying placenta'" is diagnosed when
   a. Placenta edge is >2 cm from internal os
   b. Placental edge covers internal os
   c. Placental edge is <2 cm from internal os at 12 week scan
   d. Placental edge is <2 cm from internal os at 16 week scan
5. For expectant management of placenta previa, all are correct, expect
   a. Gestation must be >34 weeks
   b. Patient must be hemodynamically stable
   c. Fetal heart should be reassuring
   d. Patient must not be in labor
6. A 28-year-pld women has a low lying placenta at 18 weeks scan, which is correct answer?
   a. Schedule delivery by CS at 38 weeks
   b. Schedule amniocentesis at 34 weeks if lung maturity present CS at 36 weeks
   c. Rescan for placental position at 32 weeks
   d. Recommend termination of pregnancy
7. Regarding abruptio placenta, which is true?
   a. It is more common in hypertensive women
   b. Its best diagnosed by USG
   c. Treatment is conservative
   d. About 50% abruption present as concealed hemorrhage
8. The following suggest placental abruption:
   a. Painless hemorrhage
   b. Tense tender uterus
   c. Empty lower segment of uterus
   d. High floating presenting part
9. High risk factor for placental abruption are all, except:
   a. Previous placental abruption
   b. Maternal hypertension
   c. Grand multipara
   d. Gestational diabetes mellitus
10. Complications of placental abruption are all, except:
    a. DIC
    b. Atonic PPH
    c. Postdate pregnancy
    d. Renal failure

Answers
1. d 2. c 3. d 4. d 5. a 6. c
7. a 8. b 9. d 10. c

8.5 PLACENTA ACCRETA SPECTRUM DISORDERS

Shrinivas N Gadappa, Ankita Rajesh Shah

INTRODUCTION

Placenta accreta was first described in the year 1937 by obstetrician Frederick C Irving and pathologist Arthur T Hertig.[1]

Over the past 40 years, cesarean delivery rates around the world have risen from less than 10% to over 30%, thus simultaneously increasing the rate of placenta accreta spectrum (PAS) disorders.[2] The incidence of PAS disorders have risen from 1 in 533 in 1998–2002 to 1 in 272 in 2016.[3] The major risk factors for PAS are history of accreta in previous pregnancy, previous cesarean delivery and other uterine surgery, including repeated endometrial curettage and also with increasing number of prior cesarean section.[4]

It would not be surprising that 80 years later, more than 90% of women presenting with a placenta accreta have had at least one prior cesarean delivery.[2]

PAS disorders were defined by Luke et al. and divided into three categories:
1. Adherent placenta accreta such as creta, vera or adherenta: Villi simply adhere to myometrium
2. Placenta increta: When villi invade the myometrium
3. Placenta percreta: When villi invade the full thickness of myometrium including the serosa and sometimes the pelvic organs.[5]

Placenta accreta spectrum disorders are also divided into focal, partial or total categories, depending on the number of placental cotyledons involved and on the variations in the lateral extension of myometrial invasion. The degree of microscopic diagnosis is limited as the degree of villous involvement is ever uniform throughout the placenta.[5]

Regarding prenatal diagnosis and screening ultrasound remains the most commonly used technique to diagnose PAS disorders. As no specific sign or set combination was diagnostic of adherent placenta, the European Working group on Abnormally Invasive Placenta (EW-AIP) an international expert group has proposed a standardized description of ultrasound signs which can be used for the diagnosis of PAS disorders.

The management of PAS has to be with adequate multidisciplinary team and at a tertiary care hospital to reduce the maternal mortality and morbidity.[6] There is a wide variation on the management of PAS ranging from spectrum of conservative management to that of radical approach.[7]

EPIDEMIOLOGY

The current hypothesis states that a defect of the endometrium-myometrial interface, typically at the site of a prior hysterotomy, leads to a failure of normal decidualization in that area, thus allowing extravillous trophoblastic infiltration and the villous tissue to develop deeply within the myometrium or at times even involving the pelvic organs.

Placenta accreta spectrum disorders are related to primary uterine anomaly or secondary damage to uterine wall structure.[8]

- *Cesarean scar:* There is strong epidemiological data suggesting increase prevalence of PAS disorders in high- and middle-income group countries, which is directly proportional to the increase in cesarean section rates, whereas no epidemiological data is currently available for low income countries.[8]

The Nordic obstetric surveillance study (NOSS) using direct clinical reports validated by the national registers found that the rate of PAS disorders at cesarean delivery and laparotomy was 3.4 per 10,000 deliveries and when vaginal deliveries with difficult to remove placenta were included the rate was found to be 4.6 per 10,000 deliveries.[8]

Table 1 enumerates the primary and secondary uterine pathologies associated with PAS disorders.

- *Placenta previa accreta and cesarean scar pregnancy:* Placenta previa is the most important risk factor in half of the PAS disorders and the risk of placenta previa increases with increasing number of prior cesarean deliveries. A retrospective cohort study of 26,987 women was conducted comparing the risk of previa in patients with prior prelabor cesarean delivery and intrapartum cesarean delivery found that prior prelabor cesarean delivery is associated with OR of 2.62. This is in contrast to only 20% of increased risk of previa associated with prior intrapartum cesarean delivery is not significant.[8]
- *Depth of villous invasion:* Prenatal evaluation for the depth of invasion is important for deciding the individual management of patient. A standardized clinical classification describing and categorizing the different forms of PAS have been proposed.

Table 2 defines the clinical grading system to assess and categorize placenta adherence or invasion at delivery.[9]

- *Surgical technique:* Surgical techniques used for entering and closing the uterus during cesarean delivery have been postulated to play a role in PAS disorders. A meta-analysis conducted of nine RCTs, including 3,969, concluded that there is no difference in incidence of cesarean scar defect or uterine dehiscence between single-layer closure and double-layer closure rather as compared to two layered closure single layer closure might require less time and less blood loss but also results in thinner residual myometrial tissue.[10]

TABLE 1: Primary and secondary uterine pathologies associated with placenta accreta spectrum (PAS) disorders.[8]

	Classification	Type of uterine pathologies
1.	Direct surgical scar	• Cesarean delivery • Surgical termination of pregnancy • Dilatation and curettage • Myomectomy • Endometrial resection • Asherman's syndrome
2.	Nonsurgical scar	• IVF procedures • Uterine artery embolization • Chemotherapy and radiation • Endometriosis • Intrauterine device • Manual removal of placenta • Previous accreta
3.	Uterine anomalies	• Bicornuate uterus • Adenomyosis • Submucous fibroids • Myotonic dystrophy

TABLE 2: A clinical grading system to assess and categorize placenta adherence or invasion at delivery.[9]

Grade	Definition
1.	• At cesarean or vaginal delivery, complete placental separation at third stage. • Normal adherence
2.	• *Cesarean/laparotomy:* No placental tissue seen invading through the surface of uterus but incomplete separation with uterotonics and gentle cord traction and manual removal of placenta- abnormally adherent placenta • *Vaginal delivery:* Manual removal of placenta required and parts thought to be abnormally adherent
3.	• *Cesarean/laparotomy:* No placental tissue seen invading through the surface of uterus. No separation with uterotonics and gentle cord traction with manual removal of placenta and whole placental bed thought to be abnormally adherent • *Vaginal delivery:* Manual removal of placenta required and whole placenta thought to be abnormally adherent
4.	*Cesarean/laparotomy:* Placental tissue seen invading through the serosa of the uterus. A clear surgical plane can be identified between the bladder and uterus to allow nontraumatic separation of urinary bladder at surgery
5.	*Cesarean/laparotomy:* Placental tissue seen invading through the serosa of the uterus. A clear surgical plane cannot be identified between the bladder and uterus to allow nontraumatic separation of urinary bladder at surgery
6.	*Cesarean/laparotomy:* Placental tissue seen invading through the serosa of the uterus and infiltrating the parametrium or any organ other than the urinary bladder

Source: Modified from Collins SL, Stevenson GN, Al-khan A. Three dimensional power Doppler ultrasonography for diagnosing abnormally invasive placenta and quantifying the risk. Obstet Gynecol. 2015;126:645-53.

DIAGNOSIS AND SCREENING

- *Ultrasound:* A systematic review and meta-analysis of ultrasound studies involving 3,707 pregnancies found that the sensitivity is 90.72% and specificity is 96.94% and diagnostic odd ratio (DOR) of 98.59.[11]

  The ultrasound signs suggestive of PAS are:
  - *2D gray-scale:*
    - Loss of clear zone underneath the placental bed
    - Abnormal placental lacunae
    - Bladder wall interruption
    - Myometrial thinning <1 mm or undetectable
    - Placental bulge
    - Focal exophytic mass
  - *Color Doppler abnormalities:*
    - Uterovesical hypervascularity
    - Subplacental hypervascularity
    - Bridging vessels
    - Placental lacunae feeder vessels
    - 3D intraplacental hypervascularity

  The specificity is highest (99.8%) with abnormalities of uterus and bladder interface and sensitivity is highest with color Doppler abnormalities (90.8%).[11]

  There is wide variation in prenatal detection rates depending on ultrasound signs, operators experience, scanning conditions, equipment used, and gestational age.

- *MRI:* The main features of placenta accreta on MRI are abnormal uterine bulging, dark intraplacental bands on T2-weighted imaging, heterogeneous signal intensity within the placenta, disorganized placental vasculature, and disruption of uteroplacental zone **(Fig. 1)**. MRI has high predictive accuracy in assessing both the depth and topography of placental invasion. MRI is only used in suspected cases and not as a screening method. A study conducted by Antonio et al. in 2014 concluded that the sensitivity and specificity of MRI in diagnosing accreta placentation varies widely between 75–100% and 65–100% respectively.[12]

- *Biomarkers of PAS disorders:* At 11–12 weeks of gestation, hCG and its free beta-subunit are lower- and PAPP-A is higher in the maternal serum of women with PAS disorders. By contrast, at 14–22 weeks serum beta-hCG and AFP are above 2.5 MoM in women presenting with placenta previa.[13]

Recommendations for prenatal diagnosis and screening of PAS disorders:
- Ultrasonography is a relatively inexpensive and widely available imaging modality and thus is the first line for the diagnosis of PAS disorders. (High and Strong)
- Women diagnosed with cesarean scar pregnancy in the first trimester should be counseled regarding the high risk and its association with PAS disorders. (High and Strong)
- The operator's interpretation for the presence or absence of each ultrasound sign will constitute that marker. (High and Strong)

MANAGEMENT

- *Nonconservative management:* The management of placenta accreta aims at reducing the maternal morbidity and mortality associated with massive obstetric hemorrhage. Due to lack of resources and research related to the management of accreta a nonconservative approach is used by most of the tertiary care centers. Hysterectomy by far remains the most definitive surgical treatment for PAS disorders, especially for its invasive forms and a primary elective cesarean hysterectomy is safest and most practical approach for low- and middle- income countries where follow-up could be a major problem and adjunctive treatment options are not available.[7]
  - *Multidisciplinary team care:*[7] The aim of having a multidisciplinary team (MDT) care is in reducing the maternal morbidity and mortality and providing standardized care to the women. The MDT has to be backed up with good surgical expertise in complex pelvic surgery. The components of MDT are enumerated as here:
    - Universal access to MDT care team 24/7 access to the care team
    - Standard care plan
    - Radiologic expertise for diagnosis
    - Experienced and senior obstetrician
    - Surgical expertise for complex surgery—urogynecologist and onco-gynecologist
    - Anesthetist
    - NICU facility

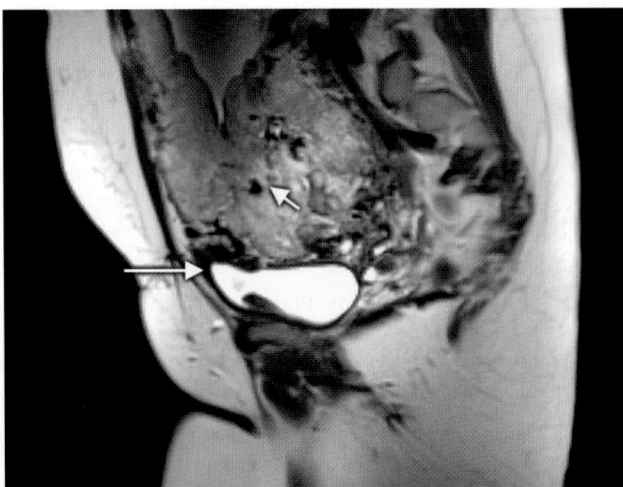

Fig. 1: MRI in placenta accreta. T2-weighted image shows a hyperintense heterogeneous placenta with multiple T2 hypointense bands (short arrow). There is interruption of the myometrial junctional zone adjacent to the bladder, which is suspicious for placenta accreta or in this case, a placenta percreta (long arrow).

- Adult ICU
- Massive transfusion capacity
- Interventional radiologist
- Cell saver and perfusionist.

• *Timing of delivery:* Scheduled nonemergent deliveries result in a significant reduction in maternal morbidity and reduction of complications related to blood loss, thus scheduling of surgical intervention with planned late preterm (35–36 weeks) or early preterm (37 weeks) delivery as a means to avoid the need of emergency surgery. An MDT care plan that decided to have a planned delivery at 34–35 weeks demonstrated a reduction in emergency deliveries from 23 to 64 % with no adverse neonatal outcome.[14]

The corollary to the above consideration of timing of delivery remains that women who are stable with no prepartum hemorrhage, preterm premature rupture of membranes (PPROM) or uterine contractions can be terminated by 36–37 weeks.[7]

• *Optimizing the hemoglobin:* Patients with suspected PAS disorders should have a hemoglobin either by iron sucrose or oral iron therapy.

• *Anesthesia:* The choice of anesthesia in a suspected case of PAS disorder will purely depend on the discretion of an anesthetist. The decision between general and neuraxial/regional anesthesia can be done through a detailed discussion with the MDT team. The highest rates of conversion from regional to general anesthesia is noted in cases where there was no prior suspicion of PAS and the diagnosis was made intraoperatively and more so in low-income countries due to the more blood loss.[15]

• *Technique of cesarean hysterectomy:* The primary aim of cesarean hysterectomy in a case of PAS disorder is to minimize the blood loss and decrease the maternal morbidity. Total hysterectomy is the recommended surgical method for emergent peripartum hysterectomy as it reduces the risk of hemorrhage and malignancy in the cervical stump and the need for regular follow-up. Subtotal hysterectomy reduces the need for blood transfusion and shorter operating time but may not be effective in cases of placenta increta and percreta with cervical involvement. **Figures 2A and B** demonstrate an accidently diagnosed hypervascular segment during a cesarean section.

The novel techniques have been reported in literature to minimize blood loss and also to reduce the inadvertent injury to the urinary tract. The technique published in literature by Selman in 11 cases of PAS disorders is posterior retrograde hysterectomy via pouch of Douglas, where after the closure of hysterotomy scar uterus is exteriorized, round ligaments divided, retroperitoneal space dissected parallel to the ureters and pelvic side wall vessels and utero-ovarian ligament are divided bilaterally.[16]

The other techniques described in the literature are modified radical hysterectomy technique and use of bipolar cautery device, linear cutting staple device for hysterotomy and use of vessel-sealing devices for peripartum hysterectomy.[7]

• *Blood conservation technique:* Massive hemorrhage during hysterectomy is the major cause of morbidity and mortality in a patient of PAS disorder. The following methods and approaches can be used in the conserving blood.
  - *Tranexamic acid:* It should be administered 1 g slowly IV immediately prior to or during cesarean delivery for PAS disorder. (Strong

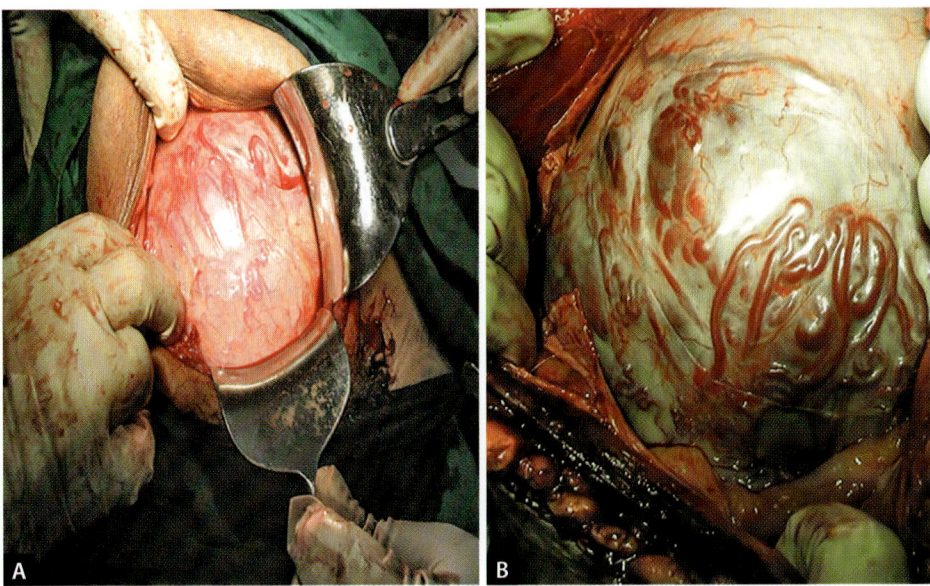

Figs. 2A and B: Accidently diagnosed hypervascular lower segment.
Courtesy: Dr SN Gadappa, Professor and Head, Department of OBGY, GMCH, Aurangabad.

recommendation). WOMAN trial demonstrated that compared to placebo, tranexamic acid administration significantly reduces death due to massive hemorrhage.
- *Balloon occlusion catheters:* Balloon devices are inserted into the aorta, common iliac, internal iliac or uterine arteries under fluoroscopic guidance and are inflated when hemorrhage is encountered. It was assumed that the use of balloon decreased blood loss and need for transfusion. Few studies postulated that empiric inflation of these balloons may actually exacerbate bleeding from the collaterals. Thus concluding that the evidence available is insufficient to make firm recommendations.[7]
- *Internal iliac artery ligation:* There is weak recommendation for the role of bilateral internal iliac artery ligation at the time of cesarean hysterectomy for PAS disorders.
- *Cell salvage:* Autologous cell salvage minimizes allogeneic red blood cell transfusion in selective patients such as those with high risk of massive obstetric hemorrhage, low preoperative hemoglobin concentration, rare blood types and Jehovah's witnesses.
- *Placental removal:* The leading cause of massive hemorrhage in a patient of PAS disorder is when attempt is made at separation of placenta at cesarean hysterectomy. Ideally no attempt should be made at manual separation of placenta as it reduces the amount of blood loss. If spontaneous partial separation of placenta occurs, management as per conservative therapy strategies could be employed. Uterotonic agents are not administered routinely unless placenta removal is imminent or complete separation of placenta occurs refuting the diagnosis of PAS disorders.[7]

Though cesarean hysterectomy aims at reducing the morbidity and mortality and decreases the need of follow-up visits it comes with certain complications like median estimation of blood loss (2–3 L), median units of packed red blood cells transfused (3.5–5.4 L), large volume of blood transfusion (>10 L), injury to bladder (2–4%), injury to ureter (0–18%), admission to ICU, bowel injury, venous thromboembolism, surgical site infection (18–32%), reoperation (4–18%) and maternal mortality (1–7%).

Figures 3 and 4 show a specimen of cesarean hysterectomy with a classical hysterotomy scar and placental removal not attempted.

Thus, considering the above complications, conservative approach for placenta accreta is importance in patients who desire to preserve their fertility and the expertise for

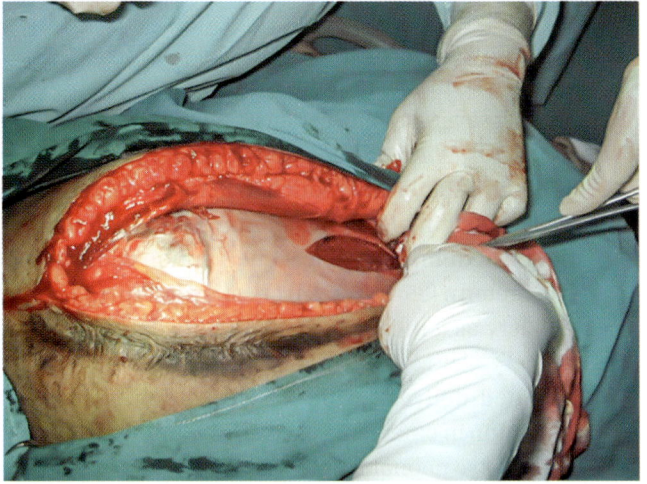

Fig. 3: Vertical skin incision and classical uterine incision.
Courtesy: Dr SN Gadappa, Professor and Head, Department of OBGY, GMCH, Aurangabad.

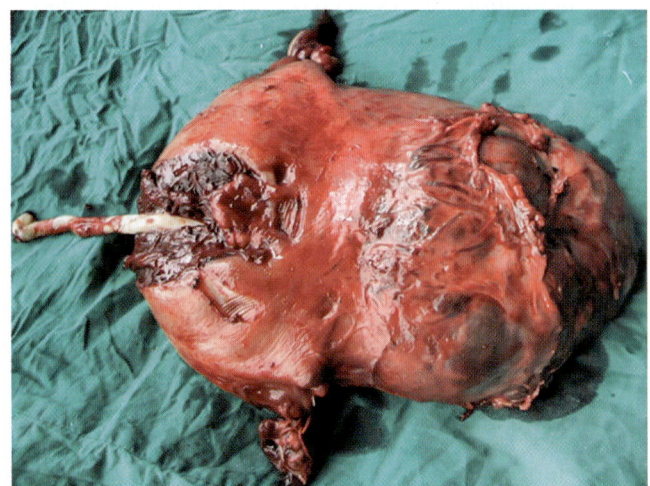

Fig. 4: Cesarean hysterectomy specimen with placenta increta.
Courtesy: Dr S N Gadappa, Professor and Head, Department of OBGY, GMCH, Aurangabad.

complex pelvic surgery is not available. The next section is concerned with the conservative approach of placenta accreta.
- *Conservative approach to PAS disorders*
  1. *Extirpative technique:* Extirpative technique means forcibly removing the placenta manually in an attempt to obtain an empty uterus but attempt to do this results in massive obstetric hemorrhage and when accreta portion is not disturbed it is associated with 50% reduction in blood loss and transfusion. The FIGO 2018 guidelines strongly recommend to abandon the extirpative approach or forcible manual removal of placenta.[17]
  2. *"Leaving placenta in situ" approach:* This technique consists of leaving the placenta in situ and waiting till complete resorption of the placenta. It has been suggested that leaving the placenta in situ after delivery of the fetus will result in decrease circulation

within the uterus, parametrium and placenta causing secondary necrosis of villous tissue and the placenta will detach from the uterus. When the diagnosis of PAS disorder is confirmed the cord should be cut near the insertion of the placenta and uterine cavity should be closed.[17]

The overall success rate of uterine preservation with the abovementioned technique is 78% and severe maternal morbidity including sepsis, septic shock, peritonitis, uterine necrosis, postpartum uterine rupture, fistula, injury to adjacent organ, acute pulmonary edema, acute renal failure, deep vein thrombophlebitis or maternal death has been reported in 10 cases (6%).

The adjunctive treatments when placenta is left in situ have been tried but none of the mentioned treatment is recommended as the literature is limited.

- Methotrexate was proposed as it hastens placental resolution but then there has been limited evidence to suggest its use. It was suggested that women treated successfully with methotrexate will have faster reduction in beta-hCG levels and Doppler vascular resistance indices of uteroplacental arterial circulation.[18]
- Systematic hysteroscopic resection of retained accreta tissue was done in a small series of 23 patients. The median size of retained placenta was 54 mm. It was concluded that hysteroscopic resection could shorten the recovery time.

Monitoring of patient when placenta is left in situ
- Serum beta-hCG on weekly basis
- Ultrasound imaging for volume and size of placental tissue
- Weekly follow up for first 2 months and then monthly till complete resorption.
- Follow-up consultation includes clinical examination (bleeding, temperature, pelvic pain), pelvic ultrasound and laboratory test for infection (hemoglobin and leukocyte count, vaginal swab)[17]

3. *One step conservative surgery:*[19] This procedure combines the benefits of "leaving placenta in situ" and minimizes the risk of secondary bleeding or infection associated with cesarean hysterectomy. The steps in this procedure are as follows:
   - Vascular disconnection if newly formed vessels and separation of invaded uterine tissues
   - Upper segmental hysterotomy and delivering the fetus
   - Resection of all invaded myometrial tissue and entire placenta in one piece, obtaining hemostasis
   - Myometrial reconstruction in two planes

4. *The Triple-P procedure*—is a novel uterine sparing technique proposed by Chandraharan et al. which constitutes the three main steps:
   I. Perioperative localization of superior edge of placenta.
   II. Pelvic devascularization with preoperative placement of balloons in the anterior division of internal iliac artery
   III. Myometrial excision and uterine repair with no attempt at removal of placenta.

The recommendations for conservative management of PAS disorders which is strongly approved by FIGO guidelines of 2018 are:
- Leaving the placenta in situ is an option for women who desire to preserve their fertility and agree for long term follow up and monitoring in centers of excellence.
- The extirpative approach or forcible manual removal of placenta should be abandoned.
- Use of methotrexate is not recommended till further evidence is available.
- Women desiring another pregnancy should be counseled about the recurrence risk of PAS disorders is high.[17]

A summary of management is depicted in **Flowchart 1**.

CONCLUSION

- Scheduled nonemergent deliveries result in a significant reduction in maternal morbidity and reduction of complications related to blood loss, thus scheduling of surgical intervention with planned late preterm (35–36 weeks) or early preterm (37 weeks) delivery as a means to avoid the need of emergency surgery.
- To enhance patient safety, it is important that the delivery be performed in an operating room by an experienced obstetric team that includes an obstetric surgeon, with other surgical specialists, such as urologists, general surgeons, and gynecologic oncologists, available if necessary.

KEY MESSAGES

Placenta accreta spectrum (PAS) disorders refer to the diseases with abnormal placentation in the form of either accreta, increta or percreta depending on the depth of trophoblastic invasion. The most accepted hypothesis in placenta accreta spectrum is the disruption of endomyometrial junction leading to the trophoblastic invasion and difficulty in separation of placenta after delivery of the fetus, attempts at removal of such placenta results in massive hemorrhage and thus increases maternal morbidity and mortality. Ultrasonography is the most useful modality in the screening of PAS disorders, MRI is done only in suspected cases. The plan for conservative versus nonconservative management of PAS disorders should be customized on the basis of individual case although the widely accepted approach is cesarean hysterectomy with placenta left in situ after delivery of the fetus. The multidisciplinary team care is a must for management of PAS disorders. Massive transfusion protocol remains the mainstay in management

Flowchart 1: Diagnosis and management of placenta accreta spectrum.

PAS disorders
(Placenta accreta spectrum (PAS) disorders refers to the diseases with abnormal placentation in the form of either accreta, increta or percreta depending on the depth of trophoblastic invasion)

Placenta accreta: Villi simply adhere to myometrium

Placenta increta: When villi invade the myometrium

Placenta percreta: When villi invade the full thickness of myometrium including the serosa and sometimes the pelvic organs

Incidence of PAS is 1 in 272 according to 2016 (ACOG Obstetric Care Consensus 2018)

Diagnosis

Ultrasonography
2D Gray Scale:
- Loss of clear zone
- Abnormal placental lacunae
- Bladder wall interruption
- Myometrial thinning
- Placental bulge
- Focal exophytic mass

Color Doppler:
- Uterovescial hypervascularity
- Subplacental hypervascularity
- Bridging vessels
- Placental lacunae feeder vessels
- 3D intraplacental hypervascularity

MRI
- Abnormal uterine bulging,
- Dark intraplacental bands on T2-weighted imaging,
- Heterogenous signal intensity within the placenta
- Disorganized placental vasculature and disruption of uteroplacental zone

Intraoperative
- Hypervascular lower segment
- Placenta not separated post-vaginal delivery
- Manual removal of placenta

Conservative:
- "Leaving placenta in situ" approach
- The Triple-P procedure
- One step conservative surgery

Nonconservative:
- Cesarean hysterectomy
- Retrograde hysterectomy via pouch of Douglas
- Linear cutting staple device for hysterotomy
- Vessel-sealing devices for Peripartum Hysterectomy

Blood conservation technique:
- Tranexamic acid
- Balloon occlusion catheters
- Internal iliac artery ligation
- Placental removal

of placenta accreta disorders. The ever increasing rise in section rate is the prime cause of increasing incidence of PAS disorders, thus providing section when needed and curtailing it when unindicated could play a major role in keeping PAS disorders in check.

REFERENCES

1. Irving FC, Hertig AT. A study of placenta accreta. Surg Gynecol Obstet. 1937;64:178-200.
2. Solheim KN, Esakoff TF, Little SE, Cheng YW, Sparks TN, Caughey AB. The effect of caesarean delivery rates on the future incidence of placenta previa, placenta accreta and maternal mortality. J Matern Fetal Neonatal Med. 2011;24:1341-6.
3. American College of Obstetricians and Gynecologists. Placenta accreta spectrum. Obstetric care consensus no. 7. Obstet Gynecol. 2018;132:e259-75.
4. Jauniaux ERM, Alfirevic Z, Bhide AG, Burton GJ, Collins SL, Silver R, et al; on behalf of Royal College of Obstetricians and Gynaecologists. Placenta Previa and Placenta Accreta: Diagnosis and Management. BJOG. 2018:27a.
5. Luke RK, Sharpe JW, Greene RR. Placenta accreta: the adherent or invasive placenta. Am J Obstet Gynecol. 1966;95:660-8.
6. Eller AG, Bennett MA, Sharshiner M. Maternal morbidity in cases of placenta accreta managed by a multidisciplinary care team compared with standard obstetric care. Obstet Gynecol. 2011;117:331-7.
7. Allen L, Jauniaux E, Hobson S, Paillon-Smith J, Belfort MA. FIGO Placenta Accreta Diagnosis and Management Expert Consensus Panel. FIGO consensus guidelines on placenta accreta spectrum disorders: nonconservative surgical management. Int J Gynecol Obstet. 2018;140:281-90.
8. Jauniaux E, Chantraine F, Silver R, Langhoff JR. FIGO Placenta Accreta Diagnosis and Management Expert Consensus Panel. FIGO consensus guidelines on placenta accreta spectrum disorders: Epidemiology. Int J Gynecol Obstet. 2018;140:265-73.
9. Collins SL, Stevenson GN, Al-khan A. Three dimensional power Doppler ultrasonography for diagnosing abnormally invasive placenta and quantifying the risk. Obstet Gynecol. 2015;126:645-53.
10. Spiezio SA, Saccone G, McCurdy R, Bujold E, Bifulco G, Berghella V. Risk of caesarean scar defect following single- versus double-layer uterine closure: Systematic review and meta-analysis of randomized controlled trials. Ultrasound Obstet Gynecol. 2017;50:578-83.
11. D'Antonio F, Lacovella C, Bhide A. Prenatal identification of invasive placentation using ultrasound. Systematic review and meta-analysis. Ultrasound Obstet Gynecol. 2013;42:509-17.

12. D'Antonio F, Lacovella C, Palacios-Jaraquemada J, Bruno CH, Manzoli L, Bhide A. Prenatal identification of invasive placentation using magnetic resonance imaging: Systematic review and meta-analysis. Ultrasound Obstet Gynecol. 2014;44:8-16.
13. Hung TH, Shau WY, Hsieh CC, Chiu TH, Hsu JJ, Hsieh TT. Risk factor for placenta accreta. Obstet Gynecol. 1999;93:545-50.
14. Shamshirsaz AA, fox KA, Salmanian B. Maternal morbidity in patients with morbidly adherent placenta treated with and without a standardized multidisciplinary approach. Am J Obstet Gynecol. 2015;212:218:e1-218.e9.
15. Munoz LA, Mendoza GJ, Gomez M, Reyes LE, Arevalo JJ. Anesthetic management of placenta accreta in a low-resource setting: a case series. Int J Obstet Anesth. 2015;24:329-34.
16. Selman AE. Caesarean hysterectomy for placenta previa/accreta using an approach via pouch of Douglas. BJOG. 2016:815-9.
17. Sentilhes L, Kayem G, Chandraharan E, Jaraquemada J, Jauniaux E. FIGO Placenta Accreta Diagnosis and Management Expert Consensus Panel. FIGO consensus guidelines on placenta accreta spectrum disorders: Conservative management. Int J Gynecol Obstet. 2018;140:291-8.
18. Lin K, Qin J, Xu K, Hu W, Lin J. Methotrexate management for placenta accreta: a prospective study. Arch Gynecol Obstet. 2015;291:1259-64.
19. Palacios-Jaraquemada JM. Placenta adhesive disorders. Berlin/Boston: Walter de Gruyter; 2012.

LONG QUESTIONS

1. How is prenatal diagnosis and screening done in a patient of placenta accreta spectrum and discuss the nonconservative surgical management in a patient of placenta accreta disorder.
2. Enumerate the risk factors for placenta accreta and discuss the conservative management in a patient of placenta accreta.
3. Discuss in details about the prenatal diagnosis and preoperative, intraoperative and postoperative management of patient of placenta percreta.

SHORT QUESTIONS

1. Discuss the Triple-P approach in management of placenta accreta.
2. Blood conservation techniques in patient of PAS disorder
3. Enumerate the risk factors of PAS disorders.
4. Clinical grading system to assess the adherence of placenta.
5. Discuss the nonconservative approaches in management of PAS disorder.

MULTIPLE CHOICE QUESTIONS

1. Which is not a common cause of placenta accreta?
   a. Previous LSCS
   b. Previous curettage
   c. Previous myomectomy
   d. Previous placenta previa/abruptio placenta
2. *Triple P procedure* has been developed for prevention of PPH in case of:
   a. Placenta previa   b. Placental abruption
   c. Traumatic PPH   d. Atonic PPH
3. What is the recommended timing of delivery in PAS disorders?
   a. 37 weeks   b. 32–33 weeks
   c. 34 weeks   d. 35–36 weeks
4. Incidence of PAS reported as in 2016?
   a. 1 in 380   b. 1 in 450
   c. 1 in 533   d. 1 in 272
5. Incidence of maternal mortality with cesarean hysterectomy is reported to be:
   a. 50%   b. 0.5%
   c. 1–7%   d. 18–29%
6. According to FIGO guidelines of 2018, which of the following is abandoned?
   a. Extirpative technique
   b. One step conservative procedure
   c. Triple- P procedure
   d. Retrograde hysterectomy via pouch of douglas
7. Which of the following modality is used for screening of PAS disorders?
   a. MRI   b. Ultrasonography
   c. CT scan   d. None of the above
8. The anesthesia of choice in a patient of PAS disorder is:
   a. Regional anesthesia   b. General anesthesia
   c. Epidural with regional d. None of the above

Answers
1. d 2. a 3. d 4. d 5. c 6. a
7. b 8. b

8.6 POST-TERM PREGNANCY

Mala Srivastava, Ankita Srivastava

DEFINITION

Pregnancy that extends beyond 42 weeks is post-term pregnancy according to the American College of Obstetricians and Gynecologists (ACOG) and World Health Organization (WHO).[1]

INCIDENCE

Post-term pregnancy is approximately 3–12%.[2] Boyd et al. states an incidence of 7.5% when based on menstrual history, 2.6% based on an early ultrasound, and 1.1% based on both menstrual history and ultrasonography.[3]

PERINATAL OUTCOMES IN POST-TERM PREGNANCIES

Perinatal mortality increases two times if the pregnancy continues beyond 42 weeks, e.g., 4–7/1,000 deliveries.[4-6]

Cotzias et al. states that the risk of intrauterine death is 1 in 926 cases beyond 40 weeks, 1 in 826 cases beyond 41 weeks and 1 in 769 cases beyond 42 weeks.[6]

The causes of fetal risks can be due to:
- Uteroplacental insufficiency
- Asphyxia - with and without meconium
- Meconium aspiration syndrome[7]
- Intrauterine infection
- Fetal macrosomia, i.e., fetal weight ≥ 4,500 g with all its complications.
- The post-term fetuses have fetal dysmaturity in 20% cases.[8-10]
- There are chances of oligohydramnios causing cord compression and non-reassuring fetal heart patterns both antenatally and during labor.
- There are risks of hypoglycemia, neonatal seizures, and difficulty in respiration.
- There are chances of neonatal encephalopathy, cerebral palsy and demise within one year after birth.[11]
- Anencephaly, though it is less seen nowadays due to modern obstetrical care.[12]

Maternal Risks

The maternal risks include:
- Increase incidence of labor dystocia.
- More chances of birth injuries both 3rd and 4th degree perineal tears maybe because of macrosomia.
- An increase in forceps or vacuum delivery, and cesarean delivery.[13-16]
- The increased risks of endometritis, chorioamnionitis, postpartum hemorrhage, and thromboembolic disease.[17]
- Mothers are more anxious while they carry the pregnancy beyond term.

ETIOLOGY

The important causes of a post-term pregnancy:
- Wrong dates[18-21]
- Primiparity
- Prior post-term pregnancy
- Male gender of the fetus
- Genetic factors[22]
- According to Laursen et al. among monozygotic and dizygotic twins the incidence is caused by father's genetic make-up in 30% of cases[23]
- Obesity[24]
- In women with irregular cycles, it is difficult to predict the estimated due date (EDD) from the last menstrual period (LMP).

PATHOGENESIS

The cause is always not clear, since the exact mechanism of labor is not yet proven. The labor is a hormonal interaction among placenta, mother and fetus and all have an important participation. The level of the peptide corticotrophin releasing hormone (CRH) is associated with the period pregnancy.[25]

The production of placental CRH gradually increases as pregnancy advances and peaks during labor. In preterm labor the levels increase quickly and earlier.[26]

This may be due to genetic factors, or the influence of the maternal tissues as occurs in an obese mother. CRH causes estriol production from placenta by stimulating the DHEAS production form fetal adrenals.[27,28]

Due to the influence of CRH the estriol level rises rapidly causing an estrogenic environment toward last weeks of pregnancy. Simultaneously, plasma progesterone levels that keep rising throughout pregnancy start falling toward the last weeks of pregnancy. This could be because CRH causes decrease in placental production of progesterone.[29]

As a result, influence of progesterone which causes the uterus to relax is overcome by the action of estriol that causes uterus to contract.

The situation in post-term pregnancies is unknown. Most probably there is alteration in these ratios which promotes post-term pregnancies.[30]

DATING OF PREGNANCY

- By LMP
- Ultrasonography early in pregnancy. But the estimation range varies depending on when the first ultrasound was done:
  - Variation from crown-rump length (CRL) is 3–5 days
  - Ultrasound done at 12–20 weeks, the variation is 7–10 days
  - Ultrasound done at 20–30 weeks, the variation is 2 weeks
  - Ultrasound done after 30 weeks, the variation is 3 weeks.

MANAGEMENT

The management plan includes:
- To induce labor
- Manage pregnancy expectantly
- Fetal surveillance.

TIMING OF DELIVERY

The important decision is when to deliver an impending post-term pregnancy. If there is a non-reassuring antenatal surveillance, oligohydramnios, growth restriction, severe PIH, IHCP and other high-risk conditions then the decision is easy. These patients should be delivered early, maybe at 39 weeks. The apprehension is that if induction of labor is done before 42 weeks, it may increase the chance of lower segment cesarean section (LSCS).

In the meta-analysis, they found that there are more chances of fetal distress and meconium-stained liquor in post-term pregnancies with or without induction of labor. There are more chances of failure of induction as well as hyperstimulation and failure to progress in labor when the labor is induced.

In the study it was also analyzed that the routine induction at 41 weeks of pregnancy does not increase the rates of LSCS.

Besides, the mother and the baby will be benefitted from a protocol to induce labor at 40 weeks routinely in properly dated low risk pregnancies. Since it causes lesser incidence of shoulder dystocia and meconium aspiration, it may in fact be more cost-effective.[31]

■ PREVENTION

It is not possible to prevent post-term pregnancy. Only way to prevent post-term pregnancy is by inducing labor. But the obstetricians and the women are worried about the consequences of failed induction. Always onset of spontaneous labor is desirable. The methods used to induce spontaneous labor include membrane stripping and having unprotected intercourse, both act by releasing endogenous prostaglandins.[32]

Some studies have suggested acupuncture as a mode to induce natural labor but it is not possible to judge the efficacy due to the lesser number of studies.[33]

■ INDUCTION OF LABOR

Once the plan to induce labor has been taken then the method has to be decided.

Approximately 80% of patients reaching post term pregnancy have a poor Bishop Score. The options available for cervical ripening include:
- Misoprost (Prostaglandin E1 oral/vaginal)
- Dinoprostone (Prostaglandin E2 for intracervical application - Prepidil)
- Dinoprostone (Prostaglandin E2 vaginal insert Cervidil). Besides, this vaginal insert can be easily removed in case of uterine hyper stimulation.
- Mechanical dilators, e.g., Foley's catheters kept in the cervix, extra-amniotic saline infusions, and laminaria tents.

The induction of labor should be carefully used in scarred uterus as there are chances of rupture of the scar during induction of labor and labor pains. In favorable circumstances maybe mechanical methods of induction of labor can be considered.

An intrapartum fetal surveillance should be done to monitor fetal wellbeing during labor. Whether continuous fetal monitoring or intermittent auscultation is used, interpretation has to be careful to prevent fetal distress and acidosis. At the slightest suspicion that the fetus is not tolerating labor, cesarean delivery is recommended.

Antepartum Fetal Surveillance

When induction of labor is not planned then antepartum fetal surveillance is done in post-term pregnancy. Though there is a scanty evidence, yet antepartum fetal surveillance is accepted as a standard of care. There is also no consensus as to which protocol of surveillance is best.[1]

The perinatal mortality increases gradually throughout pregnancy, and there is increased risk in post-term pregnancies. According to ACOG, begin antepartum surveillance once the pregnancy reaches 41 weeks.[1]

Beginning the monitoring at 41 weeks of pregnancy causes lesser complications.

The methods of antenatal surveillance include:
- Non-stress test (NST)
- Contraction stress test
- Biophysical profile (BPS)
- Combination of these methods
- Assessment of the amniotic fluid volume (AFV) is a single most important parameter to be assessed. The delivery should be planned if there is less liquor together with or without other suspicious parameters.
- Doppler ultrasound has no proven advantage for in evaluation of post-term pregnancies and should not be advocated.

The antenatal fetal surveillance should be done twice-weekly and it decreases the incidence of intrauterine deaths from 6.1 per 1,000 live births to 1.9 per 1,000.

In summary, the use of an NST and an AFV twice a week for pregnancies continuing beyond 41 weeks is acceptable. In case if there is any indication of fetal compromise during antepartum surveillance then the delivery has to be undertaken.

■ SUMMARY

The post-term pregnancies have differential management. The decision has to be individualized for expectant management with or without antepartum fetal surveillance and induction of labor.

■ KEY MESSAGES

- Post-term pregnancy extends beyond 42+0/7 weeks (294 days) according to ACOG and WHO.
- The incidence is 3–12%.
- There are significant maternal and perinatal complications of post-term pregnancies.
- The reason for post-term pregnancy is not clearly understood.
- Dating of pregnancy is done by LMP and ultrasonography early in pregnancy.
- The methods of antenatal surveillance are NST, BPS, modified biophysical profile and a combination of these modalities.
- Induction of labor is done by misoprostol, prostaglandin E2 gel, and prostaglandin E2 vaginal insert or by mechanical methods, e.g., Foley's catheters, extra-amniotic saline infusions, and laminaria tents.

■ REFERENCES

1. ACOG Practice Bulletin. Clinical management guidelines for obstetricians-gynecologists. Number 55, September 2004 (replaces practice pattern number 6, October 1997). Management of Post-term Pregnancy. Obstet Gynecol. 2004;104(3):639-46.

2. Norwitz ER, Snegovskikh VV, Caughey AB. Prolonged pregnancy: when should we intervene? Clin Obstet Gynecol. 2007;50(2):547-57.
3. Bhide A, Damania D. Arias' Practical Guide to High-Risk Pregnancy and Delivery: a South Asian Perspective. Gurugram: Elsevier India; 2015.
4. Feldman GB. Prospective risk of stillbirth. Obstet Gynecol. 1992;79(4):547-53.
5. Hilder L, Costeloe K, Thilaganathan B. Prolonged pregnancy: evaluating gestation-specific risks of fetal and infant mortality. Br J Obstet Gynaecol. 1998;105(2):169-73.
6. Cotzias CS, Paterson-Brown S, Fisk NM. Prospective risk of unexplained stillbirth in singleton pregnancies at term: population based analysis. BMJ. 1999;319(7205):287-8.
7. Kabbur PM, Herson VC, Zaremba S. Have the year 2000 neonatal resuscitation program guidelines changed the delivery room management or outcome of meconium-stained infants?. J Perinatol. 2005;25(11):694-7.
8. American College of Obstetricians and Gynecologists. Fetal Macrosomia. ACOG Practice Bulletin #22. Washington DC: ACOG; 2000.
9. Spellacy WN, Miller S, Winegar A. Macrosomia--maternal characteristics and infant complications. Obstet Gynecol. 1985;66(2):158-61.
10. Rosen MG, Dickinson JC. Management of post-term pregnancy. N Engl J Med. 1992;326(24):1628-9.
11. Shime J, Librach CL, Gare DJ, Cook CJ. The influence of prolonged pregnancy on infant development at one and two years of age: a prospective controlled study. Am J Obstet Gynecol. 1986;154(2):341-5.
12. Badawi N, Kurinczuk JJ, Keogh JM, Alessandri LM, O'Sullivan F, Burton PR, et al. Antepartum risk factors for newborn encephalopathy: the Western Australian case-control study. BMJ. 1998;317(7172):1549-53.
13. Hannah ME. Post-term pregnancy: should all women have labour induced? A review of the literature. Fetal Maternal Med Rev. 1993;5:3.
14. Rand L, Robinson JN, Economy KE, Norwitz ER. Post-term induction of labor revisited. Obstet Gynecol. 2000;96(5 Pt 1):779-83.
15. Campbell MK, Ostbye T, Irgens LM. Post-term birth: risk factors and outcomes in a 10-year cohort of Norwegian births. Obstet Gynecol. 1997;89(4):543-8.
16. Alexander JM, McIntire DD, Leveno KJ. Forty weeks and beyond: pregnancy outcomes by week of gestation. Obstet Gynecol. 2000;96(2):291-4.
17. Treger M, Hallak M, Silberstein T. Post-term pregnancy: should induction of labor be considered before 42 weeks?. J Matern Fetal Neonatal Med. 2002;11(1):50-3.
18. Eden RD, Seifert LS, Winegar A. Perinatal characteristics of uncomplicated postdate pregnancies. Obstet Gynecol. 1987;69(3 Pt 1):296-9.
19. Taipale P, Hiilesmaa V. Predicting delivery date by ultrasound and last menstrual period in early gestation. Obstet Gynecol. 2001;97(2):189-94.
20. Savitz DA, Terry JW Jr, Dole N. Comparison of pregnancy dating by last menstrual period, ultrasound scanning, and their combination. Am J Obstet Gynecol. 2002;187(6):1660-6.
21. Bennett KA, Crane JM, O'shea P. First trimester ultrasound screening is effective in reducing postterm labor induction rates: a randomized controlled trial. Am J Obstet Gynecol. 2004;190(4):1077-81.
22. Caughey AB, Nicholson JM, Washington AE. First versus Second Trimester Ultrasound: the Effect on Pregnancy Dating and Perinatal Outcomes. Am J Obstet Gynecol. 2008;198(6):703.e1–703.e6.
23. Mogren I, Stenlund H, Hogberg U. Recurrence of prolonged pregnancy. Int J Epidemiol. 1999;28(2):253-7.
24. Laursen M, Bille C, Olesen AW. Genetic influence on prolonged gestation: a population-based Danish twin study. Am J Obstet Gynecol. 2004;190(2):489-94.
25. Hickey CA, Cliver SP, McNeal SF. Low pregravid body mass index as a risk factor for preterm birth: variation by ethnic group. Obstet Gynecol. 1997;89(2):206-12. [Medline].
26. Mclean M, Bisits A, Davies J. a placental clock controlling the length of human pregnancy. Nat Med. 1995;1:460-3.
27. Ellis MJ, Livesey JH, Inder WJ. Plasma corticotrophin releasing hormone and unconjugated estriol in human pregnancy: gestational patterns and ability to predict preterm delivery. Am J Obstet Gynecol. 2002;186:94-9.
28. Smith R, Mesiano S, Chan C. Corticotropin-releasing hormone directly and preferentially stimulates dehydroepiandrosterone sulphate secretion by human fetal adrenal cortical cells. J Clin Endocrinol Metab. 1998;83:2916-20.
29. Smith R, Smith Ji, Shen X. Patterns of plasma corticotropin-releasing hormone, progesterone, estradiol, and estriol change and the onset of human labor. J Clin Endocrinol Metab. 2009;94:2066-74.
30. Yang R, You X, Tang X. Corticotropin-releasing hormone inhibits progesterone production in cultured human placental trophoblasts. J Mol endocrinol. 2006;37(3):533-40.
31. Torricelli M, Novembri R, Voltolini C. biochemical and biophysical predictors of the response to the induction of labour in nulliparous post-term pregnancy. Am J Obstet Gynecol. 2011;204:39.e1-6.
32. Kaimal AJ, Little SE, Odibo AO, Stamilio DM, Grobman WA, Long EF, et al. Cost-effectiveness of elective induction of labor at 41 weeks in nulliparous women. Am J Obstet Gynecol. 2011;204(2):137.e1-9.
33. de Miranda E, van der Bom JG, Bonsel GJ. Membrane sweeping and prevention of post-term pregnancy in low-risk pregnancies: a randomised controlled trial. BJOG. 2006;113(4):402-8.

■ LONG QUESTIONS

1. What are the implications of a postdates pregnancy on the fetus? Why does perinatal mortality increase? What monitoring schedule can be instituted in postdates pregnancy?
2. Discuss the management of a 37-year-old primigravida who has come for her antenatal visit at 40 weeks +3 days of pregnancy.

■ SHORT QUESTIONS

1. How should a pregnancy be determined as postdates?
2. The incidence of postdates pregnancy varies by dating technique. Comment on this statement.
3. What are the maternal risks of Post-term pregnancy?
4. What are the pros and cons of induction of labor compared to watchful expectancy at 40 weeks of pregnancy?

MULTIPLE CHOICE QUESTIONS

1. What is the commonest cause of post-term pregnancy?
   a. Wrong dates
   b. Multiparity
   c. Multiple pregnancies
   d. Hypertensive disorder of pregnancy
2. Most accurate method of dating a pregnancy is by:
   a. LMP
   b. CRL with variation of 3–5 days
   c. Ultrasonography at 25 weeks
   d. Ultrasonography at 30 weeks
3. In non-reassuring antenatal surveillance, e.g., Oligohydramnios, growth restriction, PIH and others. The best time to deliver is:
   a. Should be delivered by 39 weeks
   b. Should be delivered by 40 weeks
   c. Should be delivered by 41 weeks
   d. Should be delivered by 42 weeks
4. The following are perinatal risks of a postdated pregnancy, except:
   a. Fetal macrosomia
   b. Meconium aspiration
   c. Perinatal death
   d. Fetal anemia
5. The following intervention is shown to reduce the incidence of postdates pregnancy:
   a. Consumption of castor oil
   b. Squatting exercises
   c. Membrane stripping
   d. Perinneal massage

Answers

1. a 2. b 3. a 4. d 5. c

8.7 INTRAUTERINE FETAL DEMISE

Vandana Bansal, Kaizad R Damania

INTRODUCTION

Loss of a baby at any stage of pregnancy is extremely distressing for both the parents and the treating obstetrician. This sudden bereavement needs to be sensitively managed. It triggers not only good obstetric care, counseling but also guiding the parents to search for an explanation which maybe particularly valuable in determining the recurrence risk and successful management of subsequent pregnancies.

DEFINITION

The United States National Center for Health Statistics defines fetal death as the delivery of a fetus showing no signs of life, such as absence of breathing, beating of the heart, pulsation of the umbilical cord, or definite movement of voluntary muscles.[1] Intrauterine death embraces all fetal deaths occurring both during pregnancy (antepartum death) and during labor (intrapartum). The term "stillbirth" is preferred among parent groups and recently many authors have started using this term instead of "fetal death or intrauterine fetal demise".

There is, however, no uniformity in defining fetal deaths with regards to gestational age or birth weight in different countries across the globe. In the United States fetal deaths are reported at 20 weeks of gestation or greater or a weight greater than or equal to 350 g if the gestational age is unknown.[2] The cutoff of 350 g is the 50th centile for weight at 20 weeks of gestation.

UK statistics (Perinatal Mortality Surveillance Report – CEMACH) defined stillbirths as "a baby delivered with no signs of life known to have died after 24 completed weeks of pregnancy".[3]

GLOBAL BURDEN AND TRENDS OF STILLBIRTHS

Stillbirth is one of the most common adverse pregnancy outcomes in United States affecting 1 in 160 pregnancies, and is estimated to be higher than many developed countries. Approximately 23,600 stillbirths are reported annually. Stillbirth rate in United States have marginally reduced from 6.6 per 1,000 births in 2006 to 6.05 per 1,000 births in 2012 to 5.96 per 1,000 live births in 2013.[1]

As per Perinatal Mortality Surveillance report in United Kingdom (CEMACH), stillbirths are marginally less than US with 1 in 200 babies born dead and a stillbirth rate of 5.2 per 1,000 total births in 2007.[3]

Globally the stillbirth rates have declined slowly from 1990 to 2003 by an average of 1.4% per year. Since 2003, the stillbirths have not significantly declined in spite of improved obstetric and fetal care. It has been speculated that this plateauing may be due to rising obesity and advanced maternal age in modern obstetric medicine.

Global estimate of stillbirths was 2.64 million in 2009 as compared to 3.03 million in 1995. 98% of stillbirths occur in low-income and middle-income countries. Worldwide, 67% of stillbirths occur in rural families, 55% in rural sub-Saharan Africa and south Asia, where skilled birth attendance and cesarean sections are much lower than that for urban births.[4]

DIAGNOSIS OF FETAL DEMISE

History and physical examination are of limited value in the diagnosis of fetal death.

Symptoms: 50% of mothers present with decreased or absent fetal movement. Mothers may continue to feel passive fetal movements even after fetal demise. Others may present on a routine antenatal check up with fetal heart not localized on Doppler or on Ultrasound.

Signs: This may include fundal height less than the period of gestation with absent fetal heart on auscultation with stethoscope, Doppler or cardiotocograph. These methods are insufficiently accurate for diagnosis. Late fetal death may have egg shell crackling feel of fetal head. Uterus may show absence of Braxton–Hicks contraction. There may be signs of acute event causing the death like abruption or cord prolapse.

When a fetal demise is suspected it is imperative to confirm the findings as soon as possible. Fetal death must be confirmed by real time ultrasound and it should be available at all times. Ultrasonography (USG) along with color Doppler allows direct visualization of fetal heart and helps not only to establish diagnosis but helps parents accept the fact **(Fig. 1)**. Other ultrasound features of fetal death include collapse of fetal skull with overlapping bones (spalding sign) **(Fig. 2)**, hydrops **(Fig. 3)** or maceration. Intrafetal gas within the heart, blood vessels, and joints) may be associated with fetal demise.[5] Occult placental abruption may be identified as retroplacental collection in only 15% of all abruption.

Straight X-ray abdomen is rarely used but if done may show Spalding sign due to liquefaction of brain matter and softening of ligamentous structures supporting the vault occurring 7 days after demise. Hyperflexion of spine and crowding of ribs may be demonstrated. Gas shadows as described in USG may appear within 12 hours of death on X-ray as well (Robert's sign).

ETIOLOGY OF FETAL DEATH

Risk factors associated with stillbirths include nulliparity, advanced maternal age, obesity, preexisting diabetes, chronic hypertension, smoking, alcohol, pregnancy from assisted reproductive technology, multiple gestation, male fetal sex, unmarried status, and bad obstetric history. Some of the factors like smoking are modifiable while most of them are not.

Purpose of auditing and evaluating cause of death and classifying deaths is to help clinicians to understand what went wrong and to derive learning points for best clinical practice; to assist in counseling the bereaved mother and the family about the loss, the underlying reasons, and prospects for the future; and to aid public health specialist to prioritize health service resources and strategies for prevention.

It is important to establish the events that lead to the fetal death, as there may be factors that may impact her next pregnancy. In cases where a cause is clearly identified, the cause of fetal death can be attributable to fetal, maternal, or placental pathology. The understanding of these can help direct investigations.

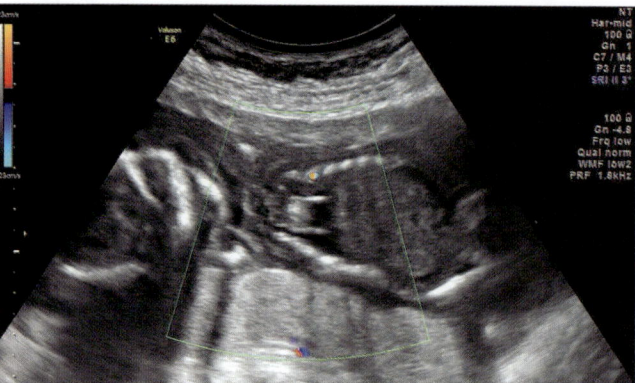

Fig. 1: Color Doppler ultrasound showing absence of color in the fetal heart.

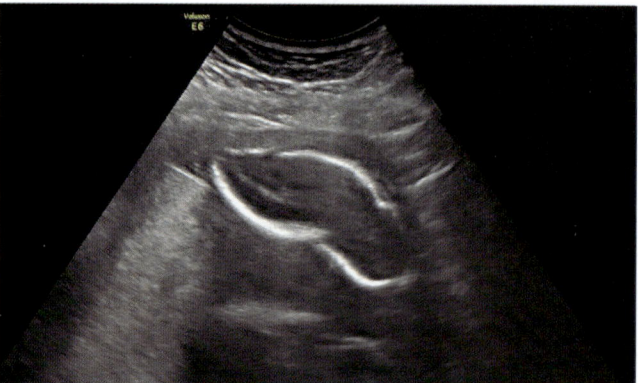

Fig. 2: Overlapping of skull bones on ultrasound (Spalding sign).

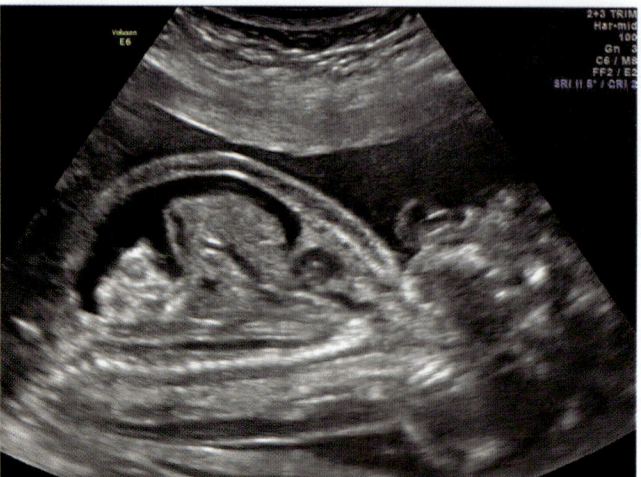

Fig. 3: USG showing fetal hydrops with demise.

Fetal

- Intrauterine growth restriction
- Fetal chromosomal abnormality or malformations
- Fetal infection
- Multiple pregnancy
- Rh incompatibility
- Nonimmune hydrops
- Anemias of fetal origin (alpha thalassemia).

Placental

- Placental insufficiency
- Abruption
- Placenta previa
- Fetomaternal hemorrhage
- Cord accidents
- Vasa previa.

Maternal

- Hypertensive disorders (preeclampsia, eclampsia, chronic hypertension)
- Diabetes (poorly controlled)
- Antiphospholipid syndrome
- Systemic lupus erythematosus
- Hereditary thrombophilias
- Prolonged pregnancy (>42 weeks)
- Extremes of reproductive age
- Maternal infections
- Hyperpyrexia

- Obstetric cholestasis
- Uterine rupture
- Asphyxia, birth trauma
- Maternal trauma
- Smoking and drug abuse
- Obesity
- Pregnancies after assisted reproductive technology
- Previous bad obstetric history (recurrence)
- Non-Hispanic black women.

Fetal Causes

Fetal growth restriction is the largest category of conditions associated with fetal demise which was previously classified as unexplained. Over one-third of stillbirths are small for gestational age with half classified as being unexplained. The most severely affected fetuses with weight below 2.5th centile are at greatest risk of fetal demise in utero (**Fig. 4**).[6] Fetal growth restriction is seen with fetal aneuploidies, fetal infections, maternal hypertension, autoimmune disorders, diabetes, obesity and maternal smoking.

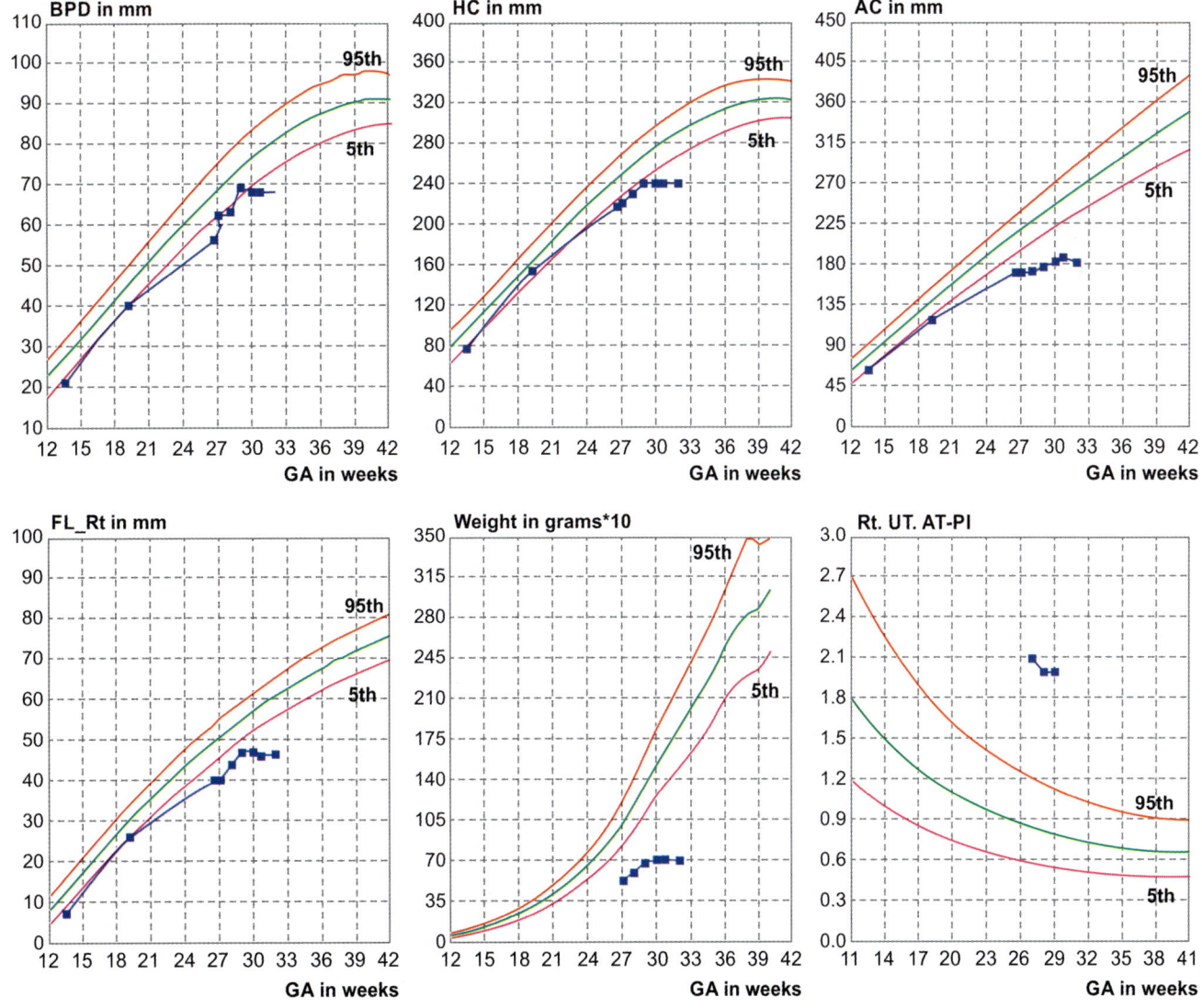

Fig. 4: Growth centile chart of a fetal demise following severe fetal growth restriction.

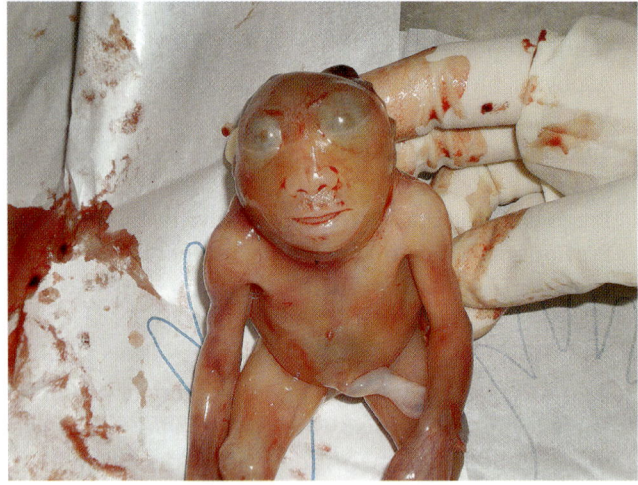

Fig. 5: Fetus with anencephaly.

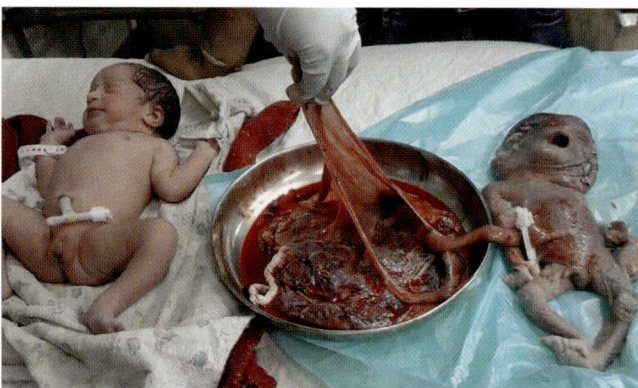

Fig. 6: Dichorionic twins with single fetal demise.

Fetal abnormalities account for 25–40% of all stillbirths. Neural tube defects **(Fig. 5)**, hydrops, hydrocephalus, and complex congenital heart disease are most often encountered and amenable to antenatal diagnosis on ultrasound. Presence of fetal demise in a symmetrically growth restricted fetus with polyhydramnios may suggest fetal cause for intrauterine fetal death (IUFD). Abnormal karyotype can be found in approximately 6–13% of stillbirths. Most common aneuploidy detected is trisomy 21 (31%), monosomy X (22%) followed by trisomy 18 and 13.[7] The chance of chromosomal abnormality exceeds 20% in fetuses with anatomical anomalies or growth restriction but is also found in 4.6% of structurally normal fetus.[7]

With the availability of microarray analysis which not only detects aneuploidy but also determines copy number variation (deletions and duplications) even in nonviable fetal tissue the diagnostic yield of genetic etiology has increased to 41.9% in all stillbirths. Microarray analysis has been incorporated as a preferred method in the stillbirth workup. Confined placental mosaicism where the fetus is euploid while the placenta has an abnormal cell lines is also associated with stillbirths. Single gene defects may also contribute to a small proportion of stillbirths but routine evaluation for microdeletion and single gene defects or a whole exome sequencing is not currently part of standard evaluation. However DNA material can be saved for later evaluation in case certain syndrome or a single gene defect is suspected on autopsy. Genetic evaluation for a specific abnormality should be guided by clinical history, dysmorphic features, skeletal abnormalities and detected fetal abnormalities.[6]

Infectious pathogens may result in stillbirth by producing direct fetal infections, placental dysfunction, severe maternal illness or by stimulating spontaneous preterm labor. Infection is associated with 10–20% of stillbirths in developed countries and much higher in developing countries. Fetal infections may occur as a result of ascending bacterial infection leading to chorioamnionitis or hematogenous spread of agents such as listeria or syphilis. Ascending infection with *Escherichia coli*, *Klebsiella*, group B *Streptococcus*, *Enterococcus* and *Chlamydia* are the more common. Preterm stillbirths are more likely to be associated with chorioamnionitis with aerobic and anaerobic bacterial species and also mycoplasma and ureaplasma.

Potentially lethal fetal pathogens include Rubella, Cytomegalovirus, Parvovirus B19, Zika, Syphilis, Varicella, *Listeriosis monocytogenes* and Toxoplasma. In the developing countries Malaria is a significant preventable cause of stillbirth. It causes death due to hyperpyrexia or due to placental parasitization causing placental insufficiency.

Rate of stillbirths are 2.5 times higher in multiple gestation (14.07 vs. 5.65 per 1,000 live births)[1,8] **(Fig. 6)**. Risk of stillbirth in twins increases with advancing gestation and is significantly greater in monochorionic twins. Higher rates are due to complications specific to multiple pregnancies such as fetofetal transfusion syndrome (TTTS), Twin reverse arterial perfusion (TRAP), aneuploidy, malformations, fetal growth restriction and higher order multiple gestations.

Rh isoimmunization can lead to excessive hemolysis of fetal blood by Rh antibodies formed in the mother resulting in fetal anemia, anoxia, cardiac failure, hydrops and death.

Placental and Cord Abnormalities

Placental abruption is the most common single identifiable cause of fetal death responsible for 14% of third trimester still births.[9] Although abruption maybe the direct cause of fetal death, it is commoner in thrombophilias, growth restriction, smoking, drug abuse and also fetal abnormalities. Placental abruption is associated with hypertension in approximately half of the cases. The rates of abruption have increased due to the use of maternal cocaine, other illicit drugs, and smoking.

Massive fetomaternal hemorrhage, a rare occurrence, can be a cause of fetal death and may have occurred hours to days before clinical presentation. Although usually spontaneous, such hemorrhage is common with severe maternal trauma. Immediate Kleihauer-Betke test even before delivery is indicated to confirm the cause.

Umbilical cord abnormalities as etiology accounts for 10% stillbirth and includes vasa previa, cord entrapment, evidence

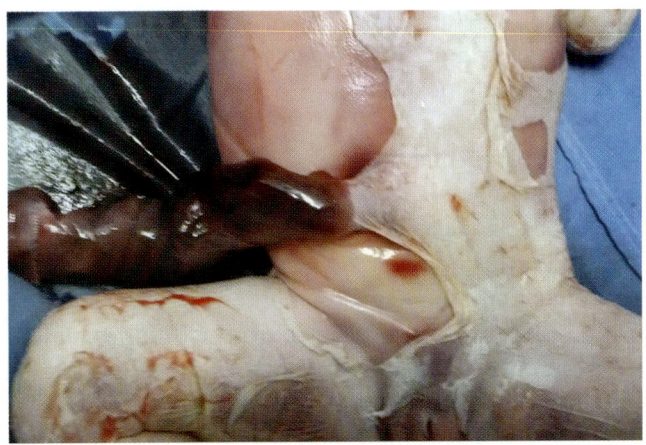

Fig. 7: Cord hematoma as the cause for stillbirth.

of cord occlusion, cord hematoma **(Fig. 7)** and fetal hypoxia, cord prolapse or stricture or thrombi or true knot and not the mere presence of nuchal cord.

Maternal Causes

Comorbid medical conditions such as hypertensive disorder and diabetes are most commonly implicated with intrauterine fetal demise.

Hypertensive disorders (Preeclampsia, eclampsia, chronic hypertension): Spasm of uteroplacental circulation causes reduced placental blood flow leading to placental insufficiency. Chronic hypertension with or without superimposed preeclampsia is particularly associated with 2–4 times higher perinatal mortality than general population.

Diabetes: Population based studies have demonstrated a two to five fold increased risk of stillbirth in women with pregestational diabetes.[10] Uncontrolled diabetes leading to fetal demise may be due to fetal hypoglycemia, hypoxia, acidosis or associated congenital malformations. With better preconceptional care and optimal glycemic control aiming for an HbA1c levels below 7%, antenatally risk of sudden fetal demise can be reduced.

Other medical disorders including systemic lupus erythematosus, renal disease, uncontrolled thyroid disease have also been implicated in risk of stillbirths.

Bimodal peak at extremes of reproductive age (<15 years and >35 years), even when corrected for known associated anomalies and medical disorders, are still independent risk factors for fetal demise.[11]

Acquired thrombophilia: Antiphospholipid syndrome is an acquired thrombophilia. Lupus anticoagulant and anticardiolipin antibodies are associated with decidual vasculopathy, placental infarction, fetal growth restriction, and fetal death.

Hereditary thrombophilias: Patients with inherited thrombophilias appear to have an increased risk of stillbirth but the association between them is weak. There is no evidence that screening an unselected population is clinically effective.[12] Screening may be indicated if evidence of fetal growth restriction or placental disease is evident with fetal death.[13] The American College of Obstetricians and Gynecologists (ACOG) and Society for Maternal-Fetal Medicine (SMFM), consensus does not recommend testing inherited thrombophilias as part of a stillbirth evaluation.[6]

Obstetric cholestasis is strongly associated with fetal death and has a recurrence of 80% in subsequent pregnancy.

About 11.7% of deaths are associated with intrapartum causes.[14] Many of these deaths are identified as having another primary condition such as fetal growth failure, highlighting the importance of growth restriction as an antecedent to birth asphyxia and intrapartum death. The antepartum care affects the fetal reserves and its ability to withstand stress of labor. But only about a quarter of small for gestational age fetuses are detected antenatally and this is considered as an important factor associated with substandard care. The strong link between fetal growth failure and still birth has important implications for preventive strategies, health policies, and subsequent care of individual patient with a previous stillbirth.

Obesity: A meta-analysis of 96 population-based studies found that maternal overweight and obesity was the highest-ranking modifiable risk factor for stillbirth.[15] Obesity defined as a prepregnancy body mass index of 30 or greater, is the fastest growing health problem in developed countries. Obesity is associated with a fivefold increased risk of stillbirth resulting from placental dysfunction. In addition obesity remains an independent risk factor for stillbirth and early fetal loss, even after controlling for smoking, gestational diabetes and preeclampsia.

Ethnicity: Non-Hispanic black women have a stillbirth rate more than twice the rate of other racial groups. This disparity may be due to higher rates of diabetes, hypertension, abruption, premature rupture of membranes. Higher stillbirth rates have also been observed in South Asian ethnic population in Australia and United Kingdom probably related to obesity.[16]

Past obstetric history of fetal demise especially women with previous adverse pregnancy outcome such as growth restriction, preterm or preeclampsia and also cases of unexplained stillbirths are at increased risk of recurrence.

Extremes of parity both nulliparous as well as multipara more than three previous pregnancies are at higher rate of stillbirth.

Male fetus has an approximately 10% higher risk than female, reason of the same remains unknown.

Substance abuse: Maternal cocaine, methamphetamine, other illicit drug uses and smoking are contributors to abruption and stillbirths. There is a clear dose related effect of tobacco smoking on stillbirth risk with 9% increased odds of having stillbirth with smoking 1–9 cigarettes a day increasing to 52% with more than 10 cigarettes a day. Risk is higher when exposure is in the first trimester.[6]

Pregnancies after assisted reproductive technology are associated with two to three fold elevated risk for stillbirth even after controlling confounding variables such as age, parity and multiple pregnancy. Increased rates of stillbirths are result of IVF or intracytoplasmic sperm injection and not the underlying infertility.

Perinatal mortality risk increases in late term and post term pregnancies. Hence induction of labor is recommended for 42 (0/7) weeks of gestation and can be considered at or after 41weeks 0/7 days of gestation.

Unexplained: Up to 60% of stillbirths have no identifiable etiology.[3] Attempting to determine the cause of fetal death remains important because it may influence estimates of recurrence and future preconceptional counseling, pregnancy management, prenatal diagnostic procedures, and neonatal management.

Of the estimated 3.2 million annual stillbirths, current method of classifying perinatal deaths (Conventional Wigglesworth classification) reports about two-thirds (66.2%) as being unexplained. A new classification system (ReCoDe: Relevant condition at death) reduced the predominance of stillbirths categorized as unexplained. The most common condition was fetal growth restriction (43%), and only 15.2% of stillbirths remained unexplained. ReCoDe identified 57.7% of the Wigglesworth unexplained stillbirths as growth restricted. Relevant condition at fetal death was identified in 85% of cases.[14]

EVALUATION OF INTRAUTERINE FETAL DEMISE

It is important to establish the cause or the events that led to the fetal demise as it may influence estimates of recurrence and future preconceptional counseling, pregnancy management and prenatal diagnostic procedures. Grieving parents need to understand that this time may be the best or only chance of finding out what happened and it will crucially influence care in the future pregnancy. Parents should also be made aware that no specific cause is found in almost half of stillbirths.

Key Components of Patient History while Evaluating Etiology (Adapted from ACOG and SMFM Consensus Care Statement)[6]

- Family history
  - Recurrent spontaneous abortions
  - Venous thromboembolism
  - Chromosomal/ structural anomalies
  - Hereditary condition or syndrome
  - Developmental delay
  - Consanguinity
- Maternal history
  - Previous venous thromboembolism
  - Diabetes mellitus
  - Chronic hypertension
  - Thrombophilia
  - Systemic lupus erythematosus
  - Autoimmune disease
  - Epilepsy
  - Severe anemia
  - Heart disease
  - Tobacco, alcohol, drugs or medications
- Obstetric history
  - Recurrent spontaneous abortions
  - Previous child with chromosomal/structural anomalies/hereditary conditions/growth restriction
  - Previous gestational hypertension/preeclampsia
  - Previous gestational diabetes
  - Previous abruption
  - Previous fetal demise
- Current pregnancy details
  - Maternal age
  - Gestational age at stillbirth
  - Medical condition complicating pregnancy (cholestasis)
  - Pregnancy weight gain and BMI
  - Complication of multiple pregnancy (TTTS, TRAP, discordant growth)
  - Placental abruption
  - Abdominal trauma
  - Preterm labor or preterm rupture of membranes
  - Abnormalities seen on ultrasound
  - Infection or chorioamnionitis.

Key Components of Diagnostic Evaluation while Determining Etiology

The **Table 1** summarizes the diagnostic tests required and the reasons for doing them. This tabulated form has been adapted from Royal College of Obstetricians and Gynecologists. Green-top Guideline No. 55.[13]

FETAL AUTOPSY

Obtain parental consent for fetal autopsy which includes placental pathology and whole body X-ray of the fetus. In case parents do not give consent, external evaluation by a perinatal pathologist should be done. Other options include photographs, X-ray, ultrasound, magnetic resonance imaging and sampling of tissues, blood or skin. Independent of fetal autopsy, placental pathology is extremely useful and must be offered even if the parents decline full autopsy **(Fig. 8)**. Dedicated perinatal pathologist should perform fetal autopsy.

Inspection of fetus and placenta:
- Weight, head circumference and length of fetus
- Weight of placenta
- Photograph of fetus and placenta—front and profile view of face, extremities, whole body
- Document findings and any abnormalities.

SECTION 8: Late Pregnancy Complications

TABLE 1: Key components of diagnostic evaluation.

	Test	Reason for the test	Comments
1a. 1b. 1c.	• Complete blood count with platelets • Bile salts • CRP	• Preeclampsia, abruption, DIC • Obstetric cholestasis • Sepsis	
2.	Coagulation profile and fibrinogen	DIC	Test needed for management purpose. Preeclampsia, abruption, sepsis and prolonged retained fetus increases the chances of DIC
3.	Kleihauer-Betke (KB) test for fetal cells in maternal circulation	• Massive fetomaternal hemorrhage screen • KB test should be recommended for all women, not only those who are Rh negative • Test should be done before birth as red cells clear quickly from maternal circulation	• In Rh -ve women, requirement of Anti-D determined by this test • In Rh +ve females this test done to determine cause of death which may be occult massive fetomaternal hemorrhage
4.	Bacteriology: Blood, urine, vaginal swab cultures	If chorioamnionitis is suspected	Indicated if maternal fever, flu such as syndrome, foul smelling liquor, prolonged rupture membranes
5.	TORCH, Parvovirus and syphilis	Occult maternal fetal infection	
6.	Blood sugar estimation (OGTT), HbA1c	Diagnose pregestational diabetes or uncontrolled gestational diabetes especially in large for gestational age fetus	Women with gestational diabetes return to prepregnancy values within few hours of fetal death
7.	Maternal thyroid function (TSH, FT3, FT4)	Thyroid disease implicated in adverse pregnancy outcomes and should be screened	
8.	Antiphospholipid antibodies	Lupus anticoagulant and anticardiolipin antibodies and beta-2 glycoprotein antibodies	If abnormal may be repeated after 6 weeks
9.	Hereditary thrombophilia	• Factor V Leiden mutation, antithrombin III, prothrombin gene mutation • Hyperhomocysteinemia, Protein C and S deficiency	• Routine testing is not recommended. Indicated if placental insufficiency or growth restriction seen in the dead fetus. Consider in cases with a personal or family history of thromboembolic disease. • If abnormal may be repeated after 6 weeks
10.	Anti-Ro, anti-La antibodies	Autoimmune disease suspected	Indicated if evidence of hydrops, endomyocardial fibroelastosis or AV node calcification on autopsy
11.	Antired cell antibodies (ICT)	Immune hemolytic anemia	Indicated if fetal hydrops diagnosed on USG or autopsy
	• Maternal alloimmune • Antiplatelet antibodies	Alloimmune thrombocytopenia	Indicated if fetal intracranial hemorrhage found on USG or postmortem
12.	Maternal urine for cocaine metabolites (toxicology screen)	For illicit drug use in pregnancy and suspected abruption	
13.	Parental karyotype	• Indicated if fetus has unbalanced translocation, other aneuploidy • If fetal genetic testing fails and history suggestive of aneuploidy/fetal abnormality/unexplained IUFD	Determine parental balanced translocation or mosaicism
14.	Fetal autopsy	• External examination, internal examination, microscopy, photographs, X-rays, placenta and cord histopathology • Fetal and placental tissues for karyotype and microarray, fetal blood and placental swab for viral and bacterial infection • Cord blood or cardiac blood in lithium heparin • Genetic material to be stored for later analysis for single gene disorders if needed	• Postmortem examination of the baby and placenta and karyotype with microarray has the highest diagnostic yield • Autopsy provides important information in 30% of cases • Placental evaluation provides additional information in 30% of cases • Infection is more common in preterm stillbirth(19% vs. 2%)

(CRP: C-reactive protein; DIC: disseminated intravascular coagulation; IUFD: intrauterine fetal death; OGTT: oral glucose tolerance test)

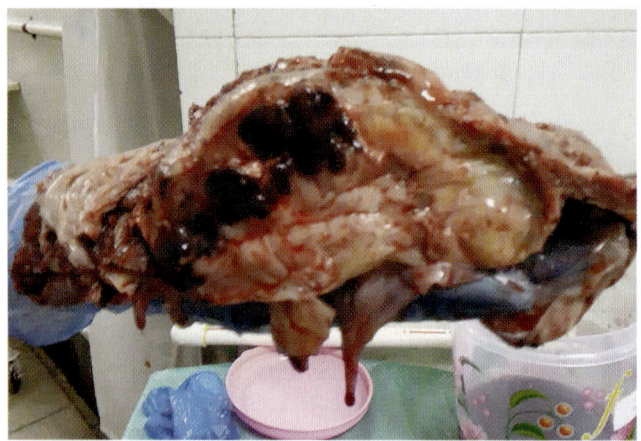

Fig. 8: Gross placenta with infarctions and hemorrhage.

Cytogenetic specimen:[6]
- Obtain parental consent for cytogenetic evaluation
- Samples from multiple tissues should be used to increase the chance of culture
- More than one cytogenetic technique (DNA based tests) should be available to maximize the chance of informative results(culture failures)
- Acceptable samples for cytogenetic specimen (at least any one)
  - Amniotic fluid by amniocentesis at the time of antenatal diagnosis of demise is a preferred sample
  - Placental block (1 × 1 cm) from below the cord insertion site from the fetal side of an unfixed placenta. (Placenta has an advantage of being the most viable tissue and most rapid cell culture but the disadvantages of maternal contamination and placental pseudomosaicism)
  - Umbilical cord segment (1.5 cm)
  - Internal fetal tissue such as costochondral junction or patella. Skin is not recommended. Skin specimens are associated with higher rate of culture failure, twice that of any other tissue (60%). If skin biopsy is taken it should be taken from the upper fleshy part of thigh and deep to include the underlying muscle. Patella is a good specimen but difficult to obtain.

Culture fluid should be stored in refrigerator and thawed thoroughly before use. Place specimen in a sterile tissue culture media of ringer lactate solution/culture fluid (if available) at room temperature when transported to the laboratory. Do not place specimen in formalin. Culture fluid containing antibiotics can reduce risk of culture failure due to bacterial contamination. Genetic material should be stored for later evaluation for any single gene disorders.[6,13]

OBSTETRIC MANAGEMENT OF CURRENT PREGNANCY

News of the diagnosis must be given to the parents sensitively but unambiguously. If the woman is unaccompanied, offer may be made to call her partner or relative.

Clinical assessment and investigations are required to assess maternal wellbeing (including coagulopathy), determine cause of death and chance of recurrence, and ensure prompt management of any potential life-threatening pregnancy complications. This would include a detailed history of events during antenatal period and clinical examination for preeclampsia, chorioamnionitis, cord accident, and placental abruption. In addition to obstetric history, exposure to drugs, medications and viral infections, a family history with a three generation pedigree should be reviewed.

Woman who is Rh D negative, blood for Kleihauer test should be taken soon after diagnosis of fetal demise, to determine the amount of fetomaternal bleed. Anti-Rh (D) immunoglobulin should be given as soon as possible after fetal death, even before delivery as effectiveness decreases after 72 hours. Babies cord blood after birth may be sent for blood group and type by conventional serology.

There is small possibility of defibrination from silent disseminated intravascular coagulation (DIC) if fetus is retained after IUFD. Risk is 10% within 4 weeks and increases to 30% thereafter.[17] It is due to gradual absorption of thromboplastin from the dead placenta into the maternal circulation. So in addition to routine test, clotting screen including platelet count and fibrinogen should be done to ensure that there is no coagulopathy.

Mode and timing of delivery would depend on gestational age, previous intrapartum history, maternal preference and her medical condition. Women with sepsis, preeclampsia, placental abruption or membrane rupture should be promptly delivered. Option of expectant management versus prompt delivery may be given to grieving mother if above is not present and no lab evidence of coagulopathy. More than 85% of women with an IUFD labor spontaneously within 3 weeks of diagnosis. The risk to the mother in the first 48 hours is low.[17] Although most desire prompt delivery, the timing of delivery is not critical and the coagulopathy associated with prolonged retention of a dead fetus are uncommon.[6]

Mothers who decide on expectant management need to be informed that short delay in labor may not be harmful but they may develop severe medical complications and suffer greater anxiety with prolonged interval. Also information obtained on postmortem may reduce with delay in delivery.[13]

Most patients would, however, opt for early induction with the potential advantage of immediate recovery and quicker return home. With the availability of better inducing agents, vaginal births can be achieved within 24 hours of induction for IUFD in 90% of women.[18]

Option of delivery of a stillborn includes dilatation and evacuation or induction of labor. Dilatation and evacuation can be an option if institutional expertise is available between 14 and 24 weeks. However this may limit the efficacy of autopsy for detection of gross fetal anomalies and does not provide opportunity of holding the fetus by the parents after birth.[6]

On the other hand, induction of labor in fetal demise between 14 and 24 weeks is less effective and associated with a higher risk of requiring a dilatation and curettage for retained placenta after fetal expulsion and increased risk of maternal infection and need for intravenous antibiotics.[6]

A combination of mifepristone and a prostaglandin preparation is recommended as first-line intervention. Misoprostol is preferred over prostaglandin E2 because of equivalent safety and efficacy with lower cost. Vaginal misoprostol is equally effective with fewer side effects as compared to oral form. Addition of mifepristone reduces the average duration of labor by about 7 hours.[18]

Dosage regime recommended by Royal College of Obstetricians and Gynaecologists and endorsed by the National Institute for Health and Clinical Excellence (NICE): Single dose of 200 mg of mifepristone given 24–48 hours before starting misoprostol. The dose of misoprostol for late IUFD should be adjusted according to gestational age (100 µg 6 hourly before 26 weeks; 25–50 µg 4 hourly at 27 weeks or more).[13]

The American College of Obstetricians and Gynecologists practice bulletin however recommends higher doses of misoprostol without mifepristone priming. 400–600 µg of misoprostol vaginally every 3–6 hours is considered effective method of induction regardless of the bishop in gestational age less than 28 weeks. Doses less than 400 µg have decreased efficacy. After 28 weeks it recommends "usual obstetric protocol" for induction.[19] The new ACOG and SMFM consensus supports the use of mifepristone (200 mg or 600 mg orally), 24–48 hours before the initiation of induction with misoprostol in the setting of stillbirth. Cesarean delivery for fetal demise should be reserved for unusual circumstances. Women with an increased risk of rupture uterus (classical hysterotomy, transfundal surgery), repeat cesarean delivery is a reasonable option.[6]

In patients with previous scar pregnancy, ACOG and SMFM consensus supports the use of vaginal misoprostol for induction before 24 weeks of gestation (400 µg every 6 hourly) but adds caution to effectiveness, safety, optimal dosage and route of administration of misoprostol in gestation between 24 and 28 weeks in whom lower dosages of 200 µg per dose may be preferred.[6]

As per the new ACOG and SMFM consensus, in patients after 28 weeks with one previous hysterotomy/LSCS, cervical ripening with transcervical Foley catheter maybe useful adjunct for trial of vaginal delivery. There is limited data to guide clinical practice in patients with classical cesarean and multiple previous LSCS and delivery plan should be individualized.[6]

In patient with prior lower segment cesarean section with late IUFD, induction of labor can be done safely with misoprostol at lower doses (25–50 µg).[13] This recommendation has been endorsed by NICE.[20] A transcervical balloon catheter technique for induction in previous LSCS can also be used with uterine rupture rates compared to spontaneous labor. These mechanical methods may increase the risk of ascending infection in the presence of fetal demise.[21] Oxytocin augmentation can be done.

Women with prior scar in labor should be closely monitored for signs of scar dehiscence in the form of maternal tachycardia, atypical pain, vaginal bleeding, hematuria or maternal collapse. The most common early sign of scar dehiscence is fetal distress which does not apply here.

Routine antibiotic prophylaxis is not recommended for prevention of maternal infection in women with IUFD. But women with sepsis should receive intravenous broad spectrum antibiotic therapy. Early artificial rupture of membranes may facilitate ascending infection and hence membranes should be left intact as long as possible. As long as the membranes are intact, infection is unlikely but once this barrier is broken, dead tissue favors growth of pathogens, especially gas forming organism such as *Clostridium welchii*.

Women in labor should have full access to labor analgesia as pain relief is particularly important for a woman with fetal death.

Postpartum hemorrhage and retained placenta are common especially with preeclampsia, abruption, prolonged fetal death or infection. Prolonged chorioamnionitis or recurrent bouts of abruptions predispose to retained adherent placenta.

Lactation is suppressed by dopamine agonists—bromocriptine (2.5 mg twice daily for 14 days) or cabergoline (1 mg single dose). These are contraindicated in women with hypertensive disorders as they increase the risk of intracerebral hemorrhage.

Women should be cared for postdelivery with adequate privacy and support. Perinatal death is associated with increased risk of postpartum depression and post-traumatic stress disorder. Counseling should be offered to all women and their partners. Medical team and the support staff should provide all the support and sympathy to the bereaved couple. Parents must be called for a follow-up to discuss result of the investigation, try to ascertain cause of death and draw a clear plan of management for next pregnancy.

Most of the above recommendations are general recommendations and would be relevant to our population. However, certain specific recommendation like role of inherited thrombophilia which remains not well studied in our population or the recommendation of genetic evaluation by incorporating microarray analysis which is costly and unavailable in many areas of our country need to be put in proper context. Needless to add that fetal autopsy and other such evaluation needs to be done by a physician who has expertise in performing the same.

CONCLUSION

Commonly associated antepartum conditions leading to fetal demise include congenital malformations, growth restriction,

BOX 1: Stillbirth recommendation.[6]

- Inherited thrombophilia has not been associated with stillbirth and testing for same as part of a stillbirth evaluation is not recommended
- Women who decline invasive testing, portion of placenta, umbilical cord segment or internal fetal tissue can be sent for genetic analysis
- Incorporation of microarray analysis in the stillbirth workup improves the success rate of the test and detection of genetic anomalies compared with conventional karyotype
- Genetic evaluation for a specific abnormality should be guided by clinical history, dysmorphic features, skeletal abnormalities and detected fetal abnormalities
- Evaluation of stillbirth should include fetal autopsy, gross and histology of placenta, umbilical cord and membranes and genetic evaluation
- Gross and microscopic evaluation of placenta, umbilical cord and fetal membranes by a trained pathologist is the single most useful component of evaluation of stillbirth
- General examination of the stillborn fetus should be done systematically noting dysmorphic features and measuring weight, length and head circumference
- Fetal autopsy is one of the most useful diagnostic tests in determining cause of death and must be offered
- Genetic analysis give a sufficient yield and should be performed in all cases of stillbirth after appropriate parental permission
- Appropriate history and physical findings should be sent in the requisition to assist the laboratory personnel to interpret cytogenetic tests
- Thorough maternal history should be taken to look for known conditions or symptoms suggestive of those that have been associated with stillbirth
- The results of autopsy, placental examination, laboratory tests and cytogenetic analysis must be conveyed to the clinician and to the family of the deceased in a timely manner
- Bereavement care should be individualized as per the personal, cultural and religious needs of the parents
- Healthcare providers should weigh the risk and benefits of each strategy in a given clinical scenario. Shared decision making plays an important role in determining the optimal method for delivery in case of fetal demise
- For women with previous stillbirth at or after 32 weeks, once or twice a week antenatal surveillance is recommended starting from 32 weeks or 1–2 weeks prior to previous stillbirth. For stillbirths prior to 32 weeks, individualized timing of antenatal surveillance may be considered

Source: Adapted from ACOG and SMFM consensus.

fetal infections, antepartum hemorrhage, preeclampsia, and maternal disease such as diabetes mellitus. Intrapartum death primarily may be due to placental abruption, maternal and fetal infections, cord prolapse, hypoxia and uterine rupture.

Death of a baby is devastating. The effect of grief can be overwhelming and parents, their family members, and friends may be left feeling guilty, remorseful, anxious, isolated and exhausted. All attempts must be made to provide emotional support as well as try providing the parents with the answer to "why" as this may be their best or only chance of finding out what happened **(Box 1)**.

REFERENCES

1. MacDorman MF, Gregory EC. Fetal and perinatal mortality, United States, 2013. Natl Vital Stat Rep. 2015;64:1-24.
2. National Center for Health Statistics. Model state vital statistics act and regulations. Atlanta, GA: Centers for Disease Control and Prevention; 1992.
3. Confidential Enquiry into Maternal and Child Health (CEMACH). Perinatal Mortality 2007. London: CEMACH; 2009.
4. Lawn JE, Blencowe H, Pattinson R, Cousens S, Kumar R, Ibiebele I, et al. Stillbirths: Where? When? Why? How to make the data count? Lancet. 2011;377:1448-63.
5. Weinstein BJ, Platt LD. The ultrasonic appearance of intravascular gas in fetal death. J Ultrasound Med. 1983;2:451-4.
6. Torri DM, Rana SB, Fretts RC, Reddy UM, Turrentine MA. American College of Obstetricians and Gynecologists and Society for Maternal Fetal Medicine Obstetric care consensus on Management of Stillbirth. Obstetrics and Gynecol. 2020;135(3):110-30.
7. Korteweg FJ, Bouman K, Erwich JJ, Timmer A, Veeger NJ, Ravisé JM, et al. Cytogenetic analysis after evaluation of 750 fetal deaths: proposal for diagnostic workup. Obstet Gynecol. 2008;111:865-74.
8. Bell R, Glinianaia SV, Rankin J, Wright C, Pearce MS, Parker L. Changing patterns of perinatal death,1982-2000: a retrospective cohort study. Arch Dis Child Fetal Neonatal Ed. 2004;89:F531-6.
9. Fretts RC, Usher RH. Causes of fetal death in women of advanced maternal age. Obstet Gynecol. 1997;89:40.
10. Casson IF, Clarke CA, Howard CV, McKendrick O, Pennycook S, Pharoah PO, et al. Outcomes of pregnancy in insulin dependent diabetic women: results of a five year population cohort study. BMJ. 1997;315:275-8.
11. Balayala J, Azoulay I, Assayag J, Benjamin A, Abenhaim HA. Effect of maternal age on the risk of stillbirth: a population based cohort study on 37 million birth in the United States. Am J Perinatol. 2011;28:643-50.
12. Wu O, Robertson L, Twaddle S, Lowe GD, Clark P, Greaves M, et al. Screening for thrombophilia in high risk situations: systematic review and cost- effectiveness analysis. The Thrombosis: Risk and Economic Assessment of Thrombophilia Screening (TREATS) study. Health Technol Assess 2006;10:1-110.
13. Royal College of Obstetricians and Gynecologists. Green-top Guideline No.55.Late intrauterine fetal death and stillbirth. London: RCOG; 2010.
14. Gardosi J, Kady SM, McGeown P, Francis A, Tonks A. Classification of stillbirth by relevant condition at death (ReCoDe): population based cohort study. BMJ. 2005;331:1113-7.
15. Flenady V, Koopmans L, Middleton P, Frøen JF, Smith GC, Gibbons K, et al. Major risk factors for stillbirth in high-income countries: a systemic review and meta-analysis. Lancet. 2011;377:1331-40.
16. Penn N, Oteng Ntim E, Oakley L, Doyle P. Ethnic variation in stillbirth risk and the role of maternal obesity: analysis of routine data from a London maternity unit. BMC Pregnancy and Childbirth 2014;14:404.
17. Silver RM. Fetal death. Obstet Gynecol. 2007;109:153-67.
18. Wagaarachchi PT, Ashok PW, Narvekar NM, Smith NC, Templeton A. Medical management of late intrauterine fetal death using a combination of mifepristone and misoprostol. BJOG. 2002;109:443-7.

19. American College of Obstetricians and Gynecologists: Management of stillbirth. Practice bulletin No.102, March 2009.
20. National Institute for Health and Clinical Excellence. Clinical guideline no. 70: Induction of labour. London: NICE; 2008.
21. Al-Zirqi I, Stray-Pedersen B, Forsen L, Vangen S. Uterine rupture after previous caesarean section. BJOG. 2010;117:809-20.

LONG QUESTIONS

1. Discuss in detail regarding risk factors and evaluation in a case of intrauterine fetal death at 28 weeks of gestation.
2. Discuss in detail regarding preconceptional care and surveillance during subsequent pregnancy following a stillbirth in previous pregnancy.

SHORT QUESTIONS

Write short notes on the following:
1. Fetal autopsy
2. Delivery in a case of intrauterine fetal death
3. Correctable causes of intrauterine fetal death

MULTIPLE CHOICE QUESTIONS

1. Which of the following are signs of intrauterine fetal death?
    a. Spalding's sign
    b. Cracking egg fetal of fetal head
    c. Intrafetal gas
    d. All of the above
2. Maternal risk factors for stillbirths include all, except:
    a. APLA
    b. Chronic hypertension
    c. Low blood pressure
    d. Postdatism
3. Fetal risk factors for stillbirths include:
    a. Intrauterine growth restriction
    b. Rh incompatibility
    c. Fetal infections
    d. All of the above
4. Which of the following is true regarding risk of intrauterine fetal death?
    a. 25% times higher in multiple pregnancies
    b. Umbilical cord abnormalities is a definite cause of intrauterine fetal death
    c. Rh Alloimmunization related risk of intrauterine fetal death occurs only in the late third trimester
    d. All of the above
5. Causes of hereditary thrombophilias:
    a. Factor V Leiden mutation
    b. Prot C/Prot S
    c. Hyperhomocysteinemia
    d. All of the above
6. Most common aneuploidy associated with stillbirths:
    a. Monosomy X
    b. Trisomy 18
    c. Trisomy 21
    d. All of above
7. Tests to detect Rh incompatibility:
    a. KB tests
    b. Rosette test
    c. Rh antibody titers
    d. All of the above
8. Fetal autopsy includes:
    a. Maternal X-ray
    b. Placental pathology
    c. Fetal hair sampling
    d. All of the above
9. Methods of delivery in a case of intrauterine fetal death include:
    a. D and E
    b. Mifepristone + Misoprostol
    c. Elective cesarean section
    d. All of the above
10. Methods for surveillance of subsequent pregnancies following stillbirth include:
    a. Preconceptional glycemic control
    b. Stringent blood pressure control
    c. Antenatal surveillance from 32 weeks or 1–2 weeks before previous intrauterine fetal death
    d. All of the above

Answers					
1. d	2. c	3. d	4. a	5. d	6. c
7. d	8. b	9. d	10. d		

SECTION 9

Labor

9.1 MECHANISM OF LABOR

Shirish N Daftary, Gaurav S Desai

INTRODUCTION

The preparation for the birth of the baby begins well before the actual onset of labor.

- *Preparatory phase:* Mechanical factors coupled with altered hormonal milieu leading to neuromuscular changes have a role to play in labor onset **(Flowchart 1)**.
- *Mechanical factors:* The increasing myometrial excitability as term approaches, coupled with progressively increasing intrauterine pressure exerted by the growing fetus and liquor leads to the defining and formation of the lower uterine segment. The fetal head often gets engaged (passive descent) well before the onset of labor—this is commonly observed in primigravidae.
- *Hormonal factors:* During the course of pregnancy, placental progesterone is the dominant hormone, it maintains uterine quiescence by promoting calcium binding, thereby reducing free intracellular calcium. As pregnancy advances—secretion of fetal and placental corticotrophin levels occurs, stimulating the fetal pituitary to release ACTH hormone. In response to it, the fetal adrenals secrete steadily increasing amounts of cortisol. The increasing cortisol levels inhibit placental synthesis

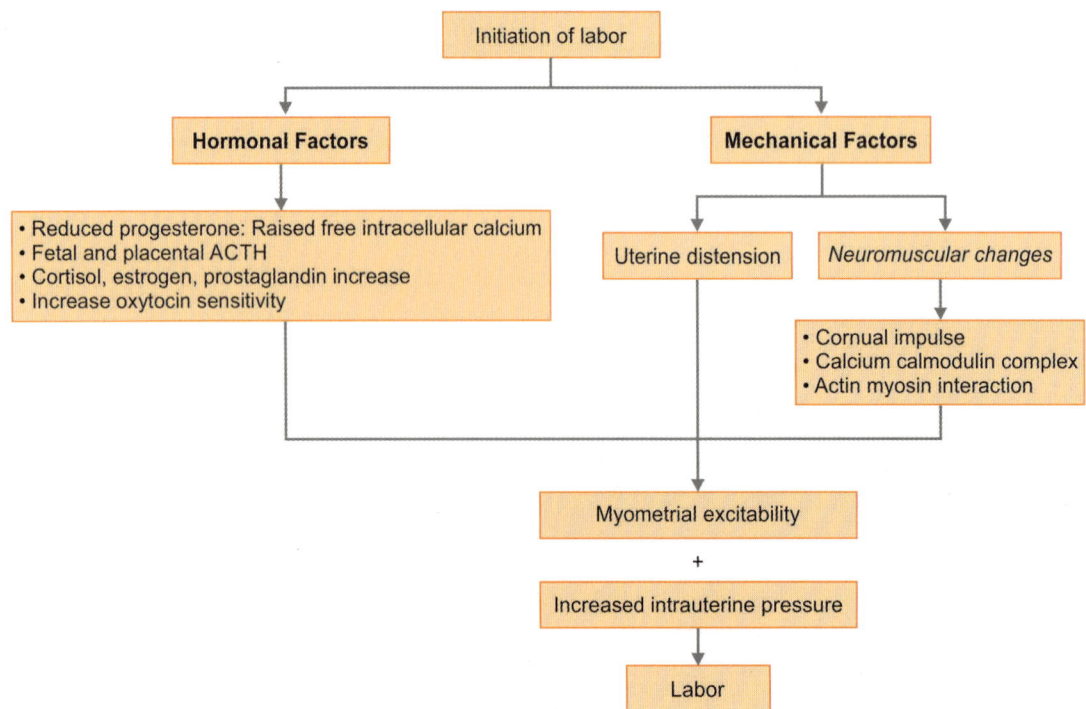

Flowchart 1: Initiation of labor.

of progesterone—fetal cortisol promotes the placental production of estrogens and prostaglandins. Thus, the prevailing *progesterone dominance* of pregnancy is replaced with *estrogen dominance*. Estrogens promote myometrial excitability by promoting sensitivity to oxytocin, and myometrial synthesis of contractile proteins *actin* and myosin through cAMP. Estrogens favor the formation of gap junctions, release of oxytocin from the maternal pituitary and promoting the synthesis of oxytocin receptors in the myometrium and decidua. Estrogens also promote prostaglandin synthesis.

CLINICAL CORRELATION

Primigravidae often feel a *lightening* sensation weeks before the onset of labor because of the *passive descent* of the fetal head and its engagement in the pelvis. The formation and defining of the lower uterine segment is particularly evident in primigravidae. Following fetal head decent, the uterus tilts forward (*shelving sign*) thereby reducing pressure on the diaphragm and easing breathing.[1]

The rising levels of endogenous circulating levels of oxytocin and prostaglandins promote *cervical ripening* (alteration in structure of the cervix – decrease in collagen, glycosaminoglycans, an increase in hyaluronic acid and decrease in dermatan sulfate). The softened cervix becomes more yielding. Clinically manifested by cervical effacement and shortening, dilation and increase in mucus discharge. As term approaches, the painless uterine contractions become increasingly painful, there may be show. On examination, there is evidence of cervical dilation and formation of the bag of waters. The uterine contractions progressively increase in intensity and frequency.

Neuromuscular changes: The uterus is in a state of minimal activity when at rest. This is known as baseline uterine tonus or tone. It is usually < 5 mm Hg in pregnancy at rest. Labor is postulated to begin from one or both uterine cornua. These cornua possess potential pacemakers near the ostia, which initiate contractions. The binding of calcium to calmodulin within the myometrial muscle results in the activation of myosin light chain kinase, which causes phosphorylation of myosin. This leads to the interaction of actin and myosin, two muscle proteins, resulting in a contraction. As a result of the contraction, the amniotic pressure within the uterus increases above 25 mm Hg reaching a peak of 45–90 mm Hg in active labor.

Uterine activity is measured in terms of Montevideo units (Barcia et al. Montivideo, Uruguay; 1960). A Montevideo unit is the pressure generated by all uterine contractions in a period of 10 minutes after subtracting baseline pressure from peak contraction pressure. Activity at the beginning of labor is 80–120 Montevideo units and 200–300 Montevideo units in established labor. During initial labor the frequency and duration of uterine contractions is between 5 and 10 minutes and 20–40 seconds respectively. Over time, frequency and duration of uterine contractions increases to 3–5 per 10 minutes and for 60–80 seconds, respectively.

MECHANISM OF NORMAL LABOR

Here the mechanism in only the most common presentation, that is, vertex is discussed.

This is described as the series movements occurring on the fetal head and its adaptation vis-à-vis the maternal pelvis during downward descent along the axis of the birth canal (J-shaped–Curve of Carus) during the process of birth **(Fig. 1)**.

Summary of landmark events:
- Descent and engagement
- Flexion
- Internal rotation
- Extension
- Restitution
- External rotation
- Lateral flexion.

Descent and Engagement

As mentioned earlier, passive descent of the fetal head occurring weeks before the actual onset of labor is a common observation in primigravida. However, in multiparae, these may only occur following true onset of labor. The process of descent is promoted by the increasing intra-amniotic pressure causing formation of the bag of waters, steadily increasing cervical effacement and dilation. The engaging fetal head diameter (suboccipitobregmatic) measuring 9.5 cm engages in the right oblique or transverse diameter of the pelvic inlet in completely flexed vertex presentation. The transverse diameter of engagement is biparietal (9.5 cm).

In normal labor, the fetal head is not exactly in the center (termed asynclitism). It can either be anterior asynclitism (Naegele's s obliquity) wherein the anterior parietal bone lies below or posterior asynclitism (Litzmann obliquity) in which the posterior parietal bone lies below. Posterior asynclitism

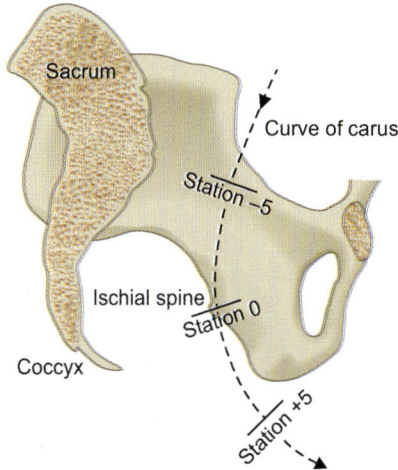

Fig. 1: Path taken by the fetus along the curve of carus.

is more common in primigravida and possibly takes place due to the strong anterior abdominal wall, which pushes the uterus posteriorly. In about a quarter of the cases synclitism (wherein the sagittal suture is exactly at the center between the symphysis and sacral promontory) may be seen.

Flexion

As the descending fetal head meets increasing resistance from the maternal soft tissues, it undergoes *flexion*. The atlanto-occipital joint of the fetal skull (fulcrum) is located off-center and is closer to the occiput. The shorter posterior arm (from the fulcrum to the occiput) descends and the longer anterior arm (from the fulcrum to the chin) ascends thereby making the occiput lower than the forehead, leading to flexion of the fetal head (Two arm lever theory). In the left occiput anterior (LOA or Vertex-1 position), the fetal head (occiput) occupies the left anterior quadrant of the pelvis **(Fig. 2)**. With further pains the head continues to descend until it reaches the pelvic floor.

The downward thrust exerted by the myometrium (fundal dominance) along the axis of the birth canal leads to passive stretching out of the lower uterine segment followed by progressive dilation of the cervix. The straightening of the fetal body enhances the effects of the downward thrust of myometrial contractions to propel and rotate the fetus along the axis of the birth canal. During the second stage of labor, maternal bearing down efforts further supplement the process of fetal descent.

Internal Rotation

Rotation of the fetal head occurs at the level of the ischial spines, when the descending fetal head meets with resistance from the sloping pelvic floor (levatores ani muscle sling, the two halves of the pelvic floor separated by the hiatus urogenitalis constitute a gutter like slope pointing downward –forward – and inward toward the midline). It causes twisting of the fetal neck to enable the engaging fetal diameter to rotate from the oblique to the anteroposterior diameter of the pelvis bringing the occiput under the pubic arch.

Additionally, the fetal head follows the law of accommodation of the maternal pelvis. The pelvic inlet is oval in the transverse plane, the midpelvis is round and outlet is oval in the anteroposterior plane. Further, the pelvic floor is deficient anteriorly under the wide pubic arch allowing the occiput to move into the area of least resistance. Differences in flexibility of fetal parts also contributes to internal rotation: law of unequal flexibility.[2]

Extension

Eventually the head of the fetus reaches the perineum causing it to bulge (crowning). The anal opening dilates, the fourchette thins out and vulval stretching takes place.

With further contraction, and maternal bearing down efforts, the occiput is born, the fetal neck pivots under the subpubic arch and the rest of the fetal head is born by extension. This occurs because of resultant vector of two forces, one which is uterine contractions pushing the head in a downward manner against the second force, the resistant pelvic floor muscles and pubic symphysis which directs the fetal head in an upward and outward manner.

Restitution

With the expulsion of the fetal head, the twisted fetal neck (torsion) untwists, the occiput thus turns to the mothers left side. This takes place by 1/8 of circle (45 degrees) in the direction opposite to internal rotation, the fetus attempting to undo the adaptations it has undergone during labor.

External Rotation

Following the delivery of the fetal head, the fetal shoulders lying in the opposite oblique diameter of the pelvis reaches the pelvic floor. The anterior shoulder rotates under the

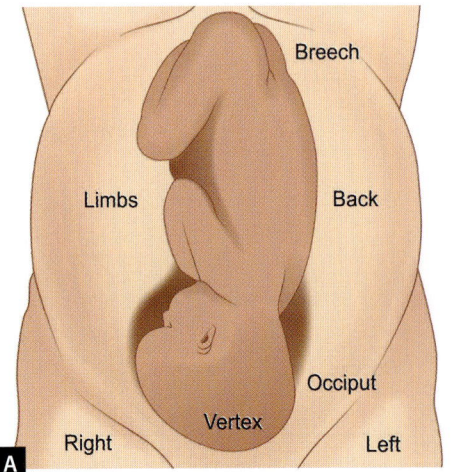
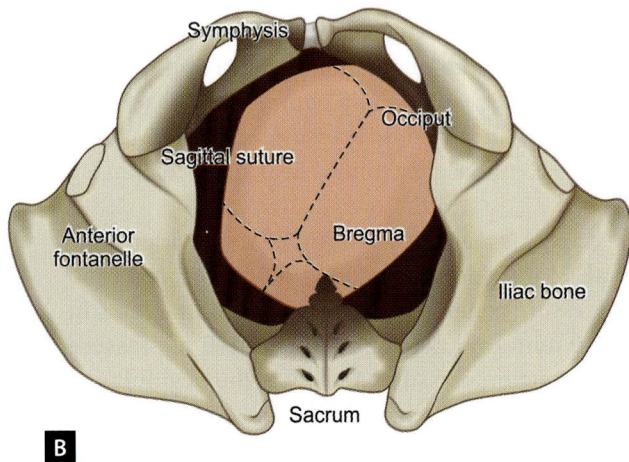

Figs. 2A and B: Left occiput anterior (LOA) vertex 1 position.

pubic arch. During external rotation, rotation by 1/8 of circle occurs in the direction of restitution. It is the counter action to internal rotation of the shoulders and results in fetal head rotating by another 45° so that the occiput lies in the left occipitotransverse position and the face toward the right thigh of the mother.

Lateral Flexion and Shoulder Delivery

After the bisacromial diameter of the fetus enters the pelvic inlet obliquely, the anterior shoulder engages in the AP diameter of the pelvic outlet and is delivered by lateral flexion, similarly followed by the posterior shoulder and the rest of the body **(Flowchart 2)**.

Influence of Pelvic Architecture on Mechanism of Labor

Caldwell and Moloy[3] described the configuration of the female pelvis and classified pelvic shapes into four basic types. Variations and combination of features have also been observed.

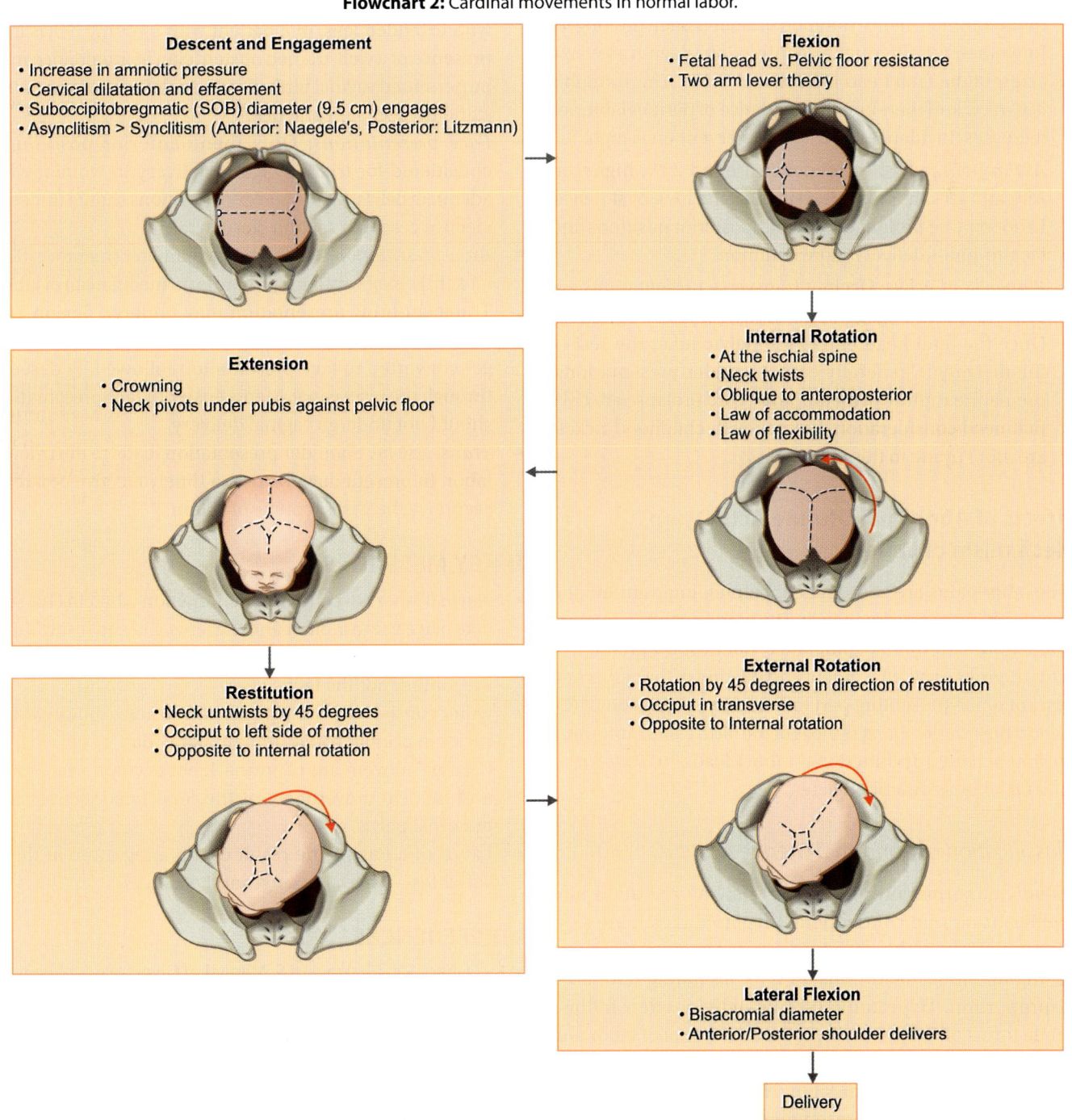

Flowchart 2: Cardinal movements in normal labor.

The pelvic shape can influence the outcome of labor. A brief review of labor outcomes in relation to pelvic configuration follows:

- *Gynecoid pelvis:* Incidence is about 50%. This is the ideal pelvic configuration to result in safe vaginal delivery. The small gynecoid pelvis displays a similar configuration except that all pelvic diameters are proportionately reduced. This is often seen in women with a short stature. If there is no cephalopelvic disproportion – normal delivery can be expected.
- *Android pelvis:* Incidence is around 25%. The forepelvis is narrow, the brim is heart-shaped, midpelvis and outlet are narrower (funnel pelvis). Occipitoposterior position are more common, hence duration of labor is often prolonged. In women with midpelvic contraction, deep transverse arrest of the fetal head is known to occur. The subpubis is narrow and therefore the incidence of perineal injuries increases. Incidence of obstetric intervention is high.
- *Anthropoid pelvis:* Incidence is around 20%, higher in African races. It is also described as the long oval pelvis. Labor may be prolonged, occipitoposterior positions and face-to-pubis delivery more common.
- *Platypelloid pelvis:* Occiput transverse presentations are common, late engagement, asynclitism are common. Once the fetal head enters the pelvic inlet, the rest of the delivery is generally easy. Shoulder presentations, premature rupture of membranes, cord prolapse are risks that need consideration. Women with childhood rickets are more prone to this disorder.

Effects of Abnormal Uterine Activity on Mechanism of Labor

True labor pains are coordinated, painful, intermittent and occur with increasing frequency. The uterine contractions are characterized by fundal dominance, diminishing gradient of activity, progressive effacement and dilation of the cervix and descent of the presenting part followed by propulsion of the fetus to the exterior along the axis of the birth canal. Abnormal uterine activity (dysfunctional labor) leads to *dystocia* or difficult labor as described here.

Classification of Abnormal Uterine Activity

Broadly abnormal uterine activity may be classified into inefficient uterine contractions (hypotonia) causing slow progress of labor. This may be corrected by amniotomy, or setting up an oxytocin infusion after excluding fetopelvic disproportion. Hypertonic uterine activity often follows subtle forms of fetopelvic disproportion. A trial of labor and close monitoring of the fetal wellbeing under well-supervised conditions may be permissible. However, timely surgical intervention is otherwise recommended.

Effects of Fetal Malposition and Malpresentations on the Mechanism of Labor

- *Occipitoposterior malposition:* In women with a roomy pelvis, the fetal head would go through a long internal rotation and deliver vaginally. However, the duration of labor would be prolonged. In women with an android pelvis, midpelvic contraction may pose a problem and cause deep transverse arrest of the fetal head necessitating obstetric intervention. In women with an anthropoid pelvis – labor may be somewhat tardy. The fetus delivers *face-to-pubis*. There is increased risk of injury to the maternal soft parts and perineum.
- *Breech presentation:* In present day practice, breech with extended legs, in a patient with a roomy pelvis and presence of a well-trained obstetrician in attendance may be permitted vaginal birth. Cesarean delivery at term is the standard accepted practice.
- *Face presentations:* Only mentoanterior position is considered for trial of vaginal delivery in women with adequate pelvis. Mentoposterior positions should undergo elective cesarean section close to term.
- *Brow presentation:* The engaging diameter (mentovertical – 14 cm) being very large—there is no mechanism of labor. Transient brow presentation may undergo flexion and convert to vertex presentation or undergo extension to get converted to face presentation followed by descent through the birth canal. Mentoposterior face presentation should not undergo vaginal delivery.
- *Transverse lie:* Shoulder presentation leads to obstructed labor. In present day practice, a timely elective cesarean section is the wisest course of action.[4-6]

KEY MESSAGES

- Normal labor is a complex phenomenon wherein changes take place in the mother and the fetus, the end result being the delivery of the fetus with no complications in either the mother nor the fetus.
- Labor consists of a latent phase and an active phase which varies in primigravidae and multigravida.
- Cardinal movements of normal labor occur in a sequence and involve movements of the fetal head against the maternal pelvis.
- Labor outcome is the result of the integration of three variables—*power, passenger* and *passages*.

REFERENCES

1. Daftary SN, Chakravarti S. Manual of Obstetrics, 2nd edition. New Delhi: Elsevier Pvt. Ltd., 1998.
2. Sharma JB. Textbook of Obstetrics, 2nd edition. New Delhi: Avichal Publishers Pvt. Ltd.; 2017.
3. Caldwell WE, Moloy HC. Anatomical variations in the female pelvis and their effect on labour with a suggested classification. Am J Obst Gynecol. 1933;26:479.

4. Oxorn H, Foote W. Human Labor and Birth, 6th edition. New York: McGraw Hill Medical; 2013.
5. Cunningham G, Leveno K, Bloom S, Hauth H, Rouse D, Spong C. Williams Obstetrics, 23rd edition. New York: McGraw Hill Medical; 2010.
6. Norwitz ER, Robinson JN, Challis JR. Control of Labor. N Engl J Med. 1999;341:660-6.

LONG QUESTIONS

1. Describe the mechanism of normal labor.
2. Describe the alterations in the mechanism of labor due to alterations in pelvic configuration.
3. Describe the mechanism of labor in occipitoposterior presentations.
4. Describe the biochemical and anatomical changes that precede the onset of labor.

SHORT QUESTIONS

1. Explain lower segment of uterus.
2. Explain curve of carus.
3. List the sequence of cardinal movements of normal labor.
4. List the causes of internal rotation.
5. What is cervical ripening?
6. Explain engagement.
7. Explain the four basic shapes of the female pelvis.

MULTIPLE CHOICE QUESTIONS

1. The engaging diameter in a brow presentation is:
   a. Mento vertical
   b. Suboccipito-bregmatic
   c. Bitrochanteric
   d. Submento-bregmatic
2. If the engaging diameter is subocciptiobregmatic, the presentation is:
   a. Breech
   b. Face
   c. Brow
   d. Vertex
3. The denominator for a face presentation is:
   a. Nasion
   b. Glabellum
   c. Occiput
   d. Mentum
4. Average duration of the second stage of labour in primigravida lasts about:
   a. 1 hour
   b. 2 hours
   c. 4 hours
   d. None of the above
5. Fetal flexibility refers to:
   a. Engagement and descent
   b. Internal rotation
   c. Restitution
   d. External Rotation
6. Suboccipitobregmatic diameter measures:
   a. 8.5 cm
   b. 9.5 cm
   c. 10.5 cm
   d. 11.5 cm
7. Pacemakers of the uterus lie in:
   a. Cornua
   b. Body
   c. Cervix
   e. Fallopian tube
8. Bisacromial diameter makes the following movement during normal labor:
   a. Oblique to AP
   b. AP to transverse
   c. AP to PA
   d. Transverse to oblique
9. Untwisting of the fetal head is:
   a. External rotation
   b. Internal Rotation
   c. Restitution
   d. Lateral flexion
10. False about Asynclitism:
    a. Posterior asynclitism is when anterior parietal bone lies below
    b. Anterior asynclitism is when anterior parietal bone lies above
    c. Both a and b
    d. None of the above

Answers
1. a 2. d 3. d 4. a 5. b 6. b
7. a 8. b 9. c 10. b

9.2 LABOR IN MALPOSITION AND MALPRESENTATIONS

Sareena Gilvaz

OCCIPITOPOSTERIOR POSITION

Introduction

Occipitoanterior and posterior positions are both vertex presentations.

In occipitoposterior (OP), the occiput is in relation to the posterior quadrant of the pelvis opposite to the sacroiliac joint. Though most OP could have a normal course, this is often referred to as malposition because it can at times cause dystocia in labor. And in that, right occipitoposterior position (ROP) occurs five times more commonly than the left because of the dextrorotation of the uterus and the presence of the sigmoid colon which occupies the left posterior segment of the pelvis.

Incidence

Occipitoposterior is seen in 25–30% of vertex presentations at the onset of labor and only 5–10% persists as OP at the time of delivery. This is because, as labor progresses, over 90% turn into an anterior position and deliver normally

Causes and Problems Associated with Occipital Posterior

- *Pelvic shape*: Two abnormal types of pelvis associated with OP (in 50% of cases) are the android and the anthropoid pelvis. In both these types of pelvis, the fore pelvis is narrow, and the back of the head with its broad biparietal diameter gets pushed to the back of the pelvis resulting in an OP position.

When OP occurs in association with an anthropoid pelvis, the occiput undergoes a reverse rotation through 45° into the hollow of the sacrum resulting in a direct OP position and the resultant delivery is by face to pubes.

When OP occurs in an android pelvis during internal rotation, due to lack of space in the anterior segment of the pelvis, labor gets arrested in the transverse position. This is often referred to as "Deep Transverse Arrest."

- *Deflexion of head seen in OP position*: Another problem apart from the pelvic shape is the deflexed attitude of the fetal head. This is because the convex curvature of the fetal spine is in apposition with the convex curvature of the maternal spine. These results are various degrees of deflexion of the fetal head. The presenting diameter is thus increased:
  - Occiptiofrontal 11.5 cm (when there is more severe degree of deflexion).
  - Suboccipito frontal 10.5 cm (with lesser degree of deflexion).

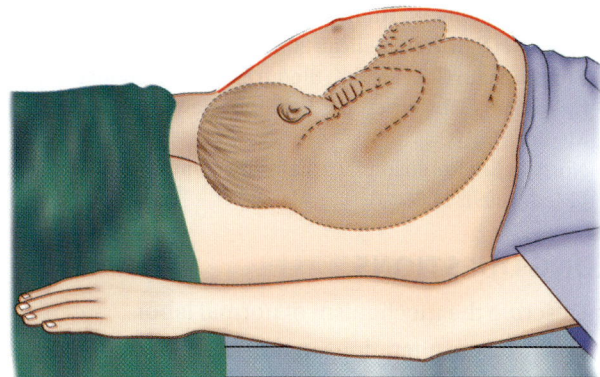

Fig. 1: Abdominal contour in occipitoposterior position.

Diagnosis of Occipitoposterior Position: On Abdominal Examination

- There is subumbilical flattening on inspection. This is because the fetal back is away from the midline and toward the flank. Hence, the curved anterior curvature of the uterus is lacking (**Fig. 1**).
- Breech occupies the fundus.
- The fetal limbs are made out more anteriorly and an either side of the midline, as the back is toward the flank.
- The head being deflexed, the occiput and sinciput are felt at the same level. This is called military attitude of the fetus.
- The anterior shoulder is also felt at a higher level and further away from the midline.
- Fetal heart sounds (FHS) are heard more posteriorly and toward the flanks.

On PV examination with the membranes ruptured, the landmarks to be noted are:

The sagittal suture is in one of the oblique diameters, e.g., in ROP, the sagittal suture is in the right oblique diameter of the pelvis. The anterior fontanelle is felt easily in one or other of the anterior quadrants of the pelvis (**Fig. 2**), while the posterior fontanelle is in the opposite posterior quadrant.

Mechanism of Labor

Mechanism of Labor involves the following movements: Engaging diameter in OP is occipitofrontal 11.5 cm—(1) descent, (2) flexion, (3) long internal rotation through 135°, (4) extension, (5) restitution, and (6) external rotation of head.

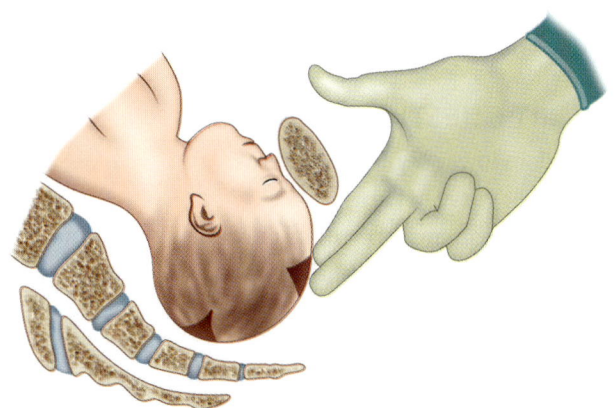

Fig. 2: In occipitoposterior, the anterior fontanelle is easily felt in the anterior quadrant on PV.

Course of Labor

The course is the same as in an occipitoanterior position, except that, there is undue delay in the progress of labor due to the deflexed attitude of the head and also because of the long internal rotation that has to take place to effect normal delivery (**Flowchart 1 and Fig. 3**). Thus, we see the following eventualities:

- *Anterior rotation*: In over 90%, the occiput rotates anteriorly through 135° and is born normally, though it takes a longer time for this, thus causing a prolonged labor.
- *Reverse rotation*: Many a times, especially when the pelvis is anthropoid and the head is deflexed, the sinciput being the leading part touches the pelvic floor first and rotates anteriorly.

The occiput thus takes a reverse rotation into the hollow of the sacrum through 45° and becomes a direct occipitoposterior and here the delivery is affected as face to pubes. In this, the root of nose or sinciput hitches under the pubic symphysis, and there is first extreme flexion whereby the occiput is born (i.e., the forehead, bregma, vertex, and occiput are born). This is followed by extreme extension and the face is born (i.e., the nose, mouth, and chin are born). In face to pubes delivery, the larger biparietal diameter of the fetal head, thus, distends the perineum causing deep perineal lacerations. Therefore,

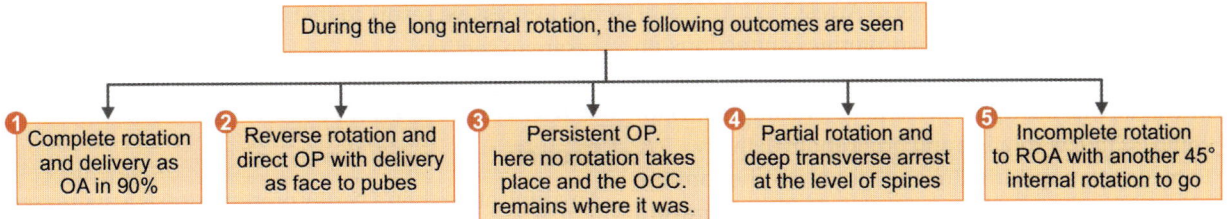

Flowchart 1: Outcomes of long internal rotation.

During the long internal rotation, the following outcomes are seen

1. Complete rotation and delivery as OA in 90%
2. Reverse rotation and direct OP with delivery as face to pubes
3. Persistent OP. here no rotation takes place and the OCC. remains where it was.
4. Partial rotation and deep transverse arrest at the level of spines
5. Incomplete rotation to ROA with another 45° internal rotation to go

(OA: occipitoanterior; OCC: occipital cortex; OP: occipitoposterior; ROA: right occipitoanterior)

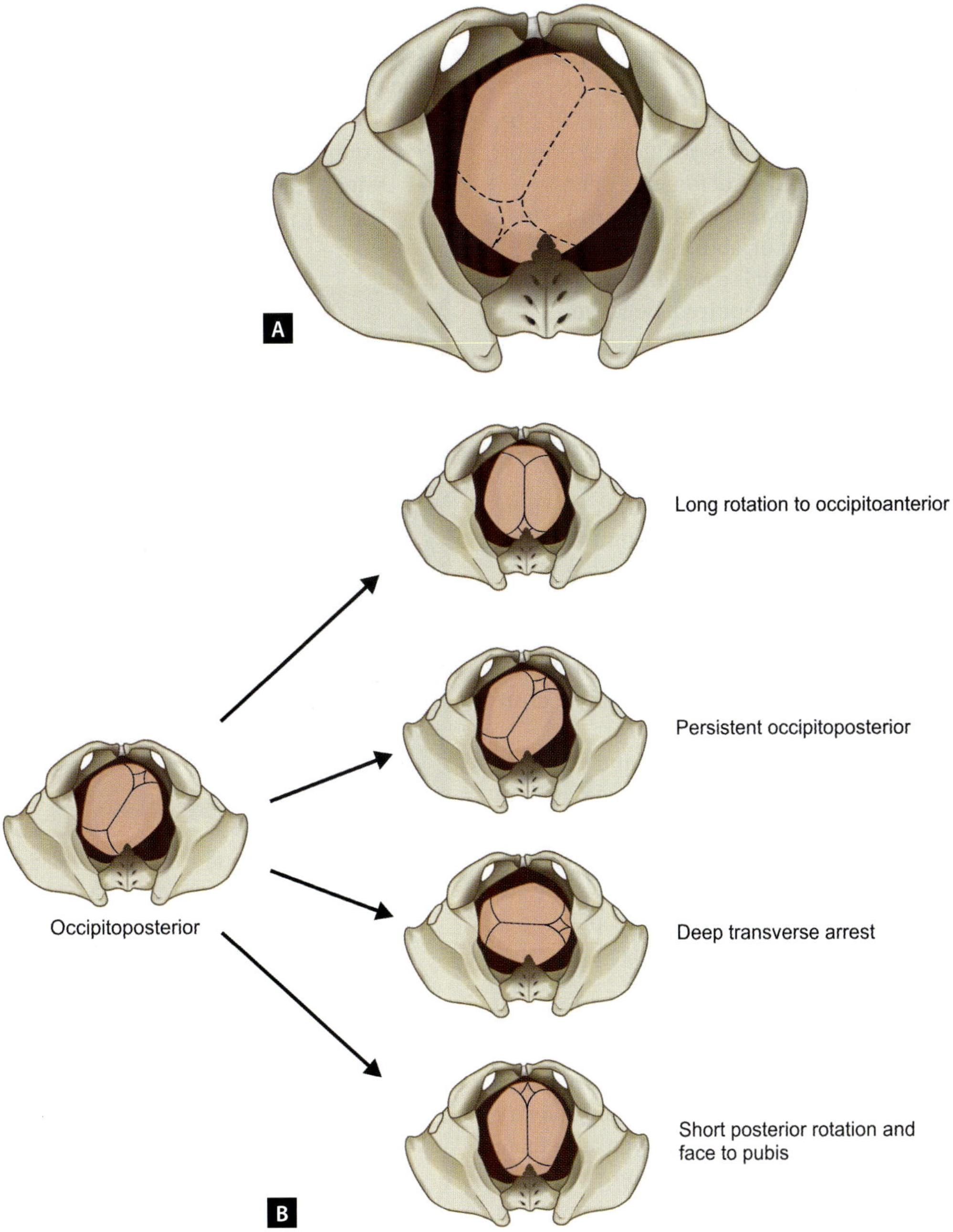

Figs. 3A and B: Vaginal view of right occiput posterior.

as a preventive measure a liberal episiotomy should be given in this situation.

- *Deep transverse arrest (DTA)*: In OP which it is associated with an android pelvis, the space available anteriorly is less due to beaking of the fore pelvis. In this situation, the head during internal rotation gets arrested in the pelvis in the transverse position. The sagittal suture is parallel to the transverse diameter of the pelvis at the level of the ischial spines and in spite of good uterine contractions and with the cervix fully

dilated, there is no progress in labor. This condition is referred to as "Deep Transverse Arrest."
- If this occurs due to inadequate uterine contractions, an oxytocin drip might help complete rotation. If it happens in a multi, who has a poor pelvic floor, a vacuum extractor could complete rotation and bring about delivery.
- Forceps rotation with Kielland's is yet another option. But if the cause is in the pelvis such as an android variety or if there is cephalopelvic disproportion due to a disproportionately large baby, then a cesarean would be a safe option. But if the baby is dead a craniotomy can also be done to effect delivery.

Management in 1st stage:
- Anticipate a longer labor than usual when it is OP. She, therefore, will also require a lot of psychological support in this situation, which we must not forget to offer.
- A partogram should also be maintained (This would help diagnosis of secondary arrest of labor).
- Adequate hydration is vital as it is a prolonged labor.
- Effective analgesia is often required because of the protracted labor and also to prevent premature straining. Pressure on the rectum by the wide occiput results in a premature desire to strain even before full dilatation. This very often exhausts the patient. Hence, an epidural analgesia would be ideal.

Management in 2nd stage: Is also prolonged as the long internal rotation occurs at this stage and many a time an arrest can also occur as has been mentioned above.

The options for operative vaginal delivery in persistent OP or in DTA in the second stage are:
- Manual rotation of fetal head under general anesthesia (GA) followed by forceps application (not often done nowadays).
- Rotational forceps delivery using the Kielland's forceps would be ideal. It is commonly used in the United Kingdom and less so in India.
- Forceps applied to a direct OP is well accepted **(Fig. 4)**. Only make sure that all the prerequisites for forceps are met, especially that no pole should be palpable per abdomen and the head should be low enough preferably at +2 stations or below.
- Rotational vacuum is a very viable option and often tried in this situation as it produces autorotation and delivery.
- The choice of the above depends on the expertise of the operator, keeping in mind that a difficult vaginal delivery should be avoided at all costs. Therefore, if you anticipate any problem, e.g., as in cephalopelvic disproportion, it would be best to resort to an immediate cesarean section for the benefit of both the mother and baby.

Neonatal outcome: The neonatal outcomes have also been adversely affected in OP position such as poor apgar scores, fetal acidosis, meconium staining of AF, increased risk of birth trauma and increased neonatal intensive care unit (NICU) admission.

Therefore in conclusion, OP positions are often associated with prolonged labor, with increased perineal trauma and increased risk of operative interventions which include both excessive resort to instrumental vaginal deliveries and cesarean section.

■ MALPRESENTATIONS IN LABOR

Breech

Anything other than a vertex presentation is a malpresentation and breech is the most common among malpresentations.

Incidence of breech at term is around 3–4%.

Types of breech:
- *Complete breech:* 5–10%, where universal flexion is maintained.
- *Incomplete breech:*
  - Extended or frank breech **(Fig. 5A)**: 70–75%
  - Knee presentation **(Fig. 5B)**
  - Footling presentation **(Fig. 5C)**.

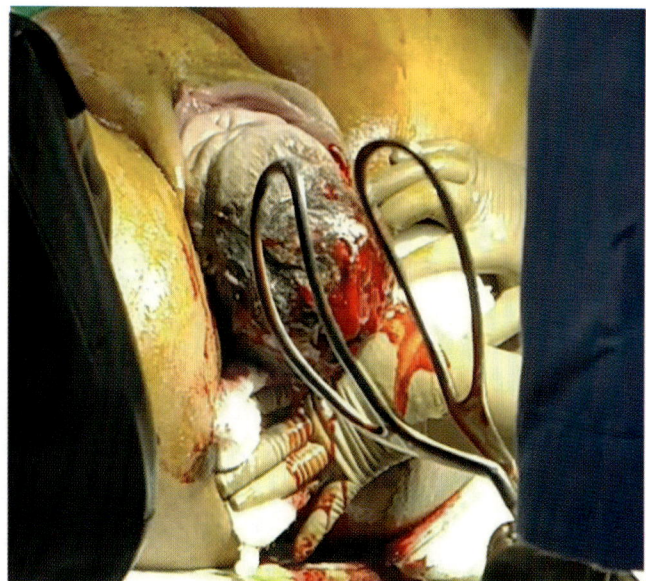

Fig. 4: Occipitoposterior position resulting in a face to pubes delivery by forceps.

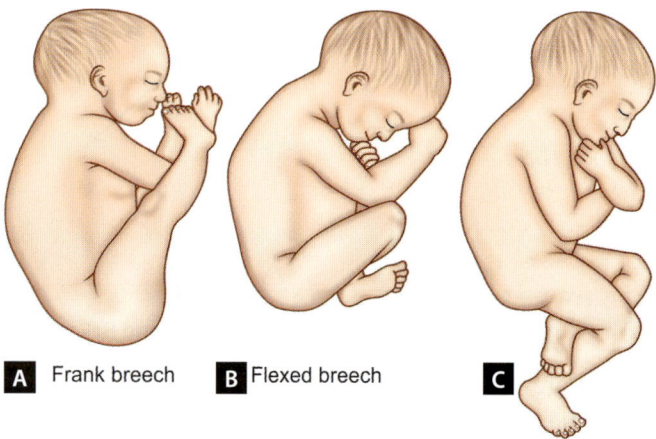

Figs. 5A to C: (A) Frank breech; (B) Flexed breech; (C) Footling presentation.

Managing a breech in labor is different from that of a vertex for the following reasons:
- Breech engages late.
- It is a poor dilator of the cervix.
- The easily compressible soft parts are born first and the unyielding head comes out later.
- There is no time for the after coming head to mold.
- In preterm babies, the disproportionately large head causes head entrapment after the body has slipped out.
- Incidence of cord compression, presentation, and prolapse is more in a breech.
  E.g.,:
  - In footling breech, 15% is the incidence of cord prolapse.
  - In flexed breech, it is 5%.
  - In extended breech, it is 0.5%.

Mechanism of delivery in a breech is divided into:
- Mechanism of delivery of buttocks
- Mechanism of delivery of shoulder
- Mechanism of delivery of head.

Mechanism of labor in breech presentation: Breech is a longitudinal lie with the podalic pole presenting at the pelvic brim. Sacrum is the denominator and presents in four positions: (1) Left sacroanterior, (2) right sacroanterior (3) right sacroposterior, (4) left sacroposterior, of which left sacroanterior is the most common.

Mechanism of delivery of the buttocks: The presenting diameter is the bitrochanteric, and is about 10 cm. And in a left sacroanterior, it occupies the left oblique diameter of the pelvis.

Descent: It is the first movement with increasing compaction of the buttocks.

Internal rotation: Then when the anterior buttocks touch the pelvic floor, it undergoes internal rotation through one eighth of a circle and it comes to lie behind the symphysis. Then the anterior buttocks hinge behind the symphysis pubis and the posterior buttocks is born followed by the anterior.

Lateral flexion: The body undergoes lateral flexion, sweeps out and is born.

Restitution of buttocks takes place.

Mechanism of delivery of the shoulder: The bisacromial diameter of the shoulder engages in the same oblique diameter as that of the buttocks, namely the left oblique diameter.

Internal rotation: Then the anterior shoulder undergoes internal rotation through one eighth of a circle thereby it comes to lie in the anteroposterior diameter of the pelvis.

Lateral flexion: The anterior shoulder hitches against the pubic symphysis then the posterior shoulder is born followed by the anterior shoulder.

Restitution of shoulders takes place next.

Mechanism of the Delivery of the Head

Engagement: The head now engages in the opposite oblique diameter namely, the right oblique diameter by the suboccipito-bregmatic diameter.

Internal rotation takes place next through one eighth of a circle and as such the occiput comes to lie under the symphysis pubis.

Delivery by flexion: The occiput hitches against the symphysis pubis and by a process of flexion the head is born.

Modes of Vaginal Breech Delivery

- *Spontaneous breech delivery:* Here, the fetus is expelled spontaneously without any assistance or manipulations. Chances of fetal complications are more in such deliveries.
- *Assisted breech delivery (partial breech extraction):* Here, the fetus is delivered spontaneously as far as the umbilicus, after which, the fetus is born with assistance. This is the most common mode of vaginal delivery.
- *Breech extraction (total breech extraction):* Here the fetus is extracted in toto by the obstetrician under GA. This might be required in situations of severe maternal distress or with acute fetal distress such as a cord prolapse. This should be carried out only in dire emergencies when a cesarean cannot be performed quickly and the baby too must be delivered immediately or following internal podalic version in second of twin.

Ideal Patients for Assisted Breech Delivery

Proper selection of cases is crucial for the success of a vaginal breech delivery.
- A patient without any maternal or fetal contraindication for vaginal birth
- Adequacy of maternal pelvis
- Average-sized baby weighing between 1.5 and 3.5 kg.
- An extended breech is preferred as it mimics a head and fits well into the pelvis.
- Fortunately, an extended breech is the most frequent and the most common variety occurring in a primi due to the good tone of the uterine muscles and the tight abdominal wall.
- It occurs in over 50–60% of breech presentation.
- Good to have a well-flexed head because when there is hyperextension of the fetal head it may cause injury to the fetal cervical spine and cord during the delivery of the after coming head.
- The success of a vaginal breech delivery is more when it is associated with spontaneous onset of pains. Augmentation of labor in breech is a much debated issue, as satisfactory progress of labor is the best indicator of pelvic adequacy.

Indications for an Elective Cesarean Section

- Complicated breech, when breech is associated with comorbidities such as hypertension, and diabetes.
- Elderly primi and patients with a bad obstetric history.
- Big breech > 3.5 kg to avoid fetopelvic disproportion.
- Premature breech < 1.5 kg is better delivered by cesarean section to avoid the risk of hypoxia in labor and an untimely cord prolapse. More than that, the danger of fetal head entrapment due to the relatively larger head in relation to the body is there with the after coming head of a premature breech.

- Footling presentation, because of the increased incidence of cord prolapse.
- Hyperextended or a star gazing head.
- Severe fetal growth restriction (FGR) in breech presentation.
- Contracted pelvis or a border line pelvis.

Management of Breech in Labor

- The risk versus benefits of a vaginal breech delivery must be discussed with the patient and her relatives.
- The success will depend upon properly selected cases and good monitoring. There should also be facilities for an immediate cesarean delivery should the need arise.
- An anesthetist should be available to ensure good analgesia/anesthesia when required.
- A good backup neonatology team to handle the newborn.
- Last but not the least, the experience and expertise of the obstetrician are vital for a successful outcome.

1st stage of labor
- The patient is best observed in the bed.
- A continuous electronic monitoring would be ideal otherwise at least every 15 minutes.
- FH monitoring is essential in the I stage.
- Hydration is better maintained by intravenous fluids instead of oral.
- Epidural analgesia would be ideal.
- Retain her membranes tell the end. But if it ruptures early, a PV must to done to rule out cord prolapse.
- The progress of labor is carefully monitored with respect to descent and cervical dilatation.
- If there is an arrest in either of these, it is best tackled by a cesarean section.

Indications for an emergency cesarean in labor would be for the following:
- Arrest in progress of labor
- Cord prolapse
- Nonreassuring fetal heart rate (FHR) pattern.

2nd stage:
- When the cervix is fully dilated, the patient is shifted to the labor table.
- Preferred position is lithotomy (i.e., the patient is brought to the edge of the table and the legs are put up on stirrups). This is the best position to assist birth and to handle complications during delivery.
- Make sure the bladder is empty.
- Good to have an IV infusion on flow and preferably with oxytocin in it, so as to have regular and effective uterine contractions.
- An experienced obstetrician and her assistant are scrubbed and ready.
- The patient is encouraged to bear down with every contraction.
- As the breech is seen climbing the perineum and the perineum is adequately thinned out under a pudendal block or under local infiltration a mediolateral episiotomy is given.
- Now comes the time for masterly inactivity. Just observe till the umbilicus is born. Once the umbilicus is born, the things that have to be done are:
  - Make sure the back of the baby is facing the obstetrician (that way, the occiput will come to an anterior position).
  - Knuckle of cord if any is pushed up to prevent it from getting compressed.
  - Next wrap the baby's abdomen with a sterile drape so that the cold air does not cause premature respiration and thereby aspiration, as the head is yet to be born.
- Now the fetus is held by the femoropelvic grip, i.e., the fingers are over the anterior superior iliac crest and the thumb over the sacrum—thus minimizing soft-tissue injury of the fetal abdominal viscera.
- The cardinal rule at this point is "DO NOT PULL." If the baby is pulled then it can lead to deflexion of the head and extension of the arms. By gentle rotatory movements, the body slips out further and further and is born.

Delivery of the shoulders: At this point, a good clue to know if the arms are flexed is, to make sure that the medial border of the scapula is parallel to the vertebral column. If the arms are extended, then there will be winging of the scapula

Next once the axilla is seen, the arms are delivered just by lifting the baby and hooking down each elbow. It makes little difference as to which shoulder is delivered first. After the arms are out, the baby is allowed to hang down so that aided by gravity and by its weight the head enters the pelvis.

Delivery of the after coming head: This is the most important and challenging stage in the delivery of a breech. The baby is allowed to hang by its own weight for 1-2 minutes.

Through all this time, an assistant gives suprapubic pressure to promote flexion of the fetal head. This is also called the Kristellar maneuver.

Once the nape of the neck is seen, the baby is grasped by its ankles with a finger between the two. With steady traction, the baby is swept over the mother's abdomen so that the head is born by flexion. This technique of delivery of the after coming head is referred to as the Marshall Burn's technique.

Other method of delivery of head is Mauriceau-Smellie-Veit technique **(Fig. 6)**: This procedure entails suprapubic pressure by an assistant while the obstetrician inserts left hand in the vagina, palpating the fetal maxilla using the index and middle finger and gently pressing on the maxilla, bringing the neck to a moderate flexion. The left palm should rest against the fetus's chest, while the right hand can grab either shoulder of the fetus and give downward traction.

Forceps application to deliver the head: Piper's forceps have long shanks with backward curve dropping the handles well below the level of the blades, are used to deliver the after coming head of the baby. This would probably be the best way to deliver the after coming head in a breech. Even though the recommended forceps is the Piper's forceps, any long forceps would do. The forceps application should be from below. So the first step is to lift the baby up and in order to prevent its hands from dangling, a sterile towel is used to wrap the trunk and the arms together and to aid in the lift of the baby up. Now the forceps can be applied from below. *Note*: The forceps is applied from above only when the head is in an OP position.

Advantages of forceps for the after coming head:
- The traction is directly on the head of the baby rather than its neck **(Fig. 7)**.
- It also allows a very controlled delivery of the head.
- Flexion of the head is maintained by this procedure.
- The baby can also breathe because of the space created by the blades.

The time interval between delivery of the umbilicus to delivery of the head should not be more than 5-7 minutes.

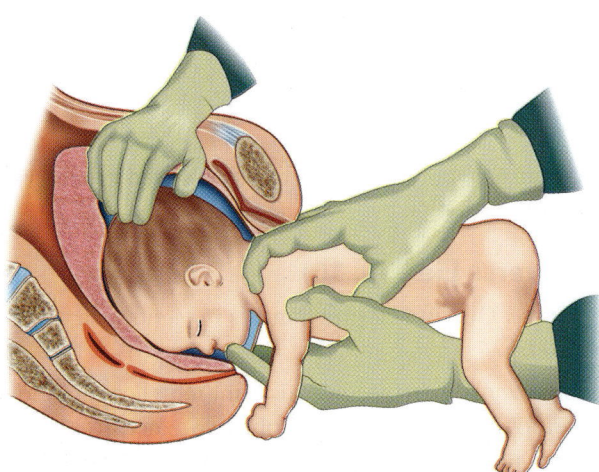

Fig. 6: Mauriceau–Smellie–Veit technique.

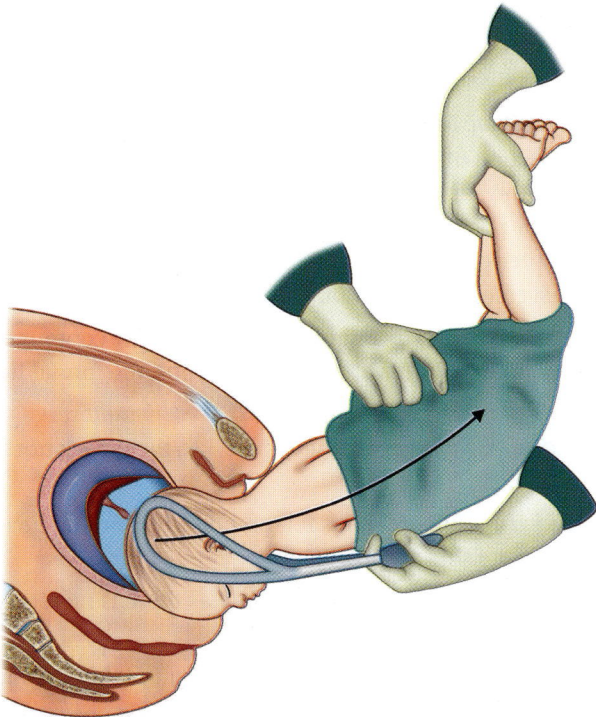

Fig. 7: Forceps application to deliver the head.

Other complications during breech delivery:
- Cord prolapse, when the cervix is not fully dilated and the cord prolapses, a cesarean is the best option. But when the cervix is fully dilated, a breech extraction can also be tried.
- *Uterine dysfunction:* In the presence of uterine dysfunction, it may be a safe option to go in for a cesarean section rather than try for oxytocin augmentation.
- *Extended legs:* If the legs are extended as in a frank breech, you can take your fingers to the popliteal fossa and give gentle pressure there and also slightly abduct the legs, wherein, the legs flex at the knee joint. Now grasp the foot and deliver the leg. Repeat this with the opposite leg. And when you have both the feet, hold them together and deliver it out of the vagina.
- *Delivery of the extended leg:* Delivery of the extended leg by Pinard's maneuver is shown in **Figures 8A and B**.

Delivery of the Extended Arms by Lovset's Maneuver (Fig. 9)

Extended Arms

The Lovset's maneuver is based on the principle that, with extended arms, when the anterior shoulder remains above the pubic symphysis, due to the inclination of the pelvis, the posterior shoulder is at a lower level than the anterior, namely below the sacral promontory. So in the first step, the baby is held and rotated through 180° keeping its back anterior and maintaining downward traction. This will bring the posterior arm to emerge from under the pubic arch, which is then hooked out. Then in the next stage, the trunk is again rotated in the reverse direction, keeping the back anterior, to deliver the erstwhile anterior shoulder which will now emerge from under the pubic symphysis.

Difficulties with the after coming head:
- *Occipito posterior position of the fetal head:* The Prague maneuver is adopted. Here, the fingers are placed over the shoulder from behind and an outward and upward traction is made over it. The legs are now grasped with the other hand and the body is swung over the mother's abdomen. By this, the occiput sweeps over the perineum and is born.

Causes for perinatal morbidity and mortality in assisted breech delivery:
- Fetal asphyxia
- Intracranial hemorrhage: Due to sudden delivery of the unmolded head
- Fetal skeletal injury fracture of the neck, long bone fracture of the femur, humerus clavicle, etc.
- Dislocation of the hip and shoulder joint
- Cervical and brachial plexus palsy
- Abdominal visceral injury (e.g., liver, adrenals) while grasping the abdomen at delivery
- Trauma to the testicles
- Hematoma of the sternomastoid muscle due to undue traction during delivering of the after coming head.

PART 1: Obstetrics and Perinatology

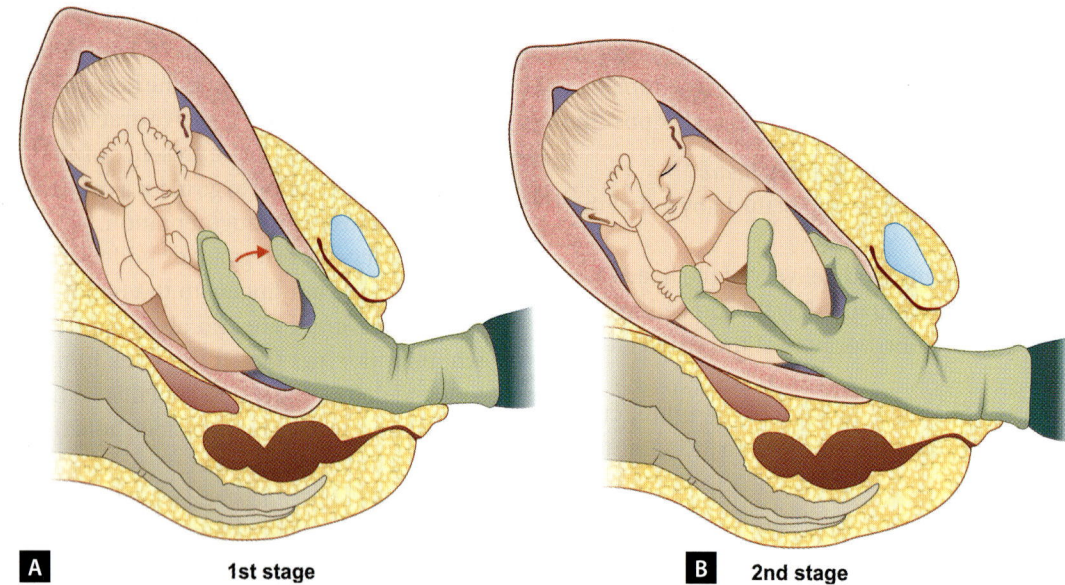

Figs. 8A and B: Pinard's maneuver: (A) 1st stage; (B) 2nd stage.

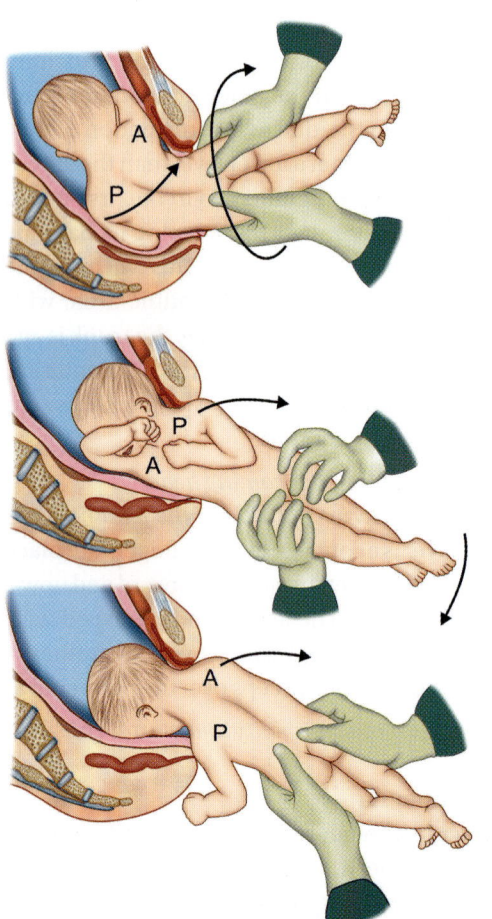

Fig. 9: Lovset's maneuver.

Therefore, breech delivery should be attempted only by an experienced personal at a center where all facilities are available to look after both the mother and her newborn baby.

Cesarean section in breech presentation: The principles to deliver a baby presenting by breech through cesarean section are same as when it is delivered by assisted breech vaginal delivery.

Transverse Lie (Fig. 10)

Incidence: One in 500 pregnancies presents as a transverse lie at term.

Introduction: When the long axis of the fetus lies perpendicular to the long axis of the maternal spine, we refer to it as transverse lie. But most often, the fetal axis may not be absolutely transverse, but may take a tilt, and most often the breech is on one side at a higher level and the heavier head is in one or either of the iliac fossa on the opposite side. To this, we refer as an oblique lie. But in both situations, when labor begins, it is the shoulder which presents at the pelvic brim and hence we collectively refer to it as shoulder presentation.

Fetal position: In a transverse lie, the position is determined by the direction of the back. The head determines if it is right or left and the back determines if it is anterior or posterior, thus, the eight positions would be dorsoanterior, dorsoposterior, dorsoinferior, or dorsosuperior, either left or right. Causes of a transverse lie are the same as in a breech.

Clinical diagnosis: In a transverse lie, the entire contour of the uterus appears transversely stretched and the fundal height is at a lower level than it should be.

Fundal grip: Neither of the fetal pole, i.e., the breech nor head is palpable.

Lateral grip: The breech is felt on one side and the head on the opposite side at a lower level.

Pelvic grip: The lower pole is empty as there is no fetal pole palpable here.

Fetal heart: FHS is heard somewhere around the umbilicus

Vaginal examination: When a vaginal examination is done in the antenatal period, there is no pole in the pelvis, i.e.,

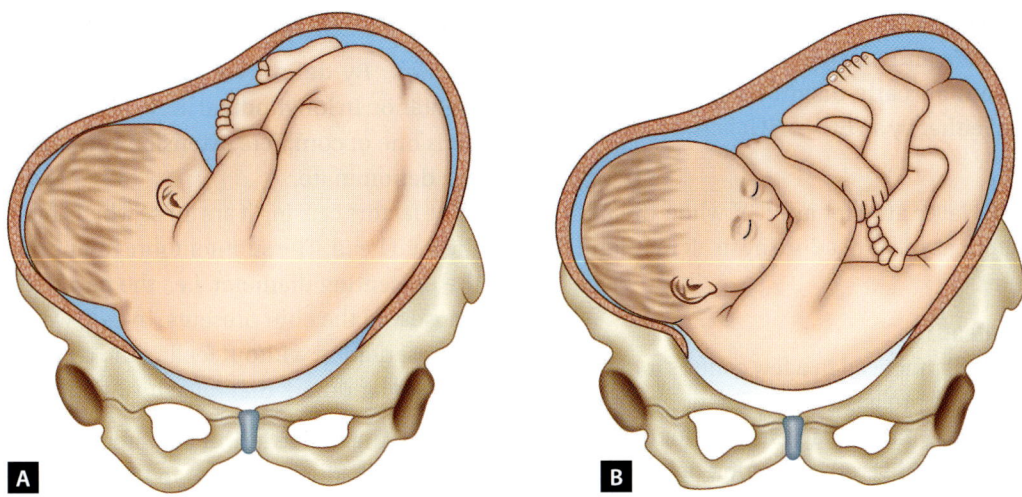

Figs. 10A and B: Transverse lie.

neither the head nor breech is felt. But when the same examination is done in labor, especially with the membranes absent, the shoulder can be identified by palpating the axilla with the scapula on one side, and the clavicle on the other, with the characteristic gridiron feel of the ribs. Rarely, an arm is prolapsed, and we can identify the side by shaking hands with the fetus and our hand identifies the side of the fetal hand. Ultrasonography further confirms the diagnosis.

Clinical course of labor: Rarely, in a transverse lie, there can be one of the following happening:
- *Spontaneous rectification*: When the baby turns and corrects itself to a cephalic presentation
- *Spontaneous version*: When it turns to a breech
- *Delivery as corpora conduplicata*: Occasionally, delivery is affected in the very premature or in a dead macerated fetus in a doubled upstate referred to as corpora conduplicata.

Outcome of pregnancy in a transverse lie: In a well cared for and supervised pregnancy when we diagnose the presentation as a transverse lie, we can convert it to a vertex presentation by an external cephalic version (ECV).

This can be followed by induction of labor often referred to as *stabilizing induction* when the lie has turned longitudinal and is cephalic.

But in an undiagnosed case or a neglected case, the outcome could be disastrous, often referred to as *neglected shoulder presentation* **(Fig. 11)**.

Sequence of events in neglected shoulder presentation: When the patient gets into labor and transverse lie goes undiagnosed, the shoulder presents itself at the pelvic brim. Since there is no mechanism of labor in a transverse lie, the shoulder gets pushed down through the pelvic brim and when the membranes rupture, the arm of that side prolapses out with or without the cord. As labor progresses, the shoulder gets wedged and impacted within the pelvis and the prolapsed arm gets swollen and edematous .The upper segment contracts and retracts, while the lower segment passively distends to

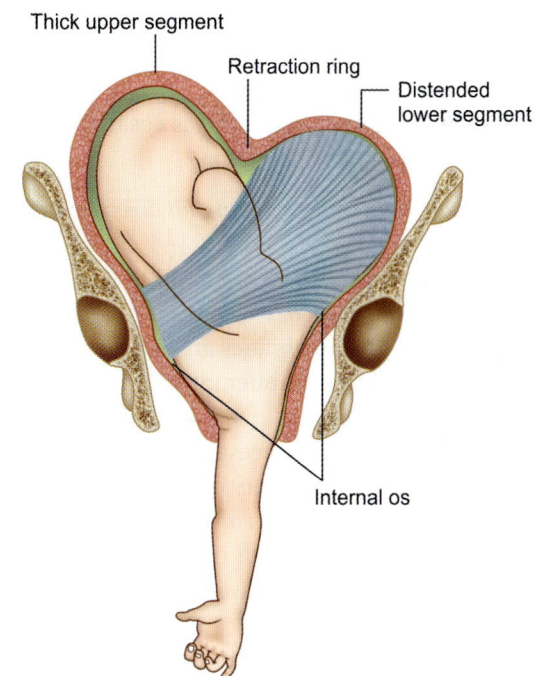

Fig. 11: Neglected shoulder presentation.

accommodate the fetus. In course of line all features of an obstructed labor sets in. A line of demarcation occurs between the upper and the lower segment often referred to as the Bandl's ring or the pathological retraction ring.

Clinical features of obstructed labor: The patient shows all features of obstructed labor. The patient is in agony. She is dry dehydrated tachypneic and febrile. Features of ketoacodosis set in and soon signs of sepsis supervene.

Any if the patient is still unattended to and the transverse lie undiagnosed, a point is reached when the lower segment is unable to distend any further, and it gives way, resulting in a rupture uterus.

This is followed by features of both hemorrhagic and septic shock.

This course of events is not so common nowadays due to good antenatal care and imaging modalities such as the ultrasound, wherein an early diagnosis is made and the patient is managed either by an ECV or if it fails, by an elective cesarean section.

A word of caution: Never attempt an ECV when the patient is in obstructed labor as the procedure by itself may land the patient in a rupture.

When the fetus is dead?
In yester years and still practiced in a few centers today, if the baby is dead with an arm prolapse, under GA the arm is pulled down to access the neck, and a decapitation is done. Then the lower half of the fetus is delivered by traction on the arm and the head is delivered by traction with an allis or vulsellum.

But when there is no arm prolapse and the baby is dead in a transverse lie, a spondylotomy can be tried and the two halves are delivered separately by pulling on each half after it is severed.

However, in modern-day obstetrics cesarean section is preferred over destructive operations.

Place of internal podalic (IP) version and breech extraction in a transverse lie:

In modern obstetrics, IP version and breech extraction are best done only in the second of a twin when it presents as a transverse lie and the membranes are intact with adequate liquor. Then under GA you can attempt an IP version followed by breech extraction.

Problems to be anticipated at cesarean with a the transverse lie, would be, difficulty in delivery of the baby, especially in dorsoinferior position. Problems may arise when there is an associated placenta previa and if there is a Bandl's ring as in an obstructed labor. In both, we may have to resort to a classical CS.

Under all other circumstances, if the fetus is term and with a transverse lie the best option would be a planned cesarean section.

FACE PRESENTATION

Definition: By definition, face presentation is a cephalic presentation in longitudinal lie, where the attitude of the fetal head is one of complete extension with the chin or mentum as the denominator.

The factors causing it are those which interfere with flexion of the fetal head. The submentobregmatic diameter of 9.5 cm is the presenting diameter, i.e., the part between the root of the nose and the chin presents. In fact, we cannot speak of a face presentation without feeling the chin as that is the most important landmark that must be identified on PV.

Incidence: Incidence is 1 in 500 pregnancies: In 70% of face presentations, the mentun is in the anterior position and in 30% the mentum is in the posterior position. In most face presentations, it is the secondary face presentation, i.e., that which occurs during labor, that is of concern to us.

Causes for face presentation:
- Multiparity: Due to the lax anterior abdominal, wall the fetus extends its spine which results in a face presentation
- Contracted pelvis
- Cord round the neck
- Tumors in the front of the neck
- Spasm of the sternocleidomastoid muscle
- Dolicocephalic head
- Anencephaly.

The factors which make a face presentation different as compared to a vertex and hence more difficult are the following:
- The face being irregular is a poor dilator of the cervix.
- The bag of membranes is not well applied to the presenting part and often results in premature rupture of membranes.
- The bones of the face being fixed cannot mould in labor.
- If the presentation is a mentoposterior **(Fig. 12)**, it requires a long internal rotation through three eighth of a circle. But in a small number of cases, it either remains as persistent mentoposterior or it rotates posteriorly into the hollow of

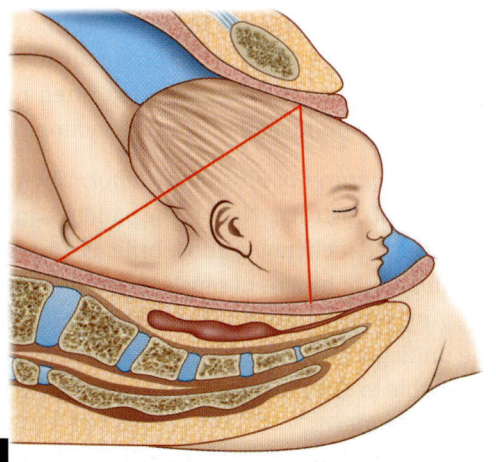
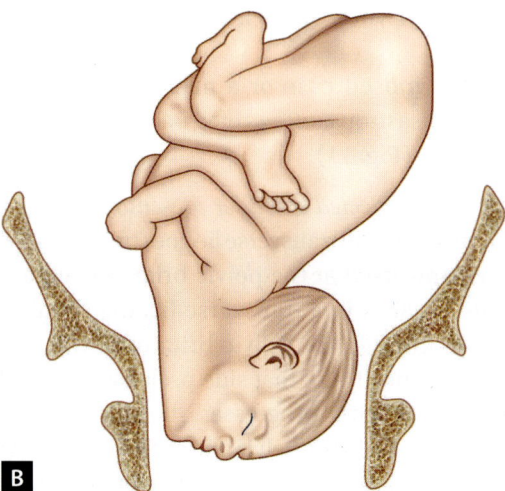

Figs. 12A and B: Mentoposterior position.

the sacrum when the head and the chest both descend into the pelvis resulting in an obstructed labor. Mentoposterior position going in for obstructed labor.

Diagnosis by abdominal examination:
- Being a longitudinal lie, the uterus is longitudinally distended, with the breech at the fundus.
- In a mentoanterior, the back being posterior is not felt easily. Instead, the fetal limbs are felt more anteriorly.
- The cephalic prominence: This is the first prominence of the fetal head, i.e., felt as we come from above down and is caused either by flexion or extension of the fetal head. In a well-flexed head, it is the siniput and it is felt on the opposite side of the back. But in a face presentation due to complete extension of the head, the cephalic prominence is the occiput, which is felt on the same side as the back.
- Due to complete extension of the fetal head in face the characteristic groove between the head and the back can be felt.
- In a face presentation, the FHS are transmitted directly through the chest wall which is thrust anteriorly as we see in a mentoanterior position.

Primary face presentations are seen before the onset of labor; when it persists or appears in labor, then it is called a secondary face presentation

Per vaginum findings in a face presentation: The first differential diagnosis at a PV examination in a face presentation is the breech, both being soft parts. The points of differentiation are given as follows:

Face	Breech
The mouth shows a sucking reflex when the finger is put inside it. But when we withdraw there is no meconium staining	The anus exhibits a sphincteric action when a finger is inserted into it and when we withdraw there is meconium staining of your fingers
The most important point of differentiation is the presence of the alveolar margin within the mouth	The smooth feel within and the absence of the alveolar margin here is an important point of differentiation
The mouth and the molar prominences make a triangle with one another	Whereas, the anus and the ischial tuberosities lie in a straight line

Points to be noted in a PV examination:
- In a face presentation, PV examination must be done gently so as not to injure the soft parts and also to be done without an antiseptic cream, as it is likely to damage the eye.
- The lack of the rounded head with its suture lines and fontanelle is worth noting and so also the presence of the irregular soft parts stands out to draw your attention.

The landmarks to identify in a face, especially when the membranes rupture are : the chin, mouth nose, the molar eminence, the root of the nose, and the supraorbital ridges.

Of these, the chin is the most important land mark, without which we cannot say it is a face presentation.

The position of the chin further tells you the position of the baby, e.g., left mentoanterior or right mentoposterior.

Mechanism of Labor in Face

This is a longitudinal lie with the head in a fully extended state. The presenting diameter is the submentobregmatic of 9.5 cm and the mentum is the denominator. Thus, there can be four positions: (1) Left mentoanterior, (2) left mentoposterior, (3) right mentoanterior, (4) right mentoposterior.

In a left mentoanterior:
First engagement takes place.
- Descent with increasing extension
- *Internal rotation*: When the chin touches the pelvic floor, it undergoes internal rotation through one eighth of a circle when the chin comes to lie behind the pubic symphysis.
- *Flexion*: The chin hitches against the pubic symphysis and by a process of flexion the head is born, i.e., the mouth, nose, forehead vertex, and last occiput is born.
- *Restitution* occurs through one eighth of a circle.
- *External rotation* also occurs through another one eighth of circle in the same direction of restitution.

Management in Labor

In a face presentation, we can have a normal vaginal delivery, as the presenting diameter which is the submentobregmatic of 9.5 cm is the same as that in a vertex.

Make sure that the pelvis is adequate and the size of the baby is not too big. The bones in a face are fixed and there is lack of molding, here so minor degrees of disproportion may become amplified problem. Also rule out congenital anomalies such as an anencephaly, as the latter often presents as face, due to the absence of a cranial vault.

Mentoanterior position:
- Labor proceeds normally, but you must remember that in face presentation internal rotation occurs late .This is because, the face has to be well applied to the pelvic floor before internal rotation is effected and this happens late in labor in face. Hence, we have to patiently wait for the same.
- Even in the event of a an instrumental delivery, the chin must be seen at the outlet, for you to say that the face is engaged and the forceps is applied. To understand this, the distance between the biparietal diameter and the chin is 7 cm in a face as compared to the distance between the biparietal diameter and the occiput in a vertex presentation which is only 3 cm. Therefore to say a face is engaged the chin should be seen at the outlet.
- In a mentoposterior, which occurs in one third of the cases of face, spontaneous rotation through three eighths of a circle occurs only in about 30% of cases. And in the remaining either it fails to rotate or it undergoes a reverse

rotation into the hollow of the sacrum and with each contraction, the head and the thorax try to enter the pelvis simultaneously eventually landing up with an obstructed labor. Therefore in a mentoposterior, it may be prudent to take an early decision about a cesarean because of these associated problems.

Even after birth the face presents an ugly picture as it is swollen and edematous and the cry of the baby is hoarse at least for the initial few days due to laryngeal edema. Hence, the patient should be reassured adequately.

■ BROW PRESENTATION (FIG. 13)

Incidence: One in 1,500 pregnancies present as brow at term.

Definition: This is a longitudinal lie, and a cephalic presentation, wherein the attitude of the head is midway between complete flexion and complete extension. As a result of this, the largest diameter, namely, the verticomental of 13.5 cm presents at the pelvic brim. This is the distance between the furtherest point on the vertex to the mentum.

Etiology: All those conditions that cause a face presentation can result in a brow. Namely, that which prevents flexion of the head can cause this presentation.

Diagnosis: The clinical diagnosis on as per abdominal examination is difficult to make out. In fact, many a time all that you will find will be a large dimension of the head at the lower pole which is often unengaged. The characteristic groove between the back and the occiput is difficult to identify.

On a PV examination: The presence of irregular soft parts would draw your first attention. The points to be noted are: The root of the nose and supraorbital ridges on one end and the anterior fontanelle at the other with the bulging forehead often obscured with a caput over it.

Course and outcome of labor: Many of the times, a brow is a transitory presentations and in over 50% it either flexes and becomes a vertex presentation or extends and becomes a face presentation. But sometimes it persists and unless the baby is small with a roomy pelvis, there is no mechanism of delivery because of its larger diameter of presentation. This results in an obstructed labor. It is often useful to think of a brow in multi when there is no progress of labor. Therefore in most situations, the best option would be to resort to a cesarean section whether the baby is alive or dead.

■ FURTHER READING

1. American College of Obstetricians and Gynaecologists. External cephalic version. Practice Bulletin No. 161. Obstet Gynecol. 2016;127(2):e54-61.
2. American College of Obstetricians and Gynaecologists, Society for Maternal-Fetal Medicine: Periviable birth. Obstet Gynecol. 2017;130(4):e187-99.
3. Hofmeyr GJ, Hannah M Lawrie TA. Planned caesarean section for term breech delivery. Cochrane Database Syst Rev. 2015;2015(7):CD000166.
4. Royal College of Obstetricians and Gynaecologists. The Management of breech presentation. RCOG Green Top Guidelines No 20b. 2006.

■ LONG QUESTIONS

1. Discuss the management of labor in a primigravida at term with occipitoposterior position. What complications should be anticipated, how are they diagnosed and managed?
2. Every breech presentation in labor should be delivered by a cesarean section. Discuss and debate this statement.
3. What are the complications of labor in a woman with a transverse lie? Discuss the management of transverse lie in labor at term and the complications that may arise.

■ SHORT QUESTIONS

1. What are the causes and problems associated with occipitoposterior position in labor?
2. What are the possible outcomes when rotation occurs with an occipitoposterior position in labor?
3. What are the maneuvers described to deliver the aftercoming head of a breech?
4. What is the Mauriceau Smellie Viet maneuver?
5. What are the indications of cesarean section in a breech presentation?
6. What are the salient features of management of labor in a vaginal breech delivery?
7. What is a Bandl's ring? In which situation do you encounter it? How do you manage labor with it?

■ MULTIPLE CHOICE QUESTIONS

1. The following is often associated with face to pubes delivery, except:
   a. Anthropoid pelvis   b. Platypelloid pelvis
   c. Reverse rotation   d. Perineal lacerations

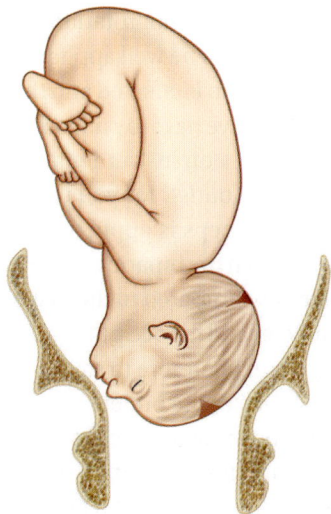

Fig. 13: Brow presentation.

2. Which of the following is the presenting diameter in occiptio posterior?
   a. Subocc bregmatic
   b. Occiptio-frontal
   c. Vertico-mental
   d. Sub-mento bregmatic
3. The causes for DTA is all, except:
   a. Poor uterine contractions
   b. Android pelvis
   c. Weak pelvic floor
   d. Platypelloid pelvis
4. Ideal forceps to tackle DTA is:
   a. The Pipers forceps
   b. Kielland's forceps
   c. Low mid cavity forceps
   d. Outlet forceps
5. Breech is associated with all of the following, except:
   a. Prematurity
   b. Poor dilator of cervix
   c. Early engagement
   d. Cord prolapse
6. Delay in the after coming head is seen in:
   a. Deflexed head
   b. Incompletely dilated cervix
   c. Hydrocephalic head
   d. All of the following
7. Maximum incidence of cord prolapse is seen in which of the following:
   a. Flexed breech
   b. Footling presentation
   c. Extended breech
   d. OP presentation
8. CS in a Breech is indicated in:
   a. A Star-gazing head
   b. Premature breech
   c. Footling presentation
   d. All of the above
   e. Non of the above
9. Kristellar's maneuver is:
   a. Swinging the baby over the mother's abdomen
   b. Suprapubic pressure
   c. Steady ankle traction
   d. Rotating the baby from anterior to posterior through 180 degree
10. The characteristic grid - iron feel is seen in:
    a. Face presentation
    b. Shoulder presentation
    c. Breech presentation
    d. Brow presentation
11. Transverse lie can be managed by:
    a. CS
    b. ECV
    c. IP Version and breech extraction
    d. Decapitation
    e. All of the above
12. Face presentation is associated with all, except:
    a. Spasm of the neck muscles
    b. Hydrocephalous
    c. Anencephalous
    d. Cord round the neck
13. Which of the following is not a cause for obstructed labor:
    a. Mentoposterior
    b. Transverse lie
    c. Deep transverse arrest
    d. Direct occ.posterior

Answers

1. a 2. b 3. c 4. b 5. c 6. d
7. b 8. d 9. b 10. b 11. e 12. b
13. d

9.3 ROUTINE INTRAPARTUM CARE AND INTRAPARTUM TESTS

Ganpat Sawant, Sachin Ajmera

INTRODUCTION

Labor though a physiological process does have a lot of emotions attached to it. Labor pains do have a dreadful connect to it aided by a lot of peer wisdom put in, women are often stressed, confused and excited about it at the same time.

The most difficult and dangerous journey any human undertakes in his lifetime is his passage from the mother's womb to her arms.

Labor has its own set of complications and it is a known fact that labor can be called as "normal'" only after it is over. The mother needs a dedicated team of care givers functioning to the best of their abilities. Also, since labor can be a long drawn out process multiple teams may be involved and hence the need for standardized care and guidelines is essential for every birthing unit.

PREPARATION

The preparation for the process of labor should start right since the antenatal period as noted in **Box 1**. The woman should

BOX 1: Preparation for labor in antenatal period.

1. Classify woman as high risk or low risk
2. Explain to the woman about the process of normal labor and the events occurring therein
3. Talk to her about labor analgesia
4. Inform her about the things she should be carrying while coming to the hospital in labor pains
5. Let her select an attendant who can be with her during labor
6. Introduce her to the doctor's and staff who will assist her during labor
7. Discuss regarding neonatal care
8. Discuss regarding shifting to a higher center in the unlikely event if any complications

be well versed with the place of delivery and the doctors as well as the staff who would be treating her during labor. She should also be explained about the process of labor and all her questions regarding the same should be answered to remove any phobias associated with it.

GENERAL MANAGEMENT

The woman in labor is under a lot of stress both physical as well as mental and hence needs a lot of empathy from her care givers. She should be greeted with a smile and your role in her care should be explained to her. A calm and confident approach will reassure the woman that all is going well. Effective communication with the woman and emotional support goes a long way in making labor a pleasant experience.

A detailed history which if already noted during antenatal period should be revisited. All the investigations done in the antenatal period should be checked and any special concerns should be addressed to. A detailed per vaginal examination should be performed with strict aseptic precautions as given in **Box 2** and findings noted as per **Box 3**. Vaginal examination during labor should be kept to a minimum. It should be done every 3–4 hours:

- To assess the progress of labor
- After rupture of membranes to rule out cord prolapse and to confirm the onset of second stage of labor.

Auscultation of the fetal heart should be done for a period of full one minute following a contraction. Baseline heart rate with acceleration or decelerations if any should be noted. If any abnormality found cardiotocography should be carried out. As of now there is insufficient evidence about whether cardiotocography as a part of initial assessment, which is also called admission test, improves perinatal outcomes in low risk women.[1] Hence, it should not be offered to all low risk women.

Based on this detailed initial assessment a low risk woman may be shifted to a high risk category as per **Box 4**. Management of high risk woman has been dealt with in subsequent chapters.

CRITERIA FOR ADMISSION

The woman presenting with true labor pains should be admitted and supported appropriately, even when in early labor, unless her preference is to await active labor at home.[2] If the woman is in latent phase of labor she should be admitted to maternity waiting area rather than labor ward. Assessment for maternal and fetal well-being should be carried out at intervals. Most of the women do not complain of much pain during this phase but few women who complain of pain can be advised breathing exercise or massages. Once the patient is in active phase of labor she should be shifted to the labor ward.

MANAGEMENT OF FIRST STAGE OF LABOR

The first stage of labor is the stage of watchful expectancy wherein labor needs to be monitored carefully but minimal interference is needed. The woman would generally complain about increasing pain and discomfort with contractions, increasing backache, indigestion, diarrhea, leg discomfort or heaviness or a general feeling of fatigue.

Enema

An enema is typically recommended in early stage of labor. However, evidences show that enemas do not have a significant effect on infection rates such as perineal wound infection or neonatal infections nor does it shorten the duration of labor. It can be given for women with a loaded rectum on per vaginal examinations to prevent soiling during second stage of labor.[3]

Mobilization

The woman in labor need not be confined to bed if membranes are intact and she can move around as per her wish and comfort.[4] While lying down supine position can be avoided to prevent aortocaval compression and lateral position may be preferred. There is clear and important evidence that walking and upright positions in the first stage of labor reduces the duration of labor, the risk of cesarean birth, the need for epidural and does not seem to be associated with increased intervention or negative effects on mother's or fetal well-being.

BOX 2: Procedure of per vaginal examination.

1. Verbal consent
2. Scrub hands and forearms
3. Use sterile gloves
4. Vulva should be cleaned with antiseptic solution like cetavlon
5. Smear gloves with cetavlon
6. Separate labia with other hand and examine with index and middle finger
7. Complete examination and only then withdraw the fingers

BOX 3: Per vaginal examination.

- Cervical dilatation
- Cervical effacement
- Presenting part and position
- Membrane status
- Abnormal discharge if any
- Station
- Pelvic assessment

BOX 4: High risk woman based on examination during labor.

Maternal examination
- Pulse more than 120 pm
- Blood pressure more than 140/90 mm of Hg
- Proteinuria of 2+
- Temperature of more than 38°C
- Vaginal blood loss other than show
- Rupture of membranes of more than 24 hours
- Meconium staining of liquor
- Abnormal pains or hypertonic uterus

Fetal examination
- Abnormal presentation or position
- High or free floating head in nulliparous woman
- Suspected IUGR or macrosomia
- Oligoamnios or polyhydramnios
- Fetal heart rate < 110 bpm or > 160 bpm
- Deceleration in fetal heart rate
- Reduced fetal movements in last 24 hours

Hydration and Oral Intake in Labor

Restriction to oral intake historically was due to the scare of aspiration if general anesthesia was required but with current obstetric anesthesia techniques this risk is negligible. Oral hydration is thus encouraged in women with spontaneously progressing labor to meet caloric and hydration needs.[5] There is a delayed gastric emptying during labor hence women should be advised to have light diet or fruit juices or isotonic drinks. Intravenous hydration though safe is not always necessary and should be considered only if woman is unable to consume orally.

Routine IV Line

Most women would be comfortable to move around during the initial phase of labor and may consider an intravenous (IV) line to be an hindrance and also painful.

Though not a compulsion[6] it is preferable to have an IV access during the phase of active labor. This can facilitate administration of medications, fluids to prevent dehydration and also blood and blood products in case of excessive hemorrhage. The IV cannula needs to be kept patent for which a saline lock or heparin lock should be used if the woman is not on fluids.

It is preferable not to collect blood from peripheral IV lines except in an emergency because there is an increased incidence of sample getting hemolyzed causing delay in obtaining the reports. So blood can be drawn for other site and can be stored for emergency cross matching during admission in the rare event of excessive hemorrhage.

Bladder Care

The woman is encouraged to pass urine at least every 4 hours during labor voluntarily as full bladder often inhibits uterine contractions.[7] Accurate urine output should be recorded on the partogram. If a woman is unable to pass urine after 4 hours a simple rubber catheterization should to be done under strict aseptic precautions.

Pain Relief

Pain relief during labor has been dealt with extensively in the chapter on Obstetric Analgesia and Anesthesia.

Assessment of Progress of Labor

The physiological process of labor lasts for many hours, hence there is need for multiple doctors as well as nurses. The problem hence often faced is the subjective assessment of different observers at different times with differing judgments leading to an iatrogenic increase in maternal and neonatal morbidity and mortality. Also in our country where many deliveries are conducted the importance for timely referral cannot be undermined. Thus, the need of the hour for any person entrusted with a pregnant woman for safe delivery is objective assessment of labor and clear guidelines as to early recognition of any complication.

The ideal way that the above can be achieved is by regular and meticulous charting of labor on a partogram.

Partogram

Partogram is a graphical representation of the progress of labor in which cervical dilatation and descent of fetal head is plotted against time in addition to maternal parameters, fetal well-being, drugs and IV fluids given to the parturient. Partograph is used synonymously as partogram. In 1954 EA Friedman described this graphicostatistical analysis of progress of labor in primigravida and multipara.[8] He showed the pattern of cervical dilatation versus time to be a sigmoid curve as shown in **Figure 1**.

As can be seen from the graph the first stage of labor consists of two phases.

1. *Latent phase:* Starts from onset of true labor pains to 3 cm dilatation. The cervix dilates slowly in this phase at around 0.6cm/hr. Mean duration of this phase is 8.6 hours in primigravidas and 5.3 hours in multiparas. Maximum duration is 20 hours in nulliparas and 14 hours in multiparas. Duration of more than 20 hours is labeled as prolonged latent phase of labor.
2. *Active phase:* This phase starts at 3 cm dilatation to full dilatation. It is further divided into:
   a. Acceleration phase: 3–5 cm dilatation. Rate of dilatation is more than 0.6 cm/h.
   b. Phase of maximum slope: 5–9 cm dilatation. Rate of dilatation is more than 1.2 cm/h in nulliparas and more than 1.5 cm/h in multiparas.
   c. Phase of deceleration: 9 cm to full dilatation.

In 1971, Philpott further developed the partogram, emphasizing on its clinical application by introducing the concept of alert line and action line.[9,10] However, the

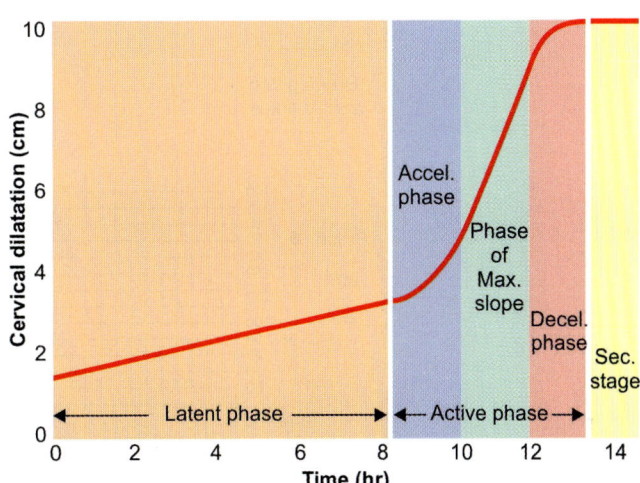

Fig. 1: Friedman's curve.
(Accel: acceleration; Max: maximum; Decel: deceleration; Sec: seondary)

suitability of action line in patients with different ethnicity and also in cases when women presented late during labor was questioned. To circumvent this, Studd introduced the concept of nomograms.[11] A nomogram has been constructed to show the normal progressive dilatation of the cervix for primigravidae admitted at different stages of cervical dilatation.

Based on various studies proving the efficacy of partograms WHO introduced the composite partograph in 1988. The first WHO partograph or "Composite partograph", as seen in **Figure 2**, covers a latent phase of labor of up to 8 hours and an active phase beginning when the cervical dilatation reaches 3 cm. The active phase is depicted with an alert line and an action line, drawn 4 hours apart on the partograph. This partograph is based on the principle that during active labor, the rate of cervical dilation should not be slower than 1 cm/hour. Since a prolonged latent phase is relatively infrequent and not usually associated with poor perinatal outcome, the usefulness of recording the latent phase of labor in the partograph has been questioned. Moreover, differentiating the latent phase from false labor is often difficult. To alleviate these disadvantages, a modified WHO "partograph" was introduced which is a simplified version and incorporated removal of the

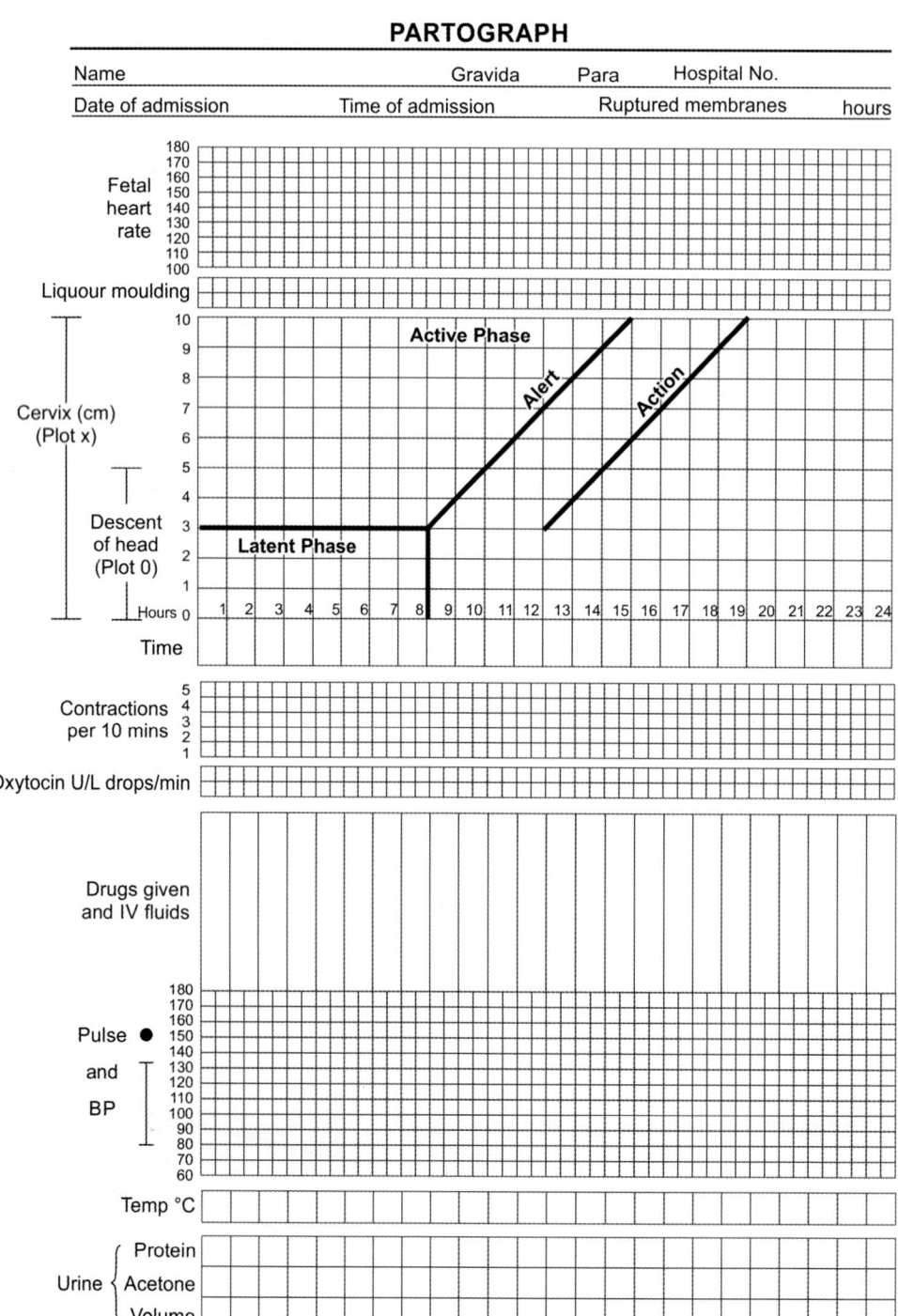

Fig. 2: WHO composite partograph.

latent phase and defined the beginning of the active phase at 4 cm cervical dilatation instead of 3 cm, i.e., from the phase of maximum slope onwards.[12]

Various other simplified partographs have been created but the standard partograph that is used the world over is the Modified WHO Partograph.

Modified WHO Partograph

As can be seen from **Figure 3**, this partograph does not have the latent phase. A line is drawn from 4 cm dilatation with a slope of 1 cm/h, which constitutes the alert line. Parallel to the alert line 4 hours to its right action line is drawn. The alert line represents the mean rate of progress in terms of cervical dilatation in the slowest of normal labors observed in nulliparas. Hence the patients' graph should remain on the left of alert line in majority of cases. If the graph crosses the alert line a reassessment of the pelvis, fetal position and uterine activity should be carried out. Augmentation of labor with oxytocin or transfer to higher center as the case may be can then be considered. If the action line is crossed

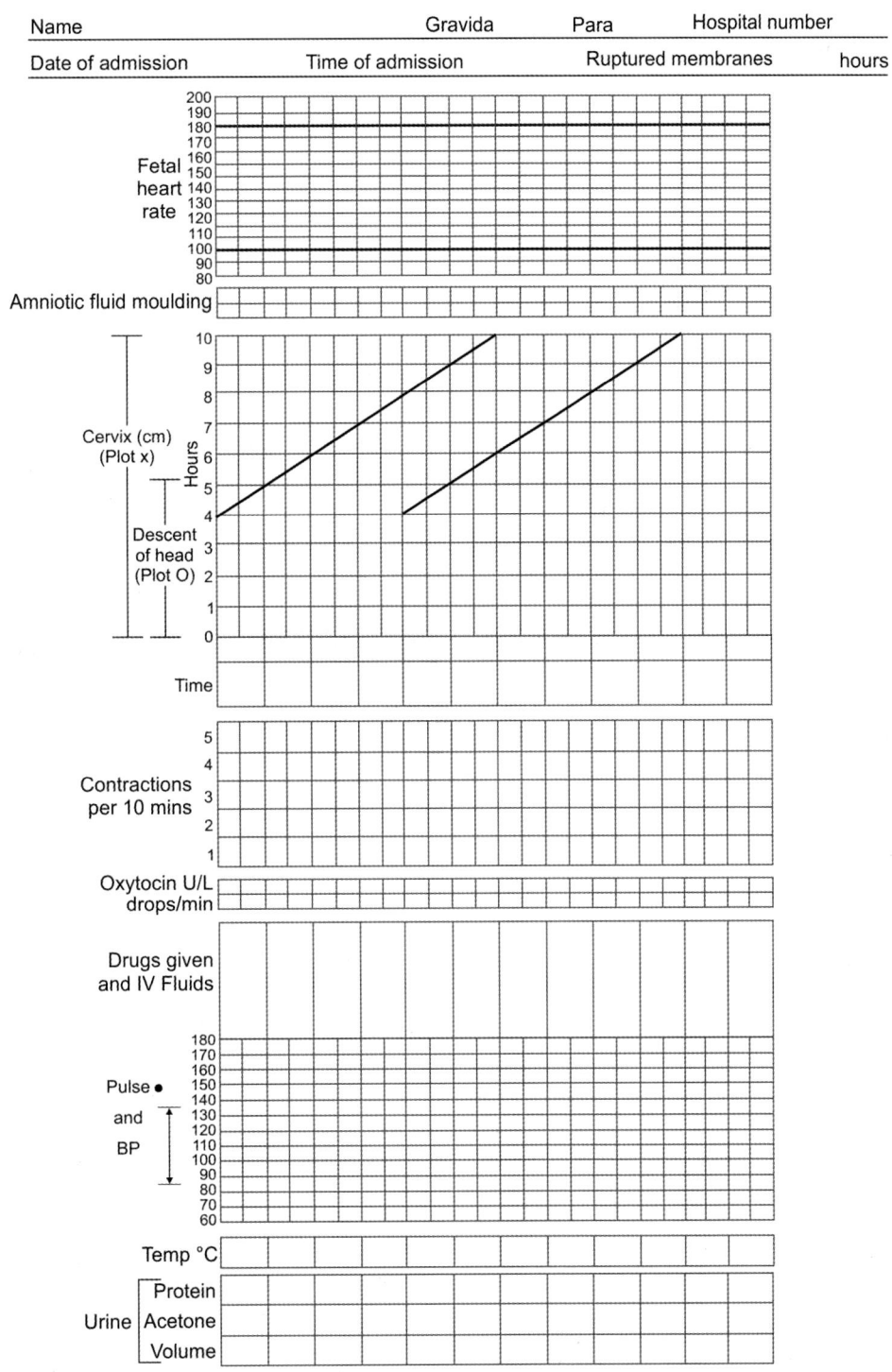

Fig. 3: Modified WHO partograph.

appropriate operative procedures need to be considered in order to prevent any morbidity or mortality. Modified WHO Partogram also includes various other components so as to provide the exact nature of labor in a particular woman on a single sheet of paper.

The five main components are:
1. Maternal identification
2. Fetal condition
3. Progress of labor
4. Maternal condition
5. Outcome

The objectives of partogram are summarized in **Box 5**.

Plotting the Partogram

World Health Organization recommends mandatory use of partogram for all women. The initial data can be filled as soon as the woman presents in labor. High-risk factor if any can be mentioned in red at the top of the partogram. Once the preliminary data is entered the actual plotting on the partogram starts when the woman is around 4 cm dilated. If the woman is already more than 4 cm dilated the plotting starts immediately.

The next component of the partogram deals with fetal well-being. Fetal heart rate is monitored every 15–30 minutes in active phase of labor. However on the partogram fetal heart rate is charted every 30 minutes. It is marked with a dot and the dots joined as the labor progresses. If electronic fetal heart monitoring is done then the mean basal rate is recorded.

The membranes if intact are labeled as "I" on the partogram. The exact time of rupture of membranes is noted as and when it happens. Liquor amnii if clear is recorded as "C", if meconium stained recorded as "M" and "B" if blood stained. Molding of fetal head is recorded as shown in **Table 1**.

Progress of labor is recorded next on the partogram starting at 4 cm or more dilatation by means of recording the descent of fetal head, cervical dilatation, and uterine contractions. Descent of head is recorded by a dot (•), as the number of fifths of head palpable above the pelvic brim (Crichton's method).

BOX 5: Aims and objectives of maintaining a partogram.
- Early detection of abnormal progress of labor
- Early recognition of cephalopelvic disproportion
- Prevent prolonged labor
- Help in early decision for transfer, augmentation or termination of labor
- Increase the quality and regularity of all observations of mother and fetus
- Early recognition of maternal or fetal problems
- Highly effective in reducing complications from prolonged labor for the mother (postpartum hemorrhage, sepsis, uterine rupture and its sequelae) and for the newborn (death, anoxia, infections, etc.).
- Reduce incidence of cesarean sections
- Facilitates handover procedure
- Medicolegal

Cervical dilatation is denoted by a cross (x). Each observation is joined to the preceding one by a straight line. Horizontal scale represents hours spent in labor with a least count of 30 minutes. Exact time is noted in the next column so as to prevent any confusion with the hours. The contraction of the uterus should be assessed every 30 minutes during labor. 3–5 regular, strong contractions in 10 minutes are usually aimed for the second stage of labor. Uterine contractions weak, moderate or good are recorded as shown in **Figure 4**.

Interpretations

There is generally no role for augmentation of labor if latent and active phases progress is normal. Dysfunctional labor can be diagnosed on partogram in the following situations:

Prolonged latent phase: According to WHO partograph, a prolonged latent phase is "cervix not dilated beyond 4 cm after 8 hours from admission and without any changes in cervical effacement or dilatation."

- *Protracted active phase:* It happens if the rate of cervical dilatation in active phase of labor is less than 1 cm/hour for a minimum of 4 hours. Causes for the same maybe fetal malpositions such as ocipitoposterior position, cephalopelvic disproportion, hypotonic uterine contractions.
- *Secondary arrest of cervical dilatation:* When the cervical dilatation stops or slows significantly for 2 hours or more prior to full dilatation of cervix. The reason most of the times is cephalopelvic disproportion.

TABLE 1: Molding of fetal head.

Observation	Degree of molding
Separated bones, sutures felt easily	0
Bones just touching each other	+
Overlapping bones (reducible)	++
Severely overlapping bones (nonreducible)	+++

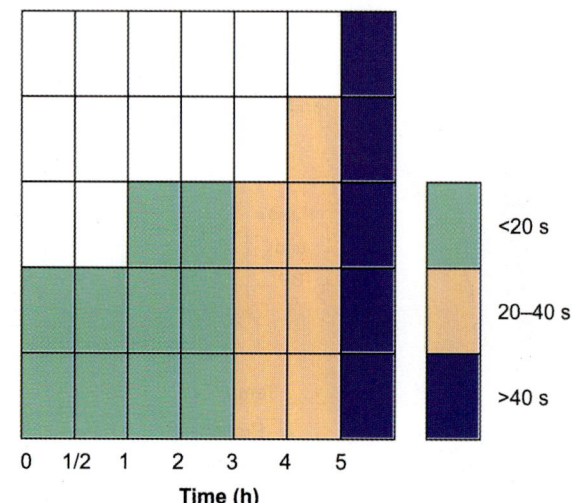

Fig. 4: Recording uterine contractions on partogram.

- *Failure of head descent:* Abnormal progress of labor may occur with normal progress of descent of the fetal head then followed by secondary arrest of descent of fetal head. The cause is generally cephalopelvic disproportion including fetal macrosomia.
- *Precipitate labor:* It is defined as a maximum slope of cervical dilatation of 5 cm/hour or more. This can lead to injuries to birth canal as well as fetal distress.

Intrapartum Fetal Heart Rate Monitoring

Fetal heart rate during labor can be monitored by:
- Intermittent auscultation
- Continuous cardiotocography
- Intermittent cardiotocography.

Intermittent Auscultation

It is offered and recommended in healthy women with an uneventful antenatal period to monitor fetal well-being.[13] In the latent phase of labor, it should be done every 1 hourly after a contraction for a period of 1 minute and in the active phase of labor every 15–30 minutes and every 5 minutes in the second stage of labor.[14]

Continuous Cardiotocography

It involves the application of a TOCO transducer which records the uterine activity and Doppler transducer which records the fetal heart rate over the women's abdomen as seen in **Figure 5**. This greatly reduces the mobility of the women during labor. Nowadays there are a few wireless monitors available and continuous CTG may be useful particularly in high-risk mothers. Cardiotocography during labor is associated with reduced rates of neonatal seizures but no clear differences in rates of cerebral palsy, infant mortality or other standard measures of neonatal well-being. It is however associated with an increase in cesarean sections and instrumental vaginal births.[15] Cardiotocography does provide a written record as well as convenience to monitor fetal heart rate.

Intermittent Cardiotocography

To circumvent the limitations of continuous cardiotocography, intermittent cardiotocography can be done as shown in **Flowchart 1**. There are a very few studies that have compared intermittent CTG with continuous CTG, but one trial comparing the two concluded than "compared with intermittent CTG, continuous CTG made no difference to the mode of delivery or neonatal outcome".[16]

Description of cardiotocographic features is given in **Table 2**. The recognition of deviations from normal is necessarily the first step to initiate appropriate interventions. The actions in case of such situations are discussed in a subsequent chapter.

Active Management of Labor

It can be done for a primigravida with singleton pregnancy, cephalic presentation in spontaneous labor and clear liquor. This is in contrast to the masterly inactivity followed by the obstetrician as described earlier. It involves active involvement of the consultant obstetrician, nurses, 2-hourly per vaginal examination, close partographic monitoring, amniotomy, oxytocin augmentation in escalating doses and compulsory delivery within 12 hours of admission.

MANAGEMENT OF SECOND STAGE OF LABOR

Patient should be informed that the second stage is guided by her own urge to push and she may adopt any position that she finds most comfortable. The various positions the women may adopt are as shown in **Figure 6**. In dorsal position, a 15° left lateral tilt should be favored to avoid aortocaval compression.[17] The obstetrician should scrub up and put

Fig. 5: Method of external fetal cardiotocography (CTG) with its monitor.

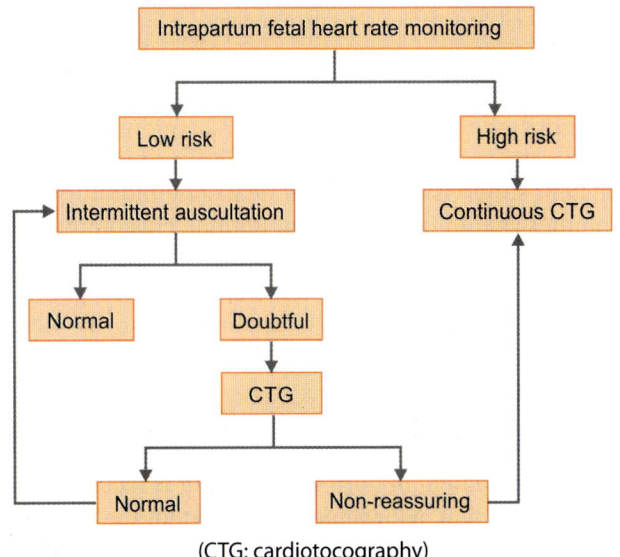

Flowchart 1: Method of intrapartum fetal heart rate monitoring.

(CTG: cardiotocography)

TABLE 2: Description of cardiotocograph trace features.[15]

Overall care
Make a documented systematic assessment of the condition of the woman and unborn baby [including cardiotocography (CTG) findings] every hour, or more frequently if there are concern

Principles for intrapartum CTG trace interpretation
- When reviewing the CTG trace, assess and document contractions and all four features of fetal heart rate: baseline rate, baseline variability, presence or absence of decelerations (and concerning characteristics of variable decelerations* if present), presence of accelerations
- If there is a stable baseline fetal heart rate between 110 and 160 beats/minute and normal variability, continue usual care as the risk of fetal acidosis is low
- If it is difficult to categorize or interpret a CTG trace, obtain a review by a senior midwife or a senior obstetrician

Accelerations
The presence of fetal heart rate accelerations, even with reduced baseline variability, is generally a sign that the baby is healthy

Description	Feature Baseline (beats/minute)	Baseline variability (beats/minute)	Decelerations
Reassuring	110–160	5–25	None or early Variable decelerations with no concerning characteristics* for less than 90 minutes
Nonreassuring	100–109† OR 161–180	Less than 5 for 30 to 50 minutes OR More than 25 for 15 to 25 minutes	Variable decelerations with no concerning characteristics* for 90 minutes or more OR Variable decelerations with any concerning characteristics* in up to 50% of contractions for 30 minutes or more OR Variable decelerations with any concerning characteristics* in over 50% of contractions for less than 30 minutes OR Late decelerations in over 50% of contractions for less than 30 minutes, with no maternal or fetal clinical risk factors such as vaginal bleeding or significant meconium
Abnormal	Below 100 OR Above 180	Less than 5 for more than 50 minutes OR More than 25 for more than 25 minutes OR Sinusoidal	Variable decelerations with any concerning characteristics* in over 50% of contractions for 30 minutes [or less if any maternal or fetal clinical risk factors (see earlier)] OR Late decelerations for 30 minutes (or less if any maternal or fetal clinical risk factors) OR Acute bradycardia, or a single prolonged deceleration lasting 3 minutes or more

*Regard the following as concerning characteristics of variable decelerations: Lasting more than 60 seconds; reduced baseline variability within the deceleration; failure to return to baseline; biphasic (W) shape; no shouldering.
†Although a baseline fetal heart rate between 100 and 109 beats/minute is a non-reassuring feature, continue usual care if there is normal baseline variability and no variable or late decelerations.

on a sterile gown, mask and gloves. The delivery should be conducted under strict aseptic precautions taking into consideration clean hands, clean surface and clean cutting. Constant supervision with fetal heart rate monitory every 5 minutes should be carried out. Routine episiotomy is not recommended during spontaneous vaginal birth and should be done selectively only.[18] Cord should be clamped after cessation of cord pulsation to facilitate transfer of 80–100 mL blood from the compressed placenta to the baby.

MANAGEMENT OF THIRD STAGE OF LABOR

Active management of third stage of labor is recommended over the expectant management as it shortens the third stage and reduces blood loss. 10U of oxytocin by intramuscular injection with delivery of the anterior shoulder or immediately after the birth of a baby and before the cord is clamped and cut is preferred over ergometrine as it has fewer side effects.

MANAGEMENT OF FOURTH STAGE OF LABOR

The mother should be monitored every 15 minutes with regards to pulse, blood pressure, uterine tone and any abnormal vaginal bleeding for a period of at least 1 hour. If found satisfactory she can be shifted out of the labor ward.

THE FUTURE

Newer methods of monitoring fetal well-being under research are:
- *Fetal pulse oximetry:* It is done by means of a sensor placed transvaginally through the cervix to rest against

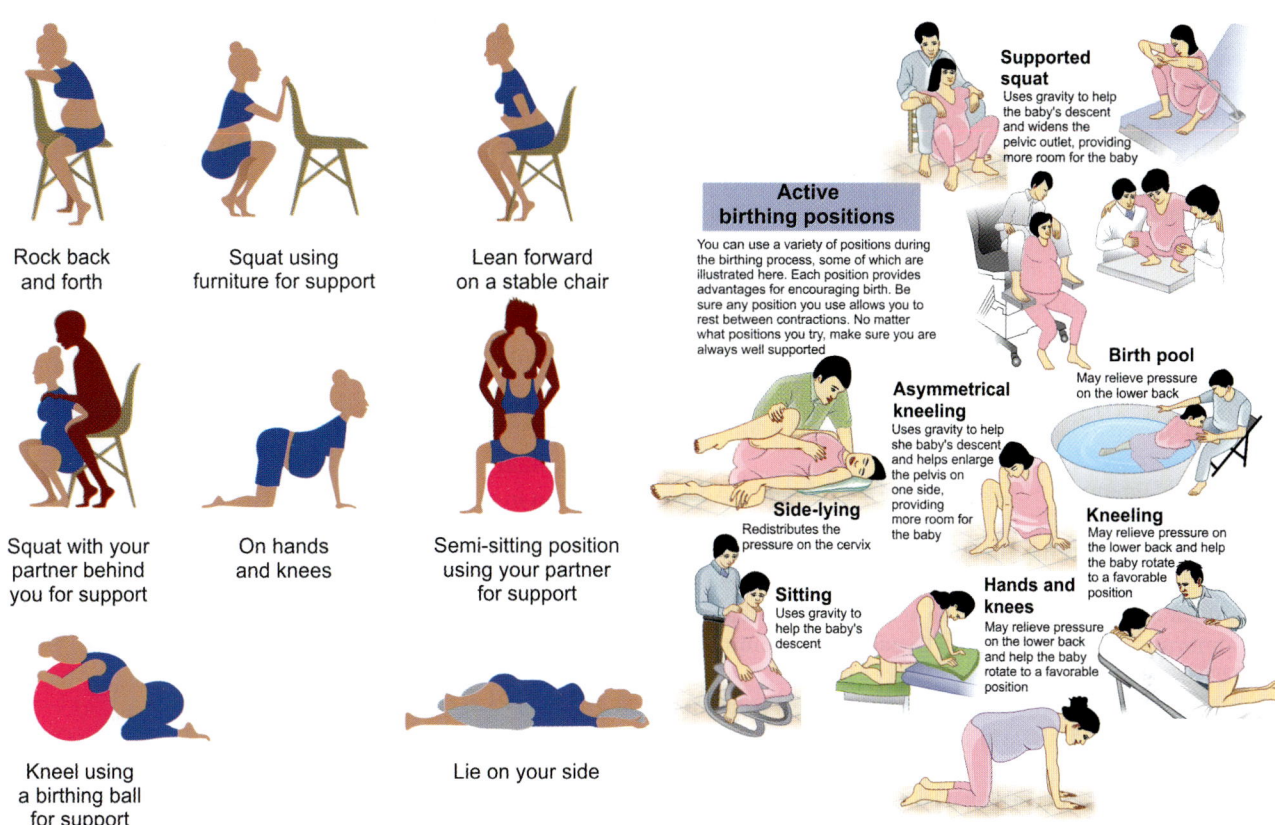

Fig. 6: Positions in labor.

fetal cheek or temple.[19] Fetal lactate levels by means of fetal scalp blood sampling to differentiate between benign respiratory acidosis and potentially dangerous metabolic acidosis.[20] Fetal electrocardiogram analysis by use of a specialized monitor can help by assessing fetal response to hypoxia insults on myocardium.[21]

- *Electronic partograph:* It is a method of monitoring the progress of labor in a mother during childbirth, by attaching a position sensor to a predetermined point on the mother's pelvic bones; monitoring the location of the position sensor in three-dimensional space relative to a reference; and monitoring the location of the fetal presenting part with respect to the predetermined point on the mother's pelvic bones.[22] The location of the fetal presenting part may be indicated by a similar position sensor, or by imaging. It can be accessed from anywhere, anytime, from within a hospital or from home.
- *Computerized labor management:* This idea has been conceived since many years but with the availability of 3D ultrasound systems, it may soon be a reality.[23] An ultrasound-based computerized labor management system with the systems in vivo generated individual partographs with real time dilatation and head station measurements. The measurements had accuracy of <5 mm. This system provides accurate continuous measurements of dilatation and station. The method is superior to digital examination and provides real time diagnosis of nonprogressive and precipitate labor.

The system is likely to reduce discomfort and infections associated with multiple vaginal examination.

KEY MESSAGES

Labor though a physiological process is associated with a plethora of complications that may result in significant maternal or neonatal morbidity or mortality. The World Health Organization (WHO) recommendations 2018, on intraparum care showed that women want a "positive childbirth experience" that fulfills or exceeds their prior personal and sociocultural beliefs and expectations. Preparation of labor should ideally start from the antenatal period both mentally as well as physically. The management of labor includes masterly inactivity in the first stage to active management of third stage. Various misconceptions regarding mobility, oral intake and monitoring in labor needs to be cleared for the mother as well as the caregiver. The importance of objective assessment of labor by means of a partogram needs to be stressed upon every obstetrician.

REFERENCES

1. Devane D, Lalor JG, Daly S, McGuire W, Cuthbert A, Smith V. Cardiotocography versus intermittent auscultation of fetal heart on admission to labour ward for assessment of fetal wellbeing. Cochrane Database Syst Rev. 2017;(1):CD005122.
2. WHO Reproductive Health Library. WHO recommendation on labour ward admission policy. (February 2018). Geneva: World Health Organization; 2018.

3. Reveiz L, Gaitán HG, Cuervo LG. Enemas during labour. Cochrane Database Syst Rev. 2013;(5):CD000330.
4. Lawrence A, Lewis L, Hofmeyr GJ, Styles C. Maternal positions and mobility during first stage labor. Cochrane Database Syst Rev. 2013;(8):CD003934.
5. ACOG. ACOG Committee Opinion No. 766: Approaches to Limit Intervention during Labor and Birth. Obstet Gynecol. 2019;133(2):e164-e173.
6. Dawood F, Dowswell T, Quenby S. Intravenous fluids for reducing the duration of labor in low risk nulliparous women. Cochrane Database Syst Rev. 2013;(6):CD007715.
7. Appleby C. Clinical Guideline for: Bladder care in labor and postnatally. Maternity Guidelines Committee Norfolk and Norwich University Hospitals. London: NHS Foundation Trust; 2020.
8. Friedman, Emanuel A. Graphic analysis of labor. AJOG. 1954;68:1568-75.
9. Philpott RH. Graphic records in labor. BMJ 1972;4:163.
10. Philpott RH, Castle WM. Cervicographs in the management of LABOR in primigravidae II. The action line and treatment of abnormal LABOR. J Obstet Gynaecol Br Commonw. 1972;79:599602.
11. Studd J. Partograms and Nomograms of Cervical Dilatation Management of Primigravid LABORing Women. Br Med J. 1973;4:451-5.
12. Kenchaveeriah SM, Patil KP, Singh TG. Comparison of two WHO partographs: a one year randomized controlled trial. J Turk Ger Gynecol Assoc. 2011;12(1):31-4.
13. Lewis D, Downe S, FIGO Intrapartum Fetal Monitoring Expert Consensus Panel. FIGO consensus guidelines on intrapartum fetal monitoring: Intermittent auscultation. Int J Gynecol Obstet. 2015;131(1):9-12.
14. WHO Reproductive Health Library. WHO recommendation on intermittent fetal heart rate auscultation during labour. (February 2018). Geneva: World Health Organization; 2018.
15. NICE guidelines CG190. Intrapartum care: care of healthy women and their babies during childbirth. London: NICE; 2014.
16. Alfirevic Z, Gyte GML, Cuthbert A, Devane D. Continuous cardiotocography (CTG) as a form of electronic fetal monitoring (EFM) for fetal assessment during labour. Cochrane Database Syst Rev. 2017;(2).
17. Gupta JK, Sood A, Hofmeyr GJ, Vogel JP. Position in the second stage of labour for women without epidural anaesthesia. Cochrane Database Syst Rev. 2017;25(5):CD002006.
18. Jiang H, Qian X, Carroli G, Garner P. Selective versus routine use of episiotomy for vaginal birth. Cochrane Database Syst Rev. 2017;2(2):CD000081.
19. East CE, Begg L, Colditz PB, Lau R. Fetal pulse oximetry for fetal assessment in labour. Cochrane Database Syst Rev. 2014;(10):CD004075.
20. East CE, Leader LR, Sheehan P, Henshall NE, Colditz PB, Lau R. Cochrane Database Syst Rev. 2015;(5):CD006174.
21. Turner J, Mitchell M, Kumar S. The physiology of intrapartum fetal compromise at term. Am J Obstet Gynecol .2020;22(1):17-26.
22. Sanghvi H, Mohan D, Litwin L, Bazant E, Gomez P, MacDowell T, et al. Effectiveness of an Electronic Partogram: a Mixed-Method, Quasi-Experimental Study Among Skilled Birth Attendants in Kenya. Glob Health Sci Pract. 2019;7(4):521-39.
23. Erlik U, Wolman I. Intrapartum sonographic assessment of labor. J Obstet Gynaecol India. 2013;63(5):297-300.

LONG QUESTIONS

1. Define labor and how will you monitor first stage of labor with the help of partogram?
2. Describe routine care given to full term pregnant woman with established labor.
3. Describe different tests done in normal labor patient.
4. What is FOGSI Manyata program and what are its principles?
5. Explain: "why giving birth to child is considered as rebirth to mother".

SHORT QUESTIONS

1. Explain criteria for admission of pregnant patient with pain in abdomen.
2. What is admission test and what is its significance?
3. Explain alert and action line with the help of diagram.
4. Define precipitate labor and significance of it.
5. Define molding and explain its significance in labor.

MULTIPLE CHOICE QUESTIONS

1. True onset of labor is determined by:
   a. Passage of bloody show
   b. Occurrence of uterine contraction
   c. Excessive fetal movement
   d. Cervical dilation and effacement
   e. Gush of vaginal fluid
2. Active management of third stage of labor includes all, except:
   a. IV oxytocin after delivery of ant shoulder
   b. Controlled cord traction
   c. Suprapubic massage
   d. Uterine massage
3. Progress in labor is determined by:
   a. Dilation and intensity of contraction
   b. Dilation and effacement
   c. Dilation and descent
   d. Frequency of contraction and descent
   e. All of the above
4. The initial assessment of the pregnant woman presenting in labor ward includes all of the following, except:
   a. Admission test   b. detailed history
   c. Per vaginal examination d. Review investigations
5. Fetal monitoring in labor for a low risk woman in spontaneous labor and clear liquor should be done by:
   a. Continuous cardiotocography
   b. Intermittent auscultation
   c. Fetal scalp blood sampling
   d. Fetal fibronectin levels
6. Active management of labor includes all of the following, except:
   a. Episiotomy   b. Oxytocin augmentation
   c. Partogram monitoring d. Amniotomy

7. All of the following are features of an Abnormal CTG, except:
   a. Persistent fetal heart rate of 90 bpm
   b. Variable decelerations lasting for 20 seconds
   c. Decreased beat to beat variability of less than 5 bpm for 50 minutes
   d. Sinusoidal pattern
8. Regarding the cardiotocograph (CTG) the following are true, except:
   a. It is assessed for four features before classifying it as normal, suspicious or pathological according to National Institute for Health and Care Excellence (NICE) guidance
   b. It is the preferred technique for monitoring fetal well-being in a low-risk labor
   c. Also records uterine contraction strength and frequency
   d. Requires the use of two transducers placed on the maternal abdomen
   e. All of the above
9. The second stage of labor is defined as which of the following?
   a. The interval from onset of contractions to the beginning of cervical dilation
   b. The time from full cervical dilation to delivery of the fetus
   c. The duration of maternal pushing efforts
   d. The time from delivery of the fetus until delivery of the placenta
10. Nonreassuring elements of intrapartum fetal heart rate monitoring patterns include which of the following?
    a. Minimal or absent variability
    b. Absence of accelerations
    c. Bradycardia or tachycardia
    d. A + B
    e. B + C
    f. A + C
11. Intermittent auscultation is adequate or preferable in all of the following conditions, except:
    a. If the CTG is of poor technical quality despite attempts at using different transducers or electrodes
    b. In a low-risk labor after an admission CTG
    c. In a low-risk labor without an admission CTG
    d. When there are two different rates of 70 bpm and 140 bpm seen on the trace
    e. When a high-risk mother is not willing to have continuous monitoring
12. The best time to listen to the fetal heart in labor is:
    a. Before a contraction   b. During a contraction
    c. After a contraction   d. All of above
    e. Both (B) and (C)
13. A few hours in labor induction CTC shows a late deceleration after episode of frequent contraction, the most likely explanation of deceleration is:
    a. Maternal position on left lateral side
    b. Uterine hyperstimulation from cervical ripening agent
    c. Compression of the fetal head mediated by vagus
    d. Umbilical cord compression
    e. All of the above

Answers
1. d 2. c 3. c 4. a 5. b 6. a
7. b 8. b 9. b 10. f 11. e 12. c
13. b

9.4 INDUCTION OF LABOR

Uday Thanawala, Manasi Venkatraman, Saloni Suchak, Nanak Bhagat

INTRODUCTION

Delivery is needed when either the maternal or fetal health is at risk, especially in complicated gestations. With advances in technology [tools such as electronic fetal heart rate monitoring (EFHRM) and ultrasonography (USG)] we are picking up the sick fetus and delivering before the intrauterine environment deteriorates. Good neonatal care back up gives us the confidence of delivering these babies earlier. Though lower segment cesarean section (LSCS) is an option, clinicians increasingly induce labor when a pregnancy may require early termination.

Induction of labor (IOL) is, thus, an important intervention in obstetrics and is offered to women with a generally a single fetus in vertex presentation with no contraindications for a vaginal delivery.

INDICATIONS OF INDUCTION OF LABOR

Some of the many clinical situations, which may warrant an induction, are discussed here.

Contraindications

Induction of labor is contraindicated where vaginal delivery is contraindicated.

Absolute contraindications to induction of labor include:[1,2]
- Cephalopelvic disproportion
- Placenta previa/vasa previa
- Transverse lie
- Active genital herpes (first episode in third trimester – not recurrent herpes)
- Previous classical uterine incision

- Fetal anatomical abnormality that contraindicates vaginal delivery.

Relative contraindications to vaginal delivery (and, therefore, induction of labor) include the important factors, which are described in **Table 1**.
- Triplet or higher order multiple pregnancy
- Breech presentation
- Two or more previous low transverse cesarean sections.

Criteria for a Successful Induction

A successful induction requires assessment of the gestational age, station of the presenting part and the status of the cervix. Chance of a successful IOL is best with a ripe cervix.
- *Evaluation of the cervix:* Cervix is considered ripe if it is dilated, effaced, soft, and anterior in position. For a ripe cervix, any/every method of IOL will work; but for an unripe cervix, IOL becomes a two-step method—the first step is to ripen cervix before going ahead with IOL.

Bishop's score is followed universally and a cervix is considered favorable for induction when the Bishop's score is high. Basically, it quantifies cervical dilatation, position, effacement, station of presenting part and consistency which gives us an idea on how much effort will be required for inducing a particular patient. IOL is likely to be successful if the score is more than 8. A score of less than 6 will require cervical ripening for an effective IOL.

Modified Bishop's score is suggested **(Table 2)**. The "effacement of cervix" is substituted with "length of the cervix".

- *The gestational age* also matters—nearer the patient to term, more likelihood of success.
- *Station:* Lower the station, higher the chance of successful induction (cephalic presentation).

Patient Counseling and Consent

Before proceeding with IOL, the obstetrician needs to have a detailed discussion with the Patient and her relatives about the situation:
- *Why deliver now (indication)*
- *The mode of delivery (CS/IOL)*
- *Method of IOL*
- *Outcomes (successful IOL with a normal vaginal/ instrumental delivery or a failed IOL which ends in an emergency LSCS)*
- *Pain relief options*
- *Condition of the baby and planned baby care*
- *The risks and benefits of induction of labor in specific circumstances and the proposed induction methods.*

All this should be documented and proper informed consent is to be taken before attempting IOL.

Induction of labor should be attempted in a maternity unit with facility for emergency CS and adequate baby care. If you are expecting an extremely preterm or compromised baby, in-utero transfer to a proper facility should be advised. The healthcare provider must:
- Allow the woman time to discuss the information with her partner before coming to a decision

TABLE 1: Relative contraindications to vaginal delivery.

Maternal:	Fetal:	Elective Induction:

• Medical disorders in pregnancy
  – Severe preeclampsia/eclampsia
  – DM
  – Cholestasis of pregnancy
  – Chronic renal disease
• PROM
	• Postdatism
	• IUGR, fetal compromise
	• Rh isoimmunization
	• Oligohydramnios
	• Polyhydramnios
	• IUFD
		• Logistic reasons: High risk patient staying far from facility
		• Patient or Doctor convenience
		• In COVID-19 pandemic, most practitioners are doing a COVID test after 38 weeks and advice delivery within 5 days of testing

(DM: diabetes mellitus; IUFD: intrauterine fetal death; IUGR: intrauterine growth restriction; PROM: premature rupture of membranes)

TABLE 2: Modified Bishop's score.

Ease of IOL = ripeness of the cervix				
	Score			
	0	1	2	3
Cervical dilatation (cm)	0	1–2	3–4	5–6
Cervical length (cm)	>4	3–4	1–2	<1
Cervical consistency	Firm	Medium	Soft	
Cervical position	Posterior	Central	Anterior	
Station (cm in relation to spine)	–3 above spines	–2 above spines	–1 to 0 above spines	Below spines
Total score 13 0–5	Favorable	Score 6–13	Unfavorable	Score

- Encourage the woman to look at a variety of sources of information
- Invite the woman to ask questions, and encourage her to think about her options
- Support the woman in whatever decision she makes.
  An induction should result in:
  - Adequate uterine activity which is defined as—3 to 5 contractions in a 10-minute period and a duration of 40–50 seconds.
  - Progressive cervical dilatation with decent of the presenting part.
  - Resulting in a vaginal delivery, which is the end point.
  Plotting a partograph is mandatory to monitor the progress of labor.

Process of Ripening the Cervix/Induction of Labor

Normal Physiology

As the gestation nears term, number of oxytocin receptors in the myometrium increase making the uterus more sensitive to oxytocics, lower segment is formed and the cervix ripens with increasing destruction of the connective tissue by hydrolysis with hyaluronidase. Erratic electric impulses in the myometrium synchronize over a period of time with establishment of polarity. As a result, the cervix becomes soft, short and yields to pressure of the presenting part with uterine contractions.

Methods for Induction

A suggested approach to induction of labor based on Bishop's score is presented in **Flowcharts 1 and 2**.

Pharmacological methods **(Table 3)**:
- Oxytocin
- *Prostaglandins:* Dinoprostone (PGE2): Transcervical Gel/intravaginal pessary
- *Misoprostol (PGE1):* Oral/vaginal.

Two drugs are not to be used together. There should be a gap of at least 12 hours before using another pharmacological agent for IOL.

In the by-gone era (1970–1980) when prostaglandins were not available - we used to start a Oxytocin drip - called a ripening drip using very low dose intravenous over many hours or at times days hoping that the cervix will ripen. With prostaglandins now this is history. So let us first talk about most widely used methods of IOL today.

Prostaglandins: The type used for induction of labor is prostaglandin E2 and E1, which acts by causing uterine contraction and softening of the cervix. IOL using prostaglandins appears to be associated with an increased likelihood of successful vaginal delivery, reduced cesarean section rates, reduced rates of epidural analgesia and increased maternal satisfaction.[3]

Prostaglandins are available in three different forms: tablets, gel and slow release pessary. Tablet, gel and pessary forms appear to be equally efficacious. The use of sustained release inserts appear to be associated with a reduction in instrumental vaginal delivery rates when compared with gel or tablets **(Figs. 1A to C)**.

Gel: PGE2 gel is available as 0.5 mg preparations. It comes with an inserter. During per vaginal examination one can guide the inserter so as to release the gel in the cervical canal. Generally 6–8 hours should elapse to note the effect of the insert. If there is no effect then the second dose is given 6 hours later. A maximum of three inserts can be done at least 6 hours apart. Oxytocin if needed can be started 6 hours after the last dose.

Ambulation of the patient is allowed after 30 minutes of insertion.

Temperature, pulse, respiratory rate, blood pressure, uterine activity and vaginal bleeding should are examined immediately after insertion then hourly for 4–6 hours.

It is a good practice to record a non-stress test (NST)/cardiotocography (CTG) 30 minutes post gel insertion. The gel should be stored in a refrigerator at 2–8°C.

Slow release pessary: PGE2 pessaries release the drug in a controlled fashion from a retrieval device. Approximately 10 mg of dinoprostone is released over 24 hours (at a constant rate of approximately 0.3 mg/hour).

If used for cervical ripening and IOL at term, one pessary (in a retrievable device) should be inserted high into the posterior fornix. It should be removed when cervical ripening is adequate/labor has become established or after 24 hours. If augmentation is needed one needs to wait at least for 60 min after removal, before starting an oxytocin drip.

Misoprostol: PGE1 (oral/vaginal) is a synthetic prostaglandin E1 analog. Misoprostol is cheap and stable at room temperature, unlike dinoprostone, which needs to be stored in a refrigerator. It can be given orally, vaginally or sublingually. (For induction it is only oral or vaginal - NOT sublingual). Its low price and easy storage makes it of potential use, particularly in resource-poor settings. However, there have been concerns about safety when used in the third trimester, particularly regarding hyperstimulation.

Dosage: Oral 25/50 µg 2 hourly - maximum 100–150 µg.

Vaginal: Maximum 25 µg 4–6 hourly (higher doses associated with increased risk of uterine hyperstimulation).

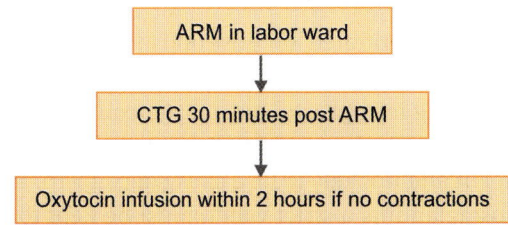

Flowchart 1: Suggested management of a patient near term with a favorable cervix (Bishop's score >4).

(ARM: artificial rupture of membrane; CTG: cardiotocography)

Flowchart 2: Suggested management of a patient with unfavorable cervix (Bishop's score <4)

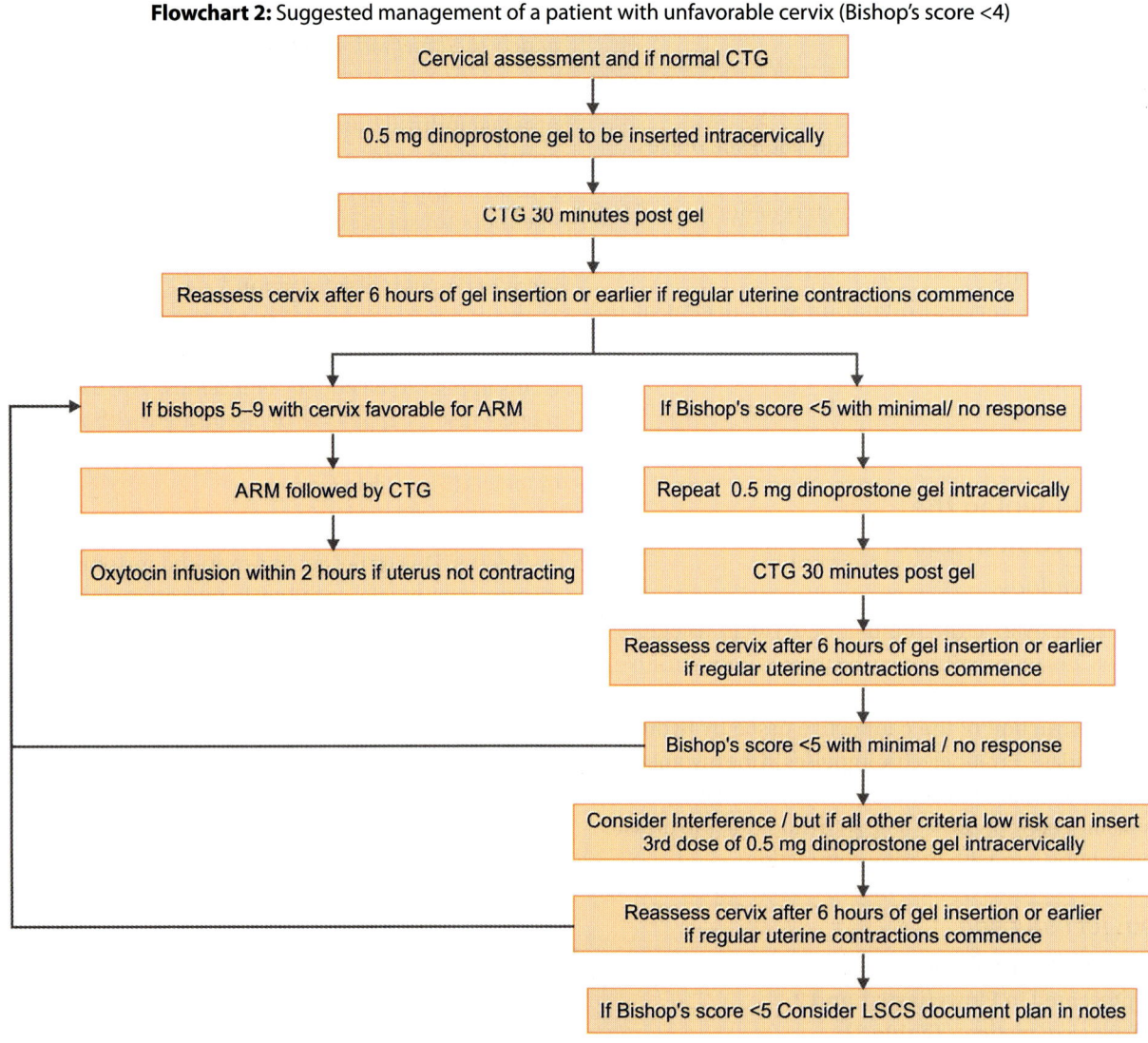

(ARM: artificial rupture of membrane; CTG: cardiotocography; LSCS: lower segment cesarean section)

TABLE 3: Pharmacological methods for induction of labor.				
Drug	**Route**	**Dosage**	**Maximum dose**	**Special note**
Oxytocin	IV infusion	10 mIU/mL in titrated doses	40 units	
Misoprostol (PGE1)	Oral	50 µg, 4 hourly 25 µg, 2 hourly	100–150 µg	May develop fever Watch for hyperstimulation
	Vaginal	25 µg, 6 hourly	100 µg	
Dinoprostone (PGE2)	Intracervical gel	0.5 mg, 6 hourly	3 doses	Watch for hyperstimulation
	Pessary	10 mg once in 24 hours	10 mg	Watch for hyperstimulation Can be removed
	Tablets	3 mg, 6–8 hourly	6 mg	(not available in our setting)

A systematic review and meta-analysis assessing the effectiveness and safety of prostaglandins (12 different agents including PGE2 gel/pessary and oral misoprostol) used for labor induction analyzed 280 RCTs of 48,068 women. Relative to placebo, this review reported that the odds of failing to achieve a vaginal delivery were lowest for vaginal misoprostol (OR 0.06, 95% CI 0.02–0.12) and the odds of cesarean section were lowest in the titrated low dose oral misoprostol (OR 0.65, 95% CI 0.49–0.83)[4]

When using misoprostol one may encounter meconium staining but that is the result of direct action of the drug on the fetal gut and unlikely to be a cause of concern. However, with prostaglandins a strict watch must be kept to prevent hyperstimulation and ensure fetal well-being.

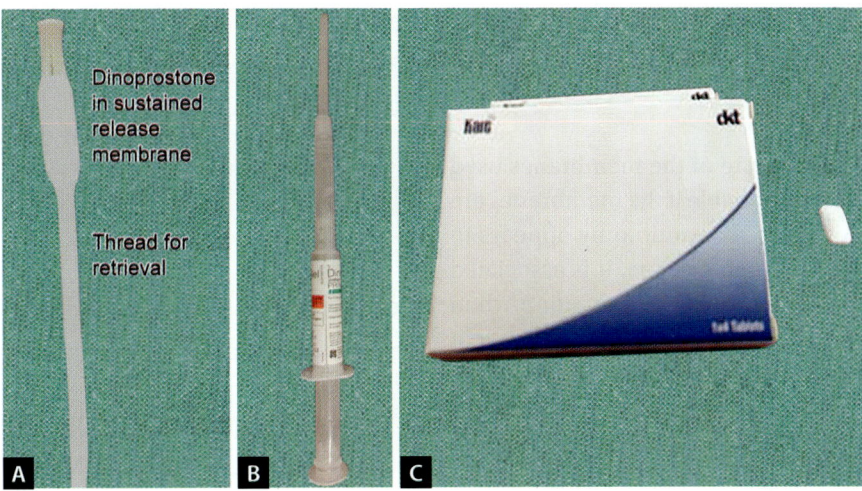

Figs. 1A to C: Prostaglandins and analogs for induction of labor. (A) Dinoprostone sustained release pessary; (B) Dinoprostone gel; (C) Misoprostol tablets.

Misoprostol is not yet approved for IOL by Drug Controller General of India. (FOGSI good clinical practice guidelines on IOL)

Oxytocin

Oxytocin is a neuropeptide hormone produced in the hypothalamus and stored in the posterior pituitary gland. In the context of IOL, it acts on specific receptors on the uterus to cause uterine contractions.

Practical Aspects of Using Oxytocin

Begin infusion with 4–6 mIU/min (Approximately 8 drops of 5 units of Oxytocin in 500 ml of RL) with dose increments of 4–6 mU/min every 30 minutes. The oxytocin infusion can be increased until labor progress is normal or uterine activity reaches 200–250 Montevideo units (i.e., good regular uterine contractions, each lasting for 40–45 seconds duration and minimum of three contractions in 10 minutes).

Upper limit of the oxytocin infusion during labor with a live fetus in the third trimester is 40 mIU/minute.

Infusion of oxytocin should be documented in mIU/minute or drops/minute with the dilution being mentioned.

Monitoring for infusion rate of oxytocin and uterine contractions and fetal heart rate by continuous CTG is preferable. In facilities where CTG is not available, fetal monitoring should be done by intermittent auscultation every 15–30 min in first stage and 5 minutes in second stage.

Blood pressure and pulse should be assessed every hour. Intake and output should be assessed every 4 hours.

Cervical status should be assessed prior to administration of oxytocin and repeated after at least four hours of moderate contractions.

A vaginal examination may also be repeated in situation of a nonreassuring fetal heart pattern to rule out the presence of meconium, abruption or a cord accident. Close watch is kept for clinical features of maternal hyponatremia, uterine hyperstimulation and uterine rupture.[5]

The biggest advantage of using an oxytocin infusion is that one can control it according to response.

Decrease oxytocin for
- Tachysystole (more than 5 contractions in 10 minutes)
- Contractions lasting more than 2 minutes
- Contractions at less than 1 minute interval from each other
- Insufficient return of uterine resting tone between contractions.

Decrease the oxytocin to half rather than stopping may correct the abnormal contraction pattern and prevent an unwarranted operative intervention.

Discontinue the oxytocin if
- Tachysystole does not resolve on decreasing the oxytocin
- Nonreassuring fetal heart rate pattern—variable decelerations/tachycardia/bradycardia/late decelerations/poor beat to beat variability
- Maternal hypotension
- Signs of impending rupture/active vaginal bleed/hyperstimulation.

The NICE guideline, therefore, recommends using prostaglandins in preference to oxytocin in women with intact membranes, irrespective of parity or modified Bishop's score.[6]

Mechanical Methods

- Membrane sweep
- Artificial rupture of the membranes (ARM or Amniotomy)
- Foley's catheter/with normal saline.

Membrane Sweep

Membrane sweeping involves the examining finger passing through the cervix to rotate against the wall of the uterus, to separate the chorionic membrane from the decidua. Membrane sweeping is regarded as an adjunct to IOL rather than an actual method of induction.

Prior to formal IOL, women should be offered a vaginal examination for membrane sweeping. At the 40 and 41 week antenatal visits, nulliparous women should be offered a vaginal examination for membrane sweeping.

Amniotomy

It is the deliberate artificial rupture of the membranes used for IOL. The procedure is only possible if the membranes are physically accessible. Although an amniotomy appears to be effective in the case of a favorable cervix, it is associated with more frequent need for oxytocin augmentation when compared with vaginal PGE2. Amniotomy with oxytocin should not be used as a primary method of IOL unless there are specific contraindications to the use of vaginal PGE2.

Role of ARM:
- May help in a favorable cervix
- May not be possible in an unripe cervix
- You are committed once ARM has been done – risk of ascending infection as time passes.

Foley's Catheter/with Normal Saline

A Foley catheter is inserted through the cervical canal and inflated. This separates the membrane applies pressure to the cervix causing it to dilate. Once the cervix is adequately dilated the catheter simply drops out. Safety is the biggest advantage of this method because it acts by the release of prostaglandins naturally by the body. This is becoming the preferred method for high risk cases such as previous LSCS and intrauterine fetal death (IUFD).

Disadvantages:
- Difficulty in inserting through an unfavorable cervix for the operator, and discomfort for the woman
- Risk of infection
- Low-lying placenta is a contraindication.

Hygroscopic dilators (laminaria tents), mifepristone, nitric oxide donors, relaxin, hyaluronidase or breast nipple stimulation are presently not recommended for IOL in view of the availability of low quality evidence for their use.

Let Us Get Practical: Whom to Induce How?

Induction of labor in women with different gestational ages is suggested in **Table 4**.

TABLE 4: Induction of labor in women by gestational age.

	Favorable cervix	Unfavorable cervix Requires a two-step process— ripening the cervix and induction
Near term	Any method including ARM and oxytocin	PGE2 Gel/PGE1 tablet PV/PO
Far from term	PGE2 Gel/PGE1 tablet PV/PO Foley's catheter	PGE2 Gel/PGE1 tablet PV/PO Foley's catheter

Failed IOL
- No onset of uterine activity or no progressive cervical changes
- The cervix fails to yield and dilate in spite of adequate uterine activity
- Fetal distress
  All these may warrant an LSCS.

Complications/Dangers/Risks of IOL

The complications of IOL are given in **Table 5**.

INDUCTION OF LABOR IN SPECIAL MATERNAL SITUATIONS

Induction of Labor for Previous Cesarean Delivery

Importance of Induction in a Case of Previous LSCS

The mode of delivery by cesarean section has been steadily rising all over the world and does not seem to plateau. A common reason for a section is *previous section.*

Any woman being induced for a trial of labor after cesarean section (TOLAC), it is imperative that she must be counseled appropriately and exhaustively as to the adverse outcomes that may result.

Risk factors that could result in increased complications, thus increasing the morbidity and mortality for women undergoing an induction for a previous section are:
- Unfavorable cervix
- Integrity of the scar (assess myometrial thickness on USG)
- Malpresentation
- Malposition
- Relative CPD (LGA/macrosomia)
- Floating head at the time of induction.

If any of the above factors are present, one should possibly avoid an induction, or if not, be very vigilant and give a short trial of labor.

TABLE 5: Complications of induction of labor.

Maternal	Fetal
• Failed induction causing higher LSCS rates • Prolonged labor • Hyperstimulation • Increased need for labor analgesia • Higher chances of operative vaginal delivery • Higher chances of PPH • Higher chances of chorioamnionitis • Uterine rupture	• Fetal distress (tachysystole with/without FHR changes) • Iatrogenic prematurity • Cord prolapse with ARM

(PPH: postpartum hemorrhage; LSCS: lower segment cesarean section)

Possible adverse outcomes:
- Uterine rupture
- Maternal morbidity
- Perinatal and neonatal morbidity and mortality.

In women with a previous LSCS, counsel for a vaginal birth after cesarean section (VBAC) on individual basis. Backup for continuous intrapartum monitoring and the facilities to deal with any possible complication especially rupture should be kept ready and made available immediately if an emergency happens.

Role of myometrial scar thickness: A recent meta-analysis by Kok et al. looked at a myometrial thickness of 2.1–4 mm as having a strong negative predictive value for uterine dehiscence or rupture whereas a thickness of 0.6–2 mm had a strong positive predictive value for the occurrence of a uterine defect.[7]

However, an ideal cut off for clinical practice has not been defined or endorsed as yet and further research needs to be conducted before it becomes standard practice.

Methods: There is no consensus on which method is ideal.

Mechanical methods like Foley's catheter, by far, are the *safest* methods for IOL in women with a previous cesarean section, as it has the least rate of uterine rupture among all methods of induction and is comparable to the risk of rupture in spontaneous labor.

The Society of Obstetricians and Gynaecologists of Canada (SOGC) clinical practice guidelines state that prostaglandins E2 (PGE2) should only be used in exceptional circumstances, and after appropriate counseling on the risk of uterine rupture, recommending that a Foley catheter be used in these women.[8]

The UK National Institute for Clinical Excellence[2] (NICE) guidelines do not make any explicit recommendations, but do not discourage the use of prostaglandin.

In contrast, practice guidelines issued by the American College of Obstetricians and Gynecologists state that the use of prostaglandins for cervical ripening or induction of labor in most women who have had a previous cesarean section should be discouraged.[9]

So, the choice of method of IOL in a patient with a previous cesarean section needs to be selected by the treating obstetrician on case to case basis and depends on the availability of the drug/device, familiarity or ease of use by the obstetrician and policy of the institute. Superiority of one method above the other is debatable and subjective.

Elective Induction of Labor and Covid-19 Pandemic

Inducing labor in the absence of a valid medical maternal or fetal indication to deliver is always a debated and controversial topic.

Indications:
- Day time obstetrics
- Social convenience for the patient or the doctor (patient residing far from facility)
- "*Mahurat timing*" (prechosen auspicious day)
- Is the Covid pandemic another valid indication for induction?

These are uncertain times and recommendations for Covid testing are changing perpetually. Patients who are going to deliver are scared, no relatives will be allowed, no birth companion! A mask has to be worn always, even when breastfeeding.

Health workers are scared – droplets, peritoneal fluid, and stools have Covid.

Do we ask all patients to do a Covid test or treat all patients as asymptomatic carriers and take universal precautions, while delivering and during hospital stay? We suppose the answers to this cannot be same for all because of the different setting we have - corporate, private and government - with varying patient population and economic status. One will have to decide what is best and safest for his/her practice (recommendations in different states also vary).

If we do a Covid-19 RT-PCR after 38 weeks for all then it may be better to induce and deliver within 5 days if the test for Covid is negative. Induction definitely has a role.

If she is Covid positive, it may be better to wait if no obstetric indication to interfere is there. But certainly we feel if one decides on an induction in these times it is worthwhile doing a Covid test before induction for everyone's safety.

If IOL for maternal request can be an alternative to a planned LSCS, it probably is worth a try!

Intrauterine Fetal Death

In the unfortunate case of an IUFD, induction of labor is the obvious choice if the blood clotting factors are normal and maternal condition stable. Prostaglandin gel, pessary or mechanical methods used to make the cervix favorable before starting oxytocin augmentation to induce labor. Many also use mifepristone especially if the patient has a poor Bishop's score 48 hours before starting misoprostol. Dinoprostone pessary can also be used.

■ CONCLUSION

Induction of labor is an art and the clinician's judgment and knowledge plays a huge role in a successful induction. With newer drugs available in different delivery forms make the task of ripening an unfavorable cervix easier. In special situation, special care is needed in selecting the method. A strict vigil on its progress and maternal/fetal wellbeing is important throughout induction. Active management of third stage is important in all the cases.

■ REFERENCES

1. Mehta A. Behavioral patterns of cervix uteri during second and third trimester of pregnancy. J Obstet Gynecol India. 1974:450-9.

2. Mehta A, Shah P. Prematurity and cervical status. J Obstet Gynecoogy of India. 1977:142-52.
3. World Health Organization. WHO Recommendations for IOL. Geneva: WHO; 2019. pp. 17-20.
4. Alfirevic Z, Keeney E, Dowswell T, Welton NJ, Dias S, Jones LV, et al. Labour induction with prostaglandins: a systematic review and network meta-analysis. BMJ. 2015;350:h217.
5. Kumari SS. Induction of Labour: Good Clinical Practice Recommendations. Mumbai: FOGSI-ICOG; 2018.
6. National Institute for Health and Clinical Excellence. Induction of Labour. Clinical Guideline 70. Manchester: NICE; 2008.
7. Kok N, Wiersma IC, Opmeer BC, de Graaf IM, Mol BW, Pajkrt E. Sonographic measurement of lower uterine segment thickness to predict uterine rupture during a trial of labor in women with previous Cesarean section: a meta-analysis. Ultrasound Obstet Gynecol. 2013;42:132-9.
8. Society of Obstetricians and Gynaecologists of Canada, Martel M, MacKinnon CJ, SOGC Clinical Practice Obstetrics Committee. Guidelines for vaginal birth after previous Caesarean birth. CPG No. 155. J Obstet Gynaecol Can. 2005;27:164-74.
9. American College of Obstetricians and Gynecologists. Vaginal Birth after Caesarean Section. ACOG practice Bulletin No.115. Obstet Gynaecol. 2010;116:450-63.

LONG QUESTIONS

1. Describe the role of oxytocin in the induction of labor.
2. Compare the various prostaglandins used in the induction of labor. Discuss advantages and disadvantages of the same.
3. Discuss the role of induction of labor in a patient with a previous LSCS.

SHORT QUESTIONS

1. Define induction of labor and discuss the indications of induction.
2. Discuss the Bishop's scoring system and the significance of the same.
3. What are the complications of induction of labor?
4. What are the various mechanical methods of labor induction? Briefly describe the same.
5. What is failed induction?

MULTIPLE CHOICE QUESTIONS

1. The following is a contraindication to induction of labor:
    a. Rh isoimmunization
    b. Oligohydramnios with AFI 6.5 cm at term
    c. Vasa previa
    d. Maternal diabetes
2. The following is not a component of Bishop's score:
    a. Cervical dilatation
    b. Cervical effacement
    c. Fetal station
    d. Fetal presentation
3. In the physiology of cervical ripening, the following statement is true:
    a. The myometrium becomes an electrical syncytium closer to term
    b. The number of oxytocin receptors reduces but become more sensitive at term
    c. The fibrous tissue component of the cervix increases
    d. Prostaglandins play a role in myometrial contractility and not in cervical ripening
4. Which of the following is true of membrane sweeping?
    a. It is painless
    b. It can cause vaginal spotting and increase unscheduled visits
    c. Number of women needing induction of labor reduces
    d. It should be offered routinely at 37 weeks of pregnancy
5. The following induction agent can be stored without refrigeration:
    a. Misoprostol
    b. Dinoprostone gel
    c. Dinoprostone vaginal inserts
    d. Oxytocin
6. The standard formulation of dinoprostone for induction of labor is:
    a. 0.5 mg dinoprostone in 3 gram of gel
    b. 3 mg dinoprostone in 3 gram of gel
    c. 0.3 mg dinoprostone in 5 gram of gel
    d. 5 mg dinoprostone in 5 gram of gel
7. The advantages of oxytocin as an induction agent are all, except:
    a. Possible to stop the effect instantly
    b. Associated with higher probability of vaginal delivery as compared to prostaglandins
    c. Low incidence of hyperstimulation and fetal distress
    d. Low cost per unit of drug
8. The possible side effects of pharmacological agents for induction of labor are:
    a. Antepartum hemorrhage
    b. Cord prolapsed
    c. Endometritis
    d. Hyperstimulation

Answers
1. c 2. d 3. a 4. b 5. a 6. a
7. b 8. a

9.5 LABOR IN SPECIAL SITUATIONS (PREVIOUS CESAREAN BIRTH, POOR PROGRESS IN LABOR, FETAL COMPROMISE IN LABOR, MECONIUM STAINED AMNIOTIC FLUID)

BS Jodha, Sudhakshi Kinger

INTRODUCTION

Most pregnancies result in delivery of a healthy infant at term without deviations from a standard course in labor. The essential features of such typical situations are listed here:
1. Singleton fetus
2. Term pregnancy (37–42 weeks)
3. Vertex presentation in a cephalic presenting part with an attitude of flexion
4. Spontaneous onset of labor and progress
5. Without complications to the mother or fetus
6. Resulting in a spontaneous and timely expulsion of the fetus and placenta.

In some pregnancies, there is a deviation from the usual pattern and this chapter deals with the most common conditions where labor care has to be modified to safely manage such kind of special situations.

VAGINAL BIRTH AFTER CESAREAN SECTION

It has been studied that an elective vaginal birth after cesarean section (VBAC) is one of the safer choices for the women with single previous lower segment cesarean delivery. This technique of providing a trial of labor after cesarean section (TOLAC) could help to reverse the growing trend in cesarean section rates and maternal morbidity. Some authors also term this management as a Trial of Scar, rather than Trial of labor.

According to The Royal College of Obstetricians and Gynaecologists (RCOG) 2015 guidelines success rate of planned VBAC is 72–75%. There is a risk for scar rupture with TOLAC/VBAC, but it is a marginal risk only. The incidence of obstetric hysterectomy is not significantly different in women planning elective repeat cesarean section (ERCS) and those VBAC. A VBAC score is used by some authors to predict the success of VBAC. Higher the score, the higher the success rate. It included five features:
1. Admission Bishop's score
2. Previous cesarean delivery indication
3. Age
4. Previous vaginal birth
5. Body mass index (BMI).

Criteria

Planned VBAC is offered to the woman with:
- A singleton pregnancy of 37 weeks or above
- Cephalic presentation
- Single lower uterine segment scar performed for a non-recurring indication with or without prior history of vaginal delivery
- Patient with previous two cesarean sections can be offered VBAC after proper counseling (RCOG 2015)
- Higher rates of successful VBAC is observed in cases where pregnancy interval between two pregnancies is more than 18 months and sonologically calibrated uterine scar >3.5 mm.

VBAC should only be attempted in the settings where facilities for the emergency cesarean section along with experienced obstetrician and anesthetists are available.

Contraindications (RCOG 2015)

- *Previous uterine rupture:* Recurrent uterine rupture is shown to be 5% or higher in women who had had a previous uterine rupture. The risk of repeat rupture was found to be 6% in a lower segment as compared to 32% with an upper segment rupture.
- *Previous uterine surgery:* Cases in which uterine cavity is breached are at increased risk of uterine rupture.
- *Classical uterine scar or with the extension of uterine scar in previous cesarean sections:* Risk of rupture relies upon the type of uterine scar which was found to be 4–95% with a classical and T scar, 1–75% with a low vertical scar and 0.2–1.5% with a transverse scar.
- Conditions with absolute contraindication of vaginal birth such as central placenta previa.

Conditions Associated with Unsuccessful Vaginal Birth after Cesarean Section

- Post-date gestation
- Multiple gestation
- Fetal macrosomia
- Maternal age above 39 years
- BMI ≥ 30
- Low Bishop's score
- Macrosomia
- Decreased ultrasonographic lower segment myometrial thickness
- Previous cesarean for recurring indications
- Short delivery interval (< 12 months).

Induction or Augmentation for Vaginal Birth after Cesarean Delivery

Induction and augmentation are to be conducted with caution in women with previous cesarean delivery. As they are associated with a two- to three-fold increased risk of uterine rupture and around a 1.5-fold increased risk of operative delivery compared with spontaneous VBAC labor. Induction using mechanical methods such as an intracervical Foley catheter are associated with low risk of rupture. Sequential use of prostaglandins and oxytocin must be avoided. Misoprostol should be avoided as far as possible in women with previous cesarean and other uterine surgery.

Intrapartum Care

All women in established VBAC labor should receive:
- Individual attention
- Intravenous access should be ensured
- Full blood count and blood group
- Continuous electronic fetal monitoring should be ensured
- Maternal symptoms and signs should be monitored
- Cervix progression should be regularly measured at an interval no less than 4 hours
- Routine use of instrumental delivery, which is commonly used to accelerate the second stage of labor, is controversial.

Clinical Features of Uterine Scar Rupture (Fig. 1)

- Severe abdominal pain, especially if persisting between contractions
- Abnormal cardiotocography (CTG), mainly fetal bradycardia
- Scar tenderness
- Vaginal bleeding
- Hematuria
- Cessation of uterine activity
- Maternal tachycardia
- Hypotension, fainting or shock
- Loss of station of the presenting part
- Change in abdominal contour
- Fetal heart rate (FHR) cannot be located at the old transducer site.

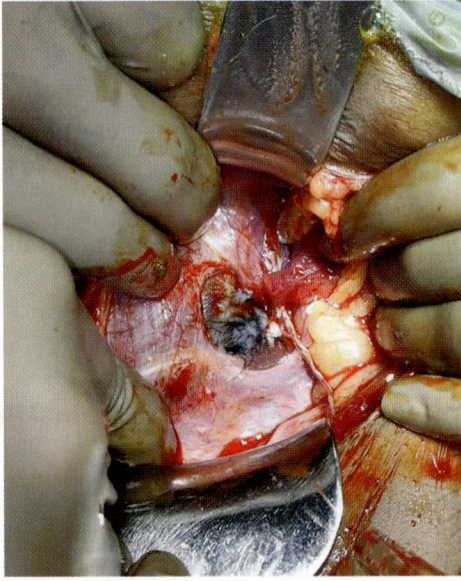

Fig. 1: Uterine rupture of a lower segment cesarean section scar.

POOR PROGRESS OF LABOR

"Failure of labor to progress/nonprogress of labor has become one of the main indications of cesarean section, especially in primiparous females."

It is quite challenging to identify the exact cause of slowly progressing labor in clinical practice. Few of the common causes include 4 Ps:
1. *Power:* Inadequate uterine contraction
2. *Passenger:* It includes malpresentation, position, attitude or macrosomia
3. *Passage:* It includes abnormal bony pelvis
4. *Push:* Suboptimal maternal efforts mainly when full cervical dilation is achieved.

Prolong First Stage of Labor

Prolong Latent Phase

The duration of the latent phase may be up to 20 hours in nulliparous and 14 h in multipara. There is no harmful effect on perinatal outcome in the case of a protracted latent period if the mother has no medical risk factors (preeclampsia, diabetes, etc.) and there are no fetal risk factors for fetal hypoxia (growth restriction, maternal pyrexia). The interventions available for the prolonged latent phase are either to sedate the patient or augmentation with amniotomy, oxytocin or both.

Prolong Active Phase

Active phase disorders have been divided into protracted active phase or primary dysfunctional labor, the second arrest of dilation, and a combination of the both **(Fig. 2)**. When there is no change in dilation for 2 hours or more after initial satisfactory progress, it is termed as secondary arrest.

Traditionally, slow progress has been identified by the experience of the obstetrician's estimate, use of estimated time of delivery clock or by a partogram. There have been many critiques of partography, but it has its advantages especially in low resource settings where decisions for the operative interventions have to be preceded by transfer of the woman to another facility. It is also an excellent method of documentation of various labor features. The partograms are designed to record the following conditions related to the progress of labor (fetal descent, frequency of uterine contraction, and duration), fetal condition (FHR, degree of caput and molding and color and amount of liquor) and maternal condition (pulse, blood pressure temperature and urinary output). If the patient is in the active phase at the time of admission, or if the woman enters the active phase at a pace of 1cm/hr. of cervical dilatation, the alert line is drawn. Action line is drawn 4 hour later to the right and parallel to the alert line. An important point to be kept in mind that partogram is drawn only when the women enters the active labor.

Prolong Second Stage of Labor

The second stage is divided into pelvic phase, also known as the phase of descent or passive phase, and perineal phase

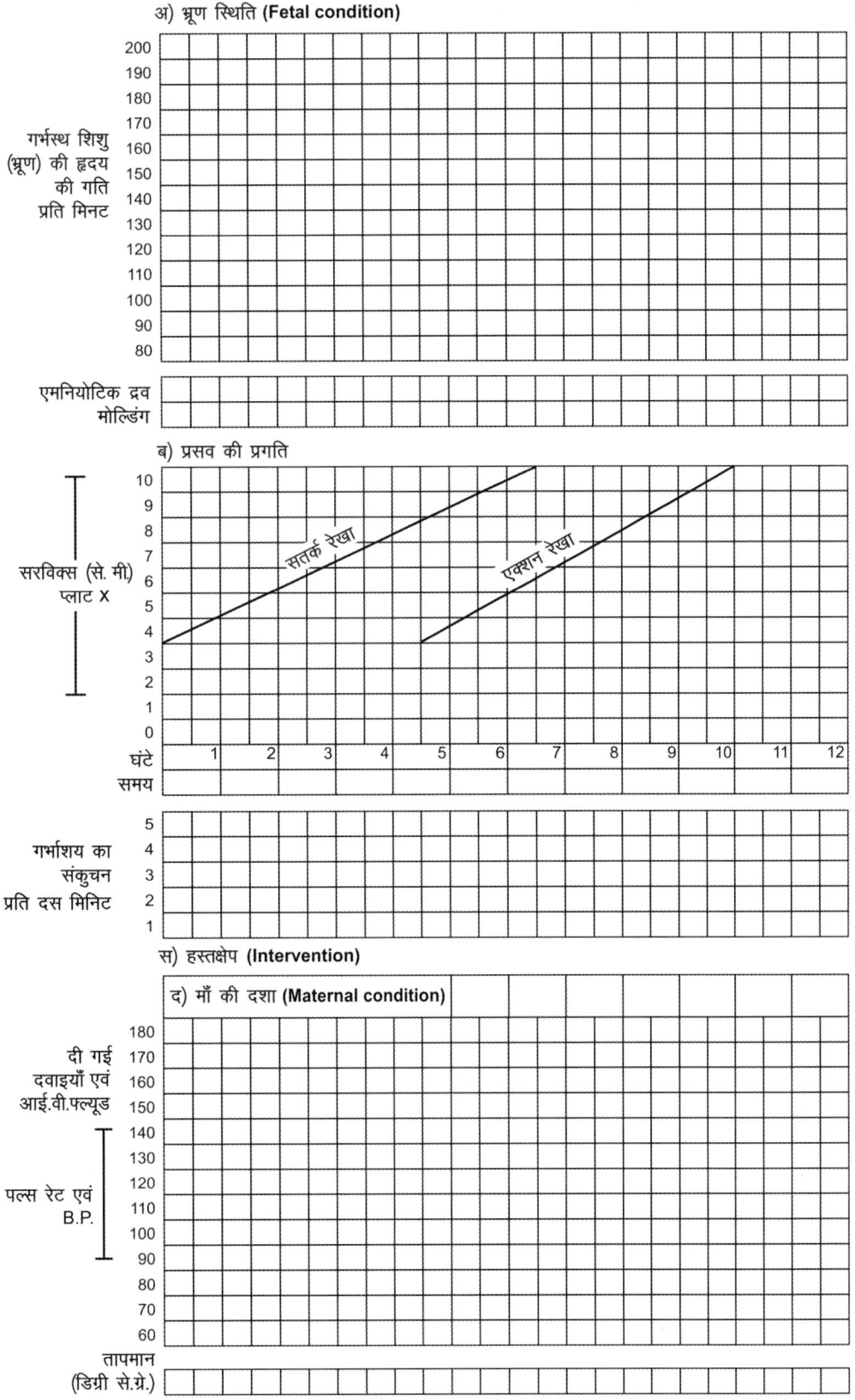

Fig. 2: Simplified partograph proforma.

also known as expulsion phase or active phase. Prolong is considered when the second stage exceeds 3 hours with epidural anesthesia and 2 hours without epidural anesthesia in a nulliparous and 2 hours and 1 hour respectively in multipara.

The pelvic phase is characterized by the descent of the presenting part of the fetus. During this phase, the uterine perfusion and fetal oxygenation is unaffected. The perineal phase starts from "bearing down" efforts and ends after the expulsion of the fetus. It is characterized by the uteroplacental insufficiency and fetal hypoxia hence its undue prolongation should be avoided **(Table 1)**.

Causes of Prolong Second Stage of Labor
- Abnormal pelvis
- Fetal macrosomia
- Cephalopelvic disproportion (CPD)
- Abnormal position such as occiput posterior (OP), occiput transverse (OT) and mentoposterior position
- Poor bearing down efforts due to anesthesia, sedation or maternal exhaustion.

■ MANAGEMENT

Oxytocin plays important role in the management of prolonged second stage. As per The National Institute for Health and Care Excellence (NICE) guideline 2014, oxytocin can be used in primiparous women under epidural if contractions are inadequate at the onset of the second stage. As per RCOG guideline 2011, caution should be exercised in multigravida patients for fear of rupture of the uterus because of undiagnosed CPD **(Table 2)**.

Cesarean section is generally indicated in these circumstances. In the past, operative vaginal delivery was attempted with special forceps if there was no obvious CPD.

TABLE 1: Complications of prolonged second stage of labor.[30-33]

Maternal complications	Neonatal complications
• Genital tract injuries	• Low APGAR score
• Increased operative delivery	• Increase admission to nursery
• Postpartum hemorrhage	• Birth trauma
• Chorioamnionitis	• Asphyxia

TABLE 2: Management of deeply engaged head and cephalopelvic disproportion (CPD).

Conditions:	Management (after excluding CPD):
• Inadequate uterine contraction	Oxytocin drip and FHR monitoring
• Use of epidural anesthesia	Use of Ventouse/Forceps to cut short second stage of labor
• Medical conditions such as cardiac diseases, hypertensive crisis, myasthenia, medulla spinalis injury, proliferative retinopathy	

This was a trial of instrumental delivery. However, with a more risk averse approach to obstetrics and lack of trained operators, this approach is generally avoided.

Complications of Cesarean Section in Late Second Stage
- Bladder injury during cesarean section
- Difficulty in delivering head
- Broad ligament hematoma due to angle extension
- Incision involving vagina
- Postpartum hemorrhage
- Puerperal infection
- Fistula formation
- Pelvic organ prolapses.

Two techniques have been described for the delivery of the deeply engaged head:
1. *Push technique:* An assistant pushed head from below once the uterine incision has been given.
2. *Pull technique:* The limbs and trunk of the baby are delivered followed by delivery of the head.

Based on the position of the back-pull technique may be of three types.
i. For back lying anteriorly, the Patwardhan maneuver is used wherein both shoulders are delivered first followed by delivery of the trunk by flexion, then the legs are delivered and finally, the head is lifted out **(Figs. 3 and 4)**.
ii. Reversed breech extraction is performed for back lying posteriorly wherein both legs are delivered first followed by delivery of trunk by flexion, then both shoulders are delivered and finally, the head is lifted out.
iii. In OT position anterior shoulder is delivered first followed by delivery of the posterior shoulder, then the trunk is delivered by flexion followed by legs and finally, the head is lifted out.

■ FETAL DISTRESS

Fetal distress is a nebulous concept. The purpose of fetal monitoring is to detect the fetus that is at a risk of hypoxia. Fetal distress is stage before hypoxia and associated acidemia set in. However, there is no definition of how early in the process should we say that a fetus is distressed (on the verge of pathological injury) rather than only stresses (displaying physiological coping mechanisms). Therefore, methods to detect "fetal distress" have to be balanced. They should be sensitive enough to detect problems in time to prevent perinatal hypoxia and asphyxia. On the other hand, they should be specific enough to restrict obstetric intervention only to situations where there is a significant risk of such an occurrence. The term "asphyxia" is derived from the ancient Greek word "a-sphyxis", meaning "no pulse". It refers to fetal compromise due to an insufficient supply of oxygen or nutrients. It manifests as:

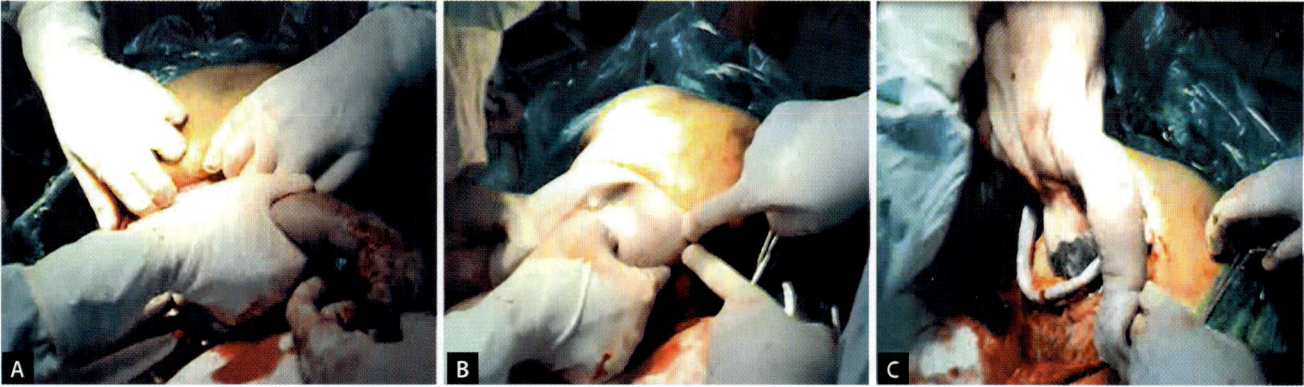

Figs. 3A to C: Patwardhan's maneuver. (A) Left arm delivered; (B) Delivery of trunk; (C) Delivery of head.

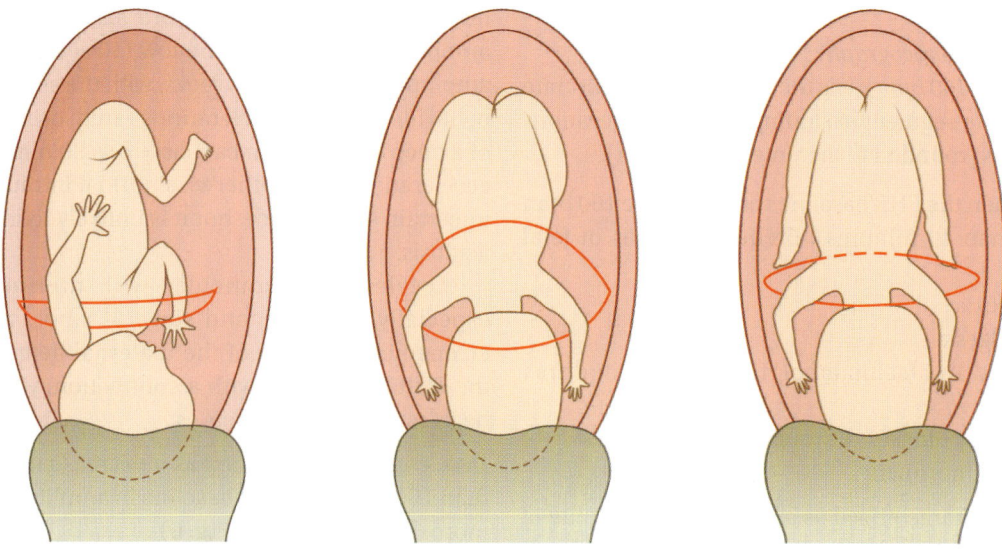

Fig. 4: Patwardhan's maneuver—diagramatic.

- Abnormal fetal heart patterns
- Reduced fetal movement
- Fetal growth restriction
- Presence of meconium stained fluid.

Perinatal asphyxia is one of the important causes of neonatal morbidity and mortality. It can cause damage to various fetal organs such as the brain, bowels, and kidney.

About one-fourth of the asphyxiated neonates faces major handicap later in life such as cerebral palsy, cognitive impairment and impaired hearing and vision. In 10–20% cases, perinatal asphyxia leads to neonatal death.

Risk Factors for Fetal Distress during Labor

Some of the risk factors for the occurrence of fetal distress are as follows:
- Maternal age
- Nulliparity
- Low placental weight
- Gestational age
- Chorioamnionitis
- Previous cesarean section
- Fetal growth restriction
- Obesity
- Diabetes
- Preeclampsia.

Methods of Intrapartum Surveillance

- Intermittent auscultation
- Electronic fetal monitoring (EFM)
- Vibroacoustic stimulation test
- Fetal scalp stimulation (FSS)
- Fetal blood sampling (FBS)
- Fetal scalp lactate
- Fetal pulse oximetry
- Electrocardiogram analysis
- Umbilical artery Doppler velocimetry.

Intermittent Auscultation

Society of Obstetricians and Gynaecologists of Canada recommended auscultation for 60 seconds immediately after contraction every, 15–30 minutes in the first stage of labor and every 5 minutes in the second stage of labor. It is important to auscultate after a contraction. This is when the FHE will manifest slowing when there are pathological changes. If there are concerns arising out of the auscultation, this should be documented by electronic fetal monitoring when it is available. Persistent and prolonged bradycardia may be acted upon instantly.

Electronic Fetal Monitoring

It is performed using a CTG. Fetal heart rate pattern can be recorded either by using an external transducer or internal transducer however former is preferred since later requires a ruptured membrane for electrode placement. Similarly, the external or internal transducer can be used to record uterine activity.

Components of Cardiotocography
Baseline FHR (110–160 bpm): It is the mean of fetal heart rate during a 10-minute segment excluding all the accelerations and decelerations (rounded to increments of 5 bpm).

Tachycardia: When the FHR baseline value is above 160 bpm (lasting more than 10 minutes). Frequent causes of fetal tachycardia are:
- Maternal pyrexia
- Epidural analgesia
- Beta-agonist drugs (salbutamol, terbutaline, ritodrine, fenoterol)
- Parasympathetic blockers (atropine, scopolamine)
- Fetal cardiac abnormality.

Bradycardia: It is characterized as an FHR baseline value of less than 110 beats per minute (lasting more than 10 minutes). It is caused due to maternal hypothermia, administration of beta-blockers, and fetal arrhythmias such as atrial-ventricular block are other possible causes.

Baseline variability: It defined as fluctuation in the FHR baseline value. Normal is 6–25 bpm between contractions.

Reduced variability: It is said to occur when the bandwidth amplitude is below 5 bpm for more than 50 minutes in baseline segments, or for more than 3 minutes during decelerations.

It can occur due to hypoxia, acidosis, infection, administration of central nervous system depressants or parasympathetic blockers. During deep sleep, variability is usually in the lower range of normality, but the bandwidth amplitude rarely under 5 bpm.

Increased variability (saltatory pattern): When bandwidth value exceeds 25 bpm, lasting for more than 30 minutes. It is caused by fetal autonomic instability/hyperactive autonomic system when hypoxia/acidosis evolves very rapidly.

Accelerations: It is defined as the sudden increase of FHR at least 15 bpm above baseline **(Fig. 5)**. The onset of the peak is within 30 seconds, of 15 seconds or more in duration and less than 2 minutes from onset to return to baseline.

Accelerations usually coincide with fetal movements and indicate neurologically responsive fetus that does not have hypoxia/acidosis. Before 32 weeks' gestation, their amplitude and rate may be low (10 seconds and 10 bpm of amplitude). After 32–34 weeks, with the establishment of fetal behavioral states, accelerations rarely occur during periods of a deep sleep, which can last up to 50 minutes. The lack of accelerations in an otherwise normal intrapartum CTG is of uncertain significance, but it is unlikely to indicate hypoxia/acidosis.

Accelerations coincides with uterine contractions, especially in the second stage of labor, suggest possible erroneous recording of the maternal heart rate, as usually the FHR decelerates with a contraction, while the maternal heart rate typically increases.

Deceleration: It is defined as a decrease in the FHR of more than 15 bpm below the baseline in amplitude, and lasting for more than 15 seconds **(Fig. 6)**.

Early decelerations are coincident with contractions. They are usually caused due to fetal head compression and does not indicate fetal compromise.

Variable decelerations (V-shaped)—decelerations that vary in size, shape and relationship to uterine contractions **(Fig. 7)**. Variable decelerations signify a baroreceptor-mediated response to increased arterial pressure and they constitute the majority of decelerations during labor. Unless they develop a U-shaped component, reduced variability within the deceleration, and/or their duration exceeds 3 minutes, they are rarely associated with serious fetal hypoxia/acidosis.

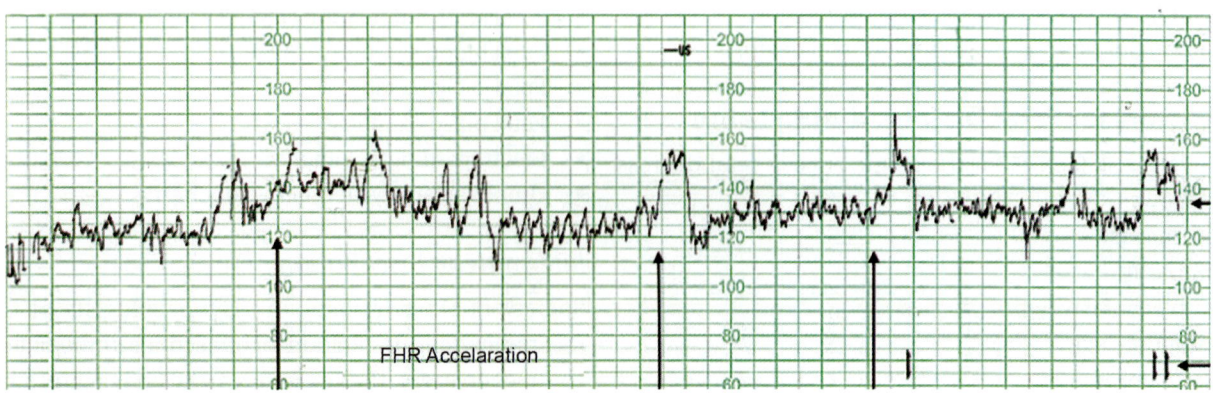

Fig. 5: Fetal heart rate (FHR) tracings acceleration with fetal movements.

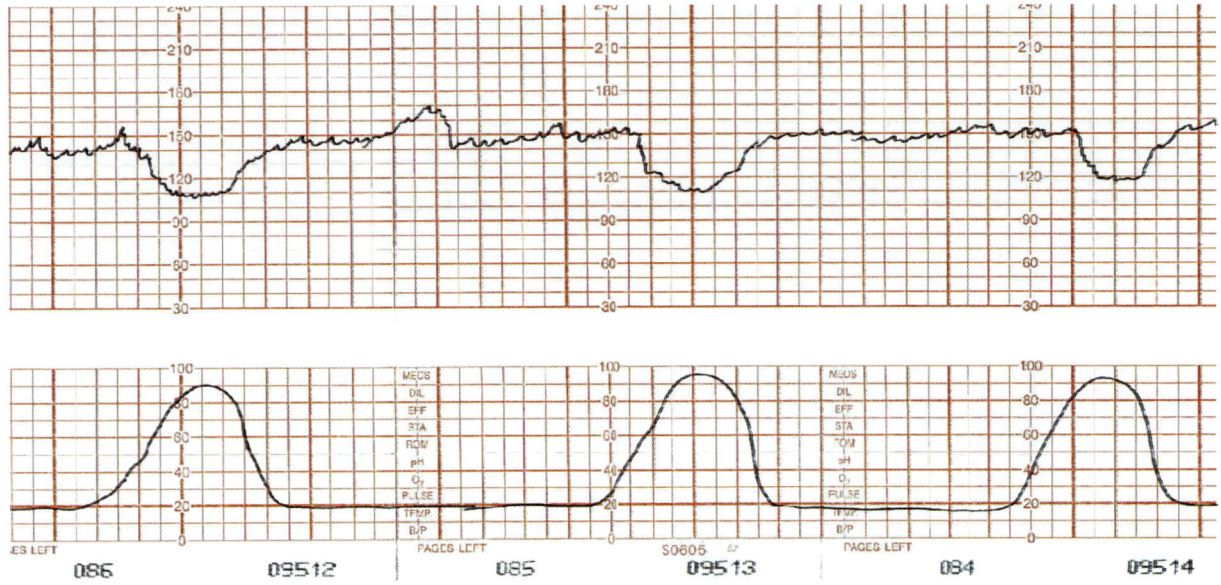

Fig. 6: Fetal heart rate (FHR) tracing showing early deceleration.

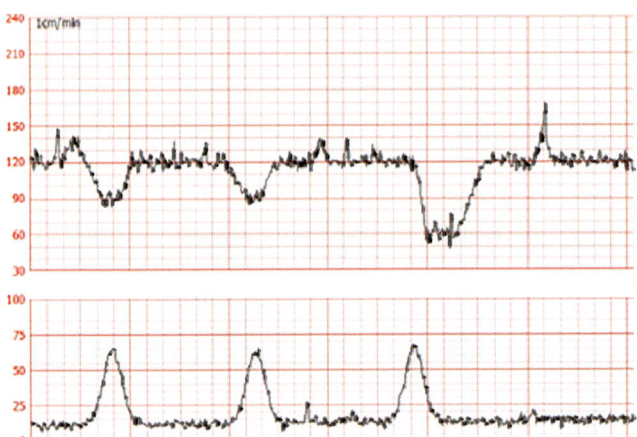

Fig. 7: Fetal heart rate (FHR) tracing showing variable deceleration.

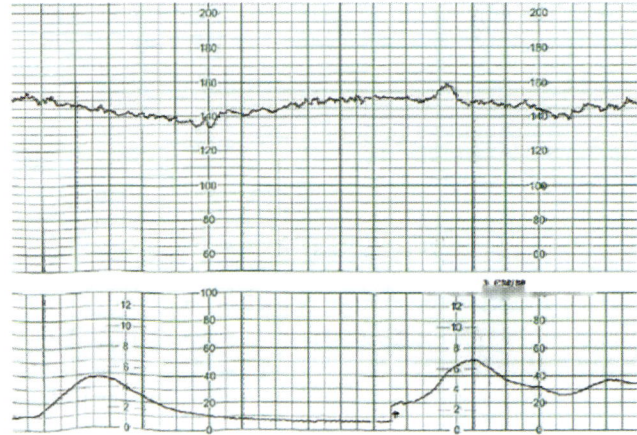

Fig. 8: Fetal heart rate (FHR) tracing showing late deceleration.

Late decelerations—begin more than 20 seconds after the onset of uterine contraction, a nadir after the acme, and a return to the baseline after the end of the uterine contraction **(Fig. 8)**. These decelerations are indicating of a chemoreceptor-mediated response to fetal hypoxemia.

Prolonged decelerations—decelerations lasting for more than 3 minutes **(Fig. 9)**. These indicate fetal hypoxemia. Decelerations of more than 5 minutes, with FHR, below 80 bpm and reduced variability within the deceleration, usually associated with acute fetal hypoxia/acidosis and require emergent intervention.

Sinusoidal pattern: Undulating signals, resembling a sine wave, which are regular and smooth, with an amplitude between 5–15 bpm, and a frequency of 3–5 cycles per minute **(Fig. 10)**. It is associated with severe fetal anemia, acute fetal hypoxia, fetal-maternal hemorrhage, twin-to-twin transfusion syndrome, cardiac malformations and ruptured vasa previa, gastroschisis, hydrocephalus and infection.

Management of abnormal fetal heart rate patterns:
- Rule out maternal infection or pyrexia in case of fetal tachycardia
- By stopping oxytocin and terbutaline, hyperstimulation can be avoided
- Hypovolemia must be treated
- In the case of oligohydramnios, amnioinfusion should be carried out
- Maternal pushing effort must be modified by asking her to bear down with every second or third contraction
- Relieve supine hypotension or cord compression by altering the position
- Oxygen administration with a face mask
- Fetal blood sampling or expedition of delivery can be done if other method fails.

Vibroacoustic Stimulation Test

The positive response seen following vibroacoustic stimulation reduces the duration of examination on admission test along with acceleration of 15 bpm for 15 seconds is a sign of fetal wellbeing.

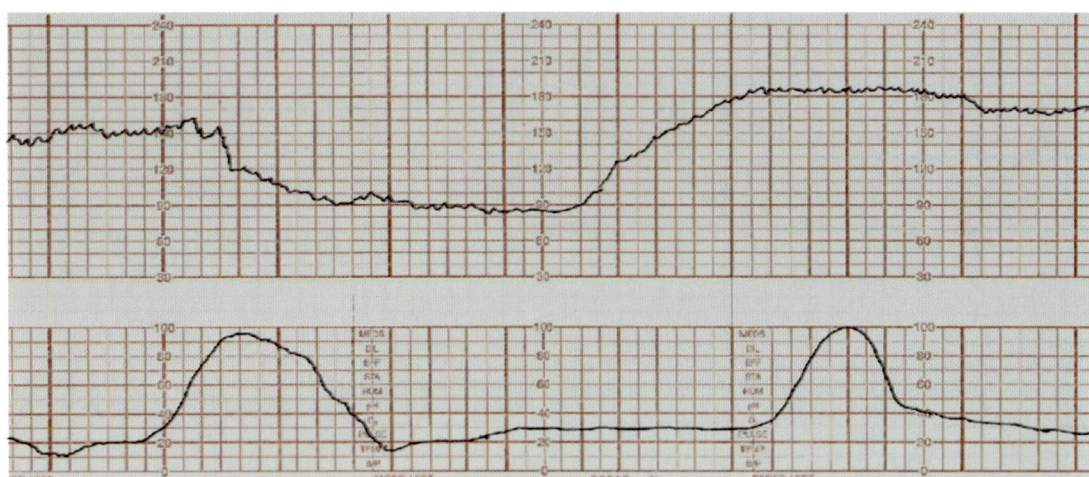

Fig. 9: Fetal heart rate (FHR) tracing prolonged deceleration.

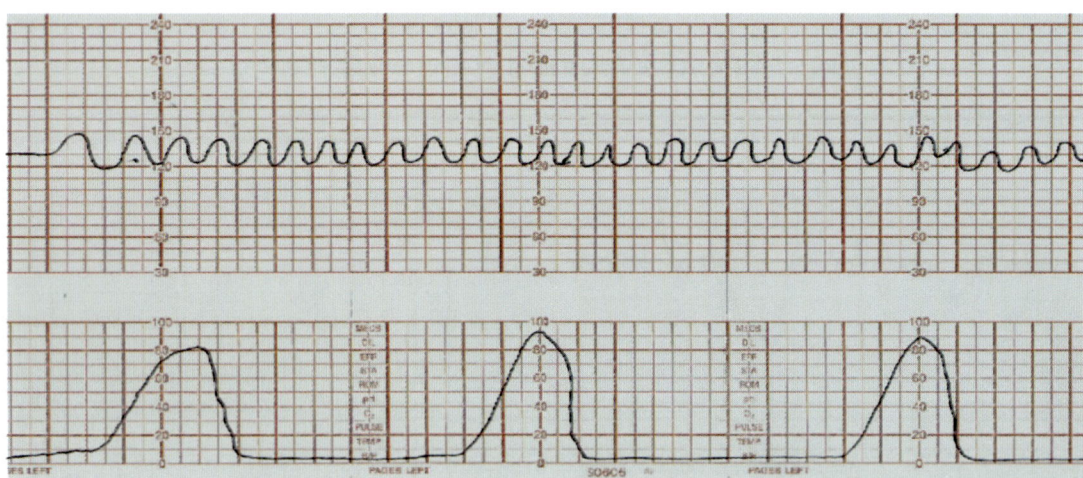

Fig. 10: Fetal heart rate (FHR) tracing showing sinusoidal pattern.

Fetal Scalp Stimulation

While doing a per vaginal examination fetal scalp is stimulated gently for 15 seconds, an acceleration in FHR by 15 bpm above baseline lasting more than 15 seconds is consistent with a fetal scalp pH>7.2.

Advantage: Fetal blood sampling can be avoided in 73%.

Disadvantage: Aggressive stimulation can produce fetal bradycardia due to vagal stimulation.

Fetal Blood Sampling

This technique was introduced by Saling in 1961. It is based on the concept that scalp pH drops as the duration and amplitude of deceleration increases.

Contraindications:
- Less than 34 weeks' period of gestation
- Face presentation
- Clotting defects
- Infections such as HIV, Hepatitis B, genital herpes.

Disadvantages: Cumbersome, require special skills and instruments and discomfort to patients.

Fetal Scalp Lactate

It is similar to FBS however much lesser quantity of blood is required. Normal fetal scalp lactate level is <2.8 mmol/L. A level >3.08 is abnormal.

Fetal Pulse Oximetry

Fall in fetal arterial pH and base excess occurred when oxygen saturation drops below 30%. However, it is not advised to use it on regular basis.

Fetal Echocardiogram Analysis

Fetal ECG is obtained using the same fetal electrode that is used for internal FHR monitoring. An increase in T wave height indicates hypoxic stress and appearance of ST depression marks severe fetal decompression.

Umbilical Artery Doppler Velocimetry

Abnormal umbilical artery Doppler is seen in severe hypoxemia. It may not be feasible during labor.

MECONIUM STAINED LIQUOR

"Meconium arion" was the term coined by Aristotle a Greek word for meconium, and is defined as the dark green liquid passes by the neonate containing mucus, bile, and epithelial cells. However, sometimes the meconium is passed when the baby is still in the womb, staining the amniotic fluid (**Figs. 11 and 12**).

Currently, 8–25% of infants are born with meconium stained liquor is and 1–3% of live births have meconium aspiration syndrome.

Theories regarding the fetal passage of meconium:
- *First:* In response to hypoxia indicating fetal compromise (Walker, 1953)
- *Second:* Neural control of normal gastrointestinal tract maturation (Mathews, 1979)
- *Third:* It follows vagal stimulation due to umbilical cord compression resulting in increased peristalsis.

Placental insufficiency, hypertensive disorders of pregnancy, oligohydramnios, and maternal drug abuse such as cocaine are some of the pathological causes in mother.

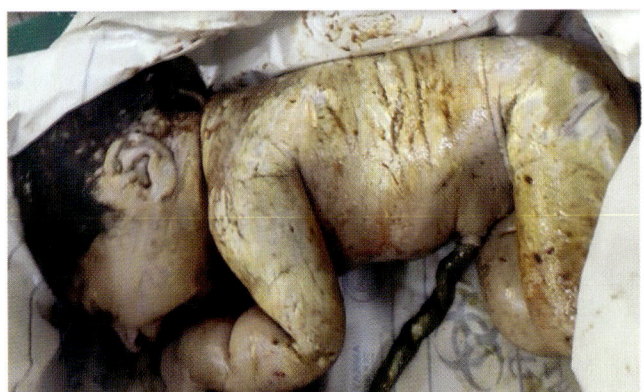

Fig. 11: Meconium smeared fetus with stained cord.

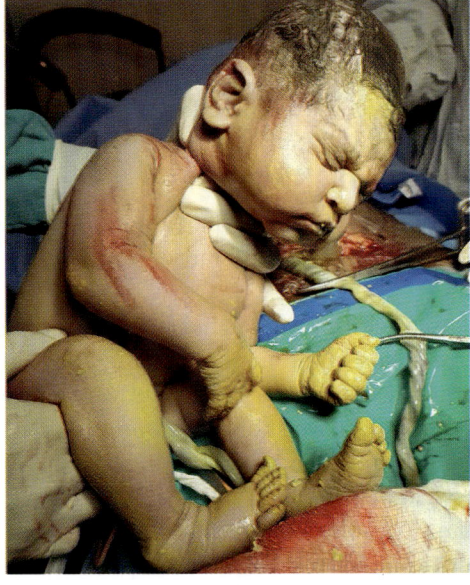

Fig. 12: Golden yellow stained fetus in postdated pregnancy.

Meconium aspiration syndrome is characterized by the presence of meconium below the vocal cord and is associated with the presence of sudden respiratory distress following birth, with radiographic findings suggestive of aspiration pneumonitis.

Intrapartum Management

- *Fetal heart monitoring:* It can either be done by continuous electronic fetal monitoring or intermittent auscultation.
- *Tocolysis:* Some study says that injection terbutaline 250 µg intravenous or subcutaneous can be used to inhibit uterine contractions and thus improving fetal oxygenation. Intravenous nitroglycerine 60–180 µg can also be used
- *Amnioinfusion:* It refers to the infusion of normal saline or ringer lactate into the amniotic cavity. Proposed benefits include dilution of thick meconium clumps and relieving cord compression.

It involves the insertion of intrauterine catheter/nasogastric tube or IV set in the uterine cavity followed by the instillation of ringer lactate (normal saline is avoided as it may cause alteration in fetal electrolyte levels).

Fluid bolus of near about 50–1,000 mL followed by constant infusion (15–225 mL) or serial bolus (200–1,000) to be instilled every 20 minutes for a period of 4 hours. There is controversy over this practice because of risk of introducing intrauterine infection and possibility of masking clinical features which would otherwise lead to an expedited delivery.

The American College of Obstetricians and Gynecologists (ACOG) does not recommend amnioinfusion.

KEY MESSAGES

"The process of labor at times challenges the expertise of obstetrician creating special situations." VBAC necessitates a thorough history, examination, and presentation as well as size of the fetus, interval from last pregnancy, the healing process, availability of experienced obstetrician and good institutional setting. The situations inviting urgent intervention as in fetal distress and meconium staining of liquor requiring antepartum fetal surveillance with electronic fetal monitoring, CTG and its interpretation, assessing fetal status with fetal scalp pH, fetal blood sampling and intervening accordingly.

Role of partography helps to assess, interpret the progress in labor prolongation and managing by medical augmentation or instrumental or cesarean delivery. Obstetricians should be trained to deal with these scenarios, such as delivering a highly involved fetus, dealing with birth canal and bladder injuries, and ligating the internal iliac arteries as necessary.

FURTHER READING

1. Al Qahtani NH, Al Hajeri F. Pregnancy outcome and fertility after complete uterine rupture: a report of 20 pregnancies and a review of literature. Arch Gynecol Obstet. 2011;284:1123-6.
2. Allen VM, Baskett TF, O'Connell CM, McKeen D, Allen AC. Maternal and perinatal outcomes with increasing duration of the second stage of labor. Obstet Gynecol. 2009;113(6):1248-58.

3. American College of Obstetricians and Gynecologists. Vaginal birth after previous cesarean delivery (ACOG practice bulletin no.115). Washington, DC: ACOG; 2010.
4. Ball RH, Parer JT. The physiologic mechanisms of variable decelerations. Am J Obstet Gynecol. 1992;166:1683-9.
5. Campo S, Campo V, Gambadauro P. Reproductive outcome before and after laparoscopic or abdominal myomectomy for subserous or intramural myomas. Eur J Obstet Gynecol Reprod Biol. 2003;110:215-9.
6. Chelmow D, Kilpatrick SJ, Laros RK Jr. maternal and neonatal outcomes after prolonged latent phase .Obstet Gynecol. 1993;81(4):486-91.
7. Chibber R, El-Saleh E, Al Fadhli R, Al Jassar W, Al Harmi J. Uterine rupture and subsequent pregnancy outcome – how safe is it? A 25-year study. J Matern Fetal Neonatal Med. 2010;23:421-4.
8. Chopra S, Bagga R, Keepanasseril A, Jain V, Kalra J, Suri V. Disengagement of the deeply engaged fetal head during cesarean section in advanced labor: conventional method versus reverse breech extraction. Acta Obstet Gynecol Scand. 2009;88:1163-6.
9. Court DJ, Parer JT. Experimental studies of fetal asphyxia and fetal heart rate interpretation. In: Nathanielsz PW, Parer JT (Eds). Research in Perinatal Medicine (I). New York: Perinatology Press; 1984. pp. 113-69.
10. Fawsitt CG, Bourke J, Greene RA, Everard CM, Murphy A, Lutomski JE. At what price? A cost-effectiveness analysis comparing trial of labour after previous caesarean versus elective repeat caesarean delivery. PLoS One. 2013;8:e58577.
11. Fong YF, Arulkumaran S. Breech extraction—an alternative method of delivering a deeply engaged head at cesarean section. Int J Gynaecol Obstet. 1997;56(2):183-4.
12. Friedman E. Labor: Clinical evaluation and management, 2nd edition. New York: Appleton-Century-Crofts; 1978.
13. Gavai M, Berkes E, Lazar L, Fekete T, Takacs ZF, Urbancsek J, et al. Factors affecting reproductive outcome following abdominal myomectomy. J Assist Reprod Genet. 2007;24:525-31.
14. Hamilton E, Warrick P, O'Keeffe D. Variable decelerations: do size and shape matter? J Matern Fetal Neonatal Med. 2012;25:648-53.
15. Holzmann M, Wretler S, Cnattingius S, Nordstrom L. Cardiotocography patterns and risk of intrapartum fetal acidemia. J Perinat Med. 2015;43(4):473-9.
16. Jadhon ME, Main EK. Fetal bradycardia associated with maternal hypothermia. Obstet Gynecol. 1988;72(3 Pt 2):496-7.
17. Jeve YB, Navti OB, Konje JC. Comparison of techniques used to deliver a deeply impacted fetal head at full dilation: a systematic review and meta-analysis. BJOG. 2016;123:337-45.
18. Kilpatrick SJ, Laros Jr RK. Characteristics of normal labor. Obstet Gynecol. 1989;74(1):85-7.
19. Kumakiri J, Takeuchi H, Itoh S, Kitade M, Kikuchi I, Shimanuki H, et al. Prospective evaluation for the feasibility and safety of vaginal birth after laparoscopic myomectomy. J Minim Invasive Gynecol. 2008;15:420-4.
20. Kumakiri J, Takeuchi H, Kitade M, Kikuchi I, Shimanuki H, Itoh S, et al. Pregnancy and delivery after laparoscopic myomectomy. J Minim Invasive Gynecol. 2005;12:241-6.
21. Landon MB, Hauth JC, Leveno KJ, Spong CY, Leindrecker S, Varner MW, et al. National Institute of Child Health and Human Development Maternal Fetal Medicine Units Network. Maternal and perinatal outcomes associated with a trial of labor after prior cesarean delivery. N Engl J Med. 2004;351(25):2581-9.
22. Le Ray C, Audibert F, Goffinet F, Fraser W. When to stop pushing: effects of duration of second-stage expulsion efforts on maternal and neonatal outcomes in nulliparous women with epidural analgesia. Am J Obstet Gynecol. 2009;201(4):361-e1.
23. Leveno KJ, Nelson DB, McIntire DD. Second stage labor: How long is too long? Am J Obstet Gynecol. 2016;214:484-9.
24. Makino S, Tanaka T, Itoh S, Kumakiri J, Takeuchi H, Takeda S. Prospective comparison of delivery outcomes of vaginal births after cesarean section versus laparoscopic myomectomy. J Obstet Gynaecol Res. 2008;34:952-6.
25. Modanlou HD, Murata Y. Sinusoidal fetal heart rate pattern: reappraisal of its definition and clinical significance. J Obstet Gynaecol Res. 2004;30:169-80.
26. Myles TD, Santolaya J. Maternal and neonatal outcomes in patients with a prolonged second stage of labor. Obstet Gynecol. 2003;102(1):52-8.
27. NICE. Intrapartum care for healthy women and babies (NICE clinical guidelines). Clinical guideline no: CG190. London: NICE; 2014.
28. Nunes I, Ayres-de-Campos D, Kwee A, Rosen KG. Prolonged saltatory fetal heart rate pattern leading to newborn metabolic acidosis. Clin Exp Obstet Gynecol. 2014;41(5):507-11.
29. Parer JT, Livingston EG. What is fetal distress? Am J Obstet Gynecol. 1990;162:1421-7.
30. Parker WH, Einarsson J, Istre O, Dubuisson JB. Risk factors for uterine rupture after laparoscopic myomectomy. J Minim Invasive Gynecol. 2010;17:551-4.
31. Reyes-Ceja L, Cabrera R, Insfran E, Herrera-Lasso F. Pregnancy following previous uterine rupture. Study of 19 patients. Obstet Gynecol 1969;34:387-9.
32. Rovio PH, Heinonen PK. Pregnancy outcomes after transvaginal myomectomy by colpotomy. Eur J Obstet Gynecol Reprod Biol. 2012;161:130-3.
33. Seracchioli R, Manuzzi L, Vianello F, Gualerzi B, Savelli L, Paradisi R, et al. Obstetric and delivery outcome of pregnancies achieved after laparoscopic myomectomy. Fertil Steril. 2006;86:159-65.
34. Silver RM, Landon MB, Rouse DJ, Leveno KJ, Spong CY, Thom EA, et al. National Institute of Child Health and Human Development Maternal–Fetal Medicine Units Network. Maternal morbidity associated with multiple repeat cesarean deliveries. Obstet Gynecol. 2006;107:1226-32.
35. Singh M, Varma R. Reducing complications associated with a deeply engaged head at caesarean section: a simple instrument. Obstet Gynaecol. 2008;10:38-41.
36. Suwanrath C, Suntharasaj T. Sleep–wake cycles in normal foetuses. Arch Gynecol Obstet. 2010;281:449-54.
37. Vousden N, Cargill Z, Briley A, Tydeman G, Shennan AH. Caesarean section at full dilatation. 2014;16(3):199-205.

LONG QUESTIONS

1. Discuss methods of intrapartum fetal surveillance in cases of fetal distress and meconium staining of liquor amnii.
2. Discuss electronic fetal heart rate monitoring and interpretation of various cardiotocography patterns.
3. Enumerate and discuss implication of biochemical methods of fetal well being in laboring women.
4. What is the role of partography in laboring women and interventions in various stages of labor?
5. Discuss Trial of Labor After Cesarean Section (TOLAC), its criteria, enumerate the complications and their management.

■ SHORT QUESTIONS

1. Vibroacoustic stimulation (VAST).
2. Classification of intrapartum fetal heart tracing.
3. Fetal blood sampling.
4. Causes of prolonged 2nd stage of labor.
5. Amnioinfusion criteria.

■ MULTIPLE CHOICE QUESTIONS

1. Which type of deceleration in fetal heart tracings are chemoreceptor mediated?
   a. Baseline FHR
   b. Early deceleration
   c. Late deceleration
   d. Variable deceleration
2. Identify the tracing and pick up the appropriate causes.

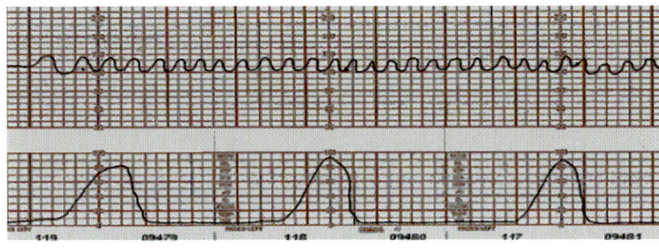

   a. Prolonged 1st stage of labor
   b. Prolonged 2nd stage of labor
   c. Fetal anemia and feto maternal hemorrhage
   d. None of the above
3. Which changes of fetal heart rate pattern coincides with:
   a. Increased myometrial contraction, Increased FHR
   b. Decreased myometrial contraction, Decreased FHR
   c. Increased myometrial contraction, Decreased FHR
   d. None of the above
4. Which of the following methods for induction of labor should not be used in patient with previous lower segment cesarean section?
   a. Prostaglandin gel
   b. Prostaglandin tablet
   c. Oxytocin drip
   d. Stripping of the membranes
5. Which statement is correct for variable deceleration pattern?
   a. Stress mediated
   b. Fetomaternal hemorrhage
   c. Cardiac anomalies in fetus
   d. Baroreceptor mediated

Answers								
1.	c	2.	c	3.	c	4.	b	5. d

9.6 INSTRUMENTAL VAGINAL DELIVERY

Haresh Doshi

■ INTRODUCTION

Instrumental vaginal delivery is also known as operative vaginal delivery and assisted vaginal delivery. Forceps and vacuum extractors are the two instruments used for vaginal delivery. They have helped millions of mankind for successful vaginal deliveries since decades.

In last two decades, the incidence of instrumental deliveries have decreased a lot and still decreasing. The main reason of this decrease is increased safety and alarming rise in the incidence of cesarean section. We have developed tolerance to high rate of cesarean section. Other reasons of decrease in instrumental delivery is lack of adequate training in residency leading to lack of skill thus leading to adverse outcomes and fear of complications as well as litigations.

■ INCIDENCE

The incidence ranges from 1.5% in some countries to 15% in other countries worldwide.[1-3] However, it differs from institute to institute within the country and not uncommon to find even less than 1%. Surprisingly, it was reported more in high income countries as compared to low and medium income countries.[4,5]

■ TYPES OF OPERATIONS

Revised American College of Obstetricians and Gynecologists (ACOG) classification (2000) is used **(Table 1)**.[6] It was originally for forceps delivery. But same can be used for vacuum extraction delivery.

■ FORCEPS

History

History of obstetric forceps is very interesting and colorful. It was invented by Peter chamberlen the eldest son of William Chamberlen. The Chamberlens were French Huguenots from Paris who migrated to England in 1569. It was used as "secret" instrument for delivery of a live child in difficult cases. It was kept as a family secret for 150 years before it was sold. Modifications since its invention have resulted in more than 700 different types and shapes of forceps by now.[7]

Types of Forceps

Different types of forceps include short forceps (e.g., Wrigley's, Simpson's short), long forceps (with or without axis traction, e.g., Simpson's long, Das'), rotational forceps (e.g., Kielland, Moolgaoker) and special forceps (e.g., Piper's for aftercoming head of breech) **(Fig. 1)**.

Parts of the Instrument (Fig. 2)

Forceps is a paired metallic instrument having two branches called blades. Each blade consists of four main parts—blade proper, shank, lock and handle.

TABLE 1: Classification of instrumental vaginal deliveries.*	
Outlet delivery	• Scalp is visible at the introitus without separating the labia • Fetal skull has reached the pelvic floor • Fetal head is at or on the perineum • Sagittal suture is in in anteroposterior diameter or right or left occiput anterior or posterior position • Rotation does not exceed 45 degrees
Low delivery	Leading point of the fetal skull is at station +2 or more and not on the pelvic floor • Rotation is 45 degrees or less left or right occiput anterior, or left or right occiput posterior • Rotation is greater than 45 degrees
Mid delivery	The station is above +2, but the head is engaged

(*High instrumental delivery was removed from the classification)

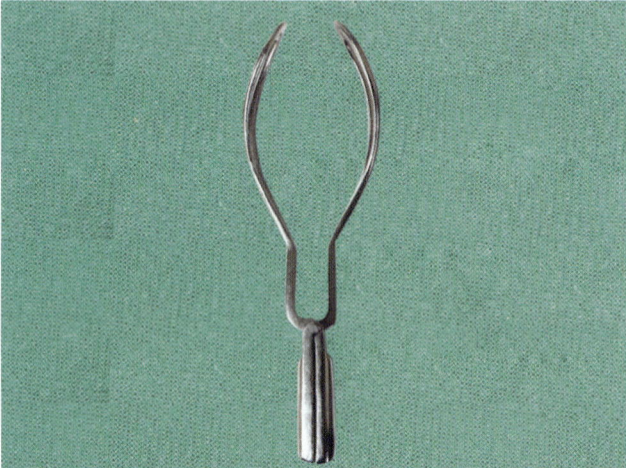

Fig. 1: Short obstetric forceps.

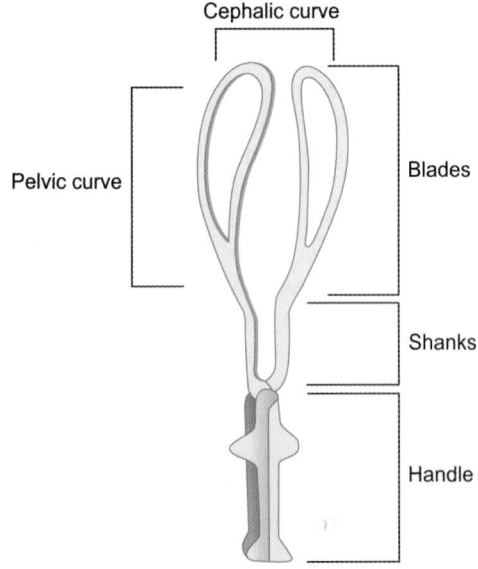

Fig. 2: Parts of forceps.[7]

- *Blades:* They are usually fenestrated for better grip on fetal head. It has two curves—cephalic curve (radius 11.25 cm) and pelvic curve (radius 17.5 cm). Pelvic curve may be absent in some short forceps. Maximum distance between 2 blades when articulated is 8.5 cm. Blades are called right and left depending upon on which side of the maternal pelvis they lie after correct application.
- *Shank:* It is the portion between the blade and the lock. It may be parallel or overlapping. It is 6.25 cm long in Simpson's long forceps.
- *Lock:* Usually it is English type, i.e., double slot lock, slot in each blade fitting with each other.
- *Handle:* It is a long metal rod, 12.5 cm long in Simpson's long forceps. It may have finger grips or rests which flare outside or fixation screw for secure grip.

Forceps with different axis traction devices are *not* used in modern times.

Functions of Forceps

- *Traction:* It is the most important function for which it was invented.
- *Rotation:* Kielland forceps is best for the purpose. Rotational forceps are rarely done at present.
- *Flexion:* Pulling in backward direction encourages flexion.
- *Compression:* Compression just enough to ensure a safe grip (to prevent slipping) is needed. When correctly applied only such is obtained.

Indications

Maternal

- *Prolonged second stage of labor:* More than 2 hours in nulliparous patient (3 hours if epidural analgesia is used) and more than 1 hour in parous patient (2 hours if epidural is used).
- Inability to bear down due to frank exhaustion, excessive sedation, epidural analgesia.
- To give less strain to mother (avoid Valsalva maneuver) in certain medical and obstetric disorders.

Fetal

- Suspected or proved fetal compromise—abnormal fetal heart rate patterns, thick meconium, abnormal fetal blood sampling results
- Failure to progress in labor due to fetal causes such as malrotation or large size fetus
- Delivery of aftercoming head of breech.

Others

- *Trial forceps:* Forceps attempted in borderline cephalo-pelvic disproportion (CPD) keeping full preparation ready for immediate cesarean section.
- In trial of labor after cesarean (TOLAC) to give less strain to the scar.

Contraindications

- More than borderline CPD
- Nonengaged head

- Malpresentation: Breech, brow, face—mentoposterior
- Cervix not fully dilated
- Fetal malformation
- Contraction ring dystocia
- Fetal bleeding disorders or a predisposition to fractures
- Pelvic tumors.

Prerequisites

All the prerequisites must be fulfilled before forceps delivery is attempted:
- Pelvis should be adequate for vaginal delivery.
- Cervix should be fully dilated.
- Head should be engaged and the station of the head accurately known.
- Position of the head should be precisely known. Ultrasound assessment of the fetal head position is recommended where uncertainty exists following clinical examination.[8]
- Estimation of fetal weight should be done.
- Membranes should have been ruptured.
- Bladder should have been emptied recently.
- Adequate anesthesia. Outlet can be done under local perineal infiltration, low forceps under pudendal block while mid forceps require epidural, spinal or general anesthesia.
- Patient and relatives should be explained about the procedure its risks, benefits and informed consent is taken.
- The operator should be skilled in instrumental delivery and familiar with the different types of instruments and their use. Backup plan should be in place in case of failure to deliver.
- Neonatologist must be present.
- Proper aseptic precautions should be taken.

Steps of Operation (Figs. 3 and 4)

- Consent is taken after proper counseling.
- After lithotomy position, painting and draping is done. Anesthesia (perineal infiltration or pudendal block) is given. Bladder is emptied by simple catheter if required.
- Pervaginal examination is done for final confirmation of all prerequisites.
- Blades are articulated in front of the patient, to decide right and left blades. Left blade is to be introduced first. It is lubricated with dilute antiseptic solution. It is held in left hand vertically, 2 fingers or whole of right hand is introduced in the vagina, and posterior vaginal wall is depressed. Blade is introduced posteriorly in the hollow of the sacrum, keeping flush contact with fetal head, till the blade becomes almost horizontal, then under guidance of internal fingers the blade is rotated to left side of the maternal pelvis.
- Hands are changed and right blade is introduced by holding it in right hand in the same manner, passing in front of the left blade.

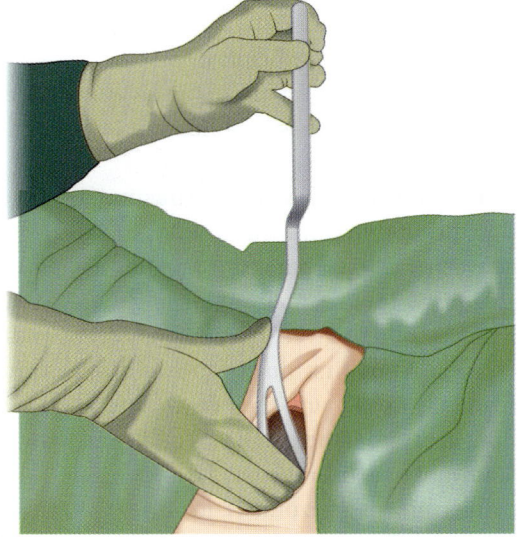

Fig. 3: Introduction of left blade.[7]

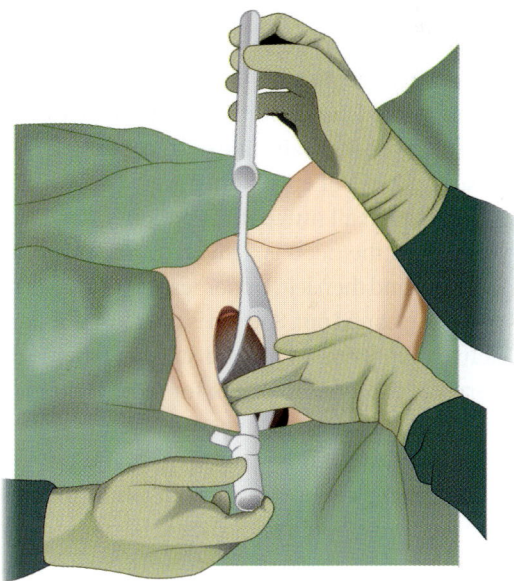

Fig. 4: Introduction of right blade.[7]

- After application in occipitoanterior position *right blade* remains on *right side of maternal pelvis,* lies on *right parietal bone of fetus* and its handle is in *right hand* of the *obstetrician.*
- Blades are slightly depressed and then locked, if application is proper there should not be difficulty in locking.

Criteria for Proper Application

- Sagittal suture throughout its length should be perpendicular to the plane of the shanks
- Lowermost part of the head should be within one inch reach from the shank
- Posterior fontanelle should not be more than one finger breadth away from the plane of the shank and should be equidistant from the side of the blades.

Traction

It is given with following principles:

- Before commencing traction criteria for proper application should be checked. Easy application and easy locking usually suggests proper application.
- Head is to be extracted slowly, and traction should be given during the uterine contraction only.
- In between traction separate the handles slightly, i.e., relax the blades, without actually unlocking them.
- Traction should be given in axis of pelvis. For midforceps and low forceps first downward and backward, then horizontally downward, then downward and forward as occiput fixes under the symphysis pubis and lastly forward and upward to deliver the head by extension.

  For outlet forceps horizontally downward, downward and forward and then forward and upward.

  In practice, this can be easily accomplished by giving traction posterior to direction of handles once the blades are locked.
- The operator should be in a comfortable position, with flexed forearms slightly below the level of delivery table. Moderate force is used for traction. The flexed elbows should not cross the waist line of the operator.
  - Restrictive use of episiotomy is advocated.[9] Usually it is required in all nulliparous patients.
  - As soon as the head is delivered, blades are removed first right and then left. Upper respiratory passages of the fetus are cleaned out. Suction is not must if liquor is clear.
  - Active management of third stage of labor is done.
  - Cervix is explored to check for tears if there is active bleeding figure of 8 stitches are taken.
  - Episiotomy wound is sutured in layers.
  - Outlet forceps are carried out in labor room, but mid and low forceps deliveries should be done in operation theater.

Complications

Maternal

- *Injuries*—genital tract injuries:
  - Extension of episiotomy, vaginal lacerations, perineal tears
  - Cervical tear, lacerations, rarely annular detachment
  - Rupture or laceration of lower uterine segment
  - Undue stretching of ligaments leading to prolapse in later life.
  - Bowel: Injury to anal sphincter, anal canal or lower rectum, i.e. third or fourth degree perineal tear
  - Lower urinary tract injuries (*uncommon*).
  - Injury to maternal pelvis (*rare*). They were found with high forceps.
- *Hemorrhage:* External (PPH)—traumatic, atonic or both
  - Internal: Vulva or vaginal hematoma, broad ligament hematoma
- *Infection:* If proper aseptic precautions are not observed, puerperal sepsis including thrombophlebitis of pelvic veins can occur.
- *Obstetric shock:* Hypovolemic—if there is severe bleeding.
  - Neurogenic if done on incompletely dilated cervix.

Fetal

- Birth asphyxia
- Intracranial hemorrhage
- Fetal scalp injuries—lacerations, pressure necrosis
- Cephalohematoma
- Blade marks on face or forehead if application not cephalic (usually self-limiting)
- Facial nerve palsies, corneal injuries
- Fracture of skull bones (rare—occurs only when excessive force is used).

Forceps in Occipitoposterior (without Rotation)

Forceps is used for face to pubis forceps delivery. Here the occiput has rotated posteriorly. Forceps blades are applied as routine. Horizontal traction should be applied until the root of the nose is under the symphysis. Then forward pull is given to deliver the vertex and occiput by flexion and finally backward pull to deliver the face by extension. Generous episiotomy is a must.

Kielland Forceps (Fig. 5)

It is long rotational forceps with overlapping shanks. It has sliding lock for correction of asynclitism of fetal head. The blades are 15 cm long and slightly thicker than usual forceps with beveled edges. The *blades* are *anterior and posterior* rather than left and right. The objective of Kielland's forceps was a biparietal application to the fetal head in any position.

Indications: (1) deep transverse arrest, (2) persistent occipitoposterior.

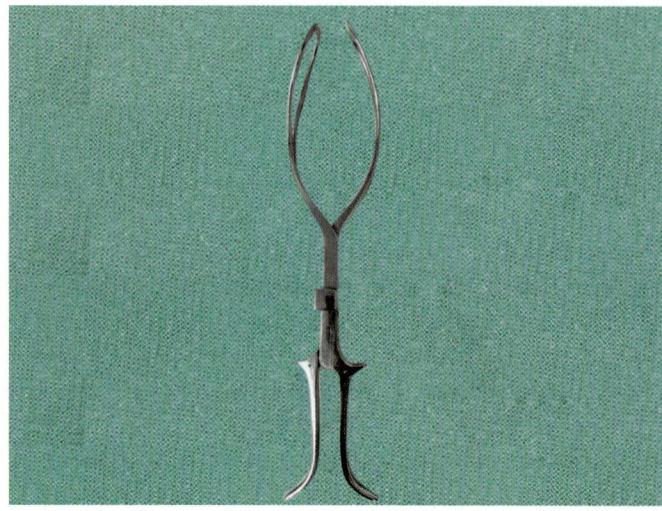

Fig. 5: Kielland forceps.

Method: Anterior blade is always introduced first. There are three methods for it.
1. *Wandering method:* Most frequently used. Blade is introduced laterally over the face side or posteriorly in the hollow of sacrum and then wandered over the face side to bring it anteriorly.
2. *Direct method:* Used when head is very low in the pelvis. Blade is introduced directly anteriorly over the fetal head.
3. *Classical or inversion method:* Obsolete.
    In any of the above method posterior blade is applied directly posteriorly.
    i. Blades are articulated by sliding lock. Asynclitism is corrected. Rotation is done in relaxation phase while traction is given during uterine contractions.
    ii. If injudiciously used it can cause injury to lower uterine segment, cervical tears, injuries at vaginal vault and spiral tears of vagina.
    iii. Although recent studies[10-12] show good outcome it is hardly used at present due to lack of training and required skill.
    vi. Muraca G M et al.[13] recently reported from their 5 years study that midcavity operative vaginal delivery is associated with higher rates of severe perinatal morbidity/mortality and severe maternal morbidity.

Prophylactic Forceps

The concept of prophylactic forceps was introduced by De Lee in 1920. It is always a low forceps delivery and it is used to shorten the second stage of labor when maternal and fetal complications are anticipated. Common indications of it are—very painful second stage of labor, heart disease, eclampsia, severe preeclampsia, post-cesarean section labor, patient under epidural analgesia.

■ VACUUM EXTRACTOR

History

Vacuum extraction was first described in 1705 by Dr James Yonge, an English surgeon. It was popularized by *Malmstrom from Sweden* in 1957. Malmstrom is considered the Father of Modern Vacuum Extractor. Although initially it was less used in English speaking countries, gradually it surpassed the forceps deliveries and by 2000 in United States 66% instrumental vaginal deliveries were by vacuum.[14]

Parts of the Instrument

It consisted of metal *suction cups* (made of steel, in four sizes 30, 40, 50 and 60 mm diameter with 20 mm depth), *traction chain* (metal chain from the metal plate to traction bar), *traction bar* (handle with lock pin) connected by rubber tube to *vacuum flask* (glass bottle with a rubber stopper) and vacuum pump.

Bird's modifications: Bird modified the original Malmstrom cup by making the traction chain and vacuum tube separate. While traction chain is still kept in the center, vacuum tube is placed eccentrically in Bird's anterior cup (used for occipitoanterior position) and shifted to the side wall of the cup in Bird's posterior cup (used for occipitotransverse and occipitoposterior positions).

Kobayashi introduced *silastic cup* in 1973. It is now commonly used instead of metal cups, because flexibility and cone shape further simplifies the use of ventouse **(Fig. 6)**. The cup is available in two sizes—60 mm and 65 mm. The cup is attached to about 20 cm long plastic shaft which is perpendicular to the axis of the cup and with the handle at the end. Different sizes and shapes of silastic cups are now available.

Mityvac vacuum assisted delivery system comprises of hand operated vacuum pump which is reusable pump and different plastic cups (from 50 to 70 mm diameter) for use in vaginal delivery as well as cesarean section **(Fig. 7)**. M-style mushroom cup of 50 mm diameter is commonly used.

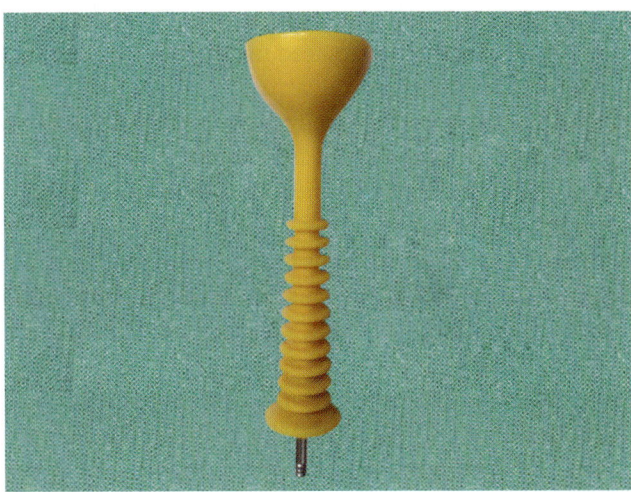

Fig. 6: Silastic vacuum cup.

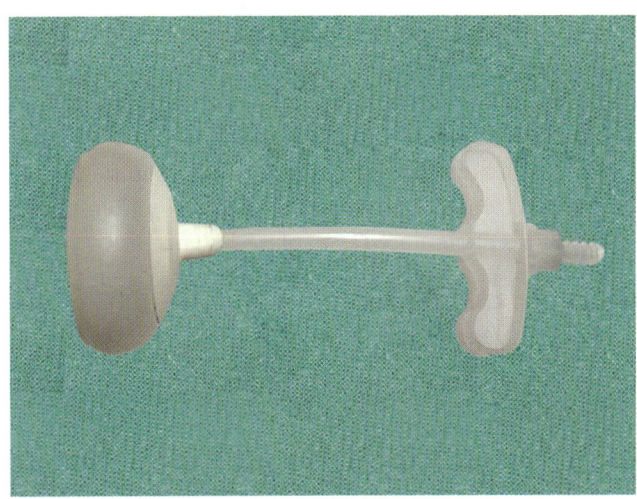

Fig. 7: Mityvac cup.

Kiwi Omni is another complete vacuum delivery system with hand operated pump. There is ease of insertion due to low profile cup and flexible stem leads to application over the flexion point of fetal head. Traction force indicator in the system measures the force exerted during traction. Like Mityvac cup it is to be disposed after single use.

Indications: They are same as mentioned in forceps.

Contraindications

- All those described under forceps.
- In addition face presentation, breech presentation (i.e., aftercoming head), less than 34 weeks maturity, congenital fetal head anomalies.
- Intrauterine death, large caput, general anesthesia and severe fetal distress are relative contraindications.

Prerequisites: Same as mentioned in forceps.

Steps of Operation

- Preliminary steps are same as described in forceps delivery.
- Metal cups of 5 and 6 cm size were used. Now silastic cups of 6–6.5 cm size have replaced metal cups.
- System is prechecked for leaking.
- Silastic cup is compressed and introduced inside the vagina after depressing the perineum.
- Cup should be applied as near the occiput as possible, to maintain flexion.
- *Application distance:* The distance between the leading edge of the cup and the anterior fontanelle is called the application distance. For flexing application it should be > 3 cm **(Fig. 8)**.
- For flexing application the center of the cup should overlie the flexion point **(Fig. 9)**. *Flexion point (or pivotal point)* lies 6 cm from anterior fontanelle on sagittal suture. Both above points imply the same thing.
- If the center of the cup is situated more than 1 cm to either side of the sagittal suture the application is described as *paramedian*. Deflexing and paramedian application lead to failure.
- Check before creating vacuum that the cervical lip or vaginal wall is not included in the cup.
- Create vacuum 0.2 kg/cm in 2 minutes initially. After checking correct application vacuum is then created rapidly to the required level of 0.8 kg/cm.

Principles of Traction

- Before starting, see that sufficient pressure is created. Check again that maternal soft tissues are not included in the cup.
- Traction is given during uterine contractions only. There is no difference in outcome whether vacuum is maintained in between contractions or released.[15]

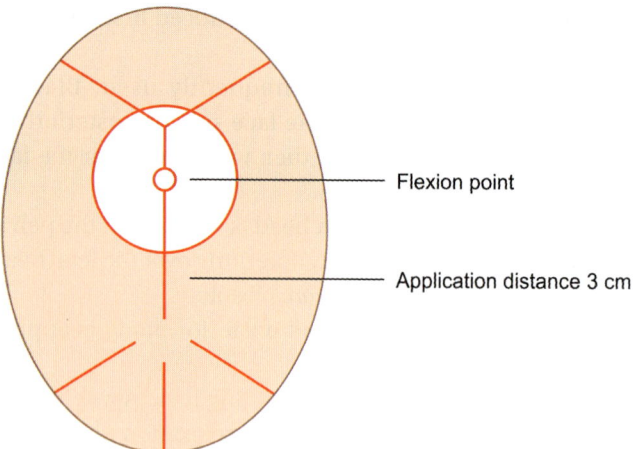

Fig. 8: Application distance and flexion point.

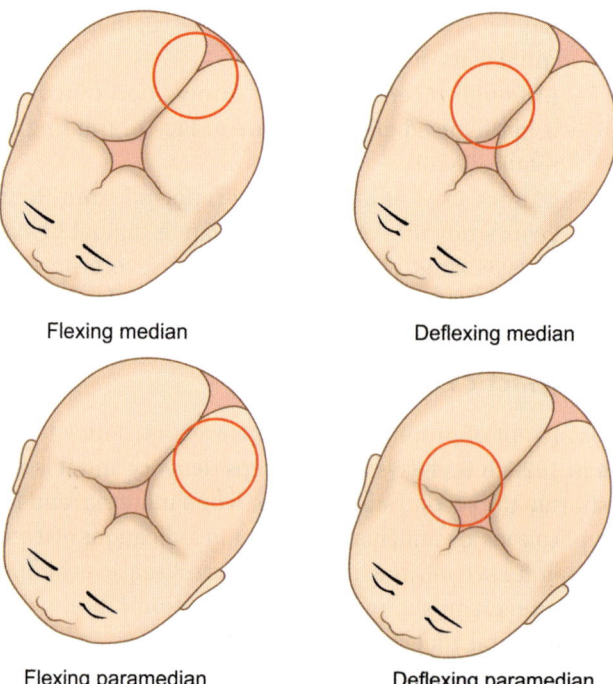

Fig. 9: Correct and incorrect positions of vacuum cup.[22]

- Traction is given perpendicular to the cup. Traction should also be given in pelvic axis to get maximum advantage. It is difficult to practice both simultaneously, so 10° off-center traction may be given. More than 10° direction will lead to leakage of vacuum and slipping of cup.
- With the left forefinger and thumb the cup (upper part) is pressed backward over the fetal head during traction.
- No rotational force is applied; the fetal head may rotate on its own with descent.
- Episiotomy may be given when the head is bulging the perineum.
  Safety rules as suggested by Bird should be observed:
  • Head should be delivered in not more than 3 pulls. With first pull head and not just the scalp must begin to move. By second pull the head must be on the pelvic floor. The head must be completely or almost completely delivered by the third pull.

- The cup should not be applied more than twice in one patient. (two pop-offs)
- Application-delivery interval should not exceed 20 minutes (except in dead fetus).

Artificial caput produced by vacuum is called *Chignon*.

Complications

If correctly performed, they are minimal.

Maternal

They are comparable to spontaneous vaginal delivery. Injury to cervix, vagina or perineum if incorrectly used.

Fetal

- Laceration, abrasion or necrosis of scalp
- Cephalohematoma
- Intracranial hemorrhage
- Subaponeurotic hemorrhage
- Hyperbilirubinemia
- Alopecia
- Retinal or subconjunctival hemorrhage
- Rarely depressed fractures of skull.

Documentation

- Complete documentation is essential in instrumental delivery.[16]
- It includes:
  - Indication for operative delivery
  - Record of informed discussion with the patient and relatives of the risks, benefits, and options
  - Assessment of maternal pelvis, fetal heart rate and contractions
  - Position and station of the fetal head, amount of molding and caput present
  - Type of analgesia or anesthesia used
  - Use of episiotomy, with details of repair.
- Ease of application of vacuum or forceps, number of attempts and duration of traction for forceps and duration of application for vacuum and force used.
- Apgar score, results of cord blood analysis, if done.
- Description of maternal and neonatal injuries, if any.

Postnatal care: Postnatal care following instrumental vaginal birth requires attention to thromboembolic prophylaxis, analgesia, voiding function, rehabilitation of the pelvic floor, and counseling regarding the index birth and future births.[16]

Advantages of Vacuum Extractor over Forceps

- Easy to use
- Much less increase in intracranial pressure during traction
- Does not interfere with internal rotation head (autorotation)
- No trauma to maternal soft tissues if correctly applied
- Minimum anesthesia is required

- Safety factor, because at some pressure (20 kg) vacuum will break and cup will pop off
- Ability to rotate fetal head without the instrument impinging upon the maternal soft tissues.

The WHO (2011)[17] suggested vacuum as the first line of instrument of vaginal delivery where there is no clear clinical indication for a specific instrument to facilitate delivery.

■ COMPARISON FORCEPS VERSUS VACUUM

In Cochrane Database of Systematic Review (2010) which included 32 studies involving 6,597 women comparing forceps with vacuum following conclusions were made.[18]

Compared to the vacuum extractor forceps were found to:
- Be less likely to fail to achieve a vaginal birth (RR 0.65, 95% CI 0.45–0.94)
- Have a trend toward fewer cases of cephalohematoma (RR 0.64, 95% CI 0.37–1.11)
- Have a trend toward fewer cases of fetal retinal hemorrhage (RR 0.6, 95% CI 0.43–1.06)
- Have a trend toward fewer cases of neonatal jaundice (RR 0.79, 95% CI 0.59–1.06)
- Have a trend toward fewer cases of shoulder dystocia (RR 0.4, 95% CI 0.16–1.04).

Compared to vacuum delivery, use of forceps was associated with a higher incidence of:
- Third or fourth degree tears of the anal sphincter (RR 1.89, 95% CI 1.51–2.37)
- Any type of vaginal trauma (RR 2.48, 95% CI 1.59–3.87)
- Incontinence/altered continence (RR 1.77, 95% CI 1.19–2.62).

There was no significant difference between instruments in the risk of:
- Low Apgar score (<7) at 5 minutes
- Low pH (<7.2) in umbilical artery at birth.

Among different types of ventouse, the metal cup was more likely to result in a successful vaginal birth than the soft cup, with more cases of scalp injury and cephalohematoma. Overall forceps or the metal cup appears to be most effective at achieving a vaginal birth, but with increased risk of maternal trauma with forceps and neonatal trauma with the metal cup.

In other studies no neurological abnormality was found at 5 and 10 years follow-up of children born by instrumental deliveries.[19,20]

Sequential use of instruments: Sequential use of vacuum extractor and forceps has been associated with increased rates of neonatal complications and should not routinely be performed.[15]

Which Instrument to be Used

Each instrument has its own advantages and disadvantages. The choice of either vacuum or forceps for instrumental vaginal delivery will depend on the judgment of the operator based on experience and training and the individual clinical circumstances.[18]

Failed Procedure

Operative vaginal delivery should be abandoned where there is no evidence of progressive descent with moderate traction during each contraction or where delivery is not imminent following three contractions of a correctly applied instrument by an experienced operator. Discontinue forceps attempted birth if the forceps cannot be applied easily, the handles do not approximate easily.[8]

Odon Device

The Odon device is a *new instrument* for assisted vaginal delivery. The device was invented by Mr Jorge Odón from Argentina. It consists of plastic sleeve which is inflated around baby's head to pull it out gently for delivery. Becton Dickinson and Company (BD) acquired the license of the device in 2013 and developed a new prototype. The device is permitted for clinical trial by WHO.[21] Initial clinical pilot study showed it feasible for clinical use. No adverse maternal or fetal outcomes were observed at 6 weeks follow-up. Randomized control trials are required before its clinical use.

Measures to Reduce the Need for Instrumental Delivery

- Continuous one to one support during labor
- Use of upright or lateral positions in the second stage of labor
- Avoiding epidural analgesia in labor. However with recent epidural techniques this is not required
- Delayed pushing in second stage of labor
- Judicious use of oxytocin infusion
- Continuous fetal monitoring may allow some more time in second stage of labor if maternal vitals are normal.

■ CONCLUSION

Instrumental vaginal birth has an important place in obstetric practice. We need to realize that though cesarean sections have become safer than 30–40 years ago it is not a natural route of delivery and it still carries a several times more short term and long-term risks as compared to vaginal delivery. Not only it compromises future obstetric carrier but also lead to increased incidence of placenta previa and dangerous PAS disorders. Also the scar in the abdomen is a problem whole life, i.e., intra-abdominal adhesions and chronic pain. Moreover, cesarean section in late second stage of labor is sometimes even more risky as compared to instrumental delivery due to difficulty in delivery of the baby, extension of incision, hemorrhage and sepsis.

If we closely look at the criteria for outlet forceps, head is as such going to deliver in next few minutes with couple of pains. Helping the mother at this junction relieves her from pain and other morbidity and avoids fetal asphyxia due to delay in delivery. This is achieved without any increase in complications meaning that Outlet and Low procedures are absolutely safe. All very recent guidelines of 2020 (RCOG, ACOG, RANCOZ) recommend instrumental delivery.[8,15,16]

Residents should achieve expertise in spontaneous vaginal birth prior to commencing training in assisted vaginal birth. They should receive appropriate training in vacuum and forceps birth, including theoretical knowledge, simulation training and clinical training under direct supervision.[8] As everything revolves around acquiring skill for the instrumental delivery senior and experienced obstetricians, i.e., teachers, need to stay in labor room, should demonstrate and train residents. Contemporary training programs face some serious limitations: a shortage of skilled faculty, reluctance of faculty to teach, the threat of litigation, patient and relatives' attitude and uninterested residents. It is the responsibility of senior obstetricians to prevent this art from dying, otherwise these instruments will soon vanish from Obstetrician's armament.

■ REFERENCES

1. Shameel F, Bava A, Nandanwar YS. Instrumental vaginal deliveries at tertiary centre. Int J Reprod Contracept Obstet Gynecol. 2016;5:4146-50.
2. Sneha BD, Ramesh CC. Trends of instrumental deliveries at tertiary care teaching hospital in Puducherry. Indian J Appl Res. 2015;5(7):2-8.
3. Hubena Z, Workneh A, Siraneh Y. Prevalence and Outcome of Operative Vaginal Delivery among Mothers Who Gave Birth at Jimma University Medical Center, Southwest Ethiopia. J Pregnancy. 2018;2018:7423475.
4. Bailey PE, van Roosmalen J, Mola G, Evans C, de Bernis L, Dao B. Assisted vaginal delivery in low and middle income countries: an overview. BJOG. 2017;124 (9):1335-44.
5. Hehir MP, Reidy FR, Wilkinson MN, Mahony R. Increasing rates of operative vaginal delivery across two decades: accompanying outcomes and instrument preferences. Eur J Obstet Gynecol Reprod Biol. 2013;171:40-3.
6. American College of Obstetricians and Gynecologists. Operative vaginal deHvery. ACOG Practice Bulletin No. 17. Washington (DC): ACOG; 2000.
7. MedScape. (2020). Forceps Delivery. [online] Available from: https://emedicine.medscape.com/article/263603-overview. [Last Accessed November, 2021].
8. Murphy DJ, Strachan BK, Bahl R, on behalf of the Royal College of Obstetricians Gynaecologists. Assisted Vaginal Birth. BJOG. 2020;127:e70-e112.
9. Anwar H. N, Gerard H.A. V , Diogo Ayres DC. FIGO Statement: Restrictive use rather than routine use of episiotomy. Int J Gynecol Obstet. 2019;146(1):17-9.
10. Burke N, Field K, Mujahid F, Morrison JJ. Use and safety of Kielland's forceps in current obstetric practice. Obstet Gynecol. 2012;120:766-70.
11. Stock SJ, Josephs K, Farquharson S, Love C, Cooper SE, Kissack C, et al. Maternal and neonatal outcomes of successful Kielland's rotational forceps delivery. Obstet Gynecol. 2013;121:1032-9.
12. Tempest N, Hart A, Walkinshaw S, Hapangama DK. A reevaluation of the role of rotational forceps: retrospective comparison of maternal and perinatal outcomes following different methods of birth for malposition in the second stage of labour. BJOG. 2013;120:1277-84.
13. Muraca GM, Skoll A, Lisonkova S. Perinatal and maternal morbidity and mortality among term singletons following midcavity operative vaginal delivery versus caesarean delivery. BJOG. 2018;125 (6):693-702.
14. Ali UA, Norwitz ER. Vacuum-assisted vaginal delivery. Obstet Gynecol. 2009;2:5-17.

15. American College of Obstetricians and Gynecologists. Operative vaginal birth. ACOG Practice Bulletin No. 219. Obstet Gynecol. 2020;135:e149-59.
16. The Royal Australian and New Zealand College of obstetrics and Gynecologists. Instrumental vaginal birth. Melbourne: RANZCOG; 2020.
17. Althabe F. Choice of Instruments for Assisted Vaginal Delivery: RHL Commentary. The WHO Reproductive Health Library. Geneva: World Health Organization; 2011.
18. O'mahony F, Hofmeyr GJ, Menon V. Choice of instruments for assisted vaginal delivery. Cochrane Database Syst Rev. 2010;11:CD005455.
19. Wesley BD, van den Berg BJ, Reece EA. The effect of forceps delivery on cognitive development. Am J Obstet Gynecol. 1993;169:1091-5.
20. Ngan HY, Miu P, Ko L, Ma HK. Long-term neurological sequelae following vacuum extractor delivery. Aust N Z J Obstet Gynaecol. 1990;30:111-4.
21. WHO. New instrument for assisted vaginal delivery. Geneva: World Health Organization; 2018.
22. MedScape. (2017). Vacuum Extraction. [online] Available from: https://emedicine.medscape.com/article/271175-overview. [Last Accessed November, 2021].

LONG QUESTIONS

1. What are the advantages and disadvantages of forceps and ventouse over each other?
2. What are the complications of instrumental vaginal delivery? Discuss the mechanisms of their occurrence with forceps and ventouse.

SHORT QUESTIONS

1. Describe the indications and contraindications of instrumental vaginal delivery in general and the forceps and ventouse individually.
2. Enlist the prerequisites for instrumental vaginal delivery.
3. What is the concept of prophylactic forceps?
4. What are the pros and cons of metallic and plastic ventouse cups?
5. What is a failed instrumental vaginal delivery?
6. What measures can be taken to reduce the need for instrumental vaginal delivery?

MULTIPLE CHOICE QUESTIONS

1. Which of the following is not *correct* as compared to the vacuum extractor forceps?
    a. It is less likely to fail to achieve a vaginal birth
    b. Have a trend toward fewer cases of cephalohematoma
    c. Have a trend toward fewer cases of fetal retinal hemorrhage
    d. Less incidence of third or fourth degree tears of the anal sphincter
2. Which of the following is correct?
    a. Vacuum requires more skill as compared to forceps
    b. Vacuum causes more increase in intracranial pressure as compared to forceps
    c. Does not interfere with internal rotation
    d. Metal cups have more failure rate than soft cups
3. Which of the following is not the safety rule of Bird for vacuum delivery?
    a. Head should be delivered in not more than 3 pulls
    b. After 2 pulls delivery should be completed by forceps
    c. The cup should not be applied more than twice in one patient (two pop-offs)
    d. Application-delivery interval should not exceed 20 minutes
4. Which is not the fetal complication of vacuum assisted delivery?
    a. Retinal hemorrhage   b. Facial injury
    c. Hyperbilirubinemia   d. Cephalohematoma
5. Which of the following forceps is used for after coming head of breech?
    a. Simpson's   b. Kielland
    c. Wrigley's   d. Piper's
6. Which of the following is not a correct prerequisite for instrumental vaginal delivery?
    a. Pelvis should be adequate for vaginal delivery.
    b. Cervix should be fully dilated.
    c. Membranes should have been ruptured.
    d. Head should be at – 1 station or below
7. Which of the following statement is *true* for instrumental vaginal delivery at present?
    a. High forceps is removed from the classification
    b. Rotational forceps are commonly done
    c. Episiotomy is must for instrumental delivery
    d. Sequential delivery can be routinely done
8. Regarding forceps and vacuum delivery, which of the following is true?
    a. Failure of instrumental delivery is more common with the vacuum
    b. Instrumental delivery requires epidural analgesia
    c. Instrumental delivery can be used after the cervix is 8 cm dilated
    d. Vacuum delivery is faster than forceps delivery
9. A woman has an instrumental delivery of a baby weighing 3.9 kg. Third degree perineal tear 3C was found. Which is the appropriate method of repair for the anal sphincter?
    a. End to end anastomosis
    b. Overlapping method
    c. Figure of 8 stitches
    d. Continuous locking stitches
10. Primigravida is in second stage of labor since 2 and ½ hours without epidural analgesia. Station is +2 and all prerequisites of instrumental delivery are fulfilled. Uterine contractions are adequate and mother is exhausted. What is the best treatment for her?
    a. Give her sedation
    b. Wait for another 1 hour
    c. Low instrumental delivery
    d. Emergency cesarean section

Answers

1. d 2. c 3. b 4. b 5. d 6. d
7. a 8. a 9. b 10. c

9.7 SHOULDER DYSTOCIA

Abha Rani Sinha, Bhawana Tiwary

■ INTRODUCTION

Shoulder dystocia (SD) is most often an unpredictable and unpreventable obstetric emergency. It continues to evoke terror and fear among physicians, nurse midwives and other healthcare providers.[1] SD is defined as a delivery that requires additional obstetric maneuvers to release the shoulders after gentle downward traction has failed. SD occurs when either the anterior or, less commonly, the posterior fetal shoulder impacts on the maternal symphysis or sacral promontory.[2]

There can be a high perinatal mortality and morbidity associated with the condition, even when it is managed appropriately.[3] Maternal morbidity is also increased, particularly postpartum hemorrhage (11%) and fourth-degree perineal tears (3.8%), and their incidence remains unchanged by the maneuvers required to effect delivery.[4] Typically SD is heralded by the classic "turtle sign": after the fetal head is delivered, it retracts back tightly against the maternal perineum.[5] In order to objectively define SD, Spong and colleagues[6] proposed defining shoulder dystocia as a "prolonged head-to-body delivery time (e.g., more than 60 seconds) and/or the necessitated use of ancillary obstetric maneuvers". The 60-second interval was selected because, in their study, it was approximately two standard deviations above the mean value for head-to-body time for uncomplicated deliveries. Despite this recommendation, SD remains an entity without a clear definition.[7]

■ INCIDENCE

There is wide variation in the reported incidence of shoulder dystocia because of clinical variation in describing SD, the patient population studied and because milder forms may be overdiagnosed or underdiagnosed. The reported incidence ranges from 0, 6 to 3% among vaginal deliveries of fetuses in the vertex presentation. Those studies involving the largest number of vaginal deliveries report incidences between 0.58 and 0.7%.[8]

PELVIC ANATOMY RELATED TO SHOULDER DYSTOCIA

The maternal pelvis is composed of series of bones forming a girdle protecting the pelvic organs. The front-most bone is the symphysis pubis. It is on this structure that a baby's anterior shoulder gets caught during a delivery complicated by shoulder dystocia. The bone at the back of the maternal pelvis is the sacrum. Because of its shape, it generally serves as a slide over which a baby's posterior shoulder can descend freely during labor and delivery. However, sometimes a baby's posterior shoulder can get caught on its slight projection into the pelvis. In normal vaginal deliveries, the head of the baby, called the "vertex", emerges first. During labor, the soft, mobile bones of the fetal head can overlap and the head as a whole can "mold"—go from perfectly round to more pointed and narrower. This facilitates the fetal head fitting into and through the maternal pelvis. The baby's shoulders, likewise being flexible, usually follow the delivery of the baby's head quickly and easily. But for this to happen, the axis of the fetal shoulders must descend into the maternal pelvis at an angle oblique to the pelvis's anteroposterior dimension. This position affords the shoulders the most room for their passage. If instead the shoulders line up in a straight anteroposterior orientation as they are about to emerge from the mother's pelvis, there will often be insufficient room for them to squeeze through. The back of the mother's pubic bone then forms a shelf upon which the baby's anterior shoulder gets caught. If this happens, the shoulders cannot deliver and a shoulder dystocia results.

Shoulder dystocia can also occur if the posterior shoulder of a baby gets caught on its mother's sacrum. This is a far less common cause of shoulder dystocia.

■ RISK FACTORS

A number of antenatal and intrapartum characteristics have been reported to be associated with shoulder dystocia. There is a relationship between fetal size and shoulder dystocia5 but it is not a good predictor. The large majority of infants with a birth weight of ≥4,500 g do not develop shoulder dystocia,[9] and equally importantly, 48% of incidences of shoulder dystocia occur in infants with a birth weight less than 4,000 g.[10] Moreover, clinical fetal weight estimation is unreliable and third-trimester ultrasound scans have at least a 10% margin for error for actual birth weight and a sensitivity of just 60% for macrosomia (over 4.5 kg).[11]

The risk factors associated with shoulder dystocia are being listed in **Table 1**.

Statistical modeling has shown that these risk factors are not independent. Although statistically associated, these clinical characteristics have a low positive predictive value both singly and in combination.[12] Conventional risk factors predicted only 16% of shoulder dystocia that resulted in infant morbidity.[12] The large majority of cases occur in the children of women with no risk factors. Shoulder dystocia is, therefore, a largely unpredictable and unpreventable event.

Sensitivity and specificity of ultrasound to detect fetal weight greater than 4,500 g were 22–69% and 98–99%, respectively. Thus, estimated fetal weight (EFW) using

TABLE 1: Risk factors associated with shoulder dystocia.	
Prelabor	**Intrapartum**
• Previous shoulder dystocia • Macrosomia • Diabetes mellitus • Maternal body mass index >30 kg/m² • Induction of labor • Multiparity • Postdates	• Prolonged first stage of labor • Secondary arrest • Prolonged second stage of labor • Oxytocin augmentation • Assisted vaginal delivery

ultrasound biometry does not appear to be more accurate than clinical estimate based upon Leopold's maneuvers. The chest to head and shoulder ratios are increased in infants of diabetic mothers thereby increasing the risk of shoulder dystocia independent of fetal weight. Maternal diabetes increases the likelihood of shoulder dystocia 2–6 folds over the nondiabetic population. There is no evidence to support induction of labor in women without diabetes at term where the fetus is thought to be macrosomic [Grade A of Recommendation, Royal College of Obstetricians and Gynaecologists (RCOG)].[2] The RCOG also affirms that elective cesarean section is not recommended to reduce the potential morbidity for pregnancies complicated by suspected fetal macrosomia without maternal diabetes mellitus (Grade C of Recommendation).[2] ACOG states upon a level B of Recommendation that "Elective IOL or elective cesarean delivery for all women suspected of carrying a fetus with macrosomia is not appropriate" due to the fact that USG is not an accurate predictor of macrosomia.[1]

MANAGEMENT

Recognition

The first step in treating shoulder dystocia is recognizing when it occurs. An experienced obstetrician should be available on the labor ward for the second stage of labor when shoulder dystocia is anticipated. However, it is recognized that not all cases can be anticipated and therefore all birth attendants should be conversant with the techniques required to facilitate delivery complicated by shoulder dystocia. Timely management of shoulder dystocia requires prompt recognition. The attendant health carer should routinely observe for (Evidence level IV, RCOG):

- Difficulty with delivery of the face and chin
- The head remaining tightly applied to the vulva or even retracting (*turtle sign*, **Fig. 1**)
- Failure of restitution of the fetal head
- Failure of the shoulders to descend.

The fifth Confidential Enquiry into Stillbirths and Deaths in Infancy (CESDI) report on SD identified that 47% of the babies died within 5 minutes of the head being delivered.[13] It is important, therefore, to manage the problem as efficiently

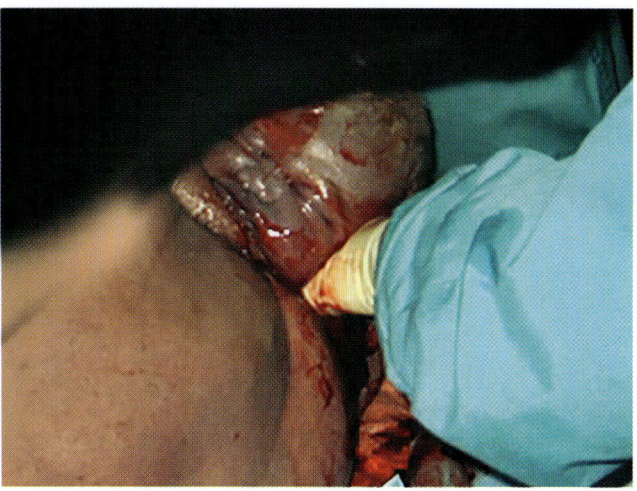

Fig. 1: Turtle sign.

as possible but also carefully: efficiently so as to avoid hypoxia acidosis, carefully so as to avoid unnecessary trauma (Evidence level III, RCOG).

Call for Help

Immediately after recognition of shoulder dystocia, extra help should be called. In a hospital setting, this should include further midwifery assistance, an obstetrician, a pediatric resuscitation team and an anesthetist. Maternal pushing should be discouraged, as this may lead to further impaction of the shoulders, thereby exacerbating the situation.[14] The woman should be maneuvered to bring the buttocks to the edge of the bed.

Fundal Pressure should not be Employed

Fundal pressure should not be used for the treatment of shoulder dystocia. It is associated with an unacceptably high neonatal complication rate and may result in uterine rupture.

Assessment for Need of Episiotomy

Some authors have advocated that episiotomy is an essential part of the management in all cases but others suggest that it does not affect the outcome of shoulder dystocia.[15] The Managing Obstetric Emergencies and Trauma (MOET) Group suggests a selective approach, reserving episiotomy to facilitate maneuvers such as delivery of the posterior arm or internal rotation of the shoulders.[16] An episiotomy should therefore be considered but it is not mandatory.

Maneuvers and Procedures

- *McRoberts maneuver:* McRoberts' maneuver is the single most effective intervention and should be performed first (Grade B of Recommendation, RCOG). This maneuver involves hyperflexion of the maternal thighs against the abdomen (**Fig. 2**). The maneuver straightens the sacrum relative to the lumbar spine, allowing cephalic rotation

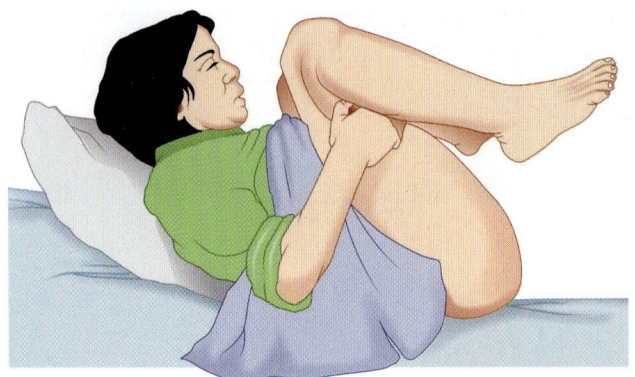

Fig. 2: McRobert's maneuver
Source (McRoberts): http://altair.chonnam.ac.kr/~tbsong/medical/sh-dyst.

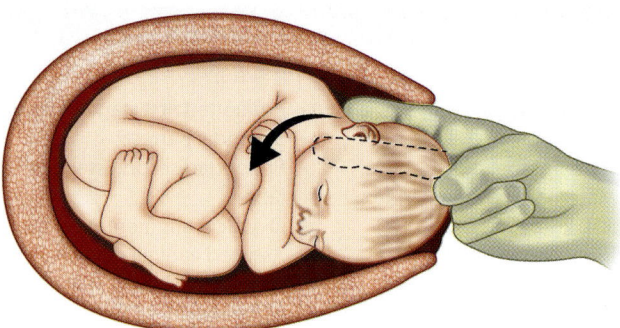

Fig. 4: Rubin's II maneuver (internal rotation).

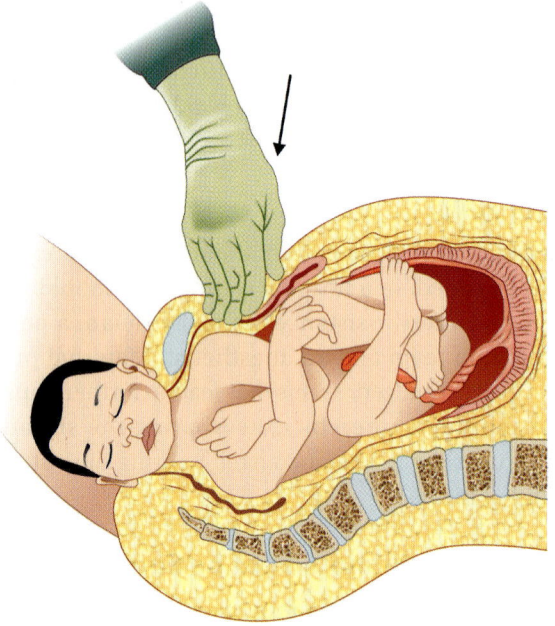

Fig. 3: Rubin's I maneuver (suprapubic pressure).
Source (Rubin I): patientsafetyauthority.org/ADVISORIES/AdvisoryLibrary/2009/dec16_6(suppl1)/Pages/18.aspx.

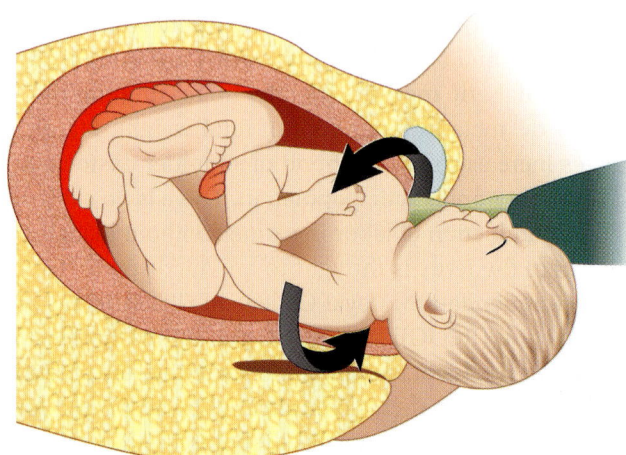

Fig. 5: Wood screw's (rotation of posterior shoulder).
Source (Rotational): http://shoulderdystociainfo.com/resolved without fetal.

of the symphysis pubis sliding over the fetal shoulder. These motions push the posterior shoulder over the sacral promontory, allowing it to fall into the hollow of the sacrum, and rotate the symphysis over the impacted shoulder.[17]

- *Rubin's maneuver:* Suprapubic pressure can be employed together with McRoberts' maneuver to improve success rates. Suprapubic pressure reduces the bisacromial diameter and rotates the anterior shoulder into the oblique pelvic diameter. The shoulder is then free to slip underneath the symphysis pubis with the aid of routine traction. External suprapubic pressure is applied in a downward and lateral direction to push the posterior aspect of the anterior shoulder toward the fetal chest **(Fig. 3)**. It is advised that this is applied for 30 seconds.
- *Rubin's II maneuver:* Adduction of the anterior shoulder by pressure applied to the posterior aspect of the shoulder.

The shoulder is pushed toward the chest, or pressure is applied to the scapula of the anterior shoulder (Rubin, 1964). These maneuvers attempt to position the shoulders to utilize the smallest possible diameter of the fetus through the largest diameter of the woman **(Fig. 4)**.

- *Wood's screw maneuver (Fig. 5):* Pressure is applied to the anterior aspect of the posterior shoulder, and an attempt is made to rotate the posterior shoulder to the anterior position. Success of this maneuver allows easy delivery of that shoulder once past the symphysis pubis. In practice, the anterior disimpaction maneuver and Wood's maneuver may be done simultaneously and repetitively to achieve disimpaction of the anterior shoulder (Woods, 1943).
- *Jacquemier's maneuver (Manual removal of the posterior arm):* The arm is usually flexed at the elbow. If it is not, pressure in the antecubital fossa can assist with flexion. The hand is grasped, swept across the chest and delivered, as shown in **Figure 6**.
- *Roll over to "all fours" position—Gaskin maneuver:* Moving the woman to "all fours" appears to increase the effective pelvic dimensions, allowing the fetal position to shift; this may disimpact the shoulders. With gentle downward pressure on the posterior shoulder, the anterior shoulder may become more impacted (with gravity), but will facilitate the

freeing up of the posterior shoulder. Also, this position may allow easier access to the posterior shoulder for rotational maneuvers or removal of the posterior arm **(Fig. 7)**.
- *Other maneuvers:* If nothing has worked to this point and all the procedures have been tried again, then some healthcare providers have suggested:
  - Deliberate fracture of the clavicle
  - *Symphysiotomy:* The cartilage of the symphysis pubis (where the pubic bones come together) may be surgically divided to increase the size of the pelvic outlet. An obsolete procedure now.
  - *Zavanelli maneuver—cephalic replacement:* This maneuver involves reversing the cardinal movements of labor. The head is rotated to occiput anterior, as shown in **Figure 8**. Flex, push up, rotate to transverse, disengage, and perform a cesarean section (Sandberg, 1999).

A common treatment mnemonic is **HELPERR** from American Life Support Organization:

H: Call for help
E: Evaluate for episiotomy
L: Legs (the McRoberts' maneuver)
P: Suprapubic pressure
E: Enter maneuvers (internal rotation)
R: Remove the posterior arm
R: Roll the patient (Gaskin's)

Another treatment mnemonic is **ALARMER**:
A: Ask for help
L: Leg hyperflexion (McRoberts')
A: Anterior shoulder disimpaction
R: Rubin's
M: Manual delivery of posterior arm
E: Episiotomy
R: Roll over on all fours (Gaskin's)

If the simple measures (the McRoberts' maneuver and suprapubic pressure) fail, then there is a choice to be made between the all-fours-position and internal manipulation. Traditionally, internal manipulations are used at this point but the-all-fours position has been described, with an 83% success rate in one case series.[18] The individual circumstances should guide the accoucheur. For a slim mobile woman without epidural anesthesia and with a single midwifery attendant, the all-fours-position is probably the most appropriate. For a less mobile woman with epidural anesthesia in place and a senior obstetrician in attendance, internal maneuvers are more appropriate.

■ COMPLICATIONS

Fetal
- Brachial plexus injury (2–16% of such deliveries)
- Clavicular fracture
- Fracture of humerus
- Fetal hypoxia
- Fetal death.

Maternal
- Postpartum hemorrhage
- Vaginal and vulval lacerations

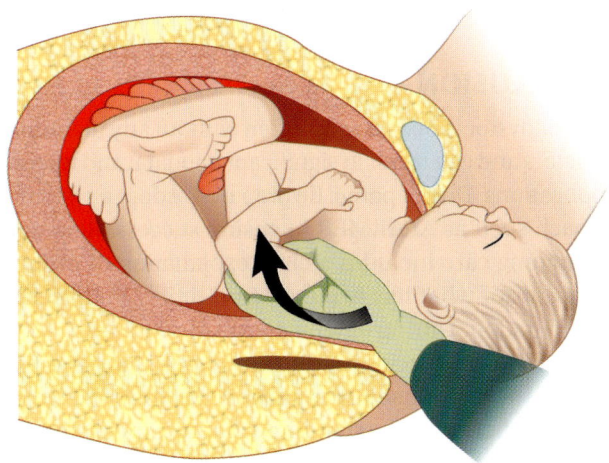

Fig. 6: Jacquemier's maneuver.
Source: (Manual delivery of posterior arm). http://www.glowm.com/resources/glowm/cd/pages/v2/v2c079

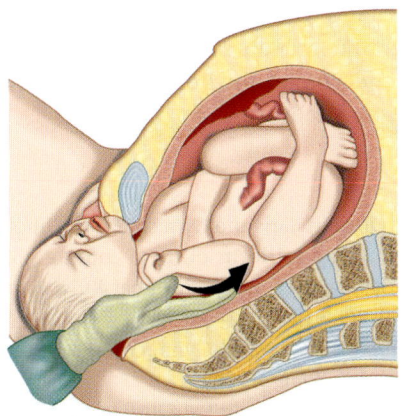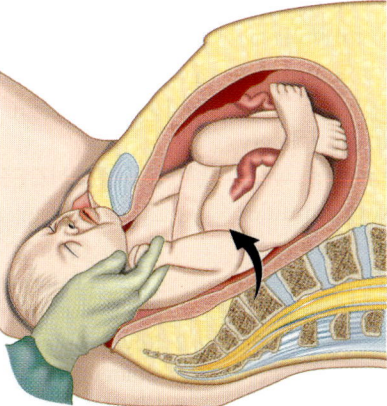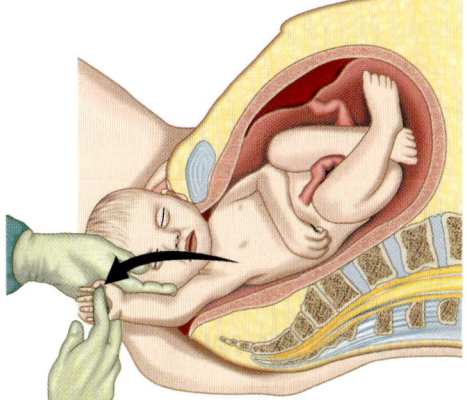

Fig. 7: Gaskin's maneuver.
Source: http://www.sciencedirect.com/science/article/pii/S0889854505700899.

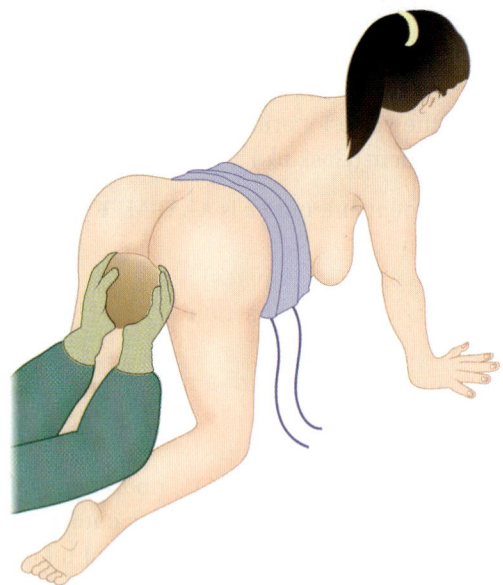

Fig. 8: Zavanelli maneuver.

- Cervical injuries
- 3 or 4th degree tears
- Obstetric fistulas
- Uterine rupture.

After Shoulder Dystocia

- Remember the *significant* risk of maternal injury (tears) and postpartum hemorrhage.
- Actively manage the third stage. Apply active management of the third stage of labor.
- Inspect for and repair tears or lacerations.
- Do cord blood gases, if this is the policy of your institution.
- Ensure appropriate neonatal resuscitation and assessment; document all actions taken to resuscitate the newborn.
- Examine the newborn for evidence of trauma. Document the occurrence of shoulder dystocia in the baby's chart. Document Apgar scores and any bruising or injuries found on the initial newborn exam.
- Re-examine the baby within 24 hours or at any time after the birth if concerns develop.
- Document and describe the maneuvers used, and, if possible, the time between the birth of the head to completion of the birth in both the mother's and the baby's charts.
- Explain to the woman and all those involved in the delivery exactly what occurred and what management steps were taken. Advise her that she is at risk for another shoulder dystocia for her next pregnancy (15% recurrence after one dystocia and 30% after two shoulder dystocias).

DOCUMENTATION

The sixth CESDI annual report highlighted inadequate documentation in obstetrics, with potential medicolegal consequences.[19] It may be helpful to use a structured proforma to aid accurate record keeping. This is a suggested format for a chart note. Detailed notes should be incorporated into both the woman's and the baby's charts. This format may also serve as a template to dictate a delivery summary. If the woman was referred from another lower-level healthcare facility, this information should be included in a report letter to be sent to the referral facility.

- Date and time of birth
- Name of healthcare provider
- Delivery of the head: spontaneous or operative. If operative, forceps or vacuum?
- Type of analgesia or anesthesia present when the shoulder dystocia was recognized and any additional anesthesia given (if any)
- Description and order of maneuvers used to deliver baby
- Estimation of traction forces used
- Use of episiotomy, description and timing, details of repair
- Estimated time from birth of head to complete birth of baby
- Apgar scores
- Results of cord blood analysis, if done
- Neonatal resuscitation activities, if needed
- Indicate which shoulder was impacted: left or right
- Description of maternal and neonatal injuries (if any)
- Recommendations for future deliveries

CONCLUSION

Shoulder dystocia occurs most often without any identifiable risk factors and can result in significant neonatal and maternal complications. Do not panic. Be prepared. Adopt a systematic approach such as ALARMER to ensure success. Remember that ongoing care includes a clear explanation of events to the parents of what has occurred and timely and accurate documentation. During antenatal care, discuss with women what major emergencies may occur during labor and birth, and how these are usually managed. In this way, women will have a better understanding what to expect; this may help to decrease anxiety. At the same time, such discussion will increase confidence in healthcare providers. After an incidence, such as shoulder dystocia, it is important to take time to talk to the woman and whoever else was present at the birth about the events that have occurred. It is important that the woman understand why the complication may have happened, and why certain procedures were done to help her and her baby. Provide the woman and her family with advice for her next pregnancy and delivery.

REFERENCES

1. American College of Obstetricians and Gynecologists. Shoulder dystocia. ACOG practice bulletin clinical management guidelines for obstetrician-gynecologists. Number 40, November 2002. Obstet Gynecol. 2002;100:1045-50.
2. Royal College of Obstetricians and Gynaecologists. RCOG Guideline No. 42. London: ROCG; 2005.
3. Gherman RB, Ouzounain JG, Goodwin TM. Obstetric maneuvers for shoulder dystocia and associated fetal morbidity. Am J Obstet Gynecol. 1998;178:1126-30.

4. Gherman RB, Goodwin TM, Souter I, Neumann K, Ouzounian JG, Paul RH. The McRobert's maneuver for the alleviation of shoulder dystocia: how successful is it? Am J Obstet Gynecol. 1997;178:656-61.
5. Gherman RB. Shoulder dystocia: prevention and management. Obstet Gynecol Clin North Am. 2005;32:297-305.
6. Spong CY, Beall M, Rodrigues D. An objective definition of shoulder dystocia: prolonged head-to-body delivery intervals and/or the use of ancillary obstetric maneuvers. Obstet Gynecol. 1995;86:433-6.
7. Amy G. Gottlirb, Henry L. Galan. Shoulder dystocia: an update. Obstet Gynecol Clin N Am. 2007:34(3):501-531.
8. Gherman RB. Shoulder dystocia: an evidence-based evaluation of the obstetric nightmare. Clin Obstet Gynecol. 2002;45:345-62.
9. Naef RW 3rd, Martin JN Jr. Emergent management of shoulder dystocia. Obstet Gynecol Clin North Am 1995;22:247-59.
10. Baskett TF, Allen AC. Perinatal implications of shoulder dystocia. Obstet Gynecol. 1995;86:14-7.
11. Rouse DJ, Owen J. Prophylactic caesarean delivery for fetal macrosomia diagnosed by means of ultrasonography-A Faustian bargain? Am J Obstet Gynecol. 1999;181:332-8.
12. Nesbitt TS, Gilbert WM, Herrchen B. Shoulder dystocia and associated risk factors with macrosomic infants born in California. Am J Obstet Gynecol. 1998;179:476-80.
13. Focus Group Shoulder Dystocia. In: Confidential Enquiries into Stillbirths and Deaths in Infancy. Fifth Annual Report. London: Maternal and Child Health Research Consortium; 1998. pp. 73-9.
14. Gonik B, Zhang N, Grimm MJ. Defining forces that are associated with shoulder dystocia: the use of a mathematic dynamic computer model. Am J Obstet Gynecol. 2003;188:1068-72.
15. Gurewitsch ED, Donithan M, Stallings SP, Moore PL, Agarwal S, Allen LM, et al. Episiotomy versus fetal manipulation in managing severe shoulder dystocia: a comparison of outcomes. Am J Obstet Gynecol. 2004;191:911-6.
16. Hinshaw K. Shoulder dystocia. In: Johanson R, Cox C, Grady K, Howell C (Eds). Managing Obstetric Emergencies and Trauma: The MOET Course Manual. London: RCOG Press; 2003. pp. 165-74.
17. Baxley EG, Gobbo RW. Shoulder Dystocia .Am Fam Physician. 2004;69(7):1707-14.
18. Bruner JP, Drummond SB, Meenan AL, Gaskin IM. All-fours maneuver for reducing shoulder dystocia during labor. J Reprod Med. 1998;43:439-43.
19. The "4kg and over" enquiries. In: Confidential Enquiries into Stillbirths and Deaths in Infancy. Sixth Annual Report. London: Maternal and Child Health Research Consortium; 1999. pp. 35-47.

LONG QUESTION

1. What is shoulder dystocia? Discuss the procedures used in the management of shoulder dystocia.

SHORT QUESTIONS

1. What are the risk factors for shoulder dystocia?
2. What are the maneuvers for shoulder dystocia?

MULTIPLE CHOICE QUESTIONS

1. Which of the following maneuvers is *not* used for management of shoulder dystocia?
   a. McRobert's maneuver
   b. Suprapubic pressure
   c. Woods Corkscrew maneuver
   d. Mauriceau Smellie Veit maneuver
2. What is true regarding shoulder dystocia?
   a. The event is considered to be predictable and therefore avoidable
   b. Most cases occur during operative delivery
   c. Three-fourths of babies weighed 4 kg and above
   d. It would have been less likely to have occurred if fundal pressure was used

Answers
1. d   2. c

9.8 CESAREAN SECTION

Suchitra N Pandit, Rakhee R Sahu

INTRODUCTION

Every woman and Obstetrician desires a healthy pregnancy and a healthy baby. This appears more fascinating and fulfilling when an obstetrician is able to assess, modify and intervene whenever needed, to counter the adversities of nature thus ensuring safe delivery of the baby. A pregnant woman expects the important lifetime event of her childbirth should be assisted appropriately by her caregiver.

Cesarean section (CS) is today the most common life-saving obstetric procedure performed worldwide. Cesarean section should be considered as one of the parameters of quality and care given during delivery. As an evolutionary gift of nature the human beings acquired the "intelligence", which propelled us to overcome the difficult labors and the associated maternal and fetal morbidity. This gave way of abdominal child birth— "the cesarean birth".

HISTORY OF CESAREAN DELIVERY

The history of cesarean birth is shrouded in enigma. It is perhaps the singular astounding human achievement in making childbirth safer.

The name of the operation is derived from the Roman emperor, Julius Caesar, who was rumored to have been delivered by an abdominal incision. However, this is not likely to be true. A related myth is that women who died in childbirth were mandated by law (The Lex Regia or Lex Caesara) to be delivered by an abdominal incision before burial in the times of Numa Pompilius in 716 BC. Early documents from Egypt, Greece and Indian civilizations also mention such deliveries.

The remarkable advances in medicine and its allied fields of surgery, anesthesia, pharmacology, blood transfusion in the last 200 years have made cesarean delivery a safe and feasible option to difficult and dangerous childbirths. Early practice of removal of the uterus and leaving the uterocervical stump unsutured or exteriorized became obsolete. Extraperitoneal cesarean was described by Frank, subsequently modified by Latzko in 1909. In 1908, Pfannenstiel performed a transperitoneal cesarean section to approach to the lower uterine segment. Osiander is given the credit for being the originator for lower segment cesarean delivery. Kerr in 1926 developed and popularized the most commonly followed approach employed throughout the world.

■ ETYMOLOGY

The use of term "cesarean section" is called a *pleonasm* meaning two words with similar meanings. The term *cesarean section* seems to originate from some form of Latin word meaning "to cut" or "to kill." The Latin verb caedo, caedere, cecidi, or ceasum means to cut or to kill. The second part of the phrase is a noun of verb seco, secare, secui, or sectum meaning to cut.

■ EPIDEMIOLOGY OF CESAREAN SECTION

The high incidence of cesarean delivery has caused a great deal of debate over the past several years among healthcare providers, third-party payers, and health policy developers. In 1985, World Health Organization (WHO) stated: "there is no justification for any region to have cesarean delivery rates higher than 10–15%".[1-3] The studies on which the WHO based the 15% recommendation 30 years ago were "limited by either having incomplete data or relying on averaged cesarean delivery rates from multiple years without accounting for year-to-year variation in these estimates".

None of the countries with a stillbirth rate of 2–4 1,000 have a Cesarean Section rate between the WHO recommended 10–15% threshold. Not surprisingly the WHO issued a new statement in 2015 with the headline, "Every effort should be made to provide cesarean sections to women in need, rather than striving to achieve a specific rate".

Over the period of time there have been changes in the indications so as to reduce the maternal and perinatal mortality rates. The possible reasons for the continued increase in cesarean section rates could be explained by the following:

- Greater percentage of nulliparity and rising average maternal age.
- Rise in induction of labor and increasing use of electronic fetal heart rate monitoring and early diagnosis of abnormal or nonreassuring fetal heart tracing.
- Most of breech presentations are delivered by CS due to concerns of fetal injury.
- The frequency of instrumental deliveries—forceps and vacuum has declined due to possible medicolegal litigations.
- Increased prevalence of medical disorders in pregnancy such as gestation hypertensive, gestational diabetes, obesity.
- Availability of well-equipped neonatal intensive care units which are able to salvage smaller babies and those which are premature which in earlier times was not possible.
- Multiple pregnancies especially with ART techniques also contributes to higher CS rates.

The incidence of CS rates in the USA has increased from 4.5% of all deliveries to 32.8%. As per the latest data [National Family Health Survey 2015–16 (NFHS-4)], the cesarean rates at population level in India is reported to be 17.2% of all deliveries. Of 195,366 total institutional births in the NFHS-4, 15,165 births (11.9%) were cesarean deliveries in public facilities, and 20,506 births (40.9%) were cesarean deliveries in private facilities. The cesarean delivery rate in public health facilities increased from 7.2% in the NFHS-1 to 11.9% in the NFHS-4, whereas in private health facilities, the rate increased from 12.3 to 40.9% during the same period. The odds ratio for cesarean deliveries in private facilities compared with public facilities increased from 1.62 (95% CI, 1.49–1.76) in the NFHS-3 to 4.17 (95% CI, 4.04–4.30) in the NFHS-4.

■ INDICATIONS OF CESAREAN DELIVERY

Indications for cesarean delivery vary depending on the clinical situation and the resources available for patient care.
- History of prior one or two cesarean section
- Abnormal placentation such as placenta previa or placental abruption
- History of prior classical CS or full-thickness myomectomy
- Multifetal gestation
- Failure of induction of labor
- Fetal malpresentation—breech, transvers lie
- Bad obstetric history, history of unexplained intrauterine fetal demise
- Failure to progress/prolonged labor which may be detrimental to fetal health
- Genital tract/pelvic obstructive mass
- Invasive cervical carcinoma
- Prior trachelectomy
- Permanent cervical cerclage
- Prior pelvic reconstructive surgery
- Pelvic bony deformity
- Active HSV lesions and HIV
- Maternal cardiac or pulmonary disease
- Cerebral Aneurysm or arteriovenous malformation
- Any pathology needing concurrent abdominal exploration
- Perimortem cesarean section

- Maternal request
- Cephalopelvic disproportion
- Failed operative vaginal delivery
- Nonreassuring fetal heart rate tracing
- Intrauterine fetal growth restriction
- Macrosomia
- Extreme preterm labor
- Fetal Congenital anomalies such as meningomyelocele and rare conditions like conjoint twins.

Robson's 10-Group Classification for analyzing cesarean section rates:
World Health Organization (2015) recommended the use of the Robson's-10 group classification as a global standard for recording and comparing cesarean section rates in all healthcare facilities **(Table 1)**.

The WHO (2015) expects that Robson's classification should help healthcare facilities to identify and analyze the women who contribute the most and least to overall cesarean section rates.

PREOPERATIVE EVALUATION

The preoperative assessment should include a detailed history and physical examination, past medical and surgical history, current medications, drug allergies, and indication for cesarean section, necessary blood investigations such as complete hemogram, urine, HIV, HbsAg, HCV and blood group. In ideal circumstances, blood should be cross matched.

Consent for Cesarean Section

- Written consent for cesarean section and anesthesia should be taken after providing evidence based information taking into consideration the clinical situation (patient's privacy, views and culture)
- Consent should always be in the language patient understands and never implied
- Patient may opt for refusal of CS though oblivious of benefits to her and baby's health. This should be recorded in the patients' indoor papers
- If consent is not signed by relatives or in case of nonavailability, signatures of two consultants are valid if surgery is life-saving.

TECHNIQUES OF ANESTHESIA FOR CESAREAN SECTION

Regional Anesthesia

Spinal anesthesia: It is the most favored technique for cesarean delivery. The advantages include faster onset of action, reliability of needle placement, relative ease of technique, reduced postoperative sequel and virtual elimination of local anesthetic toxicity. The potential complications include likelihood of hypotension and postdural puncture headache.

Epidural anesthesia: It is a good technique used especially for cesarean section following trial of vaginal delivery wherein the epidural catheter is already placed for labor analgesia or in few high-risk case where hemodynamic stability is compromised.

Combined spinal and epidural anesthesia: The level of block can be controlled by incremental epidural dosing. This has the advantage of better hemodynamic stability, fewer side effects, faster recovery at the expense of a longer preparation time for surgery.

TABLE 1: Robson's 10-Group classification for indications of cesarean section.[4]

Groups	Pregnant women
1	Nulliparous women with a single cephalic pregnancy, ≥37 weeks gestation in spontaneous labor
2	Nulliparous women with a single cephalic pregnancy, ≥37 weeks gestation who either had labor induced or were delivered by cesarean section before labor 2a: Labor induced 2b: Prelabor CS
3	Multiparous women without a previous uterine scar, with a single cephalic pregnancy, ≥37 weeks gestation in spontaneous labor
4	Multiparous women without a previous uterine scar, with a single cephalic pregnancy, ≥37 weeks gestation who either had labor induced or were delivered by cesarean section before labor 4a: Labor induced 4b: Prelabor CS
5	All multiparous women with at least one previous uterine scar, with a single cephalic pregnancy, ≥37 weeks gestation 5.1: With one previous CS 5.2: With two or more previous CSs
6	All nulliparous women with a single breech pregnancy
7	All multiparous women with a single breech pregnancy, including women with previous uterine scars
8	All women with multiple pregnancies, including women with previous uterine scars
9	All women with a single pregnancy with a transverse or oblique lie, including women with previous uterine scars
10	All women with a single cephalic pregnancy <37 weeks gestation, including women with previous scars

The complications of regional anesthesia are total spinal or high block, intravenous injection, subdural block, hypotension, shivering, postdural puncture headache.[5]

Contraindications to regional anesthesia: Bleeding disorder, uncorrected hypovolemia and shock, major hemorrhage, anticoagulation severe preeclampsia induced thrombocytopenia, disorders of the spine, local anesthetic drug allergy, local infection, maternal disease (cardiac disease) and refusal to consent.

General Anesthesia

It has the advantage of rapid induction, less association with hypotension and cardiovascular stability and there is better control of airway and ventilation. Morbidity is usually due to hypoxia secondary to tracheal intubation or from aspiration pneumonitis.

Surgical Techniques for Cesarean Delivery

Many different practitioners use the benefits of various techniques of skin incision, uterine incision, uterine closure, and individualize it as per convenience.

Choice of the Skin Incision

A number of skin incisions have been used in abdominal deliveries. Traditionally midline vertical incision was used because of its advantage in proper and adequate exposure of the operative field, less vascularity and rapid entry.

However, over the period of time there is increased awareness regarding the safety and cosmetic value of suprapubic transverse incisions such as Pfannenstiel incision, Joel Cohens incision, Maylard, Cherney and the low transverse incision.

Rarely vertical paramedian incision may be used.

Pfannenstiel incision: It is made transversely in the maternal abdomen approximately 3 cm above the symphysis pubis and is curvilinear about 15 cm in length, with the lateral apices of the incision smiling up toward the anterior superior iliac spines. This incision is given upto the level of the anterior rectus fascia. The anterior rectus fascia is then sharply incised with the scalpel in a transverse manner in the midline to expose the belly of the rectus muscle on either side of the midline. At this time, the incision in the anterior rectus fascia may be extended laterally using either the scalpel or the Mayo scissors.[6]

Care must be taken not to cut the underlying rectus muscles. During this dissection, care must be taken to identify and ligate or electrocoagulate the perforating vessels between the rectus muscles and the anterior fascia; this can be performed at entry, or in the event of an emergency cesarean delivery, at the time of closure. Regardless of which manner is chosen, the entry point should be high in the operative field to avoid injury to the maternal bladder. Opening of the peritoneum may be performed by elevating the peritoneal membrane between two hemostats, palpating the opposing pieces of membrane for evidence of entrapped bowel, and making incision with a scalpel or by bluntly introducing a finger through the peritoneum at the level of the umbilicus. Once the peritoneal cavity is entered, the peritoneal incision is extended by stretching the opening or using scissors to maximize surgical exposure.

Maylard incision: With the Maylard incision, once the anterior rectus sheath is incised in a transverse fashion, the fascia is not dissected free from the underlying rectus muscles; instead, the inferior epigastric arteries are identified and ligated,[7] and the rectus muscles are incised, usually with electrocautery to minimize bleeding. The posterior rectus sheath and the peritoneum are then incised in a transverse fashion. It is used originally in radical pelvic surgery. It is recommended when certain risk factors such as macrocosmic fetus or twins needing maximal exposure. But due to more tissue dissection postoperative discomfort is likely.[8]

Cherney incision: It is performed in the same manner as the Pfannenstiel and the Maylard incisions except that the rectus fascia is not entered; instead, the rectus muscles are cut free from the symphysis pubis at their tendinous insertion and reflected superiorly. There are few if any indications for the use of this type of incision for an abdominal delivery.

Joel-Cohen incision: It is performed in a transverse manner 2 finger breadth cm above the location of a Pfannenstiel incision and is linear, not curvilinear. The fascia is not dissected off of the rectus muscles, and the peritoneum is entered transversely, as in the Maylard incision. An advantage of this type of incision includes decreased operating time; however, there are no maternal or fetal advantages other than speed.

In the moderately obese patient, a variation of the Pfannenstiel incision is performed several cm higher than the true Pfannenstiel to avoid placing the incision in the fold created by the abdominal pannus and thereby decreasing the rate of wound complications.

Vertical incisions: Vertical incisions remain useful in situations such as cesarean section for fetal bradycardia and in the morbidly obese patient in whom a transverse incision may not allow for adequate exposure of the operative field. The incision is performed vertically from just below the umbilicus and extended to just above the symphysis pubis and can easily be extended around the umbilicus if exposure of the upper abdomen is required. The incision is carried sharply down to the level of the rectus sheath, which is then incised sharply with the scalpel in a vertical direction. This incision may be completed with the scalpel or by using the Mayo scissors. The fascial edge closest to the midline is then grasped with a pair of Kocher clamps, and sharp and blunt dissections are used to separate the rectus muscles from the overlying fascia.

The rectus muscles are then separated in the midline, and the peritoneum is entered vertically as described previously.

Approach to Lower Uterine Segment

Blunt dissection of fascia of Scarpa's and Campers is advisable as it is associated with decreased intraoperative bleeding. During dissection of anterior rectus sheath from the underlying muscle, care should be taken as perforating vessels might get cut and subsequently bleed. Such a bleeding does not occur in Joel-Cohen technique, as it does not include the dissection. Rectus muscle should be split vertically and not transversely. Care should be taken to avoid injury to the vessels on the undersurface of the muscle bellies. Peritoneum should be opened as high as possible. It can be cut transversely in order to avoid injury to bladder. If opened in any other way care should be taken to avoid bladder injury. Dextrorotation of uterus should be noted prior to opening the vesicouterine space. Development of bladder flap should entail dissection in the midline and not laterally to avoid vessel injury.

Uterine Incision

There are several types of uterine incisions **(Fig. 1)** with each one having its own advantages and disadvantages.
- Lower segment transverse (Kerr incision)
- Lower segment vertical (Kronig incision)
- Classical incision
- Variations of transverse incision, e.g., J-shaped incision, U-shaped or trap door incision, T-shaped incision.

Lower segment transverse (Kerr incision): It is most commonly used incision for cesarean birth. For making a lower segment transverse incision, a 2–3 cm incision is made in the center, with scalpel, till the membranes are reached. At this stage, caution is must to avoid injury to fetal parts. The incision can be extended on both sides with either sharp dissection with scissors or blunt fashion with fingers. Blunt separation is preferable when lower segment is thin and effaced, while sharp dissection is preferred when lower segment is not well formed.[9] The direction of widening the incision with fingers should be upwards to avoid angle extension.

Lower segment vertical incision: This incision is employed in preterm patients in whom lower segment is not well formed and fetus is in transverse lie.[10] More downward displacement of bladder is required than required in lower segment transverse incision. It has obvious risk of downward or upward extension into the urinary bladder or rarely vagina and into the upper segment respectively. Many trials have concluded that there is increased chance of scar rupture in this type of incision.

Classical incision: The classical upper segment vertical incision was the standard uterine incision used for cesarean delivery. In this technique, an initial incision is made with scalpel 1–2 cm above the bladder reflection. After the fetus or membranes are visualized, the incision is extended upwards with scalpel or scissors. The upward extension depends on the estimated fetal size.[10] Classical incision is associated with more intraoperative hemorrhage from the cut edges. It is associated with increased

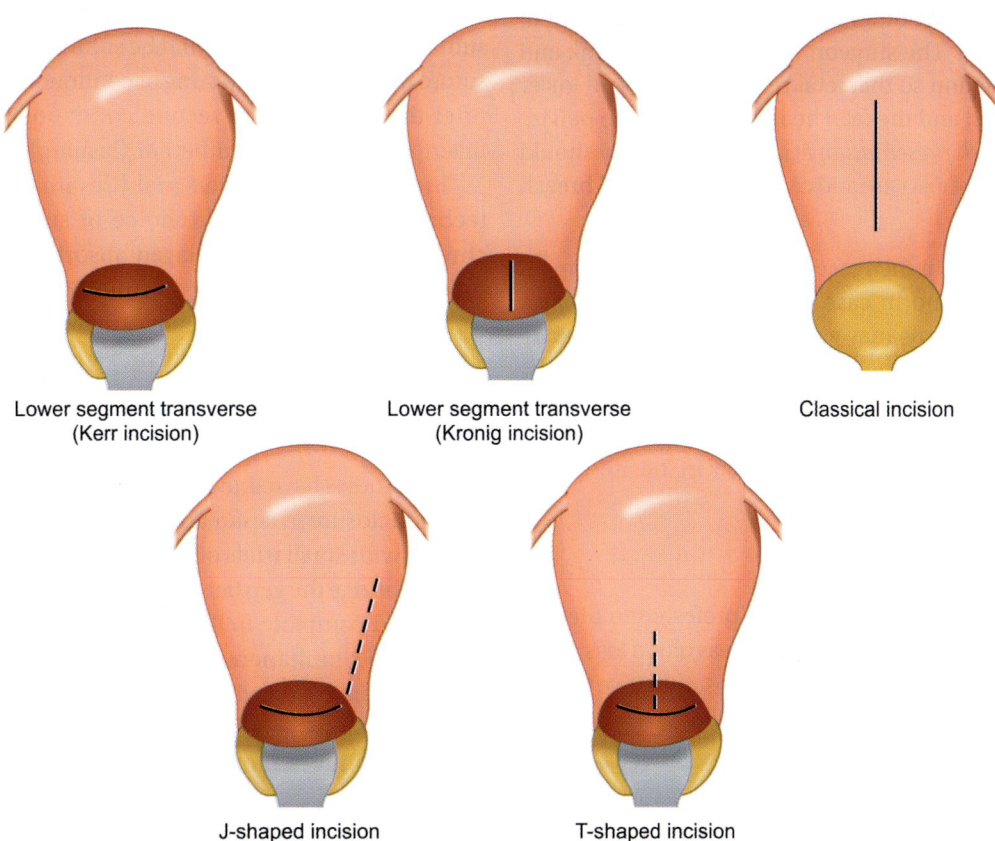

Fig. 1: Uterine incisions for cesarean delivery.

risk of infection, poor healing leading to increased risk of scar rupture in subsequent gestation. It is employed in extremely premature (28 weeks), large cervical fibroid which makes the lower segment incision difficult, in cases of severe adhesions in lower segment making it inaccessible and in anterior placenta previa.

Variations: Sometimes, as a desperate measure for baby delivery, few modifications in the uterine incisions have to be done, like J-shaped incision, U-shaped incision or trap door incision and inverted T-shaped incision.

Technique of Baby Delivery

This is the most crucial step in the surgery. Induction to delivery interval should not be more than 8 minutes and incision to delivery time should not be more than 5 minutes as it adversely affects the Apgar score and perinatal outcome.[11] The flexion of the fetal head should be maintained. Floating head can be delivered by conventional method after allowing drainage of amniotic fluid, so that the fetal head descends in the uterine incision, vacuum or forceps.[12] Deeply engaged fetal head can be disengaged by pushing up through vagina and then extracted by vertex, Patwardhan method or rarely by reverse breech extraction.

Patwardhan's maneuver needs expertise but has minimal complications if done skillfully. In Patwardhan's maneuver, if the fetal back is anterior, the fetal upper limb closer to midline is grasped and delivered out of incision and gentle traction is applied so that opposite upper limb comes near midline. The axilla is hooked and the other upper limb is delivered out of the uterine incision. The surgeon now holds fetal trunk and applies gentle traction so that fetal trunk, buttock and lower limbs are delivered and the fetal head slips out of the pelvis.

Fetuses in breech presentation at cesarean delivery should be delivered with utmost care and caution as in vaginal breech delivery.[13]

Fetus in transverse lie: In such cases, the lower uterine segment is not well formed and in case the membranes have also ruptured then the uterus may grip the baby. After adequate uterine incision is made, the fetal spine is traced to grasp the lower limb and deliver out of the incision. The rest of delivery is accomplished as a breech delivery. If the fetal upper limb come out of the incision it is reposited back in the uterus and subsequently lower limb is grasped.

Placental Delivery

Spontaneous placental delivery should preferred to manual removal of placenta as the former causes less blood loss and is associated with a decreased incidence of postoperative wound infection.[15]

Uterine Exteriorization

Uterine exteriorization at CS allows ease of suturing, manual uterine massage, observation of uterine tone and routine examination of adnexa.[16] It also allows easy performance of tubal ligation. There is slight increase incidence of nausea, vomiting, and peritoneal irritation and in some cases possibly a venous air embolism.[17] But these adverse effects are not commonly seen with improved anesthetic techniques. In situ repair in expert hands does not cause increased blood loss and is without any technical complications. It should be practiced more often.

However, as a routine, adnexa should be palpated to rule out any pathology before closure of the abdomen.

Uterine Closure

Uterine incision should be meticulously inspected for bleeding points and extension prior to suturing. Angles of uterine incision should be held with Allis forceps or Green Armytage clamps. Lateral limit of the incision must be identified. The suturing is done starting from one angle to the other in a continuous or continuous interlocking fashion. The uterine incision may be sutured in double or a single layer. Two layer closures is the conventional way of suturing. The single layer closure, introduced by Pritchard and MacDonald (1976) was also found satisfactory by many surgeons. A double layer closure is not superior to single layer closure as regards homeostasis, postoperative endometritis and requires more operating time. But single layer closure does lead to increased risk of scar dehiscence in a subsequent gestation, hence can be used only when patient is never subjected to trial of labor in subsequent pregnancy.[18] While performing a double layer suturing, the first layer should be sutured with an absorbable suture in a continuous locking or continuous running fashion. After the first layer the second continuous layer is used to invert the first layer (Lambert or Cushing).

In a large randomized trial [Cesarean section surgical techniques (CORONIS)], choice of suture material [e.g., chromic catgut versus delayed absorbable synthetic (e.g., polyglactin 910, poliglecaprone 25)] did not result in statistically significant differences in maternal outcome. Most surgeons prefer No. 1 Polyglactin for uterine suturing.[19]

Peritoneal Closure

Various studies have shown no advantage of peritoneal closure over nonclosure in cesarean section. Peritoneal wound starts healing with small islets of peritoneal cells approaching each other to bridge the gap between each other beginning in 48–72 hours and complete in 5–6 days. The process starts all over the wound simultaneously as compared to tissue healing in the epithelial tissue where it starts at margins and proceeds toward the center. Closure of peritoneum with chromic catgut introduces more suture material in the wound site, leading to more fibrosis. Also the normal peritoneal which is already traumatized by suturing, lose their ability to lyse the fibrin, leading to excessive fibrosis and adhesion formation.

Also the suturing of visceral peritoneum advances the bladder and vesicouterine fascia to lower segment. Peritoneal nonclosure is associated with less operative time, reduced need for postoperative analgesia, decreased postoperative morbidity, and quicker return of bowel cavity and associated with decreased adhesion formation.[20] But various other studies have shown controversial results. To prevent the disadvantages of closure as stated earlier, if peritoneum is sutured, only Polyglactin should be used and suturing should be loose enough so as to only approximate the peritoneal edges.

Abdominal Closure

All the structure of the abdominal wall is important and should be appropriately dealt with during closure of abdominal wall. Muscle bellies do not need to be sutured. If they are sutured, only gentle apposition is to be done, tight suturing should to be avoided. The rectus sheath is the most vital structure of abdominal wall. It should be closed with bites 1 cm apart as well 1 cm away from the incision on either side. If continuous suture is used, a cobbler knot should be taken at every few throws. Vertical incision is at best closed with monolayer suture. Chromic catgut should not be used for suturing the rectus sheath. Delayed absorbable sutures like Polyglactin should be used. The rectus sheath stiches should be placed 1 cm apart and 1 cm away from the edges. The closure of subcutaneous tissue in nonobese patients may not be done, however if depth of subcutaneous tissue is 2 cm or more it should be done. Skin closure should be done with meticulous care, so as to provide maximum cosmetic benefits to the patients. Monocryl 2-0 or Prolene 3-0 or Ethilon 2/3-0 can be used for subcuticular skin closure.

CARE OF THE BABY

- Well trained neonatologist should attend the CS
- Thermal care of newborn is essential as these babies are likely to have lower body temperature
- Early skin to skin contact between mother and baby
- Cord care
- Offer additional support to these women to start breastfeeding early.

Postoperative Care

- Use of oxytocics to prevent or control PPH—oxytocin, ergometrine, PGF2 alpha, Misoprostol 600 µg per-rectal can be used
- Patient can be started on clear liquids after resumption of bowel movements as assessed by presence of intestinal sounds on auscultation and if there is no nausea and vomiting, patient should be given soft diet
- Monitoring: Temperature, pulse, BP, RR ½ hourly for first 2 hours and hourly thereafter if these are normal. Watch for excessive bleeding per vaginum
- Nonsteroidal anti-inflammatory agents for analgesia on demand
- Remove catheter as soon as possible (after 12 hours)
- Antibiotics: Prophylactic/routine
- Early ambulation enhances circulation, encourages deep breathing and stimulates return of normal gastrointestinal function
- Hospital stay is increased after cesarean by 3–4 days. Patient is advised follow-up after 7 days for wound check.

Infection Control Policy

- Timely admission of high risk cases
- Rigorous hand washing and preoperative skin preparation
- A single IV dose of antibiotics after clamping of cord may suffice in a low risk cases (Cochrane studies)
- Foley's catheterization with aseptic precautions and early removal
- Avoid manual removal of placenta, meticulous hemostasis
- Limiting number of people in theater: Regular cleaning of theater, operation table, trolleys and swab checking
- Drills, audits and periodic evaluation are must to ensure quality and monitoring of outcomes.

REFERENCES

1. World Health Organization. Appropriate technology for birth. Lancet. 1985;2(8452):436-7.
2. Molina G, Weiser TG, Lipsitz SR, Esquivel MM, Uribe-Leitz T, Azad T, et al. Relationship between caesarean delivery rate and maternal and neonatal mortality. JAMA. 2015;314:2263-70.
3. World Health Organization. WHO Statement on Caesarean Section Rates. Geneva: World Health Organization; 2015.
4. Robson M, Murphy M, Byrne F. Quality Assurance, The 10 group classification system (Robson Classification), induction of labour and Caesarean delivery. Int J Gynaecol Obstet. 2015;131(S1):S23-7.
5. Morgan B. Unexpectedly extensive conduction blocks in obstetric epidural analgesia. Anesthesia. 1990;45:148-52.
6. Sippo WC, Burghardt A, Gomez AC. Nerve entrapment after Pfannenstiel incision. Am J Obstet Gynecol. 1987:157:420-1.
7. Maylard AE. Dircection of abdominal incisions. Br Med J. 1907;2:895.
8. Rayburn WF, SwartzWJ. Refinements in performing cesarean delivery. Gynecol Obstet Surg. 1996:51:445-51.
9. Shipp TD, Zelop CM, Repke JT, Cohen A, Caughey AB, Liberman E. Intrapartum uterine rupture and dehiscence in patients with lower uterine segment vertical and transverse inciosions. Obstet Gynecol. 1999;94;735-40.
10. Depp R. Cesarean delivery and other surgical procedures. In: Globbe SG, Niebyl JR, Simpson JL (Eds). Obstetrics: Normal and abnormal pregnancies, 4th edition. pp. 635-92. Philadelphia: Churchill Livingstone; 2002.
11. Depp R. Cesarean delivery and other surgical procedures. In Globbe SG,Niebyl JR, impson JL (Eds). Obstetrics: Normal and abnormal pregnancies, 4th edition. pp. 635-92. Philadelphia: Churchill Livingstone; 2002.

12. Datta S, Ostheimer GW, Weiss JB, Brown WU Jr, Alper MH. Neonatal effects of prolonged anesthetic induction for Cesarean section. Obstet Gynecol. 1981;58:331-5.
13. Locksmith GJ, Gei AF, Rowe TF, Yeomans ER, Hanikins GD. Teaching the Laufe-Piper forceps technique at cesarean delivery. J Reprod Med. 2002:22(4):375-8
14. Pelosi MA, Apuzzio J, Fricchone D, Gowda VV. The intrabdominal version technique for delivery of transverse lie by low-segment cesarean section. Am J Obstet Gynecol. 1979;135(8):1009-11
15. McCurdy CM Jr, Magnann EF, McCurdy CJ, Saltzman AK. The effect of placental management at cesarean delivery on operative blood loss. Am J Obstet Gynecol. 1992:167:1363-7.
16. Hershey DW, Quilligan EJ. Extra-abdominal exteriorization at cesarean section. Obstet Gynecol. 1978:52:189.
17. Lowenwrit IP, Chi DS, Handwerker SM. Nonfatal air embolism during cesarean section: a case review report and review of literature. Obstet Gynecol Surv. 1994;49:72-6.
18. DiSpiezio Sardo A, Saccone G, McCurdy R, Bujold E, Bifulco G, Berghella V. Risk of Cesarean scar defect following single- vs double-layer uterine closure: systematic review and meta-analysis of randomized controlled trials. Ultrasound Obstet Gynecol. 2017;50(5):578.
19. CORONIS Collaborative Group, Abalos E, Addo V, Brocklehurst P, El Sheikh M, Farrell B, Gray S, et al. Caesarean section surgical techniques (CORONIS): a fractional, factorial, unmasked, randomised controlled trial. Lancet. 2013;382(9888):234-48.
20. Rayburn WF, Schwartz WJ. Refinements in performing cesarean delivery. Obstet Gynecol Surv. 1996;51:445-51.

LONG QUESTIONS

1. What are the various types of uterine incisions during Cesarean section? Discuss the application of these in various surgical situations.
2. What are the difficulties that a surgeon may encounter during delivery of the fetal head? What measures can reduce or avoid such difficulties?

SHORT QUESTIONS

1. What are the most common indications for cesarean section?
2. What is cesarean delivery on maternal request?
3. What are the pros and cons of regional and general anesthesia for cesarean section?
4. Enumerate the common intraoperative and postoperative complications of cesarean section.
5. What is the role of antibiotic therapy in cesarean section? What are the principles and commonly accepted regigmens?

MULTIPLE CHOICE QUESTIONS

1. Extraperitoneal cesarean section was pioneered by:
   a. Pfannenstiel   b. Ossiander
   c. MunroKerr   d. Frank and Latzko
2. The rising rates of cesarean birth may be attributed to all of the following, except:
   a. Increasing number of multiparous women giving birth
   b. Increasing number of women with previous cesarean deliveries
   c. Medicolegal considerations
   d. Women having children at a later age
3. The advantages of general anesthesia over regional anesthesia for cesarean section are:
   a. Lower postoperative morbidity and mortality
   b. Can be used in case of coagulopathy
   c. Less postoperative pain
   d. Lower blood loss
4. The following incisions can be used to open the abdomen for cesarean section, except:
   a. McBurney incision   b. Joel Cohen incision
   c. Cherney incision   d. Midline incision
5. The following maneuvers can ease the delivery of a deeply engaged head at cesarean, except:
   a. Pushing up the baby's head from the vagina
   b. Patwardhan's maneuver
   c. Shirodkar's procedure
   d. Application of vectis
6. Awaiting spontaneous placental expulsion at cesarean section is associated with:
   a. Lesser blood loss
   b. Higher infective morbidity
   c. Pain during surgery
   d. Uterine rupture

Answers
1. d 2. a 3. b 4. a 5. c 6. a

9.9 RUPTURE UTERUS

Vidya Thobbi, Priyanka S Deshpande

INTRODUCTION

Rupture uterus is an obstetrician's nightmare come true. Though statistically rare, rupture uterus poses a high morbidity and risk of mortality to the mother and the unborn fetus. It has been quoted that from the time of diagnosis, only a couple of minutes are available before significant fetal morbidity sets in. Hence, knowledge about this obstetric catastrophe is essential for timely detection and management.

DEFINITION AND TYPES OF UTERINE RUPTURE[1]

- *Uterine dehiscence/incomplete uterine rupture:* Separation of the uterine muscle but the visceral peritoneum is intact **(Fig. 1A)**.
- *Complete uterine rupture:* Separation of all layers of the uterine wall **(Fig. 1B)**.

RISK FACTORS

The greatest risk factor for either form of rupture is prior cesarean delivery.[1]

Risk factors for uterine rupture can be classified and are described in **Table 1**.

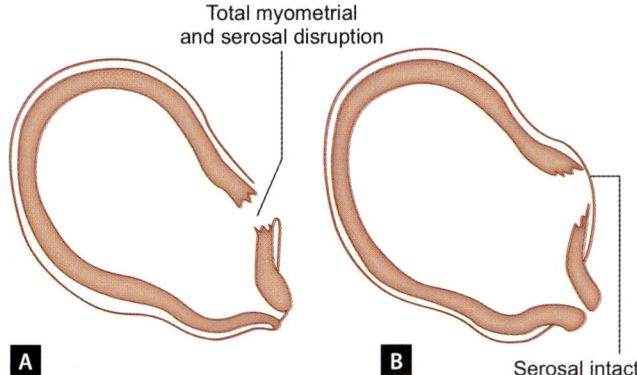

Figs. 1A and B: Uterine dehiscence and uterine rupture.

Some of the important risk factors and their salient features are as follows:

- *Previous cesarean section:* It is currently the single most important risk factor for uterine rupture **(Fig. 2)**. The risk for uterine rupture in cases of previous cesarean section depends on:
  - *Prior incision type* **(Table 2)**:[1]
  - *Prior incision closure:* The debate between single- and double-layer closure and the risk of rupture in further pregnancies continues. However, the balance tilts in favor of double layer closure to prevent future rupture. NICE guidelines on "Cesarean Section" also recommend double layer closure.[3]
  - *Number of prior cesarean sections:* Numerous studies have shown that the risk of rupture increases with number of prior cesarean sections by two-fold.
  - *Interdelivery interval:* Interdelivery interval <6 months increases the risk of rupture by 4-fold.[4]
  - *Other factors:* Factors that potentially increase the risk of uterine rupture post-date pregnancy (>41 weeks), maternal age of 40 years or more, obesity, lower prelabor Bishop score, macrosomia (> 4 kg) and decreased ultrasonographic lower segment myometrial thickness (< 2 mm).[5]
- *Previous uterine surgeries:*
  - Previous uterine surgeries that increase the risk of rupture are previous myomectomy (open/

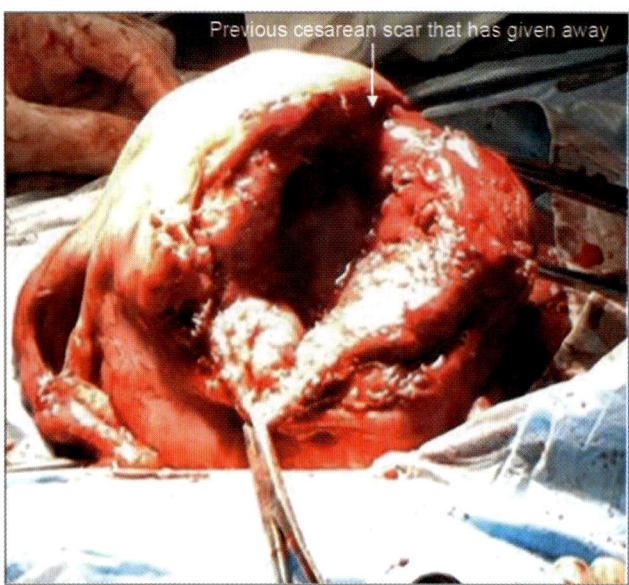

Fig. 2: Intraoperative rupture in a case of previous cesarean section.

TABLE 1: Risk factors for uterine rupture.[2]

Antenatal	Intrapartum	Postpartum
• Previous classical CS • Previous myomectomy • Placenta accreta • Mullerian anomalies • Motor vehicle accidents • Hysteroscopic metroplasty • Difficult curettage for miscarriage • Previous hysterotomy • Ehlers-Danlos syndrome • Chronic steroid use • Use of cocaine • Injury by animal hits • Domestic violence	• Previous cesarean section • Previous myomectomy • Grand multiparity • Malpresentation: Unrecognized brow, face and shoulder presentation • Obstructed labor and unrecognized cephalopelvic disproportion • Prostaglandin and oxytocin use • Instrumental delivery • Assisted breech deliveries • Tumors obstructing birth canal • Pelvic deformity	• Precipitate labor • Manual removal of placenta • Uterine manipulation (intrauterine balloon)

(CS: cesarean section)

TABLE 2: Effect of prior incision type on risk of uterine rupture.

Prior incision	Estimated risk of rupture (%)
Classical	2–9
T-shaped	4–9
Low vertical	1–7
One low transverse	0.2–0.9
Multiple low transverse	0.9–1.8

laparoscopic), hysteroscopic metroplasty for uterine anomalies, previous difficult curettages, multiple previous curettages and previous hysterotomy.

- Patients with previous history of myomectomy need to be evaluated and counseled very thoroughly. Trial of labor after myomectomy is associated with a 0.47% risk of uterine rupture. Uterine rupture after prior myomectomy occurred mainly before 36 weeks and before labor.[6] Uterine rupture after myomectomy is not related to the surgical technique (laparotomy or laparoscopy), myoma size or location.
- Uterine ruptures during pregnancy after hysteroscopic septoplasty are very rare (0.02%). Septoplasty by monopolar electrocautery has higher risk than endoscopic resection by scissors. The damage to the vascular supply from electrosurgery may cause weakness in the myometrium. Intraoperative uterine rupture during septoplasty is also considered a risk factor for uterine rupture during pregnancy.[7,8]
- Other factors that can predispose to uterine rupture are history of previous curettages and history of manual removal of placenta. There is weakening of the myometrium in these procedures and hence the risk of future uterine rupture.

- *Intrapartum factors:* It is very rare to have a uterine rupture, whether in scarred or unscarred uterus before the onset of labor. *More than 90% of the ruptures occur during labor (maximum at 4–5 cm cervical dilatation), with around 18% occurring in the second stage of labor and 8% being identified post vaginal delivery.*[5]

Thus, intrapartum factors play a very important role in the etiology of rupture uterus.

- *Risk of rupture in spontaneous labor versus induced labor:* Spontaneous labor in cases of previous cesarean sections carries a 0.5% risk of uterine rupture. There is a two- to three-fold increased risk of uterine rupture in induced and/or augmented labor compared with spontaneous vaginal birth after cesarean section (VBAC) labor.
- *Use of drugs:* Use of oxytocin and prostaglandins are associated with increased risk of uterine rupture in both scarred and unscarred uterus. Higher dose oxytocin (exceeding 20 milliunits/minute) during VBAC augmentation increases the risk of uterine rupture by around four-fold or greater. Risk of rupture with oxytocin increases with dose and duration of labor. All the inducing agents increase the risk of uterine rupture including mechanical methods (Foley's catheter), oxytocin and use of prostaglandins (PGE2 and PGE1). According to the latest American College of Obstetricians and Gynecologists (ACOG), some studies state that PGE2 is safe in cases of previous cesarean section. However, the use of PGE1 (misoprostol) is contraindicated in a term uterus with a scar.[10] Drugs such as misoprostol are also commonly used for second trimester abortions. While they are safe in unscarred uteruses, there is a reported increased risk of rupture by almost 10-fold in cases of scarred uterus.[9] However, ACOG recommends that misoprostol can be considered for second trimester abortions.
- *Risk associated with operative vaginal delivery:* Instrumental delivers increase the risk of uterine rupture, especially the injudicious use of Kielland's forceps.[2,5]
- *Obstructed labor and unrecognized cephalopelvic disproportion,* unrecognized brow, face and shoulder presentations remain very important causes of rupture of uterus in developing countries and in women with unscarred uterus.
- *Uterine manipulation maneuvers:* Both external cephalic version and internal podalic version have been reported to increase the risk of uterine rupture. Also, maneuvers for assisted breech delivery increase chances of rupture.

- Other important causes
  - *Congenital uterine malformations:* For pregnancies that implant in a rudimentary horn of a uterus, a particularly high risk of uterine rupture is associated with the induction of labor. 80% of ruptures involving these types of rudimentary horn pregnancies occurred before the third trimester, with 67% occurring during the second trimester. Although the uterine rupture rate for unscarred anomalous uteri during pregnancy is increased relative to that for normal uteri, the precise increase in risk associated with the different types of uterine malformations remains uncertain. The walls of the abnormal uteri tend to become abnormally thin as pregnancies advance, and the thickness can be inconsistent over different aspects of the myometrium (uterine musculature).
  - *Grand multiparity:* Grand multiparas are increased risk of fetal malposition and malpresentations and fetal macrosomia. Along with this, injudicious augmentation of labor with oxytocin increases the chance of rupture in these cases.

DIAGNOSIS

Signs and Symptoms

Abnormal cardiotocography (CTG) is the most consistent finding in uterine rupture and is present in 66–76% of these events.

- The classic triad of a complete uterine rupture (pain, vaginal bleeding, and fetal heart rate abnormalities) may present in less than 10% of cases.
- Around 48% of scar dehiscence is asymptomatic.[5]

The clinical features associated with uterine scar rupture include:[5]
- Abnormal CTG
- Severe abdominal pain, especially if persisting between contractions
- Acute onset scar tenderness
- Abnormal vaginal bleeding
- Hematuria
- Cessation of previously efficient uterine activity
- Maternal tachycardia, hypotension, fainting or shock
- Loss of station of the presenting part
- Change in abdominal contour and inability to pick up fetal heart rate at the old transducer site.

Role of Cardiotocography

- Prolonged, late, or recurrent variable decelerations or fetal bradycardias are often the first and only signs of uterine rupture.
- Most of the studies have reported rates of around 80% or more as first signs of rupture uterus.
- Prolonged decelerations and fetal bradycardias are the most commonly reported fetal heart rate abnormalities.
- Thus, continuous CTG monitoring is recommended in all cases of TOLAC (trial of labor after cesarean section).[10]

Role of Radiology

- It has been suggested that measurement of lower uterine segment (LUS) thickness antenatally in women with a previous cesarean delivery could be used to predict the occurrence of a uterine defect in women undergoing VBAC.
- According to the study, a myometrial thickness (the minimum thickness overlying the amniotic cavity at the level of the uterine scar) cut-off of >2 mm provided a strong negative predictive value for the occurrence of a uterine defect during VBAC.[5]

MANAGEMENT (FLOWCHART 1)

Uterine Rupture is an Obstetric Emergency

Team approach is needed for appropriate and timely management of cases of uterine rupture. The following members of the team must be summoned immediately as resuscitation and mobilization of the patient for proper surgical management continues.
- Senior obstetric consultant
- Senior anesthesia consultant
- Neonatologist
- Senior staff nurse
- Blood bank staff for blood and blood products as needed.
The main aspects of treatment in the case of uterine rupture are:
- Timely diagnosis

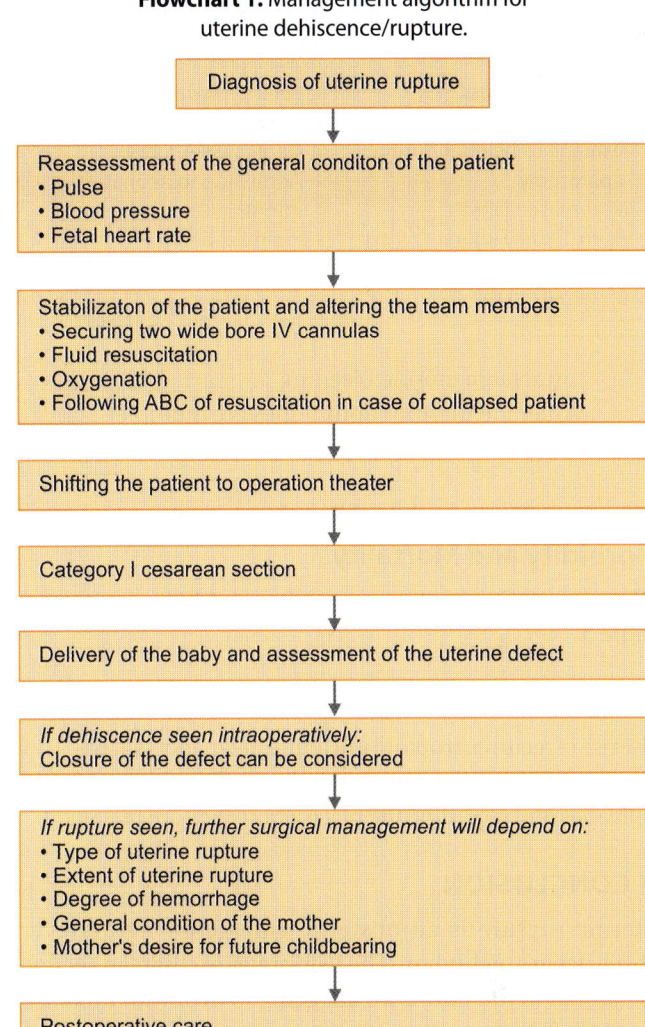

Flowchart 1: Management algorithm for uterine dehiscence/rupture.

- Minimizing the time from the onset of signs and symptoms until the start of definitive surgical treatment.

Numerous studies have shown that the time available for successful intervention after frank uterine rupture is only a couple of minutes. Thus, Category I cesarean section needs to the done as soon as possible after the diagnosis for favorable outcomes of the mother and the baby.

Surgical Management

- Conservative surgical management involving uterine repair should be reserved for women who:
    - Want future childbearing
    - Low transverse uterine rupture
    - No extension of the tear to the broad ligament, cervix, or parametrium
    - Uterine hemorrhage controlled easily
    - Stable general condition
    - No clinical or laboratory evidence of an evolving coagulopathy.
- Hysterectomy should be considered the treatment of choice when

TABLE 3: Effects of uterine rupture on mother and baby.

Effects on mother	Effects on baby
• Severe blood loss • Need for blood transfusion • Damage to bladder during laparotomy • Maternal collapse • Acute kidney injury • Need for intensive care unit • Maternal death	• Fetal hypoxia or anoxia • Acidosis • Depressed Apgars • Admission to neonatal intensive care unit • Perinatal death

- Intractable uterine bleeding
- When the uterine rupture sites are multiple
- Longitudinal or low-lying rupture.

Effect on Maternal and Fetal Morbidity and Mortality

Effects of uterine rupture on mother and baby are given in **Table 3**.

Effect on Future Pregnancies

The risk of recurrent rupture in a future pregnancy is 5–6%. Thus, this should always be kept in mind regarding mode of further deliveries and regarding the place where they are managed.

CONCLUSION

Uterine rupture is an obstetric emergency and is every obstetrician's nightmare. The rising rates of cesarean sections mean that in the future we are going to deal with increased number of pregnancies with a scarred uterus.

In patients with risk factors for uterine rupture, always maintain a high level of suspicion regarding the diagnosis as the time frame for a successful intervention is very small.

When in doubt the response has to be quick and definitive for food maternal and fetal outcome.

KEY MESSAGES

- The probability of uterine rupture must always be kept in mind in laboring patients with risk factors for a rupture.
- Previous cesarean section is the most important risk factor for rupture of uterus.
- Patients willing to undergo a TOLAC should be counseled properly and delivered at a center where emergency facilities are available.
- Continuous CTG monitoring of patients for TOLAC is necessary for early diagnosis of uterine rupture.
- Fetal bradycardia and decelerations are the first sings on CTG for a suspected rupture.
- Clinical signs and symptoms of rupture uterus must always be kept in mind during labor in cases at high risk for rupture.
- Drugs for induction and augmentation of labor should be used judiciously in cases at high risk for rupture.
- The definitive management of uterine rupture is a category I cesarean section.
- Maternal resuscitation is important along with definitive surgical intervention.
- Early diagnosis and quick management are the key factors for a good outcome.

REFERENCES

1. Cunningham FG, Levono KJ, Bloom SL, Spong CY, Dashe JS, Hoffman BL, et al. Prior caesarean delivery. Williams Obstetrics, 24th edition. New York: McGraw Hill; 2014. pp. 609-19.
2. Manoharan M, Wuntakal R, Erskine K. Uterine rupture: a revisit. Obstet Gynaecol. 2010;12:223-30.
3. National Institute for Health and Care Excellence. Caesarean section [Clinical guideline (CG132)]. London: NICE; 2011 (updated 2019).
4. Esposito MA, Menihan CA, Malee MP. Association of interpregnancy interval with uterine scar failure in labor: a case-control study. Am J Obstet Gynecol. 2000;183(5):1180-3.
5. Royal College of Obstetricians and Gynaecologists (RCOG). Birth after Previous Caesarean Birth. Green-top Guideline No. 45. London: RCOG; 2015.
6. Kim HS, Oh SY, Choi SJ. Uterine rupture in pregnancies following myomectomy: a multicenter case series. Obstet Gynecol Sci. 2016;59(6):454-62.
7. Dural O, Yasa C, Bastu E, Ugurlucan FG, Can S, Yilmaz C, et al. Reproductive outcomes of hysteroscopic septoplasty techniques. JSLS. 2015;19(4):e2015.00085.
8. Nouri K, Ott J, Huber JC, Fischer EM, Stögbauer L, Tempfer CB. Reproductive outcome after hysteroscopic septoplasty in patients with septate uterus—a retrospective cohort study and systematic review of the literature. Reprod Biol Endocrinol. 2010;8:52.
9. Daniel Seow Choon K, Eek Chaw T, Hester Chang QL, Mor Jack N, Wan Shi T, Kok Hian T. Incidence and contributing factors for uterine rupture in patients undergoing second trimester termination of pregnancy in a large tertiary hospital - a 10-year case series. Eur J Obstet Gynecol. 2018:227:8-12.
10. American College of Obstetricians and Gynecologists. ACOG Practice Bulletin No. 205. Obstet Gynecol. 2019;133:e110-27.

LONG QUESTIONS

1. A G5P4L2NND1IUFD1 has come in labor at progresses rapidly to 9 cm. She is at 9 cm, with cervix 90% effaced since 1.5 hours. She is getting contractions of 3-4/10/30-35. Suddenly the fetal heart drops to 90 bpm and the patient starts getting tachycardia and tachypnea.
   Mention the differential diagnosis and management of this patient.
2. Describe the risk factors and management of rupture uterus.

3. Prepare a management plan for the care of a women with history of two myomectomies and one curettage for infertility with regards to:
   a. Antenatal counseling
   b. History taking
   c. Antenatal investigations
   d. Intrapartum management
   e. Management of complications if any
   f. Postpartum advice

SHORT QUESTIONS

1. Enumerate the risk factors for rupture of uterus.
2. Mention the signs and symptoms of rupture of uterus.
3. What are the pre-requisites for a safe TOLAC?

MULTIPLE CHOICE QUESTIONS

1. The most important risk factor for rupture uterus is:
   a. History of curettage
   b. History of myomectomy
   c. History of previous cesarean section
   d. Congenital uterine malformation
2. In the following image, the parameter that is measurement has a safe cutoff for TOLAC as:

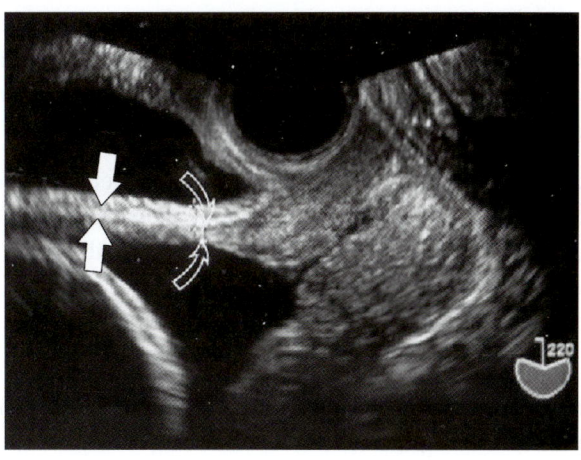

   a. 5 mm
   b. 5–7 mm
   c. 2–3.5 mm
   d. <1 mm
3. The risk of rupture in a case of previous one cesarean section is:
   a. 1/500
   b. 1/100
   c. 1/1,000
   d. 1/200

Answers
1. c   2. c   3. d

9.10 OBSTETRIC ANALGESIA AND ANESTHESIA

Siddesh Iyer, Shanthakumari S, M Krishna Kumari

INTRODUCTION

Obstetrics has evolved over the years and safety has increased greatly from the days of ether and chloroform, to modern day anesthesia with improved techniques, technology and medication.

LABOR ANALGESIA

Childbirth is physiological and yet it may probably be one of the most painful experiences a woman has ever faced. A number of factors influence the degree of pain. Her gravid status, complex psychosocial factors such as fear and anxiety, prior experience of labor pain, cultural beliefs, ethnicity, emotional support, antenatal check-ups and educational attainment are a few of them.[1] Pain previously considered a part of the process of pregnancy and delivery, however in modern day obstetrics, is not a necessary feature of childbirth.

Pain can be either visceral or somatic and originates from various sites during labor and childbirth. In the first stage of labor, the spinal nerves of T10–L1 transmit the pain that results from uterine contractions and dilatation of the cervix. The stretching of the pelvic ligaments causes pain via the pudendal nerve. This originates from the S2–S4 nerve roots in the second stage of labor.[2,3]

The experience and tolerance to pain is very individualized and it is difficult to quantify the intensity of pain and the need for analgesia.

Informed consent of the different methods and associated risks are essential.

There are different pain management strategies for women in labor, which include non-pharmacological, pharmacological and regional analgesia.

Non-pharmacological Methods

Early or mild pain can be managed by adjuvant or non-pharmacological ways. They are inexpensive, easy to institute and low risk; however, there is not very good quality evidence supporting their effectiveness in reducing moderate to severe labor pain.

Continuous one-to-one support in labor and the care provider: The attitude and behavior of the woman's caregiver is probably the single most important factor in a woman's perception of pain during labor and childbirth.[4-6] A designated midwife in labor is associated with a lower analgesic requirement, lower rates of dissatisfaction with childbirth and reduced instrumental delivery.[7] Women in labor can be taken care of by a companion (or "doula") to provide nonmedical care.

Prenatal counseling and information: Good prenatal counseling about the likely labor experience including analgesic options has been shown to reduce pain levels during labor.[8,9]

Music and aroma therapy: Music reduces anxiety levels and distracts the pain[10] during labor.[11] Application of essential oils to the skin or inhalation of the scents is aromatherapy with essential oils which is said to increase the production of the body's sedative, stimulant and relaxing neurotransmitters.[11-15]

Birthing balls and postures: A birthing ball is an air-filled rubber ball (roughly 60 cm in diameter), on which a woman can sit on during labor, thereby assisting her to adopt an upright position, and also allowing a rocking movement during labor thereby reducing her pain sensation.[16-18]

Breathing/relaxation techniques and massage: "Respiratory autogenic training" means progressive muscle relaxation and focused slow breathing and "traditional psychoprophylactic course" which is an alternative form of relaxation training, are two relaxation techniques used in labor. Breathing exercises and relaxation techniques help reduce labor pain with no adverse effects on maternal or neonatal outcomes.[13]

Acupuncture and acupressure: Acupuncture[16,19] and acupressure involve the insertion of fine needles or application of pressure to specific areas of the body that work through the stimulation of touch fibers. These block pain impulses at the "pain gates"[20-22] within the spinal cord and the modification of endorphin release, which alters pain perception.[2]

Transcutaneous electrical nerve stimulation: Transcutaneous electrical nerve stimulation (TENS)[20] involves the application of low-voltage electrical impulses to the lower back at the vertebral levels T10 to S2. This is where nerve pathways from the uterus, vagina and perineum enter the spinal cord and this works by stimulating the body to produce endorphins.

Sterile water injections: It is believed that sterile water injected subcutaneously into the area of the lumbosacral spine inhibits the transmission of pain by stimulating large afferent nerve fibres.[21] About 4–6 injections of water (0.1 mL) can be administered over the painful area and the therapy can be repeated with minimal adverse effects.[22,23]

Warm water immersion: Warm water immersion causes physiological increase in uterine perfusion, which may promote endorphin and oxytocin release. The temperature of the pool should be checked hourly to ensure the woman is comfortable and not becoming pyrexial. The water temperature should also not exceed 37.5°C. It can be used during any stage of labor and for any duration of time.[24]

Hypnobirthing: During labor, hypnosis (or "hypnobirthing") is a method that can be used to focus attention on calm and comforting influences, increase a woman's receptivity to positive "suggestions" and reduce the awareness of external stimuli. It not only helps to relieve pain but also helps to enhance feelings of relaxation, safety and control.[25] It is said to affect the anterior cingulate gyrus of the limbic system and can suppress the neural activity between the sensory cortex and the amygdala–limbic system. It can be delivered either by a practitioner-led method or by self-hypnosis with audio instruction.

Biofeedback: It is a form of behavioral therapy that aims at training women in labor to recognize various body signals such as changes in heart rate, muscle tension or temperature and to change their body responses with the aid of electronic instruments.[26,27]

Pharmacological Methods

There are not too many pharmacological options because they have dose-dependent maternal and fetal adverse effects and would likely require large cumulative doses if used in labor. Pharmacological options can be classified by their route of administration and can be further subdivided into opioid and nonopioid options.

Nitrous oxide (gas and air): Entonox (gas and air) is a mixture of inhaled nitrous oxide and oxygen in a fixed 1:1 ratio. It has been available since 1962. At high concentrations, it acts as a very weak anesthetic and as an analgesic and anxiolytic at lower concentrations. It suppresses activity within the reticuloendothelial system. It increases the release of endogenous endorphins, corticotrophins and dopamine which activate descending pain pathways.[28] Entonox can be self-administered, has a short half-life of 2–3 minutes and is cleared rapidly via the lungs. It does not interfere with endogenous oxytocin and does not affect the labor process or spontaneous vaginal birth rate. It crosses the placenta readily, but does not affect the fetal heart rate or respiratory rate in the newborn.[29] Side effects include light-headedness, nausea, vomiting and hallucinations, hyperventilation and tetany are also seen but less commonly.

Nonopioid analgesics: Paracetamol, nonsteroidal anti-inflammatory drugs (NSAIDs), sedatives and antispasmodics are the nonopioid analgesics available. Paracetamol is a cyclo-oxygenase-2 inhibitor that reduces the inflammatory response and pain by blocking the production of prostaglandins.[30-32]

Opioids: Dihydrocodeine, pethidine, diamorphine, fentanyl and remifentanil are the opioids available. Pethidine is the most commonly used opioid worldwide for labor analgesia. Opioid receptors are mainly located in the periaqueductal gray area of the brain and spinal cord, whose activation leads to a reduction in neuronal cell excitability and transmission of nociceptive impulses.[33,34] Adverse effects include drowsiness, hypoventilation, urine retention, nausea/vomiting and a risk of aspiration due to increase in gastrointestinal transit time

A neonate may take as long as 6 days to eliminate pethidine from its system. Respiratory depression, hypothermia, poor feeding, altered crying and decreased alertness are the recognized adverse effects.[35-38] Naloxone is the antagonist of choice if the neonate develops respiratory depression.

Women given diamorphine were also more likely to be satisfied with their analgesia than pethidine.

Patient-controlled Analgesia

Delivery of drugs through a preprogramed pump is called patient-controlled analgesia (PCA) and it offers an alternative to regional anesthesia where patient self-administers boluses of the drug. The only one widely used for labor pain is remifentanil.

Remifentanil PCA: Remifentanil is a rapidly acting synthetic opioid, which is rapidly metabolized by tissue esterases. It has a half-life of 3 minutes.[39,40]

It takes just 5 minutes to work and provides on demand pain relief. It requires an intravenous (IV) access attached to a PCA pump. It is used for those in established labor and continuous fetal monitoring is not required. It cannot be used if morphine or pethidine have been used in the past 4 hours.

Respiratory depression is reported in up to one-third of patients and 5% encounter oxygen saturations below 90%.[41-43]

Hence, continuous oxygen saturation monitoring is mandatory during its use. Other common adverse effects include maternal pruritus, nausea and vomiting. Potential tolerance may occur after just 60 minutes of use, resulting in a reduction in efficacy.[44] A bolus dose of the drug has a peak effect 1–3 minutes after administration, and this often results in suboptimal analgesia for contraction pain because it is used either too early or late. Also the effect on respiration is also delayed by some 2–4 minutes from administration and so respiratory depression can sometimes be missed.[45] A bolus dose of remifentanil of 0.15–1 µg/kg with a 2-minute lock out and a background infusion of 0.025–0.05 µg/kg/minute is an acceptable dose.[46,47] A maximum bolus dose of no more than 0.7 µg/kg remifentanil is recommended.

Relative contraindications to remifentanil PCA include morbid obesity, clinical features of a chest infection and primigravida who are at risk of prolonged labor.[48]

Regional Analgesia[5]

It is still the gold standard for pain relief in labor and includes epidural, combined spinal–epidural and spinal analgesia. Epidural anesthesia involves the use of local anesthetics with or without an opioid. The drug is injected into the epidural space by a fine plastic tube into the epidural space L4–L5 or L5–S1 and produces a reversible loss of sensation and motor function. Local anesthetics block sodium channels in nerve cell membranes, thereby preventing the propagation of nerve impulses.[49-51]

It takes 20 minutes to set up and 20 minutes to work. It provides most complete pain relief of all. It, however, needs continuous blood pressure and fetal monitoring and it is easy to provide a top up in case a cesarean section is required.

Failure to work, pruritus, headache, severe hypotension, nerve damage and meningitis are the side effects.

The lower concentration of local anesthetic solutions combined with a variety of opiates (such as 0.0625–0.1% bupivacaine and 2 µg/mL fentanyl) has vastly reduced the adverse effects of epidural anesthesia in labor and has improved maternal satisfaction.

Noteworthy improvements include the retention of more motor function and even the ability to walk during labor (known as a "mobile epidural"), better ability to bear down and a reduction in hypotension and its accompanied adverse effects.

Maintenance regimens containing a low concentration of local anesthetic with opioid solutions, are administered by one of three methods:
1. Intermittent top-ups
2. Patient-controlled epidural pump (PCEA)
3. Continuous infusion with or without PCEA

The use of the PCEA allows the woman to administer self top ups and be in control of her pain. PCEA pumps are preprogramed with a set dose and lock out time (usually 30 minutes). This avoids high blocks and toxicity. The use of PCEA is associated with lower pain scores, less motor block and better maternal satisfaction.

Epidural analgesia is associated with a prolonged second stage of labor and increased instrumental delivery rates.[52] There is no association with a prolonged first stage of labor, increased risk of cesarean section or long-term back problems, for which epidurals have been commonly blamed.

Combined Spinal and Epidural

Combined spinal–epidural (CSE) involves a single injection of local anesthetic and/or opioid into the subarachnoid space (spinal). An epidural catheter is inserted and used as per usual once the effects of the spinal analgesia wear off. CSE provides rapid onset of pain relief as compared with conventional epidural and it can be useful in women with very severe labor pain. The hole in the dura from a CSE results in spread of epidural local anesthetic into the subarachnoid space and the epidural space, increasing the effectiveness of analgesia.[53-55]

A disadvantage of CSE is that it is difficult to ascertain whether the epidural is working immediately because of the initial effects of the spinal injection. CSE has now replaced epidural anesthesia as the primary form of regional analgesia offered to laboring women in many institutions worldwide.

A special mention about epidural in obese parturients—the American Congress of Obstetricians and Gynecologists, recommends an early insertion of epidural anesthesia in obese mothers to alleviate or prevent issues[56] such as multiple attempts at insertion, longer epidural needles as well as higher rates of dural puncture and epidural migration into the fatty subcutaneous tissue.[57] Ultrasound guidance (both real-time and pre puncture) can be used to facilitate catheterization of the epidural space to overcome such difficulties.[58]

Recommendations for regional analgesia:
- To secure IV access prior to commencing regional analgesia
- Routine preloading and maintenance fluid to not be administered
- Blood pressure to be checked every 5 minutes for 15 minutes during establishment or after further boluses
- A review, by anesthetist after 30 minutes if woman is not pain-free
- Sensory block to be checked hourly
- Continuous electronic fetal monitoring for 30 minutes during establishment or after boluses of 10 mL or more.

As per the American College of Obstetricians and Gynecologists, "Maternal request is a sufficient indication for analgesia during labor" provided there are no contraindications. However, the decision to offer regional anesthesia should be individualized where vaginal delivery is imminent, to avoid the potential risks of regional anesthesia. This decision will depend on the woman's parity, the fetal condition on cardiotocograph and on whether a prolonged or difficult second stage is anticipated.[59]

Other than labor, there is a wide scope of anesthesia in obstetrics:
- *Local anesthesia during episiotomy:* Episiotomy is the most frequent procedure in obstetrics done to increase the introitus to enhance safe vaginal delivery.[60] Lignocaine is the most commonly used anesthetic agent for local infiltration. Ropivacaine has been shown to be superior to lignocaine for various reasons. The accidental overdose of local anesthetics may be fatal. Intravenous lipid emulsions can be used as a rescue in local anesthetic-cardiotoxicity, and anesthetic organizations over the globe, have developed guidelines on the use of this drug.[61]
- *Pudendal block:* Operative delivery is associated with a lot of pain and so efficient anesthesia is prudent. Local anesthesia by pudendal block is a safe and easy way to provide pain relief. With epidural anesthesia, forceps can be directly applied. However, where epidural is not used, this pudendal block is a boon to obstetricians.
  Technique: 20 mL 1% lidocaine is drawn into a syringe. A special needle where the point is guarded is used. The depth of penetration is limited to 1 cm (where the pudendal nerve is located) and helps avoid needle stick injuries.
  When performing a left-sided block, the ischial spine is palpated with the index or middle finger of the left hand and vice-versa for a right-sided block. The syringe is held with the other hand and then the guarded needle is guided between the index and middle fingers.
  There are two accepted methods for performing a paravaginal pudendal block.
  a. The index finger is positioned on the ischial spine and the needle guard is run between the index and middle fingers. The needle guard is placed 1 cm posterior and medial to the ischial spine. The guard can then be unhooked and the needle advanced a centimeter into the tissue.
  b. The middle finger is positioned on the ischial spine and needle guard is run in between the index and middle fingers. The end of the needle guard is placed 1 cm anterior and medial to the ischial spine. The guard can then be unhooked and then the needle advanced a centimeter into the tissue.

  As large pudendal vessels lie in close proximity to the nerve, it is very important to aspirate the syringe (to check that the tip of the needle is not in a vessel) prior to injecting local anesthetic. After aspiration, up to 7 mL of lidocaine 1% can be injected.
  The block can be repeated on the other side. The remaining 6 mL of lidocaine should be used to infiltrate the perineum.[62]
- Spinal/Regional/Saddle anesthesia for cesarean sections: More than 95% of elective cesarean deliveries and more than 85% of emergency cesarean deliveries should be performed using regional anesthetic technique, as proposed by The Royal College of Anaesthetists in the United Kingdom.[63]

Apart from these, cerclages, hysterotomies and many procedures can be done under regional anesthesia.

The advantages of regional anesthesia include avoiding the problem of a difficult airway, avoidance of multiple drugs required for general anesthesia and also letting the parturient be awake to witness the delivery of her baby thereby enabling her to participate and enjoy the birthing experience.

Common and minor complications include:
- Nausea and vomiting
- Mild hypotension
- Bradycardia
- Urinary retention
- Postdural puncture headache or postspinal headache
- Most of these minor complications can be managed with adequate fluids and hydration.

The following are some major complications:
- Severe hypotension, total spinal anesthesia
- Cardiac arrest
- Nerve injuries: Cauda equina syndrome, radiculopathy
- Spinal epidural hematoma, with or without subsequent neurological sequelae due to compression of the spinal nerves

- Epidural abscess
- Infection (e.g., meningitis).

High spinal and total spinal anesthesia can be a disaster at cesarean and quick identification and resuscitation is the key to patient safety.

- *General anesthesia:* The indications for general anesthesia are medical termination of pregnancy, os tightening, cesarean sections with failed regional anesthesia, maternal request and conditions where regional anesthesia is contraindicated. These include coagulopathy, life-threatening fetal compromise when there might not be adequate time to perform a regional technique.

  It is the method of choice for manual removal of placenta and internal podalic version, where halothane is the preferred agent to relax the uterus to allow digital manipulation.

Challenges with general anesthesia: Anatomical and physiological changes during pregnancy make airway problems more common in pregnancy than in the general population. These include upper airway edema, breast enlargement and excessive weight gain. There is an association between difficult intubation and a short neck, obesity, receding mandible and protruding maxillary incisors as per a study. A well thought-out difficult obstetric airway algorithm with availability of airway adjuncts to deal with airway emergencies during difficult or failed intubation is therefore mandatory.

Aspiration pneumonitis is one of the concerns of general anesthesia in obstetric patients. Risk factors include a prolonged gastric emptying time in labor, increased intra-abdominal pressure due to the gravid uterus and relaxation of the lower esophageal sphincter due to hormonal changes. Prophylaxis against acid aspiration is therefore administered prior to anesthesia. The use of rapid sequence induction with thiopental/propofol/succinylcholine helps to decrease the incidence of pulmonary aspiration. Maintenance is usually with nitrous oxide or sevoflurane.

One must remember that general anesthesia, although is the mode of choice in severe preeclampsia, heart disease, etc., general anesthetics do cause uterine relaxation and adequate preparedness with uterotonics must be available.

When faced with maternal hemorrhage, sustained fetal bradycardia or severe thrombocytopenia general anesthesia might be the only feasible option. Whenever general anesthesia is warranted, an anesthetist must take precautions to avoid swings in blood pressure, especially during laryngoscopy and airway manipulation. A difficult airway should be anticipated and difficult airway equipment must be handy thus making it vital for the obstetric anesthetist to be very familiar with failed intubation drills.

Post-cesarean Analgesia

Postoperative pain may increase the incidence of thromboembolism, postpartum depression, post-traumatic stress disorder and chronic pelvic pain. Good postoperative analgesia with neuraxial opioids helps the mother to better care for the neonate and be more mobile. Intravenous opioids or multimodal analgesia that minimizes individual drug effects are alternatives.

The science of obstetric analgesia and anesthesia continues to evolve with the primary focus being patient centric care with the best maternal and neonatal outcomes.

REFERENCES

1. Lowe NK. Self-efficacy for labor and childbirth fears in nulliparous pregnant women. J Psychosom Obstet Gynaecol. 2000;21:219-24.
2. Jones L, Othman M, Dowswell T, Alfirevic Z, Gates S, Newburn M, et al. Pain management for women in labour: an overview of systematic reviews. Cochrane Database Syst Rev. 2012;(3):CD009234.
3. Association of Anaesthetists of Great Britain and Ireland, Obstetric Anaesthetists' Association. OAA/AAGBI Guidelines for Obstetric Anaesthetic Services 2013. London: AAGBI; 2013.
4. National Institute for Health and Care Excellence. Intrapartum Care: Care of Healthy Women and Their Babies during Childbirth. NICE clinical guideline 190. London: NICE; 2014.
5. Niven CA, Murphy-Black T. Memory for labor pain: a review of the literature. Birth 2000;27:244-53.
6. Rooks JP. Labor pain management other than neuraxial: what do we know and where do we go next? Birth. 2012;39:318-22.
7. Hodnett ED, Gates S, Hofmeyr GJ, Sakala C, Weston J. Continuous support for women during childbirth. Cochrane Database Syst Rev. 2011;(2):CD003766.
8. Melzack R, Taenzer P, Feldman P, Kinch RA. Labour is still painful after prepared childbirth training. Can Med Assoc J. 1981;125:357-63.
9. LabourPain. Obstetric Anaesthetists' Association. Pain relief in labour. [online] Available from: http://www.labour pains.com/ui/content/content.aspx?id=45. [Last Accessed November, 2021].
10. Vickers A. Complementary medicine or antagonistic medicine? Complement Ther Med. 1999;7:125.
11. Pelletier CL. The effect of music on decreasing arousal due to stress: a metaanalysis. J Music Ther. 2004;41:192-214.
12. Allaire AD, Moos MK, Wells SR. Complementary and alternative medicine in pregnancy: a survey of North Carolina certified nurse-midwives. Obstet Gynecol. 2000;95:19-23.
13. Stevenson C. Complementary medicine. All things considered. Nurs Times. 1995;91:44-5.
14. Smith CA, Collins CT, Crowther CA. Aromatherapy for pain management in labour. Cochrane Database Syst Rev. 2011;(7):CD009215.
15. Kaviani M, Azima S, Alavi N, Tabaei MH. The effect of lavender aromatherapy on pain perception and intrapartum outcome in primiparous women. Br J Midwifery. 2014;22:125-8.
16. Cho SH, Lee H, Ernst E. Acupuncture for pain relief in labour: a systematic review and meta-analysis. BJOG. 2010;117:907-20.
17. Gau ML, Chang CY, Tian SH, Lin KC. Effects of birth ball exercise on pain and self-efficacy during childbirth: a randomised controlled trial in Taiwan. Midwifery. 2011;27:e293-300.
18. Lawrence A, Lewis L, Hofmeyr GJ, Styles C. Maternal positions and mobility during first stage labour. Cochrane Database Syst Rev. 2013;(10): CD003934.

19. Gupta JK, Hofmeyr GJ, Shehmar M. Position in the second stage of labour for women without epidural anesthesia. Cochrane Database Sys Rev. 2012;(5):CD002006.
20. Dowswell T, Bedwell C, Lavender T, Neilson JP. Transcutaneous electrical nerve stimulation (TENS) for pain relief in labour. Cochrane Database Syst Rev. 2009;(2):CD007214.
21. Melzack R, Wall PD. Pain mechanisms: a new theory. Science. 1965;150:971-9.
22. Martensson L, Stener-Victorin E, Wallin G. Acupuncture versus subcutaneous injections of sterile water as treatment for labour pain. Acta Obstet Gynecol Scand. 2008;87:171-7.
23. Fogarty V. Intradermal sterile water injections for the relief of low back pain in labour: a systematic review of the literature. Women Birth. 2008;21:157-63.
24. Cluett ER, Burns E. Immersion in water in labour and birth. Cochrane Database Syst Rev. 2009;(2):CD000111.
25. Madden K, Middleton P, Cyna AM, Matthewson M, Jones L. Hypnosis for pain management during labour and childbirth. Cochrane Database Syst Rev. 2012;(11):CD009356.
26. Barragan Loayza IM, Sola I, Juando Prats C. Biofeedback for pain management during labour. Cochrane Database Syst Rev. 2011;(6):CD006168.
27. Nursing and Midwifery Council. Standards for Medicines Management. London: NMC; 2008.
28. Sanders RD, Weimann J, Maze M. Biologic effects of nitrous oxide: a mechanistic and toxicologic review. Anesthesiology 2008;109:707-22.
29. Rooks JP. Safety and risks of nitrous oxide labor analgesia: a review. J Midwifery Womens Health. 2011;56:557-65.
30. Axelsson G, Ahlborg G Jr, Bodin L. Shift work, nitrous oxide exposure, and spontaneous abortion among Swedish midwives. Occup Environ Med. 1996;53:374-8.
31. Likis FE, Andrews JC, Collins MR, Lewis RM, Seroogy JJ, Starr SA, et al. Nitrous oxide for the management of labor pain: a systematic review. Anesth Analg. 2014;118:153-67.
32. Othman M, Jones L, Neilson JP. Non-opioid drugs for pain management in labour. Cochrane Database Syst Rev. 2012;(7):CD009223.
33. Bricker L, Lavender T. Parenteral opioids for labor pain relief: a systematic review. Am J Obstet Gynecol 2002;186 (5 Suppl Nature): S94-109.
34. AnaesthesiaUK. (2007). Pharmacology of Opioids. [online] Available from: http://www.frca.co.uk/article.aspx?articleid=100933. [Last Accessed November, 2021].
35. Hogg MI, Wiener PC, Rosen M, Mapleson WW. Urinary excretion and metabolism of pethidine and norpethidine in the newborn. Br J Anaesth. 1977;49:891-9.
36. Ullman R, Smith LA, Burns E, Mori R, Dowswell T. Parenteral opioids for maternal pain relief in labour. Cochrane Database Syst Rev. 2010;(9): CD007396.
37. Obstetric Anaesthetists' Association. Analgesia for Labour and C-section. [online] Available from: http://www.oaa-anaes.ac.uk/ui/content/content.aspx?id=194. [Last Accessed November, 2021].
38. Wee MY, Tuckey JP, Thomas PW, Burnard S. A comparison of intramuscular diamorphine and intramuscular pethidine for labour analgesia: a two-centre randomised blinded controlled trial. BJOG. 2014;121:447-56.
39. Munoz H, Guerra S, Perez-Vaquero P, Valero Martinez C, Aizpuru F, Lopez-Picado A. Remifentanil versus placebo for analgesia during external cephalic version: a randomised clinical trial. Int J Obstet Anesth. 2014;23:52-7.
40. Howie KM, Millar S. Usage of remifentanil patient controlled analgesia in labour in the UK. Int J Obstet Anesth. 2011;20:S36.
41. Van de Velde M. Controversy. Remifentanil patient-controlled analgesia should be routinely available for use in labour. Int J Obstet Anesth.2008;17:339-42.
42. Bonner JC, McClymont W. Respiratory arrest in an obstetric patient using remifentanil patient-controlled analgesia. Anaesthesia. 2012;67:538-40.
43. Kranke P, Smith AF. Cardiac arrest and remifentanil PCA. Anaesthesia. 2013;68:640.
44. Douma MR, Verwey RA, Kam-Endtz CE, van der Linden PD, Stienstra R. Obstetric analgesia: a comparison of patient-controlled meperidine, remifentanil, and fentanyl in labour. Br J Anaesth. 2010;104:209-15.
45. Shen MK, Wu ZF, Zhu AB, He LL, Shen XF, Yang JJ, et al. Remifentanil for labour analgesia: a double-blinded, randomised controlled trial of maternal and neonatal effects of patient-controlled analgesia versus continuous infusion. Anaesthesia. 2013;68:236-44.
46. Muchatuta NA, Kinsella SM. Remifentanil for labour analgesia: time to draw breath? Anaesthesia. 2013;68:231-5.
47. Tveit TO, Halvorsen A, Seiler S, Rosland JH. Efficacy and side effects of intravenous remifentanil patient-controlled analgesia used in a stepwise approach for labour: an observational study. Int J Obstet Anesth. 2013;22:19-25.
48. Bhatia K. Unknowns in the use of remifentanil PCA for labour analgesia. Anaesthesia. 2013;68:641-2.
49. Liu ZQ, Chen XB, Li HB, Qiu MT, Duan T. A comparison of remifentanil parturient-controlled intravenous analgesia with epidural analgesia: a meta-analysis of randomized controlled trials. Anesth Analg 2014;118:598-603.
50. Obstetric Anaesthetists' Association. (2003). Epidural Information Card. [online] Available from: http://www.labourpains.com/assets/_managed/editor/File/Info%20for%20Mothers/EIC/2008_eic_english.pdf. [Last Accessed November, 2021].
51. The Royal College of Anaesthetists. 3rd National Audit Project (NAP3). London: RCOS; 2009.
52. Anim-Somuah M, Smyth RM, Jones L. Epidural versus non-epidural or no analgesia in labour. Cochrane Database Syst Rev. 2011;(12): CD000331.
53. Simmons SW, Taghizadeh N, Dennis AT, Hughes D, Cyna AM. Combined spinal-epidural versus epidural analgesia in labour. Cochrane Database Syst Rev. 2012;(10):CD003401.
54. Abrão KC, Francisco RP, Miyadahira S, Cicarelli DD, Zugaib M. Elevation of uterine basal tone and fetal heart rate abnormalities after labor analgesia: a randomized controlled trial. Obstet Gynecol. 2009;113:41-7.
55. Kinsella M. Obstetrics. In: Raising the Standard: a compendium of audit recipes, 3rd edition. London: Royal College of Anaesthetists; 2012. pp. 205-29.
56. American College of Obstetricians and Gynecologists. Obesity in pregnancy. Committee Opinion Number 549. Washington DC: ACOG; 2013.
57. Rao DP, Rao VA. Morbidly obese parturient: Challenges for the anaesthesiologist, including managing the difficult airway in obstetrics. What is new? Indian J Anaesth. 2010;54:508-21.

58. National Institute for Health and Care Excellence. Ultrasound-guided Catheterisation of the Epidural Space. NICE interventional procedure guidance 249. London: NICE; 2008.
59. American College of Obstetricians and Gynecologists. Pain relief during labor. Committee Opinion Number 295. Washington DC: ACOG; 2004.
60. Pritchard JA, Gant NF. William's Obstetrics. Norwalk: Appleton-Century-Crofts; 1985. pp. 17.
61. Bern S, Weinberg G. Local anesthetic toxicity and lipid resuscitation in pregnancy. Curr Opin Anaesthesiol. 2011;24(3):262-7.
62. Royal College of Obstetricians and Gynaecologists. Performing a pudendal block. [online] Available from: https://elearning.rcog.org.uk//easi-resource/preparing-instrumental-delivery/analgesia/performing-pudendal. [Last Accessed November, 2021].
63. Russell IF. Raising the standard: a compendium of audit recipes. In: Technique of Anaesthesia for Caesarean Sections. London: Royal College of Anaesthetists; 2006. pp. 166-7.

LONG QUESTIONS

1. What are the options of non-pharmacological management of pain in labor? What are the pros and cons of these methods as compared to pharmacological methods?
2. What is the role of opioids in the management of labor pain? Discuss the concept of patient controlled analgesia.
3. Discuss the technique, indications, contraindications, pros and cons of regional analgesia in labor.

SHORT QUESTIONS

1. What is the origin of pain in labor?
2. What is the Lamaze method?
3. What is the role of inhalation analgesia in labor?
4. Write a short note on pudendal block.
5. What is local anesthetic toxicity? How should it be prevented?

MULTIPLE CHOICE QUESTIONS

1. The following is true about pain in labor:
   a. It arises from a single point of origin
   b. Pain is somatic only
   c. In the first stage, pain is conducted by nerve roots T5-T8
   d. In the second stage, pain is conducted by nerve roots S2-S4
2. The following are true about non-pharmacological pain management in labor:
   a. There is minimal risk to the mother
   b. There is a high risk of fetal injury
   c. They are highly effective methods in later stages of labor
   d. Labor duration is prolonged
3. Which of the following is true about inhalation anesthesia:
   a. It suppresses release of endogenous endorphins
   b. Nitrous oxide and oxygen are used in a ratio of 1:1
   c. The half life of inhalation agents is 2 to 3 hours
   d. Fetal heart rate decelerations are common
4. The following are contraindications to a spinal anesthesia for cesarean delivery, except:
   a. Meningitis
   b. Severe hypotension
   c. Platelet count of 50,000/mL
   d. Preeclampsia
5. The following are good practice recommendations regarding spinal anesthesia, except:
   a. Establish intravenous access
   b. Phenylephrine bolus to maintain blood pressure
   c. Check blood pressure
   d. Use the thinnest possible gauge of spinal needle

Answers
1. d   2. a   3. b   4. d   5. b

SECTION 10
Postpartum Issues: Maternal and Neonatal

10.1 NORMAL PUERPERIUM

Indrani Roy

■ DEFINITION

"Puerperium", this word comes from the Latin word—"puer", child + "parus", to bring forth. It is defined as the period following delivery during which the psychological and anatomical changes induced during pregnancy regress and return to the near non-pregnant state with the exception being the lactating breasts. Its duration is considered to be between 4 and 6 weeks.[1]

■ PHYSIOLOGICAL CHANGES

General Changes

Temperature

Temperature remains normal but a reactionary rise may occur if there is a difficult labor. It usually does not exceed 38°C and drops within the first 24 hours.[2] A slight rise may be seen on the third day due to breast and engorgement.

Pulse

There may be mild tachycardia for a few hours postdelivery, which is followed by a normal pulse rate. Increase in pulse rate must lead to a suspicion of hemorrhage or infection.

Blood Pressure

It may be normal or mild rise post-delivery because of the increased venous return and also may be due to administration of methylergometrine after delivery to minimize blood loss.

After Pains

Painful uterine contractions occur in early puerperium which increases with suckling due to the release of oxytocin.[3] Analgesics may be used to alleviate after pains.

Urine and Urinary Tract

There is increase in diuresis by the second and fourth day, lasting for 3–4 days, which adds to the weight loss.[4] Retention of urine may occur due to atony of the bladder, laxity of the abdomen, recumbency, reflex inhibition if the perineum is sutured and compression of the urethra by vulval edema or hematoma. As a result there is increased incidence of urinary tract infection. Dilated uterus and renal pelvis return to normal size within 6–8 weeks.[4]

Bowel and Gastrointestinal Tract

There is increased thirst in the early puerperium due to loss of fluid during labor. Also increased tendency to constipation due to atony of the intestine, laxity of abdomen and perineum, anorexia, loss of fluids.

Loss of Weight

This is due to evacuation of uterine contents (5–6 kg), due to fetal expulsion and placenta, liquor and blood. A further loss of around 2 kg is attributed to diuresis due to loss of fluid in urine and sweat.[5] Weight loss may continue up to 6 months postpartum.

Blood

There is increased coagulability of the blood for the first 2 weeks in spite of decrease in the coagulation factors. All changes of the cardiovascular system induced by pregnancy, such as increased blood volume, increased cardiac output, mild tachycardia and reduced peripheral resistance gradually revert back to prepregnant state by 4–6 weeks.[6,7]

Blood examination reveals marked leukocytosis soon after labor (about 20,000 per mm^3) due to granulocytosis with relative lymphopenia. Hemoglobin and hematocrit levels show considerable variations and return to normal by 8 weeks.

Menstruation and Ovulation

Menstruation is regained by 6–8 weeks after delivery but lactating women may present with variable period of amenorrhea.[8,9]

Ovulation may also precede the first menstrual period, but on an average after 10 weeks.

Emotional Instability

Many women may experience stress and anxiety to fulfill the new demands and changes in her lifestyle and the term "postpartum blues" or "puerperal blues" is used to describe such a condition.

Anatomical Changes

Birth Canal

Vagina gradually diminishes in size and there is reappearance of the rugae in the vaginal wall by third week. The hymen is replaced by small tissue tags, and the vaginal outlet is relaxed. Once there is restarting of the production of ovarian estrogen, the vaginal epithelium proliferates. Damage to pelvic floor following difficult delivery may predispose to pelvic organ prolapse or urinary incontinence.

Involution of Uterus

Weight: Immediately after delivery the uterus weighs about 1,000–1,200 g. By first week there is further decrease by 500 g and by the end of the second week the uterus weighs about 300 g. The process completes by 5–6 weeks and by the end of 6 weeks the weight comes back to around 50 g **(Fig. 1)**.[10]

Size: The length of the uterus immediately after delivery is around 20 cm and is at the level of the umbilicus. By end of first week the size is midway between the umbilicus and pubic symphysis. By the end of second week it is at the level of pubic symphysis. The process is completed by 6 weeks and by that time it is around 7.5 cm long. The uterine ligaments are also involuted and subinvolution predisposes to prolapse and retroversion.

The mechanism of involution is by the reduction in size of the uterine muscular fibers and not by the reduction of the number of muscle fibers. This is achieved by these three processes:
- Autolysis of the excess muscle fibers
- The blood vessels are obliterated by thrombosis and becomes regenerated while the remnants are transformed into elastic tissue
- The decidua except the basal layer is separated.

The venous sinuses undergo thrombosis at the placental site. The involution of the placental site is by the process of exfoliation. Exfoliation consists of regeneration of the decidua from the glandular remnants and interglandular stroma and also from extension and down growth of endometrium from the margins of the placental site. The process of regeneration is completed by 4–6 weeks postpartum. The placental site is the last part of the uterus where involution occurs. The sloughing of decidual lining of the uterus along with the secretions from the uterine cavity, cervix, and vagina postpartum give rise to the discharge, which is called "lochia". Lochia is alkaline initially but becomes acidic progressively and it has a fishy odor.

Lochia: This is the discharge from the genital tract due to the sloughing of the decidua in the first 15 days of puerperium. It is composed of blood, decidual fragments, cervical mucus, vaginal transudate and bacteria.
- *Lochia rubra (red):* Days 1–4, consists of blood, leukocytes, sloughed decidua and mucus
- *Lochia serosa (pale):* Days 5–10, due to relative decrease in RBCs and predominance of leukocytes
- *Lochia alba (white):* Days 10–15, consist of mucus, serous exudate, granular epithelial cells, leukocytes and cholesterol crystals
- Average duration of low seal discharge ranges from 24 to 36 days.[11] The character of local discharge is of clinical importance. Offensive order of lochia signifies infection and retained cotton swab. In case there is persistence of lochia rubra, subinvolution may be suspected. In severe septicemia with infection, the lochia is scanty and not offensive.

Involution of Other Pelvic Organs

Cervix: Cervix begins to contract soon after delivery but remains patulous for a few days postpartum period **(Figs. 2A and B)**. By 1 week it reforms, thickens, tubular, but may still admit the examining finger. By 6 weeks involution is completed.

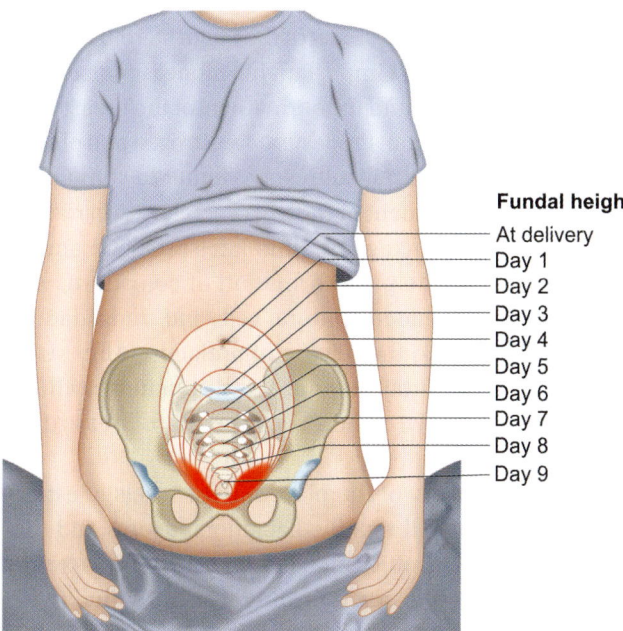

Fig. 1: Involution of uterus.

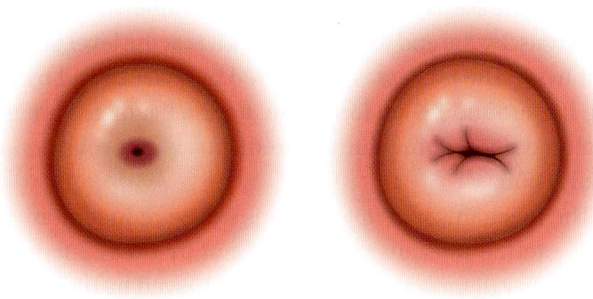

| A | Nulliparous cervix | B | Parous cervix |

Figs. 2A and B: Cervical.

Pelvic musculature: The facial planes and pelvic musculature which undergo stretching and are partially torn at times are engorged with blood and serum immediately after birth. These fluids get rapidly reabsorbed in the next few days. By the end of 6 weeks the muscle tone returns, but some degree of relaxation may always manifest in the perennial tissue due to damage sustained during childbirth.

Peritoneum and abdominal wall: The round ligaments and broad ligaments take additional time for recovery. The wall of the abdomen remains flabby and soft due to loss of skin elasticity. An abdominal binder may be of benefit in this situation. Some post natal exercise can be advised only after 6 weeks to regain the tone of the abdominal wall.

■ BREAST AND LACTATION

The breast secretes a thick, sticky yellowish color liquid called colostrum in the first 2–3 days.[12] Colostrum is rich in immunological components and contains more amino acids and minerals **(Tables 1 and 2)**. Also the protein contents are more, with more of globulin and less of fat and sugar. This secretion persists for five days to upto 2 weeks with gradual conversion to mature milk by 4–6 weeks. The immunoglobulin A (Ig A) content in the colostrum offers the newborn protection against enteric pathogens. Colostrum also contains other host resistance factors such as macrophages, lymphocytes, complement, lactoferrin, lysozyme and lactoperoxidase.

Mature milk is a complex and dynamic biological fluid which includes fat, proteins, carbohydrates, bio active factors, minerals, vitamins, hormones and many cellular products.[13] The concentrations and contents of human milk change even during a single feed and are influenced by maternal diet, age of the infant, health and needs. A lactating mother produces around 600 mL of milk daily.

Physiology of Lactation

The physiology of lactation is divided into four phases:
1. *Mammogenesis*: Preparation of breasts
2. *Lactogenesis:* Induction of secretions from the breast alveoli
3. *Galactokinesis:* Ejection of milk
4. *Galactopoiesis:* Sustaining lactation.

TABLE 1: Composition of breast milk and colostrum.

	Protein	Fat	Carbohydrate	Water
Breast milk	1.2	3.2	7.5	87.0
Colostrum	8.6	2.3	3.2	86.0

TABLE 2: Comparison of composition of human milk and cow's milk.

	Mature human milk (30 days)	Cow's milk
Energy (kcal)	70	69
Total solids (g)	12	12.7
Lactose (g)	7.5	4.8
Protein (g)	1.1	3.3
Cesium (g)	–	2.8
Whey protein	0.5	0.19
Lactalbumin	0.167	–
Lactoferrin	0.162	–
IgA	0.152	–
Total fat (g)	3.7	3.2
Polyunsaturated	2.9	–
Long chain fatty acids (%)	–	–
Minerals (g)	0.4	2.2
Calcium (mg)	28	125
Phosphorus (mg)	15	96
Iron (mg)	40	100
Vitamin A (IU))	137	–

The precise humoral and neural mechanisms involved are complex and nature's preparation for effective lactation begins during pregnancy. Most of the major steroid hormones play a role but the most important hormone is prolactin.[14] Its role is both secretory and mitotic activity of the breast during pregnancy and lactation. Progesterone, estrogen and placental lactogen, cortisols, and insulin act together to stimulate the growth and development of the milk secretary apparatus.

The combined lactogenic stimulates prolactin and HPL during pregnancy helps in formation of colostrum, which consists of desquamated epidural cells and transudate. The major stimulation to the release of prolactin is by estrogen and together with progesterone acts as a potent stimulator to promote the growth and development of breast during pregnancy.

After the delivery of the placenta, the levels of estrogen and progesterone fall rapidly. Lactation ensures and this is perpetuated by episodic bursts of release of prolactin by a neural reflex in response to suckling. The hormone oxytocin is released from the paraventricular and supraoptic nuclei of the maternal hypothalamus in response to the stimulus of suckling. This is transported via the neurons to the posterior pituitary and reaches the breast tissue through blood. The oxytocin hormone helps in contraction of myoepithelial cells in the glandular alveoli of the breast and helps in propulsion of the milk to eject from the nipples.

Preparation for Lactation and Breastfeeding

Preparation of breasts for successful nursing includes advice about a diet which is balanced and adequate to provide 500 kcal extra. During the antenatal period proper breast care should be advised to all the patients and also look out for retracted nipple so that proper care can be taken to avoid feeding difficulties in the postpartum period **(Figs. 3A and B)**. Postpartum, nipple care is an important aspect in care toward cracked or fissured nipples should be taken to prevent entry of pyrogenic bacteria.[14] To alleviate pain, topical lanolin or nipple shield may be used for a breast pump in case of severe cases. A mother should be taught about the correct technique of attachment that is "latch on" technique.

The advantages of breastfeeding are:
- Nutrition is of the utmost natural form and is easily digestible for the infant.
- It contains all essential nutrients and is free of pathogenic organisms and has antibodies which prevent infection in the infants.
- Breastfeeding always promotes additional bonding between the mother and infant.
- It contains IgA antibodies to safeguard the infant against allergens.
- Suckling promotes proper development of the baby's jaws in teeth.
- It helps in involution of the uterus due to the release of oxytocin following suckling.
- It acts as a natural contraception and delays the return of fertility.

Contraindications for Breastfeeding

- Mother on cytotoxic drugs such as cyclophosphamide, cyclosporine, doxorubicin, methotrexate and mycophenolate
- Women on alcohol and illicit drugs
- Infants with galactosemia
- Women undergoing breast cancer treatment
- Radioactive isotopes of iodine, indium
- HIV infection
- Active or untreated tuberculosis

Suppression of Lactation

Drugs used are bromocriptine 2.5 mg once or twice daily for a week or two.

Also cabergoline 0.5 mg which is a more preferred drug can be used to suppress lactation.

Breast Engorgement

It is common in women who do not breastfeed and is characterized by pain which peaks 3–5 days postpartum. Analgesics are recommended along with breast binder to alleviate pain.

Other Issues with Lactation

Inverted nipple: The lactiferous ducts open directly into a depression at the center of the areola and causes difficulty in feeding. Breast pump may be used or daily attempts during the last few months of pregnancy to tease the nipple out with fingers.

Polymastia: Extra breasts.

Polythelia: Extra nipples may develop along the former embryonic mammary ridge. Polymastia has no obstetrical significance.

Galactocele: It is a milk duct which becomes obstructed by inspissated secretions. May resolve spontaneously or require aspiration.

Agalactia: Complete lack of mammary secretion.

Disadvantages of Cow's Milk

As compared to mother's milk, the disadvantages of cow's milk are:
- Cow's milk has a higher solute content and increased sodium. This leads to fretful infant and thirst, so increased tendency to feed more and may result in hypernatremia
- Cow's milk has higher phosphate content leading to hypocalcemia and hypomagnesemia leading to neonatal convulsions.
- Babies tend to be overweight if top fed. The tendency to add more sucrose and to feed concentrated milk increases the problem.

Baby friendly hospital: The "baby friendly hospital initiative" is an international program to increase the exclusive breast-feeding rates and to increase the duration of breastfeeding.[15] This is granted by World Health Organization (WHO) and

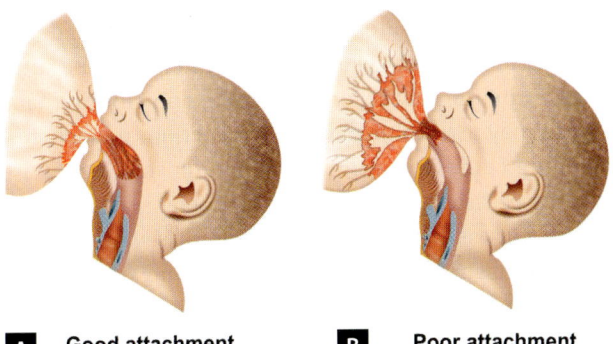

A Good attachment   **B** Poor attachment

Figs. 3A and B: Proper attachment at breast.

United Nations Children Fund (UNICEF) to worldwide hospitals who meet certain stringent criteria.

Ten Steps to Successful Breastfeeding (Revised 2018 version):

1a. *The International Code of Marketing of Breast-milk Substitutes:* Comply fully with the *International Code of Marketing of Breast-milk Substitutes* and relevant World Health Assembly resolutions.
1b. *Infant feeding policy*: Have a written infant feeding policy that is routinely communicated to staff and parents.
1c. *Monitoring and data management systems:* Establish ongoing monitoring and data management systems.
2. *Staff competency:* Ensure that staff have sufficient knowledge, competence and skills to support breastfeeding.
3. *Antenatal information:* Discuss the importance and management of breastfeeding with pregnant women and their families.
4. *Immediate postnatal care:* Facilitate immediate and uninterrupted skin-to-skin contact and support mothers to initiate breastfeeding as soon as possible after birth.
5. *Support with breastfeeding:* Support mothers to initiate and maintain breastfeeding and manage common difficulties
6. *Supplementation:* Do not provide breastfed newborns any food or fluids other than breast milk, unless medically indicated.
7. *Rooming-in:* Enable mothers and their infants to remain together and to practice rooming-in throughout the day and night.
8. *Responsive feeding:* Support mothers to recognize and respond to their infants' cues for feeding.
9. *Feeding bottles, teats and pacifiers:* Counsel mothers on the use and risks of feeding bottles, teats and pacifiers.
10. *Care at discharge:* Coordinate discharge so that parents and their infants have timely access to ongoing support and care.

The advantages of breastfeeding and dangers of top feeds are discussed with mothers in the antenatal clinic. Aim is to make the mothers more confident in breastfeeding.

Rooming In: Immediately after birth the mother and baby are allowed to stay together which is called rooming in.[16] The baby must spend maximum time together with the mother. This practice helps the mother to get used to the needs of the baby earlier and increases bonding between the baby and the mother.

The advantages of rooming in are that it enables a mother to respond to the baby whenever the baby is hungry, which helps in bonding and breastfeeding. Babies are less likely to cry and also bottle feeding is discouraged. Rooming in also enables a mother to breast feed on demand and this continues even after discharge from the hospital. A baby should get feeds whenever the baby wants and not just during specified times that is demand feeding is practiced.

Hospital care: Post-delivery vitals such as pulse and blood pressure to be monitored at 15 minute interval till stable. Also temperature assessment is to be done 4 hourly for the first 8 hours. Patient is kept under observation for the first 2 hours and then shifted out of the labor room after assuring her vitals, the uterus should be well contracted and bleeding should be within normal limits. Patients are encouraged to void urine in the toilet and if required bed pan to be given. Patients are encouraged to breastfeed immediately after birth.

Rest and exercise: Early ambulation is encouraged in uncomplicated vaginal delivery and breathing exercises to minimize the risk of deep vein thrombosis (DVT). Pelvic floor exercises can be encouraged early if there is no perineal wound by contraction and relaxation alternatively of the pelvic floor muscles. Abdominal exercises are encouraged after 6 weeks.

The advantages of exercise are:
- Diminish respiratory and vascular complications
- Minimize future prolapse and stress incontinence
- Give a better cosmetic appearance later.

Hospital stay: Early discharge from hospital is encouraged, within 24–48 hours for a normal delivery and 4–7 days following cesarean section. Proper perineal care where in the vulva and perineum are washed with antiseptic lotion from before backward after each micturition and defecation and a sterile vulval pad is used. Antiseptic cream is to be applied locally if there are perineal stitches. Change of pads to be encouraged every 6 hours or earlier if required. Increase in postpartum bleeding on lochia, or if the odor is offensive may be a sign of puerperal sepsis.

Diet: No dietary restrictions are advised post normal delivery. Increased intake of fluids and easily digestible diet is advised. The diet should be rich in proteins, vitamins, and minerals. Milk, green leafy vegetables, fresh fruits are advised. For cesarean section normal diet can be started after 24 hours, but feeding can be started within 6 hours following cesarean section.

Sleep: Adequate rest and sleep is advised to the mother. Mother should be encouraged to sleep when the baby is also sleeping.[17]

Bowel care: Constipation can occur, hence diet with sufficient fluids and green vegetables are advised. When indicated, mild laxative may be started.

Bladder care: Bladder atonicity and insensitivity after delivery along with diuresis may lead to urinary retention. The sutures in the perineum may be an additional contributing factor, all these may lead to urinary tract infection. In such cases, indwelling catheter to drain the bladder may be advised. Following cesarean section, Foley's catheter is kept for 12–24 hours and in cases of extensive bladder dissection for repeat section, or obstructed labor, prolong second stage, catheter may be kept for a longer duration.

Breast care: Breastfeeding is to be encouraged as early as possible. There may be engorged breasts, painful breasts if early feeding is not initiated. Analgesics, cold fomentation and breast support is encouraged for relief of pain. Mothers should be taught about the correct positioning to assist nursing. The breasts should be manually emptied if they are heavy after feeding. Nipple and areola should be cleaned properly with warm water. Emollient can be used for sore nipples.

Mood and cognition: Some degree of mood variations may be fairly common for a few days post-delivery. "Postpartum blues" are a consequence of emotional disturbance following the fear and excitement during pregnancy and delivery, discomforts of the early puerperium, anxiety, and sleep deprivation. Effective treatment includes most importantly reassurance, recognition and counseling. Usually it is self-limiting in 2–3 days, but may last up to 10 days. If these symptoms persist, evaluation and psychiatric consultation is warranted. Postpartum hormonal changes may also affect brain functions.

Neuromusculoskeletal Problems

Muscular skeletal injuries: Pelvic girdle pain, hips and pains in the lower extremities maybe do you to tearing or stretching injuries sustained in difficult deliveries. Most injuries resolve with anti-inflammatory agents and rarely there may be septic pyomyositis or psoas abscess. MRI may be helpful to diagnose such conditions. Separation of pubic symphysis during labor may lead to pain and interference with locomotion. Conservative treatment with pelvic binder is used.

Obstetrical neuropathies: It is a relatively infrequent condition. Pressure on the lumbosacral nerve plexus during labor may cause cramp like pain in both legs. If there is nerve injury, there may be some degree of sensory loss. Foot drop may also occur secondary to injury at the level of lumbosacral nerve. Nerve injuries with cesarean delivery include iliohypogastric and ilioinguinal nerves.

Immunization: Anti-D immunoprophylaxis is given to Rh –ve mother when the baby is Rh +ve. 300 µg of anti-D is given seventy 2 hours within delivery. Rubella vaccine is advised to all nonimmune women. If tetanus toxoid is missed earlier a booster dose is given.

Baby care: Women, soon after delivery, should be explained about the baby care and direct her to the pediatrician for advice regarding vaccination and well-baby care.

Contraception: Contraceptive advice to both partners should be initiated in the hospital. It is advised to avoid oral contraceptive pills after delivery, but progesterone only pill (POP) may be prescribed. Depot medroxyprogesterone or progesterone implants do not affect quantity or quality of milk and can be advised. Intrauterine device can be advised at 6 weeks postpartum.[18] Multiparous woman, completing family, can have the option of surgical sterilization done at 24 to 48 hours post-delivery.[19]

Medications

- Iron and calcium supplements to continue till inclusive breastfeeding as these are helpful for the infants
- Laxatives as and when indicated
- Analgesics as paracetamol if required
- Uterotonics if uterus not well contracted post delivery
- Thromboprophylaxis with low molecular weight heparin in high risk cases, especially after cesarean section.

Follow-up Care and Discharge Advice

Examination of the mother and child thoroughly at the time of discharge from hospital. Advice is given regarding:
- Breastfeeding care of newborn
- Iron and vitamin tablets
- Contraceptive advice
- Gradual return to normal activity at home
- Postnatal checkup in the outpatient.

Coital advice: Coitus may be resumed after 2 weeks based on desire and comfort. Too soon intercourse may be painful and unpleasant due to episiotomy wound. Also due to the hypoestrogenic state following delivery, the vaginal epithelium is thin and very little lubrication follows sexual stimulation.[20]

Postnatal checkup: This is scheduled at the end of 6 weeks.

Objectives are:
- Maternal problem if any
- Breastfeeding issues
- Immunization of the baby
- Clinical examination to record pulse, blood pressure, weight, pallor, breast examination.

Also a proper pelvic examination to determine the position of uterus and involution. Speculum examination to see the cervix for erosion, cervicitis, vaginal wall laxity.

Sub-involution of the uterus: The uterus in such cases does not regress to the prepregnant size by the end of the puerperium. Causes are:
- Retained placental fragments
- Infection
- Retroversion causing infection
- Myomas.

Laboratory test for hemoglobin estimations, urine for albumin, and blood sugar estimation for gestational diabetes. Any other special test if indicated.
- Ensure that patient continues her iron and calcium supplements
- Review contraceptive decision of the couple.

KEY MESSAGES

- Puerperium is defined as a period of 6 weeks post-delivery during which the reproductive organ return to their prepregnant state.

- The uterus is at the level of umbilicus soon after delivery and weighs 1,000 g.
- Involution occurs rapidly and becomes a pelvic organ weighing 300 g after 2 weeks and 50 g by the end of 6 weeks.
- Uterine discharge occurs up to about 15 days from lochia rubra to lochia serosa and finally lochia alba as the end of second week after delivery.
- Menstruation is regained by 6–8 weeks after delivery, but in lactating women a variable period of amenorrhea may be present.
- Care during puerperium includes emotional and psychological support, encouraging mother and infant bonding, education to mothers on breastfeeding and care of newborn, exercise, medication, contraceptive advice and well-baby care.

REFERENCES

1. Cunningham FG, Leveno KJ, Bloom SL, Spong CY, Dashe SJ, Hoffman LB, et al. The Puerperium. In: Williams Obstetrics, 24th edition. New York: McGraw Hill Education; 2014. pp. 668-81.
2. Geneva Foundation for Medical Education and Research. The Puerperium. [online] Available from: https://www.gfmer.ch/Obstetrics_simplified/puerperium.htm. [Last Accessed November, 2021].
3. Holdcroft A, Snidvongs S, Cason A. Pain and uterine contractions during breast feeding in the immediate post-partum period increase with parity. Pain. 2003;104:589.
4. Daftary NS, Chakravarty S, Pai VM, Kushtagi P. Normal Puerperium. In: Holland and Brews Manual of Obstetrics, 4th edition. Gurgaon: Elsevier; 2016. Pp. 395-402.
5. Schauberger CW, Rooney BL, Brimer LM. Factors that influence weight loss in the puerperium. Obstet Gynecol. 1992;79:424.
6. Hunter S and Robson SC. Adaptation of the maternal heart in pregnancy. Br Heart J. 1992;68:540-3.
7. Robson SC, Dunlop W, and Hunter S. Haemodynamic changes during the early pueperiunm. BMJ. 1987;294:1065.
8. Jackson E, Glasier A. Return of ovulation and menses in postpartium, nonlactating women: a systematic review. Obstet Gynecol. 2011;117:657-62.
9. Wang IY, Fraser IS. Reproductive function and contraception in the postpartum period. Obstet Gynecol Surv. 1994;49:56-63.
10. Cluett ER, Alexander J, Pickering RM. What is the normal pattern of uterine involution? An investigation of postpartum uterine involution measured by the distance between the symphysis pubis and the uterine fundus using a paper using tape measure. Midwifery. 1997;13:9-16
11. The World Health Organization multinational study of breast-feeding and lactational amenorrhea IV. Postpartum bleeding and lochia in breastfeeding women. Fertil Steril. 1999;72:411-7.
12. Ballad O, Morow AL. Human milk composition: nutrients and bioactive factors. Pediatr Clin North Am. 2013;60(1):49.
13. Walker M. Breastfeeding Management for the Clinical: Using the Evidence, 2nd edition. Sudbury, MA: Jones and Bartlett; 2011.
14. Riordan J, Wambach K. Breastfeeding and Human Lactation, 4th edition. Sudbury, MA: Jones and Bartlett; 2010.
15. World Health Organization. Implementation guidance: protecting, promoting and supporting breastfeeding in facilities providing maternity and newborn services – the revised Baby-friendly Hospital Initiative. [online] Available from: https://www.who.int/nutrition/publications/infantfeeding/bfhi-implementation-2018.pdf. [Last Accessed November, 2021].
16. Foster DA, McLachlan HL. Breastfeeding initiation and birth setting practices: a review of the literature. J Midwifery Womens Health. 2007;52:273-80.
17. Hunter LP, Rychnovsky JD, Yount SM. A selective review of maternal sleep characteristics in the postpartum period. J Obstet Gynecol Neonat Nurs. 2009;38:60-8.
18. Centers for Diseases Control. United States Medical Eligibility Criteria for Contraceptive Use. Washington DC: CDC; 2010
19. Pollack A. American College of Obstetricians & Gynecologists Practice Bulletin No. 46: Benefits and Risks of Sterilization. Obstet Gynecol. 2003;102:647-58.
20. Palmer AR, Likis FE. Lactational atrophic vaginitis. J Midwifery Womens Health. 2003;48:282.
21. Liberal Dictionary. Image of parous cervix. [online] Available from: URL https://www.liberaldictionary.com/parous/. [Last Accessed November, 2021].

LONG QUESTIONS

1. Define puerperium. Describe the physiological and anatomical changes in puerperium.
2. Describe the physiology of milk let down. What is early initiation of breast feeding and what are the steps to promote successful breast feeding?
3. Describe in detail the advice to be given to post natal mothers at the time of discharge.
4. Describe the process of involution of uterus.

SHORT QUESTIONS

1. Write a short note on postpartum contraception.
2. What is postpartum blues? Describe in brief the treatment approach for postpartum depression?
3. What is sub-involution of uterus? Enumerate its causes.
4. What are the ten steps to successful breastfeeding according to WHO?
5. Describe the different types of lochia in the normal puerperal period.

MULTIPLE CHOICE QUESTIONS

1. The average duration of puerperium is:
   a. 2 weeks b. 48 hrs
   c. 4–6 weeks d. 6 months
2. Which of the following is not true of puerperium?
   a. There is decreased coagulability of blood in the first 2 weeks
   b. There is leukocytosis after labor
   c. There is increased tendency to constipation
   d. Retention of urine is not uncommon
3. Immediately after delivery, the weight of the uterus is:
   a. 500 g b. 2,000–3,000 g
   c. 100 g d. 1,000–1,200 g

4. A 21-year-old P 2, calls her gynecologist 7 days postpartum because she is still concerned that she is still bleeding from the vagina. She describes the bleeding as light pink in color and less heavy than the first few days post delivery. She has no history of fever or pain. On examination, she is afebrile and has an appropriately sized nontender uterus. The vagina contains about 10 cc of old blood clot with a closed cervix. Which of the following is the most appropriate treatment?
   a. Antibiotics for endometritis
   b. Oxytocin for uterine atony
   c. Reassurance
   d. Suction and curettage for retained placenta
5. Lochia comprises of all of the following, except:
   a. Cervical mucus
   b. Decidual fragments
   c. Bacteria
   d. Pus
6. Galactokinesis denotes:
   a. Preparation of breasts
   b. Ejection of milk
   c. Sustaining lactation
   d. Induction of secretions from breast alveoli
7. Oxytocin is secreted from:
   a. Posterior pituitary
   b. Anterior pituitary
   c. Hypothalamus
   d. Breast myoepithelial cells
8. Which hormone remains elevated in the postpartum period of a breast feeding woman?
   a. Estrogen
   b. Prolactin
   c. Progesterone
   d. Human placental lactogen
9. A woman gave birth to a healthy neonate 5 days ago. What type of lochia is expected?
   a. Lochia rubra
   b. Lochia alba
   c. Lochia serosa
   d. Lochia sangra
10. A woman gave birth to a 4 kg neonate 2 hours ago. The nurse determines that the woman's bladder is distended because the fundus is now 3 cm above the umbilicus and to the right of the midline. The most serious consequence in the immediate postpartum period due to bladder distension is:
    a. Urinary tract infection
    b. Ruptured bladder
    c. Excessive uterine bleeding
    d. Bladder wall atony

Answers
1. c 2. a 3. d 4. c 5. d 6. b
7. a 8. b 9. c 10. b

10.2 EPISIOTOMY AND PERINEAL TRAUMA

Picklu Chaudhuri, Arindam Halder, Hiralal Konar

■ OVERVIEW

Episiotomy is the most common surgical procedure in obstetric practice worldwide. The rate of episiotomy is variable in different part of the globe ranging from 8% in Netherlands, 14% in UK, 50% in USA and 99% in Eastern European countries.

Different degrees of perineal trauma affects majority of women having vaginal birth. A report from UK shows 85% of women sustain perineal injury after vaginal birth and 69% require repair.[1]

Although repair of episiotomy and perineal trauma are technically simple procedures, faulty technique of repair by unskilled providers, lack of aseptic measures, inappropriate suture material, and instruments may lead to serious short- and long-term morbidity. Therefore, standard evidence-based methodology should be practiced.

■ EPISIOTOMY

Definition: A planned incision on the perineum and posterior vaginal wall during second stage of labor is called episiotomy. The term episiotomy is a misnomer as it means incision of pudendum. The literally correct terminology would be perineotomy.

Purpose: The main objective is to enlarge the vaginal introitus to facilitate easy passage of the fetus and to prevent or minimize trauma to the perineum.

Indications

Restrictive versus Routine Episiotomy

There has been a reduction in the percentage of women undergoing episiotomy over the last 25 years all over the world. A study in USA by Weber and Meyn, 2002 found a reduction of incidence of episiotomy from 65% in 1979 to 39% in 1997.[2] Martin and associates (2005) found the incidence to be only 18% in their cohort.[3]

Contrary to popular belief, routine episiotomy was found to be associated with anal sphincter and rectal tears more often than those without episiotomy in a number of studies.[4-6]

Signorello and associates, 2000, in a randomized trial found four to six-fold increase in fecal and flatus incontinence in women with episiotomy than with intact perineum.[7]

There is little evidence to show that "prophylactic" episiotomy prevents pelvic organ prolapse or stress urinary incontinence. On the contrary, Rockner and associates, 1991 found less strength of pelvic floor muscles in women with episiotomy in comparison to women who had vaginal deliveries without episiotomy.[8]

Cochrane database systematic review (2009) compared restrictive and routine episiotomy policies and concluded that restrictive use is beneficial in terms of reduction of complications[9] **(Table 1)**.

The international bodies (NICE guideline,[10] ACOG guideline[11]) recommend that restricted use of episiotomy is preferable to routine use.

Episiotomy should therefore be performed in presence of definite clinical indication:
1. To prevent perineal injuries as in instrumental delivery, assisted breech delivery, shoulder dystocia, face to pubis delivery, fetal macrosomia, rigid inelastic perineum.
2. To expedite delivery as in fetal compromise.

Episiotomy should not be routinely performed in women with history of third or fourth degree perineal tear in previous birth.

Types of Episiotomy

Mediolateral and median are the two commonly performed types. Two other types have been also described in earlier textbooks, i.e., lateral and J shaped, are hardly performed nowadays. The median episiotomy is an incision made from the midpoint of fourchette going downward in the midline toward the anus, but stopping well short of it. Mediolateral episiotomy is the recommended type in which the incision starts from the midpoint of fourchette and extends diagonally downward at an angle 45–60 degrees with the vertical axis up to 2.5 cm lateral to the anus (midpoint between anus and ischial tuberosity).

Advantages and disadvantages of the two types are given in **Table 2**.

Steps of Episiotomy

Step I: Preliminaries

Perineum is swabbed with antiseptic solution (povidone-iodine) and draped. The proposed site of incision is infiltrated with 10 mL of 1% solution of lignocaine.

Step II: Incision

Timing of episiotomy incision: Timing of episiotomy is important as an early episiotomy cause unnecessary blood loss while a late episiotomy fail to prevent perineal trauma. The ideal time for episiotomy is when the perineum is thinned and bulged during a uterine contraction with 3–4 cm of fetal head is visible. During forceps delivery, episiotomy should be given preferably after application of the blades except in cases of rigid and inelastic perineum.

Method: Two fingers are positioned in the vagina between the presenting part and the posterior vaginal wall. One blade of a curved or straight blunt pointed scissors is placed in between the fingers and the posterior vaginal wall and the other blade on the skin along the proposed line of incision. The incision should be given at the height of uterine contractions and should be adequate enough to serve the purpose.

Structures cut are—posterior vaginal wall mucosa, superficial and deep transverse perineal muscles, bulbospongiosus and few fibers of levator ani along with their

TABLE 1: Restricted use of episiotomy: Results of Cochrane review.

Clinically relevant morbidities	Relative risk	95% CI
Posterior perineal trauma	0.88	0.84–0.92
Need for suturing	0.74	0.71–0.77
Healing complications at 7 days	0.69	0.56–0.85
Anterior perineal trauma	1.79	1.55–2.07

(CI: confidence interval)
Note:
1. No increase in incidence of major outcomes (e.g., severe vaginal or perineal trauma nor in pain, dyspareunia or urinary incontinence).
2. Incidence of 3rd degree tear reduced (1.2% with episiotomy, 0.4% without).

TABLE 2: Mediolateral versus median episiotomy.

	Median	Mediolateral
Advantages	• Easier to give the incision and easier to repair • Muscles are not cut and therefore blood loss is minimal • Healing is better • Postoperative comfort is maximum • Wound disruption is rare • Dyspareunia is rare	• Incision can be extended if situation demands • Relatively safe in terms of extension leading to third and fourth degree perineal trauma
Disadvantages	• Cannot be extended if needed • Accidental extension leads to third or fourth degree perineal trauma • Not suitable for operative and manipulative vaginal deliveries	• Technically more difficult and requires skill in incising and repairing • Apposition of tissue may be suboptimal • Blood loss is more • Postoperative discomfort is more • Incidence of wound disruption is more • Incidence of dyspareunia is more

fascia, transverse perineal branches of pudendal vessels and nerves, subcutaneous tissue and skin.

Step III: Repair

Timing of repair: The repair should be done soon after expulsion of placenta ensuring its completeness. Repair earlier to placental expulsion may lead to disruption in case manual removal of placenta or exploration of genital tract is needed. Any spurting vessel from the wound may be crushed with artery forceps or oozing surface may be subjected to pressure by sterile gauze swab during this period.

Preliminaries: The woman is placed in lithotomy position. Good light source is required for visualization. Perineum is cleansed and draped as described before.

Method: Basic principles of repair are:
- Good hemostasis
- Anatomical apposition without excessive tension
- Obliteration of dead space.

Absorbable suture material such as No. 0 or 2-0 atraumatic catgut or polyglactin (Vicryl) sutures are used for repair. Polyglactin 910 (Vicryl rapid), a rapidly absorbable synthetic suture has been compared with the standard absorbable suture in a randomized controlled trial and the use of the former was associated with lower rate of suture removal after 3 months.[12]

Repair is done in three layers in the following order—vaginal mucosa, muscle, and skin.

Suturing of vaginal mucosa: Apex of the incised vaginal mucosa is identified and the first stitch should be applied just above it. Continuous non-locking stitches should be applied for vaginal mucosa from apex down to the hymenal ring. If there are large mucosal bleeders, sutures may be locked as needed.

Suturing the muscles: Depending upon the depth of the cut muscles (deep and superficial perineal), one or two layers of continuous non-locking stitches should be applied to approximate them. It is a common practice to also suture the muscle with interrupted sutures. This is labor intensive and not necessary. Kettle and coworkers (2002) compared repair by interrupted versus continuous suturing techniques and found that continuous suturing is associated with less perineal pain.[12]

Suturing the skin: Skin should be approximated by continuous subcuticular stitches from inferior perineal margin to hymen. Subcuticular sutures are associated with less pain and better cosmetic results but may have a marginal increase in wound disruption.

Postoperative Care

The episiotomy wound should be cleaned with cotton swab soaked in antiseptic solution after each act of urination and defecation followed by application of antiseptic powder or ointment. Ice packs may be used if there is swelling. Compress with magnesium sulfate or infrared heat is the alternatives to reduce pain and inflammation. Women are instructed to be ambulatory as early as possible and sit with thighs apposed. Analgesics (Paracetamol, Ibuprofen) may be prescribed to allay pain and discomfort. As the suturing is mostly done with absorbable material, there is no need to cut the stitches and women can be discharged after 48–72 hours.

Complications

Immediate/Early Complications

Extension of incision and injury to anorectum (third and fourth degree lacerations): The incidence of third and fourth degree laceration is 11.6% following midline episiotomy as reported by Harris (1970).[13] This can also happen following mediolateral episiotomy during forceps delivery or "face to pubes" delivery.

Vulval Hematoma

Vulval hematoma arising as a complication of episiotomy wound is usually infralevator type.

This complication arises due to improper hemostasis during repair of episiotomy or perineal lacerations especially failure to secure hemostasis at the apex of the vaginal mucosa and in the perineal muscle. Patient complains of severe pain in the perineum, rectal tenesmus and or voiding difficulty. The diagnosis can readily be made on finding variable degree of shock and local examination revealing tense, fluctuant, purple or dusky swelling.

In general, hematomas usually require surgical intervention due to pain and the risk of forming an abscess. In rare circumstances, where the hematoma is very small and the woman is asymptomatic, a conservative management may be considered with close monitoring of general condition and change in the size of swelling. Larger hematomas demand prompt surgical intervention along with correction of shock by fluid and blood transfusion. This should be done under anesthesia in an operation theater. The hematoma is incised to evacuate blood clots and bleeding points are secured by sutures. Cautery should not be used. Sometimes, there are no identified bleeding points. The cavity is then obliterated by mattress suture and a corrugated rubber drain can be kept for 24 hours. A tight vaginal pack can be given for 24–48 hours and the woman should be catheterized with an in-dwelling catheter.

Infection

Infection occurs due to lack of perineal care and unhygienic practices like use of unclean napkins. Presence of hematoma also favors infection. Symptoms as throbbing pain in the perineum, rise of temperature, foul smelling discharge should raise suspicion. Local examination shows edema. Induration, redness and offensive purulent or serosanguinous discharge clinches the diagnosis. Routine blood count and wound swab for gram stain and culture should be done. Systemic broad spectrum antimicrobial, analgesics along with local dressing with antiseptic powder or ointment and magnesium sulfate compress is the treatment. A few stitches may have to be removed to facilitate drainage of purulent discharge. Usually, surgical debridement is not necessary.

Dehiscence

Incidence of wound dehiscence following episiotomy is fortunately not very high (0.5%).[14] A higher incidence (4.6–10%) is reported after repair of third and fourth degree lacerations.[15]

Infection, hematoma and faulty repair lead to dehiscence in most of the cases. Opinions are divided regarding the timing of repair. However, recent trend favors early repair.

Early Repair

Hauth and colleagues (1986), were the first to advocate early repair.[16] Subsequently other reports supported the benefits of early repair.[14,17] *The prerequisite of repair are: the woman should be afebrile; wound needs to be free of infection and exudates; wound covered by healthy pink granulation tissue.* Therefore prior to attempting early repair, broad spectrum systemic antibiotic and thorough wound care in the form of twice daily scrubbing with povidone-iodine along with debridement of necrotic tissue under local anesthesia are mandatory. Often, one may note significant healing with a few dressings and healing by secondary intention may proceed.

Late Repair

Repair after 6 weeks or 3 months were done in the past to allow time for revascularization and healing of the wound and improvement of general condition of the women. However, this causes inconvenience to the patient in terms of fecal incontinence and loss of sexual activity. Late repair is not supported by current evidence based opinion.

Technique of Secondary Repair

First step of successful secondary repair is removal of all devitalized granulation tissue. Second step is adequate dissection for mobilization of tissue so that they can reapproximated without tension. Finally, layered repair (as in primary repair) with proper hemostasis is performed.

Necrotizing Fasciitis

It is a rare but dangerous complication in which the severe infection by virulent organism (as beta hemolytic streptococci) involves deep soft tissue, fascia and muscles. It occurs in diabetic and immunocompromised women. The myofascitis spreads rapidly to thighs, buttocks and abdominal walls. Septicemia and septic shock ensues unless the condition is suspected and diagnosed early and aggressively treated by antimicrobials, extensive surgical debridement, and intensive care.

Late/Remote Complications

Flatus/Fecal Incontinence and Rectovaginal Fistula

This occurs if a third or fourth degree perineal tears remain undiagnosed or repaired in a faulty manner. Surgical intervention is required after proper preparation.

Dyspareunia

This occurs if vaginal introitus is narrowed due to faulty technique of repair or due to scarred perineum as a result of extensive laceration.

Scar Endometriosis

It is a rare condition arising due to ectopic endometrial tissue in the scar site. The treatment is primarily surgical and accomplished by wide excision of the affected tissue and repair.

■ PERINEAL TEARS

Classification

Laceration to the vagina and perineum can be classified into four degrees [Royal College of Obstetricians and Gynaecologists (RCOG, 2007)]:[18]

- *First degree:* Injury to perineal skin only
- *Second degree:* Injury to the perineal muscles but not the anal sphincter
- *Third degree:* Injury to the perineum involving the anal sphincter complex:
  - *3a:* Less than 50% of external anal sphincter (EAS) thickness torn
  - *3b:* More than 50% of EAS thickness torn
  - *3c:* Internal anal sphincter (IAS) torn
- *Fourth degree:* Injury to the perineum involving the anal sphincter complex (external and internal anal sphincter) and anal epithelium.

Buttonhole tear: If the tear involves only anal mucosa with intact anal sphincter complex. This has to be documented as a separate entity.

Risk Factors

The risk factors to perineal trauma are: big baby (≥4 kg), rigid inelastic perineum in nulliparous women, outlet contraction with narrow pubic arch, manipulative and instrumental delivery, shoulder dystocia, face to pubis delivery (persistent occipitoposterior), precipitate labor, midline episiotomy, scarred perineum following previous perineorrhaphy second stage of labor >1 hour and epidural analgesia.

Management

Prevention

Perineal trauma can be prevented by modifying some of the risk factors. Performing mediolateral episiotomy in indicated cases instead of median episiotomy, preferring Ventouse over Forceps[19] can reduce major perineal trauma. Other methods as perineal massage in the antenatal period,[20] water birth, different positions during delivery, delayed and controlled pushing during second stage, perineal stretching and support of perineum during second stage have been proposed to reduce trauma. However, no conclusive opinion could be derived regarding the use of these interventions.

Identification of the Injury

All women having a vaginal birth are to be examined systematically post birth by a midwife or doctor trained and competent in the identification and classification of perineal trauma. Rectal examination should be performed to detect anal sphincter and mucosal defects. A written informed consent is compulsory before undertaking repair.

Timing of Repair

Perineal tears should be repaired immediately following delivery of placenta. This reduces the chance of infection and minimizes blood loss. Perineal lacerations especially of third and fourth degree if not repaired within 24 hours should be delayed for 3 months.

Method of Immediate Repair of Third and Fourth Degree Tear (First and Second Degree Repair is same as Episiotomy Repair)

Preliminaries

Woman is placed in lithotomy position. Local area is cleaned with antiseptic solution as povidone-iodine. Bladder catheterized. Proper illumination by bright light source and suitable instruments are prerequisites. General or regional anesthesia is preferable. In resource poor setups, local infiltration with 1% lignocaine and pudendal block should be given.

Technique and Suture Materials

Anal Epithelium

The torn edges of anorectal mucosa are identified and approximated with running or interrupted sutures placed in the submucosa 0.5 cm apart using fine absorbable suture material as 3-0 polyglactin (Vicryl) or polydioxanone (PDS) with atraumatic needle (26 mm round bodied) with the knots tied in the anal lumen.

Internal anal Sphincter

A second reinforcing layer of continuous or interrupted sutures is applied in the rectal muscularis and fascial layer. This should include internal anal sphincter which is identified as thickening of circular muscle fibers at distal 2–3 cm of anal canal.

The recommended sutures include fine 3-0 PDS or 2-0 Vicryl as it may cause less irritation and discomfort.

External Anal Sphincter

The torn ends of the EAS should be fully mobilized and repaired using either an overlap or end-to-end technique using the same suture material as in IAS. Burying of surgical knots beneath the superficial perineal muscles is recommended to prevent knot migration to the skin.

In traditional end to end method, 4–6 interrupted sutures are placed at 3, 6, 9, 12 O'clock positions .Overlapping method of approximation of EAS does not appear to be better than the traditional method as evidenced in different studies.[9,21]

Perineal muscles, vaginal mucosa, and perineal skin are sutured in the same way as in episiotomy.

Rectal examination has to be performed after the repair to ensure the intactness of rectal mucosa and the establishment of sphincter tone. Documentation of the type of injury and the details of repair is mandatory.

Postoperative Care Following Repair of Third and Fourth Degree Lacerations

Apart from routine care (rest, ice pack, analgesics) *broad spectrum antibiotic* should be given to prevent infection and dehiscence.

Women with fourth degree tear are given intravenous fluid for 24 hours and liquids for another 24-48 hours. Low residue diet is allowed from 3rd postoperative day.

Laxatives or stool softeners (lactulose) are recommended in the postoperative period for 7-10 days as hard stool can cause dehiscence. *With 4th degree tears, postoperative laxatives are delayed* because of the rectal mucosal injury. Enema should not be given.

Women are advised to come for follow-up after 6 weeks. *A pelvic floor muscle rehabilitation* program under the guidance of physiotherapist should be commenced as soon as comfortable, usually at about 2–3 days post birth and to be continued up to 6–12 weeks.

Management of Subsequent Pregnancy

There were no systematic reviews or randomized controlled trials to suggest the best method of delivery following obstetric anal sphincter injury. However, RCOG guideline, 2007 suggests that women who have sustained an obstetric anal sphincter injury in a previous pregnancy and who are symptomatic or have abnormal endoanal ultrasonography and/or manometry should have the option of elective cesarean birth. Women who had an obstetric anal sphincter injury in a previous pregnancy should be counseled about the risk of developing anal incontinence or worsening symptoms with subsequent vaginal delivery and they should also be informed that there is no evidence to support the role of prophylactic episiotomy in subsequent pregnancies.

CONCLUSION

- Perineal trauma is sustained by majority of women following vaginal delivery and episiotomy is the most common obstetric procedure.
- Third and fourth degree of trauma can be prevented by prior risk assessment and conducting delivery properly.
- Mediolateral episiotomy is preferred and should be given in selective cases.
- Repair of episiotomy and major degree of perineal trauma should be done by trained care provider. Adequate anesthesia, proper instruments, good light source, suitable suture material and optimum postoperative care are the keys to successful repair.
- Faulty repair technique and infection leads to considerable morbidity in the form of hematoma and dehiscence.

REFERENCES

1. McCandlish R, Bowler U, van Asten H, Berridge G, Winter C, Sames L, et al. A randomized controlled trial of care of perineum during second stage of normal labour. Br J Obstet Gynecol. 1998:105:1262-72.
2. Weber A M, Meyn L. Episiotomy use in United States, 1979-1997. Obstet Gynecol. 2002;100:1177.
3. Martin JA, Hamilton BE, Sutton PD, Entura SJ, Menacker F, Munson ML. Births: final data for 2002. Natl Vital Stat Rep. 2003 Dec 17;52(10):1-113.
4. Angioli R, Gomez-Marin O, Cantuaria G, O'sullivan MJ. Severe perineal lacerations during vaginal delivery: the University of Miami experience. Am J Obstet Gynecol. 2000;182: 1083.
5. Eason E, Labrecque M, Wells G, Feldman P. Preventing perineal trauma during childbirth: a systematic review. Obstet Gynecol. 2000;95:464.
6. Negar CW, Helliwell JP. Episiotomy increases perineal laceration length in primiparous women. Am J Obstet Gynecol. 2001;185:444.
7. Signorello LB, Harlow BL, Chekos AK. Midline Episiotomy and anal incontinence: Retrospective cohort study.Br Med J. 2000;320:86.
8. Rockner G, Jonasson A, Blund A. The effect of mediolateral episiotomy at delivery on pelvic floor muscles strength evaluated with vaginal cones. Acta Obstet Gynecol Scand. 1991;70(1):51-4.
9. Beckmann MM, Stock OM. Antenatal perineal massage for reducing perineal trauma. Cochrane Database Sys Rev. 2009:1: CD005123.
10. NICE. (2007). Intrapartum Care. NICE clinical guideline. Guideline 55. [online] Available from: www.nice.org.uk/CG055. [Last Accessed November, 2021].
11. American Colleges of Obstetrician and Gynaecologists. Episiotomy: ACOG Practice bulletin No.71. Washington DC: ACOG; 2006.
12. Kettle C, Hills RK, Jones P, Darby L, Gray R, Johanson R. Continuous versus interrupted perineal repair with standard or rapidly absorbed sutures after spontaneous vaginal birth: a randomized controlled trial. Lancet. 2002;359:2217.
13. Harris RE. An evaluation of median episiotomy. Am J Obstet Gynecol. 1970:106(5):660-5.
14. Ramin SM, Ramus R, Little B, Gilstrap 3rd LC. Early repair of episiotomy dehiscence associated with infection. Am J Obstet Gynecol. 1992:167:1104.
15. Goldaber KG, Wendel PJ, Mc Intire DD, Wendel GD. Postpartum perineal morbidity after fourth degree perineal tear. Am J Obstet Gynecol. 1993;168:489.
16. Hauth JC, Gilstrap LC III, Ward SC, Hankins GD. Early repair of an external sphincter ani muscle and rectal mucosal dehiscence. Obstet Gynecol. 1986;67:806.
17. Hankins GDV, Hauth JC, Gilstrap LC, Hammond TL, Yeomans ER, Snyder RR. Early repair of episiotomy dehiscence. Obstet Gynecol. 1990;75:48.
18. RCOG. Green-top Guideline No. 29: The management of third and fourth degree perineal tears. London: RCOG Press; 2007.
19. Johansson RB, Menon V. Vacuum extraction versus Forceps for assisted vaginal delivery. Cochrane Database Sys Rev. 1999:2:CD000224.
20. Goh J, Carey M, Tjandra J. Direct end-to-end or overlapping delayed anal sphincter repair for anal incontinence: long term results of prospective randomised study. Neurourol Urodyn. 2004;23:412-4.
21. Williams A, Adams EJ, Tincello DG, Alfirevic Z, Walkinshaw SA, Richmond DH. How to repair an anal sphincter injury after vaginal delivery: results of a randomised controlled trial. BJOG. 2006;113:201-7.

LONG QUESTIONS

1. Classify perineal lacerations. Enumerate the risk factors of perineal trauma after vaginal birth. Describe the management of fourth degree perineal tear.
2. What is episiotomy? What are the types of episiotomy? Which type is recommended and why? Describe the complications of episiotomy.
3. A 23-year-old primipara who delivered vaginally with episiotomy 3 hours back complains of severe pain in the perineum. What are the possible causes? How will you manage such a case?

SHORT QUESTIONS

1. Justify the statement: "Restrictive or selective use of episiotomy is preferable to routine episiotomy."
2. Write a short note on "vulval hematoma".

MULTIPLE CHOICE QUESTIONS

1. Which of the following statements regarding perineal trauma is most accurate?
    a. Perineal massage after 35 weeks gestation reduces the risk of perineal trauma in first vaginal deliveries
    b. Restricting the use of episiotomy reduces the risk of anterior perineal trauma

c. Forceps delivery has a lower risk of third degree tears than vacuum delivery
   d. Midline episiotomy reduces the risk of third degree tears
2. Mediolateral episiotomy is preferred to median episiotomy because of all, except:
   a. Operative delivery can be performed
   b. Less chance of extension to involve anal sphincter
   c. Bleeds less
   d. It can be extended if required
3. Episiotomy is a planned perineal injury of:
   a. First degree
   b. Second degree
   c. Third degree
   d. Fourth degree
4. Incidence of fourth degree perineal tear is:
   a. 0.5%
   b. 5%
   c. 10%
   d. More than 10%
5. Predisposing factors to fourth degree perineal tear are all, except:
   a. Pelvic outlet contraction
   b. Instrumental vaginal delivery
   c. Mediolateral episiotomy
   d. Face to pubis delivery.
6. Measures to prevent fourth degree perineal tear are all, except:
   a. Making a mediolateral episiotomy while delivering the aftercoming head of breech
   b. Augmenting labor with oxytocin
   c. Avoiding difficult instrumental vaginal delivery
   d. Controlled delivery of head
7. Measures recommended in the management of fourth degree perineal tears are all, except:
   a. Suture the injury under anesthesia and good light source to secure proper tissue approximation
   b. Perioperative antibiotic prophylaxis
   c. Stool softeners to prevent constipation
   d. Daily enema to keep the bowel moving
8. Recent trend suggest that dehiscence of episiotomy should be repaired:
   a. As soon as detected
   b. Within a week
   c. Within 2 weeks
   d. When the wound is free of infection
9. Compared with midline episiotomy, mediolateral episiotomy is associated with all of the following, except:
   a. An increased risk of rectal tear
   b. More blood loss
   c. More postpartum pain
   d. More difficult repair
10. At the time of forceps delivery, an episiotomy reduces the risk of:
    a. Rectal sphincter tear
    b. Rectal mucosal tear
    c. Hemorrhage
    d. None of the above

Answers
1. a 2. c 3. b 4. a 5. c 6. b
7. d 8. d 9. a 10. d

10.3 POSTPARTUM HEMORRHAGE AND ITS MANAGEMENT

Parul J Kotdawala, Sapana Shah, Sunil Shah

INTRODUCTION

Postpartum hemorrhage (PPH) is the most treacherous obstetric condition that can strike an obstetrician. Hemorrhage has remained a leading cause of maternal death in developing countries in Africa (33.9%) and in Asia (30.8%).[1] Severe PPH following vaginal births is reported in about 3% of women in spite of pertinent management.[2] Overall, 13% of all maternal deaths are due to hemorrhage and PPH accounts for two-thirds of these deaths, making it the culprit in almost 11% of all maternal deaths and accounting for about a half million maternal death every year globally! These are very high rates and pose a significant risk to every pregnant woman in those countries. Unfortunately, it has failed to prompt the obstetricians to establish necessary and appropriate skills among the labor ward nursing care staff. Keeping that in mind, each and every member of obstetric team should have complete understanding of this complication and appropriate management plan to act upon. Each and every obstetrician should have the following questions at the back of their minds while dealing with PPH: Whether the blood loss is significant? What could be the reason? How can I manage it? Was there any high-risk factor for prediction?

DEFINITION

Postpartum hemorrhage is traditionally defined as primary PPH when the amount of blood loss, within 24 hours after a vaginal delivery, is more than 500 mL.[3,4] Secondary PPH is defined as same amount of blood loss noticed after 24 hours and up to 7th day postpartum. This definition is used to operate in times when assessment of blood loss was quite inaccurate. Subsequently, with very precise measurement of blood loss as well as with better understanding of hemodynamic physiology of pregnancy and labor, the definition has been revised to a blood loss of 1,000 mL irrespective of mode of delivery. The cut-off value of 1,000 mL approximates the increased volume of blood gained during pregnancy. There is physiological hemodilution due to blood volume expansion but conditions such as preeclampsia and fetal growth restrictions are associated with significantly lesser blood volume expansion.[3] A similar amount of blood loss in such conditions may lead to ischemic injury as compared to normal patients. The real definition in terms of clinical value, however, would be, a blood loss leading to hemodynamic instability and compromised oxygen carrying capacity. The simplest clinical parameter to assess this is the presence of tachycardia (pulse rate >100/min or 10% rise from baseline).

After the acute blood loss, the hemoglobin levels do not coordinate well with the blood loss and RBC volume deficits.[5] This can be attributed to the fact that there is proportional decrease in volume of red cells and plasma with the loss of whole blood. Decreased hematocrit in the beginning is due to the dilution effects of infused crystalloids. It takes approximately 8–12 hours for the manifestation of physiological response to reduced hematocrit once the kidney begins sodium conservation.[6] Hence, this situation requires the clinical methods of hemodynamic monitoring.

The plus point of pregnancy is that the 30% increased blood volume at term gives a cushion against ill-effects of sudden blood loss at delivery. But this is coupled with a high flow of blood in pregnant uterus, and may lead to quick exsanguinations if there is any prevarication or delay in treating the PPH.

BACKGROUND PHYSIOLOGY

The physiological mechanism to avert hemorrhage after a delivery is primarily the constriction of blood vessels supplying the placental bed by uterine contraction. The crisscross pattern of uterine muscle acts as a living ligature and the uterine contraction compresses spiral arterioles passing through the interlacing fibers (mechanical hemostasis). The subsequent hemostasis is also achieved by vasoconstriction, platelet aggregation and clot formation. The placental bed blood flow varies with duration of pregnancy, and at term it is approximately 750 mL/min. There is a physiological rise in blood volume (hypervolemia of pregnancy) and at term it is approximately 7 liters (100 mL/kg). In spite of this rise in blood volume, a blood loss of 30% may quickly become life-threatening if it remains uncorrected. A mother can become critical within few minutes if the blood flow to the placental bed is not arrested quickly following the placental separation.

CAUSES OF POSTPARTUM HEMORRHAGE

- Uterine atony
- Trauma and lacerations of genital tract
- Coagulation disorders.

Myometrial contractions and clotting are important for postpartum hemostasis. During the 3rd stage of labor, the myometrial contractions constrict the spiral arteries and the placental bed vessels. In postpartum period, inadequate uterine contractions can lead to atonic PPH in conditions such as over distended uterus due to polyhydroamnios and twins, induced or augmented labor with uterotonics, chorioamnionitis and the drugs such as magnesium sulfate, calcium channel blockers and inhalation anesthetic agent like halothane.[7,8] Rare but significant event of uterine inversion leads to PPH due to altered ability of myometrium to contract the placental bed vessels.

Lacerations in any part of the genital tract can lead to significant amount of blood loss. In placenta accreta spectrum disorders, disruption of newly formed blood vessels may lead to torrential hemorrhage and can also be classified as lacerations to genital tract.

There is increased incidence of PPH with inherited or acquired coagulopathy that suggest the importance of having normal clotting mechanism for postpartum hemostasis.[9,10] PPH is commonly seen in inherited coagulopathies such as factor VIII deficiency (hemophilia), von Willebrand's disease and factor XI deficiency. Most of the times thrombocytopenia is idiopathic in nature and it is another common condition in India leading to PPH.[9,11,12] von Willebrand's disease causes primary PPH in up to 22% women and secondary PPH in 28% of women. Women with carrier of hemophilia are associated with primary PPH in up to 18.5% women and secondary PPH in 11%.[9,11,12]

Acquired coagulopathy leads to PPH in cases of preeclampsia and sepsis. Also, PPH itself due to hemodilution with vigorous use of crystalloids and/or consumption of coagulation factors can lead to acquired coagulopathy.

In number of situations, all of the above-mentioned three mechanisms can coexist and the best notable condition is placental abruption. In placental abruption, blood infiltration of the myometrium interferes with uterine contractility, disruption of uteroplacental blood vessels and disseminated intravascular coagulation all together are responsible for postpartum hemorrhage.

PREDICTING BLOOD LOSS

The risk factors for PPH can help us to predict in which patients, PPH can develop as a complication and thus allow us to prepare the required resources, staff personnel and counsel the woman and her family. The risk factors for the PPH have been identified by various studies documented in literature. As these studies were including diverse population from different countries (USA, Zimbabwe, Nigeria, UK), different definition of PPH and various modes of deliveries, the results of the studies should be interpreted with caution. These risk factors are listed in **Table 1** in order of their significance and consistency with PPH.[13-17]

The various modes of delivery also predispose to PPH, which was beautifully highlighted in the study which included over 37,000 women in UK. PPH was defined as greater than 1,000 mL of blood loss and incidence was 1.33%. The independent risk factors which were strongly associated with PPH are grouped together in **Table 1**—independent of management [abruptio placenta, placenta previa, multiple gestation, big baby (weight >4 kg), obesity] and related to management [retained placenta, episiotomy, labor induction, mode of delivery].[8] The impact of mode of delivery on the occurrence of PPH also is quite interesting **(Table 2)**.

HOW TO PREVENT HEMORRHAGE?

Several studies have evaluated the ways to prevent the complication of PPH as it occurs most often in absence of any risk factors. The active management of third stage of labor (AMTSL) includes immediate use of prophylactic oxytocics after birth of baby, delayed clamping of cord, and controlled cord traction. These are directed towards decreasing the postpartum blood loss and for prevention of PPH. Recent meta-analysis in literature compiling the three randomized trials including more than 45,00 women which compared active versus expectant third stage management by gravity or nipple stimulation.

In contrast to expectant management, active management demonstrated:
- Reduced blood loss (mean blood loss was 79 mL less)
- Reduced risk of PPH> 500 mL
- Reduced risk of severe PPH > 1,000 mL
- Reduced risk of postpartum anemia
- Reduced need for puerperal transfusion
- Reduced therapeutic use of oxytocics.

Active management of third stage of labor should be offered to all the women as those decreases the probability of PPH and need for blood transfusion. Prophylactic oxytocics help to reduce the risk of PPH by 50% in a vaginal or cesarean birth. Manual removal of placenta should be avoided during a cesarean delivery, and one should employ controlled cord traction (CCT) as a preferred technique for placental delivery at cesarean section to prevent PPH.

Active Management of Third Stage of Labor

The World Health Organization recommendation (2012):
- Oxytocin 10 IU IM or misoprostol 600 μg rectal (if oxytocin not available or not possible) immediately after delivery (Recommended)
- Delayed (1-3 min after birth) cord clamping (Recommended).
- Controlled cord traction for delivery of placenta (Optional)
- Uterine massage after delivery of placenta (Optional)
- Regular and frequent assessment of uterine tone by palpation of the uterine fundus after delivery of placenta (Recommended).

When ergometrine was used earlier in place of oxytocin, adverse effects such as headache, nausea, vomiting and hypertension were common.[18] AMTSL prevents approximately 60% of PPH and the role of each component of management protocol to the benefit and the superiority of one type of oxytocic over other is still to be determined.

TABLE 1: Risk factors for postpartum hemorrhage (>1,000 mL).

Risk factor	Risk of PPH	
	Retrospective studies Odds Ratio [range]	Prospective studies Relative Risk (99% CI)
Prior PPH	2.9–8.4	
Multiple pregnancy	2.8–4.5	4.5 (3.0–6.6)
Preeclampsia	2.2–5.0	1.2 (0.3–4.2); 1.7 (1.2–2.5)*
Prolonged 3rd stage	3.5–7.6	
Prolonged 2nd stage (>20 min)	2.9–5.5	
Prolonged active phase	2.4–4.4	
Episiotomy	1.6–4.7	2.1 (1.4–3.1)
Maternal age >35	3.0	1.4 (1.0–2.0)
General anesthesia	3.0	
Obesity	3.1	1.6 (1.2–2.2)
Chorioamnionitis	2.7	
Prior cesarean section	2.7	
Forceps or vacuum extractor	1.7	
Multiparity	1.5	1.1 (0.6–2.1)
Ethnicity Native American Hispanic Asian	6.4 1.7–1.8 1.7	
Placental abruption	–	12.6 (7.6–20.9)
Placenta previa	–	13.1 (7.5–23.0)
Retained placenta	–	5.2 (3.4–7.9)
Labor >12 h	–	2.0 (1.4–2.9)
Pyrexia in labor >38°C	–	2.0 (1.03–4.0)
Birth weight >4 kg	–	1.9 (1.4–2.6)
Labor induction	–	1.7 (1.7–3.0)

*Pregnancy-induced hypertension without proteinuria
Source: References 13–17

Prostaglandins (PG) are superior to other oxytocic drugs for preventing PPH and its role in preventing PPH has been studied extensively.[19,20] Several studies are published which compare the effectiveness of PG with other oxytocics and also injectable PG with rectal PG. There was notable reduction in the duration of third stage with PG and also the lesser incidence of severe PPH (>1,000 mL blood loss). PGs are associated with mild but frequent adverse effects. One study demonstrated coronary artery spasm and MI, which led to the stoppage of trial by their supplier. Other study compared the benefits of injectable form of PG with respect to its higher cost, requirement of refrigeration and their safety.

TABLE 2: Mode of delivery and risk of postpartum hemorrhage (PPH) of ≥1,000 mL.

Mode of delivery	Relative risk of PPH (99% CI)
Emergency cesarean section	
vs. elective	2.2 (1.4–3.5)
vs. operative vaginal delivery	3.7 (2.5–5.4)
vs. spontaneous vaginal delivery	8.8 (6.74–11.6)
Elective cesarean section	
vs. operative vaginal delivery	1.7 (0.98–2.8)
vs. spontaneous vaginal delivery	3.9 (2.5–6.2)
Operative vaginal delivery	
vs. spontaneous delivery	2.4 (1.6–3.5)

(CI: confidence interval)
Source: Stones RW, Paterson CM, Saunders NJ. Risk-factors for major obstetric haemorrhage. Eur J Obstet Gynecol Reprod Biol. 1993;48:15-8.

Rectal and oral administration of PG is significantly cheaper than injectable form of PG and also does not require any refrigeration, thus making it a probable alternative to other oxytocics in resource poor countries. It has been demonstrated that the decrease in blood loss and PPH rates with oral and rectal misoprostol were similar to other oxytocics and lesser than the placebo.[19,21-24] Further clinical trials are needed for confirmation of this findings for implementation of misoprostol in routine management of third stage of labor.

Carbetocin, a new oxytocin analog, has a greater biological effect and longer and sustained half-life than oxytocin. It is also more heat stable, with obvious advantage in resource poor situations. A single dose of 100 µg (1 mL) of carbetocin injection should be administered intravenously as a bolus injection, slowly over 1 minute after delivery of the baby. It can be administered either before or after the delivery of placenta. It is costlier than oxytocin, and hence, it is recommended currently for prevention of PPH after cesarean delivery. The side effect profile is similar to oxytocin, and has lesser diuretic effects.[25] A large trial of this drug in collaboration with WHO has recently concluded in India, and it is likely to be made available soon.

Treating Excessive Bleeding

For the successful management of PPH, treatment plan must be well understood and put into action immediately by the team members of labor ward. Management plan includes three parallel pathways:
1. Resuscitation
2. Differential diagnosis of underlying cause
3. Initial management targeted to most common cause of PPH.

The resuscitation starts with establishment of two large bore (16–18G) IV lines for crystalloids and/or colloids, and insertion of indwelling Foley's catheter to evacuate the bladder and to monitor urine output. Clinical status of clotting system should be done by observing spontaneous bleeding site and evaluating clotting by tapping of test tube with patient's blood for 5 minutes. Regarding the superiority of crystalloids over colloids is still debateable.[26] With colloids, larger expansion of intravascular volume is achieved compared to crystalloids, but it may cause anaphylactic reactions, interfere with cross matching of blood (Dextran) and may lead to prolonged partial thromboplastin time (Hetastarch).[27,28] The studies have shown that resuscitation with the colloids has not been associated with improved survival rate compared to crystalloids in women with hypovolemic shock. Transfusion of packed RBC (PRBC), fresh frozen plasma (FFP) and cryoprecipitate must be given in cases of prolonged bleeding and severe PPH after evaluating clotting status, invasive and/or noninvasive testing.

The blood loss is often underestimated and imprecise and thus making it vital for monitoring of hemodynamic status in cases of PPH and it also provides an effective measure regarding the respond to resuscitation. However, it is also necessary to know the limitations of methods that are available for monitoring. As the blood pressure may remain normal till the loss of blood volume by 30–40%, it is insensitive method for monitoring and it may remain falsely low on measuring by arm cuff.[27] Significant hypovolemia in patients requires the monitoring by intra-arterial recording.

Other methods of invasive monitoring include the measurement of cardiac filling pressure by either pulmonary capillary wedge pressure or central venous pressure. When the blood loss is <30%, there is poor correlation with invasive monitoring. The sensitivity of cardiac filling pressures can be improved by carrying out orthostatic manuevers.[29]

Apart from volume resuscitation in management of cases of PPH, both the differential diagnosis and primary treatment are important. These include the number of steps which are targeted at ruling out the probable causes of PPH which may vary among the different centers **(Flowchart 1)**.

If the clinical examination suggests uterine inversion, it should be reposited back. Several methods for uterine inversion management are in literature and a large review has been published recently.[30] Further evaluation in the steps of management of PPH is by excluding the uterine atony by palpating the firmness of uterine fundus as atonic PPH is responsible for 90% cases. Evacuation of bladder and oxytocic drugs should be administered after the failure of uterine massage.

Over last few decades, some very potent uterine ecbolics have been added to our armamentarium, making an obstetrician's life very easy. Oxytocin, Ergometrine and Prostaglandins are all good quality uterine stimulants and help significantly in treating as well as preventing the atony of uterus. The mantra should be to anticipate atonic PPH in conditions such as multiple pregnancies, accidental hemorrhage, prolonged and/or induced labors, precipitate labors, grand multipara, etc. All experienced obstetricians would agree that half of the PPH cases are the ones where it was least expected.

There are no contraindications for oxytocin and it should be given as infusion in 1 L of normal saline (10–40 U/L, up to 500 mL in 10 minutes) which is effective in majority of cases.

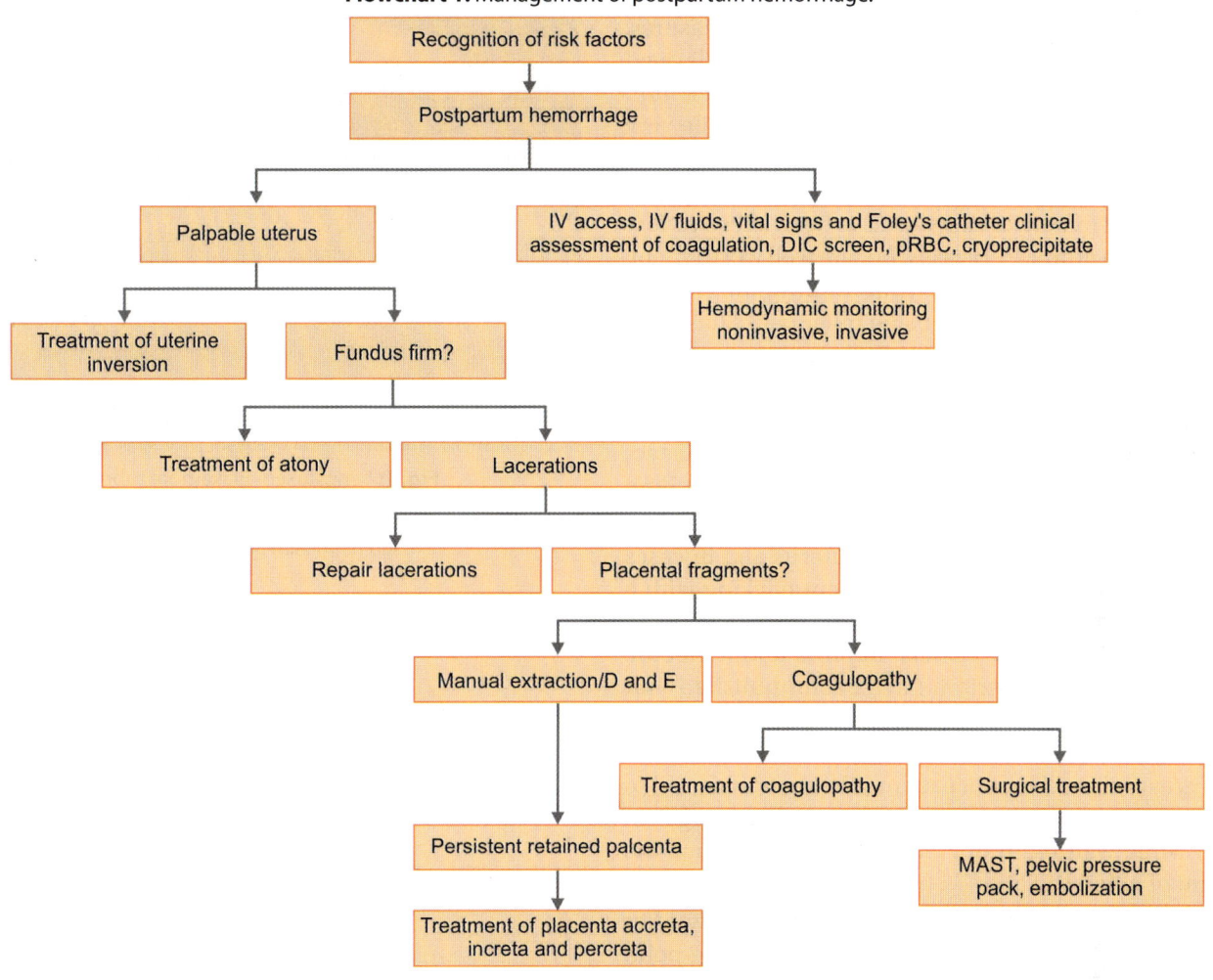

Flowchart 1: Management of postpartum hemorrhage.

There is significant risk of water intoxication with the greater doses of oxytocin due to its antidiuretic effect. However, the small dosage of 5 IU of IV oxytocin bolus leads to maternal hypotension which may lead to further worsening of PPH in patients.[28,31-33]

The next step in management of atonic PPH is 0.2 mg of Ergometrine (IM or IV or intramyometrial injection) and it can be repeated every 2–4 hours. The IV administration of Ergometrine should be used with caution as it has been attributed to greater risk of stroke and hypertension and intravenous administration is not recommended. Hypertension, asthma and Raynaud's syndrome are contraindications for ergometrine administration.[34]

Prostaglandins are the last modality of medical management in cases of persistent bleeding in PPH.[35] The dosage of Carboprost (PGF2α) is 250 μg IM or intramyometrium every 15 minutes and can be repeated up to 8 times. In a study in literature, 86% patients ($n = 44$) responded to carboprost which are unresponsive to other measures, and out of 14% ($n = 7$) non-responders to PG, 7.8% ($n = 4$) were having chorioamnionitis.[36] Nausea, vomiting, fever, chills and diarrhea are the frequent side effects of carboprost and can also cause pulmonary vasoconstriction, bronchospasm, arterial oxygen desaturation and hyper or hypotension. Hence, carboprost should be used cautiously in cases of renal disorders and bronchospasm as well as in cases with arterial or pulmonary hypertension.

Prostaglandin E (PGE) analogs have been successful in effective treatment of PPH and it is also effective in pessaries form inserted into uterus.[37] Recent study in literature demonstrates that the 1000 μg of PGE1 (misoprost) administered rectally are effective in controlling bleeding in patients not responding to oxytocin and ergometrine.[38-40] Further studies are needed for evaluating the efficacy and safety of this drug in management of PPH.

THE SURGICAL MANAGEMENT OF POSTPARTUM HEMORRHAGE

The surgical management of PPH is not a measure of first choice, but surgery can be life-saving. This entails that all obstetricians have the requisite skills to deal with this urgent situation, almost always in trying conditions.

There are some mechanical measures that help one tide over the time to prepare for surgery. The elevation of uterus high up in abdomen by putting a whole fist in the vagina leads to angulation and kinking of uterine vessels. This may be achieved to a little extent by pressing the lateral fornix with a swab on a holder. This diminishes the blood flow to the uterus and gains precious seconds for other measures. Compression, anteversion and massaging over this elevated uterus may bring in contractions of the myometrium. Douching with warm water, although claimed to be very effective by few colleagues, has not proved as effective in personal experience. Packing the uterine cavity with gauze, roller pack and inflatable balloons have been effective very occasionally in atonic PPH cases, but are well worth trying as a preliminary measure or while waiting for surgical intervention. Uterine packing using miler packs has been reported to control PPH. Bakri balloon is tamponade devices with promising results in controlling PPH. This has to be inflated with up to 500 mL of normal saline and left inside uterine cavity for 24 hours. Then it is slowly deflated. Foley's catheter, Sengstaken-Blakemore tube or condom catheter can also be used in place of Bakri balloon **(Fig. 1)**.[41]

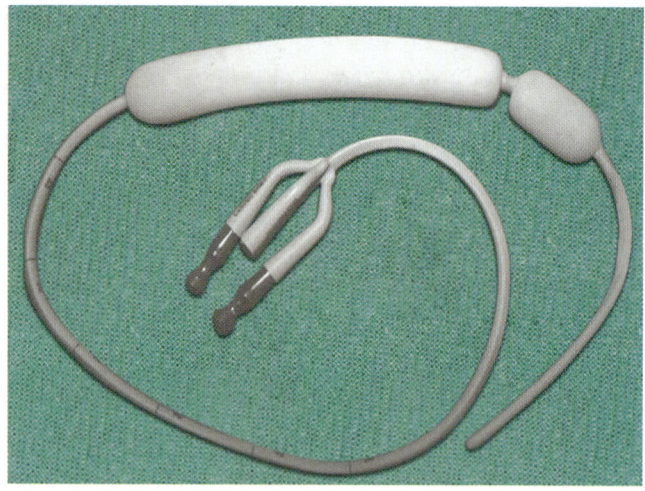

Fig. 1: Sengstaken–Blakemore tube

Packing works well in Couvelaire uterus and in cases of placenta previa where lower segment packing with a couple of mops at cesarean section helps the clogging and occlusion of these large vessels. Reports about electric stimulations of myometrium have been published, but seem to be a desperate measure. Military antishock trousers (MAST) can divert the blood to vital organs and are of great value when the patient is being transferred to other location. Even direct compression of aorta against spine, while waiting in operating room can reduce the amount of blood lost.

In cases of secondary PPH from pelvic cavity after hysterectomy, we do not find any specific bleeding point to ligate or cauterize. There is a general oozing from the entire pelvic bed and one is at his wits end to manage these occasional but very difficult cases. The Umbrella Pack (more famously known as Logo Pack from its inventor's name—Logothetopulos[42]) can be life-saving. A review of literature from 1985–2000 revealed nine cases successfully treated out of 10 attempted with Logo pack.

Dr VN Purandare from Mumbai has developed an indigenous technique based on the principles of Logo pack, wherein he used a couple of condoms filled with 1.5 L of warm saline **(Fig. 2)**. He used a metal ring at vulva and the fluid filled condoms are fixed by the ring to maintain pressure on the pelvic walls. This technique is quite effective as we have witnessed personally, in a bad case of protracted PPH and surprisingly inexpensive!

In cases of post-hysterectomy when bleeding cannot be controlled by conventional measures and when specific bleeders cannot be caught pelvic pressure packing is done by placing a large pressure pack in pelvic cavity through the vagina. Though effective, this technique should be used as a last resort as it is associated with high mortality.[39]

Postpartum hemorrhage in a firm, contracted uterus raises suspicious of hemorrhage due to trauma such as genital tract laceration traumatic PPH is a second most common cause of PPH. The entire genital tract is to be inspected and examined for hematomas or any other sign of trauma. Sometimes, the degree of hemodynamics collapse is more than the amount of visible blood loss. It can be due to internal hemorrhage, broad ligament hematoma or retroperitoneal hematoma. Such condition requires laparotomy for exploration or sometimes, embolization as an alternative method.

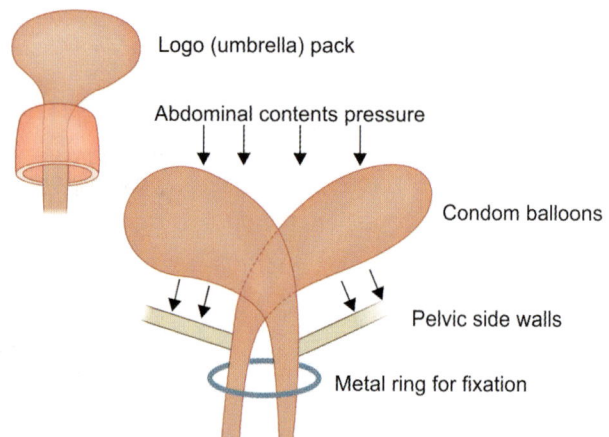

Fig. 2: Purandare's system.

When atonic PPH and traumatic PPH have been ruled out, retained placental tissue or adherent placenta might be causing PPH when retained placental tissues are diagnosed by ultrasonography or expelled placenta is missing some of its cotyledon, manual exploration or curettage will prove to be of benefit as the bleeding will stop and uterus will contract. In case when bleeding continues even after this steps, placenta accreta, increta or percreta suspected and surgical intervention is required. Usually hysterectomy is indicated in cases with average blood of 4 liters. Conservative surgical approach – manual removal of placenta with packing or oversewing the bleeding site can be attempted. But it is associated with high mortality and morbidity.

Large amount of blood loss cause consumption of clotting factors and thus leading to acquired coagulopathy. In a study of 70 cases of postpartum hysterectomy, 43%

were due uterine atony, 30% due placenta accreta and 13% due uterine rupture and 10% were as result of extension of uterine incision during lower segment cesarean section.[40] A similar study at Ahmedabad revealed a slightly different proportion – having higher number of cases of uterine ruptures compared to placenta accreta (**Fig. 3**). These studies were reported two decades ago and medical treatment of uterine atony today may be more successful.

The technique of obstetric hysterectomy is slightly different than a conventional hysterectomy. One is generally in haste and the anesthetist is breathing down one's neck. The quick thing to do is to employ clamp cut and drop technique. At least 5–6 good quality, heavy Kocher's clamps should be on the trolley when we start the surgery. Rather than wasting precious moments in tying the clamps, one should keep on putting clamps, cutting the pedicle and applying the next clamp, till the uterine vessels are clamped. Only then should one attend to tying these clamps. A subtotal hysterectomy should be seriously considered when reaching the lower part of cervix is difficult, or when the margins of cervix and vagina are blurred.

A hysterectomy is a last resort procedure to save the life of a woman, and whenever fertility preservation is required, conservative procedures such as uterine artery ligation and uterine compression sutures (surgical tamponade) should be employed as far as possible.

Ligation of Uterine Arteries

Bilateral uterine artery ligation is performed 2–3 cm below the uterine incision for cesarean section, by passing the single suture through lateral myometrial wall of uterus. The stitch would go from anterior surface of lateral wall of uterus to the posterior wall behind the broad ligament. A finger guard here is imperative to avoid inadvertent pricking of intestines with the needle. The needle is brought back through avascular area of the broad ligament to the front and is then ligated with the free end. This will compress the uterine vessels against the lateral uterine wall and would avoid avulsion of small branches if it is attempted in the broad ligament alone. If performed at the time of cesarean section, two stitches—one above the scar and one below the scar—are required. One study of 265 patients has reported only 10 failures (3–7% failure rate).[43] Thus, proving its efficacy, the safety of bilateral uterine artery ligation can be proved by regular menstruation after procedure and post-surgery successful pregnancy.[44]

Dr Ajit Rawal (personal communication) has improvised this technique to avoid taking needle to the posterior aspect during cesarean section cases. He recommends that by pulling on to the lateral angle of the CS scar, the uterine vessels can be brought forward and then can be ligated through the uterine cavity.

Uterine Artery Ligation (O'Leary Method and Ajit Rawal Method) (Figs. 4A and B)

Generally, the ovarian arteries also need to be ligated to cut off the collateral blood supply and arrest the bleeding. This is done at the junction of ovarian ligament and ovary. The vessel at this level, even if ligated has given off the blood supply to the fallopian tube and the ovary. By lifting the ovarian ligament by a Babcock forceps one can isolate the mesovarium and the vessel can be clamped and ligated easily. The bilateral procedure takes hardly 10 minutes.

Ovarian Artery Ligation

A stepwise uterine devascularization technique has also been reported. It involves a sequential ligation of uterine and ovarian arteries on both the sides of uterus (**Fig. 5**). To start with, unilateral uterine ligation, followed by bilateral uterine vessel ligation, followed by low bilateral uterine vessel ligation after mobilization of the bladder, and unilateral or bilateral ovarian vessel ligation is performed. In one study, this technique succeeded in at least 80% of cases and has resulted in normal menstruation and pregnancy.[45]

Uterine devascularization is a stepwise technique involving sequential ligation of uterine and ovarian arteries on both sides of uterus. Success rate of 80% has been recorded with normal menstruation and pregnancy post-procedure.

Obstetricians are generally reluctant to opt for a laparotomy to control atonic bleeding in cases of vaginal delivery. The analysis of our own institute showed that 75% of vessel ligation was done at CS although the rate of vaginal deliveries was 75%!

These underscores both the facts that the incidence of PPH is higher at CS compared to vaginal delivery, and also that the decision to ligate is easy as no special consent, and the necessary explanations to the patient are needed! Under such situations a novel technique of vaginal uterine artery ligation described by Swiss group is quite a useful option. The initial report showed success in 12 out of 13 attempted cases.[46] In this technique both the lips of cervix are held firmly by a swab holder. The bladder is dissected away by cutting the anterior pouch of vagina. A retractor

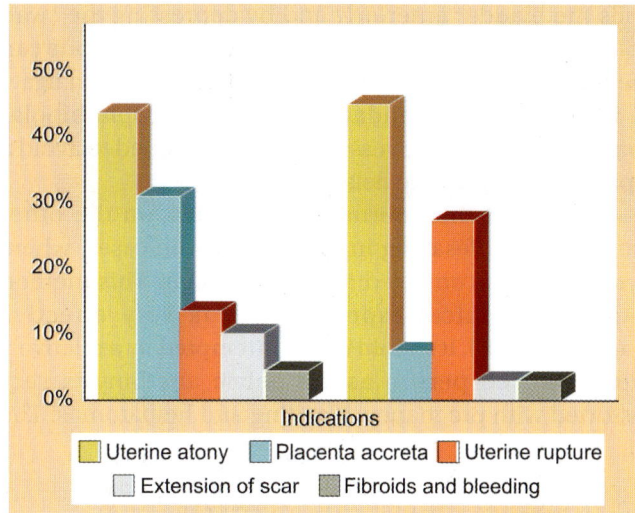

Fig. 3: Etiology of postpartum hemorrhage.
Courtesy: Dr NM Patel, VS Hospital.

pulls the bladder anteriorly and by depressing the swab holder and pulling the cervix to the opposite side one can see the angle of uterine artery under vision one can ligate it. In protracted secondary PPH, laparoscopic bipolar coagulation of uterine vessels can be attempted to avoid a laparotomy to manage delayed PPH.

Ligation of the internal iliac arteries, on the other hand, can be lifesaving in some desperate cases, where hysterectomy is objected to by the patient. This method requires technical expertise, but is very effective **(Figs. 6A and B)**. It should not be attempted by a relatively inexperienced person as the pelvic anatomy is very distorted with pregnancy, bleeding and hematomas. The pressure of doing it quickly in a critical patient is likely to result in a serious complication. The complications we have witnessed each of these complications on more than one occasions, usually they were made by the non-gynecology colleagues unaware of the effects of pregnancy in the pelvis and the bubbling greenhorns in the profession!

Classically, ligation is performed by opening the posterior leaf of broad ligament lateral to the ureter near the bifurcation of common iliac arteries. The internal iliac artery is skeletonized by sharp cutting of fascia covering the vessel. This will produce a cleavage between the artery and the vein. A right angle artery (Mixter forceps) or an aneurism needles then passed around the artery and the silk suture is tied twice around the vessel **(Figs. 7A and B)**. Two stitches will ensure the accidental loosening of the single stitch due to pulsatile pressure in the artery.

Uterine Compression Techniques

Hemostatic multiple square sutures technique for uterine bleeding during cesarean section described by Cho et al. from Korea is very simple **(Fig. 8)**. Cho sutures are large box type sutures that control PPH by compressing the anterior wall to the posterior wall of uterus. This technique has proven to be successful and hysterectomy has been avoided in 23 women with severe PPH in cesarean delivery. Normal menstruation was reported to have resumed in 100% and 4% achieved further pregnancies.[47]

B-Lynch suture is another technique in which large suture is taken compressing the whole body of uterus. B-Lynch has reported its efficacy in five cases **(Fig. 9)**.[48] This technique looks quite fantastic as outlined, but is likely to fail as we have gathered from personal communication from colleagues, and incidentally, the average blood units required in the original report was eight per patient persists after hysterectomy, and in cases of genital tract lacerations.[49,50]

Uterine artery embolization has shown great potential in avoiding the relatively complicated surgery at critical juncture **(Fig. 10)**. Developed initially to treat fibroids, it has been successfully used to arrest the PPH. This technique is helpful if bleeding persists after hysterectomy or in cases of genital tract laceration also UAE can be used as an alternative to nonconserving surgery-hysterectomy. The concept is quite

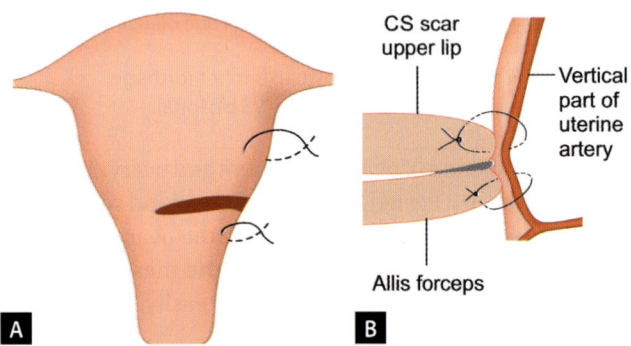

Figs. 4A and B: Uterine artery ligation.
(A) O'Leary method; (B) Ajit Rawal Method.

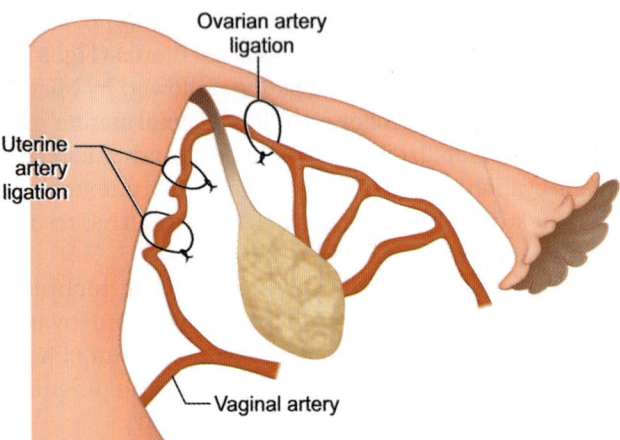

Fig. 5: Ovarian artery ligation.

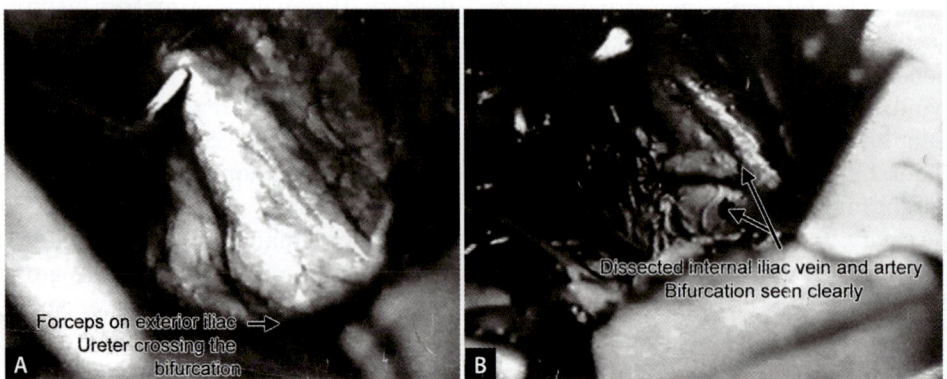

Figs. 6A and B: Anatomy and dissection of internal iliac artery.

SECTION 10: Postpartum Issues: Maternal and Neonatal 649

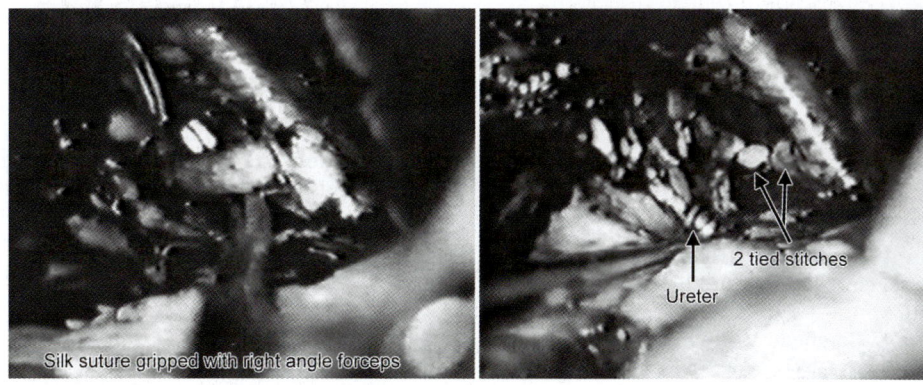

Figs. 7A and B: Ligation of internal iliac artery.

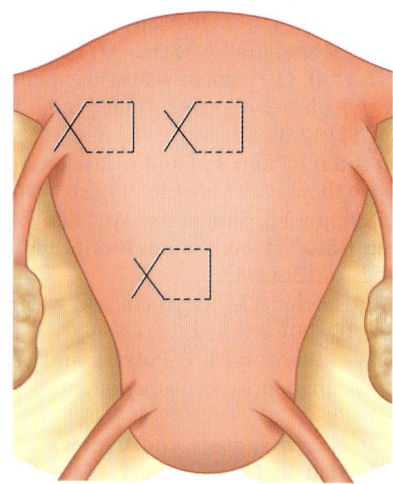

Fig. 8: Cho technique of box stitches.

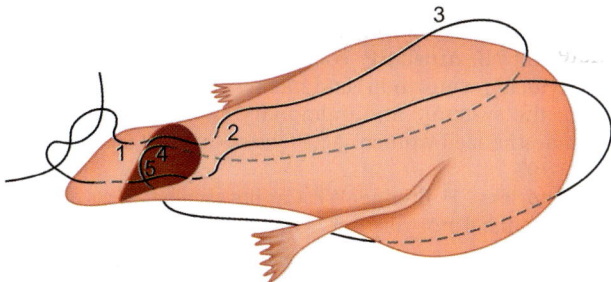

Fig. 9: B-Lynch suture: Brace suturing of uterus.

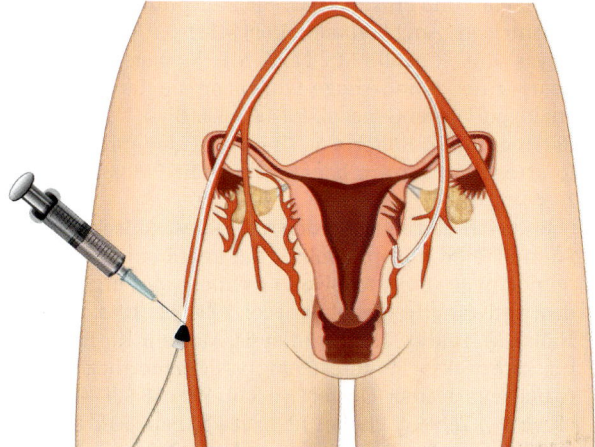

Fig. 10: Retrograde uterine artery embolization.

simple, but the procedure is in relatively early stage and we shall know more in times to come. We use the retrograde femoral artery catheter enter the internal iliac and inject the occlusion particles at the origin of uterine artery. Gelatin foam and polyvinyl alcohol particles (size 150–250 and 300–600) are used with an idea that this will occlude the larger arterioles of myometrium bring about cessation of bleeding, without affecting the tissue perfusion through capillaries and smaller vessels.

Several tertiary care centers have reported promising results with UAE.[51-54] Immediate cessation of bleeding was observed in all cases in a study involving 35 patients—25 with primary and 10 with secondary PPH (2.8%). Only in one patient, a delayed hysterectomy was required.[51] Although results regarding efficacy and safety are awaited, findings obtained are quite promising.

A major concern here is that if the particles used are of smaller size, they may occlude the microcirculation and result in necrosis of the tissues. Recent reports of complete uterine necrosis after arterial embolization for PPH have tempered the initial enthusiasm generated.

Uterine artery embolization is not practical for primary massive hemorrhage for organizational reasons. The patient needs to be shifted to the radiology department where the units are generally installed. Availability of skilled imaging personnel round the clock is another limitation. This procedure is a good option in cases of protracted primary PPH and in cases of secondary PPH in hospitals where facilities are available, but may not cater to a mass of PPH cases due to obvious limitations. The pregnancy after uterine artery embolization is regarded as high-risk pregnancy as revealed by a recent analysis of 50 such cases.

■ CONCLUSION

We reiterate that PPH is a major complication that all obstetricians dread to handle. With good uterine ecbolic medicines available a sense of complacency and ill found confidence is noticed especially among the inexperienced colleagues. One needs to ensure adequate stocks of these medicines while conducting any delivery. An attitude of anticipation in high-risk cases may improve the quickness of medical response in event of PPH. All obstetricians should be well-versed in the basic skills for the surgery of uterine artery ligation and obstetric hysterectomy. All referral hospitals should have at least one experienced and skilled person available to undertake internal iliac artery ligation when needed.

■ REFERENCES

1. Cottier JP, Fignon A, Tranquart F, Herbreteau D. Uterine necrosis after arterial embolization for PPH. Obstet Gynecol. 2002;100(5 Pt 2):1074-7.
2. Goldberg J, Pereira L, Berghella V. Pregnancy after uterine artery embolization: an analysis of 50 cases. Obstet Gynecol. 2002;100(5 Pt 1):869-72.
3. Ueland K. Maternal cardiovascular dynamics. VII. Intrapartum blood volume changes. Am J Obstet Gynecol. 1976;126: 671-7.
4. Pritchard JA, Baldwin RM, Dickey JC, Wiggins KM. Blood volume changes in pregnancy and puerperium and Red blood cell loss and changes in apparent blood volume during and following vaginal delivery, cesarean section, and cesarean section plus hysterectomy. Am J Obstet Gynecol. 1962;84:1271-82.
5. Cordts PR, LaMorte WW, Fisher JB, DelGuercio C, Niehoff J, Pivacek LE, et al. Poor predictive value of hematocrit and hemodynamic parameters for erythrocyte deficits after extensive elective vascular operations. Surg Gynecol Obstet. 1992;175:243-8.
6. Stamler KD. Effect of crystalloid infusion on hematocrit in nonbleeding patients, with applications to clinical traumatology. Ann Emerg Med. 1989;18:747-9.
7. Mark SP, Croughan-Minihane MS, Kilpatrick SJ. Chorioamnionitis and uterine function. Obstet Gynecol. 2000;95:909-12.
8. Stones RW, Paterson CM, Saunders NJ. Risk-factors for major obstetric haemorrhage. Eur J Obstet Gynecol Reprod Biol. 1993;48:15-8.
9. Kadir RA, Economides DL, Braithwaite J, Goldman E, Lee CA. The obstetric experience of carriers of haemophilia. Br J Obstet Gynaecol. 1997;104:803-10.
10. Kadir RA. Women and inherited bleeding disorders: pregnancy and delivery. Semin Hematol. 1999;36:28-35.
11. Briet E, Reisner BM, Blatt PM. Factor IX levels during pregnancy in a women with hemophilia B. Haemostasis. 1982;11:87-9.
12. Kadir RA, Lee CA, Sabin CA, Pollard D, Economides DL. Pregnancy in women with von Willebrand's disease or factor XI deficiency. Br J Obstet Gynaecol. 1998;105:314-21.
13. Combs CA, Murphy EL, Laros RK Jr. Factors associated with postpartum hemorrhage with vaginal birth. Obstet Gynecol. 1991;77:69-76.
14. Combs CA, Murphy EL, Laros RK Jr. Factors associated with hemorrhage in cesarean deliveries. Obstet Gynecol. 1991;77:77-82.
15. Tsu VD. Postpartum haemorrhage in Zimbabwe: a risk factor analysis. Br J Obstet Gynaecol. 1993;100:327-33.
16. Naef RW 3rd, Chauhan SP, Chevalier SP, Weber BM, Martin RW, Morrison JC. Prediction of hemorrhage at cesarean delivery. Obstet Gynecol. 1994;83:923-6.
17. Selo-Ojeme DO, Okonofua FE. Risk factors for primary postpartum haemorrhage. A case control study. Arch Gynecol Obstet. 1997;259:179-87.
18. Prendiville WJ, Elbourne D, McDonald S. Active versus expectant management in the third stage of labour. Cochrane Database Syst Rev. 2000;(3):CD000007.
19. Gulmezoglu AM, Forna F, Villar J, Hofmeyr GJ. Prostaglandins for prevention of postpartum haemorrhage (Cochrane Review). Cochrane Database Syst Rev. 2002;(3):CD000494.
20. McDonald S, Prendiville WJ, Elbourne D. Prophylactic syntometrine versus oxytocin for delivery of the placenta. Cochrane Database Syst Rev. 2000;(2):CD000201.
21. Amant F, Spitz B, Timmerman D, Corremans A, Van Assche FA. Misoprostol compared with methylergometrine for the prevention of postpartum haemorrhage: a double-blind randomised trial. Br J Obstet Gynaecol. 1999;106:1066-70.
22. Bamigboye AA, Merrell DA, Hofmeyr GJ, Mitchell R. Randomized comparison of rectal misoprostol with Syntometrine for management of third stage of labor. Acta Obstet Gynecol Scand. 1998;77:178-81.
23. Bamigboye AA, Hofmeyr GJ, Merrell DA. Rectal misoprostol in the prevention of postpartum hemorrhage: a placebo-controlled trial. Am J Obstet Gynecol 1998;179:1043-6.
24. el-Refaey H, O'Brien P, Morafa W, Walder J, Rodeck C. Use of oral misoprostol in the prevention of postpartum haemorrhage. Br J Obstet Gynaecol. 1997;104:336-9.
25. Larcipret G, Montagnoli C, Frigo M, Panetta V, Todde C, Zuppani B, et al. Carbetocin versus oxytocin in caesarean section with high risk of post-partum haemorrhage. J Prenat Med. 2013;7(1):12-8.
26. Falk JL, O'Brien JF, Kerr R. Fluid resuscitation in traumatic hemorrhagic shock. Crit Care Clin. 1992;8:323-40.
27. Shippy CR, Appel PL, Shoemaker WC. Reliability of clinical monitoring to assess blood volume in critically ill patients. Crit Care Med. 1984;12:107-12.
28. Whalley PJ, Pritchard JA. Oxytocin and water intoxication. JAMA. 1963;186:601-3.
29. Amoroso P, Greenwood RN. Posture and central venous, pressure measurement in circulatory volume depletion. Lancet. 1989;2:258-60.
30. Kochenour NK. Diagnosis and management of uterine inversion. In: Hankins GDV, Gilstrap LC, Cunningham FG (Eds). Operative Obstetrics. Norwalk: Appleton and Lange; 1995. pp. 273-81.
31. Eggers TP, Fliegner JR. Water intoxication and Syntocinon infusion. Aust N Z J Obstet Gynaecol. 1979;19:59-60.
32. Secher NJ, Arnsbo P, Wallin L. Haemodynamic effects of oxytocin (syntocinon) and methyl ergometrine (methergin) on the systemic and pulmonary circulations of pregnant anaesthetized women. Acta Obstet Gynecol Scand. 1978;57: 97-103.
33. Hendricks CH, Brenner WE. Cardiovascular effects of oxytocic drugs used postpartum. Am J Obstet Gynecol. 1970;108: 751-60.
34. Browning DJ. Serious side effects of ergometrine and its use in routine obstetric practice. Med J Aust. 1974;1:957-9.
35. Buttino L Jr, Garite TS. The use of 15 methyl F2 alpha prostaglandin (Prostin 15M) for the control of postpartum hemorrhage. Am J Perinatol. 1986;3:241-3.
36. Hayashi RH, Castillo MS, Noah ML. Management of severe postpartum hemorrhage-with a prostaglandin F2 alpha analogue. Obstet Gynecol. 1984;63:806-8.
37. Barrington JW, Roberts A. The use of gemeprost pessaries, to arrest postpartum haemorrhage. Br J Obstet Gynaecol. 1993;100:691-2.
38. O'Brien P, El-Refaey H, Gordon A, Geary M, Rodeck CH. Rectally administered misoprostol for the treatment of postpartum hemorrhage unresponsive to oxytocin and ergometrine: a descriptive study. Obstet Gynecol. 1998;92:212-4.
39. Hallak M, Dildy GA 3rd, Hurley TJ, Moise Jr KJ. Transvaginal pressure pack for life-threatening pelvic hemorrhage secondary to placenta accreta. Obstet Gynecol. 1991;78:938-40.
40. Clark SL, Yeh SY, Phelan JP, Bruce S, Paul RH. Emergency hysterectomy for obstetric hemorrhage. Obstet Gynecol. 1984; 64:376-80.

41. Katesmark M, Brown F, Raju KS. Successful use of a Sengstaken-Blakemore tube to control massive postpartum haemorrhage. Br J Obstet Gynaecol. 1994;101:259-60.
42. Logothetopulos K. Eine absolut sichere blutstillungsmethode bei vaginalen und abdominalen gynakologischen operationen. [An absolutely certain method of stopping bleeding during abdominal and vaginal operations.] Zentralbl Gynakol. 1926;50:3202-4.
43. O'Leary JL, O'Leary JA. Uterine artery ligation for control of postcesarean section hemorrhage. Obstet Gynecol. 1974;43:849-53.
44. O'Leary JA. Pregnancy following uterine artery ligation. Obstet Gynecol. 1980;55:112-3.
45. AbdRabbo SA. Stepwise uterine devascularization: a novel technique for management of uncontrolled postpartum hemorrhage with preservation of the uterus. Am J Obstet Gynecol. 1994;171:694-700.
46. Hebisch G, Huch A. Vaginal Uterine Artery Ligation, University Hospital, Zurich. Obstet Gynecol. 2002;100(3):574-8.
47. Chou YC, Wang PH, Yuan CC, Yen YK, Liu WM. Laparoscopic bipolar coagulation of uterine vessels to manage delayed postpartum hemorrhage. J Am Assoc Gynecol Laparosc. 2002;9(4):541-4.
48. Cho JH, Jun HS, Lee CN. Hemostatic suturing technique for uterine bleeding during cesarean delivery. Obstet Gynecol. 2000;96:129-31.
49. B-Lynch C, Coker A, Lawal AH, Abu J, Cowen MJ. The B-Lynch surgical technique for the control of massive postpartum haemorrhage: an alternative to hysterectomy? Five cases reported. Br J Obstet Gynaecol. 1997;104:372-5.
50. Nizard J, Barrinque L, Frydman R, Fernandez H. Fertility and pregnancy outcomes following hypogastric artery ligation for severe post-partum haemorrhage. Hum Reprod. 2003 Apr;18(4):844-8.`
51. Pelage JP, Le Dref O, Jacob D, Soyer P, Herbreteau D, Rymer R. Selective arterial embolization of the uterine arteries in the management of intractable postpartum hemorrhage. Acta Obstet Gynecol Scand. 1999;78:698-703.
52. Pelage JP, Soyer P, Repiquet D, Herbreteau D, Le Dref O, Houdart E, et al. Secondary postpartum hemorrhage: treatment with selective arterial embolization. Radiology. 1999;212:385-9.
53. Merland JJ, Houdart E, Herbreteau D, Trystram D, Ledref O, Aymard A, et al. Place of emergency arterial embolisation in obstetric haemorrhage about 16 personal cases. Eur J Obstet Gynecol Reprod Biol. 1996;65:141-3.
54. Hansch E, Chitkara U, McAlpine J, El-Sayed Y, Dake MD, Razavi MK. Pelvic arterial embolization for control of obstetric hemorrhage: a five-year experience. Am J Obstet Gynecol. 1999;180:1454-60.

LONG QUESTIONS

1. Define postpartum hemorrhage. What are the major causes of postpartum hemorrhage? How will you manage a case of atonic PPH?
2. Describe conservative surgical management of postpartum hemorrhage.
3. Discuss preventive strategies for reducing maternal mortality due to postpartum hemorrhage.

SHORT QUESTIONS

1. What are the important risk factors for PPH ?
2. Short note on Carbetocin.
3. Discuss AMTSL.
4. Role of uterine artery embolization in management of PPH.
5. Short note on obstetric hysterectomy.

MULTIPLE CHOICE QUESTIONS

1. Uterine artery blood flow at term is:
   a. 300 mL/min	b. 200 mL/min
   c. 400 mL/min	d. 700 mL/min
2. All are uterine compression or brace sutures, except:
   a. B Lynch	b. Hayman
   c. Cho	d. Worms
3. All can be used for prevention of PPH as per WHO guideline, except:
   a. Misoprostol
   b. Combination of oxytocin and ergometrine
   c. Carbetocin
   d. Prostaglandin F 2 alpha (Carboprost)
4. Uterine artery is a branch of:
   a. Anterior division of internal iliac artery
   b. Posterior division of internal iliac artery
   c. External iliac artery
   d. Abdominal aorta
5. The most common type of shock in uterine inversion is:
   a. Hypovolemic
   b. Septic
   c. Neurogenic
   d. Hypovolemic and neurogenic
6. Suture materials used for brace sutures are all, except:
   a. Catgut
   b. Vicryl (Polyglactin 910)
   c. Monocryl (Poliglecaprone 25)
   d. Prolene (Polypropelene)
7. Maximum dose of injection ergometrine (0.2 mg) for treatment of PPH is:
   a. 3 doses	b. 4 doses
   c. 5 doses	d. 8 doses
8. Carbetocin dose for prophylaxis of PPH is:
   a. 100 µg IM	b. 50 µg IV
   c. 150 µg IV	d. 250 µg IM
9. All are done in massive PPH, except:
   a. Hysterectomy
   b. Thermal endometrial ablation
   c. Internal iliac A. ligation
   d. Balloon tamponade
10. AMTSL includes all, except:
    a. Early cord clamping	b. Controlled cord traction
    c. Oxytocin 10 IU I/IM	d. Delayed cord clamping

Answers									
1. d	2. d	3. d	4. a	5. d	6. d
7. c	8. a	9. b	10. a		

10.4 OBSTETRIC HYSTERECTOMY

Ajit C Rawal, Janki Pandya

INTRODUCTION

Obstetric hysterectomy is a procedure devised around a century back, as a surgical attempt to manage life-threatening obstetric hemorrhage and infection. This operation has its champions and critics since its inception. Eduardo Porro documented the first case of cesarean hysterectomy with patient survival in 1876. Godson [who pioneered the lower segment incision for cesarean section (LSCS)] and Lawson Tait introduced further refinements of the procedure which improved survival of mothers.

Does it have any role in modern obstetrics? Yes, it does have a major life-saving role even today as a terminal step, in cases where obstetric hemorrhage is not controlled with all other measures. Continuous respect has been given to this procedure over these many years, looking at it as a terminal solution for dealing with the most challenging obstetric problems. It is a well-recognized surgical procedure, with a limited set of indications. All obstetricians should be well versed with obstetric hysterectomy, as it may be the only option left, and may make a difference between life and death. Improved surgical skills and back up in form of availability of blood products, have contributed significantly toward reducing morbidity and mortality.

OBSTETRIC HYSTERECTOMY: POSTOPERATIVE PROBLEMS

Every surgical procedure comes with a set of possible postsurgical problems that may arise. Patient who undergoes obstetric hysterectomy may suffer from urinary tract infection, cuff infection and vault hematoma. Abdominal wall infection and wound dehiscence may occur in 5% of cases. Pneumonia, paralytic ileus, intestinal obstruction, pulmonary embolism are immediate and early complications. Repeat laparotomy might be the possibility in around 0.5–3.3% of the cases. Bladder laceration, vesicovaginal fistula, uterovaginal fistula and psychological trauma are long-term complications. Maternal mortality is noted in only 0.66% of cases, due to improved care and adequate provision of blood and blood products **(Table 1)**.[1]

The near-miss events that are marked in these settings are blood transfusion, need for intensive care and probability of bladder and ureter trauma.

Incidence and Risk Factors

Obstetric hysterectomy is the last option, only when other conservative measures fail. A fine balance is needed between taking premature decision of obstetric hysterectomy and delay by ineffective applications of conservative measures.

TABLE 1: Long-term complications of obstetric hysterectomy.

Complications	Percentage
UTI	17.7%
Cuff infection, hematoma	14.1%
Abdominal wall infection/dehiscence	5%
Bladder laceration	2.6%
VVF	0.88%
UVF	0.22%
Pneumonia	4.9%
Paralytic ileus, obstruction	0.33%
Pulmonary embolism	0.22%
Exploration	0.5–3.3%
Psychological trauma	10%
Maternal mortality	0.66%

(UTI: urinary tract infection; UVF: ureterovaginal fistula; VVF: vesicovaginal fistula)

The decision of obstetric hysterectomy depends on age of the patient, parity, desire of future fertility, amount of blood already lost and the clinical background that the woman is delivering in.

Incidence varies, in view of reports of last 25 years, ranging from 1:331 to 1:6978 deliveries. Developed countries have reported incidence around 1:2,000 deliveries. Incidence in Canadian province was 0.53/1,000 deliveries. Incidence in USA was noted to be around 0.6–2.8 per 100 live births.[2]

In developed countries, the incidence of emergency obstetric hysterectomy is about 0.2–1.6 per 1,000 deliveries per year.[3] In developing countries, the incidence varies from 0.4 to 0.7%.[4] In India, the reported incidence is in range of 0.04–0.38%. (Banale M et al., 2015)

Compared to vaginal birth, obstetric hysterectomy is strongly associated with cesarean birth. This could be a function of the indications for which delivery has to be undertaken by Cesarean rather than only the fact that it is a cesarean birth. Cesarean section rates are rising over last few decades, thus increasing rates of obstetric hysterectomy from 0.26/1,000 deliveries to 0.46/1,000 deliveries. Overdistension of uterus leading to atonic postpartum hemorrhage (PPH) is a known risk factor for obstetric hysterectomy. Multiple gestation, known to cause overdistension has been associated with 6-fold increase in chances of obstetric hysterectomy. With the advent of artificial reproductive technology (ART), an association has been found between obstetric hysterectomy with pregnancies conceived by ART. Pregnancy following oocyte donation has been associated with higher rate of obstetric hysterectomy. Many elderly patients are getting conceived with the help of ART, and they are prone to develop PPH, and thus, are having chances of undergoing obstetric hysterectomy.[5]

Various studies in India have been published with regards to incidence. It varies between 0.05–0.38%. Rural setting has reportedly higher incidence as compared to urban setting. Metro cities reported lowermost incidence. Other associated factors may be poverty, illiteracy, ignorance and limited access to health care. Multiparity, pregnancy with anemia, improper management of third stage of labor, and misoprostol usage have contributed as risk factors.

Decision Making

Decision is taken by the obstetrician as an emergency measure to save patient. The decision making for obstetric hysterectomy is a delicate balance. The decision should not be so delayed that the patient goes into extreme or irreversible stage. It is easier to take a decision in case of multiparous women, as compared to primigravida, as the latter's desire of fertility is to be weighed against decision of saving life.

The obstetrician should call for additional help. Getting a second opinion if time and circumstances allow is a helpful practice. It reinforces the decision and boosts morale. Multidisciplinary team approach in form of senior obstetricians, anesthetists, surgical help, hematologist and the blood bank is needed. Maternal mortality may range from 0 to 10% according to time of taking decision, availability of manpower and resources. Mortality can be high due to hemorrhage, blood transfusion, disseminated intravascular coagulation (DIC), infection and potential injuries to lower urinary tract.

Indications of Obstetric Hysterectomy

Earlier, atonic PPH used to be the most common indication for obstetric hysterectomy, but over a period of time, abnormal placentation has become the most common indication, rising from 25 to 41%.[6] Adherent placenta in form of placenta accreta, increta and percreta are the most common. Following is the list of the indications for obstetric hysterectomy.

- Normally situated placenta, placental bed does not retract.
- Retained placenta or cotyledons.
- *Abruptio placenta:* Couvelaire uterus when DIC sets in where placental bed is culprit—release of thromboplastin and activators.
- Placenta previa.
- Placenta previa with previous LSCS **(Fig. 1A)**.
- Placental adherent syndrome (accreta, increata, percreta). It is best to proceed for classical cesarean section and to go for total obstetric hysterectomy with the placenta in situ **(Figs. 1B and 2)**.
- *Uterine atony refractory to all applications:* Medical and surgical.
- *Traumatic injury to uterus:* Rupture of uterus, lower segment trauma, and cervical trauma.
- Sepsis-in the era of modern antibiotics it is not a common reason. But secondary hemorrhage due to lower segment scar infections, A-V fistula and endomyometritis needs removal of uterus.
- Uterine inversion rarely, despite successful manual replacement, it may recur or may end up in PPH, requiring obstetric hysterectomy **(Figs. 3 and 4)**.

Surgical Technique

Surgical technique is similar to hysterectomy in gynecological patient. However, there are many pregnancy-induced, profound anatomical and physiological changes in the uterus and the pelvis in general, which, if not taken into account, can create difficulties. The uterus is greatly enlarged. Round ligament and fallopian tube and ovarian ligament are at different levels, requiring separate clamping **(Fig. 5)**. Pelvic tissues are edematous and friable. Broad ligament is widened,

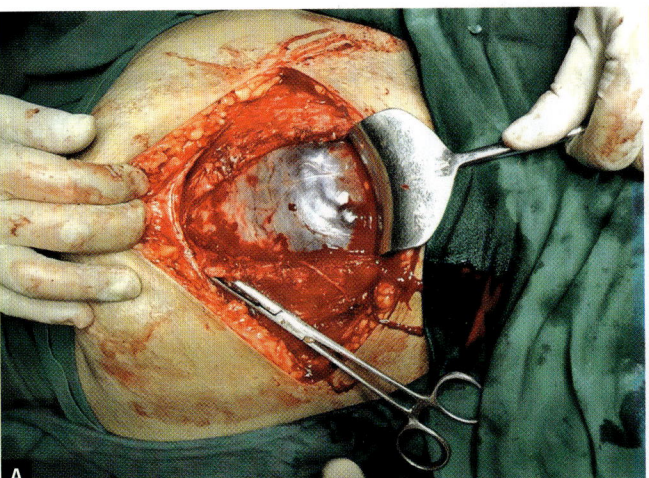
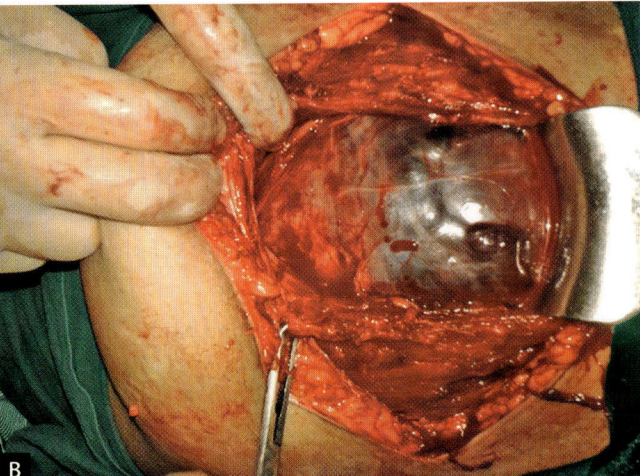

Figs. 1A and B: Placenta previa in case of previous lower segment cesarean section.

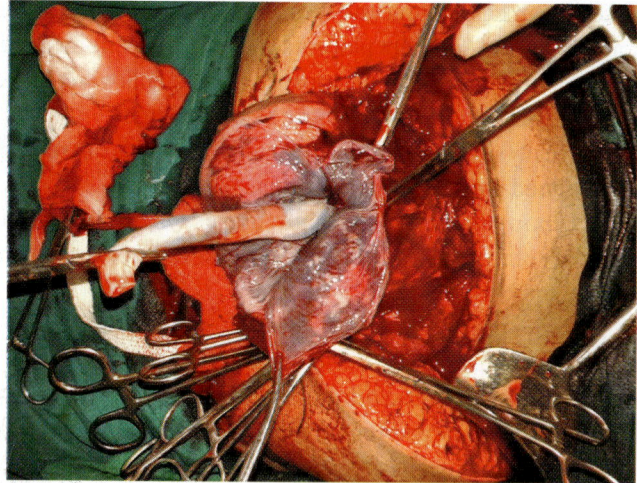

Fig. 2: Classical cesarean section.

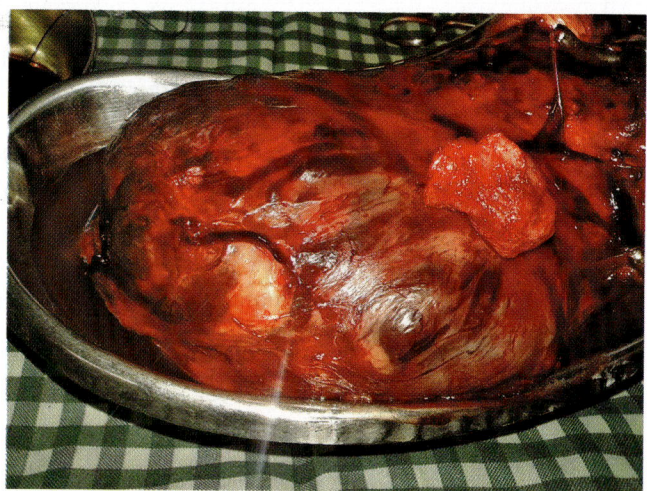

Fig. 3: Total obstetric hysterectomy.

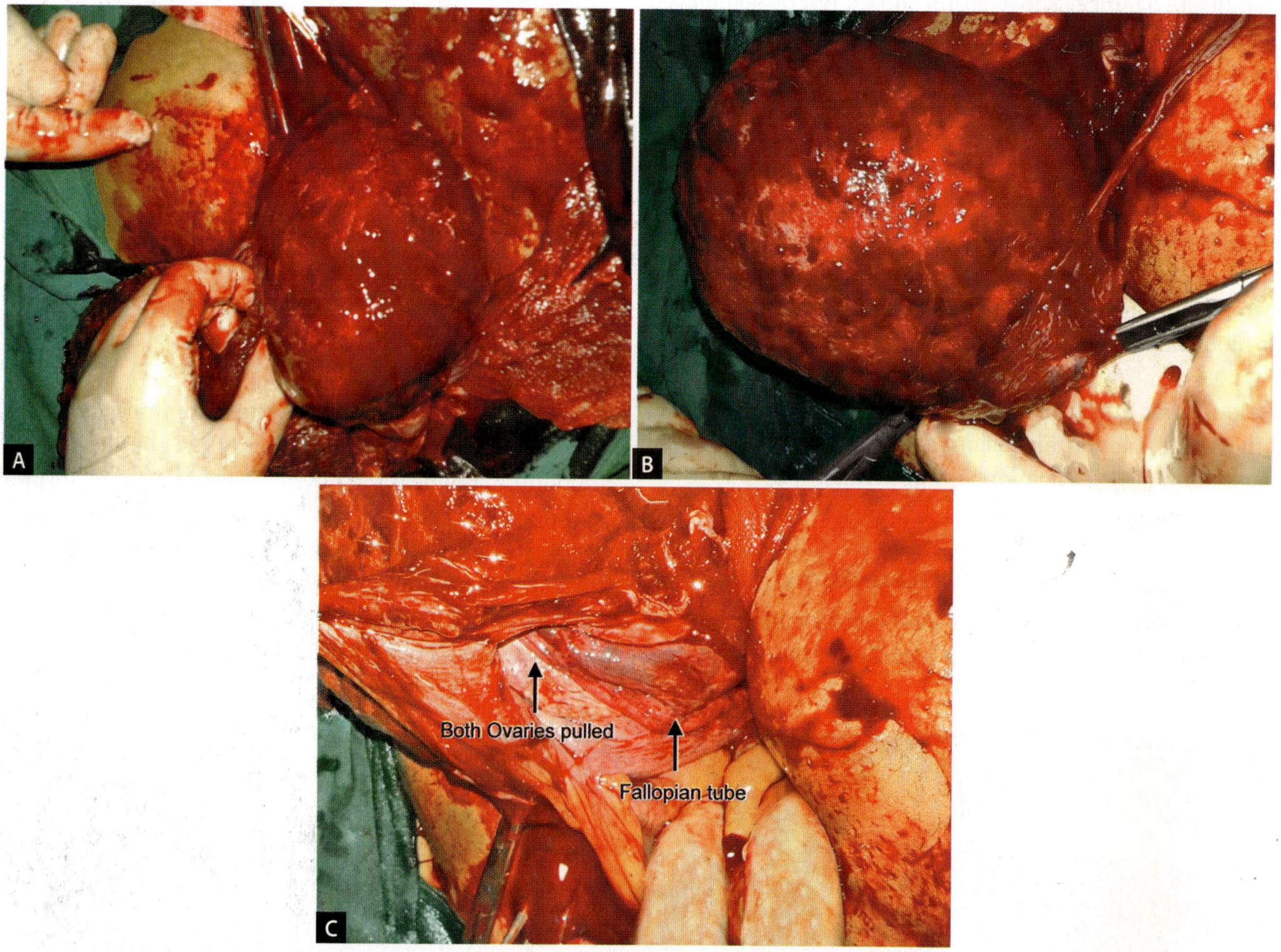

Figs. 4A to C: Technique of inversion of unicornuate uterus–CS.

needing special care for hemostasis. Large blood vessels run in the broad ligaments, including the branches of Sampson's artery **(Fig. 6)**. Delineating the lower segment and cervix becomes difficult when the patient is in advanced labour, with thinning of the lower segment and effacement and dilation of the cervix.

Lower urinary tract is closer to uterus and it is more prone to get injured. Uterine and ovarian vessels are enlarged almost five times the prepregnant state in caliber, and they are engorged and tortuous.[7] In case of previous LSCS, bladder may be adherent, which can be damaged during surgery, thus making it mandatory to separate bladder properly **(Fig. 7)**.

SECTION 10: Postpartum Issues: Maternal and Neonatal

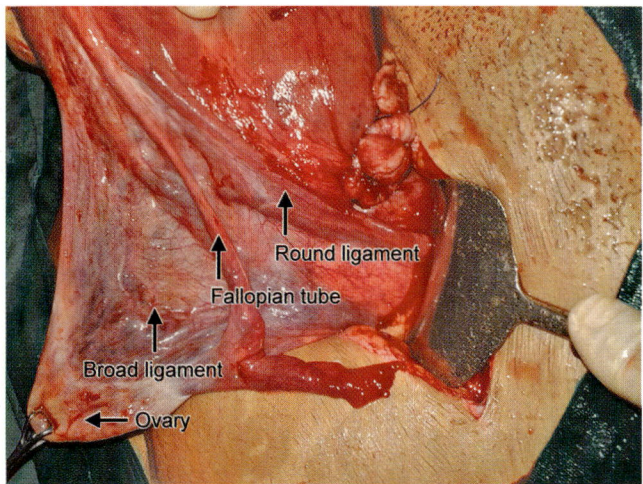

Fig. 5: Identification of anatomical structures for proceeding with obstetric hysterectomy.

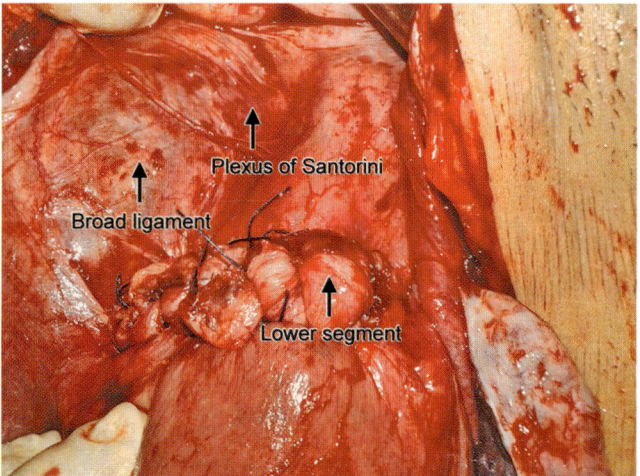

Fig. 6: Identification of anatomical landmarks.

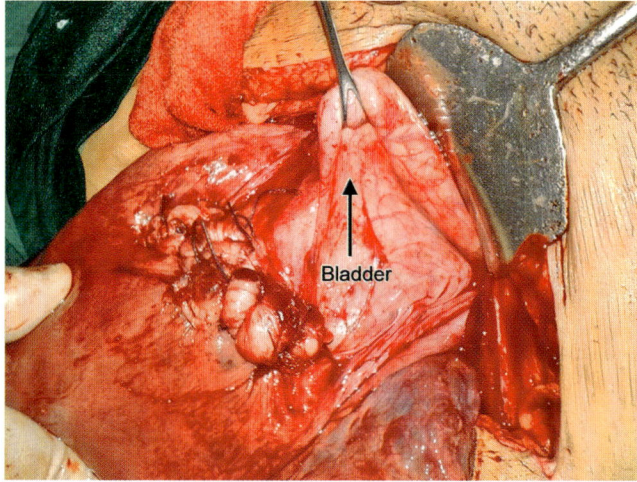

Fig. 7: Identification of bladder.

Ligaments and pedicles are hypertrophic and edematous, thus making encircling sutures dangerous, as they may slip off once edema subsides, leading to postoperative hemorrhage.

Thus, double clamp technique, along with double ligation/transfixation is required.[8]

These edematous ligaments are friable enough, requiring gentle handling, or else, they may tear off if manipulated in a rough manner. As the vascularity increases immensely during pregnancy, and is maximum at term, vessels of Santorini which lie just lateral to cervix, at bladder pillars, are greatly dilated, and need to be handled properly while dissecting the bladder.

Bleeding is notorious at the "bloody angle" of the upper vagina at the cardinal ligament and angle of the vagina.[9] Great care must be taken to incorporate the vaginal epithelium to prevent postoperative vaginal cuff bleeding and hematoma.

Method of Tying Pedicles

An occluding ligature is one that entirely cuts off the blood supply to the part distal to the ligature which is always better (white infarction) **(Figs. 8A to F)**.

Suboccluding ligatures are where in which the main blood supply to the portion distal to Ligature is cut off, but a tract of capillary anastomosis remains (red infarction). It is also good but has some disadvantages. As capillary circulation continues, it may lead to pedicle oozing, hematoma, hemorrhage, infection, adhesions formation **(Figs. 9A and B)**.

The choice between total and subtotal hysterectomy will depend upon the indication for the procedure. If bleeding is confined to the upper uterine segment as seen with atony, placental site bleeding of a normally located placenta or rupture of a classical previous cesarean scar, one may consider a subtotal hysterectomy. It is quicker, simpler, safer, associated with less blood loss and least risk of trauma to ureter and bladder.

One of the faster ways is "clamp, cut and drop technique" which helps in removing the pathological uterus fast.[10] Subtotal hysterectomy may not be effective for controlling bleeding from lower uterine segment, cervix and fornicial trauma, making it necessary to go for total obstetric hysterectomy.

Total obstetric hysterectomy is indicated in patient with previous LSCS, who has central placenta previa and morbidly adherent placenta in lower uterine segment. Perfect diagnosis is needed to be done in such cases, by ultrasonography and/or MRI for grading/staging/location of placenta, followed by classical cesarean section, and elective obstetric hysterectomy. Every effort must be made to reduce morbidity and mortality. Patient and relatives must be properly counseled and informed consent must be taken, and properly documented.

Finer Aspect of Technique

Figures 10 to 19 are self-explanatory, with regards to the steps of obstetric hysterectomy.
- In case of vaginal vault trauma, cervical tear and lower segment tears, (traumatic PPH),[11] hypogastric artery

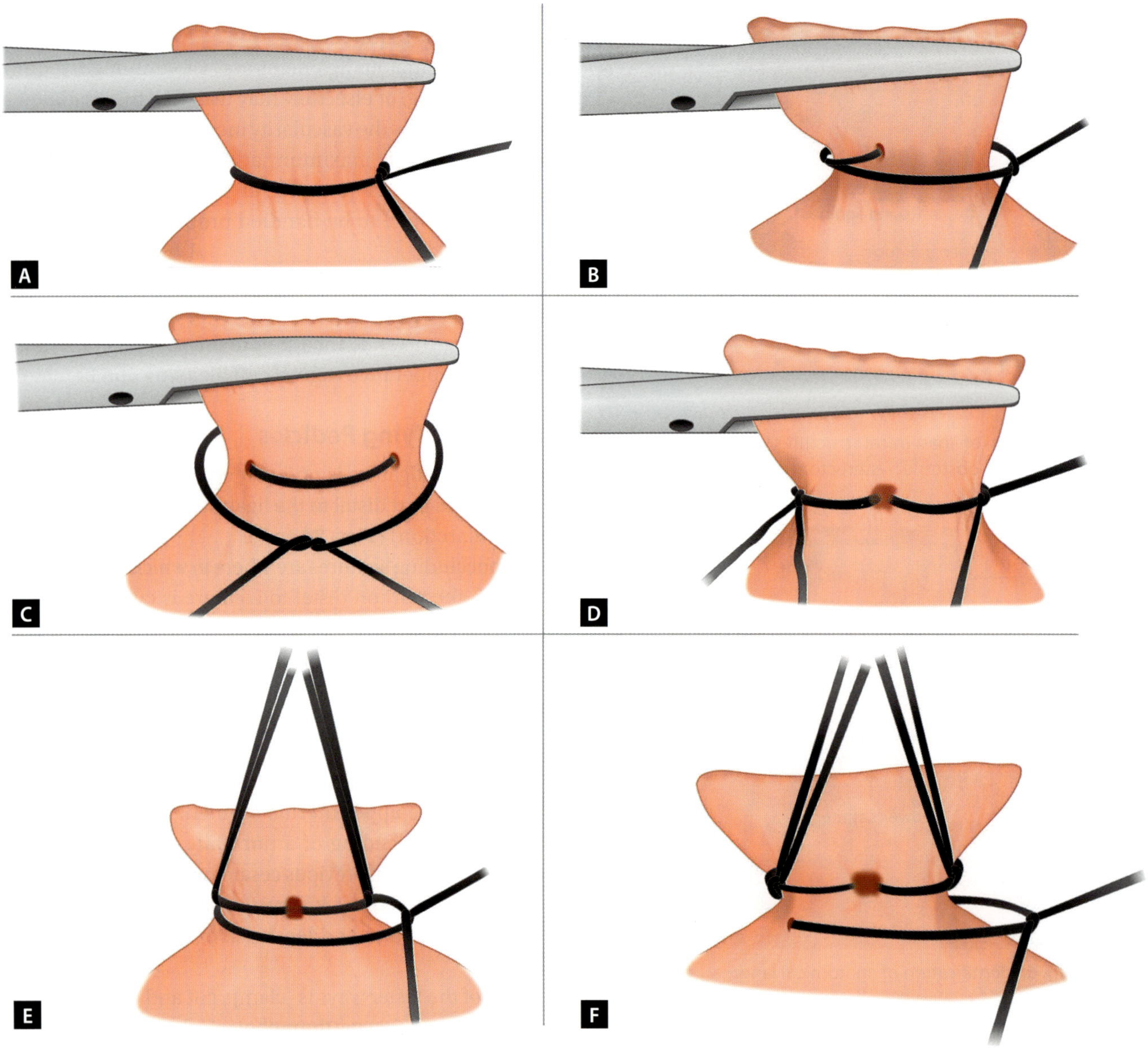

656 **PART 1:** Obstetrics and Perinatology

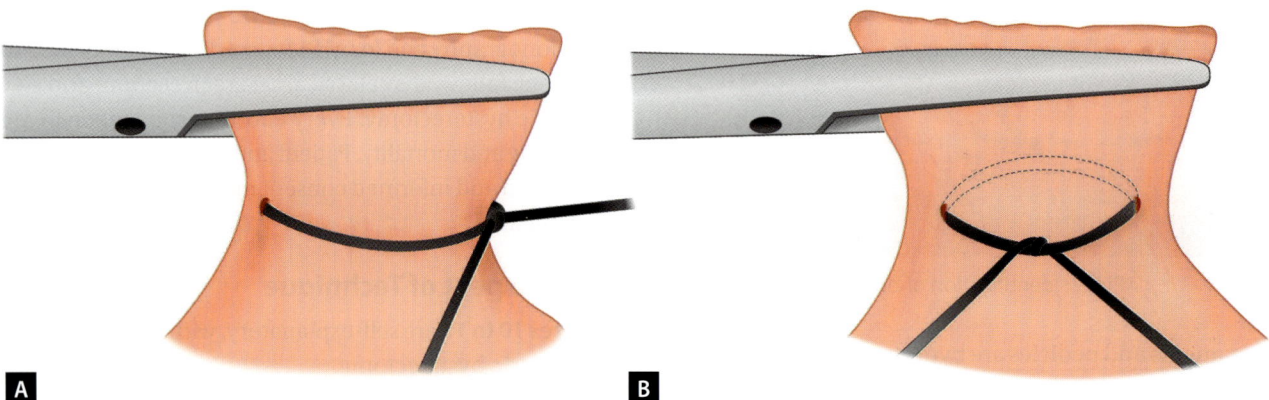

Figs. 8A to F: Occluding ligature.

Figs. 9A to B: Suboccluding ligature.

ligation to reduce the blood flow and suturing of the tears must be done, rather than going for obstetric hysterectomy.
- Subtotal hysterectomy for central placenta previa is to be avoided.
- A transverse or midline vertical Incision for opening the abdomen is preferred.
- Round ligaments are clamped separately, followed by fallopian tube and ovarian ligament, after opening broad ligament. Care must be taken while ligating these pedicles, as they are hypertrophic and congested.
- A small artery (Sampson's artery) that runs beneath the round ligament and its branches in the leaves of broad ligament which are ordinarily unobtrusive in nonpregnant patient, may require separate ligation.
- The bladder mobilization should be adequate and uterine vessels on each side are clamped close to the uterus and divided.

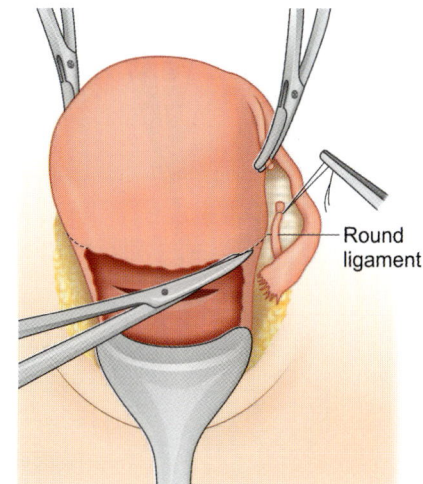

Fig. 12: Opening vesicouterine peritoneum after clamping round ligament.

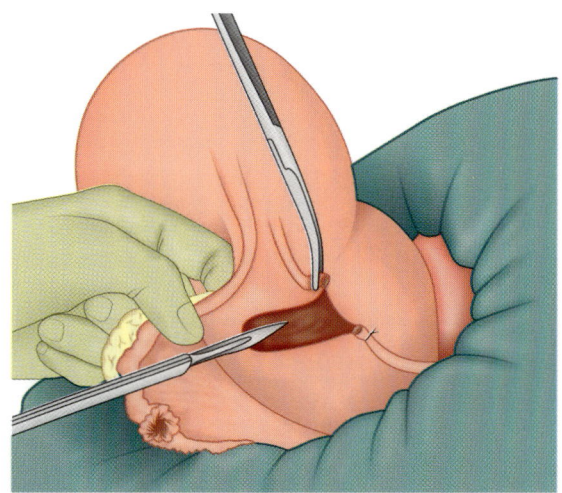

Fig. 10: Ovarian ligament, fallopian tube and portion of broad ligament – clamp and cut.

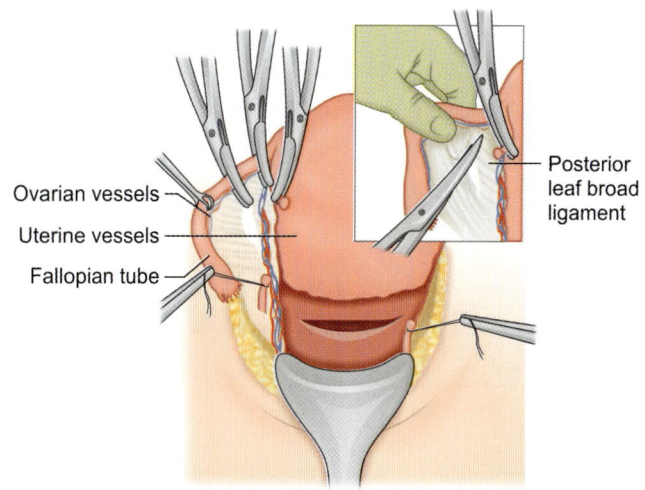

Fig. 13: Clamping upper pedicles.

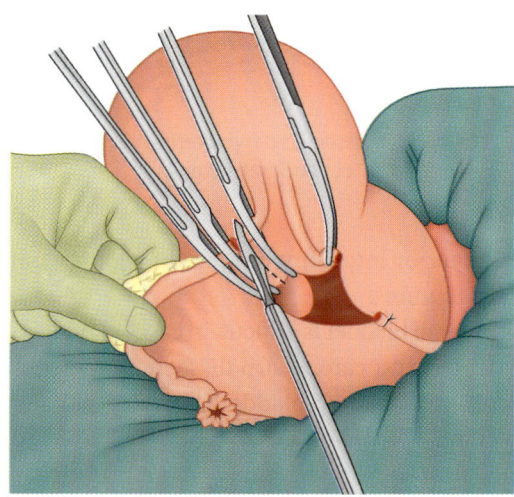

Fig. 11: The round ligament is clamp separately, broad ligament opened.

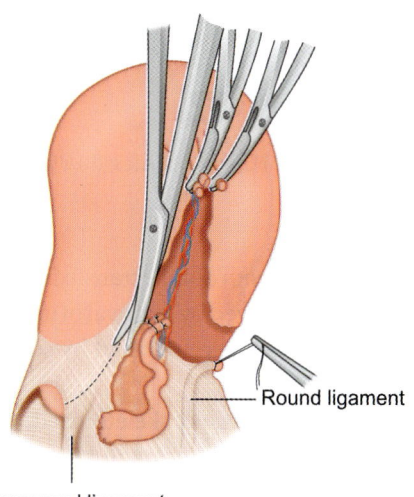

Fig. 14: Area of broad ligament is broad.

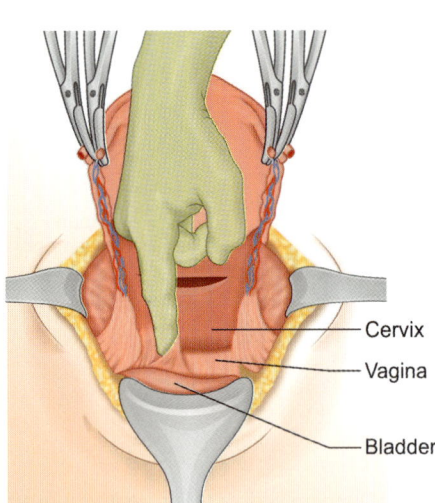

Fig. 15: Dissection of bladder sharp dissection may be necessary. Accidently opened up bladder may be helpful in further dissection of bladder down.

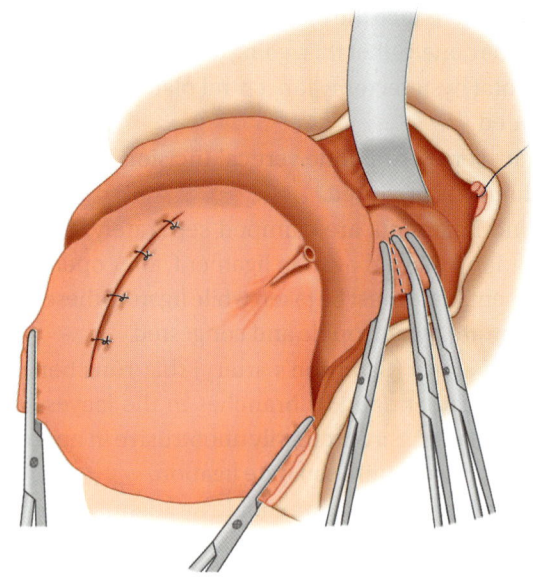

Fig. 17A: Bladder dissected down. Uterine vessels clamped, cut and transfixed.

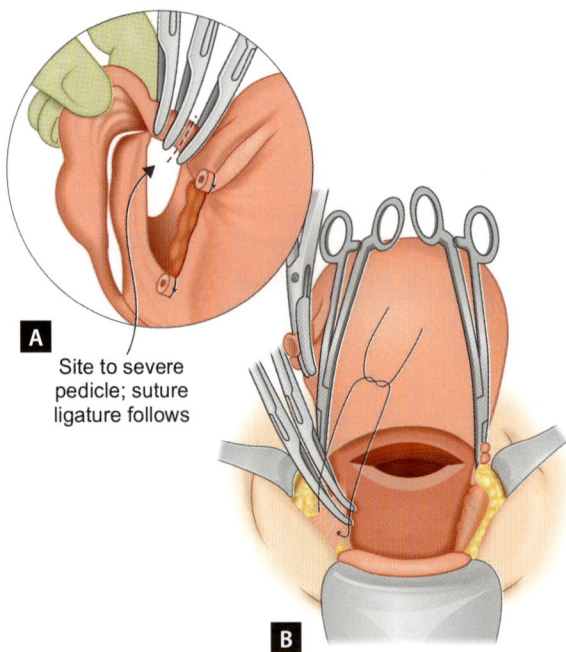

Figs. 16A and B: (A) Upper pedicles; (B) Uterine vessels.

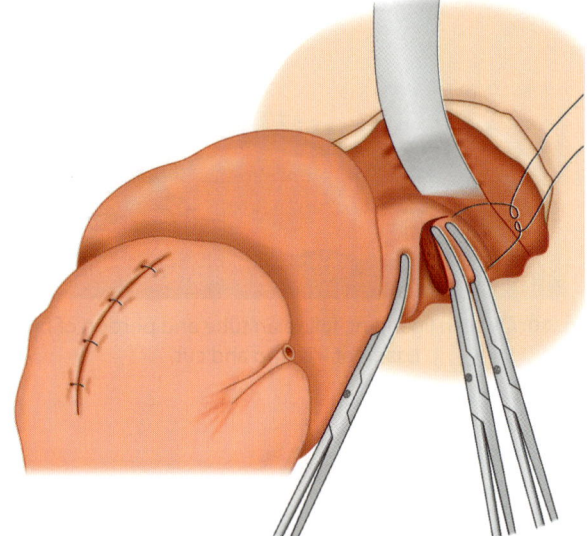

Fig. 17B: Bladder dissected down uterine vessels clamped, cut and transfixed.

- Ligation of pedicles with double transfixing—an occluding ligature is done, followed by removal of uterus at this level in subtotal hysterectomy, followed by suturing of lower segment.
- Uterine vessels are partially skeletonized, and care must be taken not to damage large parauterine veins.
- Angles of lower segment are sutured separately.
- Various ways of suturing the lower segment, such as continuous interlocking anterior, posterior wall separated or together or interrupted figure of eight or transverse mattress sutures.
- Dissection of bladder is difficult in cases of previous LSCS, and needs extra care. Sharp dissection and sometimes, accidently opened up bladder is very helpful for further dissection.
- In total obstetric hysterectomy, identification of cervix is more important particularly in cases of dilated and effaced cervix, if you go on applying clamp, as in a hysterectomy

SECTION 10: Postpartum Issues: Maternal and Neonatal

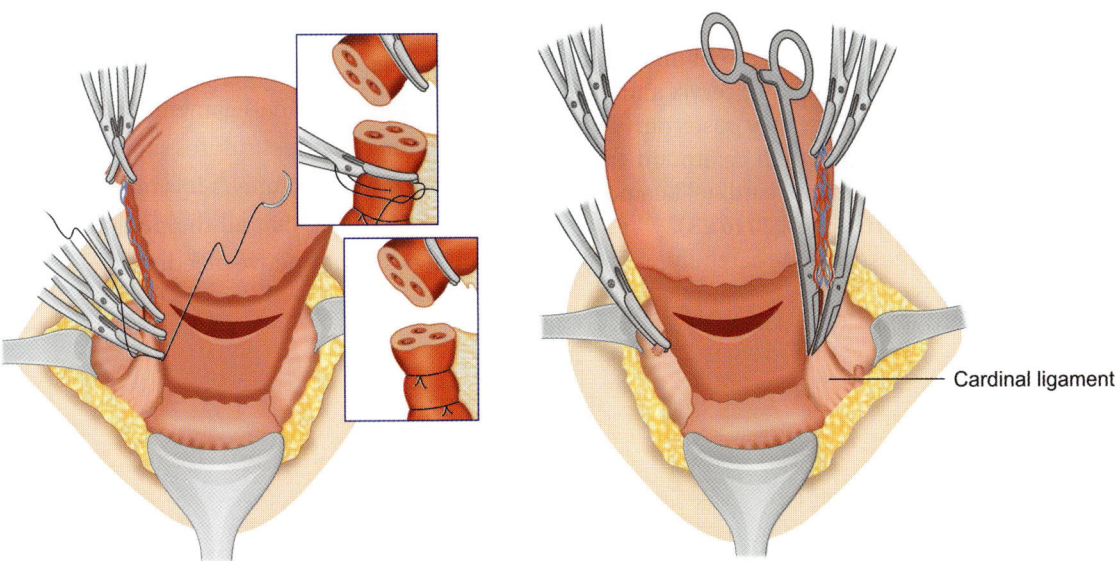

Fig. 18: Uterine pedicles and cardinal ligaments.

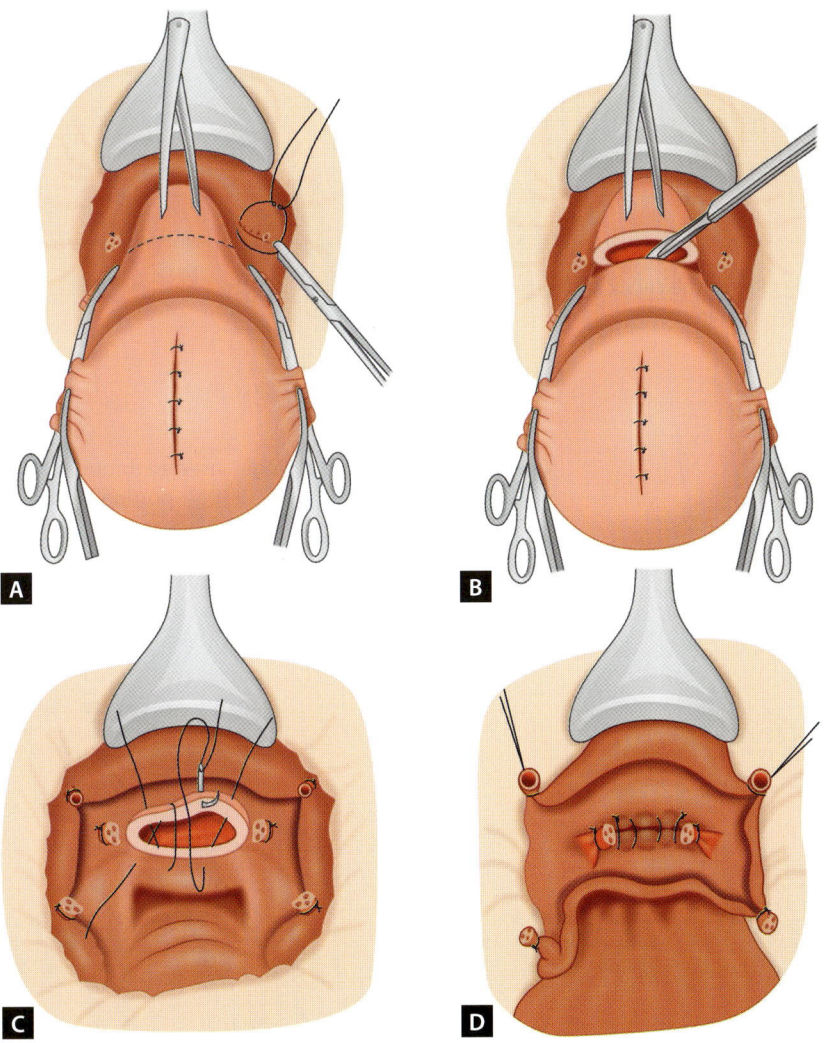

Figs. 19A to D: (A and B) Subtotal obstetric hysterectomy—dotted line indicates level of incision at lower segment; (C and D) Suturing of the lower segment.

in gynecological cases, you are likely to remove the upper part of vagina and ureter is in danger.
- So you have to enter into lower segment and go down to palpate and identify the margin of cervix and vaginal fornices and put a cut at fornix usually posteriorly as close as to cervix to open the vagina then go around catching or clamping uterosacral ligament, cardinal ligament and vagina to remove the uterus **(Figs. 20 to 23)**.
- Ligation of ligaments must be done carefully.

Closure of the vagina can be done in a continuous locking anterior edge and posterior edge separately or both edges together **(Figs. 24 to 27)**. Angle of vagina is taken separately and secured to cardinal ligaments or interrupted figure of eight or transverse mattress sutures same at lower segment in case of subtotal hysterectomy.[12] It is not necessary to reperitonize the pelvis. Check that all the pedicles are intact and there should not be any active bleeding.

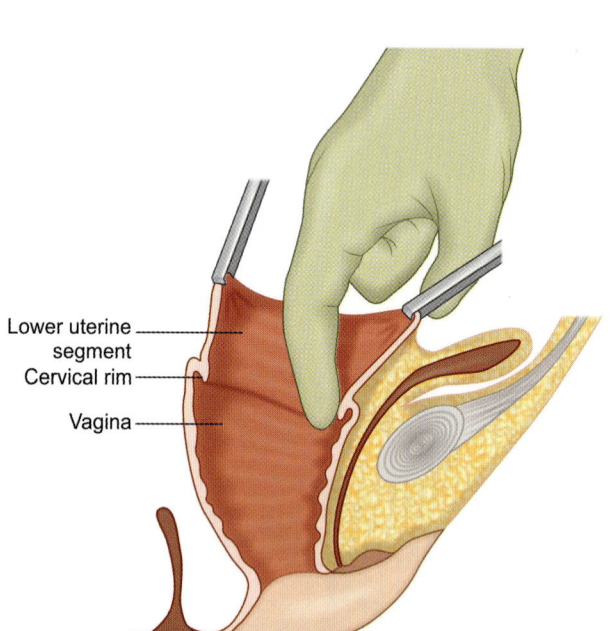

Fig. 20: The finger can readily identify the cervix and fornices for total obstetric hysterectomy.

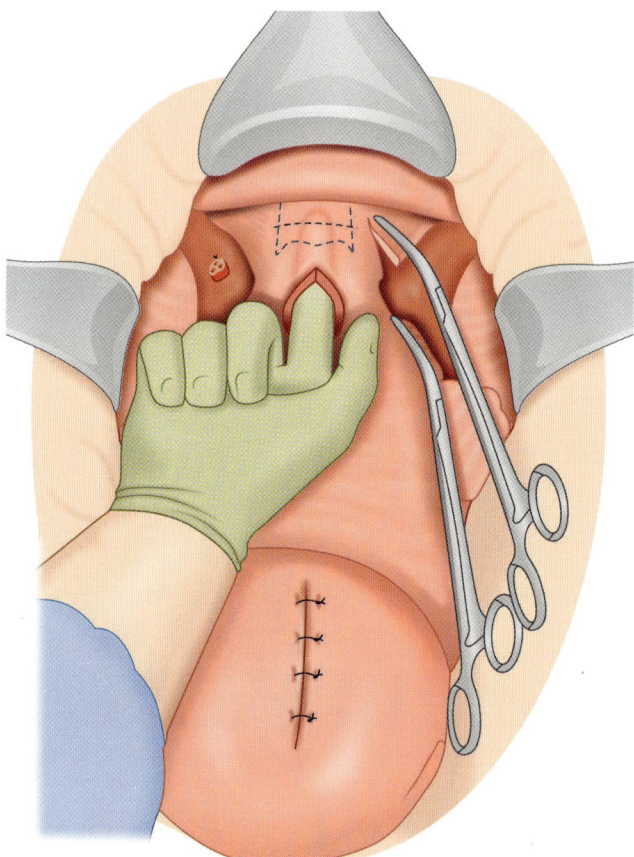

Fig. 22: Finger inserted through lower segment to identify the portion of the cervix.

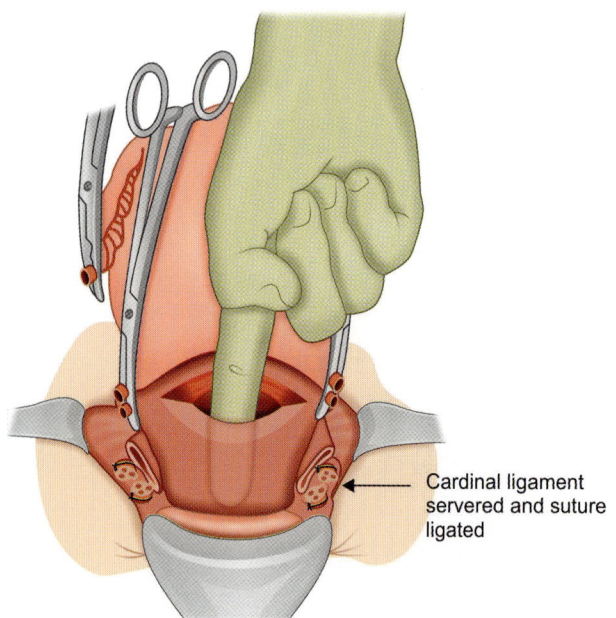

Fig. 21: Finger going down for identification of cervical edge.

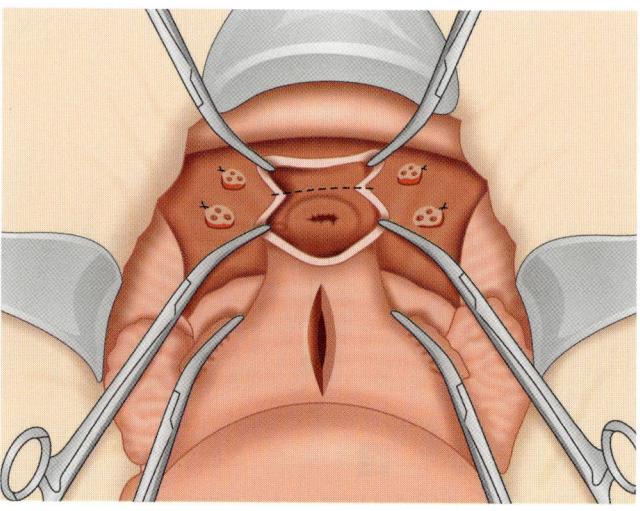

Fig. 23: Opening of the vagina as close as to cervix.

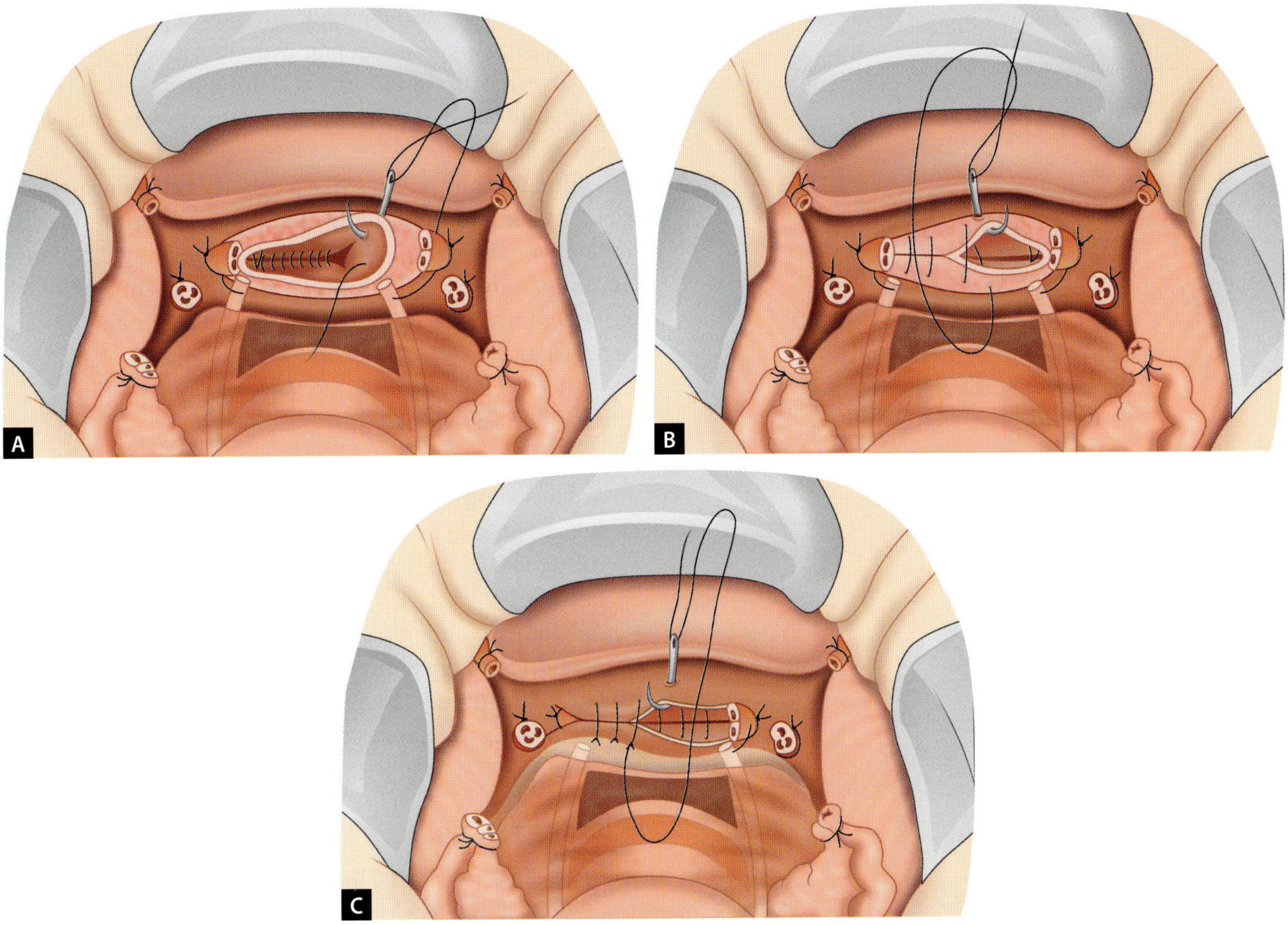

Figs. 24A to C: Suturing the angle of vagina with suturing cardinal and uterosacral ligament and suturing of vagina.

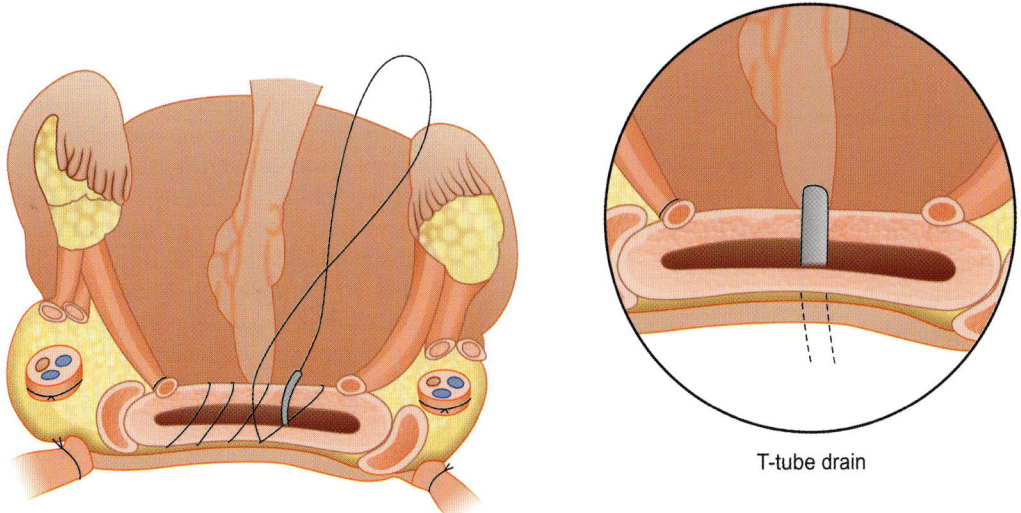

Fig. 25: Cuff run with continuous suture (T-tube drain can be kept, as and when required).

Vaginal swabbing should be done to see that there is no vaginal bleeding before closure of abdomen. Abdomen should be closed in layers, putting intraperitoneal drain (ADK). Postoperative antibiotics are to be given. If the patient requires intensive care, she should be shifted to ICU/HDU. Opinions of intensivist and hematologist can be taken for their inputs in further management.

Proper documentation in form of detailed notes to include the preoperative events, indications and decision-making for hysterectomy and surgical details.

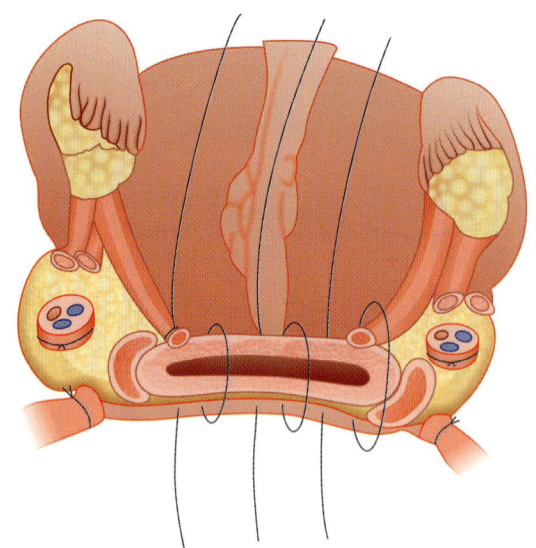

Fig. 26: Closure of cuff with figure of eight sutures.

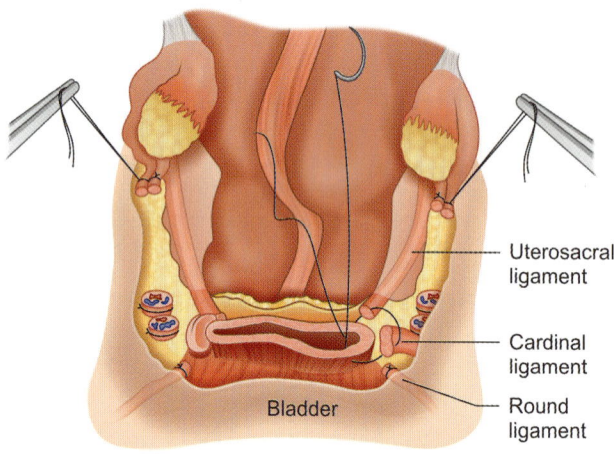

Fig. 27: Vaginal vault.

After the initial postoperative recovery, the woman should receive a comprehensive outline of events.

If the obstetric hysterectomy was not anticipated preoperatively, counseling and documentation of informed consent are of prime importance. The family should be closely counseled concerning the clinical problems that occurred and postoperative recovery and complications.

In a number of series, as many as 25% of women who received an emergency obstetric hysterectomy were primigravida for whom the fertility ending nature of the procedure was devastating. Adequate attempts of uterine conservation and control of hemorrhage should be considered or performed in this group of women.

Bladder injury may be anticipated in case of pervious LSCS. In 1–4% of cases the bladder is inadvertently entered, particularly in case of previous cesarean section and in total obstetric hysterectomy. It is less likely with sharp dissection but even with good technique, bladder injury may occur. Recognize the injury and repair it at same time.

Inadvertent ureteric injury at clamping of uterine vessels, cardinal and vaginal vault in total obstetric hysterectomy may occur.

Ultimately one has to strike a balance between spending excessive time on alternative techniques that are proving ineffective leading to delay, further hemorrhagic collapse, DIC and moving to definitive and life-saving obstetric hysterectomy. Such is the art of obstetric judgment in trying circumstances.

■ KEY MESSAGES

- Obstetric hysterectomy comes as an emergency. Preservation of uterus is first goal but do not wait till patient goes in extreme condition.
- Anticipate in high risk patients, blood availability is the key.
- Ask for help and make a decision about subtotal or total obstetric hysterectomy.
- Skill of the procedure comes with experience.
- Counseling to relatives and documentation have a great value.

■ REFERENCES

1. Plauche WC. Cesarean hysterectomy indications, techniques, and complications. Charity Hospital of New Orleans (CHNO), Louisiana State University School of Medicine (LSU). Clin Obstet Gynecol. 1986;29,(2):324.
2. Kaster ES, Figueroa R, Garry D, Maulik D. Emergency peripartum hysterectomy: experience at a community teaching hospital. Obstet Gynecol. 2002;99:971-5.
3. Temizkan O, Angın D, Karakuş R, Şanverdi İ, Polat M, Karateke A. Changing trends in emergency peripartum hysterectomy in a teriary obstetric center in Turkey during 2000-2013. J Turk Ger Gynecol Assoc. 2016;17:26-34.
4. Nisar N, Sohoo NA. Emergency peripartum hysterectomy: frequency, indications and maternal outcome. J Ayub Med Coll Abbottabad. 2009;2:48-51.
5. Cromi A, Candeloro I, Nicola M, Casarin J, Serati M, Agosti M, et al. Risk of peripartum hysterectomy in births after assisted reproductive technology. Fertil Steril. 2016;106(3): 623-8.
6. Zorlu CG, Turan C, Isik AZ, et al. Emergency hysterectomy in modern obstetric practice. Acta Obstet Gynecol Scand. 1998;77(2):186-90.
7. Baskett TF. Peripartum hysterectomy. In: Lynch B (Ed). A Textbook on Postpartum Hemorrhage. New Delhi: Jaypee Brothers Medical Publishers (P) Ltd; 2006. pp. 313.
8. Arulkumaran S, Robson M. Obstetric hysterectomy. In: Munro Kerr's Operative Obstetrics, 13th edition. Gurugram: Elsevier India; 2019. p. 311.
9. Plauche WC. Cesarean hysterectomy: Indications, technique, and complications. Clin Obstet Gynecol. 1986:325.
10. Mickal A, Plauche WC. Cesarean hysterectomy. Mediguide Ob Gyn. 1984;4(1):2-9.

11. Arulkumaran S. Postpartum hemorrhage (PPH). In: Warren R, Arulkumaran S (Eds). Best Practice in Labour and Delivery. Cambridge: Cambridge University Press; 2010. p. 167.
12. Plauche WC. Peripartal hysterectomy. Obstet Gynecol Clin North Am. 1988;15(4):783-97.

FURTHER READING

1. Douglas G, Stromme WB. Operative Obstetrics. New York: Appleton-Century-Crofts; 1976.
2. O'Grady JP, Gimovsky ML, Bayer-Zwirello LA, Giordano K. Operative Obstetrics. Cambridge: Cambridge University Press; 2008.

LONG QUESTION

1. Enumerate various indications for Obstetric Hysterectomy. How will you evaluate adherent placenta in full term primigravida patient?

SHORT QUESTION

1. Name the regions supplied by plexus of santorini.

MULTIPLE CHOICE QUESTIONS

1. Subtotal hysterectomy can be done in case of placenta previa:
   a. True
   b. False
2. Following complications may occur while performing obstetric hysterectomy, except:
   a. Ureteric injury
   b. Bladder injury
   c. Intestinal injury
   d. Vesicovaginal fistula
3. Which type of uterine incision is to be kept in case of central placenta previa with placenta accrete?
   a. Lower uterine segment
   b. Upper uterine segment (classical cesarean)
4. Lower uterine segment tear is first managed by:
   a. Subtotal obstetric hysterectomy
   b. Total obstetric hysterectomy
   c. Internal iliac artery ligation
   d. Ovarian artery ligation

Answers
1. b   2. d   3. b   4. c

10.5 POSTPARTUM PYREXIA

Indranil Dutta, Dilip Kumar Dutta

INTRODUCTION

Postpartum pyrexia is a common condition that is sometimes associated with serious maternal morbidity and occasional mortality. Mostly these are due to underlying infection in the genital tract but there are a wide variety of other possible causes that may not always be clinically obvious. The topic is very important and relevant as there was a wide number of maternal deaths attributable to group A streptococci (GAS) in the 2000s. Various studies in UK had also documented deaths attributable to endometritis that is infection within the uterus. Indian statistics shows that puerperal infections contribute to 12% of maternal mortality. It is a largely preventable cause of maternal death.

The history of puerperal sepsis is a classic example of observation, analysis, and application of common sense technology to a difficult problem. The story of Ignaz Semmelweiss is central to the puerperal sepsis. He is regarded as the pioneer of research in the field. His name is immortalized with puerperal fever or childbirth fever as it was known in those times.

Various advancements in diagnosis, medical managements have not been able to fully prevent puerperal pyrexia. In rural areas and less developed countries of the world, there is a lack of access to infrastructure, clean childbirth practices, and trained personnel for delivery. These are obvious reasons for the prevalence of puerperal sepsis. Even in the West, where healthcare facilities are more advanced, puerperal sepsis is a potential problem. In the UK, it accounts for 10 deaths every year. The mortality from severe sepsis with organ dysfunction is 20–40% and it may be as high as 50% in case of septicemic shock.

DEFINITIONS AND TERMINOLOGY

Puerperal pyrexia is defined as the presence of a fever, which is ≥38°C in a woman within 6 weeks of her having given birth. *Puerperal fever* is a sign and not a diagnosis. It should be further evaluated to find the potential reason for the fever. Fever could be due to puerperal sepsis (discussed later), extragenital or incidental infections and other noninfective causes.

At present, there is no universally agreed upon definition of sepsis in obstetric practice. It can be looked upon as a continuum of infection-related illness ranging from minor, localized features and progressing (if unchecked) to a systemic state causing organ dysfunction, failure and shock. The working definition of puerperal sepsis is an infection of the genital tract after delivery.

Puerperal sepsis is the infection of the genital tract occurring at any time from the rupture of membranes or onset of labor to 6 weeks after delivery in which two or more of the following features are present:
- Fever
- Pelvic pain

- Abnormal vaginal discharge (purulent) or foul vaginal odor
- Abnormal bleeding
- Incomplete or delayed uterine involution.

RISK FACTORS

Puerperal sepsis is more likely to occur when certain risk factors exist. These factors may be in the host (medical or obstetric conditions), infrastructure for delivery and obstetric practice or events in labor/delivery. They may be classified as given in **Table 1**.

CAUSES OF PUERPERAL PYREXIA

Puerperal fever should be considered to be due to an infectious etiology until proven otherwise. There are a few noninfectious conditions which give rise to puerperal fever. These should be "diagnosis of exclusion" rather than the primary line of thought when a woman presents with puerperal fever. The most common site of infection is the genital tract or the operative wound site. Other sites of infection are the urinary tract and the breasts. The causes to be considered are outlined in **Table 2**.

MICROBIOLOGY AND ETIOPATHOGENESIS

Most puerperal infections are due to organisms that are commonly found bacterial flora in the genital tract or skin. The process of labor, delivery and the interventions conducted during these times allow for a breach in the continuity of the epithelium allowing entry of the bacteria into the skin or infected organ. As such, pregnancy and labor/delivery should not be considered as immunocompromised states in this context unless there are preexisting conditions such as uncontrolled diabetes, HIV infection, cancer, renal failure, steroid use.

The **Table 3** outlines the predominant bacterial organism and mechanisms that drive the etiopathogenesis of the infection at various sites.

PRESENTATION AND HISTORY

- As the name suggests, the main presenting feature of puerperal pyrexia is fever. The fever should be measured by a thermometer. A woman may feel a sensation of warmth during breastfeeding which is physiological. Ambient temperature may also influence this sensation. A measured and documented temperature above the criteria of greater than or equal to 38°C should prompt further clinical evaluation.
- The history of fever in terms of onset, duration and progress should be taken. The accompanying temperature related changes such as chills, rigors and shivering should be noted. Fever patterns are typical for certain conditions as outlined here. It should be noted that these are described patterns and not diagnostic or exclusive of the disease. The use of antibiotics and antipyretics influences the patterns.
  - *Periodic fevers:* Quotidian, tertian and quartan patterns are suggestive of malaria (vivax or ovale). Very high tertian patterns suggest falciparum malaria.
  - *Hectic fevers:* Very high spikes of fever with normal interval readings of temperature could indicate bacteremia from an abscess, pyelonephritis or infected thrombophlebitis.
  - Step ladder pattern is associated with typhoid.
  - Low evening rise of temperature is a characteristic of tuberculosis.
- The associated complaint is very important to explore. Usually, the patient will give a leading history of the associated feature. Some of the important associated

TABLE 1: Risk factors in the predelivery, labor and delivery phases for puerperal sepsis.

Predelivery risk factors	Risk factors arising in labor/delivery
Anemia, malnutrition	Prelabor rupture of membranes
Diabetes—preexisting or gestational and other factors of compromised immune function	Repeated vaginal examinations, internal fetal monitoring
Carriage of infective focus before labor begins—genital and extragenital	Home births, untrained birth attendants, low quality obstetric care in terms of sepsis prevention protocols
Obstetric procedures in pregnancy such as reduction of high order multiple pregnancy, amniocentesis, cervical cerclage	General anesthesia, cesarean delivery, operative vaginal delivery, retained placenta, hematomas, fourth degree perineal tears

TABLE 2: Causes of puerperal pyrexia.

Genital tract infections	Other infections and infestations	Noninfective causes of fever
Uterine infection—endometritis, myometritis, pelvic abscess	Urinary tract infection—cystitis, pyelonephritis	Thrombosis complicated by thrombophlebitis in the leg or pelvic vasculature
Operative site—uterine incision, episiotomy, abdominal wound	Mastitis, breast abscess	Spinal anesthesia drugs or infection
	Respiratory infections—pharyngitis, COVID, influenza, pneumonia, tuberculosis	Drug induced fever
	Other infections and infestations—malaria, dengue, typhoid, hepatitis	

TABLE 3: Predominant bacterial organism and mechanisms that drive the etiopathogenesis of puerperal infections.

Site	Bacteria (predominant)	Etiopathogenetic mechanisms
Genital tract infection / puerperal sepsis	Group A *Streptococcus* (GAS) (also known as *Streptococcus pyogenes*) and *Staphylococcus* spp. Anaerobes such as *Clostridium welchii* play a role after initial aerobic infection	Seeding of the genital tract by vaginal flora Loss of the cervical mucus barrier Rupture of membranes allows exposure of the upper genital tract to the bacterial flora Availability of a raw surface (placental site, abrasions on the mucosa, uterine wound, episiotomy) for bacterial culture
Mastitis and breast abscess	*Staphylococcus* spp.	Engorgement, incomplete emptying of the breasts Increased vascularity Nipple trauma (usually induced by incorrect latching)
Urinary tract infection—cystitis, pyelonephritis	*Escherichia coli*, *Proteus* spp. and *Klebsiella* spp.	Exposure of the urethral mucosa during labor and delivery Catheterization
Operative site—uterine incision, episiotomy, abdominal wound	*Staphylococcus* spp.	Presence of wounds especially with untrained attendants not employing good aseptic practice Preoperative shaving Not administering prophylactic antibiotics before cesarean
Respiratory tract infections	Pharyngitis: *Streptococcus pneumoniae* Other viral and bacterial organisms: COVID, influenza, tuberculosis	

complaints which should be sought and the possible diagnosis are mentioned in the next section of physical evaluation.

- History taking should include details of labor process including duration of rupture of membranes, length of the labor, whether any instrumentation was done, whether placenta was expelled completely, whether there was any postpartum hemorrhage (PPH) associated, whether repeated blood transfusions were required and what medications, especially antibiotics have been already taken by the woman.
- Any recent illness/exposure to illness in close contacts, particularly streptococcal infections, and Coronavirus disease (COVID) should be noted.
- An enquiry into the health of the neonate is necessary to determine if there are associated features and if pediatric referral is needed.

PHYSICAL EXAMINATION

Examination plays an important role in formulating a working diagnosis. The vital parameters are important guidelines to the general condition of the woman and this will determine the site of care needed (home, hospitalization or intensive care). The woman should be examined systemically and systematically. This should necessarily include an examination of the respiratory system, throat, breasts, abdomen, and wound sites. The legs should be examined for possible thromboses.

The important causes of puerperal pyrexia, their presentation and symptoms with clinical signs are detailed in **Table 4**.

INVESTIGATIONS

Some investigations are standard and should be performed for every hospital admission of puerperal fever. These include:

Complete Blood Count and Peripheral Smear, Hematology

- Anemia is a risk factor for puerperal sepsis as would be seen with low hemoglobin and alteration of the red cell parameters.
- High total leukocyte count with neutrophilic shift goes in favor of a bacterial infection. There is a mild leukocytosis in the puerperal period, especially in the first week of delivery. In the clinical context of fever, this physiological leukocytosis should be viewed critically and should be considered as an evidence of infection. Leukocytosis may be suppressed when the woman has already taken antibiotics.
- A low platelet count is suggestive of viral infections, malaria, dengue or severe sepsis.
- Peripheral smear may reveal parasites such as *Plasmodium*
- Inflammation markers such as C-reactive protein (CRP) are more sensitive than total count to pick up early infection. But they are raised in nonspecific situations also.
- Coagulation parameters should be assessed if the presentation includes secondary hemorrhage, there is clinical evidence of abnormal bleeding or if surgical intervention is needed.

Biochemistry

Renal and liver parameters should be assessed at least once as a baseline so as not to miss organ involvement.

TABLE 4: Causes of puerperal pyrexia, their presentation and symptoms with clinical signs.

Condition	Predominant associated symptoms	Clinical signs
Genital tract infection / puerperal sepsis	Abdominal and pelvic pain Foul smelling vaginal discharge Vaginal bleeding (secondary PPH)	Uterine tenderness Subinvoluted uterus Abnormal color and smell of lochia Open cervical canal with material in the canal Bogginess and tenderness in fornices suggest pelvic hematomas, collections or abscess
Operative site—uterine incision, episiotomy, abdominal wound	Pain at the site Discharge from the wound site	Features of inflammation (redness, warmth, tenderness, swelling and restricted movement) are classic features. The degree of features will depend on the extent of the tissue involved and is then called a surgical site infection (SSI), cellulitis or in unusual circumstances there may be necrotizing fasciitis The wound and suture line may be disrupted There may be a purulent discharge from the wound. If an abdominal wound is disrupted and if there is a pinkish watery discharge from it, abdominal wall dehiscence should be suspected
Urinary tract infection—cystitis, pyelonephritis	Urinary burning, pain and frequency	If there is pyelonephritis, there may be renal angle pain and tenderness
Mastitis and breast abscess	Breast pain, redness and discharge	Skin over the breast shows redness, becomes shiny and tense Nipples may be cracked An abscess presents as a well-defined indurated fluctuant lump
Respiratory tract infections	Cough, breathlessness, hoarseness, throat pain, chest pain	Pharyngitis, pus pockets or tonsillitis, tachypnea, desaturation, rales and rhonchi
Gastroenteritis	Vomiting, diarrhea, blood and excessive mucus in stools, abdominal cramps, bloating	Abdominal tenderness may be present Look for features of dehydration
Thrombophlebitis	Leg and calf pain, pelvic pain	Unilateral swelling of the leg, calf or ankle with throbbing pain, redness Pain on flexion of the ankle and squeezing the calf may be elicited (Homan's sign).
Viral fevers	Myalgia, arthralgia, skin rash	Skin rashes are usually nonspecific in the form of transient widespread macules. Some diseases have a typical rash. Some examples are: • Pleomorphic, centrifugal rash in varicella • Slapped cheeks appearance may be noticed in light skin colored women with parvovirus infection

Swabs and Cultures

Specimens should be collected as appropriate to the clinical presentation and the working diagnosis.
- Blood culture should be collected before starting antibiotic therapy. However, first line antibiotic therapy should be initiated immediately. The results of the blood culture will give a result after 24–72 hours and should be used to modify the antibiotic regimen and not to initiate antibiotic cover.
- Urine routine and culture should be sent.
- Swabs from the genital tract may be sent for identification of specific organisms. However, this is often of only academic interest.
- If there is evidence of respiratory features, a throat and nasopharyngeal swab should be sent for COVID or flu test.

Imaging

- Ultrasound of the abdomen and pelvis should be done early in postoperative patients and in women who present with secondary PPH. It will help to identify pelvic hematomas or abscess, abdominal collection (pus or from organ damage) and retained products of conception. A CT scan of the abdomen or pelvis may help to further define the lesion when there is a suspicion on ultrasound.
- X-ray or CT scan of the chest is indicated for women who present predominantly with respiratory features.

Other Investigations

The clinical presentation will dictate other tests that may be needed such as
- Widal test in suspected typhoid in a woman with predominant gastrointestinal features
- Spinal puncture and CSF evaluation for spinal abscess, meningitis.

CLINICAL MONITORING

As the diagnosis of puerperal pyrexia includes various serious and potentially life-threatening conditions, along with an early

> **BOX 1:** Important signs that warrant admission at tertiary care unit (Red Flag Signs).
>
> - Fever (≥ 38°C)
> - Sustained tachycardia (≥ 100/min)
> - Respiratory rate > 20
> - Abdominal tenderness/perineal tenderness
> - Diarrhea/vomiting
> - Chest pain
> - Patient is anxious/disoriented

start to the treatment, the woman's condition should be closely monitored. The presence of red flag symptoms listed in **Box 1** should necessitate hospitalization and a change in the general condition, vital parameters, and organ specific features should trigger a shift to a high dependency unit or intensive care unit. There are various types of criteria. It would be prudent to use a modified obstetric early warning system (MOEWS) to identify critical conditions early. There are a number of such systems which encompass vital parameters and clinical signs which are assigned scores or colors. Crossing a certain score or the presence of color criteria should trigger further level of care and involvement of other specialists. Some important features are:

- Deteriorating general condition
- Persistent tachycardia above 120/minute
- Persistent tachypnea above 30/minute
- Persistent hypotension (systolic BP < 90 mm Hg for over an hour)
- Urine output < 30 mL/hour over 2 hours
- Oxygen desaturation with levels below 95
- Metabolic acidosis suggested by high lactate levels (>4 mmol/L)
- Features of end organ damage
  - *Hepatic:* Jaundice, high liver enzymes, coagulopathy
  - *Renal:* Oliguria, altered color of urine
  - *Neurological:* Convulsions, altered sensorium.

■ MANAGEMENT

The management of puerperal pyrexia is based on the clinical condition of the woman and the reason for the fever. Considering the chief diagnosis as puerperal sepsis, the management should be considered along the following:
- Resuscitation and supportive medical care
- Antibiotic therapy
- Surgical intervention.

Resuscitation and Supportive Medical Care

- The woman should be aggressively resuscitated if there is evidence of hypoxia or hypotension. The initial fluid administration should be done with crystalloids such as Ringers lactate or normal saline. Dextrose based fluids should be avoided. The volume of administration for an averagely built woman is 1 liter in the first hour followed by 1 liter every 2–4 hours depending on the general parameters. Technically, this works out to 20 mL/kg/hour.
- If there is hypotension, early intervention with vasopressors such as dopamine or noradrenaline infusion is beneficial in settings of septic shock. The woman should be in an HDU or ICU and these infusions should be monitored closely. The pressor response is usually seen in the first hour of treatment. The dose is titrated as per the response.
- If there is anuria or oliguria with rising renal parameters, the woman will need dialysis.
- The woman will need antipyretics and analgesics. Fever should be controlled with adequate antipyretic use. Paracetamol is the first choice for both these purposes. Opioid based analgesics can also be used. NSAIDs should be avoided as they impede the ability of polymorphs to fight streptococcal infections.

Antibiotic Therapy

Antibiotic treatment should be started without waiting for blood or culture results. Once sepsis is identified, every hour of delay of starting antibiotic therapy is associated with a worsening in the maternal outcomes. Antibiotics should be commenced after taking blood and culture specimens. Women who need hospitalization should be treated with parenteral antibiotics. Initial therapy should be started with a combination of second or third generation cephalosporin and metronidazole. Cefotaxime 1 g every 12 hours and metronidazole 500 mg every 8 hours is a commonly used combination. If there is suspicion of urinary sepsis, Amikacin (1 mg/kg/day) as a single dose should be added. Do not change the antibiotic for at least 48 hours. RCOG suggests a combination of either piperacillin/tazobactam or a carbapenem plus clindamycin provides one of the broadest ranges of treatment for severe sepsis. In severe sepsis or nonresponsive situations, newer antibiotics such as Meropenem, cefepime and tazobactam should be considered. Immunoglobulin G (IVIG) is recommended for severe invasive streptococcal or staphylococcal infection if other therapies have failed. Breastfeeding limits the use of some antibiotics. This should be discussed with the pediatrician. Antibiotics can cause allergies. This should be determined by a test dose.

Surgical Intervention

Surgical intervention is needed in the following situations:
- Retained products in the endometrium
- Breast abscess
- Pelvic or episiotomy collections, hematomas, abscess.

In such situations, surgical procedures are high risk due to the possibility of deteriorating maternal general condition and a higher than usual probability of surgical complications. The surgical intervention should be undertaken by an experienced practitioner with adequate infrastructure and personnel backup.

Uterine evacuation is a seemingly simple procedure. But it is also a blind one. It should be performed in the operation theater, under anesthesia. Blood should be cross matched and available for transfusion at immediate notice. Suction evacuation with a manual vacuum aspiration syringe is a simple and safe technique. It should be preferred over an electrical suction. Curettage should not be done in a puerperal uterus. The risks of perforation, bleeding and requiring a laparotomy are higher with a curettage. In the long-term, curettage is associated with a higher risk of intrauterine adhesions.

A laparotomy may be needed to manage a pelvic hematoma or abscess. This should be done sooner rather than later. There could be a tendency toward complacence as antibiotics may control the obvious clinical features. However, antibiotic therapy is not a long-term solution as the picture deteriorates when antibiotic penetration is limited and antibiotics cannot be continued ad infinitum. Therefore, drainage of the pus is essential. If the collection is small and most liquid (as evidenced by imaging), a CT scan guided drainage with insertion of a pig-tail catheter may be considered. However, this may not always work as pelvic collections tend to get organized and infected. A laparotomy is the recommended, definitive surgical intervention. If the woman has been delivered by a cesarean, the same scar can be opened again. This incision is suitable for collections limited to the pelvis. If there is widespread fluid/pus collection and there is a suspicion of organ injury, a midline incision is more practical. At the time of the laparotomy, the essential elements are to evacuate the collection completely. This should be achieved by finger evacuation, suction and copious warmed saline lavage until the returning fluid is clear. The bladder, uterus and bowel should be examined and repairs should be undertaken as needed. Hysterectomy may be a last resort in the face of uncontrolled hemorrhage with sepsis. The surgery is difficult due to the friable tissues, distorted anatomy, possibility, of organ injury and slippage of ligatures. A subtotal hysterectomy reduces surgical risk as compared to a total hysterectomy. However, a total hysterectomy will be needed in case there is cervical trauma, pathology or retained adherent lower segment placenta.

COMPLICATIONS

The common complications include:
- Septicemia, septic shock, maternal death
- Genital tract infection may lead to abscess formation, adhesions, peritonitis, hemorrhage and subsequent infertility if not treated early and aggressively
- Urinary tract infection may progress to pyelonephritis and renal scarring if left untreated
- Mastitis may lead to the formation of breast abscesses if treatment is not started early
- Pulmonary embolus
- Disseminated intravascular coagulation
- Pneumonia.

PROGNOSIS

The prognosis depends on correct and quick diagnosis followed by prompt treatment; if treatment is late then prognosis can be poor. The majority of patients will make a full recovery with no lasting effects if treated fast enough with antibiotics and other supportive medicines. However, the possibility of septicemia and lasting sequelae or even death mean it is important to treat all cases of puerperal pyrexia early and aggressively.

PREVENTION

- Hygiene and cleanliness should be maintained throughout delivery process. Frequent per vaginal examination should be avoided.
- Prophylactic antibiotic should be given as per guidelines in case of prelabor rupture of membranes and before surgical procedures.
- Catheterization should be done under aseptic precautions and avoided where possible.
- Perineal wounds should be cleaned and sutured as soon as possible after delivery.
- All blood losses and the completeness of the placenta should be recorded at all deliveries.
- Early mobilization of delivered mothers will help to protect against venous thrombosis.
- New mothers should be helped to acquire the skills required for successful breastfeeding in order to reduce the risk of mastitis.

CONCLUSION

Puerperal pyrexia is a condition that deserves careful and early medical attention. The diagnosis of the pyrexia is the key feature to further care. The default diagnosis should be considered as puerperal sepsis until proven otherwise. Early detection, aggressive antibiotic therapy, resuscitation, and appropriate surgical intervention can reduce morbidity and mortality in puerperal sepsis. Other causes of puerperal pyrexia should be assessed and managed to optimize maternal outcomes.

FURTHER READING

1. Centre for Maternal and Child Enquiries (CMACE). Saving Mothers' Lives: reviewing maternal deaths to make motherhood safer: 2006–08. The Eighth Report on Confidential Enquiries into Maternal Deaths in the United Kingdom. BJOG. 2011;118 (Suppl 1):1-203.
2. Dellinger RP, Levy MM, Carlet JM, Bion J, Parker MM, Jaeschke R, et al. Surviving Sepsis Campaign: international guidelines for management of severe sepsis and septic shock. Crit Care Med. 2008;36:296-327. Erratum in Crit Care Med. 2008;36:1394-6.

3. Khlifi A, Kebaili S, Hammami M. Postpartum ovarian vein thrombophlebitis: report of a case and review of the literature. N Am J Med Sci. 2010;2(8):389-91.
4. Lewis G. The Confidential Enquiry into Maternal and Child Health (CEMACH). Saving Mothers' Lives: Reviewing Maternal Deaths to Make Motherhood Safer 2003–2005. The Seventh Report on Confidential Enquiries into Maternal Deaths in the UK. Obstet Med. 2008;1(1):54.
5. Maharaj D. Puerperal pyrexia: a review. Part I. Obstet Gynecol Surv. 2007;62:393-9.
6. Maharaj D. Puerperal pyrexia: a review. Part II. Obstet Gynecol Surv. 2007;62:400-6.
7. Palaniappan N, Menezes M, Willson P. Group A streptococcal puerperal sepsis: management and prevention. Obstet Gynecol. 2012;14:9-16.
8. RCOG. Bacterial sepsis following pregnancy. Green-top Guideline No. 64b. London: Royal College of Obstetricians and Gynaecologists; 2012.
9. Sinha P, Otify M. Genital tract sepsis: early diagnosis, management and prevention. Obstet Gynecol. 2012;14:106-14.
10. Smaill FM, Gyte GM. Antibiotic prophylaxis versus no prophylaxis for preventing infection after cesarean section. Cochrane Database Syst Rev. 2010;20(1):CD007482.
11. Stefonek KR, Maerz LL, Nielsen MP, Besser RE, Cieslak PR. Group A streptococcal puerperal sepsis preceded by positive surveillance cultures. Obstet Gynecol. 2001;98:846-8.
12. Tang HJ, Lin HJ, Liu YC, Li CM. Spinal epidural abscess – experience with 46 patients and evaluation of prognostic factors. J Infect 2002;45:76-81.
13. UKOSS. A national system to study rare disorders of pregnancy. [online] Available from: https://www.npeu.ox.ac.uk/ukoss. [Last Accessed November, 2021].

LONG QUESTIONS

1. What is puerperal pyrexia? What are the causes of puerperal pyrexia? How do you manage puerperal sepsis?
2. What are the complications of puerperium? What are the causes of puerperal pyrexia? How do you prevent puerperal sepsis?
3. Define puerperal sepsis. Enumerate clinical finding associated with puerperal pyrexia. How will you investigate a case of puerperal fever?

SHORT QUESTIONS

1. What are the predisposing factors of puerperal sepsis?
2. Explain briefly about medical management of puerperal pyrexia.
3. What are the complications of puerperal sepsis?
4. What are risk factors and complications of puerperal sepsis?
5. Enumerate the prevention of puerperal sepsis.

MULTIPLE CHOICE QUESTIONS

1. A person is said to have a fever during puerperium when the temperature is:
   a. 99°F or higher
   b. 100°F or higher
   c. 101°F or higher
   d. 102°F or higher
2. A woman has had a recent uncomplicated vaginal delivery but has developed a significant postpartum pyrexia and tachycardia. She is thought to be allergic to penicillin. You suspect puerperal sepsis and are keen to commence treatment prior to the investigations coming back.
   What is the antibiotic regime of choice?
   a. Cefuroxime
   b. Clindamycin
   c. Co-amoxiclav
   d. Erythromycin
   e. Metronidazole
3. With regards to risk factors for puerperal sepsis, which of the following is/are true?
   a. The single most important risk factor for postpartum infection is PROM
   b. The use of prophylactic antibiotics in preventing puerperal sepsis following PROM is well established
   c. Maternal sepsis is commonly associated with gram negative infections, reflecting colonization of the urogenital tract
   d. In severe cases of puerperal pyrexia, Group B beta-hemolytic streptococcus should be suspected as the most likely pathogen
   e. Repeated vaginal examinations predispose to maternal infection
4. An infection of the genital tract 3 weeks after delivery with rise in temperature, foul smelling lochia, pain and tenderness in the lower abdomen is likely to be:
   a. Puerperal sepsis
   b. Thrombophlebitis
   c. Acute glomerulonephritis
   d. Ureteric calculi
5. A postpartum woman has acute puerperal mastitis. Which of the following statements is true?
   a. The initial treatment is penicillin
   b. The source of the infection is usually the infant's gastrointestinal (GI) tract
   c. Frank abscesses may develop and require drainage
   d. The most common offending organism is *Escherichia coli*
   e. The symptoms include lethargy
6. What are the causes of puerperal pyrexia?
   a. Genital tract infection
   b. Cholelithiasis
   c. Mastitis or breast abscess.
   d. I and III
   e. I and II
7. Red flag signs of puerperal pyrexia include all, except:
   a. Fever (≥ 38°C)
   b. Sustained tachycardia (≥100/min)
   c. Respiratory rate > 20
   d. Intermittent pain abdomen
8. The common complications of puerperal pyrexia, except:
   a. Septicemia

b. Genital tract infection may lead to abscess formation, adhesions, peritonitis, hemorrhage and subsequent infertility if not treated early and aggressively
c. Perineal tenderness associated with frequent loose stools
d. Mastitis may lead to the formation of breast abscesses if treatment is not started early

9. Prevention methods of puerperal pyrexia include all, except:
   a. Hygiene and cleanliness should be maintained throughout delivery process. Frequent per vaginal examination should be avoided
   b. Any GAS identified during pregnancy should be treated aggressively
   c. Prophylactic antibiotic should be given as soon as the membranes rupture
   d. Catheterization should be changed frequently to avoid infections

10. To control Infections in labor room following method should be adopted:
    a. Suspected women to be kept together in ward
    b. Healthcare workers need not wear extra protective gear/PPEs when in contact with patient suspected to have some infectious condition
    c. Fluid repellent surgical masks with visors must be used at operative debridement/change of dressings
    d. Break in skin of infected patient to be kept open for better healing

Answers										
1.	c	2.	a	3.	All	4.	a	5.	c	6. d
7.	d	8.	c	9.	d	10.	c			

10.6 PROBLEMS WITH BREASTFEEDING

Sarita Agrawal, Rajeshwari G

"No safer place in the entire world, No better place to rest
No calmer harbour can be found, than that of mother's breast
No poetry brings it justice, No rhyme or ancient verse
One word only can love describe, Love, that is, to nurse."

— (Anonymous)

INTRODUCTION

Breastfeeding is the first fundamental right of the child. Breastfeeding, indeed, is an essential component of nutrition, child health, and development of a child; and for the mother, it helps in involution, prevents postpartum depression, and creates a bond that is pure, selfless, and divine. Despite this understanding, breastfeeding, which is a natural and primitive reflex, is declining significantly in the recent years due to various social and economic reasons. In order to pause this trend, the World Health Assembly (WHA), in 2014, has set a goal to achieve an exclusive breastfeeding rate of >50% by 2025; only 23 countries have achieved around 60% of exclusive breastfeeding,

Why does breastfeeding matter?

While breastfeeding is a natural act, it is also a learned behavior. It is obvious that by encouraging breastfeeding alone we could save 823,000 lives per year among children of <5 years. Evidences show that breastfeeding reduces the risk of noncommunicable diseases and obesity in later life. Breastfeeding protects the child against diarrheal disease and respiratory infections to a great extent, as evident in low- and middle-income countries. Recommendations have been laid by the World Health Organization (WHO) and United Nations Children's Fund (UNICEF) to start breastfeeding within 1 hour of birth and to continue the exclusive breastfeeding for 6 months followed by adding complimentary feeds to it till 24 months at least. It is found that by practicing breastfeeding within 1 hour of birth could prevent 20% of neonatal deaths; there is 15 times more risk of infant mortality due to pneumonia and 11 times more risk due to diarrhea in infants who are not breastfed. The statistics presented by the Rapid Survey on Children (RSOC) 2014 states that 44.6 % of mothers initiate breastfeeding within 1 hour of birth, though 78.7 % of them are institutional deliveries. Around 64.9% of babies are exclusively breastfed up to 6 months and only 50.5% of babies are given complementary feeds.

COMMON PROBLEMS DURING BREASTFEEDING

Breastfeeding is a wonderful and a satiating experience that completes womanhood; still, it is not an easy task, as every child and mother have their unique way to communicate. The commonly encountered problems are discussed in the following text.

INADEQUATE MILK INTAKE

The problem of inadequate milk is mostly perceived rather than real and results in early initiation of top feeding and termination of breastfeeding. Excessive cry of the baby is usually perceived as insufficient milk; however, the reasons are usually baby seeking maternal warmth or wet nappy pads. True inadequate milk intake can be due to insufficient production or infant factors preventing it to extract milk; the conclusion can be drawn from the history, urine output, and frequency of stools per day and weight gain of the infant. On an average, an infant with adequate intake will micturate about six to eight times a day and pass stools about three times a day. Usually, the infant regains the birth weight by 1-2 weeks of life after an initial loss in the first 3-5 days. If there is no proper weight gain or there is a loss of 10% of the birth weight, inadequate milk intake is suspected. Inadequate milk may be due to failure of the infant to extract milk or insufficient milk production, determining the primary problem is important. The diagnosis is made clinically based on a nursing history, infant urine and stool output, and weight gain of the infant. By the fifth day of life, infants with adequate intake; urinate six to eight times daily, have three or more stools daily and regains the birth weight by 1-2 weeks of life after initial loss of 7% in first 3-5 days. If an infant loses 10% of its weight or fails to regain appropriately, inadequate intake should be considered. Inadequate milk or infant's inability to extract milk usually responds to maternal education and support. But if specific maternal and/or infant factors are identified, specific interventions depending on the cause need to be addressed.

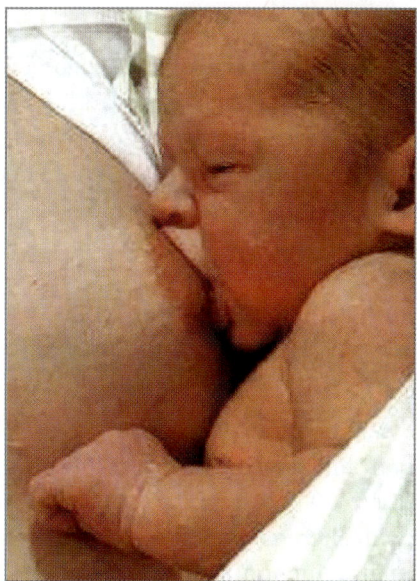

Fig. 1: Correct positioning and latching.

Nipple Pain (Latching Pain)

Persistent nipple pain or latching pain: Most of the mothers avoid exclusive breastfeeding due to a persistent pain in the nipples and tend to use artificial feeds. At times, this can lead to a great psychological distress to the mother and affects her physical and emotional balance interfering with the bonding between the mother and child. The most common cause of nipple pain is suboptimal positioning and latching of infant to the breast. Improper latching can cause nipple abrasion, bruising, nipple cracks, and rarely, blisters in the mother. The infant factors that may cause nipple pain are ankyloglossia (tongue tie), palatal anomalies such as high-arched palate are risk for trauma. Nipple cracks are most common cause of nipple pain and they predispose to breast abscess as well. If the baby is pulled out while suckling, creates circumferential crack at the base of the nipple. Dryness of nipple precipitated by frequent washing of nipple will also result in cracks. It is believed to remove the natural oily substance. Other frequently encountered conditions causing nipple pain are flat or inverted nipples, strong infant suction, nipple bite, milk blisters, infections (*Candida albicans, Staphylococcus aureus*, Herpes simplex, Herpes zoster) psoriasis, dermatitis, and Raynaud's phenomenon. Sometimes, normal nipple sensitivity is perceived as nipple pain which usually subsides within few minutes of suckling and diminishes after fourth day and usually completely resolves within 1 week, whereas the pain due to trauma persists or even worsens.

Management

The first step would be to educate the mother on proper positioning **(Fig. 1)** and attachment; this simple process improves the duration of feeding and reduces few of the problems. Nipple shield is a temporary measure for preterm infants and in few cases of sore nipple, but long-term use of it is not advisable. Application of hind milk, highly purified anhydrous lanolin or vitamin A ointments may be used to alleviate the pain. Frenotomy for ankyloglossia has been shown to be effective in relief of pain and increasing milk transfer. Nipple pain due to confirmed bacterial infection needs treatment with antibiotics, or an antifungal for *Candida* infection. Dermatitis and psoriasis present as sore itchy and painful burning of areola and nipple during acute condition with vesicles crusting and erosions; whereas, when chronic generally dry erythematous, lichenified, and scaling these are treated by advising the mother to avoid irritants and at times may require a course of topical corticosteroids. The pain due to Raynaud's phenomenon typically presents as burning and paresthesia on cold exposure and is characterized by classical tricolor change of pallor, cyanosis, then erythema as circulation returns. Usually, it responds to warmth and abstinence of vasoconstrictors such as nicotine and caffeine, sometimes require nifedipine. In case of Herpes simplex and Herpes zoster lesions of breast, all breastfeeding is to be avoided until the lesions resolves for the risk of transmission to the infant.

Engorgement of Breast

In the 18th century, engorged breast with fever was called "milk fever". Primary engorgement of breast occurs with lactogenesis phase II on day third to fifth postdelivery. Secondary engorgement occurs when there is mismatch between production and extraction of the milk usually in later weeks; it usually follows infant's illness, early weaning, intake of galactagogues, scheduled feeding, missed feeds, and feeding from one breast every time.

Diagnosis

A fullness of breast may be similar to an engorgement, except for fever. In the former, the breast appears hot and heavy but not associated with fever, there is free flow of milk, while in the later the breast is hard, shinny, lumpy, with venous dilatation; there is no paucity in milk ejection and is associated with low-grade fever.

Management

Prevention
- Frequent breastfeed every 1 1/2 to 2 hours during the day and every 2–3 hours at night.
- Let the baby finish on one breast before switching to the second.
- Starting with alternate breast.
- Timely management of painful/sore nipple and ensure proper latching

Treatment
- Manual expressions of small amount of milk before feeding that softens the areola and facilitates proper latching.
- If baby is unable to breastfeed, expressed breast milk (EBM) and then feed using spoon, feeding cup, or syringe.
- Use gentle massage from the chest wall to the nipple area in a circular fashion.
- Between feeds, applying ice for 15–20 minutes decreases swelling and discomfort.
- Just before a feed, applying moist warmth to the breast helps in milk let down.
- *Reverse pressure softening (RPS)*: RPS uses gentle positive pressure to soften a 1–2-inch area of the areola surrounding the base of the nipple. It works by moving fluid away from the nipple **(Fig. 2)**.
- Adequate breast support.
- Use of breast pump should be restricted to soften the breast immediately before feeding, in an engorged breast as this causes the nipple-areolar area very tough.
- There are insufficient evidences to the widely used measures including acupuncture, cabbage leaf application, protease kinase, gua sha (scrapping therapy).
- Analgesics such as acetaminophen may be used to relieve from pain.

Plugged Ducts

Plugged milk ducts or clogged milk ducts: These are localized areas of milk stasis within the mammary ducts and presents as tender and palpable lump without signs of inflammation. Sometimes a small bleb or white spot is seen on the nipple which is due to obstruction of the nipple pores **(Fig. 3)**; these are called "milk blisters." The conditions which may precipitate a clogged milk duct are previous breast surgery or biopsy, poor feeding technique, tight clothing including tight brassieres, sudden decrease in feeding, engorgement, and bacterial intraductal infections.

Management

The principle behind the management is to open up the blocked ducts and drain the area distal to blockage. Topical lecithin massaged into the nipple after each feeding has been recommended; however, oral lecithin preparation is not recommended.

Galactoceles

Galactoceles are retention cyst usually seen beneath the areola, resulting from occlusion of lactiferous duct, seen in pregnancy, lactation, and after weaning **(Fig. 4)**. They are painless until infection sets in; they may be single or multiple and can occur in one or both the breast. The content is milk; initially thin, as it progresses, the fluid becomes thick oily and creamy. Ultrasound shows a spectrum of appearance from cystic-to-solid well-circumscribed mass. On color Doppler interrogation, there are no vascular pickups. An aspiration of milky fluid will be confirmatory. The differential diagnoses are other breast masses such as adenoma, fibroadenoma,

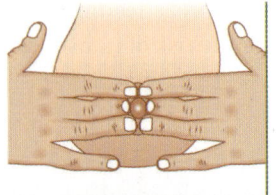 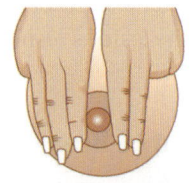 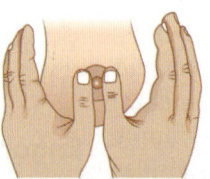 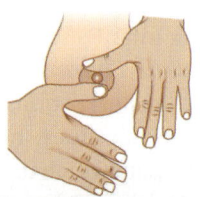 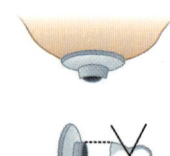

Two handed, one-step method	Two handed, two-step method	Two thumbs, two-step method (Step 2)	Two thumbs, two-step method (Step 1)	Soft ring method
Fingernails short, fingertips curved; each one touching the side of nipple	Using 2 or 3 straight fingers on each side, first knuckles touching nipple. Move ¼ turn. Repeat above and below nipple	Move ¼ turn. Repeat above and below nipple.	Using straight thumbs, base of thumbnail even with side of nipple.	Cut off bottom half of an artificial nipple to place on areola to press with fingers.

Fig. 2: Reverse pressure softening.

papilloma, lipoma, abscess, fibrocystic disease, and rarely malignancies. It is a benign lesion; most of the patients have spontaneous resolution and few may have a residual collection. A gentle massage may release the blocked ducts and lying on the opposite side of the galactocele may help in resolution.

Management

Gentle massage to release the blocked ducts and change of posture lying on opposite site of galactocele usually leads to resolution over the time.

Breast Infections (Mastitis and Breast Abscess)

Mastitis: As the name suggests, it is an inflammatory condition of breast tissue; it may or may not be associated with infection. It is referred to as lactational mastitis or puerperal mastitis when it occurs during lactation, but because of its presenting features, it is often mistaken for an infection and the mother is asked to abstain from breastfeeding the child. About 20 % of lactating women present with mastitis, most commonly in the second and third weeks of their postpartum period, though it can occur at any time during lactation, few cases are reported even at 2 years postdelivery. Recent research suggests that mastitis may increase the risk of transmission of HIV through breastfeeding.

Causes of mastitis: Gunther in 1958 recognized that mastitis results from stagnation of milk within the breast. This stasis of milk becomes a nidus for infection and progress to infective mastitis and then to an abscess, expression of the breast milk would prevent abscess formation. The organism gains entry into the breast tissue through the nipple at the site of a fissure or abrasion, from nursing infant's nose and throat, rarely hematogenous. It involves the parenchymatous breasts tissues first causing cellulitis, then spreads to the lactiferous duct leading to development of primary mammary adenitis.

Clinical presentation: In the first 2–4 weeks, the onset is acute and fulminant with severe breast pain, high grade fever with chills, flu-like symptoms and on examination, part of the breast becomes red swollen and tender **(Fig. 5)**.

Thomsen et al. proposed the following classification based upon leukocytes and bacterial load in milk from patients with mastitis.

- *Milk stasis:* <106 leukocytes and <103 bacteria
- *Non-infectious mastitis:* >106 leukocytes and <103 bacteria
- *Infectious mastitis:* >106 leukocytes and >103 bacteria.

In a randomized study, they found that milk stasis improved with continued breastfeeding alone; noninfectious mastitis could be treated by additional expression of milk after a feed, and infectious mastitis was treated effectively with removal of milk and systemic antibiotics.

Breast abscess: Breast abscess, a localized collection of pus within the breast, preceded by infected mastitis. The incidence ranges from 0.4 to 11%, majority within the first 12 weeks postpartum. Initially, the infection tends to be confined to

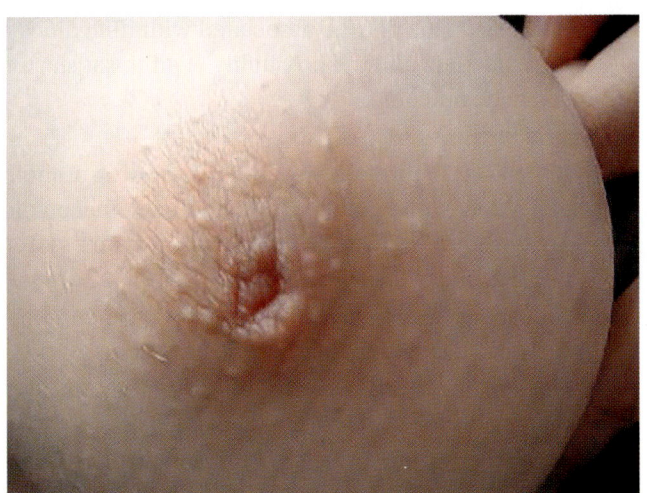

Fig. 3: Retracted nipple with blocked duct.

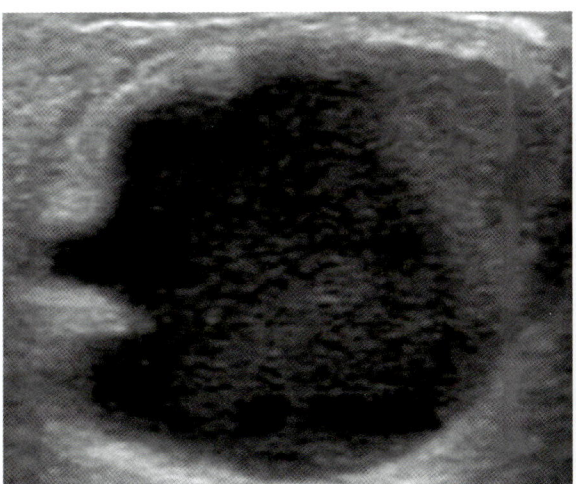 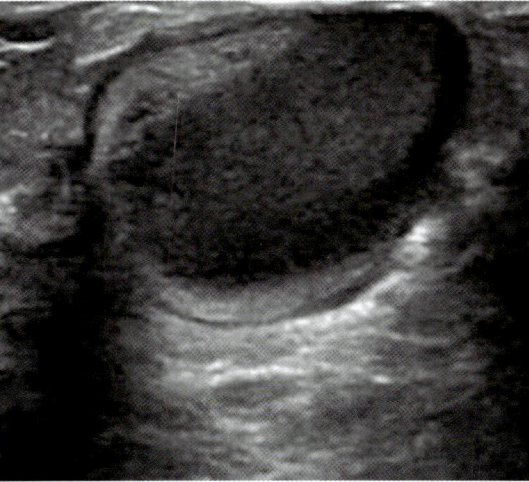

Fig. 4: Galactocele ultrasonography.

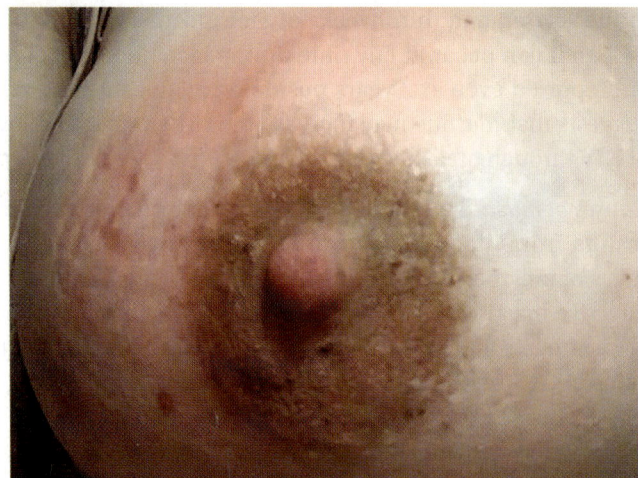

Fig. 5: Mastitis.

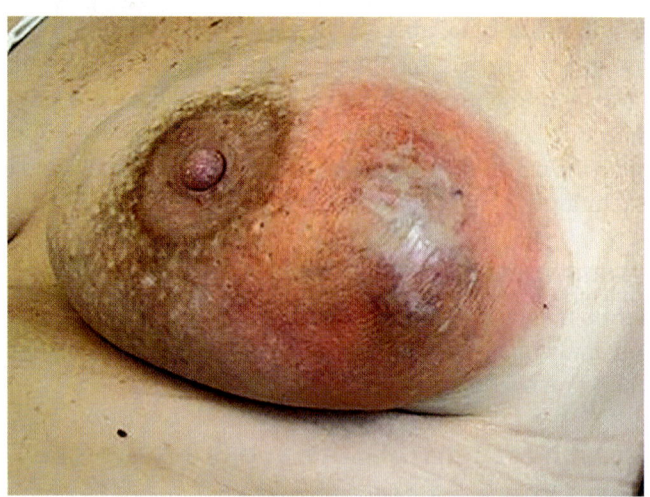

Fig. 6: Breast abscess.

single segment of the breast but the loose parenchyma of the lactating breast allows the infection to spread rapidly both within the stroma and through the lactiferous ducts and if unchecked, the bacteria are excreted in the milk. Benson and Goodman in a study found that majority of infections were due to *S. aureus*; and of these, only 50% had penicillin-sensitive organisms. Other organisms identified were *Streptococcus* spp, gram-negative bacilli (*Escherichia coli*, *Salmonella*) and *Mycobacteria*, fungi (*Candida* and *Cryptococcus*) in rare instances. Breast abscess is seen more commonly in the first month of lactation and often encountered in first pregnancy; due to inexperience, the nipples are more likely to be damaged and at weaning, when the breasts are more likely to become engorged or nipple trauma by erupting teeth.

Clinical Features

The patient presents with intense breast pain and systemic symptoms similar to mastitis; in addition, there is a fluctuant, tender, and palpable mass; sometimes with enlarged axillary lymph nodes **(Fig. 6)**. Occasionally, breast abscesses may also occur without fever or breast redness.

Management

Surgery is reserved for huge fluctuant mass and cases not responding to medications. In the early phase with cellulitis, surgery may be destructive but prolonged antibiotic therapy without drainage when pus is formed may lead to deterioration. A test-needle aspiration preferably ultrasound guided should be performed and even if no pus is aspirated, the aspirate should be subjected to bacteriological and cytological examination to rule out rare case of inflammatory carcinoma.

- *Specific measures*:
  - *Aspiration of pus*: Needle aspiration is recommended for abscesses less than 3 cm; ultrasound-guided aspiration is preferred over palpatory method as it helps in recognizing multiloculation and adequacy of drainage. In cases with large abscesses, a suction drain insertion into the abscess cavity is recommended to avoid refilling after aspiration.
  - *Incision and drainage*: Drainage of abscess is done by radial or circumareolar incisions, breaking all loculi and ensuring complete drainage followed by regular dressings. This may be associated with difficulties in breastfeeding and the possibility of an unsatisfactory cosmetic outcome.
- *General measures*:
  - *Analgesics*: Ibuprofen is regarded as the drug of choice as it reduces inflammation; tramadol and other opioids are avoided as they have central nervous system depressant effect on newborn.
  - Breast support garment, by relaxing the stretched Cooper's ligament, relieves pain and edema.
  - Hot and cold compresses are effective; they are better than cold cabbage leaves in relieving pain.
  - *Breast emptying*: As the root cause for the infection and abscess is milk stasis, frequent emptying of breast is an important aspect of management of mastitis. The breast may be emptied either by suckling or by expression. This condition is not a contraindication for breastfeeding even though the milk has bacteria; there is no harm to the infant rather mother's milk protects against the causative organism as the specific antibody and immunocompetent cells are secreted in the mother's milk hence provides immunological protection.
  - *Antibiotics*: The antibiotic chosen should be secreted and concentrated in milk, should remain active in acidic pH of milk and should not harm the suckling baby. The beta-lactamase-resistant penicillins (cloxacillin, dicloxacillin, or flucloxacillin) are found to be effective and are recommended. Erythromycin, being alkaline, is well concentrated and remains active in human milk. Judicious use of antibiotics and

avoiding combination such as co-amoxiclav for the fear of inducing methicillin-resistant *Staphylococcus aureus* (MRSA). The recommended duration of antibiotic therapy is 10 days.

Bloody Nipple Discharge (Rusty Pipe Syndrome)

Some women experience blood discharge from the nipple usually on birth of first baby in first few days of lactation resulting probably due to increased vascularity of alveoli and lactiferous ducts. It usually resolves in few days; however, if persists beyond 1 week, it needs evaluation to rule out subacute mastitis, intraductal papilloma, and very rarely *Serratia marcescens* colonization of breast milk. Persistent blood-tinged breast milk requires cytological examination, mammography, and breast ultrasound with surgical consultation in suspected cases.

Hypergalactia or Hyperlactation

The 10th International Classification of Diseases uses the terms hypergalactia, hyperlactation, and increased lactation wherein, there is increased production of milk or forceful ejection reflex. It is usually associated with maternal intake of galactagogues traditional or pharmaceutical and in some women with hypo- or hyperthyroidism. The flow of milk is not managed by the infant so they may either have an increased weight gain or, paradoxically, poor weight or the infant is not receiving hind milk with its higher caloric content. Overproduction of milk typically resolves over the first few weeks of lactation. Persistence makes mothers vulnerable for a fast let down, acute mastitis, plugged ducts, chronic breast pain, infant fussiness, and early weaning.

Management

- *Alternate nursing position*: Feeding in a more upright position, leaning back, or in the side lying position allows the infant to better control the flow of milk.
- *Block feeding*: This behavioral strategy involves the mother nursing from alternate breast in 3-hour blocks (±30–60 minutes). This allows one breast to remain undisturbed for 3 hours or more at one time, so that local control from an increase in 5-HT will provide feedback to lactocytes to decrease the milk supply.
- *Manual reduction of flow*: Mechanical obstruction either by using a scissors-hold on the areola or pressing on the breast with the heel of the hand may restrict flow.
- *Medications*: Instruct to stop if on any galactagogues. The use of pharmacologic intervention is not well studied. Low-dose oral contraceptives or pseudoephedrine may be helpful but should be used with caution.

Breast Milk Jaundice

Breast milk jaundice is defined as the persistence of benign neonatal hyperbilirubinemia (total bilirubin levels > 5 mg/dL) beyond the first 2–3 weeks of age. It is essential to distinguish this naïve condition from breastfeeding failure jaundice; the latter is due to suboptimal fluid and caloric intake during the first 7 days of life. The pathophysiology of "breast milk jaundice" is not conclusively known; presence of high concentrations of beta-glucuronidase, causing degradation of beta-D-glucuronic acid is thought to promote an increase in intestinal absorption of unconjugated bilirubin. Breast milk jaundice is a self-limiting condition, usually mild and typically does not require intervention. However, jaundice is to be investigated when the bilirubin levels begin to raise or there is a significant raise of conjugated bilirubin. For management, beta-glucuronidase inhibitors, such as enzymatically hydrolyzed casein or L-aspartic acid, which is contained in casein hydrolysate formula, have been used; however, there appears to be no benefit for the use of these agents.

Lactation Failure

Lactation failure is diagnosed when top feeds are to be started for the baby within 3 months of delivery because of inadequate breast milk supply. Total lactation failure is defined as either a total absence of milk flow or secretion of just a few drops of breast milk following suckling for at least 7 days.

Primary Lactation Failure

When mother is unable to reach copious milk production stage (lactogenesis II), it is called "primary lactation failure" or "primary milk insufficiency syndrome" and is due to intrinsic factors.

Etiology
- Severe postpartum hemorrhage with Sheehan's syndrome
- Undiagnosed retained placenta
- Breast hypoplasia, congenital insufficient glandular tissues
- Breast surgery such as mastectomy, breast reduction, cyst removal, implants and nipple piercing, etc., can disrupt the ductal and neurological pathways
- Breast irradiation
- Delayed lactogenesis is common in women with prepregnancy obesity, insulin resistance, pregnancy-induced hypertension, PCOD, and other conditions associated with high androgen levels during pregnancy. This is managed with breastfeeding support and increased frequency of feeding to stimulate lactogenesis as the suckling reflex is the best secretagogue.

Secondary Lactation Failure

When an initial normal milk supply rapidly diminishes, it is called "secondary lactation failure" or "secondary milk insufficiency syndrome." This reduction in milk production and supply is mainly due to extrinsic factors, as successful lactation is a complex interplay of hormonal, emotional, physical and dietary factors; it is bound to be affected by all the components. This is the most common preventable and treatable cause.

Etiology
- Inappropriate feeding practices: Prelacteals, bottle feeding, incorrect positioning, delayed start, fixed schedule feeding, infrequent feeds, and no night feeds
- Maternal worry, stress, embarrassment, doubt, lack of self-confidence, and previous poor experiences
- Pain during breastfeeding due to sore and cracked nipple, inverted nipple, engorged breast, mastitis, and abscess
- Lack of support system from family, friends, health professionals, employers, etc.
- Early maternal infant separation, illness of infants
- Lack of understanding of the process of lactation
- Lack of knowledge of infant behavior and infant cues
- Maternal medical conditions: Endocrinopathies (thyroid, pituitary, ovarian dysfunction), chronic maternal illness, psychiatric disorder
- Maternal medications: Calcitonin, diuretics—loop, thiazide, dopamine receptor agonist, ergotamine, levodopa, contraceptives, pseudoephedrine, pyridoxine, tamoxifen, etc.
- Early subsequent pregnancy
- Poor milk extraction due to specific infant factors such as prematurity, neuormotor delay, neurologic, sucking percentage, swallowing disorders or anatomic abnormalities such as cleft palate, ankyloglossia, short frenulum, micrognathia, and choanal atresia.

Management of Lactation Failure (Flowchart 1)

Primary prevention:
- Antenatal:
  - Antenatal screening for risk factors
  - Evaluation of systemic illness
  - Maternal general condition and dietary habits
  - Breast examination and lactation assessment in third trimester
  - Antenatal counseling sessions with mother and family: Education should be given regarding advantages of breastfeeding, disadvantages of top feeds, refuting misconception, breastfeeding techniques. Attitude and knowledge of mother as well as her near ones should be changed to have successful breastfeeding; awareness among the family members is very essential to establish breastfeeding practice
  - Display and provide reading material about breast feeding.
- Natal and immediate postnatal:
  - Avoiding maternal exhaustion during labor.
  - Presence of birth companion during labor makes mother more comfortable hence more conductive to breastfeeding.
  - Mode of delivery has no bearing on breastfeeding provided it is well managed; however, difficult traumatic delivery may not have mother and/or baby in optimal condition for breastfeeding.
  - Practicing "breast crawl" soon after birth.
  - Teach mothers to recognize early feeding cues and how to wake up sleeping baby.
  - Implementing baby-friendly hospital initiative 10 steps including written breastfeeding policy, training of healthcare staffs.
  - Initiate breastfeeding as soon as possible within 1 hour of birth.
  - Breastfeeding on demand.
  - Show mothers how to breastfeed and to maintain lactation even if they are separated.
  - Rooming in and encourage "kangaroo mother care".
  - No artificial teats or pacifiers or prelacteal feeds to the baby.
  - Mother support group
  - Address local breast problems at the earliest.
  - Counseling regarding diet of mother.

Treatment: To ensure and increase breast milk supply, an integrated approach is required involving physical, dietary, and medications; improving water intake is the best and most successful method of increasing the breast milk supply. It should be managed in joint consultation with neonatologist, lactational specialist, obstetrician, and midwife with involvement of family members.

Role of galactagogues: Galactagogues (or lactogogues) are medications or other substances believed to assist initiation, maintenance, or augmentation of maternal milk production. There are limited evidence to support their efficacy, and due to safety concerns, routine use is not recommended. Commonly used galactagogues are: (1) Pharmaceutical drugs, (2) anecdotal herbal drugs, and (3) lactogenic diet.

Pharmaceutical drugs:
- *Metoclopramide:* A dopamine antagonist can boost milk production by about 40%. Dose is 10–20 mg thrice daily given for 7–14 days then taper off in next 5–7 days. Side effects are anxiety, tiredness, gastrointestinal and extrapyramidal symptoms. It is not advised for routine use as it causes drastic reduction in the protein concentration of breast milk and changes the electrolyte composition of breast milk.
- *Domperidone:* It is also a dopamine antagonist with negligible side effects as reported. It is given in a dose of 10, three times daily for 3–8 weeks. Its risky for mothers who are at risk for prolonged QT syndrome or on CYP3A4 inhibitors.
- *Sulpiride:* Antipsychotic drug has galactagogue effect by augmenting the hypothalamic prolactin-releasing hormone concentration, used in doses of 50 mg 2–3 times daily. Side effects include extrapyramidal effects and weight gain.

SECTION 10: Postpartum Issues: Maternal and Neonatal

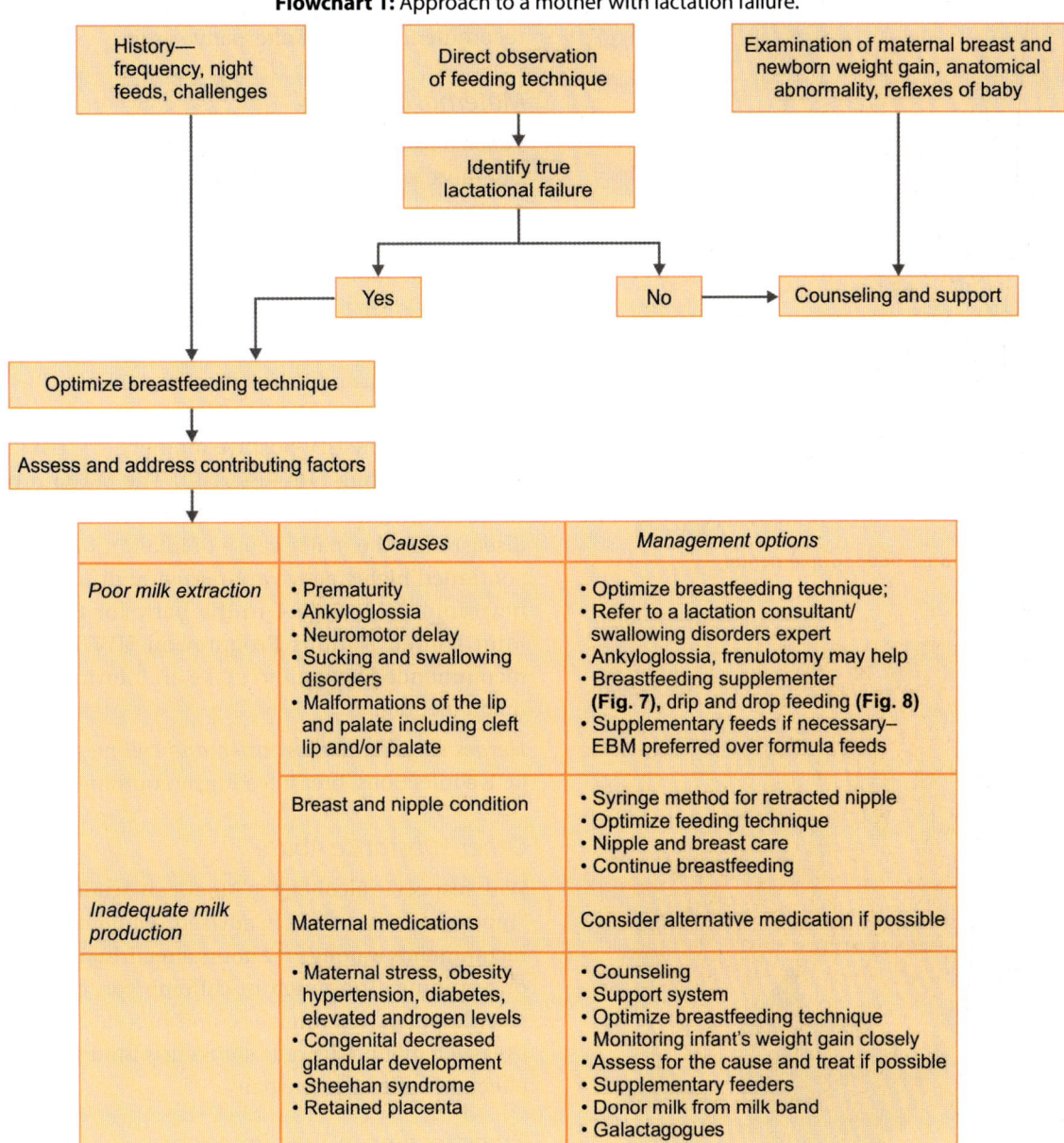

Flowchart 1: Approach to a mother with lactation failure.

Uncommonly used drugs are chlorpromazine, haloperidol, and risperidone
- *Metformin:* The exact mechanism by which metformin increases milk production is not clear but it is believed that by reducing the insulin resistance mainly in polycystic ovary syndrome (PCOS) patients it helps in increasing milk production.

Hormones: Oxytocin nasal spray (1 spray in each nostril prior to pumping milk), recombinant human growth hormone (0.1 IU/kg/day subcutaneously), recombinant human prolactin, thyrotropin-releasing hormone have also been used successfully.

Anecdotal herbal galactagogues: Fenugreek, fennel seeds, anise seed, sweet cumin, chaste berry, bellflower, Nettle leaf, etc.

Lactogenic diet: Diet plays a major role in lactogenesis, a diet rich in protein, vitamins, and essential fatty acids are essential to milk production, especially proteins play a major role in increasing the milk secretion. Traditional lactogenic food are: Oatmeal, spinach, carrots, papaya, asparagus, brown rice, apricot, salmon, flax seeds, chick peas (chhole /kabli chana), lentils, green beans, garlic etc. Milk is 97% water and so increasing intake of water improves the milk production.

Complementary therapies: Relaxation, hypnosis, audio tapes, acupuncture, acupressure, reflexology, etc. have shown variable efficacy.

Breastfeeding in Special Situations

Maternal Use of Medication

Most of the medications commonly used, though not all of them, are relatively safe for breastfeeding; the amount of drug secreted in breast milk and hence transferred to the child is

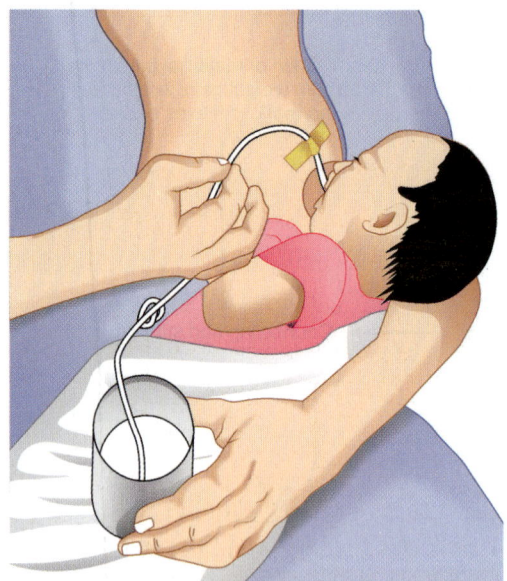

Fig. 7: Breastfeed supplementer.

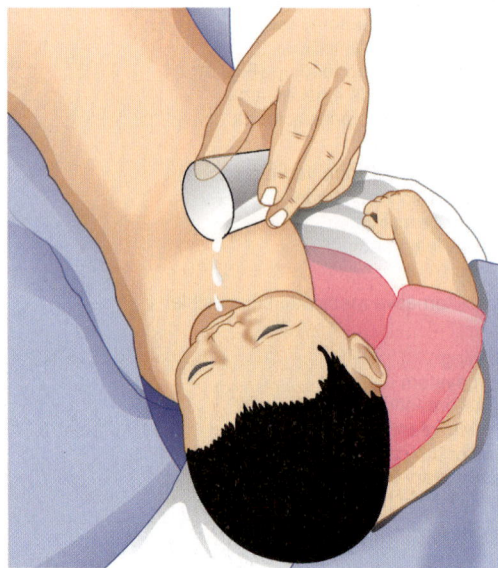

Fig. 8: Drip-drop feeding.

much lower than safe doses of the same drug. The benefits of breastfeeding for both the infant and mother need to be weighed against the potential risks of drug exposure to the infant. It is a better practice to advise the dosing of medication after nursing and before prolonged infant sleep. Lactation compatibility for prescription needs to be checked while prescribing during breastfeeding. For a drug to be transferred into the breast milk depends on the size of the molecule, protein binding capacity, lipid solubility, tissue distribution, time course of maternal plasma-drug concentration, and degree of ionization. Drugs which are highly protein bound, with low lipid solubility, and larger molecular weight do not enter breast milk significantly. The LactMed database authoritative reference which provides data on drug levels in human milk and infant serum, potential adverse effects and recommendations for alternative drugs.

Maternal Infections

Tuberculosis: Women who have been treated appropriately for 2 or more weeks for tuberculosis and who are not considered contagious may breastfeed. *Mycobacterium tuberculosis* rarely causes mastitis or a breast abscess. The WHO has laid recommendation for mothers with tuberculosis to continue breastfeeding in the setting where BCG vaccination is part of the routine immunization schedule.

Human immunodeficiency virus (HIV): Research has highlighted a lower risk of HIV transmission with exclusive breastfeeding by HIV-positive mothers (4% risk), compared to mixed feeding (10-40% risk). The WHO recommends breastfeeding in areas where malnutrition and infectious diseases are the major cause of infant mortality along with continued highly active antiretroviral drugs to mother and nevirapine/zidovudine to the baby for 6–12 weeks. The Joint United Nations Program on HIV/AIDS (UNAIDS) recommended women to make an informed choice about infant feeding.

Herpes simplex, herpes zoster, and cytomegalovirus: During active infections, breast feeding is contraindicated.

Other Substance Abuse

With respect to alcohol, the American Academy of Pediatrics, "moderation is definitely advised" while breastfeeding and recommends waiting for 2 hours after drinking before nursing or pumping. Too much of caffeine can cause irritability, sleeplessness, nervousness, and increased feeding in the breastfed infant. Cigarette smoking is thought to increase the effects of caffeine in the baby.

Breastfeeding in Twin Pregnancy

Reassure the mother that she can produce enough milk for two babies, help her to find best method for her babies (football hold position, double cradle or cross cradle hold, saddle or parallel hold) and get family support.

Breastfeeding Preterm/Low Birth Weight Babies

Baby <34 weeks or weight <1,600 g may have poor or uncoordinated suckling and swallowing may need feeding of EBM through nasogastric tube or spoon feed. One must remember that the preterm milk contain more protein than mature milk hence mother's own preterm milk to be preferred than donated milk; when necessary EBM can be fortified with calcium and other nutrients.

■ CONCLUSION

Imbibing supportive and effective breastfeeding policies in hospital constitute the foundation for initiation of successful breastfeeding by mothers, constant encouragement and support to all lactating mothers is essential to maintain lactation. Suckling is the best galactagogue.

FURTHER READING

1. Abou-Dakn M, Fluhr JW, Gensch M, Wockel A. Positive effect of HPA lanolin versus expressed breast milk on painful and damaged nipples during lactation. Skin Pharmacol. Physiol. 2011;24:27-35.
2. American Academy of Pediatrics. Transmission of Infectious Agents via Human Milk. In: Red Book: 2018 Report of the Committee on Infectious Diseases, 31st, Kimberlin DW, Brady MT, Jack son MA, Long SS (Eds), American Academy of Pediatrics, Itasca, IL. 2018. p.115.
3. Amir LH, Harris H, Adriske L. An audit of mastitis in the emergency department. Journal of Human Lactation. 1999;15 (32):221-4.
4. Amir LH. Managing common breastfeeding problems in the community. BMJ. 2014;348.
5. Anderson JE, Held N, Wright K. Raynaud's phenomenon of the nipple: a treatable cause of painful breastfeeding. Pediatrics 2004;113:360-4.
6. Anderson PO, Valdés V. A critical review of pharmaceutical galactagogues. Breastfeed Med. 2007;2:229.
7. Anderson PO. Domperidone: the forbidden fruit. Breastfeed Med. 2017;12:258.
8. Available at: https://www.verywellfamily.com/how-to-breastfeed-twins-together-4114638
9. Available at: https://www.who.int/nutrition/publications/infantfeeding/global-bf-scorecard-2017.pdfI
10. Baker TP, Lenert JT, Parker J, et al. Lactating adenoma: a diagnosis of exclusion. Breast J. 2001;7:354.
11. Banapurmath S, Banapurmath CR, Kesaree N. Initiation of Lactation and Establishing Relactation in Outpatients. Indian J Pediatr. 2003;40:343-7.
12. Barankin B, Gross MS. Nipple and areolar eczema in the breastfeeding woman. J Cutan Med Surg. 2004;8:126-30.
13. Berry J, Griffiths M, Westcott C. A double-blind, randomized, controlled trial of tongue-tie division and its immediate effect on breastfeeding. Breastfeed. Med. 2012;7:189-93.
14. Campbell-Yeo M L, Allen A C, Joseph K S, Ledwidge JM, Caddell K, Allen VM, et al. Effect of Domperidone on the Composition of Preterm Human Breast Milk. Pediatrics. 2010;125:e107-14.
15. Carlsen SM, Jacobsen G, Vanky E. Mid-pregnancy androgen levels are negatively associated with breastfeeding. Acta Obstet Gynecol Scand. 2010;89:87.
16. Coovadia HM, Rollins NC, Bland RM, Little K, Coutsoudis A, Bennish ML. "Mother-to-child transmission of HIV-1 infection during exclusive breastfeeding in the first 6 months of life: an intervention cohort study". The Lancet. 2007;369(9567):1107-16.
17. Cotterman KJ. Reverse pressure softening: a simple tool to prepare areola for easier latching during engorgement. J Hum Lact. 2004;20:227-37.
18. Dener C, Inan A. Breast abscesses in lactating women. World J Surg. 2003;27:130-3.
19. Foong SC, Tan ML, Foong WC, et al. Oral galactagogues (natural therapies or drugs) for increasing breast milk production in mothers of non-hospitalised term infants. Cochrane Database Syst Rev. 2020;5:CD011505.
20. Jeanne Spencer MD. Common problems of breastfeeding and weaning, https://www.uptodate.com/contents/common-problems-of-breastfeeding-and-weaning.
21. John G, Nduati R, et al. Correlates of perinatal HIV-1 transmission in the Kenyan breast feeding study. 1999. (Abstract 13ET5-1. XIth International Conference on AIDS and STDs in Africa, September 1999, Lusaka, Zambia.).
22. Joint United Nations Program on HIV/AIDS. HIV and infant feeding. Wkly Epidemiol Rec. 1996;71:289-91.
23. Jones W, Breward S. Use of domperidone to enhance lactation: what is the evidence? Community Practitioner. 2011;84(6):35-7.
24. Kvist LJ, Rydhstroem H. Factors related to breast abscess after delivery: a population-based study. BJOG. 2005;112(8):1070-4.
25. Lawrence RA, Lawrence RM. Breastfeeding: A Guide for the Medical Profession, 5th edition CV Mosby. 1999. p. 369.
26. Lawrence RA, Lawrence RM. Breastfeeding: A Guide for the Medical Professions, 7th edition, Elsevier Mosby, Maryland Heights, 2011. p. 268.
27. Lawrence RA, Lawrence RM. Breastfeeding: A Guide for the Medical Professions, 7th edition, Elsevier Mosby, Maryland Heights. 2011. p. 253.
28. Livingstone V, Stringer LJ. The treatment of Staphyloccocus aureus infected sore nipples: a randomized comparative study. J Hum Lact. 1999;15:241-6.
29. Mangesi L, Zakarija-Grkovic I. Treatments for breast engorgement during lactation. Cochrane Database Syst Rev. 2016;CD006946.
30. Marshall BR, Hepper JK, Zirbel CC. Sporadic puerperal mastitis. An infection that need not interrupt lactation. JAMA 1975;233:1377-9.
31. McClellan HL, Hepworth AR, Garbin CP, Rowan MK, Deacon J, Hartmann PE, et al. Nipple pain during breastfeeding with or without visible trauma. J Hum Lact. 2012;28:511-21.
32. McKechnie AC, Eglash A. Nipple shields: a review of the literature. Breastfeed. Med. 2010;5:309-14.
33. Meek J, Tippins S. American Academy of Pediatrics New Mother's Guide to Breastfeeding, Bant am Books, 2011. p. 150.
34. Moorhead AM, Amir LH, O'Brien PW, Wong S. A prospective study of fluconazole treatment for breast and nipple thrush. Breastfeed. Rev. 2011;19:25-9.
35. Righard L. Are breastfeeding problems related to incorrect breastfeeding technique and the use of pacifiers and bottles? Birth. 1998;25:40-4.
36. Schwarz RJ, Shrestha R. Needle aspiration of breast abscesses. Am J Surg. 2001;182(2):117-9.
37. Scott J, Binns C, Oddy W. Predictors of delayed onset of lactation. Maternal and child nutrition 2007;3(3):186-93.
38. Tait P. Nipple pain in breastfeeding women: causes, treatment, and prevention strategies'. Midwifery Womens Health. 2000;45: 212-5.
39. Tewari M, Shukla HS. Effective method of drainage of puerperal breast abscess by percutaneous placement of suction drain. Indian J Surg. 2006;68(6):330-3.
40. The WHO Archived November 7, 2006, at the Wayback Machine on Breastfeeding and maternal tuberculosis; acquired. 2006-08-19.

41. Thomsen AC, Espersen T, Maigaard S. Course and treatment of milk stasis, noninfectious inflammation of the breast, and infectious mastitis in nursing women. Am J Obstetrics Gynecol. 1984;149(5):492-5.
42. Whitaker-Worth DL, Carlone V, Susser WS, Phelan N, Grant-Kels JM. Dermatologic diseases of the breast and nipple. J Am Acad Dermatol. 2000;43:733-51.
43. Wilson-Clay B. Milk oversupply. J Hum Lact. 2006;22:218-20.

LONG QUESTIONS

1. Discuss the prevention and management of breast infections – mastitis and abscess – during the lactation period.
2. Discuss the approach and interventions in lactation failure.
3. Discuss the rationale of breastfeeding advise in situations where the mother carries viral infections such as HIV or hepatitis B.

SHORT QUESTIONS

1. Enlist the common problems that are faced with breastfeeding.
2. What is a galactocele?
3. What are the various galactagogues available?
4. What is the usual etiology and management of blood stained discharge while breastfeeding?
5. Discuss the guidelines on breastfeeding for a baby whose mother is infected or suspected to be infected with coronavirus.

MULTIPLE CHOICE QUESTIONS

1. All of the following neonatal infections can be prevented by breastfeeding, except:
   a. Pneumonia
   b. Diarrhea
   c. Urinary tract infections
   d. Hemorrhagic disease of newborn
2. An indicator of inadequate breastfeeding in an infant is:
   a. Baby sleeping for 2–3 hours after feed
   b. Urine 5–7 times/day
   c. Stool 4 times/day
   d. Weight loss >7 % of birth weight
3. All are measures to prevent breast engorgement, except:
   a. Frequent breastfeeding every 1 1/2hr-2hr during day and every 2–3 hrs at night
   b. Reverse pressure softening
   c. Let the baby finish on one breast before switching to other
   d. Drip drop method
4. Galactogogues—all, except:
   a. Metoclopramide   b. Domperidone
   c. Metformin   d. Sulpiride
5. Primary breast engorgement occurs during which phase of lactation?
   a. Mammogenesis   b. Lactogenesis phase I
   c. Lactogenesis phase II   d. Lactogenesis phase III
6. A 26 years old primigravida with severe preeclampsia was delivered by cesarean section due to uncontrolled blood pressure at 33 weeks gestation, baby was shifted to NICU due to prematurity. All are true regarding preterm breast milk, except:
   a. Baby less than 34 weeks have poor or uncoordinated suckling and swallowing
   b. Early and frequent milk expression in the first 2 weeks following delivery can help in establishing adequate milk volume
   c. Vitamin D and iron supplementation required in preterm infants who are breastfed
   d. Preterm milk contain less protein than mature milk
7. A 22 years old, P1L1, following normal delivery, baby was shifted to NICU after 6 hrs of birth in view of persistent grunting, As the baby is in NICU, expressed breast milk stored in refrigerator can be used up to how many hours?
   a. 6 hours   b. 12 hours
   c. 24 hours   d. 48 hours
8. Which of the following statement is false?
   a. Protein content of human milk is more than cow's milk
   b. Lactose content of human milk is more than cow's milk
   c. Casein content of cow's milk is more than human milk
   d. Calorie content of human milk is more than cow's milk
9. Which of the following are wrongly matched?

Breast milk content	Protection against
a. Lysozyme	Escherichia coli infection
b. Bifidus factor	Plasmodium falciparum infection
c. Lactoferrin	Salmonella infection
d. Low levels of PABA	Plasmodium infection

10. Breastfeeding promotion network of India (BPNI) theme for the year 2020 is?
    a. Breastfeeding: Just 10 steps. The baby friendly way
    b. Empower parents, enable breastfeeding: Now and for the future
    c. Support breastfeeding for a healthier planet
    d. Sustaining breastfeeding: Building alliances without conflicts of interest

11. A 26 years old nursing mother presents with fever and pain in her left breast. She had difficulty with breastfeeding previously, and now examination reveals her left breast is warm, red, swollen, and painful to palpation. What advice should be given to the mother regarding breastfeeding?
    a. Complete cessation of breastfeed
    b. Continue feeding from both the breasts
    c. Continue feeding from only right breast
    d. Continue feeding from only left breast
12. All are true regarding breastfeeding in a COVID-19 positive mother, except:
    a. Expressed breast milk can be given in case of mother and baby separation
    b. Breastfeeding is contraindicated till the mother is having positive status
    c. Infant may receive passive antibody protection since breast milk is source of antibodies and other anti-infective factors
    d. Should follow strict wash hand, wear mask, wipe surface protocols
13. HIV and breastfeeding: all are, except:
    a. Mastitis and breast abscess have been associated with an increased risk of HIV transmission
    b. Infant antiretroviral use is important as short term post exposure prophylaxis after delivery
    c. WHO recommends combination exclusive breastfeeding and maternal HAART
    d. HIV infection in infants during the first two weeks of life may represent transmission that occurred due to breastfeeding.
14. Contraindication to breastfeeding are all, except:
    a. HTLV infection
    b. Active herpetic breast lesion
    c. Active TB within 2 weeks of starting ATT
    d. Maternal hepatitis due to hepatitis B virus after immunoprophylaxis
15. Causes of primary lactation failure are:
    a. Severe PPH
    b. h/o breast irradiation
    c. Undiagnosed retained placenta
    d. All of the above
16. A 24 year primigravida delivered a 3.2 kg baby vaginally after which she had atonic PPH and was transfused with 2 pint PRBC, following which her condition was stable. Breastfeeding was initiated after 2 days, but there was no/very little secretion, both breasts grossly normal. What could be the probable reason?
    a. Primary lactation failure
    b. Secondary lactation failure
    c. Poor suckling of the baby as feeding started late
    d. Inexperienced mother
17. Following a normal delivery a 32 yr P2L2 mother has developed bloody discharge from her left nipple after four days, what is the most probable cause of such a discharge?
    a. Intraductal papilloma   b. Subacute mastitis
    c. Rusty pipe syndrome   d. Breast malignancy
18. A 22 year old mother of a female baby, who was delivered vaginally 4 weeks ago started complaining of beast bite by baby and cracked nipples since 1 week following which she had developed fever and breast pain, on examination her general condition was stable with 101.2°F fever and 108/min pulse rate, on bilateral breast examination tenderness and redness and a localized lump noted in right breast. What is your probable diagnosis?
    a. Breast abscess   b. Mastitis
    c. Hypergalactia   d. Engorged breast
19. Which of the following statements is/are true about smoking can affect breastfeeding?
    a. Suppresses milk production
    b. Alters the composition of breast milk
    c. Suppresses milk production
    d. All of the above
20. All are true about breast milk jaundice, except:
    a. Breast milk jaundice is defined as the persistence of benign neonatal hyperbilirubinemia (total bilirubin levels >5 mg/dL)
    b. Jaundice persist beyond the first two to three weeks of age
    c. Presence of high concentrations of beta-glucuronidase
    d. Significant component is conjugated bilirubin

Answers

1. d	2. d	3. d	4. c	5. c	6. d
7. c	8. a	9. b	10. c	11. c	12. b
13. d	14. d	15. d	16. a	17. c	18. b
19. d	20. d				

10.7 NEONATAL ADAPTION TO EXTRAUTERINE LIFE

Ruchi Nimish Nanavati, Suman Rao PN

INTRODUCTION

India contributes to one-fifth of global live births and more than a quarter of neonatal deaths. About three fourths of all neonatal deaths occur in the first week of life. The first 24 hours accounting for more than one-third of the deaths.[1] Thus, serious, concentrated efforts have to be made to address the needs of a newborn in its first days to facilitate extrauterine transition in order to reduce neonatal mortality. 90% of newborns achieve intrauterine to extrauterine adaptation with little or no assistance. In neurobiology, it is understood that experience can change the mature brain but experience during the critical period of early childhood organizes brain systems. Therefore supporting the neonates, both normal and high risk, for successful adaptation to extrauterine life is of utmost importance and the duty of all healthcare personnel involved with mother and child care.

MECHANISMS OF PHYSIOLOGICAL ADAPTATION

Thermal Adaptation

The newborn at birth has to make a successful transition from the warm in utero environment to the cold, wet, extrauterine environment. Humans being precocial homeotherms, the newborn has to maintain a constant body temperature in the normal range, i.e., 36.5–37.5°C. In utero, the fetus maintains a body temperature 0.5°C greater than the mother. In addition to producing heat as a byproduct of various biochemical processes vital to the growth and function, the fetus has the capacity to generate heat solely for purpose of maintaining core body temperature. However, fetal thermogenesis is suppressed in utero by placental adenosine and prostaglandin E.[2] The thermogenetic processes are capable of being activated immediately at birth. *Brown adipose tissue (BAT)*, the specialized adipose tissue with the uncoupling protein 1(UCP 1), has the sole function of thermogenesis. BAT is highly vascular and rich in triglycerides and mitochondria. In the newborn, it is found around the kidneys and in the interscapular area of the back, extending up the dorsal neck. The key stimulus for thermogenesis by BAT is norepinephrine. Thyroid hormone (T_3 and T_4), cortisol and possibly leptin and prolactin also regulate BAT activity.

Mechanisms of Thermogenesis[3]

- *Nonshivering thermogenesis*: At delivery, cord clamping removes the inhibitors of thermogenesis from the placenta. The cold sensors in the skin activate the sympathetic nervous system resulting in increased circulating concentrations of epinephrine and nor epinephrine. Activation of the β_3 receptors results in release of free fatty acids and stimulation of UCP 1. The cortisol surge prior to birth increases UCP 1 and releases T_4. BAT lipolysis generates heat and also releases two major biochemical products—glycerol and fatty acids, which act as important metabolic fuel in the highly active organs such as the heart, brain, diaphragm, and skeletal muscles resulting in prolonged thermogenic response. Thus triggered by temperature sensation of the skin, the glycogen and brown fat reserves in the term newborn increases infant metabolic rate two- to three-fold and thus maintain body temperature for a period of several hours.
- *Shivering thermogenesis*: In newborns shivering, thermogenesis is the second line of defense. The newborn is capable of shivering but the temperature at which it is activated is much lower than in adults and shivering does not contribute to heat production, except in severe hypothermia.

This thermogenic response in newborns utilizes significant amounts of oxygen and fuel. The oxygen use increases by 100% or more.

Cardiopulmonary Adaptation[4]

Placenta is the organ of gas exchange in fetal life. The fetal lungs do not function as a route to transport oxygen into the blood or to excrete CO_2 as fetal lungs are filled with fluid rather than air. In addition, the arteries that perfuse fetal lungs are markedly constricted.

Normally, three major changes begin immediately after birth:
1. The fluid in the alveoli is absorbed into pulmonary lymphatics and replaced by air.
2. With clamping of umbilical cord, umbilical artery and vein functionally close. This removes low resistance placental circulation and results in increasing systemic blood pressure.
3. As a result of increased oxygen levels in alveoli, the blood vessels in the lungs are relaxed, decreasing resistance to blood flow.

This decreased resistance, together with the increase systemic blood pressure, leads to a dramatic increase in pulmonary blood flow and a decrease in flow through the ductus arteriosus. The oxygen from the alveoli is absorbed by the blood in the pulmonary vessels, and the oxygen-enriched blood returns to the left side of the heart, where it is pumped to the tissues of the newborn's body. In most circumstances, air provides sufficient oxygen (21%) to initiate relaxation of the pulmonary blood vessels. As blood levels of oxygen increase and pulmonary blood vessels relax, the ductus arteriosus begins to constrict. Blood previously diverted through the ductus arteriosus now flows through the lungs, where it picks up more oxygen to transport to tissues throughout the body.

At the completion of this normal transition, the baby is breathing air and using his lungs to transport oxygen into his blood. His initial cries and deep breaths have been strong enough to help move the fluid from his airways. The oxygen and gaseous distension of the lungs are the main stimuli for the pulmonary blood vessels to relax. As adequate oxygen enters the blood, the baby's skin gradually turns from gray/blue to pink.

Although the initial steps in a normal transition occur within a few minutes of birth, the entire process may not be completed until hours or even several days after delivery. For example, studies have shown that, in normal newborns born at term, it may take up to 10 minutes to achieve an oxygen saturation of 90% or greater. Functional closure of the ductus arteriosus may not occur until 12–24 hours after birth, and complete relaxation of the lungs vessels does not occur for several months.

The respiratory rate during early transition ranges from 60 to 100 bpm and then slows to 50–60 bpm. This is particularly true for infants born of an elective cesarean section. Healthy infants may continue to breathe well above 60 bpm, they do not appear distressed and can slow their rate enough to feed successfully. Infants with hyperventilation to compensate for metabolic acidosis, to increase O_2 intake or to eliminate CO_2 are unlikely to slow their rate enough to feed successfully.

Metabolic Adaptation

Fetus exists in a complex, dynamic, and yet intriguing symbiosis with its mother as far as fuel metabolism is concerned. The neonate must become independent after birth, transitioning from a continuous intravenous supply of predominantly glucose as fuel to a variable and intermittent exogenous intake orally that is the hallmark of the neonatal period.[5] This successful adaptation requires not only an immediate catabolic cascade but also adaptation to enteral feeding.

A normal term fetus has adequate stores in the form of glycogen in the liver and adipose tissue. It is capable of glycogenolysis, gluconeogenesis, and lipolysis, though these processes are suppressed in utero. At birth, the surge of cortisol and adrenergic hormones during labor followed by the surge in glycogen at cord clamping initiate the metabolic cascade. This mobilizes hepatic glycogen and adequate glycogen stores are available to sustain fuel supply in the first 12 hours. By this time, activation of phosphoenolpyruvate carboxykinase (PEPCK) initiates gluconeogenesis. Lipolysis, fatty acid ?-oxidation with generation of ketone bodies, and proteolysis generate lactate and other substrates for gluconeogenesis. Ketone bodies and lactate serve as alternative fuels with glucose-sparing effects, and are especially important in maintaining cerebral energy. The fetus and neonate have a high lipoprotein lipase activity in the liver in contrast to the adult. 50% of the caloric intake of the newborn is from lipids. Blood glucose concentration falls rapidly after birth, reaching a nadir by 1 hour of age and then rising to stabilize by 3 hours of age. The normal term fetus is able to make this transition well. Routine monitoring of sugar is unnecessary in a healthy term infant.

Transition from fetal to newborn life is associated with major changes in water and electrolyte homeostatic control. Reduction in extracellular compartment of body water resulting in weight loss of 5–10% and up to 15% in both term and preterm infants, respectively during the first days of life is physiologic and not associated with electrolyte imbalance. Physiologic diuresis and insensible water loss through skin and respiratory system is mainly responsible.

Neonates who encounter perturbations in this normal transitional physiology are at risk of developing perinatal asphyxia, hypothermia, hypoglycemia, shock, respiratory distress syndrome, transient tachypnea of newborn, patent ductus arteriosus, necrotizing enterocolitis, meconium aspiration syndrome (MAS), persistent pulmonary hypertension (PPHN), and their consequences.

■ NEONATES AT RISK OF MALADAPTATION

Preterm/Low Birth Weight Infant

The preterm infant behaves more like an altricial animal with little thermogenic capacity in the immediate newborn period. The preterm infant has reduced fat stores (1% in a 28 weeks preterm vs. 16% at term) especially BAT, larger surface area/weight ratio, immature skin with increased trans epidermal evaporative water loss, extended posture, rapid breathing, increased risk of hypoxia—all of which predisposes to hypothermia.

Extremely preterm infants have structurally immature lungs, absence of pulmonary surfactant, and insufficient muscle strength to make strong initial respiratory efforts and may be difficult to ventilate. Their small blood volumes make them more susceptible to hypovolemic effects of blood loss.

Preterms are vulnerable to neurologic injury. Before 32 weeks' gestation, preterm babies have a fragile network of capillaries in germinal matrix. Rapid changes in blood carbon dioxide (CO_2) levels, blood pressure, or blood volume as well as obstruction of the venous drainage from the head, may increase the risk of rupturing these capillaries. Bleeding in the germinal matrix may cause an intraventricular hemorrhage, hydrocephalus, and a lifelong disability. Inadequate blood flow and oxygen delivery may cause damage to the white matter of the brain, resulting in cerebral palsy, even in the absence of hemorrhage. Excessive oxygen administration may cause damage to the developing retina, resulting in retinopathy of prematurity and visual loss.

Small energy stores, glycogen and fat, delayed maturation of gluconeogenesis, hyperinsulinemia, or increased demands as in a sick infant may hamper the normal metabolic transition and lead to hypoglycemia. Under these conditions, the most vital organ—the brain tries to maintain the metabolism by increasing blood supply and glucose transfer to brain, using alternate fuels such as lactate, fatty acids, and ketone bodies.

Fetal Growth Restriction

Perinatal mortality amongst fetal growth restriction (FGR) infants is 10 to 20 times as compared to appropriate-for-gestational age (AGA) infants. Chronic fetal hypoxia, perinatal asphyxia, multisystem disorders associated with asphyxia, and lethal congenital anomalies are mainly responsible. Uterine contractions add on additional hypoxic stress on the chronically hypoxic fetus with marginally functioning placenta. Depleted myocardial glycogen stores further limit fetal cardiopulmonary adaptation. Limited stores of BAT make them vulnerable to cold stress. Hypoglycemia develops in infants who are FGR more than any other neonatal category due to reduced hepatic glycogen stores, impaired gluconeogenesis and decrease in hepatic glucose production. Fetal hypoxia increases erythropoietin secretion leading to the hyper viscosity—polycythemia syndrome which adversely affects neonatal hemodynamics.

Postmaturity

Dysmaturity syndrome affecting 20% of postterm pregnancies occurs when placental function is reduced. It is associated with perinatal asphyxia, meconium aspiration syndrome (MAS), hypothermia, hypoglycemia, polycythemia—hyperviscosity, persistent pulmonary hypertension of the newborn (PPHN), hypocalcemia, and congenital anomalies.

Multiple Gestation

Animal models exhibit inverse relationship between litter size and birth weight and gestation. The consequence of prematurity is a true challenge faced by this group making postnatal adaptation at times very stormy. Most texts cite a two-to-three-fold increased risk of malformation and increase in cerebral palsy (CP) with the number of fetuses seems to be exponential.[6]

Congenital Anomalies

Congenital anomalies do affect neonatal adaptation. Soon after birth, infant with choanal atresia would need insertion of an oral airway to allow air to pass through while those with pharyngeal airway malformation as in Robin's sequence may pose difficulty in endotracheal tube placement. Prone position and nasopharyngeal tube are often sufficient to maintain airway. Congenital diaphragmatic hernia mandates selective intubation and placing of large orogastric catheter to evacuate stomach. Apart from the anomalies encountered in delivery room (DR), other systemic anomalies involving cardiopulmonary, nervous, gastrointestinal systems make adaptation difficult. Prompt identification and appropriate timely action is vital.

■ SUPPORT FOR NORMAL ADAPTATION

Prevention of Heat Loss in Delivery Room

"Newborn Care Corner" is a space within DR and maternity operation theater where immediate care is provided to all newborns. This area is mandatory for all health facilities where deliveries take place in order to provide acceptable environment to all infants after birth.[7] DR should be warm and temperature < 25°C is not advisable when anticipating a preterm birth. At delivery, evaporation of the amniotic fluid may result in a drop of the infant's body temperature at a rate of 0.2–1.0?C/minute with heat loss of 0.58 kcal/mL of water loss.[8] Increasing DR temperature and use of a prewarmed radiant warmer facilitates positive radiant heat transfer. Receiving the infant in warm sterile towels, covering the cold weighing machine plate with a warm towel reduce conductive heat losses. Delivering in a draught-free room and switching off the fan reduce convective heat losses. Prompt drying of the infant and in the case of extreme preterm infant, covering with a cling wrap can reduce evaporative heat loss. Preservation of vernix caseosa also may contribute to this. Drying of infant's body, except hands, is advisable as presence of amniotic fluid on baby's hands facilitates breast crawl. Babies born prematurely should have all steps taken to reduce heat loss, even if they do not initially appear to require resuscitation.

The newborn infant at all times must be managed in a Thermo Neutral Environment (TNE), that range of environmental temperature at which the metabolic rate and oxygen consumption is at the lowest **(Fig. 1)**.[8] TNE depends on various factors such as weight, gestational age, and day of life of the infant. "Rooming In" must be practiced in postnatal period. Slightly premature infants (32–35 weeks) or FGR infants may appear to have normal body temperature at the expense of metabolically generated heat. Nursing these infants in TNE either in an incubator, or under a radiant warmer or preferably in continuous skin to skin contact with the mother is vital. Kangaroo mother care (KMC) is initiated soon after birth fosters their health and well-being by promoting effective thermal control, breastfeeding, infection prevention, and bonding.

Timing of Umbilical Cord Clamping

Cord clamping should be delayed for at least 30–60 seconds for most vigorous term and preterm newborns. A meta-analysis of 15 trials (3,911 women and infant pairs) comparing early versus delayed cord clamping (DCC) in term neonates showed that DCC was beneficial up to 6 months of age in the form of

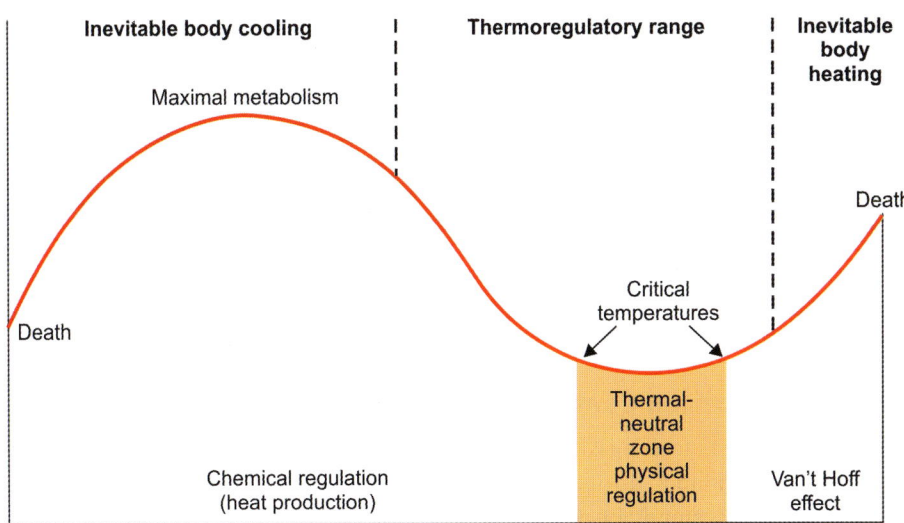

Fig. 1: Thermoneutral Environment (TNE). Environmental temperature on horizontal axis and minimal metabolic rate on vertical axis.
Source: Friedman M, Baumgart S. Thermal regulation. In: Mhairi MG, Seshia MMK, Mullett MD, (eds). Avery's Neonatology, 6th edition. Philadelphia: Lippincott Williams & Wilkins; 2005. pp. 445-57.

improved iron status.[9] DCC has more benefits for preterm neonates. A recent meta-analysis of 48 studies, involving 5,721 preterm babies has shown that DCC reduces mortality [average risk ratio (aRR) 0.73, 95% confidence interval (CI) 0.54–0.98], any intraventriuclar hemorrhage (aRR 0.83, 95% CI 0.7–0.99), and may also reduce the number of babies who die or have neurodevelopmental impairment in early years (aRR 0.61, 95% CI 0.30–0.96).[10]

Resuscitation

The Neonatal Resuscitation 2015 Guidelines by the American Academy of Pediatrics and the American Heart Association should be followed. At every delivery, at least 1 person trained in neonatal resuscitation should be present. It is not sufficient to have someone "on call" as no delay is acceptable when resuscitation is required. The following precautions apply to babies of all gestational ages, but are particularly important when resuscitating a preterm baby.

- Handle the baby gently.
- Avoid placing the baby in a head-down (Trendelenburg) position.
- Avoid delivering excessive positive pressure during ventilation or CPAP (continuous positive airway pressure).
- Use an oximeter and blood gases to adjust ventilation and oxygen concentration gradually and appropriately
- Do not give rapid infusions of fluid.

Additional trained personnel should be present at birth to perform complex resuscitation with preterm births. If preterm baby is breathing spontaneously, and HR > 100 bpm, but has labored respiration, is cyanotic or has low SpO_2, CPAP administration is helpful **(Table 1)**. Studies have shown that infants < 30 weeks gestation may benefit from early treatment with CPAP soon after resuscitation.[4]

TABLE 1: Targeted preductal SpO_2 (%).

Time after birth (minutes)	Targeted preductal SpO_2 (%)
1	60–65
2	65–70
3	70–75
4	75–80
5	80 - 85
10	85–95

Healthy term infants are generally awake and alert for 30–60 minutes immediately after birth with intermittent gross body movements and then asleep for several hours. Term infants without period of wakefulness before sleep may be lethargic and term infants who fail to go into quite sleep may be neurologically irritable. Preterm infant may not demonstrate above states.

Early Feeding

The interactions between mothers and their newborns that result in nursing are the single most important behaviors in the hours following birth for the survival of the newborn. The fetus at full term is swallowing approximately 50 mL of amniotic fluid every hour. Early initiation of feeding is therefore in continuum of normal fetal physiology. Help mothers initiate breastfeeding within one half-hour of birth. In case of cesarean section, breastfeeding should be initiated as soon as mother has recovered from anesthesia and definitely within 4 hours of birth. Immediately after delivery, the infant is most alert, active, with good sucking and rooting reflexes. Early feeds not only help prevent hypothermia and hypoglycemia, but also provide the first "immunization" to the infant.

The immunoglobulin concentration in colostrum is maximum on day 1. Early initiation of feeds helps in establishing and maintaining lactation, improves exclusive breastfeeding rates at 6 months and thereby reduces infant mortality. With preterm delivery, the mother should be encouraged to express and feed colostrum to the infant. Nonnutritive sucking and KMC are useful adjuncts. Monitoring of at-risk infants, prevention, and early treatment of hypoglycemia are critical to prevent adverse neurodevelopmental outcome. The target blood glucose should be >50 mg%.

Breast Crawl and Early Skin-to-Skin Contact

The preferred method of initiating breastfeeding is The Breast Crawl (TBC).[11] The current recommendation during neonatal resuscitation is that "all healthy infants should be placed and remain in skin-to-skin contact with their mothers *immediately* after delivery *until the first feeding occurs.*" TBC is when a newborn, left undisturbed and skin to skin on the mother's trunk following delivery, moves toward his mother's breast for the purpose of locating and self-attaching for the first feeding. The neonatal reflexes and release of oxytocin in the mother and the infant aid in this process. Smell of amniotic fluid preserved on the hands facilitates breast crawl. The primary benefits of TBC are initiating and establishing effective breastfeeding, thermoregulation, physical stabilization of the healthy newborn and improving mother's confidence. Indeed, the breast crawl is nothing short of a continuation of the miracle of birth!

The meta-analysis on early skin-to-skin contact including 46 trials with 3,850 women and their infants has shown that skin-to-skin contact at birth improves breastfeeding; infants have better stabilization scores and higher glucose levels.[12]

Neonatal Transport

As per the National Family Health Survey (NFHS 4), approximately 21% deliveries in India still occur at home. Organized neonatal transport is an integral component of perinatal care. In critically ill babies, the outcome does depends on the effectiveness of transport system. Unfortunately, very less attention is paid to this modality in India. It is the responsibility of the primary physician. *Pretransport stabilization* is the key to intact survival. Available models for pretransport stabilization and care during transport are:

- STABLE: *S*ugar, *T*emperature, *A*irway, *B*lood pressure, *L*aboratory work, *E*motional support.
- SAFER: *S*ugar, *A*rterial circulatory support, *F*amily support, *E*nvironment, *R*espiratory support.
- TOPS: *T*emperature, *O*xygenation (Airway and Breathing), *P*erfusion, *S*ugar

KEY MESSAGES

- "Newborn Care Corner" is a space within DR and maternity operation theater where immediate care is provided to all newborns. This area is mandatory for all health facilities where deliveries take place.
- At every delivery, at least 1 person trained in neonatal resuscitation should be present.
- The current guidelines NRP 2015 suggest use of pulse oximeter and oxygen blender in DR to achieve targeted saturation.
- Thermoregulation and prevention of hypothermia are a vital and unique aspect of neonatal adaptation.
- Breastfeeding should be initiated in the first half hour of delivery. The preferred method of initiating breastfeeding is TBC.
- Nonnutritive Sucking and KMC are useful adjuncts to maintain and enhance lactation.
- Pretransport stabilization is the key to successful transport.

REFERENCES

1. Sankar MJ, Neogi SB, Sharma J, Chauhan M, Srivastava, Prabhakar PK, et al. State of newborn health in India. J Perinatol. 2016;36:S3-8.
2. Power GG, Blood AB. Perinatal thermal physiology In: Polin RA, Fox WW, (eds). Fetal and Neonatal Physiology, 4th edition. Philadelphia: Saunders; 2011. pp. 615-24.
3. Sahni R, Schulze K. Temperature control in newborn infants. In: Polin RA, Fox WW, (eds). Fetal and Neonatal Physiology, 4th edition. Philadelphia. Saunders; 2011:624-48.
4. Kattwinkel J. Overview and principles of resuscitation. Textbook of Neonatal Resuscitation, 1st edition. New Delhi. Jaypee Brothers Medical Publishers (P) Ltd.; 2012. pp. 1-36.
5. Ward Platt M, Deshpande S. Metabolic adaptation at birth. Semin Fetal Neonatal Med. 2005;10:341-50.
6. Blickstein I, Shinwell ES. Obstetric Management of Multiple Pregnancies and births. In: Martin RJ, Fanaroff AA, (eds). Neonatal Perinatal Medicine Diseases of the Fetus and Infant, 8th edition. Philadelphia: Mosby; 2006. pp. 375-82.
7. National Neonatology Forum, UNICEF. (2010). Toolkit For Setting Up Special Care Newborn Units, Stabilization Units & Newborn Care Corners. [online] Available from: https://www.healthynewbornnetwork.org/hnn-content/uploads/UNICEF_Toolkit-for-Setting-Up-Special-Care-Newborn-Units-Stabilisation-Units-and-Newborn-Care-Corners.pdf. [Last accessed November, 2021].
8. Friedman M, Baumgart S. Thermal regulation. In: Mhairi MG, Seshia MMK, Mullett MD, (eds). Avery's Neonatology, 6th edition. Philadelphia: Lippincott Williams & Wilkins; 2005. pp. 445-57.
9. McDonald SJ, Middleton P, Dowswell T, Morris PS. Effect of timing of umbilical cord clamping of term infants on maternal and neonatal outcomes. Cochrane Database Syst Rev. 2013;(7): CD004074.
10. Rabe H, Gyte GM, Diaz-Rossello JL, Duley L. Effect of timing of umbilical cord clamping and other strategies to influence placental transfusion at preterm birth on maternal and infant outcomes. Cochrane Database Syst Rev. 2019;9:CD003248.
11. Henderson A. Understanding the breast crawl: implications for nursing practice. Nurs Womens Health. 2011;15:296-307.

12. Moore ER, Bergman N, Anderson GC, Medley N. Early skin-to-skin contact for mothers and their healthy newborn infants. Cochrane Database Syst Rev. 2016;11:CD003519.

LONG QUESTIONS

1. Explain the interventions that help the newborn to adapt to extrauterine life.
2. Describe the thermal adaptation of the newborn at birth. Add a note on the importance of skin-to-skin contact at birth.
3. Describe the neonatal adaptation to extrauterine life.
4. Which are the fetuses at risk for mal adaptation at birth? Describe how you would support these newborns to make the transition to extrauterine life.
5. Describe safe neonatal transport. Add a note on stabilization of a baby during transport.

SHORT QUESTIONS

1. What are the mechanisms of thermogenesis?
2. Write a short note on cardiopulmonary adaptation of the newborn at birth.
3. What is the breast crawl?
4. Write a short note on metabolic adaptation of the newborn at birth.
5. What is warm chain?

MULTIPLE CHOICE QUESTIONS

1. The number of newborns who need assistance to make the transition to extrauterine life is approximately:
   a. 5%
   b. 10%
   c. 15%
   d. 20%
2. The normal temperature range of a newborn is:
   a. 35–37°C
   b. 36–37°C
   c. 36.5–37.5°C
   d. 36–37.5°C
3. Thermogenesis at birth is dependent on:
   a. Brown fat
   b. Thyroid hormones
   c. Nor epinephrine
   d. Glycogen stores
   e. All of the above
4. All are part of the warm chain at birth, except:
   a. Warm delivery room
   b. Drying the baby
   c. Skin-to-skin contact at birth
   d. Warm bath
5. The main mechanism for thermogenesis at birth is:
   a. Shivering thermogenesis
   b. Nonshivering thermogenesis
   c. Muscle activity
   d. Specific dynamic action of feeds
6. All are parts of cardiopulmonary adaptation at birth, except:
   a. Decrease in systemic vascular resistance
   b. Decrease in pulmonary vascular resistance
   c. Fluid in alveoli replaced by air
   d. Rise in oxygen saturation.
7. The oxygen saturation in the newborn reaches >90% by:
   a. 2 minutes
   b. 5 minutes
   c. 10 minutes
   d. 20 minutes
8. Functional closure of the ductus arteriosus may not occur by:
   a. 1–2 hours
   b. 3–6 hours
   c. 6–12 hours
   d. 12–24 hours
9. All are part of metabolic adaptation at birth, except:
   a. Gluconeongenesis
   b. Glycogenesis
   c. Lipolysis
   d. Use of ketone bodies and lactate
10. The nadir of blood sugar after birth:
    a. Half hour
    b. 1 hour
    c. 3 hours
    d. 6 hours
11. The following are benefits of skin-to-skin contact at birth:
    a. Maintains temperature
    b. Improves exclusive breastfeeding rates at 6 weeks
    c. Improves mothers confidence
    d. All the above
12. All are problems of a preterm newborn at birth, except:
    a. Hypothermia
    b. Intraventricular hemorrhage
    c. Meconium aspiration syndrome
    d. Hypoglycemia
13. Regarding cord clamping at birth, identify the correct statement:
    a. Cord should be clamped after 5 minutes
    b. Early cord clamping interferes with resuscitation at birth
    c. Delayed cord clamping reduces anemia
    d. Delayed cord clamping reduces hypoglycemia
14. While resuscitating a preterm neonate, identify the wrong statement:
    a. Avoid fluid boluses
    b. Extreme preterm neonate not to be dried but should be placed in a plastic bag.
    c. Place the baby in skin-to-skin contact.
    d. If the baby has labored breathing, provide CPAP.
15. All are part of pretransport stabilization, except:
    a. Electrolytes
    b. Sugar
    c. Perfusion
    d. Oxygenation

Answers

1. b 2. c 3. e 4. d 5. b 6. a
7. c 8. d 9. b 10. b 11. d 12. c
13. c 14. c 15. a

10.8 NEONATAL RESUSCITATION

Sonali Tank

INTRODUCTION

Neonatal resuscitation, also known as newborn resuscitation, is an emergency procedure focused on supporting the newborn children who do not readily begin breathing at birth putting them at risk of irreversible organ injury and death. Globally, about one quarter of all neonatal deaths are caused by birth asphyxia, birth asphyxia being defined simply as the failure to initiate and sustain breathing at birth.[1]

Approximately 10%[2] of newborns require some assistance to begin breathing at birth. Less than 1% require extensive resuscitation measures,[3,4] such as cardiac compressions and medications. Although most newly born infants successfully transition from intrauterine to extrauterine life without special help, a significant number will require some degree of resuscitation.

Why do newborns require a different approach to resuscitation than adults?

Unlike adults, wherein cardiac arrest is a complication of trauma or existing heart disease, most newborns requiring resuscitation have a healthy heart and the problem is with respiration leading to inadequate gas exchange.

Hence, the focus of neonatal resuscitation is effective ventilation of the baby's lungs.

FETAL PHYSIOLOGY[5]

Understanding the fetal physiology of transition from extrauterine to intrauterine life will help in understanding the steps of neonatal resuscitation.

Before birth, the fetus is dependent on the placenta for gas exchange. The fetal lungs are expanded in utero but the potential air sacs (alveoli) are filled with fluid. The pulmonary arterioles are constricted, most of the blood bypasses the lungs and enter the aorta through the ductus arteriosus.

A series of physiologic changes occur after birth that culminates in a successful transition from fetal to neonatal circulation. The process begins within a few minutes but may not be completed for hours or even days.

The following three important changes take place:
1. When the baby breathes and the cord is clamped and cut, the newborn uses its lungs instead of the placenta for gas exchange.
2. The baby's initial cries and deep breaths help to move out fluid from the airways and replace it with air.
3. The air in the alveoli causes the blood vessels in the lungs to dilate increasing the pulmonary blood flow and constriction of the ductus arteriosus.

What can go wrong?
- Compromise of uterine or placental blood flow—deceleration of fetal heart rate (FHR)
- *Weak cry:* Inadequate ventilation to push out the alveolar fluid
- *In utero hypoxia:* Meconium passage—may block airways
- *Fetal blood loss (abruption):* Systemic hypotension
- *Fetal hypoxia/ischemia:* Poor cardiac contractility and fetal bradycardia—systemic hypotension
- Pulmonary arterioles remain constricted—PPHN.

Clinical findings of abnormal transition:
- Apnea or tachypnea
- Bradycardia or tachycardia
- Decreased muscle tone
- Low oxygen saturation
- Low blood pressure.

PREPARING FOR RESUSCITATION

Readiness for neonatal resuscitation requires assessment of perinatal risk, a system to assemble the appropriate personnel based on that risk, an organized method for ensuring immediate access to supplies and equipment, and standardization of behavioral skills that help assure effective teamwork and communication.

Every birth should be attended by at least 1 person who can perform the initial steps of newborn resuscitation and PPV, and whose only responsibility is care of the newborn. In the presence of significant perinatal risk factors that increase the likelihood of the need for resuscitation,[6,7] additional personnel with resuscitation skills, including chest compressions, endotracheal intubation, and umbilical vein catheter insertion, should be immediately available.

Furthermore, because a newborn without apparent risk factors may unexpectedly require resuscitation, each institution should have a procedure in place for every birth. A standardized checklist to ensure that all necessary supplies and equipment are present and functioning may be helpful **(Table 1)**. The following guidelines are a summary of the evidence presented in the 2015 International Consensus on Cardiopulmonary Resuscitation and Emergency Cardiovascular Care Science With Treatment Recommendations (CoSTR).[8,9]

What questions should you ask before every birth?
It is important for the obstetric and newborn care provider to coordinate care by establishing effective communication.

The following prebirth questions should be asked:
1. What is the expected gestational age?
2. Is the amniotic fluid clear?

TABLE 1: Equipment checklist.[10]	
Warm	• Preheated warmer • Warm towels or blankets
Clear airway	• Bulb syringe or suction • 10-F or 12-F suction catheter, attached to wall suction, set at 80–100 mm Hg • Meconium aspirator
Auscultate, ventilate	• Stethoscope • Flow meter set to 10 L/min • Oxygen blender set to 21% (21–30% if <35 weeks gestation) • Term and preterm-sized masks • 8F feeding tube and large syringe
Oxygenate	• Equipment to give free-flow oxygen • Pulse oximeter • Target saturation table
Intubate	• Laryngoscope with size-0 and size-1 straight blades (size 00, optional) • Stylet (optional) • Endotracheal tubes (sizes 2.5, 3.0, 3.5) • CO_2 detector • Measuring tape • Sticking tape • Scissors • Laryngeal mask 9 (size 1) and a 5-mL syringe
Medications	Access to: • 1:10,000 (0.1 mg/mL) epinephrine • Normal saline • Supplies for placing umbilical venous catheter • ECG monitor

(ECG: electrocardiography)

3. How many babies are expected?
4. Are there additional risk factors?

Timing for clamping of umbilical cord:[11] At the time of birth, a large volume of blood remains in the placenta and majority of this placental blood transfusion occurs during the first minute of life. The ideal time for clamping the cord is the subject of ongoing research. Potential benefits of delayed cord clamping for preterm neonates are decreased mortality, higher blood pressure and volume, less need for blood transfusion after birth, fewer brain hemorrhages and a lower risk of necrotizing enterocolitis. In term neonates, it may decrease the chance of developing iron deficiency anemia and may improve neurodevelopment outcomes. Potential adverse effects are increased risk of polycythemia and jaundice and delaying resuscitation for compromised newborns.

The current evidence suggests that clamping should be delayed for at least 30–60 seconds for most vigorous term and preterm neonates.

If the placental circulation is not intact, such as after a placental abruption, bleeding placenta previa, bleeding vasa previa or cord avulsion, the cord should be clamped immediately after birth. There is currently not enough evidence to evaluate the safety of delayed cord clamping in cases of multiple gestation, fetal intrauterine growth restriction (IUGR), abnormal umbilical artery Doppler measurements, abnormal placentation and situations where uteroplacental perfusion or cord blood flow are affected.

What is the Neonatal Resuscitation Program (NRP) flowchart?[4]

The NRP flow diagram describes the steps that are to be followed to evaluate and resuscitate a newborn **(Flowchart 1)**.

The pink blocks indicate assessments and the green/blue ones show actions that may be required, depending on the result of the assessment.

How do you assess the newborn immediately after birth?
As soon as the baby is born, the following three questions should be answered:
1. Term gestation?
2. Good muscle tone?
3. Crying/breathing?

If the answer to all the questions is YES, then the baby does not require active resuscitation.

Provide warmth, dry the baby after cutting the cord, change the wet linen, position the head and neck so that the airway is open and clear the airway of secretions and providing gentle tactile stimulation. Observation of breathing, activity, and color should be ongoing.

In *case, the answer to any of the questions is NO,* the infant should receive one or more of the following four categories of actions in sequence:
1. Initial steps in stabilization
2. Ventilation
3. Chest compressions
4. Administration of epinephrine and/or volume expansion.[13,14]

In case, the answer to any of the questions is NO, the baby is placed under a preheated *warmer* (temperature 36.5–37.5°C), the basic steps are carried out as above. To *clear airway*, suction mouth first and then nose and in case of copious secretions, turn the head to one side and use a suction catheter. Note that the maximum time for suction should not exceed 15 seconds. Also, vigorous suctioning is avoided as it may stimulate the posterior pharynx leading to bradycardia or apnea secondary to vagal response.

If the respiratory effort is poor, then *tactile stimulation* by flicking or tapping the soles and rubbing the back briefly but firmly, is done.

The baby's heart rate (HR) and respiration is checked:
- If breathing well, pink—observe.
- If breathing well, HR > 100, but cyanosed—give free flow oxygen *
- If not breathing well, HR < 100—provide positive-pressure ventilation (PPV)**

---

*The goal of providing free-flow oxygen is to prevent hypoxia or hyperoxia.
** *Indications for PPV* are if the baby is apneic or gasping, has a HR under 100 even if breathing well, has persistent cyanosis despite 100% O_2 or if the baby is nonvigorous born via meconium-stained liquor. A diaphragmatic hernia is a contraindication to PPV. An orogastric tube is inserted if PPV is needed for a longer period.

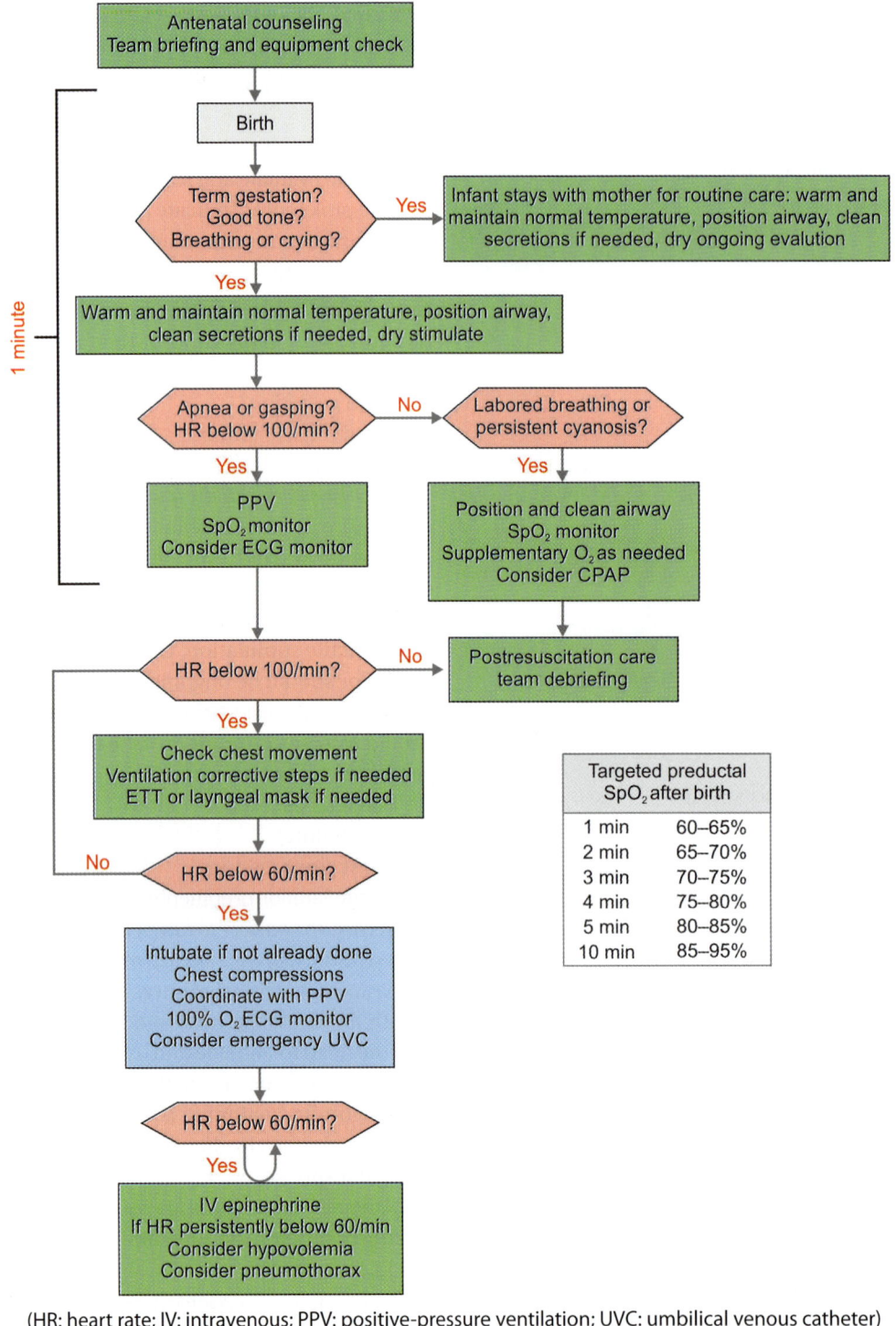

Flowchart 1: Neonatal Resuscitation Algoritm–2015 update.

(HR: heart rate; IV: intravenous; PPV: positive-pressure ventilation; UVC: umbilical venous catheter)

60 seconds ("golden minute") are allowed for completion of the initial steps, reevaluation and beginning of ventilation, if needed.

For resuscitation of babies >35 weeks, 21% oxygen (room air) is sufficient. For babies <35 weeks, resuscitation begins with 21–30% oxygen.

Several recent studies have suggested that resuscitation of newborns with 21% oxygen (room air) is just as successful as resuscitation with 100% oxygen. There is also some evidence that exposure to 100% oxygen during and following perinatal asphyxia may be harmful.[15,16] This is very important in a country like ours wherein oxygen may not be freely available or a delivery has taken place in a remote place.

Free-flow oxygen can be provided by flow-inflating bag and mask, by oxygen tubing or by face mask.

The frequency of ventilation should be 40-60 breaths per minute, starting with 21% O_2 and increased as per target saturation (**Flowchart 2**).

Free-flow oxygen: Effective ventilation can be achieved with the help of an oxygen mask, either a flow-inflating or self-inflating bag or with a T-piece mechanical device.[16,17] An oxygen tubing held close to the baby's mouth and nose (cupping the hand increases oxygen concentration) can also provide free-flow oxygen. Laryngeal mask airways (LMAs) that fit over the laryngeal inlet have been tried in near-term and term infants in cases where facemask ventilation and/or tracheal intubation is not feasible or unsuccessful.[4,13,18,19]

The *self-inflating bag (Ambu bag)* is found more commonly in the delivery room. It remains fully reinflated unless it is being squeezed. Once you release the bag, it recoils and draws fresh gas into the bag (if attached to an O_2 source, it fills with gas at the supplied O_2 concentration; else it fills by drawing room air—21% O_2).

It has a pressure-release valve which makes overinflation less likely. Because it self-inflates, it does not require a compressed gas source and when used with a mask forming a tight seal and an oxygen reservoir, it delivers sufficient oxygen to the baby (90–100%). The *mask* should be cushioned, round, or anatomically shaped, made from soft flexible material and form a good seal (rests over the chin, covers the mouth and nose but not the eyes).

The *flow-inflating bag* (used by anesthetists) inflates only when a compressed gas source is flowing into the bag and the outlet is sealed, such as when the mask is applied. It can deliver 100% oxygen but requires a compressed gas source and a pressure gauge to monitor the pressure being delivered at each breath. It takes more practice to use this bag effectively and as there is no safety valve, the degree of chest movement has to be watched each time to prevent over-/underinflation of the lungs. A manometer should always be used to ensure appropriate pressure is used.

T-piece resuscitator is a device that uses valves to regulate the flow of compressed gas directed to the patient and also needs a compressed gas source. A breath is delivered by using a finger to alternately occlude and release a gas escape opening on top of the T-piece cap so as to direct the gas to the patient or for it to escape respectively. It has two control dials to limit the inspiratory pressure and a pop-off valve to prevent increasing the pressure beyond a preset value.

The HR is assessed after 30 seconds and an improvement is indicated by an increase in HR, spontaneous respiration, good tone, and improving color.

An initial inflation pressure of 20 cmH_2O may be effective, but ≥30 to 40 cm H_2O may be required in some term babies.[4] *In summary, assisted ventilation should be delivered at a rate of 40-60 breaths per minute to promptly achieve or maintain a HR > 100 bpm.*

If:
- HR > 100 bpm, spontaneous respiration—discontinue PPV.
- HR = 60–100 bpm—continue bag and mask ventilation. Endotracheal intubation is needed at this point.
- HR < 60 bpm, begin chest compression, but first use corrective ventilation steps **(Flowchart 2)**.

Chest compressions (CCs) are begun if the HR < 60 bpm after 30 seconds of PPV. The theory is that a rhythmic compression of the sternum will compress the heart against the spine, increasing the intrathoracic pressure and circulating blood, thereby mechanically pumping blood to the vital organs. Intubation *must* be done at this time. It is important to remember the CCs are always accompanied by PPV and hence two people are needed. Both should NOT be given simultaneously but must be coordinated such that there must be one ventilation interposed after every third compression (30 breaths and 90 compressions per minute).

Chest compressions can be done using two techniques, viz., (1) *thumb technique* (where the two thumbs are used to depress the sternum while the hands encircle the torso and fingers support the spine) or (2) the *two-finger technique* (where the tips of the middle finger and either ring or index finger of one hand are used to compress the sternum, while the other hand is used to support the baby's back). *The thumb technique is preferred* as one can control the depth of compression and consistent pressure is applied. The *site* is the lower one third of the sternum, which lies between the xiphoid and a line drawn between the nipples. Only enough pressure to depress the sternum to a depth of approximately one-third the anterior-posterior diameter of the chest is used.[4,13,20,21]

Once the HR > 60 bpm, CCs can be discontinued, but the PPV needs to be continued till the HR rises above 100 bpm and there is spontaneous respiration.[4,13]

Indications for endotracheal intubation[4,13] are a need for prolonged or ineffective bag and mask ventilation, suspected or known diaphragmatic hernia, surfactant administration or in case of extreme prematurity. Timing of endotracheal intubation also depends on the skill of the available providers. The tube size varies with the age (**Flowchart 2**) and the laryngoscope blade depends on the baby's gestation (No. 0—preterms, No. 00—extreme preterms, No. 1—term babies). *Before attempting intubation*, always check the light by clicking the blade open, make sure that the suction equipment, the bag to deliver PPV, a stethoscope, scissors, and tape are accessible.

After endotracheal intubation and administration of intermittent positive pressure, a prompt increase in heart rate is the best indicator that the tube is in the tracheobronchial tree. Exhaled CO_2 detection is effective for confirmation.[22] Other clinical indicators of correct endotracheal tube placement are condensation in the endotracheal tube, chest movement, and presence of equal breath sounds bilaterally, but these have not been systematically evaluated in neonates.[22]

If initial attempts at intubation fail or are not successful in improving the HR and respiration, remember that it is better to resume PPV with a bag and mask and then try again.

If the baby still does not improve, an umbilical catheter is inserted and drugs are administered. In 99% cases, babies improve without medications.

Flowchart 2: Neonatal Resuscitation Program–reference chart.

Neonatal resusciatation program–reference chart
The most important and effective action in neonatal resuscitation is ventilation of the baby's lungs

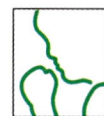

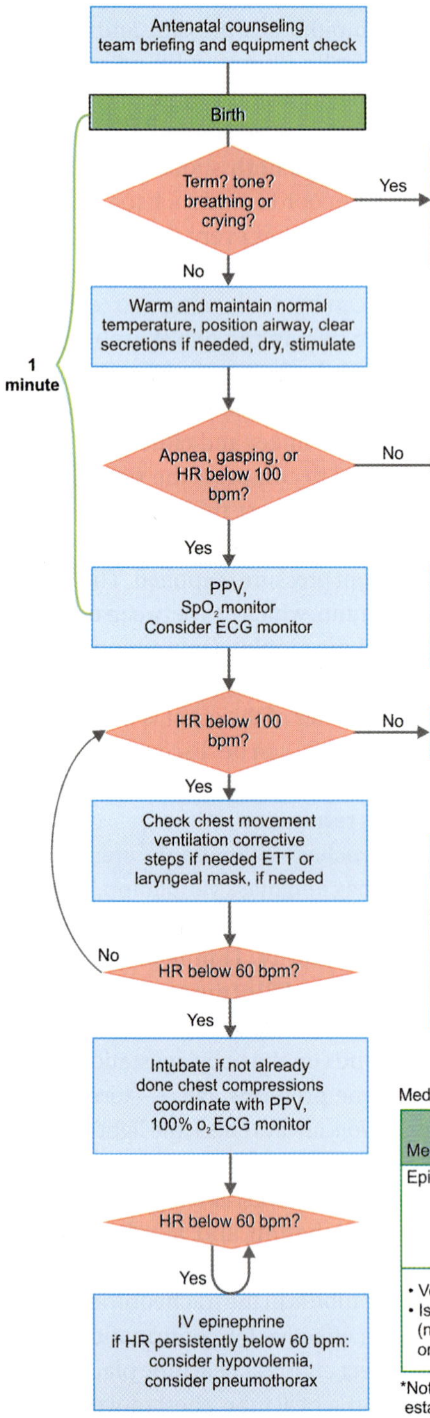

```
Antenatal counseling
team briefing and equipment check
           ↓
         Birth
           ↓
  Term? tone?                    Stay with mother for routine care:
  breathing or    ── Yes →       warm and maintain normal
  crying?                        temperature, position airway,
           │                     clear secretions if needed, dry,
          No                     ongoing evaluation
           ↓
  Warm and maintain normal
  temperature, position airway, clear
  secretions if needed, dry, stimulate
           ↓
  Apnea, gasping, or              Labored breathing
  HR below 100    ── No →         or persistent
  bpm?                            cyanosis?
           │                           │
          Yes                         Yes
           ↓                           ↓
    PPV,                         Position and clear airway
    SpO₂ monitor                 SpO₂ monitor,
    Consider ECG monitor         Supplemental o₂ as needed.
           ↓                     Consider CPAP
   HR below 100     ── No →      Post-resuscitation care
   bpm?                          Team debriefing
           │
          Yes
           ↓
  Check chest movement
  ventilation corrective
  steps if needed ETT or
  laryngeal mask, if needed
           ↓
   HR below 60 bpm?  ── No ┐
           │               │
          Yes              │
           ↓               │
  Intubate if not already  │
  done chest compressions  │
  coordinate with PPV,     │
  100% o₂ ECG monitor      │
           ↓               │
   HR below 60 bpm?  ──────┘
           │
          Yes
           ↓
  IV epinephrine
  if HR persistently below 60 bpm:
  consider hypovolemia,
  consider pneumothorax
```

1 minute

A Airway
- Put baby's head in "sniffing" position
- Section mouth, then nose
- Suction trachea if meconium-stained and not vigorous

B Breathing
- PPV for anpnea gasping, or pulse <100 bpm
- Ventilate at rate of 40 to 60 breaths / minute
- Listen for rising heart rate, audible breath sounds
- Look for slight chest movement with each breath
- Use CO₂ detector after intubation
- Attach a pulse oximeter

C Circulation
- Start compressions if HR is <60 bpm after 30 seconds of effective PPV
- Give (3 compressions: 1 breath) every 2 seconds
- Compress one-third of the anterior-posterior diameter of the chest

D Drugs
- Give epinephrine if HR is <60 bpm after 45 to 60 second of compressions and ventilation
- Cautions epinephrine dosage is different for ET and IV routes

Corrective steps

M	Mask adjustment
R	Reposition airway
S	Suction mouth and nose
O	Open mouth
P	Pressure increase
A	Airway alternative

Pre-ductal SpO₂ Target

1 min	60–65%
2 min	65–70%
3 min	70–75%
4 min	75–80%
5 min	80–85%
10 min	85–95%

Endotracheal intubation

Gestational age (weeks)	Weight (kg)	ET tube size (ID, mm)	Depth of insertion* (cm form upper lips)
<23	<1.0	2.5	6–7
23–34	1.0–2.0	3.0	7–8
34–35	2.0–3.0	3.5	8–9
>35	>3.0	3.5–4.0	9–10

*Depth of insertion (cm) = 6 + weight (in kg)

Medicatoins used during or following resuscitation of the newborn

Medicatoins	Desage / Route*	Concentration	Wt (kg)	Total IV volume (mL)	Precautions
Epinephrine	• IV(UVC preferred route) 0.1 to 0.3 mL/kg • Nigher IV doses not recommended endotracheal 0.5 to 1 mL / kg	1:00,000	1 2 3 4	0.1–0.3 0.2–0.6 0.3–0.9 0.4–1.2	• Give rapidly • Repeat every 3–5 minutes if HR <60 with chest compressions
• Volume expanders • Isotonic crystalloid (normal saline) or blood	10 mL/kg IV		1 2 3 4	10 20 30 40	• Indicated for shock • give over 5–10 minutes • Reassess after each bolus

*Note: Endotracheal dose may not result in effective plasma concentration of drug, so vascular access should be established as soon as possible. Drugs given endotracheal require higher dosing than when given IV.

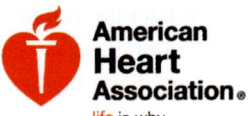

(ECG: electrocardiography; HR: heart rate; IV: intravenous; PPV: positive-pressure ventilation)

Medications[4,13,23] are rarely needed and are given only if the HR < 60 bpm despite adequate PPV and CC for 60 seconds with 100% O_2. They can be given via the umbilical vein, intraosseous route or endotracheally.

- *Epinephrine* is a cardiac stimulant, used in 1:10,000 dilution and can be given through intravenous or intraosseous route (dose: 0.1–0.3 mL/kg) or endotracheally (dose: 0.5–1 mL/kg).
- *Volume expanders* in the form of normal saline or Rh-negative packed red blood cells (PRBC) are given if the baby is not responding to resuscitation and appears to be in shock or if there is fetal blood loss. The dose is 10 mL/kg, given over 5–10 minutes. The expected response would be and increase in HR, stronger pulses, lesser pallor and increase in BP. A repeat dose can be given if needed.
- *Naloxone* is no longer recommended.[9]

In case there is no improvement even after medications, recheck, reevaluate, and consider special situations (airway malformations, lung problems such as pneumothorax or diaphragmatic hernia, and congenital heart disease).

Flowchart 2 should be put above every *resuscitation bed* for quick reference.[12]

POSTRESUSCITATION CARE

Babies who require resuscitation are at risk for deterioration after their vital signs have returned to normal. Once adequate ventilation and circulation have been established, the infant should be kept or transferred to an environment where close monitoring and anticipatory care can be provided.

If despite everything, there is no HR, then one should consider discontinuing resuscitation.

Management of Babies Born with Meconium-stained Liquor[11]

A special mention of meconium-stained liquor is made as this is frequently encountered and there are changes in the approach to a baby born with meconium-stained liquor.

In case of meconium-stained liquor with a vigorous baby, if the respiratory effort is strong, muscle tone is good and the HR is >100 bpm, then the mouth and nose are cleared with a bulb syringe or a large-bore suction catheter (Avoid vigorous suctioning).

If the baby is born through meconium-stained liquor and is not vigorous, only then is tracheal suctioning recommended. In such cases, 02 is administered while monitoring the HR, a laryngoscope is inserted; the mouth is cleared with a 12-F or 14-F suction catheter; the endotracheal tube is inserted into the trachea and the enotracheal tube is attached to the suction source. Suction should be applied while the tube is being withdrawn. This can be repeated as needed.

THE INDIAN SCENARIO

The NRP instructor programs have been conducted by the National Neonatology Forum (NNF) since 1990 with the aim of ultimately increasing the pool of trained NRP providers.[24] However to develop a cost-efficient, sustainable system in NRP training on a large scale in a populous country like ours and to achieve the Millennium Development Goals (MDG4), the Indian Academy of Pediatrics (IAP) launched the NRP-First Golden Minute (IAP-NRP-FGM) in 2009. This curriculum is based on the Academy of Pediatrics (AAP) manual of NRP and is sponsored by Later-Day Saint Charities (LDSC) with academic grant from Johnson & Johnson, India. With the launch of IAP-NRP-FGM, it was envisaged at that time, that along with the Federation of Obstetrics and Gynecological Society of India (FOGSI) and NNF members, it may be possible to have an NRP-trained skilled birth attendant for every delivery.[25]

Though NRP is the most widely used curriculum, many other organizations around the world have developed neonatal resuscitation standards. In technology and resource-restricted settings, NRP may not be practical. Hence in 2009, the AAP in collaboration with the World Health Organization (WHO), US Agency for International Development (USAID), etc., initiated a new educational program entitled "Helping Babies Breathe," (HBB) aimed at local nurses, midwives, and traditional birth attendants in developing countries.[26]

In 2012, the WHO published guidelines on basic newborn resuscitation for use in first referral and higher level in low resource-limited settings.[1]

In India, HBB initiative has been integrated into the Navjaat Shishu Suraksha Karyakram (NSSK).[27]

What's new?[28]
- Delayed cord clamping for 30–60 seconds for most preterm and term neonates
- Resuscitation begins with 21% O_2 in babies ≥35 weeks' gestation
- At least 30 seconds PPV must be given through a properly placed endotracheal tube
- CCs are administered for 60 seconds before checking HR
- CCs are administered using a two-thumb technique
- An electronic cardiac monitor is preferred to assess HR
- No tracheal suctioning for a vigorous baby born through meconium.

KEY MESSAGES

- Most newly born babies are vigorous. About 10% require some kind of assistance and only 1% need major resuscitative measures.
- The most important and effective action in neonatal resuscitation is to ventilate a newborns lungs.
- Lack of ventilation results in sustained constriction of the pulmonary arterioles preventing systemic arterial blood to be oxygenated. Prolonged lack of adequate perfusion and oxygenation to the baby's organs can lead to brain damage, damage to other organs, and even death.

BOX 1: Perinatal risk factors increasing the likelihood of neonatal resuscitation.[10]

Antepartum risk factors:

Maternal diabetes	Fetal Hydrops
Preeclampsia or eclampsia	Fetal macrosomia
APH	IUGR
Poly/Oligohydramnios	Multiple gestation
PROM	No prenatal care
Gestational age (GA) <36.7 or >41.7 weeks	Maternal infection

Intrapartum risk factors:

Emergency cesarean delivery	Intrapartum bleeding
Forceps or Vacuum assisted delivery	Chorioamnionitis
Breech or other abnormal presentation	
Abnormal FHR pattern	Shoulder dystocia
Maternal GA or magnesium therapy	MSAF
Placental abruption	Prolapsed umbilical cord

(APH: antepartum hemorrhage; FHR: fetal heart rate; IUGR: intrauterine growth restriction; MSAF: meconium-stained amniotic fluid; PROM: premature rupture of the membranes)

- Many, but not all, babies who will require neonatal resuscitation can be anticipated by identifying ante/intrapartum risk factors **(Box 1)**.
- Every birth should be attended by one person who is skilled in all the aspects of resuscitation.
- Approximately 60 seconds ("the Golden Minute") are allotted for completing the initial steps, reevaluating, and beginning ventilation. The decision to progress beyond the initial steps is determined by simultaneous assessment of two vital characteristics: (1) *Respirations* (apnea, gasping, labored or unlabored breathing) *and (2) HR* (greater than or less than 100 bpm). Assessment of HR should be done by intermittently auscultating the precordial pulse. When a pulse is detectable, palpation of the umbilical pulse is more accurate.
- Once positive-pressure ventilation or supplementary oxygen administration is begun, assessment should consist of evaluation of three vital characteristics: (1) HR, (2) respirations, and (3) the state of oxygenation, the latter optimally determined by a pulse oximeter. The most sensitive indicator of a successful response to each step is an increase in HR.
- If one cannot detect audible breath sounds and see no perceptible chest expansion during assisted ventilation, check or correct the following:
  - *****M**- Mask adjustment
  - *****R**- Reposition airway
  - *****S** -Suction mouth and nose
  - *****O**- Open mouth
  - *****P**- Pressure increase
  - *****A**- Airway alternative.
  *(remember the mnemonic **Mr. Sopa**).
- If the above steps are checked and there is no increase in the heart rate or no perceptible chest expansion, insert an endotracheal tube and begin PPV at a rate of 40–60 breaths per minute for 30 seconds.
- If the heart rate still remains below 60 bpm, begin CCs and continue simultaneous PPV in a ratio of 3:1.
- Consider intravenous epinephrine via umbilical vein in cases where the HR remains below 60 bpm, despite 30 seconds of effective assisted ventilation and chest compression. (Dose is 0.1–0.3 mL/kg of 1:10,000 concentration solution, given rapidly). Volume expansion is considered in cases of shock (pale color, weak pulses, persistent low HR, no improvement in circulatory status despite resuscitation) or fetal blood loss in the form of normal saline, Ringer's Lactate or O Rh-negative blood (dose 10 mL/kg via umbilical vein over 5–10 minutes).
- The baby should be transferred to a neonatal intensive care unit for further observation and management.

REFERENCES

1. World Health Organization (WHO). (2012). Guidelines on basic newborn resuscitation. [online] Available from: https://apps.who.int/iris/handle/10665/75157. [Last accessed November, 2021].
2. Merck Manuals Professional Edition. Neonatal Resuscitation—Pediatrics". [online] Available from: https://www.msdmanuals.com/en-in/professional/pediatrics/perinatal-problems/neonatal-resuscitation. [Last accessed November, 2021].
3. AHA/AAP Neonatal Resuscitation Program Steering Committee. Textbook of neonatal resuscitation, 4th edition. Elk Grove Village, Il: American Academy of Pediatrics; 2000.
4. Kattwinkel J, Perlman JM, Aziz K, Colby C, Fairchild K, Hazinski MF, et al. Part 15: neonatal resuscitation: 2010 American Heart Association Guidelines for Cardiopulmonary Resuscitation and Emergency Cardiovascular Care. Circulation. 2010;122(Suppl 3):S909-19.
5. Weiner GM. Textbook of neonatal resuscitation, 7th edition. New Delhi: CBS publishers and distributors; 2016. pp. 3-8.
6. Aziz K, Chadwick M, Baker M, Andrews W. Ante- and intra-partum factors that predict increased need for neonatal resuscitation. Resuscitation. 2008;79:444-52.
7. Zaichkin J (ed). Instructor Manual for Neonatal Resuscitation. Chicago, IL: American Academy of Pediatrics; 2011.
8. Perlman JM, Wyllie J, Kattwinkel J, Wyckoff MH, Aziz K, Guinsburg R, et al; on behalf of the Neonatal Resuscitation Chapter Collaborators. Part 7: Neonatal resuscitation: 2015 International Consensus on Cardiopulmonary Resuscitation and Emergency Cardiovascular Care Science With Treatment Recommendations. Circulation. 2015;132(suppl 1):S204-41.
9. Wyllie J, Perlman JM, Kattwinkel J, Wyckoff MH, Aziz K, Guinsburg R, et al; on behalf of the Neonatal Resuscitation

Chapter Collaborators. Part 7: neonatal resuscitation: 2015 International Consensus on Cardiopulmonary Resuscitation and Emergency Cardiovascular Care Science With Treatment Recommendations. Pediatrics. 2015;136 Suppl 2:S120-66.
10. Weiner GM. Textbook of neonatal resuscitation, 7th edition. New Delhi: CBS Publishers and Distributors; 2016. pp. 18-25.
11. Weiner GM. In: Foundation of neonatal resuscitation. Textbook of neonatal resuscitation, 7th edition. New Delhi: CBS Publishers and Distributors; 2016. pp. 36-7, 51.
12. Wyckoff MH, Aziz K, Escobedo MB, Kapadia VS, Kattwinkel J, Perlman JM, et al. Part 13: neonatal resuscitation: 2015 American Heart Association guidelines update for cardiopulmonary resuscitation and emergency cardiovascular care. Circulation. 2015;132(suppl 2):S543-60.
13. Shah NK, Mathur NB, et al. Neonatal resuscitation. IAP-NNF guidelines 2006 on level II neonatal care. 2006;3-13.
14. Kattwinkel J, McGowan JE, Zaichkin J. Overview and principles of resuscitation. Textbook of neonatal resuscitation, 6th edition. New Delhi: Jaypee Brothers Medical Publishers (P) Ltd; 2012. pp. 1-36.
15. Davis PG, Tan A, O'Donnell CP, Schulze A. Resuscitation of newborn infants with 100% oxygen or air: a systematic review and meta-analysis. Lancet. 2004; 364:1329-33.
16. Rabi Y, Rabi D, Yee W. Room air resuscitation of the depressed newborn: a systematic review and meta-analysis. Resuscitation. 2007;72:353-63.
17. Finer NN, Rich W, Craft A, Henderson C. Comparison of methods bag and mask ventilation for neonatal resuscitation. Resuscitation. 2001;49:299-305.
18. Benett S, Finer NN, Rich W, Vaucher Y. A comparison of three neonatal resuscitation devices. Resuscitation. 2005;67:113-8.
19. Kattwinkel J, McGowan JE, Zaichkin J. Use of resuscitation devices for positive-pressure ventilation. Textbook of neonatal resuscitation, 6th edition. New Delhi: Jaypee Brothers Medical Publishers (P) Ltd; 2012. pp. 71-132.
20. Orlowski JP. Optimum position for external cardiac compression in infants and young children. Ann Emerg Med. 1986;15:667-73.
21. Braga MS, Dominguez TE, Pollock AN, Niles D, Meyer A, Mylkebust H, et al. Estimation of optimal CPR chest compression depth in children by using computer tomography. Pediatrics. 2009;124:e69-74.
22. Repetto JE, Donohue PK, Baker SF, Kelly L, Nogee LM. Use of capnography in the delivery room for assessment of endotracheal tube placement. J Perinatol. 2001;21:284-7.
23. Barber CA, Wycoff MH. Use and efficacy of endotracheal versus intravenous epinephrine during neonatal cardiopulmonary resuscitation in the delivery room. Pediatrics. 2006;118:1028-34.
24. Deorari AK, Paul VK, Singh M, Vidyasagar D. The national movement of neonatal resuscitation in India. J Trop Pediatr. 2000;46:315-7.
25. Choudhury P. Neonatal Resuscitation Program: First Golden Minute. 2009;46:7-9.
26. Niermeyer S. For the Global Implementation Task Force Helping Babies Breathe. Elk Grov Village: American Academy of Pediatrics; 2009.
27. Kak LP, Johnson J, McPherson R, Keenan W, Schoen E. (2015). Helping Babies Breathe. Lessons learned guiding the way forward. [online] Available from: https://www.healthynewbornnetwork.org/resource/helping-babies-breathe-lessons-learned-guiding-the-way-forward/. [Last accessed November, 2021].
28. Weiner GM. In: Foundation of neonatal resuscitation. Textbook of neonatal resuscitation, 7th edition. New Delhi: CBS Publishers and Distributors; 2016.

LONG QUESTIONS

1. What are the risk factors that could point toward a need for neonatal resuscitation?
2. What are the physiologic changes that occur during transition from intrauterine to extrauterine life? How do they present at birth in a compromised neonate?
3. How should one equip the neonatal workstation?
4. Discuss the different ways in which oxygen can be delivered to the newborn?
5. How are chest compressions given and how do you assess the response?

SHORT QUESTIONS

1. What four questions should you ask before every birth?
2. What is the role of delayed cord clamping in a neonate?
3. What are the indications for endotracheal intubation?
4. Name the drugs used in neonatal resuscitation, along with their uses.
5. Name the corrective ventilation steps to be checked before starting chest compressions.

MULTIPLE CHOICE QUESTIONS

1. What percentage of births requires neonatal resuscitation?
   a. 1%   b. 10%
   c. 18%   d. 30%
2. The following statement is false about the transition from intrauterine to extrauterine environment:
   a. In utero, the fetal alveoli are filled with fluid.
   b. The expansion of the alveoli and gas exchange depends on surfactant.
   c. The pulmonary arterioles are dilated in utero.
   d. Umbilical cord clamping raises neonatal systemic blood pressure.
3. Which of the following statements is true about preparing for neonatal resuscitation?
   a. With adequate screening, all births requiring neonatal resuscitation can be identified
   b. The risk of endotracheal intubation is higher with cesarean section birth at 39 weeks as compared to a vaginal delivery at the same gestational age
   c. Narcotics administered 6 hours before birth are likely to affect neonatal breathing
   d. A trained person should be assigned to neonatal care at every birth.
4. Which of the following is not a part of the initial assessment block as per the NRP protocol?
   a. Term gestation   b. Crying / breathing
   c. Muscle tone   d. Heart rate

5. The following statement about initial resuscitation is true:
   a. Fetal mouth should be cleared of secretions first and then the nose
   b. The usual operation theater suction apparatus can be used to clear neonatal secretions
   c. The fetal neck should be placed in a position of hyperextension
   d. Neonatal temperature does not play a role in resuscitation
6. The indications for positive-pressure ventilation are all except
   a. Heart rate of 80 bpm   b. Apnea
   c. Gasping respirations   d. Acrocyanosis
7. The following statement about initial breathing and ventilation is false.
   a. Initial breathing creates a functional residual capacity
   b. The primary measure of adequate ventilation is improvement in heart rate
   c. The usual inflation ventilation pressure required is 50 cmH$_2$O for neonatal resuscitation.
   d. Positive-pressure ventilation should be delivered at about 40 to 60 breaths per minute
8. The following can be used for assisted ventilation of the neonate except
   a. Ambu bag
   b. Flow inflating bag
   c. High-pressure oxygen delivery
   d. Continuous positive airway pressure devices (CPAP)
9. Resuscitation in term infants should be done at this oxygen concentration:
   a. 30%   b. 21%
   c. 80%   d. 100%
10. All are the potential benefits of delayed cord clamping for preterm neonates, except:
   a. Lower risk of necrotizing enterocolitis.
   b. Less need for blood transfusion after birth
   c. Fewer brain hemorrhages
   d. Low incidence of jaundice.

Answers
1. b   2. c   3. d   4. d   5. a   6. d
7. c   8. c   9. b   10. d

10.9 PERINATAL ASPHYXIA

Ashish Mehta

INTRODUCTION

When there is an impaired gas exchange in the human body, it leads to hypoxia, hypercarbia and acidosis. The degree of impairment correlates to the extent of damage. This condition in extremis is called asphyxia. In the perinatal period, it can variably affect fetal and neonatal outcomes. The degree of neonatal damage and future dysfunction is dependent on a number of factors. The most widely used definition of fetal acidosis is an umbilical artery pH of 7 or lower. However, this is not the only criteria or sole determinant of brain injury. The pathophysiology of perinatal asphyxia is complex and multifactorial. At the outset of the chapter, it should be noted that birth and labor related events are a minority of causes of perinatal asphyxia.

NORMAL FETAL CIRCULATION (FIG. 1)

The human fetus lives in a hypoxemic state but this is not considered as a pathological hypoxia. Oxygen diffuses readily from the maternal to fetal circulation due to high binding affinity of fetal hemoglobin. The blood from the placenta goes from umbilical vein has a PO$_2$ of 40 to 50 mm Hg. It mixes with less oxygenated blood coming through inferior vena cava while entering right atrium. More oxygenated blood goes to left side of heart through foramen ovale and it exits the left ventricle through the aorta to carotid and coronary arteries. Thus, fetal heart and brain are supplied through more oxygenated blood. In utero, the fetus has some additional factors to sustain the hypoxemic state. These are necessary to meet the oxygen and hemoglobin requirements. These adaptations are:
- Hemoglobin levels are higher in fetal life than in adults
- Fetal hemoglobin has a higher affinity for oxygen, allowing oxygen transfer to tissues at a lower gradient
- Better tissue perfusion rates
- Minimal energy usage on thermoregulation and respiration.

The vital changes that lead to adaptation on birth are:
- Drop in pulmonary vascular resistance due to the rapid lung expansion
- Marked rise in pulmonary blood flow
- Closure of the ductus arteriosus
- Rise in systemic vascular resistance.

CAUSES OF PERINATAL ASPHYXIA

The most common final pathway leading to in utero asphyxia is interruption of placental blood flow. This interruption can be from either maternal, placental, or neonatal cause. **Table 1** enlists selective causes of perinatal asphyxia.

ADAPTIVE MECHANISMS AFTER ASPHYXIA (FLOWCHART 1)

Circulatory Changes after Asphyxia

Following asphyxia redistribution of cardiac output occurs to vital organs (brain, heart) from other nonvital organs (intestines, kidney, skin, etc.) due to "diving reflex". This is mediated by the release of catecholamines due to hypoxemia. Adaptive cerebral mechanisms decrease cerebral vascular resistance to increase cerebral blood flow. When systemic blood pressure falls, very low compensatory mechanism fails which leads to decrease cerebral blood flow, less oxygen delivery and brain injury.

Noncirculatory Response to Asphyxia

Several biological factors aid in preserving viability during and after asphyxia. These are—decrease in cerebral metabolic rate, use of alternate energy source such as ketones and lactate, and the fetal and neonatal myocardium which is resistant to hypoxia-ischemia compared to adult myocardium.

Impaired Gas Exchange and Acidosis

The hallmark of perinatal asphyxia is a diminished exchange of oxygen and carbon dioxide across the placenta. Both of these contribute to hypoxemia. The fetus is adapted to a mild hypoxic state as described earlier. However, when fetal oxygen demands are not met by the placental oxygen delivery, anaerobic respiration is initiated for fetal survival. This leads to the accumulation of lactic and metabolic acidosis, which is the pathway to brain injury and damage to other organs. Generally, an umbilical artery pH of 7.0 or less is considered as severe fetal acidemia and correlates to adverse neurological outcomes including cerebral palsy. However, this is not a conclusive level. Fetuses have been known to have severe injury with pH above 7 and some fetuses may not have any significant effects at lower umbilical artery pH. However, from the study by Perlman et al., we can conclude that severe acidemia in the context of significant bradycardia requiring intense resuscitation should be looked upon as a major risk factor for hypoxic ischemic encephalopathy (HIE).

PATHOLOGICAL BRAIN INJURY AFTER PERINATAL ASPHYXIA

Neuronal trauma and brain injury vary based on the type and duration of hypoxemia/acidemia as well as the gestational age at birth. In addition, postdelivery factors such as adequacy of resuscitation, hypothermia and general condition of the fetus will affect the long-term outcomes. The classic patterns of brain injury are outlined in **Table 2**.

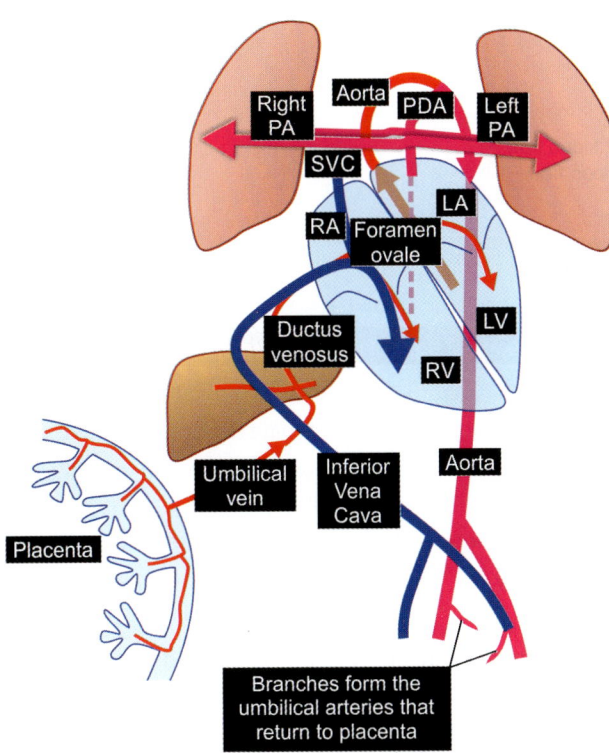

Fig. 1: Overview of fetal circulation.

TABLE 1: Selective causes of perinatal asphyxia.		
Maternal	**Placental/umbilical cord**	**Neonatal**
Sudden maternal hypotension due to neurogenic or cardiac events	Placental abruption	Cardiac anomalies causing circulatory failure
Maternal hemorrhage from the uterus (uterine rupture) or other sources (injury, accidents, massive bleeding varices) causing hypovolemia or hypotension	Fetomaternal hemorrhage due to antepartum hemorrhage, accidents, abdominal trauma	Airway or neurological abnormalities causing respiratory failure
Chronic maternal disease leading to poor uterine perfusion such as severe anemia, hypertension, vascular disease from diabetes or autoimmune conditions	Cord prolapse or tightening of a true knot of the umbilical cord	Infection
	Velamentous cord insertion, vasa previa with membrane rupture leading to fetal hemorrhage	Medication effect
	Infection/inflammation	
	Uterine hyperstimulation	

Flowchart 1: Adaptive mechanism and systemic consequences of perinatal asphyxia.

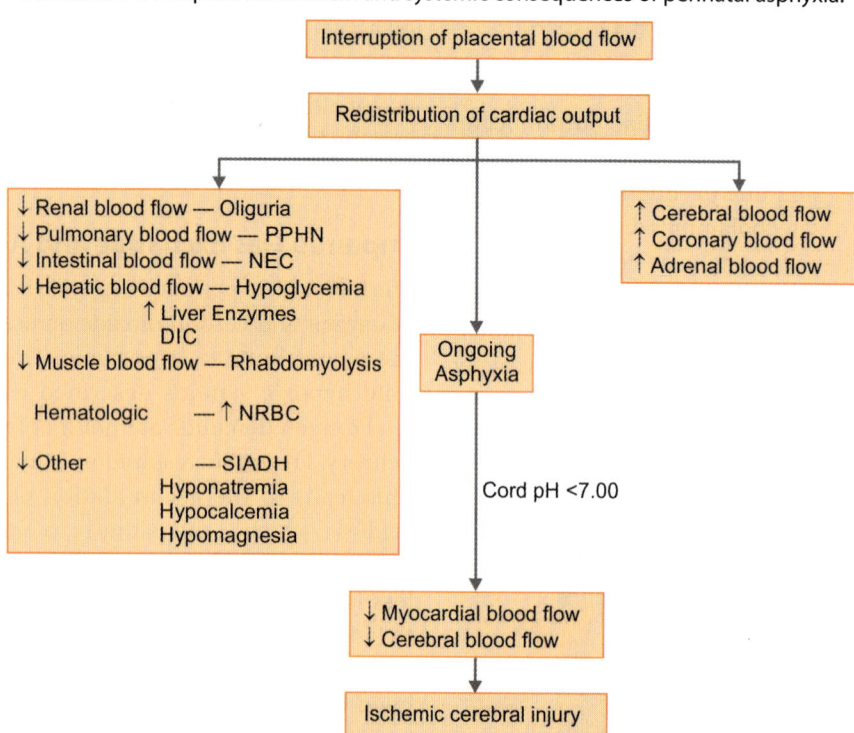

TABLE 2: Classic patterns of brain injury.			
Selective neuronal necrosis	Parasagittal cerebral injury	Periventricular leukomalacia	Focal ischemic necrosis
Can subtyped based on location as diffuse, cortico-deep nuclear or deep nuclear brainstem	Occurs in the end arterial watershed area of the parieto-occipital cortex and subcortical white matter		

TABLE 3: Neonatal signs of perinatal asphyxia.	
APGAR score	Less than 5 at 5 and 10 minutes of life
Umbilical artery gas	<7.0 and/or base deficit ≥12 mmol/L
Neuroimaging	Deep nuclear gray matter or watershed cortical injury
Organ dysfunction	Multisystem organ failure
Cerebral palsy	Spastic quadriplegic or dyskinetic type

Magnetic resonance imaging (MRI) findings, which are associated with poor outcome, include involvement of the basal ganglia and thalamus, posterior limb of internal capsule, and loss of gray-white matter differentiation.[2,3]

TIMING AND DURATION OF PERINATAL ASPHYXIA

The timing and duration of perinatal asphyxia events are a focus of enquiry when an infant or child has significant birth asphyxia. It is also a source of litigation. In acute events, the marker event such as trauma, uterine rupture, cord prolapse are self-evident. The time to delivery from such events will give the duration of the damage. However, in events, which are more insidious such as an abnormal fetal heart rate pattern in the duration of a prolonged labor or in even more chronic circumstances such as severe fetal growth restriction, identifying such marker events and durations are not always possible. In general, severe and prolonged hypoxic insults lead to more diffuse brain injury. When the hypoxic insult is moderate to severe and prolonged, there is cortical and deep nuclear (thalamus, basal ganglia) affection. Severe, abrupt events lead to deep nuclear and brainstem injury.

PERINATAL ASPHYXIA FROM OBSTETRIC STANDPOINT

Perinatal asphyxia with acute hypoxia-ischemia may result in neonatal signs, which occurred before delivery. The APGAR score, umbilical cord gas, neuroimaging and multiorgan dysfunction can be used to decide whether injury is consistent with peripartum event **(Table 3)**.

Antenatal Wellbeing Tests as Screening Tests for Perinatal Asphyxia

A number of tests have been devised to identify the fetus at risk of perinatal asphyxia. These have been discussed in detail in a separate chapter of this textbook. These tests are daily fetal movement counting, fetal cardiotocography (CTG), biophysical profile (BPP) or modified BPP and color Doppler evaluation. The tests are based on identifying an abnormal fetal response or fetal state in a high-risk pregnancy. All the tests have their utility. The level of sensitivity and specificity in identifying perinatal asphyxia or predicting fetal death varies. In general, they have a high negative predictive value, i.e., a normal test indicates a healthy fetal state. This should not preclude further testing. If an abnormal test result is obtained, further action will depend on the degree of deviation from normal, gestational age and clinical background. The next step could be more testing, observation or repeating the test or delivery. Broadly, ultrasound based tests such as amniotic fluid assessment, BPP and color Doppler are useful for medium to long-term assessment and prediction while fetal heart rate based CTG is useful for the short term.

Intrapartum Monitoring as a Screening Test for Perinatal Asphyxia

Intrapartum monitoring is an integral part of obstetric care and the purpose of fetal monitoring in labor is to identify events that could lead to perinatal asphyxia with a view to prevent the inciting factors or achieve accelerated delivery. At the outset of the chapter, it was emphasized that intrapartum events contribute to small proportion of perinatal asphyxia. However, these events are important to study and care for because they are potentially preventable. Toward this end, electronic fetal monitoring (EFM) was supposed to be a major scientific advance. However, this method may not be able to predict or prevent all instances of birth asphyxia. Also, there is evidence that its use in low risk labor is associated with an increase in cesarean rates and no reduction in perinatal asphyxia or mortality. Newer modalities such as fetal ECG, ST segment analysis (STAN) are under study.

Postpartum Screening for Perinatal Asphyxia

After delivery, the umbilical artery blood gas levels are important markers for perinatal asphyxia. The umbilical artery pH level of 7 or below has been discussed earlier in the chapter. Other tests could include placental histopathology to look for features or infarction, inflammation or infection.

Strategies to Reduce Risk of Perinatal Asphyxia

In the antenatal period, the standard care includes identification of high risk factors, which may exist even from the preconceptional period. Some of these are modifiable and efforts should be made to optimize maternal health in the preconceptional or at least in the antenatal period. Chronic diseases such as hypertension, diabetes, renal disease and autoimmune conditions are major contributors here. Obstetric conditions such as multiple pregnancy and preterm labor also raise the risk for perinatal asphyxia. A number of risk reduction strategies have been proposed to prevent fetal death, damage in utero and perinatal asphyxia. These strategies are directed toward:

- *Optimizing the maternal condition:* Control of blood pressure, blood sugar, etc.
- *Elimination or neutralizing the risk factor:* Cervical cerclage, progesterone for preterm birth prevention, etc.
- Early identification of placental dysfunction or uteroplacental circulatory disturbance, monitoring or delivery. In this category, care has to be exercised in order to prevent overzealous obstetric interventions.

The essence of risk reduction strategies in labor and in the immediate postpartum period are good obstetric protocols and monitoring. These have been discussed in detail in other chapters of this textbook.

■ DIAGNOSIS

Perinatal asphyxia typically occurs in settings where the child has been born with a low APGAR score, requires ventilation at birth and continues to have a low APGAR of ≤3 for ≥ 10 minutes. For a term neonate, the possible differential diagnoses in such situations are:

- Birth asphyxia
- Maternal or fetal infection
- Neonatal anomalies (cardiac, respiratory) or neuromuscular dysfunction
- Maternal medications including anesthesia, analgesia.

If APGAR is >6 by 5 minutes, perinatal asphyxia is not likely. pH and base deficit on the cord or first blood gas is helpful for determining which neonate needs evaluation for the development of HIE.

The typical features of birth asphyxia and HIE reasonably include:

- Prolonged (>1 h) antenatal acidosis
- Fetal heart rate <60 beats/minute
- APGAR score ≤3 at ≥10 minutes
- Need for positive pressure ventilation for >1 minute or first cry delayed >5 minute
- Seizures within 12–24 hours of birth
- Burst suppression or suppressed background pattern on EEG or amplitude-integrated electroencephalography (EEG) (aEEG).

Sarnat and Sarnat Stages of HIE

Sarnat adapted three stages of encephalopathy, which can be used in early neonatal period. It is also used to decide about therapeutic hypothermia. It is well-correlated with long-term neurodevelopmental outcome **(Table 4)**.

Laboratory Evaluation of Asphyxia

There is no specific test which is gold standard to diagnose perinatal asphyxia.

Laboratory tests are mainly related to label oxygen deprivation to various organs.

TABLE 4: Sarnat and Sarnat classification of hypoxic ischemic encephalopathy.

Criterion	Stage I	Stage II	Stage III
Consciousness	Hyperalert	Obtunded	Stuporous
Tone/posture	Good tone, mild distal flexion	Hypotonic, strong distal flexion	Flaccid, occasionally decerebrate
Stretch reflexes	Increased	Increased	Decreased or absent
Suck	Weak	Variably weak to absent	Absent
Moro	Strong	Weak	Absent
Pupils	Mydriatic	Miotic	Variable, anisochoria, poor light response
Heart rate	Tachycardia	Bradycardia	Variable
Respiratory secretions	Sparse	Profuse	Variable
Gastrointestinal motility	Normal or decreased	Increased	Variable
Seizures (clinical)	None	Common	Uncommon

- *Neurologic markers of brain injury:* Increased serum CK-BB.
- *Renal evaluation:* Elevated blood urea nitrogen and creatinine, typically is seen after 2–4 days of birth.
- *Cardiac evaluation:* Elevated cardiac troponin1 (cTN1), cardiac troponin T (cTnT) and serum CK-MB (creatine kinase myocardial bound).

Neuroimaging and Other Diagnostic Tests in Neonatal Encephalopathy

Prediction, prognostication of brain injury and long-term outcomes are the important steps in the care of the neonate affected by perinatal asphyxia. These considerations are important for the clinician to stratify babies according to the need for intensive care and neuroprotective strategies. They are also important for the parents and families to understand long-term implications. The tests that are used for this purpose are neuroimaging (cranial ultrasound, MRI), EEG and near infrared spectroscopy (NIRS).

Cranial Ultrasound

This is a simple, bedside, noninvasive modality which makes it a first line assessment tool. Ongoing care of the sick neonate need not be interrupted. The features of damage include brain edema demonstrated as a loss of gray-white matter differentiation. This is more clearly after the first day of life. Resistive index of middle cerebral artery is considered to be important correlation in assessing brain edema.

Magnetic Resonance Imaging

It has become feasible in modern ICU settings with the development of MR-compatible incubators. It is now the modality of choice for assessing brain injury. The most sensitive technique is MRI with diffusion weighted imaging (DWI). It is the gold standard to detect abnormalities associated with other causes of neonatal encephalopathy such as cerebral dysgenesis, infection, stroke, and metabolic disorders. MRI based neuroimaging has revealed patterns of injury following hypoxic ischemic insult that are unique to the immature brain and it depends on the age at which it occurs and the severity and duration of the insult. Acute and profound asphyxia produces injury in the basal ganglia and thalamus, prolonged and partial asphyxia causes diffuse injury in the white matter. The basal ganglia predominant pattern involves the basal ganglia, thalamus and perirolandic cortex while the watershed pattern predominantly involves the vascular watershed, from the white matter and extending to the cerebral cortex.

Determining the onset and progression of injury: Diffusion MR (DWI) techniques have facilitated the identification of the onset and progression of injury. DWI detects alterations in free water diffusion. Injured areas will be seen as increased signal intensity areas on DWI. There is an evolution of the brain injury after birth. The optimal time to conduct the examination is 3–5 days of life. Early or late examinations may miss these findings.

MRI and outcome prediction: Miller SP et al. showed that 56% of 173 surviving infants with injury predominantly in the basal ganglia/thalamus had spastic quadriplegia, whereas only 11% of infants with the watershed pattern of injury had severe cerebral palsy. In the absence of motor problems, cognitive deficits were more appreciable at 30 months of life than at 12 months with a watershed pattern of injury. Abnormal signal intensity in the posterior limb of the internal capsule (PLIC) as associated with neurodevelopmental impairment at the first year of life as per the analysis of Rutherford et al. Further evidences on the correlation of brain injury patterns and neurodevelopment have been published by Hayes et al. More than three-fourths of neonates with basal ganglia or thalamus injury on MRI died or developed cerebral palsy at the first year of life. The predictive value of MRI is not affected by hypothermia treatment as shown by a recent meta-analysis. Hypothermia is a modality of treating neurological injury in the neonate and infants who were cooled were more likely to have normal scans.

Advanced magnetic resonance techniques: Advanced MR techniques, such as diffusion and spectroscopy imaging are useful. Diffusion tensor imaging (DTI) may help to detect microstructural brain developments, which may appear earlier than typical lesions. Such examinations are under study and could be useful as ongoing monitoring tools.

Quantitative diffusion weighted imaging and diffusion tensor imaging: The basis of DTI technique is to study the apparent diffusion coefficient (ADC) and the direction of water motion. As the brain matures, the cell membranes develop and the ADC decreases in gray and white matter. Modern software allows brain mapping according to ADC-areas of interest. Reduced ADC values in the PLIC are found to be associated with a greater risk of poor neurodevelopment parameters.

Diffusion tensor imaging has given rise to another derivative technique—the diffusion tensor tractography. This provides information on resilience of microstructure and specific functional pathways. When HIE infants were studied with this technique, impaired microstructure and corpus callosum pathways were found to be predictors for poor neurodevelopment parameters at 21 months of age according to the study by Massaro et al.

MR spectroscopy: Magnetic resonance is also being used to study physiology and biochemistry by incorporating spectroscopy. Brain metabolites have specific signatures on spectroscopy. These signatures and their interpretation can be obtained from specific brain regions. In a normal brain, the strongest signals are from choline, creatine, N acetylaspartate (NAA). In an injured brain, lactate predominates in the first 24 hours. It has been shown that significant brain injury can be predicted by high lactate levels and low NAA levels when imaging is done in the first 3 days of life.

Amplitude Integrated Electroencephalogram

The raw electroencephalogram signal has numerous artifacts. When this raw signal is amplified and passed through a filter to minimize artifacts and time compressed, the result is an aEEG. This is obtained in modern machines by single channel (3 electrodes) or 2 channels (5 electrodes). aEEG has been classified based on either voltage or pattern to determine the background as listed in **Box 1**. aEEG may be affected by the use of anticonvulsants and readings should not be taken for 60 minutes after they have been administered. Hypothermia does not affect aEEG readings.

aEEG was found to have a pooled sensitivity of 0.91 in predicting brain injury in a recent meta-analysis of 8 studies. Time to recovery of background seems to be important; even infants with a severely abnormal background pattern (burst suppression) in the first 6 hours of life had a good likelihood of survival without significant disability if the pattern normalized within the first 24 hours of life. Time of onset of sleep wake cycles (SWC) also may be predictive of later outcomes.

> **BOX 1:** Amplitude integrated electroencephalography classification system.
>
> *Classification by voltage:**
> - Normal (upper >10 µV, lower >5 µV)
> - Moderately abnormal (upper >10 µV, lower ≤5 µV)
> - Severely abnormal (upper <10 µV, lower <5 µV)
>
> *Classification by pattern:***
> - Continuous normal voltage
> - Discontinue voltage
> - Burst suppression
> - Continuous low voltage
> - Flat tracing

*The first method uses voltage of the upper and lower margin of the aEEG signal to classify amplitude as normal, moderately abnormal, or severely abnormalities.
**The second method distinguishes five different patterns. Flat tracing, continuous low voltage, burst suppression are considered significantly abnormal.

TREATMENT OF HYPOXIC ISCHEMIC ENCEPHALOPATHY

Perinatal Management

The obstetric management of labors in women with high-risk factors outlined earlier should be conducted in accordance to standard protocols. Safe labor ward practices should be the cornerstone in identifying labors where problems such as preterm birth, abnormal CTG patterns and thick meconium may complicate outcomes. In such situations, in utero resuscitation with a view to limiting hypoxia and hypovolemia related injury are important steps and should be used until definitive management – usually an expedited delivery – can be achieved.

Delivery Room Management

A prompt resuscitation by neonatologist or those who are trained in neonatal resuscitation is desirable. Initial care of neonate in DR includes care of temperature, breathing and circulation. Avoid hypocarbia due to overzealous tube/bag ventilation. If required a bolus of normal saline to improve circulation can be useful.

Postnatal Management

- *Ventilation:* Keep CO_2 in normal range. High levels of CO_2 will amplify the "steal phenomenon" and cause cerebral acidosis and vasodilatation. Low levels of CO_2 from overzealous ventilation and washout can result in cerebral vasoconstriction and decrease cerebral blood flow.
- *Oxygenation:* A balance has to be kept in the administration of oxygen to the sick neonate. The purpose of supplying oxygen is to treat hypoxemia and adequate flow rates are needed. However, hyperoxia can cause free radical injury.
- *Temperature:* In a neonate with HI insult, passive cooling by turning off warming lights can be tried. Low and high temperature variations should always be avoided.

- *Perfusion:* Hemodynamic stability and adequate mean systemic arterial blood pressure are important to maintain adequate cerebral perfusion pressure.
- *Electrolytes and metabolic issues:* The monitoring and maintenance of biochemical parameters is an important step in the management. Hypocalcemia is associated with decreased myocardial contractility and seizures. Hypoglycemia increases cerebral blood flow and increases energy deficit whereas hyperglycemia causes increased brain lactate, damage to cellular structure and cerebral edema.
- *Fluid management:* The volume of infused fluids should be critically adjusted. Hypovolemia will cause an inadequate circulating and overloading the system may result in cerebral and pulmonary edema. Fluid restriction helps in minimizing cerebral edema.
- Syndrome of inappropriate antidiuretic hormone (SIADH) secretion is often seen 3–4 days after the hypoxic ischemic event. It manifests as hyponatremia with hypo-osmolarity with low urine output and inappropriately concentrated urine. Renal function can also be affected by acute tubular necrosis (ATN) which can result from "diving reflex".
- Control of seizures and management of injury to other organs are described here.

Seizures generally start within 12 hours of birth, increases in frequency, and then resolve in few days. Seizures in HIE are can be extremely difficult to control and may not be possible to stop completely. Seizures are sometimes subclinical and difficult to identify. Here, EEG is useful in detection and prognostication. Metabolic disturbances (hypoglycemia, hypocalcemia, and hyponatremia) can cause or exacerbate seizure activity and should be simultaneously corrected.

In the acute management of seizures, the drug of choice is phenobarbital. A loading dose of 20 mg/kg is given and if seizures persist then additional loading dose of 5–10 mg/kg can be given. A maintenance dose of 3–5 mg/kg divided into two doses should be started 12–24 hours after loading dose. Neonates should be monitored for respiratory depression. Because of prolonged half-life therapeutic levels (15–40 mg/dL) should be monitored in case of hepatic or renal dysfunction. Phenytoin can be added (loading dose 15–20 mg/kg followed by 4–8 mg/kg maintenance dose divided 8 hourly) if seizures are not controlled with phenobarbital. Benzodiazepines are considered third-line drugs and it includes lorazepam (dose 0.05–0.1 mg/kg/dose IV). Data regarding safety and efficacy are limited.

Levetiracetam has been tried recently due to its safety and efficacy in other childhood epilepsy. Anticonvulsant drugs can be weaned when clinical and EEG indicate seizure free state. Weaning should be done in the order of initiation (if multiple anticonvulsants are started) and phenobarbital should be weaned last. Newborns with persistent neurologic deficit and with abnormal EEG are at high risk of recurring seizures in infancy or childhood.

Other organ dysfunction that may manifest in early neonatal life is cardiac and renal. The heart function needs to be optimized by correction of acidosis, hypoxemia and metabolic disturbances. Babies with HI will require continuous monitoring of mean arterial blood pressure and urine output (UOP). Renal dysfunction manifests as oliguria or anuria. A good balance of fluid administration is critical in this matter. Avoid fluid overload by limiting free water administration to replacement of insensible losses and urine output (60 mL/kg/day) and low dose dopamine (2.5 µg/kg/min) can be considered. Volume status should be checked before starting fluid restriction. 10–20 mL/kg saline bolus followed by a loop diuretic like furosemide may be helpful. To avoid fluid overload and hypoglycemia concentrated glucose solution should be delivered through central line. Feeding should be withheld till blood pressure is stable and active bowel sounds are audible.

NEUROPROTECTIVE STRATEGIES

It is shown to be beneficial in decreasing risk of brain injury in newborns exposed to perinatal hypoxic ischemic condition. Therapeutic hypothermia methods include whole body cooling and selective head cooling. Both methods showed similar effects regarding long-term neurologic outcomes. Many RCTs and Cochrane reviews demonstrated that therapeutic hypothermia resulted in less death and better neurodevelopmental outcome at 18 month of age who survived. It is shown to increase survival without increasing disability in survivors. At 6 or 7 years, children treated with therapeutic hypothermia (TH) had significant higher frequency of survival with an IQ score of 85 or higher compared with children who did not receive cooling.

Criteria for Therapeutic Hypothermia

Inclusion

- Gestational age ≥36 weeks and Birth weight ≥2000 g.
- Evidence of fetal distress as evidenced by at least one of the following:
  - History of acute perinatal event (abruptio placentae, cord prolapse, fetal HR abnormality, variable, or late deceleration)
  - Biophysical profile <6/10 within 6 hours of birth
  - Cord pH ≤7.0 or Base deficit ≥16 mEq/L
- Evidence of neonatal distress by one of the following:
  - APGAR score ≤5 at 10 minutes
  - Postnatal blood gas pH at <1 hour ≤7.0 or base deficit ≥16 mEq/L
  - Continued need for ventilation initiated at birth and continued for at least 10 minutes.
- Evidence of neonatal encephalopathy by physical examination
- Abnormal EEG with minimum of 20 minutes recording shows one of the following:

- *Severely abnormal:* Upper margin <10 µV
- *Moderately abnormal:* Upper margin >10 µV and lower margin <5µV
- Seizure identified by aEEG.

Exclusion

Patient can be excluded from this protocol according to the judgment of attending neonatologist. Following are the exclusion criteria:

- *Normal initial aEEG tracing:* No seizures, lower margin >5µV
- Inability to initiate cooling by 6 hours of age
- Presence of lethal chromosomal abnormality (e.g., Trisomy 13 or 18.)
- Presence of severe congenital malformations (e.g., complex cyanotic heart disease, major CNS anomaly)
- Symptomatic systemic congenital viral infection (e.g., hepatosplenomegaly, microcephaly)
- Symptomatic systemic bacterial infection (e.g., meningitis, DIC)
- Bleeding diathesis (platelet count <50,000/mm^3, spontaneous clinical bleeding)
- Major intracranial hemorrhage.

Cooling should be started before 6 hours of age so early recognition is essential. The target per rectal temperature goal should be 33.5°C. Arterial access and central venous access should be obtained prior to initiation of TH protocol.

Safety monitoring of newborn during 72 hours of TH and rewarming temperature:

- *Temperature:* Monitor skin and per rectal temperature continuously. Check for areas of skin breakdown and reposition newborn frequently given the risk of subcutaneous fat necrosis. The hypothermia blanket should be kept dry.
- *CVS/respiratory system:* Use pulse oximetry cautiously as reading may be inaccurate. Follow arterial blood gases and lactate levels.
- *Renal/GI/FEN:* Monitor serum electrolytes, BUN, creatinine, AST/ALT to avoid cerebral edema Na$^+$ should be maintained between 140 and 148.
- *Heme:* Monitor PT/PTT/INR, fibrinogen, platelets and treat as clinically indicated.
- *Infection:* Monitor CBC, differential counts, and blood culture results. Antibiotics can be used prophylactically during the period of hypothermia.
- aEEG to monitor seizure activity. Head ultrasound in first 24 hours to rule out any major intracranial hemorrhage.

At the end of 72 hours of induced hypothermia, the newborn is rewarmed at a rate of 0.5°C every 2 hours till temperature reaches 36.5°C which may take 10 hours. An MRI should be done at 7–10 days of age or later to detect the full extent of any HI brain injury.

CONCLUSION

Modern neonatal practice in perinatal asphyxia is based on good delivery room management to optimize resuscitation of the sick infant. The early initiation of protective strategies and managing the overall condition of the infant will help in minimizing neuronal injury. Modern prognostic methods including MRI and aEEG are excellent tools for prognostication. The principles of supportive care are well established and should be backed by neonatal care infrastructure. The care of such infants may lead to future medicolegal issues, and documentation and communication should be done meticulously.

FURTHER READING

1. Ahearne CE, Boylan GB, Murray DM. Short and long term prognosis in perinatal asphyxia: An update. World J Clin Pediatr. 2016;5(1):67-74.
2. Azzopardi D, Strohm B, Marlow N, Brocklehurst P, Deierl A, Eddama O, et al. TOBY Study Group. Effects of hypothermia for perinatal asphyxia on childhood outcomes. N Engl J Med. 2014;371(2):140-9.
3. Gillam-Krakauer M, Gowen Jr CW. Birth Asphyxia. 2021 Aug 27. In: Stat Pearls [Internet]. Treasure Island (FL): StatPearls Publishing; 2021 Jan. PMID: 28613533.
4. Groenendaal F, de Vries LS. Fifty years of brain imaging in neonatal encephalopathy following perinatal asphyxia. Pediatr Res. 2017;81(1-2):150-5.
5. Herrera CA, Silver RM. "Perinatal Asphyxia from the Obstetric Standpoint." Clinics in Perinatology. 2016.
6. Matthew A. Rainaldi, Jeffrey M. Perlman. "Pathophysiology of Birth Asphyxia", Clinics in Perinatology, 2016.
7. McGuire W. Perinatal asphyxia. BMJ Clin Evid. 2007;2007:0320.
8. Stephanie L. Merhar, Vann Chau. "Neuroimaging and Other Neurodiagnostic Tests in Neonatal Encephalopathy", Clinics in Perinatology, 2016.
9. van Handel M, Swaab H, de Vries LS, Jongmans MJ. Long-term cognitive and behavioral consequences of neonatal encephalopathy following perinatal asphyxia: a review. Eur J Pediatr. 2007;166(7):645-54.

LONG QUESTIONS

1. Discuss the causes of perinatal asphyxia. Elaborate on the obstetric aspects of perinatal asphyxia.
2. What is the Sarnat staging of hypoxic ischemic encephalopathy? What differential diagnosis should be considered in a neonate presenting with such features?
3. Discuss neuroimaging and diagnostic tests in perinatal asphyxia. What is the clinical relevance and prognostic value of such tests?
4. Discuss the important management aspects of perinatal asphyxia. What is the role of hypothermia in such neonates?

SHORT QUESTIONS

1. Mention the factors that allow the fetus to survive in a state of relative hypoxia in utero.
2. What are the adaptive responses seen in the neonate to perinatal asphyxia?
3. What are the patterns of brain injury seen with perinatal asphyxia according to timing and duration of hypoxic insult?
4. What features in the neonate suggest birth asphyxia?
5. Enumerate the strategies available for neuroprotection in the infant with perinatal asphyxia.

MULTIPLE CHOICE QUESTIONS

1. Which of the following is true about the fetal circulation?
   a. Hemoglobin levels are higher in fetal life than in adults
   b. Fetal hemoglobin has a lower
   c. Lower tissue perfusion rates
   d. High energy usage on thermoregulation and respiration
2. The vital changes that lead to adaptation on birth are all, except:
   a. Drop in pulmonary vascular resistance due to the rapid lung expansion
   b. Marked drop in pulmonary blood flow
   c. Closure of the ductus arteriosus
   d. Rise in systemic vascular resistance
3. The following conditions can cause perinatal asphyxia due to maternal hypovolemia, except:
   a. Placental abruption
   b. Uterine rupture
   c. Cord prolapse
   d. Maternal vehicular accident with pelvic fracture
4. Which of the following is true about adaptive responses to perinatal asphyxia:
   a. Diving reflex leads to a drop in blood flow to the brain
   b. Diving reflex is mediated by interleukins
   c. There is an increase in lactate production
   d. Brain metabolic rate increases
5. The typical features of hypoxic ischemic encephalopathy in a neonate are all, except:
   a. Fetal heart rate < 60 beats/minute
   b. Apgar score 8 at ≥ 5 minutes
   c. Need for positive pressure ventilation for > 1 minute or first cry delayed > 5 minute
   d. Seizures within 12 to 24 hours of birth
6. Which of the following is not an inclusion criteria for hypothermia therapy?
   a. Gestational age ≥ 36 weeks and birth weight ≥ 2000 grams.
   b. Evidence of neonatal encephalopathy by physical examination
   c. Postnatal blood gas pH at <1 hour ≤ 7.0
   d. Lethal chromosomal anomaly

Answers
1. a 2. b 3. c 4. c 5. b 6. d

10.10 BIRTH INJURIES

Upendra Kinjawadekar, Anjali Otiv

INTRODUCTION

Birth trauma is defined as preventable and unavoidable mechanical or ischemic damage to the newborn's tissues or organs during labor and delivery, resulting in either functional deterioration or underlying structural destruction. The spectrum of birth injuries ranges from mild (lacerations) to severe (spinal cord injuries). These can lead to severe neonatal morbidity or mortality. Birth injuries are also considered to be caused by putting the fetal scalp electrodes and intrauterine heart rate monitor, but those following neonatal resuscitation procedures are excluded.

This reflects the level of standard of obstetric care. The number of cases of birth injury decreases with improvements in obstetric care and prenatal diagnosis. Injuries commonly occur during labor, delivery, or after delivery.

The estimated incidence is 2–7 cases per 1,000 live births and accounts for 2–3% of neonatal deaths.

Table 1 depicts the interventions that may act as risk factors and their associated injuries.

RISK FACTORS

Although birth injuries are frequently associated with traumatic delivery, they can often occur without any risk factors.

The risk factors that may be related to the fetus, mother, and obstetrical instruments used during labor and delivery are given in the following text.

Fetus

- *Macrosomia:* Birth injury is directly related to fetal weight >4,000 g.
- Preterm infants with very low birth weights <1,000 g.
- *Abnormal fetal presentation:* Fetal presentations, particularly face and breech presentations, are at more risk as compared to a vertex position.

TABLE 1: Interventions that may act as risk factors and their associated injuries.	
Intervention	**Probable injury**
Breech presentation	Brachial plexus palsy, intracranial hemorrhage, gluteal lacerations, long bone fractures
Forceps delivery	Facial nerve injuries
Vacuum extraction	Depressed skull fracture, subgaleal hemorrhage
Forceps/vacuum/ forceps and vacuum	Cephalohematoma, intracranial hemorrhage, shoulder dystocia, retinal hemorrhages
Abnormal presentation (face, brow, transverse, compound) Macrosomia	Excessive bruising, retinal hemorrhage, lacerations Shoulder dystocia, clavicle and rib fractures, cephalohematoma, caput succedaneum
Prematurity	Bruising, intracranial and extracranial hemorrhage
Precipitous delivery	Bruising, intracranial and extracranial hemorrhage, retinal hemorrhage

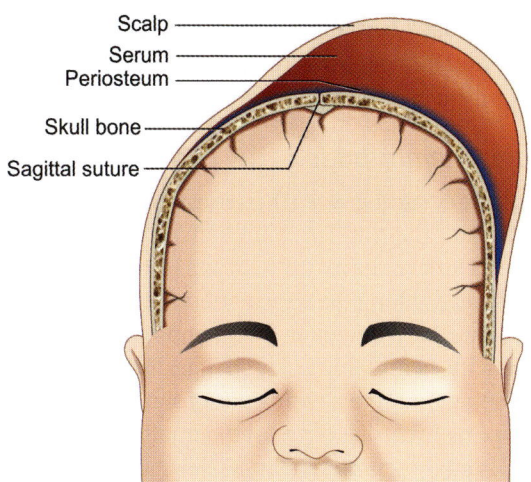

Fig. 1: Caput succedaneum

Mother

- *Maternal factors:* Small maternal stature, e.g., cephalopelvic disproportion
- *Maternal obesity:* These mothers are at an increased risk of having a large-gestational-age baby with shoulder dystocia hence increase in the use of instruments during delivery.

Mode of Delivery

- Operative vaginal delivery (use of forceps and vacuum) has a higher risk of birth injuries as compared with nonoperative vaginal delivery.
- The C-section: It was found that the risk of birth trauma is lower in comparison with vaginal delivery.

■ CLASSIFICATION

Soft-tissue Injury

It is the most commonly seen birth injury. These include easy bruising, petechiae, subcutaneous fat necrosis, and laceration.

Easy Bruising and Petechiae

They are usually self-limiting and observed on the presenting part of the body where the device was applied. Infant delivered especially with a face presentation may have petechiae of head and neck. These petechiae do not advance and are not associated with any other bleeding events. If the bleeding and petechiae continue, one must determine the platelet count to rule out thrombocytopenia. The significant bruises have a significant risk factor for severe hyperbilirubinemia.

Subcutaneous Fat Necrosis

As a result of ischemia to the adipose tissue, well-circumscribed firm nodules with purplish discoloration are seen following a traumatic delivery. They resolve spontaneously over weeks to months and some babies may develop hypercalcemia.

Lacerations

The most common birth injury attributed to emergency cesarean delivery. The majority of fetal lacerations are mildly restricted only to the skin; however, they can be moderately extended to muscles or severely extended up to the bones and nervous tissue requiring suturing and prevention from secondary bacterial infection. Most common are facial lacerations seen with a cephalic presentation followed by the transverse or breech presentation.

Extracranial Injuries

Injuries leading to swelling or bleeding in different areas of the scalp and the skull are as follows:

Caput Succedaneum (Fig. 1)

Swelling of the soft tissues on the presenting part of the scalp underneath the skin and above the periosteum, which is occasionally hemorrhagic. It is ill defined, diffuse, edematous, boggy, pitting, and nonfluctuant swelling which crosses the suture lines. The high pressure of the walls of the vagina and the uterus on the head of the fetus leads to an accumulation in the blood and serum. As a general rule, this is a benign condition with spontaneous recovery within a few days.

Cephalohematoma (Fig. 2)

Cephalohematoma is a subperiosteal collection of blood beneath the periosteum. It is more common after the use of the vacuum and forceps during the delivery. It is unilateral fluctuant, well and sharply demarcated swelling limited to a single bone and does not cross suture lines. The spontaneous resolution does occur over few weeks without any intervention. Complications include anemia, calcification, infection, osteomyelitis, sepsis, and hyperbilirubinemia.

The absence of discoloration of the overlying skin and the longer period for resolution differentiates cephalohematoma from caput succedaneum

Subgaleal Hemorrhage

Hemorrhage occurs between the periosteum of the skull and the aponeurosis as the emissary veins between the scalp and dural sinus are sheared or have ruptured as a result of traction on the scalp. It spreads along the subcutaneous plane of the layers of the soft tissue. Early detection is very important. It is fluctuating swelling in the head, which may change during the motion. An affected infant may have early signs of shock. The classic triad consists of tachycardia, decreased hematocrit, and increased occipital frontal circumference (OFC) in the first 24–48 hours of birth. OFC can be increased to 1 cm with each of the 30–40 mL of blood collection. The treatment covers a wide range of use of packed red blood cells, fresh frozen plasma, depending on the ongoing bleeding and correction of coagulopathy. In rare cases, hematoma evacuation surgery is required.

Scalp Electrode Injuries

The location of the application of electrodes can be a site of infection in 1% of cases. Usually benign, but in preterms can lead to hypotension due to bleeding.

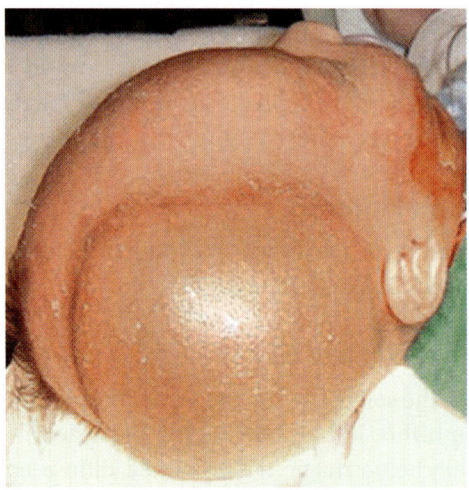

Fig. 2: Cephalohematoma.

Facial Injury

Nasal Septal Dislocation

It occurs due to compression of the nose, from the pubic symphysis or sacral promontory. The newborn may present with difficulty in breathing due to airway obstruction. There is the deviation of the nose to one side with the asymmetric nares and flattening on the dislocated side. The diagnosis is made by rhinoscopy.

Ocular Injuries

They are commonly found and resolved spontaneously without affecting the baby. They are secondary to a sudden increase in intrathoracic pressure during the passage through the birth canal. Minor injuries include swelling of the eyelids, retinal, and subconjunctival hemorrhage. Significant damage includes a hyphema, bleeding within the eye, lacrimal duct tear and fracture of the orbital ridge.

Intracranial Injuries

Intracranial hemorrhage (ICH), as a result of birth trauma, has subdural, subarachnoid, epidural, and intraventricular hemorrhages (**Figs. 3A and B**). They occur due to the sudden compression and decompression of the head.

Epidural Hemorrhage (Fig. 4A)

Epidural hemorrhage is very rarely seen in newborn babies. It occurs between the dura mater and the inner surface of the skull. The middle meningeal artery is usually injured. It is often accompanied by a linear skull fracture and is located in the parietal-temporal region. The clinical presentation is irritability, lethargy, and convulsions which progress to signs of raised intracranial pressure and ultimately uncal herniation.

Subdural Hemorrhage (Fig. 4B)

Subdural hemorrhage (SDH) occurs as a result of damage to the superficial veins, where the vein of Galen and the inferior sagittal sinus connects to form a straight vein. The most common intracranial hemorrhage is seen in full-term neonates

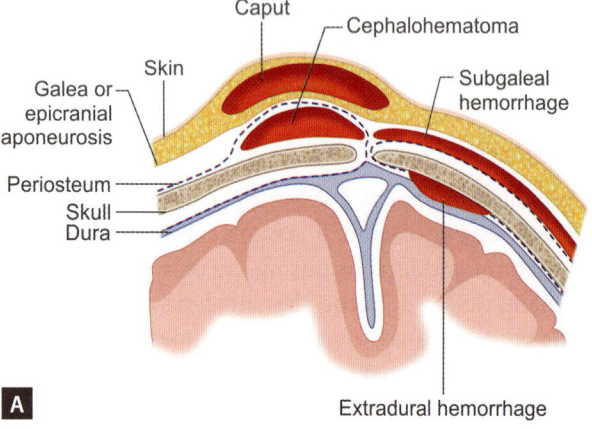
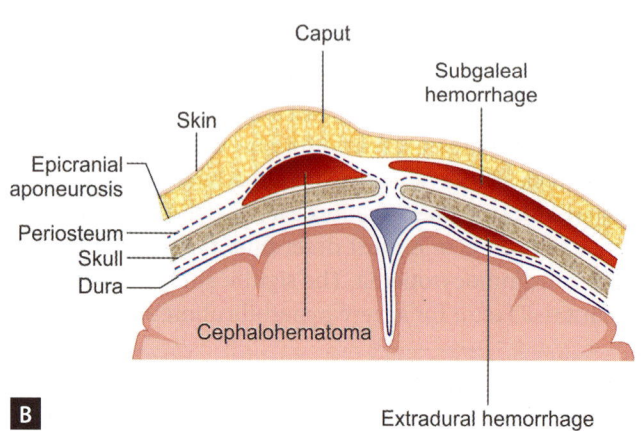

Figs. 3A and B: Intracranial injuries.

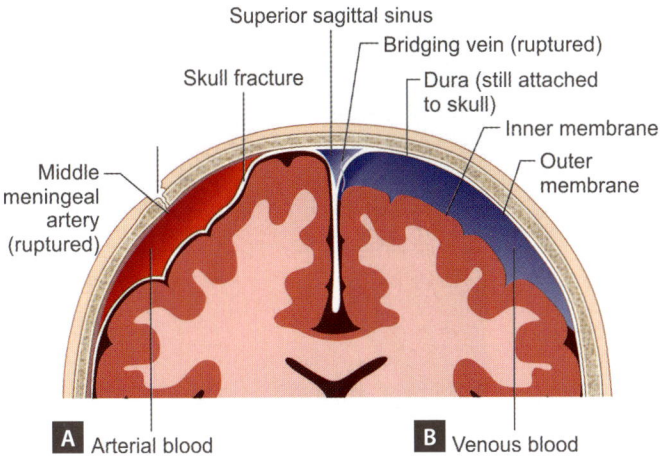
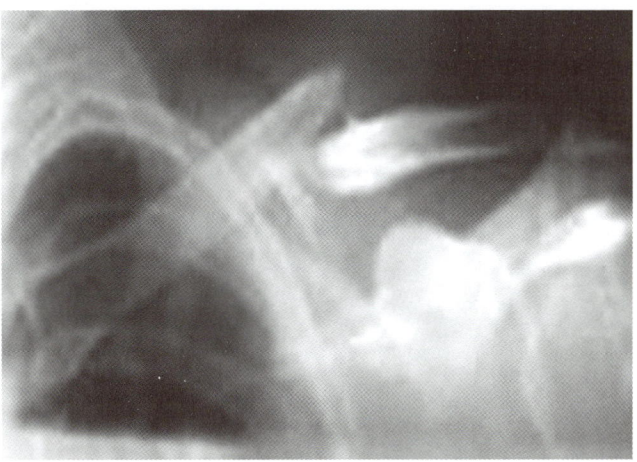

Figs. 4A and B: (A) Epidural hematoma; (B) Subdural hematoma.

Fig. 5: Clavicular fracture.

and the most common site of SDH is the interhemispheric or the tentorial region. It is often, characterized by pallor, lethargy, irritability, and a decreased Moro's reflex with the development of focal cerebral signs. Symptoms can occur within hours or a day. The bulging of the anterior fontanelle may be a sign of an acute hemorrhage. This may manifest itself as apnea, bradycardia, altered mental status, and seizures. The diagnosis is made by ultrasound or computed tomography (CT) scan.

Subarachnoid Hemorrhage

Subarachnoid hemorrhage is a very common injury as a result of damage to the veins that pass through the subarachnoid space. This type of injury can manifest as seizures. The diagnosis is made by obtaining blood-tinged cerebrospinal fluid on lumbar puncture. On examination, the anterior fontanel is tense and bulged. Infant presents with altered level of consciousness, convulsions, nausea, vomiting, and irregular periodic breathing with high-pitched cry. The condition usually resolves spontaneously and hence no treatment is needed.

Intraventricular Hemorrhage

Intraventricular hemorrhage (IVH) is more seen in preterm deliveries, but it can also be seen in full-term labor. IVH in full-term infants will resolve spontaneously with no long-term effect but close monitoring is required because of the risk of the spread of the hemorrhage into the surrounding parenchyma. There are usually no clinical symptoms. In severe cases, the clinical symptoms include periods of apnea, abnormal breathing, a high-pitched cry, pallor or cyanosis, inability or failure to suck well, muscle spasms, seizures, reduced muscle tone, and a tense bulging anterior fontanelle. IVH classification includes a grading system that is following increasing severity. Diagnosis is suspected on basis of history (events at birth, weight and gestational period of newborn) and clinical findings.

Retinal Hemorrhage

Retinal hemorrhage occurs in approximately 75%, 33%, and 6.7% during vacuum, spontaneous vaginal and C-section deliveries, respectively. Lower rates in the context with C-sections probably suggest that the reason may be that the pressure on the head as it passes through the birth canal. The fundoscopic examination should be performed within the first 24 hours after birth.

Fracture

Clavicle

The most commonly reported fractures during delivery and the chance increases with the use of vacuum/forceps. The other risk factors are: advanced maternal age and birth weight of more than 4 kg. Clavicular fracture **(Fig. 5)** is often associated with difficult vaginal delivery with shoulder dystocia in vertex presentations and of the extended arms in breech deliveries. The arm is not freely moved by the infant on the affected side. Moro's reflex is absent on the affected side. Displaced (complete) clavicular fracture is accompanied by physical findings. These include crepitus, edema, lack of movement of the affected extremity, asymmetrical bone contour, and crying with passive motion.

Nondisplaced clavicular fractures are usually delayed for days or weeks until there is a visible formation or palpable callous. The neonate is usually asymptomatic. Diagnosis made with an X-ray of the clavicle. In addition, it also warrants clinical evaluation for brachial plexus injury. Clavicular fractures in infants heal spontaneously with the callous formation with no long-term sequelae. Parenteral reassurance, gentle handling, and analgesics are all that is required for management. The prognosis is excellent.

Humerus

The most common long bone to get fracture is a proximal third of the humerus, which are transverse and complete.

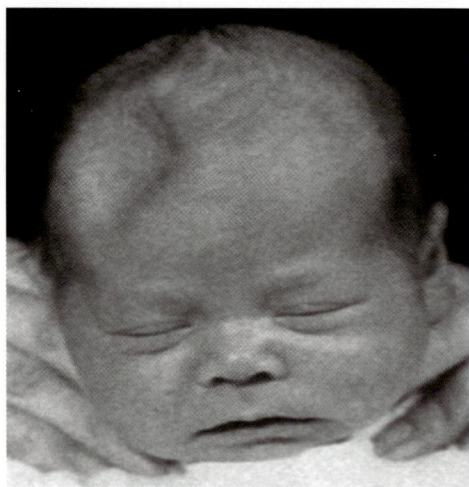

Fig. 6: Depressed skull fracture.

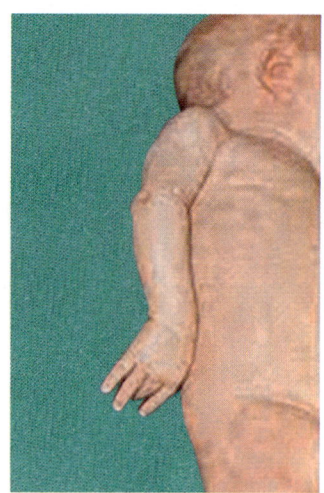

Fig. 7: Erb's Duchenne palsy.

The major risk factors for fractures are shoulder dystocia, macrosomia, and breech presentation during delivery. Clinical manifestations of fracture in the newborn include decreased movement and increased pain response to the touch of the affected arm, decreased Moro's reflex, localized swelling and crepitations. One should look for evidence of brachial plexus injury.

A plain radiograph of the arm will aid the diagnosis. Treatment of humeral fractures consists of immobilization of the affected arm with the elbow in 90° flexion to prevent rotational deformities. The outcome result is very good with evidence of callus formation seen in radiography by 7–10 days.

Femur

Fractures of the femur are rare. The fracture is usually spiral and involves the proximal half of the femur. Risk factors include twin pregnancies, breech presentations, prematurity, and diffuse osteoporosis. Neonates are asymptomatic with only an increased pain response upon manipulation of the affected extremity. Diagnosis can be done by a plain radiograph. The Pavlik harness is used to treat the neonatal femoral fracture. The results are very good with evidence of callus formation commonly seen in radiography at 7–10 days.

Skull

Cranial fractures due to traumatic birth include linear and depressed skull fractures **(Fig. 6)**, often with cephalohematoma. Depressed skull fractures are due to the inward buckling of the skull bones and are often associated with forceps-assisted delivery or spontaneous unassisted and elective cesarean delivery. The diagnosis is made by a plain radiograph of the head. Neurological sequelae are rarely seen with fractures of unassisted vaginal births. In contrast, there is an increased risk of intracranial bleeding and/or cephalohematoma in forceps-assisted delivery. Further evaluation with CT imaging is required to determine the presence or absence of intracranial lesions. If the fracture is <1 cm, depressed, and there is no neurodeficit, it can be managed or treated with close monitoring. SDH is the most common with depressed fracture. Neurosurgical consultation is a must within 12–24 hours of diagnosis in those with evidence of increased intracranial pressure and if the depression is >1 cm.

Nerve Injuries

Peripheral Nerve Injury

Brachial plexus injuries: Injury is caused by stretching or rupture of the cervical nerve roots from traction on the neck during delivery. Incidence is 0.5–2.5 per 1,000 live births. The risk factor for the injury is the birth weight of >4,500 g, shoulder dystocia, extended arms in the breech, and assisted delivery.

Erb's Duchenne palsy is the most common palsy due to the injury to the upper roots of the brachial plexus (5th and 6th cervical nerve) **(Fig. 7)**. The child presents with adduction, internal rotation, extended elbow, pronated forearm and wrist flexion (policeman tip appearance). Moro's biceps and radial reflexes are absent. It is frequently associated with phrenic nerve injury. An adequate grasp reflex in Erb palsy excludes total arm paralysis.

Klumpke's palsy is rare and involves the lower roots of the brachial plexus (7th and 8th cervical and 1st thoracic nerve). Wrist drop or claw hand is presented as hand muscles and long flexors of hand are paralyzed. Deep tendon reflexes are present. Klumpke's palsy is frequently associated with ipsilateral Horner's syndrome. The grasp reflex is absent. Management involves intermittent immobilization of the arm with gentle massage. Neuroplasty or nerve grafting must be considered if no recovery beyond 6 months.

Facial nerve injury: Incidence is 0.1–0.7% of live births. The peripheral nerve gets compressed by forceps or a prominent maternal sacral promontory. Usually, only the mandibular branch of the facial nerve is affected, and the baby will have

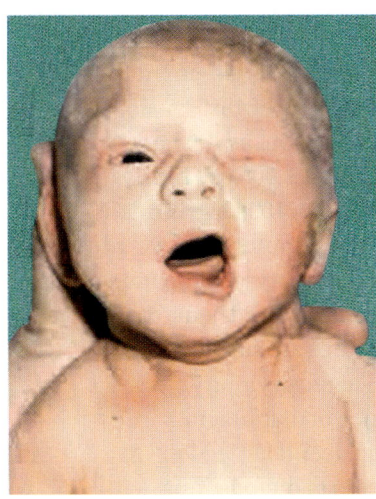

Fig. 8: Facial palsy.

reduced mobility on the affected side of the face. Often, there is a loss of the nasolabial fold, partial closure of the eye, and inability to move facial muscles on the affected side, giving an appearance of a "drooping" mouth **(Fig. 8)**. Within the first 2 weeks of life, there is an excellent outcome with no residue.

Phrenic Nerve Injury

Symptoms of phrenic nerve injury are often associated with brachial plexus injury and seen on the first day of life.

Lateral hyperextension of the neck causes overstretching or avulsion of the 3rd, 4th, and 5th cervical roots which supply the phrenic nerve. The infant presents with respiratory distress, elevated hemidiaphragm, and paradoxical diaphragmatic movement. Recovery is unlikely if no improvement is seen within 1 month.

Laryngeal Nerve Injury

Laryngeal nerve damage can cause vocal cord paralysis. The baby presents with stridor and respiratory depression. Direct laryngoscopy helps in diagnosis. Depending on the severity, resolvent occurs over time, usually within 4–6 weeks.

Spinal Cord Injury

The incidence of injury is 0.14 per 10,000 live births. Due to the traction and rotation of the upper cervical spine during childbirth, there is a high risk of injury to the cord. Spinal epidural hematoma, vertebral artery injury, and traumatic cervical hematomyelia are the most common injuries seen.

Visceral Injuries

Visceral injuries primarily involve the internal organs of the abdomen which include rupture of the liver, spleen, and adrenal gland. The presentation of the baby will depend on the amount of blood loss. Hepatic and splenic ruptures may present as sudden pallor, abdominal discoloration, and signs of shock. With a unilateral adrenal hemorrhage, an abdominal mass is seen.

Ultrasonography is the best way to diagnose visceral injuries. Useful diagnostic information can be obtained from abdominal CT scan. Treatment includes fluid resuscitation and control of bleeding. Hemodynamically unstable infants with hepatic or splenic rupture may need laparotomy.

■ KEY MESSAGES

- Incidence of birth injuries is about 2–7/1,000 live births.
- The risk of birth injuries are related to fetal, maternal factors, and the mode of delivery.
- The most common form of traumatic birth injuries are soft-tissue injuries.
- The extracranial injuries usually resolve spontaneously without any intervention. In contrast, subgaleal hemorrhage may result in massive blood loss that may lead to shock and death.
- For intracranial hemorrhages, the decision for neurosurgical intervention is based upon the evidence of increased intracranial pressure.
- Clavicular and humeral fractures are common limb injuries.
- The most common neurologic injury is the brachial plexus injury.
- Visceral injuries due to birth trauma are rare.

■ FURTHER READING

1. Agrawal M. Textbook of Paediatrics, 1st edition. Mumbai: Bhalani Publication; 2009. p. 261.
2. Alexander JM, Leveno KJ, Hauth J, Landon MB, Thom E, Spong CY, et al. Fetal injury associated with cesarean delivery. Obstet Gynecol. 2006;108(4):885.
3. Amar AP, Aryan HE, Meltzer HS, Levy ML. Neonatal subgaleal hematoma causing brain compression: report of two cases and review of the literature. Neurosurgery. 2003;52(6):1470.
4. American Academy of Pediatrics Subcommittee on Hyperbilirubinemia. Management of hyperbilirubinemia in the 7 newborn infant 35 or more weeks of gestation. Pediatrics. 2004;114(1):297.
5. Davis DJ. Neonatal subgaleal hemorrhage: diagnosis and management. CMAJ. 2001;164(10):1452.
6. Gault DT. Extravasation injuries. Br J Plast Surg. 1993;46:91-6.
7. Ghai OP. Ghai Essential Pediatrics, 7th edition. New Delhi: CBS Publishers and Distributors; 2009. p. 488.
8. Kliegman RM, Marcdante K, Behrman RE, Jenson HB. Nelson Textbook of Pediatrics. 18th edition. Philadelphia: Elsevier; 2007. pp. 714,720.
9. Looney CB, Smith JK, Merck LH, Wolfe HM, Chescheir NC, Hamer RM, et al. Intracranial hemorrhage in asymptomatic neonates: prevalence on MR images and relationship to obstetric and neonatal risk factors. Radiology. 2007;242(2):535.
10. Moczygemba CK, Paramsothy P, Meikle S, Kourtis AP, Barfield WD, Kuklina E, et al. Route of delivery and neonatal birth trauma. Am J Obstet Gynecol. 2010;202(4):361.e1.
11. Nassar AH, Usta IM, Khalil AM, Melhem ZI, Nakad TI, Abu Musa AA, et al. Fetal macrosomia (>or =4500 g): perinatal outcome of 231 cases according to the mode of delivery. J Perinatol. 2003;23(2):136.
12. Singh M. Care of the Newborn, 7th edition. New Delhi: Sagar Publications; 2010. p. 421.

13. Uhing MR. Management of birth injuries. Pediatr Clin North Am. 2004;51(4):1169.
14. Wilkins CE, Emmerson AJB. Extravasation injuries on regional neonatal units. Arch Dis Child Fetal Neonatal Ed. 2004:89:F274-5.

LONG QUESTIONS

1. A 3-day-old home-delivered preterm infant brought to an emergency room by grandparents with complaints of vomiting and refusal of feeds. On examination, she has subtle convulsions and looked pale.
   a. Enumerate the differential diagnosis of the case.
   b. Define birth injury.
   c. Describe investigations and management of such case.
2. Classify neonatal birth injuries and describe the etiology, investigation, and management of intraventricular hemorrhage.

SHORT QUESTIONS

1. Define and discuss the risk factors associated with birth injury.
2. Differentiate between cephalohematoma and caput succedaneum.
3. Answer the following questions according to the given image:
   a. What is the likely diagnosis?
   b. What is the etiology?
   c. What is the most common associated complication?

MULTIPLE CHOICE QUESTIONS

1. Incidence of birth injury in India is:
   a. 2–7/1,000 live births
   b. 2–7/100 live births
   c. Less than 2/1,000 live births
   d. More than 7/1000 live births
2. A neonate was noted to have adduction and internal rotation of left arm with pronation of the forearm. A chest X-ray revealed a raised hemidiaphragm on the same side. These findings are suggestive of:
   a. Brachial plexus injury
   b. Absence of diaphragm
   c. Transplacental Infection
   d. Defect in gametogenesis
3. Pitting and nonfluctuant swelling which crosses the suture lines is:
   a. Cephalohematoma
   b. Caput succedaneum
   c. Subgaleal hemorrahge
   d. Intraventricular
4. Cephalohematoma usually disappears within:
   a. 3–5 months   b. 3–5 weeks
   c. 5–7 weeks   d. 10–15 days
5. The most frequently fractured bone in new born during delivery is:
   a. Femur   b. Humerus
   c. Clavicle   d. Skull

Answers
1. a   2. a   3. b   4. c   5. c

10.11 COMMON NEONATAL PROBLEMS

Bakul Jayant Parekh

INTRODUCTION

The neonatal problems perceived by a mother or a doctor immediately after a child's birth or in the first 28 days are either transient or physiological, not requiring any intervention, except for the assurance to the parents or they may be pathological or may require intervention for further management.

RESPIRATORY DISTRESS IN NEWBORN BABIES

Respiratory difficulties constitute the most common cause of morbidity in infants and postexamination results may suggest pulmonary pathology, which is the diagnosis of lung disorder in newborn babies. When the respiratory rate in an infant in resting position is >60 per minute, as well as there are grunting sounds during breathing and difficulty in breathing, it suggests respiratory distress.

Breathing issues or respiratory problems can arise as a symptom for several reasons and it is even more complex to identify the exact diagnosis for newborn babies as they have a limited capacity to express through their signs and symptoms what they are feeling. Respiratory distress may be due to several reasons such as congenital heart disease, respiratory distress syndrome (RDS), pneumonia, pneumothorax, and meconium aspiration syndrome (MAS), hence it is critical to correctly identify the symptoms and make the diagnosis of respiratory distress in an infant.

The neonatal problems perceived by a mother or a doctor immediately after a child's birth or in the first 28 days are either transient or physiological, not requiring any intervention, except for the assurance to the parents. In certain cases, however it may be pathological and require intervention for further management.

BREAST ENGORGEMENT (MASTITIS) (FIGS. 1A AND B)

The infection of the breast tissue, also known as *mastitis*, causes the breasts to engorge. Both the breasts may become fuller and the skin around the breast may be sensitive to touch, have redness and be warm. Sometimes, a white liquid discharge may happen from the breasts which is also referred to as "witch's milk."

This is not related to cancer and the symptoms may improve on its own without any medication. Usually, the breast engorgement happens due to the breast tissue stimulation due to the high levels of maternal hormones. Touching, pressing, or massaging the breasts or nipples may aggravate the situation and cause infection hence it should be avoided. Usually, if medication is required, it can be treated with antibiotics and analgesic tablets.

CAPUT SUCCEDANEUM (FIGS. 2A AND B)

Caput succedaneum is a common and usually harmless condition in newborns caused from the pressure on the newborn's head during the vaginal delivery. It is observed as a soft swelling and bruises on the scalp which resolves by itself within a few days. There is no treatment or tests necessary to manage caput succedaneum. This condition occurs during birth and is different from cephalohematoma.

Caput succedaneum is the formal medical term for the area of localized swelling or edema which is commonly present on the head of a newborn baby following vaginal delivery. More simply, it is fluid under the skin on the baby's head.

Caput succedaneum is usually a benign neonatal condition resulting from normal pressure and compression on the baby's head as it passes through the birth canal. Caput succedaneum itself is harmless as the swelling is limited to the scalp and is not a symptom of a deeper injury to the skull or brain. Although caput succedaneum itself is nothing to worry about and quickly resolves, it can lead to other complications including newborn jaundice.

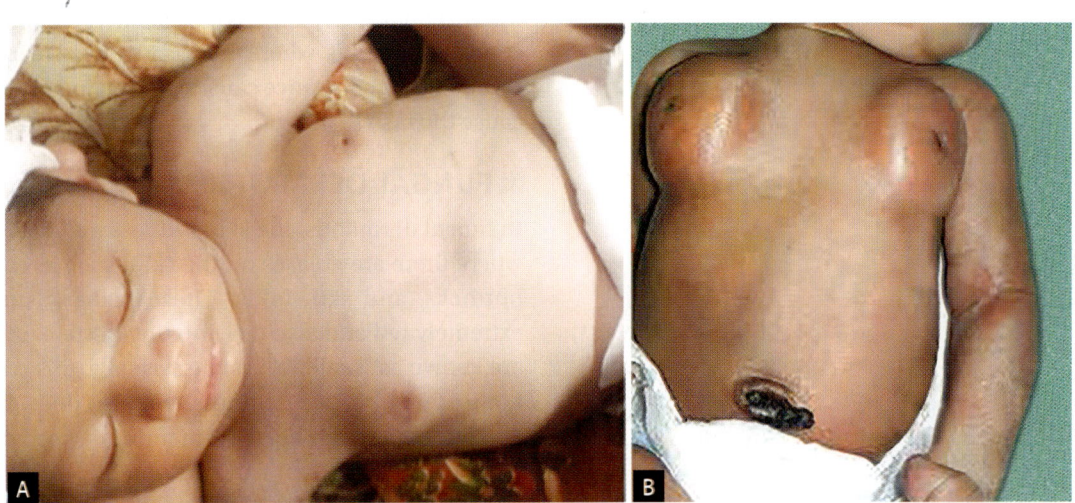

Figs. 1A and B: Breast engorgement.

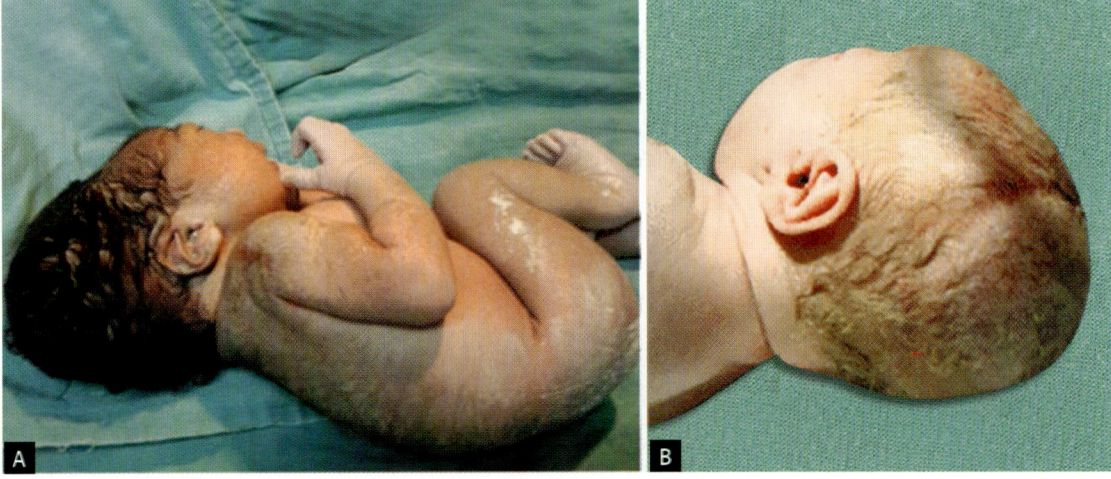

Figs. 2A and B: Caput succedaneum.

CEPHALOHEMATOMA (FIG. 3)

Cephalohematoma is a neonatal condition wherein there is a hard swelling in the scalp due to blood being accumulated between the newborn's scalp and the skull. The swelling has clear edges and does not cross the suture lines. With time, the swelling becomes calcified, with a softer center and gradually subsides in a few months.

It is not a rare condition and is also usually not risky as there is no brain damage. In some cases, the baby may develop anemia, jaundice, or hypotension. In case skull fracture is suspected, computed tomography (CT) scan or skull X-ray can be done for diagnosis. Due to an enhanced risk of infection, aspiration is not recommended.

VAGINAL DISCHARGE/VAGINAL BLEEDING (FIG. 4)

The development of menstrual-like withdrawal bleeding may occur in about one fourth of female babies after 35 days of birth. It occurs due to fall in the level of sex hormones after birth when baby is disconnected from the placenta. The discharge and bleeding is not heavy and lasts for 2–4 days and it is recommended that local aseptic cleaning of the genitalia be done. Additional vitamin K will not be necessary.

The baby girl here has a vaginal discharge that is thick and has a creamy texture. It can happen on and off for the first few days after birth. This condition does not require any treatment procedures as it is a self-limiting condition that occurs as the maternal hormones are withdrawn. Parents need to be assured as this condition reduces within the first few weeks.

CONTACT DERMATITIS (FIG. 5)

Dermatitis, in general, refers to an inflammation of the skin. Irritant contact dermatitis, specifically, is an inflammation of the skin caused by contact with a foreign substance. This can be any chemical substance, including soaps, detergents, and fabric softeners. The reaction can look like a burn. Infants experiencing irritant contact dermatitis will usually be fussy. There may be obvious skin irritation, including inflammation, swelling of the area, and warmth. The rash will be confined to the specific area that came into contact with the offending agent. The onset of the skin reaction in irritant contact dermatitis is immediate, as opposed to allergic contact dermatitis, where there is a delayed reaction in which the offending substance causes production of antibodies that cause the rash to develop.

FUNGAL DERMATITIS

In fungal dermatitis, the skin redness and rashes that occur where there are creases on the skin, such as the groin area, buttocks, and skin folds. These rashes usually become extremely red and also develop tiny blisters or sports which are known as "satellite" lesions. Usually, this condition does not irritate or cause itchiness and also does not hurt. This condition, unlike contact dermatitis, may occur in the groin region. The treatment can be done by applying antifungal ointments. Further, the affected area should be kept dry and often exposed to air.

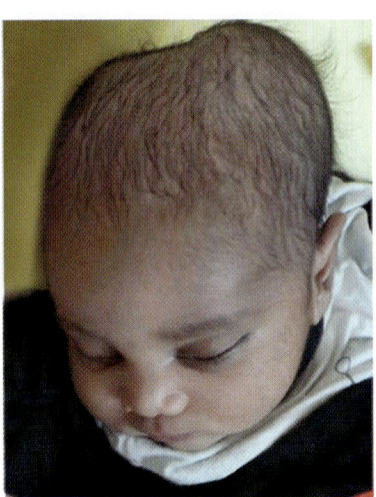

Fig. 3: Cephalhematoma.

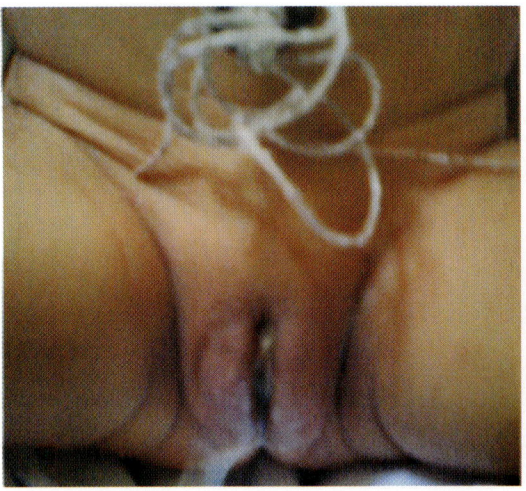

Fig. 4: Vaginal discharge/Vaginal bleeding.

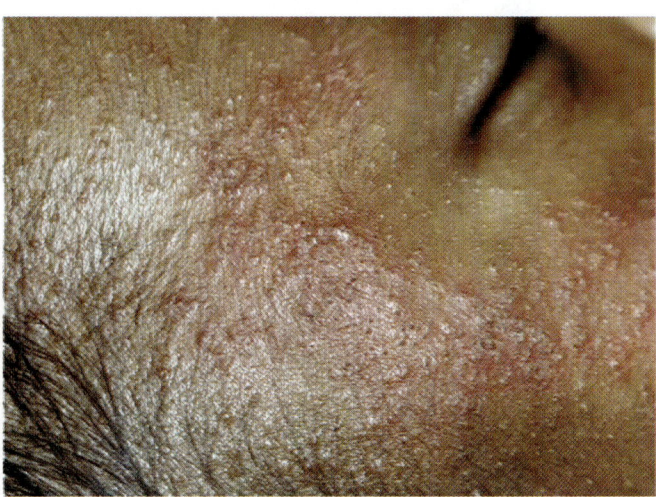

Fig. 5: Contact dermatitis.

SEBORRHEIC DERMATITIS (CRADLE CAP)

A newborn baby, in the first 4 weeks, may develop yellow and greasy scales or plaques on the scalp and also have some level of hair loss. This does not cause itchy skin or irritation, unlike the condition of atopic dermatitis. Such patches are common during the first few weeks of birth and may also affect the areas where the skin folds and creases.

Cradle cap usually clears up on its own within a few months. Treatment can be done by the application of mild shampoo that contains cetrimide or cetavlon. The doctor may also prescribe antifungal medicine.

ERB'S PALSY (FIG. 6)

The waiter's tip deformity is a sign of Erb's palsy which causes weakness in the arm and loss of motion. The arm loses movement and hangs by the side and can be rotated medially. The baby cannot raise its arm and the forearm becomes extended and pronated, which is facing downward. In the same way, the forearm cannot be turned upward or be supinated and the power of flexing or bending the elbow and deep tendon reflexes is lost. The hand and the wrist are not affected. These symptoms are observed in 90% of all brachial plexus injuries.

Another condition known as Klumpke's paralysis has a bigger impact wherein the hand becomes clawed and the baby does not have the ability to grasp or flex and bend the wrist. Usually, this condition improves on its own and babies may recover within 2–4 weeks. If "antigravity" movement is observed in the affected part by the end of the third month, it is a good sign of recovery. For Klumpke's palsy and total plexus injuries, if improvement in the condition is not observed in 3–6 months, then surgical treatment should be evaluated.

INFANT OF DIABETIC MOTHER (FIG. 7)

Infant of diabetic mother (IDM) are newborns whose mothers are diabetic, which can affect the baby. The baby is often much larger in size than normal birth weight and has higher fat deposits in the cheeks, torso, limbs, and neck. Such babies also may be hairy around the ears which indicate that the mother may be diabetic.

The cord blood glucose evaluation should be done post birth to predict the condition of hypoglycemia. The condition should be monitored and managed by early and frequent feeding; close clinical tracking to look out for any complexities and treatment of hypoglycemia.

PRETERM

A preterm baby, or a baby which is born before 37th week of pregnancy, is usually tiny and has a skin texture that is thin, smooth, and looks pink across the body. The breast buds may not be present or barely seen, as is the case with the ear recoil as well. The area around the ears is also smooth and may have very less or absent ear cartilage. The baby may have substantial body hair on the torso, forehead, and back. In baby girls, the labia minora may be visible, and labia majora is spread out, while in males, the scrotum has less rugosity. The testes may also be outside the scrotal sac. Various techniques such as using the New Ballard score or Modified Dubowitz score can be utilized for diagnosis. Some of the medical complications associated with preterm birth include hypothermia, RDS, below optimum motor coordination, heart defect such as patent ductus arteriosus, gastrointestinal disease such as necrotizing enterocolitis and intraventricular hemorrhage.

INTRAUTERINE GROWTH RESTRICTION (FIG. 8)

Intrauterine growth restriction (IUGR) is a condition wherein the baby does not grow as per the normal levels expected in the mother's womb. The baby looks smaller than expected

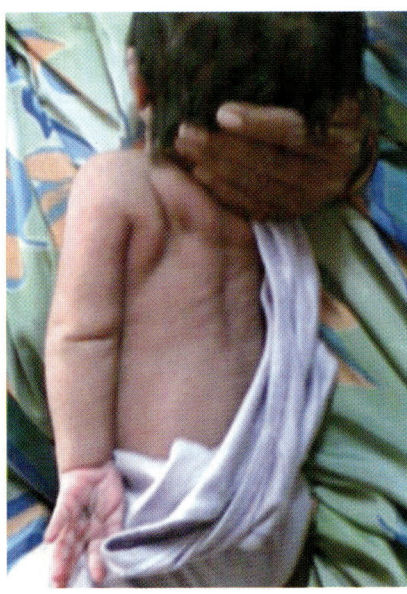

Fig. 6: Erb's palsy.

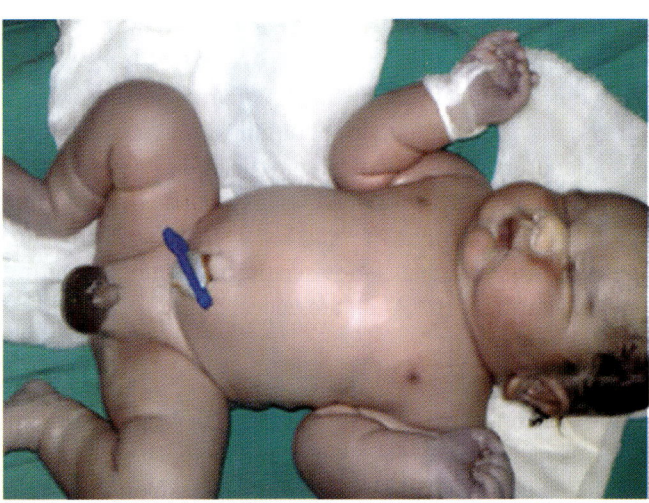

Fig. 7: Infant of a diabetic mother.

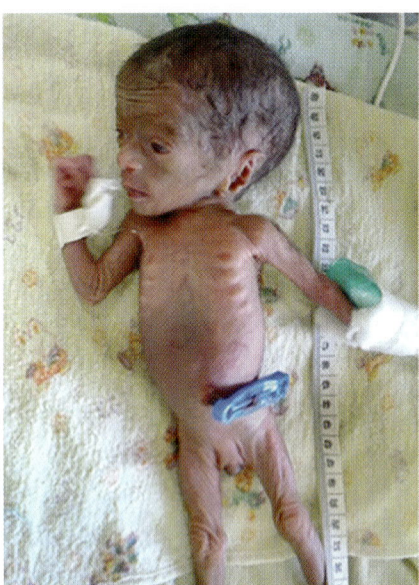

Fig. 8: Intrauterine growth restriction (IUGR).

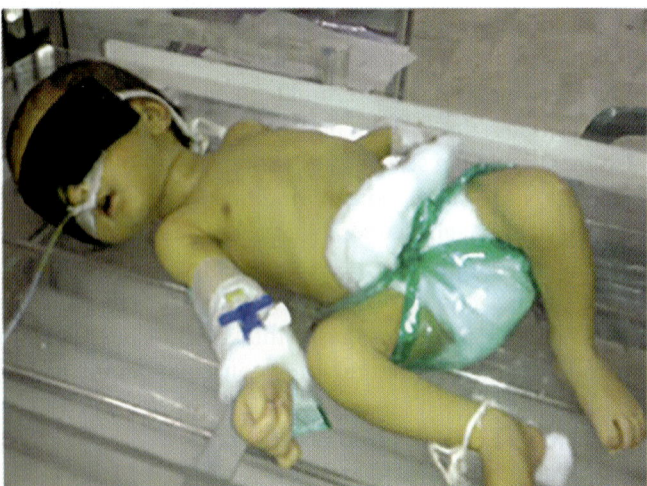

Fig. 9: Jaundice.

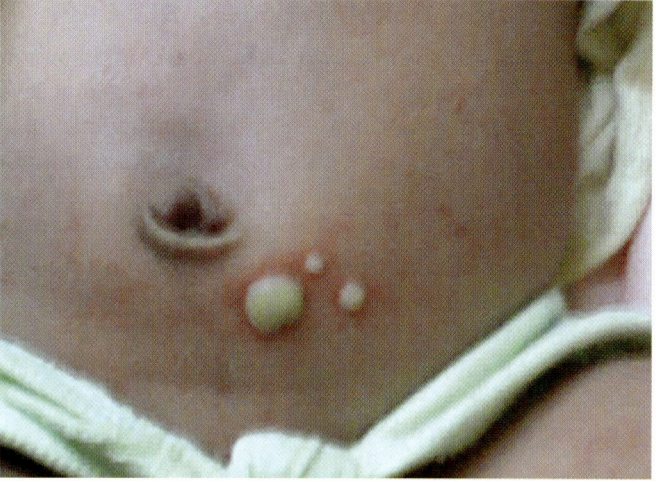

Fig. 10: Pustules.

and also may seem to have lost subcutaneous fat. The baby is underweight and the limbs are thin and the newborn appears malnourished even if alert. The baby's head appears to be larger compared to the body.

If the weight of the baby is <10% of predicted fetal weight for gestational age, then the condition is known as small-for-gestational age (SGA). Medical complications related to IUGR include blood glucose-related issues such as hypothermia, hypoglycemia, polycythemia, as well as jaundice and meconium aspiration. It is advised that close monitoring and early diagnosis of the issues are necessary.

■ JAUNDICE (FIG.9)

Jaundice in newborn infants appears as yellowish skin over the body, especially, the thighs, limbs, and torso. The condition is evaluated in bright light by applying pressure on the skin or blanching the skin with the fingers to look for the underlying skin discoloration. The assessment of jaundice in newborns receiving phototherapy may not be correct.

However, only the visual or physical examination may not be the right indicator of the level of jaundice. This should be done by estimating the total serum bilirubin (TSB). If the TSM > 95th percentile for the age in hours, then according to the guidelines of the American Academy of Pediatrics (AAP), further diagnosis is essential.

Physiological Jaundice

In almost two thirds of term babies, physiological jaundice appears on the second day of birth, reaches peak on the 4th or 5th day and disappears by 10–14 days. The jaundice is not deep and it causes mild yellow staining of the trunk. The physician attending on the newborn should be alert and look for other causes of jaundice in the neonatal period.

■ PUSTULES (FIG. 10)

In this condition, the periumbilical area or the area around the navel develops blisters or pustules. The surrounding skin shows erythema, which is redness of the skin. In some cases, pustules may discharge pus as well as lead to hardening of the adjacent skin.

For mild cases, topical antibiotics and oral therapy can be administered. For more severe occurrences, or of pustules condition in preterm babies, intravenous treatment may be needed. Pustules are most commonly caused due to the bacteria, *Staphylococcus aureus*.

■ UMBILICAL GRANULOMA

In a newborn baby, sometimes a moist, crumbly pink or red lump of tissue can be observed in the belly button which is known as umbilical granuloma. It may get infected and have a discharge that can irritate the adjacent skin of the baby. This condition is different from an umbilical polyp which appears to be redder than a granuloma and cannot be treated via silver nitrate catheterization.

Umbilical granuloma that is small can be treated by applying silver nitrate or crystal salt. Larger ones or those that do not get healed may need surgical treatment.

AMBIGUOUS GENITALIA

This is not a very common condition wherein the baby has darker skin and pigmentation around the genitals, navel, and belly button and the external genital organs do not appear to be clearly male or female as there is clitoral hypertrophy and impalpable testes. It can lead to salt wasting or excessive loss of sodium from the body, as well as metabolic acidosis (excess acid in body fluids), hyponatremia (sodium deficiency), and hyperkalemia (excess potassium). The main cause of this condition is congenital adrenal hyperplasia (CAH). Diagnosis can be done by baseline tests such as 17-hydroxyprogesterone (reference range < 6 nmol/L), adrenocorticotropic hormone assay (reference range 2–11 pmol/L) which are inflated and karyotyping (46XX female) that confirms the diagnosis of salt wasting type of congenital adrenal hyperplasia (CAH). Replacement therapy with glucocorticoids (hydrocortisone 10–20 mg/m^2 day) and mineralocorticoids (fludrocortisone 100–200 μg/day) will be necessary.

UNDESCENDED TESTIS (FIG. 11)

In this condition, the scrotum or scrotal sac looks empty and does not have complete overlying rugosity which means that one or both the testes has not moved to its proper position in the scrotum. This is different from retractile testes which can move between the groin and the scrotum.

To diagnose the issue, a physical examination of the infant is to be done to check if the testis is present in the scrotal sac. Surgical evaluation should be done by 3 months of birth in cases where undescended testes is detected. If the baby has bilateral testes that is nonpalpable, then an endocrine evaluation needs to be done to eliminate sex development disorders such as anorchia or intersex. Surgical treatment called orchiopexy can be done but gonadotropin-releasing hormone (GnRH) and human chorionic gonadotropin (hCG) are used, with the success rate between 30 and 50%

ANAL AGENESIS

In this condition, a male newborn has no anal opening that indicates a birth defect wherein the anus and rectum have not developed properly. There may be an abnormal connection or fistulae between the rectum urinary or genital tracts. Newborn babies with this condition will show swelling in the abdomen soon after birth and will not be able to pass meconium, which is the first stool of the baby. Physical examination needs to be done to check if anal opening is present. In the first 24 hours postbirth, a lateral pelvic radiography or invertogram has to be performed and to address the condition, surgery will be required.

POLYCYTHEMIA

This is a condition wherein the soles of the feet of the newborn baby appear red and flushed. The baby looks to have excess blood and the body looks red. Diagnosis of polycythemia is confirmed when hematocrit is >65%. This is observed more in cases of placental insufficiency, placental transfusion, and IUGR. Hematocrit is to be performed 6–8 hours post birth for high-risk newborns, such as SGA. If hematocrit is 70% in an asymptomatic baby and 65% in symptomatic baby, then partial exchange transfusion needs to be done.

CYANOSIS (FIG. 12)

In this condition, the soles of the baby's feet become discolored and look blue. This happens due to the increased concentration of reduced hemoglobin in the blood, i.e., >5 g%. The main symptom of central cyanosis is presence of mucus membranes and dusky skin, while peripheral cyanosis does not affect the mucous and the central body and in fact impacts the hand and feet.

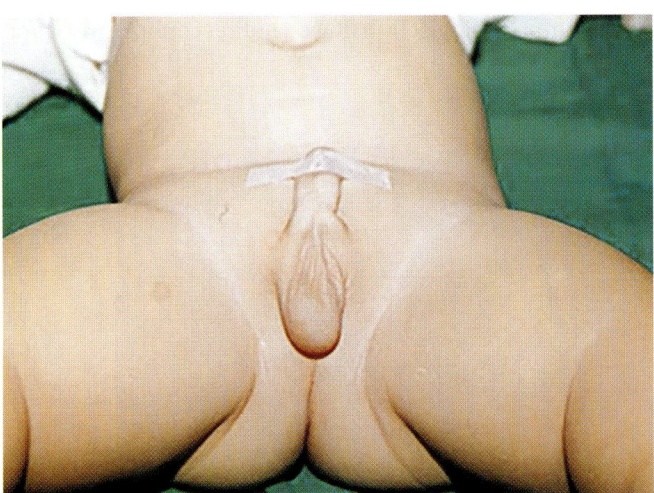

Fig. 11: Undescended testis.

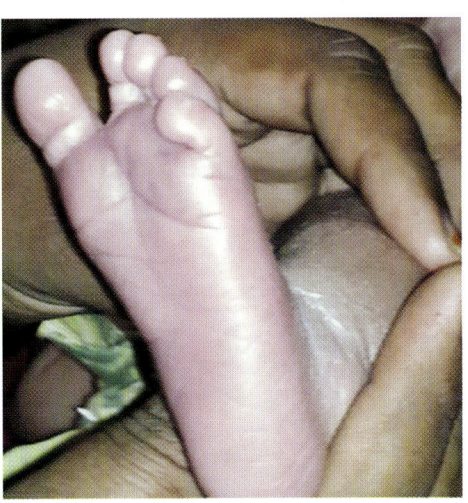

Fig. 12: Cyanosis.

The diagnosis of central cyanosis is a cause of concern and can be risky. Cyanosis can lead to several medical issues such as cardiac issues, hypothermia, metabolic disorders, parenchymal/nonparenchymal pulmonary issues as well as neurological problems. Newborn babies with this condition require immediate medical intervention and assessment of the problem and treatment to be initiated on an urgent basis.

■ INGUINAL HERNIA

Inguinal hernia causes a swelling and bulge on the left side of the groin or inguinal area that may expand into the scrotal sac. The bulge does not cause any pain and there are no indications of soreness and inflammation. It does not affect the right side of the groin. This condition develops when the content of the abdomen protrudes outside the peritoneal cavity via the inguinal canal.

After physical examination and study of the clinical history, the diagnosis can be made but, in some instances, tests such as inguinal ultrasonography may be necessary. Surgery is recommended as early as possible to avoid complications arising due to the obstruction of the hernia.

■ MENINGOMYELOCELE (FIG. 13)

Meningomyelocele is a birth defect or a neural tube defect which affects the lumbar spine. An abrasion can be found on the skin over the spine. The skin remains intact, and has no discharge but indicates that the baby's spinal cord did not develop properly. In such cases, the nerves of the bowel and bladder and lower limbs of the body may get impacted. In case the defect is severe, the impact will be higher and can also lead to paralysis. It may be an isolated condition or may occur with other congenital defects such as defects relating to the midline.

To treat this condition, the open meningomyelocele must be closed as early as possible to avoid infections. A ventriculoperitoneal shunt could be required to treat associated hydrocephalus. To avoid neural tube defects, folic acid supplement is advised before pregnancy. A multidisciplinary strategy is required for the long-term.

■ CLUBFOOT-CONGENITAL TALIPES EQUINOVARUS (FIG. 14)

A structural or postural deformity where in both the feet of the infant are impacted and causes it to rotate internally at the ankle is termed as clubfoot-congenital talipes equinovarus (CTEV). Such abnormality can also be observed for spina bifida; therefore, it is recommended that the spinal dysraphism be also checked for such babies.

About 50% of such cases may be treated without surgery and can be managed by gentle stretches and frequent casting of the feet within 2 weeks of birth. Post that, a special brace can be worn nearly all the time from 3 months to 3 years of age. The procedure of tenotomy may also help. In extreme cases, surgery will be necessary.

■ RETINOPATHY OF PREMATURITY SCREENING

The examination for retinopathy of prematurity (ROP) is done by an ophthalmologist by using an indirect ophthalmoscope.

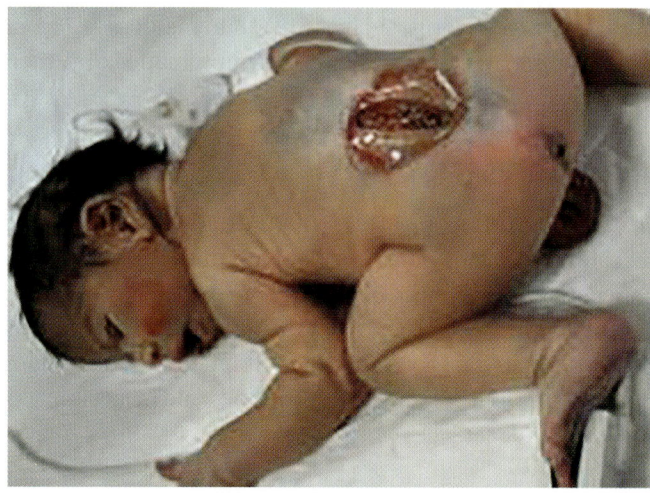

Fig. 13: Meningomyelocele.

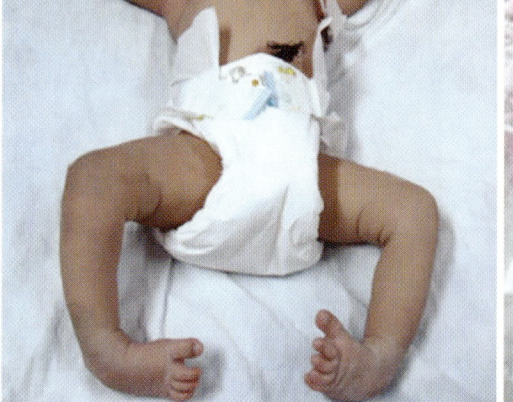 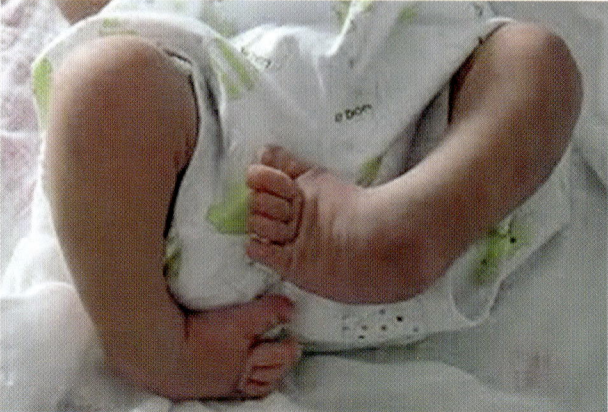

Fig. 14: Clubfoot—congenital talipes equinovarus (CTEV).

Tropical drops are used to dilate the pupils along with local anesthesia. The screening for ROP should be done on all preterm babies as well as newborns weighing <1,750 g at birth at 4 weeks postbirth age.

Retinopathy of prematurity is a disorder that affects the eye generally in preterm babies due to incomplete retinal vascularization, which means that the retinal blood vessels which grow from the optic nerve, and travel to the inner retina at about 16 weeks of gestation, and eventually reach the temporal peripheral retina at approximately 40 weeks of gestational age do not get the chance to develop completely.

In severe cases, ROP may lead to blindness. Oxygen toxicity as well as relative hypoxia can lead to the formation of ROP. The severity and occurrence of ROP are directly related to the gestational age during birth and birth weight and the treatment is guided by prethreshold and threshold diseases to prevent severe impact like blindness.

■ VOMITING

It is normal for babies to throw up and vomit on the first day of their birth due to the irritation in the stomach caused due to swallowing of amniotic fluid. If the vomiting does not subside, the stomach should be washed with 100 mL normal saline. Improper technique of feeding as well as aerophagia may result in vomiting soon after a baby is fed. The regurgitation is nonprojectile and adequate weight gain is maintained. The proper advice regarding feeding and burping, whether solicited or not, should be given to all mothers.

In case vomiting does not recede and is stained with bile and projectile, along with failure to pass the first stool or meconium or abdominal inflammation, then the baby should be examined for intestinal obstruction. In cases of gastroesophageal reflux (GER) and hiatus hernia, when the baby is laid down, the incidence of vomiting is seen, and it does not occur when the infant is held up. Pylorospasm may also be a cause of vomiting in some newborns. In the case of hypertrophic pyloric stenosis, vomiting usually occurs after the baby is 2 weeks old. It is more likely to occur in a first-born male infant and is characterized by nonbilious projectile vomiting, poor weight gain, and constipation. Vomiting can point to multiple medical conditions including birth asphyxia, systemic infection, meningitis, cardiac arrest, raised intracranial tension caused by intracranial hemorrhage as well as metabolic issues such as galactosemia and congenital adrenal hyperplasia due to loss of salt. In case of GER, treatment is semireclining position and antiemetic drops to be administered.

■ FAILURE TO PASS MECONIUM AND URINE

It is possible that newborns pass meconium in the uterus or soon after birth but all babies should pass meconium in the first 24 hours of birth. Meconium is the blackish tarry stool which newborns pass in the first 2–3 days post birth. This is followed by the passing of stool that is greenish in color or transitional stool for the next couple of days. The baby should be examined in case meconium does not happen in the first 24 hours to rule out medical issues including intestinal obstruction.

After 12 weeks of gestational age, the fetus discharges urine in the uterus regularly. On the first day of birth, most babies pass urine but it is critical that all babies must urinate in the first 48 hours post birth. In most cases of alleged nonpassage of urine, the baby has actually passed urine which has been overlooked. In actual cases, the baby should be examined to check for obstructive uropathy and agenesis of kidneys. Normally, the infant will pass urine after each feed and between 6 and 12 times in a day. It is normal for babies to cry before passing urine due to feeling uncomfortable because of a full bladder, be silent and dazed while passing urine, and again cry post passing urine due to the irritation caused by wet diapers or cloth on the skin. The stream of urine should be good and forceful and there should be no straining during micturition or dribbling in the end.

■ DIARRHEA

Breastfed babies often pass 15–20 motions in 24 hours and it may be semiwatery, frothy with sour smell, varying in colors, but they gain weight adequately. These are to be taken as normal stools and donot require treatment. But if motions are large and watery with loss of weight or if there is visible blood, then treatment with antibiotics is advised along with routine and microscopic examination of stools.

■ EXCESSIVE CRYING

One should not worry about a baby who is crying but can be consoled by cuddling or changing the wet nappies or by feeding. But if there is an inconsolable cry, then one should think of serious causes such as otitis media, meningitis, or septic arthritis.

■ EVENING COLIC

It is a distinct clinical entity of uncertain etiology. The clinical picture is characterized by sudden bouts of unexplained crying spells in the evening after a few days of birth. It will be observed that always at a particular time in the evening the crying and screaming spell or the frowning and flushing of the face occurs and lasts for anything between a few minutes to hours. This is supposed to be caused due to the condition of intestinal colic because of excessive gurgling or peristaltic sounds on palpation or auscultation of the abdomen. This becomes a vicious cycle of colic crying leading to crying again as excessive crying leads to swallowing of air. The condition is more common among first born wiry and active babies of anxious parents and grandparents. The incidence of disorder is equal among breast-fed and formula-fed infants.

Nothing seems to provide relief to the baby who cries with full vigor and the whole family is extremely upset and demoralized by these unexplained shrieking episodes. Holding the baby against skin, rocking, taking him for a drive, cuddling, patting, kissing, prone positioning, etc., may provide temporary relief.

Providing antispasmodic drops half hour before colic is anticipated and keeping the baby in a prone position so that the wind can be released from above and below offers relief to most cases. Avoid making unnecessary changes in the feeding regime of the baby. The condition spontaneously resolves after 1–2 months. There is a need to conduct follow-up studies to assess the later behavior and personality profile of these colicky infants versus the noncolicky placid babies.

MILIA

Milia is a condition wherein yellow-white spots develop on the nose. This happens due to the presence of sebum and is very common in all newborn babies. They reduce and go away on their own without any treatment.

MONGOLIAN BLUE SPOTS

It has been observed that infants of African and Asian descent may show nonuniform blue patches of skin pigmentation on the buttocks and sacral region of the body. It is also possible for these spots to appear on other parts of the torso as well. Mongolian blue spots have no relation to Down syndrome and usually disappear by the age of 6 months. They should not be confused with bruising seen in babies delivered by breech presentation.

TONGUE-TIE

Tongue-tie is a condition that is observed as a form of broad membrane or layer of skin, or as a thick fibrous fold of mucous membrane under the tongue. It can create a notch at the tip of the tongue due to traction. The tongue cannot be protruded beyond the hr margins. Tongue-tie seldom interferes with sucking or causes delay in the development of speech. It may affect the clarity of speech. The condition is uncommon and is often overdiagnosed. The genuine tongue-tie may be snipped after 1 year if it is a source of anxiety to the parents.

NONRETRACTABLE PREPUCE

The foreskin or prepuce of male infants is normally nonretractable and should not be confused with phimosis. The urethral opening is tiny and can be seen with difficulty and it is suggested that the baby's mother should not use force to pull back the foreskin in the neonatal stage.

After 2 years of age, while bathing, mother should gently retract the prepuce. The diagnosis of phimosis should be considered if prepuce is fibrosed and nonretractable, stream of urine is not forceful and interrupted and when there is history of recurrent urinary tract infections. Ballooning of foreskin during urination is normal. Circumcision is contraindicated in infants with hooded prepuce, hypospadias, ambiguous genitalia, and bleeding disorder.

Fever:
- Infections are common in neonates and tend to spread rapidly.
- They are not easy to identify and hence it is important that diagnosis is done early.
- Infections are a common cause of death and morbidity; therefore; prompt and adequate treatment is necessary.
- There is no role of prophylactic antibiotics in preterm, asphyxiated neonates, lower segment cesarean section (LSCS) deliveries, etc.
- More babies can be saved by prevention of infection rather than by use of antibiotics.
- The most common organisms responsible for systemic infections are staphylococci and gram-negative organisms.
- Symptoms and signs are nonspecific and investigations must be carried out to exclude infection.
- Definitive diagnosis is made by the culture of organisms from specific sites.
- On suspicion of infection, antibiotics should be started. They can be omitted if cultures are negative and reliable and the baby is asymptomatic.
- A cerebrospinal fluid (CSF) examination must be done in all cases of proven sepsis to rule out meningitis.

Signs and symptoms:
- Not taking feeds
- Failure to gain weight/weight loss
- Lethargy/hypotonia/irritability/seizures
- Fever/hypothermia
- Abdominal distension/vomiting/loose stools/increased gastric aspirate
- Respiratory distress/apneic attacks/cyanosis/acidosis
- Late or persistent jaundice/purpura/liver, spleen enlargement
- Tachycardia/congestive cardiac failure (CCF)/hypotension
- Sclerema
- Signs of meningitis—head retraction, full AF
- Signs of disseminated intravascular coagulation (DIC): Gastrointestinal tract (GIT) bleeding, purpura, bleeding from any site
- Local infection: Conjunctivitis, skin infection, umbilical sepsis.

Management:
- Proper maintenance of thermoregulation, fluid and electrolyte balance
- Correction of acidosis and adequate ventilation
- Use of appropriate antibiotics in correct dosages and for an adequate period of time.

FURTHER READING

1. Fernandez A, et al. Manual of Neonatal Care, 1993.
2. Illing worth RS (ed.) The Normal Child. London, Churchill Livingstone, 10th edition; 1991.
3. Parthasarathy A, et al. IAP Color Atlas Of Pediatrics, 1.2 Common Neonatal Problems. pp. 6-10.
4. Singh M. Care of the newborn, 7th edition.
5. Singh M. Common neonatal problems and their management, Indian Practitioner. 1970;23:65.

LONG QUESTIONS

1. Discuss the common skin problems and dermatitis seen in the neonate with an approach to diagnosis and management.
2. What is icterus? What are the mechanisms of physiological jaundice in the neonate? How should a neonate with jaundice be assessed and managed?
3. Discuss the common gut related problems that are seen in neonates.

SHORT QUESTIONS

1. What are the common reasons for respiratory distress in the first hour of life?
2. What is acrocyanosis?
3. What are the reasons of swelling of the neonatal scalp? How can a caput and a cephalhematoma be distinguished?
4. What is the etiology and management of vaginal discharge in neonate?
5. How should the cord stump be managed in a healthy neonate? What is an umbilical granuloma?

MULTIPLE CHOICE QUESTIONS

1. Respiratory rate above .... suggest respiratory distress in a newborn.
   a. 15 breaths per minute   b. 30 breaths per minute
   c. 45 breaths per minute   d. 60 breaths per minute
2. Neonatal breast engorgement should be usually treated with:
   a. Reassurance   b. Antibiotics
   c. Surgical drainage   d. Hormone therapy
3. The following is true about nerve injuries and palsy in the neonate:
   a. Erb's palsy is a result of injury to nerve roots C8-T1
   b. In Erb's palsy, the arm lies supinated
   c. Klumpke's palsy leads to the position of the upper limb described as a claw hand
   d. Klumpke's palsy has a better prognosis than Erb's palsy
4. The following statement is true about neonatal jaundice:
   a. Neonatal jaundice usually starts on day 15 of life
   b. Mother's ABO blood group influences prognosis
   c. The first line of treatment is an exchange transfusion
   d. Jaundice is the leading cause of neonatal mortality
5. In a fetus with undescended testes, which of the following is true:
   a. The neonate should be operated in the first week of life
   b. In the future, there will be azoospermia
   c. Medical management is useful in 30% of neonates
   d. The surgery of choice is orchidectomy
6. In a neonate with ambiguous genitalia:
   a. The commonest cause is congenital adrenal hyperplasia
   b. In CAH, the 17 hydroxyl progesterone level is low
   c. CAH affected babies with ambiguous genitalia usually have a 46 XX genotype
   d. Salt wasting CAH is associated with hypernatremia and hypokalemia
7. All the following neonatal swellings are physiological, except:
   a. Umbilical hernia   b. Inguinal hernia
   c. Hydrocele   d. Caput succedaneum

Answers
1. d 2. a 3. c 4. b 5. c 6. a
7. b

SECTION 11

Social Obstetrics

11.1 PERINATAL MORTALITY, SURVEILLANCE AND RESPONSE

Manju Puri, Kanika Chopra

INTRODUCTION

The World Health Organization (WHO) defines perinatal death as a late fetal death at or after (≥) 28 completed weeks of gestation or fetal weight of more than or equal (≥) to 1,000 g if gestation is not known or a death of a newborn within 7 days of life. Globally, there is a wide variation in the upper and lower limits for defining perinatal death. Intercountry and intracountry variations exist based on the variations in the age of viability ranging between 20 and 28 weeks of gestation. Many developed countries consider the lower limit at 22 completed weeks or a birth weight of 500 g. The National Center of Health Statistics (NCHS) in United States defines perinatal deaths as sum of fetal deaths from 20 completed weeks of gestation and neonatal deaths up to 28 days after birth. This is an inclusive definition but not practical for international comparisons.

Peller in 1940s introduced the term perinatal mortality.[1] The WHO defines perinatal mortality rate (PNMR) as number of deaths in fetuses ≥28 completed weeks of gestation or weighing ≥1,000 g if gestational age is not known, up to 7 completed days postdelivery per 1,000 total births (live and still birth).[2,3] This definition is used for uniformity in data collection globally and for international comparisons. The causes of late fetal and early neonatal deaths are likely to be similar; hence, the PNMR reflects both the quality of antenatal care and neonatal care. Many perinatal deaths are preventable; hence, it is an important health indicator of a country.

MAGNITUDE OF PROBLEM

The world is facing a huge burden of neonatal and still births with 2.6 million and 2.7 million cases every year,[4] majority occurring in low- and middle-income countries. Majority of neonatal deaths occur in the first week of birth with three fourths of these in first 24 hours.[5] The actual numbers are likely to be higher as many perinatal deaths go missing due to significant number of babies delivering and dying at home. Moreover, there is nonavailability of any uniform system for reporting these cases across facilities in most of the developing countries including India.[6]

The Indian National Neonatology Forum launched the National Neonatal-Perinatal Database initiative in 1995. In 2004, the program "Save the Children Saving New-born Lives" was initiated which amongst other activities, periodically released "State of India's newborns (SOIN)" reports.[7] According to the 2014 report, the national PNMR was 28/1,000 total births; 5/1,000 stillbirths and 23/1,000 early neonatal deaths with marked interstate variability with Kerala at 10/1,000 total births, and Odisha at 37/1,000 total births.[8] The WHO General Assembly in 2014 adopted "Every Newborn Action Plan" which called for the stillbirth rate to be a core indicator of progress and set a global target of 12 or fewer stillbirths per 1,000 births for all countries by 2030. Furthermore, stillbirths were incorporated in the UN's Global Strategy for Women, Children, and Adolescents' Health (2016-30), which included ending preventable stillbirths by 2030.[9]

The next step in dealing with such an enormous problem is to make efforts in determining the cause of each perinatal death. Majority of perinatal deaths are preventable by providing quality care to mothers during pregnancy and delivery, and to newborns at birth, hence, the importance of surveillance of perinatal deaths. One meta-analysis showed a 30% reduction in perinatal deaths after introduction of death review meetings.[10]

Currently, there are multiple classification systems available for defining the cause of perinatal death. It is not necessary that a system that works in developed countries will work in developing countries due to differential availability of resources such as autopsy. Hence, the need of the hour is to establish a uniform classification system with clear guidelines to identify the associated problems and their solutions in order to limit the number of perinatal deaths.

CAUSES AND DETERMINANTS OF PERINATAL MORTALITY

The causes of perinatal deaths can be maternal, fetal, placental, or unexplained. About 30% or more are unexplained[11] **Box 1**. In developing countries, the common causes of perinatal deaths are prematurity, infections, and intrapartum hypoxia. These are strongly associated with poor socioeconomic status and poverty. It is important to understand that there are many modifiable social contributory factors affecting perinatal deaths.

CLASSIFICATION OF PERINATAL DEATH (ICD-PM)

The WHO has applied International statistical classification of disease and health-related problems 10th revision (ICD 10) to classify perinatal deaths (ICD-PM). The ICD-PM provides a standardized system for classifying perinatal mortality (including stillbirths) based on time of death (antepartum or intrapartum) into fetal and maternal causes thereby enabling comparisons within and between diverse settings and context. It is used worldwide to maintain uniformity.[12] The ICD-PM application for classifying a perinatal death is a three-step procedure.[12] **Box 2** depicts the three-step procedure for classification of perinatal death.

This has been successfully used in many countries UK, South Africa, and sub-Saharan Africa.[13]

MODIFIABLE FACTORS

Modifiable or avoidable factors are those missed opportunities within the health system which when identified may help in forming policies to reduce perinatal deaths. These social determinants can be divided into structural and intermediary. Structural factors include socioeconomic status, education, gender, religion, culture, and policy gaps, whereas intermediary factors may be related to the community, family, individual, or health system. The community-related factors include place of residence, caste, factors influencing access to healthcare services such as lack of transport, and migration status. Family-related factors include family structure, size, and quality of relationships within the family. Individual-related factors include baseline health status, knowledge, awareness, healthcare-seeking behavior and psychosocial factors such as fear of admission to hospital. Health system-related factors include availability of services, accessibility, competence, skill and behavior of providers and quality of care provided.[14]

The modifiable factors can also be described as per the delay model[15] **(Box 3)**.

PERINATAL DEATH SURVEILLANCE AND RESPONSE

Most perinatal deaths such as maternal deaths are preventable. To reduce preventable perinatal deaths, it is essential to capture accurate information on how many late stillbirths and early neonatal deaths occur at a facility, to analyze and assign the cause and factors contributing to those deaths.

Perinatal death surveillance and response (PDSR) is a process like maternal death surveillance and response (MDSR) that facilitates collecting relevant and accurate information by

---

BOX 1: Causes of perinatal deaths.

- *Maternal*:
    Race
    Obesity
    Age < 19 or >35 years
    Hypertension
    Diabetes mellitus
    Intrahepatic cholestasis in pregnancy
    Infections
    Autoimmune disease
    Smoking
    Complication of labor such as obstructed labor/PROM
- *Fetal*:
    Gestational age: Preterm/post-term
    Structural defect
    Syndromes
    Growth disorder
    Infections
    Multiple pregnancy
- *Placental/Cord*
    Placental abruption
    Placental insufficiency
    Chorioamnionitis
    Cord prolapse
    Vasa previa

(PROM: prelabor rupture of membranes)

BOX 2: ICD-PM application for classification of perinatal death

- *Classifying type of death based on its timing*:
    Antepartum
    Intrapartum
    Unknown timing of stillbirth
    Neonatal
- *Identifying the main disease-causing stillbirth or neonatal death*:
    Congenital
    Antepartum
    Intrapartum
    Prematurity
    Infection
    Other causes or unknown
- *Identifying underlying maternal cause leading to stillbirth or neonatal death*:
    M1: Maternal complications of pregnancy
    M2: Complications of placenta/cord/membranes
    M3: Complications during labor/delivery
    M4: Medical/surgical conditions
    M5: No maternal conditions

(ICD-PM: International statistical classification of disease and health-related problems—perinatal deaths)

BOX 3: Three delays in seeking care.
- *Delay 1:* Delay in decision to seek care, e.g., woman may labor at home for long before seeking medical help
- *Delay 2:* Delay in reaching heath facility, e.g., lack of transport facilities
- *Delay 3:* Delay in receiving the care at facility due to poor facilities and behavior of providers

BOX 4: Steps of PDSR.
- Recording of all deliveries, births, stillbirths, early and late neonatal deaths at a facility
- Identifying designated data collectors at all levels, i.e., facility/community/state, and national level
- Perinatal data certification to avoid underreporting
- Systematic review of all or defined cases of perinatal deaths both at facility and community levels based on institutional policy
- Encouraging and designing a system of linking community deaths with facility-based audit system
- Training of data collectors in interview techniques in community-based deaths where medical records relating to deaths are not available. The interviewer should be sensitive enough so that in-depth information can be received
- Training of audit teams to analyze the data related to perinatal deaths
- Setting up of enthusiastic teams which work toward collecting data and analyzing it systematically to plan recommendations, work on solutions and maintenance of the same

(PDSR: Perinatal Death Surveillance and Response)

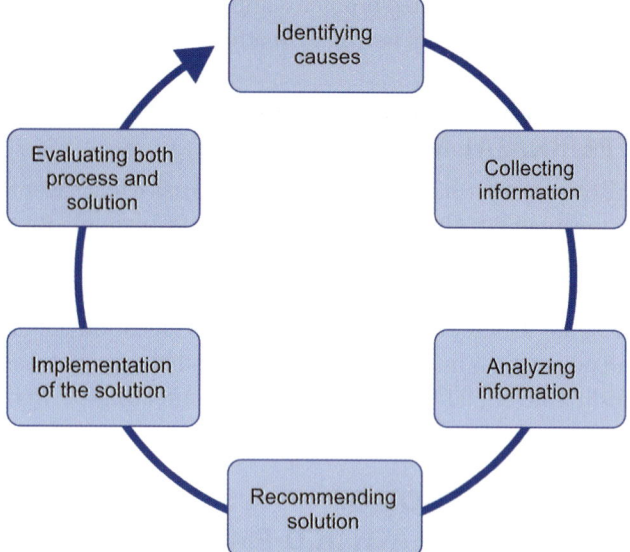

Fig. 1: Six-step mortality audit cycle can be planned.

BOX 5: Strategies to increase the effectiveness of PDSR.
- Linking of perinatal mortality audits to existing maternal mortality audits
- Linking perinatal mortality audits to quality improvement initiatives
- Positive enabling environment and supportive administration at health facility, both regional and national levels
- Ensuring "No blame" environment[18]
- Mapping of cases: Geographical mapping of cases is a time-consuming task, but if recognized can help by facilitating changes in the existing system such as lack of transportation facilities, trained health staff at primary health center level leading to faulty management and delayed referral
- Formulation of guidelines based on recommendations as suggested by audit meets
- Organization of CME, drills, and simulations for healthcare workers (doctors, nurses, and paramedical) on a regular basis
- Setting up of community-based "Identifier reporters and reviewers" for community perinatal deaths
- Involvement of trained interviewers with expertise in verbal or social autopsy is a must especially for community-based perinatal deaths. This can help by exploring information about social, cultural, behavioral, and health system issues contributing to death.[19] Maternal and perinatal death inquiry and response approach has helped communities in India by decreasing deaths and formulating focused interventions[20,21]
- Dissemination of minutes of meeting of audits to multiple levels including policy makers and community via community representatives
- Communication of changes suggested to community may help in developing trust between public health system and community

promoting routine identification and timely notification of perinatal deaths, review of these deaths, implementation and monitoring of steps to prevent similar deaths in the future. The steps of PDSR are listed in **Box 4**.

ACTION PLAN AND IMPLEMENTATION

The prerequisite for successful development of action plans and its implementation is development of an efficient steering committee. It should include all those who are enthusiastic and willing to work in the direction of decreasing the enormous burden of perinatal deaths. It should include representatives from district health office, facility administrators, obstetricians, neonatologists, pediatricians, nursing officers, anesthesiologists, pathologists, pharmacists, statistician and community leaders, or representatives. The committee should conduct regular audit cycles[16] **(Fig. 1)**.

A root-cause analysis that will help in identifying all the probable contributing factors leading to stillbirth/neonatal deaths may help in formulating necessary strategies and recommendations.[17]

Strategies to increase the effectiveness of PDSR are listed in **Box 5**.

Solutions provided after audit meets must be SMART, i.e., specific, measurable, appropriate, relevant and time bound. Changes suggested must be channelized as per facility or community. They are facility based such as formulation of standard operating protocols or community based such as improvement of infrastructure and promotion of health-based educational program.

Quartile trial suggested that a multifaceted approach is required to translate recommendations into actions and include involving efficient leaders for finding changes in healthcare facility and designing actions. Engagement of quality improvement committee is helpful in determining the efficiency of the recommendations suggested and strengthening capacity of healthcare professionals in terms of their clinical knowledge.[22,23] Quality improvement methodology using point of care quality improvement (POCQI) methodology is an effective way of fixing modifiable causes and sustain the changes. The steps of a Model Quality improvement project for a facility to reduce perinatal deaths using POCQI methodology are listed in **Box 6**.

COVID-19 PANDEMIC AND PERINATAL MORTALITY

During coronavirus disease 2019 (COVID-19) pandemic, a marked increase in perinatal deaths has been observed and documented all over the world. It is interesting to note that COVID-19 disease per se has not contributed significantly to an increase in number of perinatal deaths, except on account of prematurity, but other pandemic-related factors with resultant delays at all three levels have contributed significantly to an increase in PNMR.

Delay in decision to seek care by the women due to lockdown and fear of contracting infection among them on visiting health facility and lack of antenatal care due to restricted registrations in order to follow social distancing.[24,25] Many pregnant women preferred to visit untrained birth attendants in close vicinity. Delay in reaching the health facility due to lack of money and transport facilities due to lockdown. Delay in receiving care at facility as many hospitals were converted into COVID-dedicated facilities hence many COVID-negative and COVID-untested women were denied care in these hospitals. Booked pregnant women of many such centers were at loss and did not know where to seek care in emergency. At many facilities, care providers were reluctant in providing care for the fear of contracting infection or lack of personal protective equipments (PPEs).[26]

In an analytical case-control study conducted in Lady Hardinge Medical College, a tertiary-level hospital in New Delhi, India comparing the causes of stillbirths in March to September 2020 during COVID pandemic (cases) with those in March to September 2019 (controls). It was found that COVID-19 infection was present in only 1.5% of the study group and nearly three-fourth of the stillbirths in the study group were preventable stillbirths. Modifiable factors were noted in 76.1% cases and 59.6% controls, the difference was found to be highly significant with p value < 0.001, relative risk (RR) 1.8.[27] The delay 2 and 3 were significantly higher in COVID pandemic (cases) as compared to controls in pre-COVID times. Level 2 delay was found in 12.7% cases and none in control (p value < 0.0006, RR-47.7). Level 3 delay was found in 31.3% cases and 11.5% controls (p value < 0.001, RR-2.7).

In pandemics such as COVID, regular perinatal death review meetings help us understand the impact of pandemic on PNMR. Certain change ideas that were developed and implemented after perinatal audits to reducing perinatal deaths in COVID pandemic at this tertiary level hospital included:

- Introducing telemedicine to antenatal women
- Explaining them about danger signs with the advice to contact emergency room telephonically
- Referring the low-risk women to primary and secondary level facilities closer to their homes at the time of registration with the reassurance that they will be cared at tertiary level if need
- Initiating the practice of a growth scan between 34 and 36 weeks to identify average for gestational age growth restriction and monitoring of high-risk pregnancies on day care basis.

CONCLUSION

We should believe and aim that every perinatal death is preventable. Regular perinatal death audits (PDSR), identifying the modifiable factors, working in the direction of best possible solutions, and their implementation are a key to success. An efficient and dedicated leader to lead the process of surveillance in a no-blame environment makes the audits meaningful. Involvement of all involved in the process of improvement will help sustenance of changes.

KEY MESSAGES

- The WHO defines perinatal death as a late fetal death at or after (≥) 28 completed weeks of gestation or fetal weight of ≥1,000 g if gestation is not known or a death of a newborn within 7 days of life.

BOX 6: Steps of POCQI methodology.

1. Do a baseline analysis of perinatal deaths every week or 2 weeks to list out the common causes
2. Line list the important contributors to perinatal deaths
3. Do prioritization and list the contributing factors according to their importance and ease to fix the problem
4. Identify one problem
5. Make an aim statement
6. Make a team comprising all those involved around that problem
7. Do the detailed analysis of the problem with the team using methods such as process flow chart, fishbone analysis, brainstorming, 5 whys and Pareto principle. Make a list of contributing factors and possible change ideas that can fix those factors
8. Implement each change idea one after the other as Plan-Do-Study and Act (PDSA) cycle. The changes can be adopted, adapted, or abandoned according to the results obtained
9. Each problem may require multiple change ideas or PDSA cycles to be implemented
10. Hardwire the change ideas implemented for sustenance
11. Pick up the next problem to be fixed and repeat the steps to fix the next problem

(POCQI: point of care quality improvement)

- The world has a huge burden of reported and unreported neonatal and still births every year.
- The WHO has applied 10th revision (ICD 10) to classify perinatal deaths (ICD-PM), a standardized three-step system for classifying perinatal mortality (including stillbirths).
- Most perinatal deaths are preventable and to reduce these perinatal deaths, audits are essential to capture accurate information on how many perinatal deaths occur at a facility, to analyze and assign the cause and factors contributing to those deaths.
- The PDSR is a process that facilitates collecting relevant and accurate information by promoting routine identification and timely notification of perinatal deaths, review of these deaths, implementation, and monitoring of steps to prevent similar deaths in the future.
- The POCQI is an effective way of fixing modifiable causes and sustain the changes.

REFERENCES

1. Peller S. Studies on mortality since Renaissance, twins, and singleton. Bull Hist Med. 1944;16:362-81.
2. Moxon SG, Ruysen H, Kerber K, Amouzou A, Fournier S, Grove J, et al. Count every new-born; a measurement improvement roadmap for coverage data. BMC Pregnancy Childbirth. 2015;15(Suppl. 2):S8.
3. Laun J, Kerber K (eds). Opportunities for Africa's newborns: practical data, policy and programmatic support for newborn care in Africa. Cape Town: partnership for maternal, newborn and child health, Save the children, United Nation Population fund. United Nation Children's fund, United State agency for International Development, WHO; 2006.
4. UNICEF. UNICEF data: Monitoring the situation of children and women. 2016.
5. Blencowe H, Cousen S, Jassir FB, Say L, Chou D, Mathers C, et al. Nation and worldwide estimates of still birth rates in 2015 with trends from 2000: a systematic analysis. Lancet Glob Heal. 2015;4(2):e98-108.
6. Sarkar MJ, Neogi SB, Sharma J, Chauhan M, Srivastava R, Prabhakar PK, et al. State of newborn health in India. J Perinatol. 2016;36:S3-8.
7. Zodpey S, Paul VK, (eds); Public Health Foundation of India; All India Institute of Medical Sciences.(2014). Save the children.. State of India's Newborn (SOIN) 2014-A Report. [online] Available from: https://www.newbornwhocc.org/SOIN_PRINTED%2014-9-2014.pdf. [Last accessed November, 2021]..
8. Registrar General of India. Sample Registration system. Statistical report 2012. New Delhi: Registrar General of India; 2013.
9. World Health Organization. (2014). Every newborn: an action plan to end preventable newborn deaths. [online] Available from: https://cdn.who.int/media/docs/default-source/mca-documents/advisory-groups/quality-of-care/every-new-born-action-plan-(enap).pdf?sfvrsn=4d7b389_2. [Last accessed November, 2021].
10. Pattison R, Kerber K, Waiswa P, Day LT, Mussell F, Asiruddin SK, et al. Perinatal mortality audit: countability, accountability and overcoming challenges in scaling up in low- and middle-income countries. Int J Gynaecol Obstet. 2009;107(suppl):S113-22.
11. Hoyert DL, Gregory ECW. Cause of death. Data from the fetal death file, 2015-2017. Nat Vital Stat Rep. 2020; 69(4):1.
12. World Health Organization. (2016). The WHO application of ICD-10 to deaths during the perinatal period: ICD-PM. [online] Available from: https://www.who.int/reproductivehealth/publications/monitoring/icd-10-perinatal-deaths/en/. [Last accessed November, 2021].
13. Dase E, Wariri O, Onuwabuchi E, Alhassan JAK, Jalo I, Muhajarine N, et al. Applying the WHO ICD-PM classification system to stillbirth in a major referral centre in Northeast Nigeria: a retrospective analysis from 2010-2018. BMC Pregnancy childbirth. 2020;20(1):383.
14. Solar O, Irwin A. (2010). A conceptual framework for action on the social determinants of health. Social determinants of Health Discussion Paper 2(Policy & Practice). [online] Available from: https://www.who.int/sdhconference/resources/ConceptualframeworkforactiononSDH_eng.pdf. [Last accessed November, 2021].
15. Thaddeus S, Maine D. Too far to walk: Maternal mortality in context. Soc Sci Med. 1994;38(8):1091-110.
16. World Health Organization. (2016). Making every baby count: audit and review of stillbirth and neonatal deaths. [online] Available from: https://www.who.int/docs/default-source/mca-documents/maternal-nb/making-every-baby-count.pdf?Status=Master&sfvrsn=6936f980_2. [Last accessed November, 2021].
17. Buchman EJ. Towards greater effectiveness of perinatal death audits in low- and middle-income countries. BJOG. 2014; 121(Suppl 4):134-6.
18. Piette JD, Lun KC, Moura LA, Fraser HSF, Mechael PN, Powell J, et al. Impacts of e-health on the outcomes of care in low and middle-income countries: Where do we go from here? Bud World Heath Organ. 2019;90(5):365-72.
19. Kallender K, Kadobera D, Williams TN, Nielsen RT, Yevoo L, Mutebi A, et al. Social autopsy: in DEPTH network experiences of utility, process, practices and challenges in investigating causes and contributors to mortality. Popul Health Metr. 2011;9(1):44.
20. Biswas A. Maternal, newborn, child and adolescent health. Maternal and perinatal death reviews: experience in Bangladesh. WHO. 2015.
21. Biswas A, Rahman F, Halim A, et al. Maternal and Neonatal Death Review (MNDR): a useful approach to identifying appropriate and effective maternal and neonatal health initiative in Bangladesh. Health. 2015;6:1669-79.
22. Ndour C, DossouGbete S, Brun N, Abrahamowicz M, Fauconnier A, Traoré M, et al. Predicting in hospital maternal mortality in Senegal and Mali. Plos ONE. 2013;8(5):e64157.
23. Dumont A, Fournier P, Abrahamowicz M, Traoré M, Haddad S, Fraser WD, et al; QUARITE research group. Quality and care, risk management and technology in obstetrics to reduce hospital based maternal mortality in Senegal and Mali (QUARITE): a cluster randomized trial. Lancet 2013;382(9887):146-57.
24. Khalil A, Kalafat E, Benliogle, O'Brien P, Morris E, Draycott T, et al. SARC-COV 2 infection in pregnancy: a systematic review and meta-analysis of clinical features and pregnancy outcome. EClinical Med. 2020;25:100446.
25. Ashish KC, Gurung R, Kinney MU, Sunny AK, Moinuddin M, Basnet O, et al. Effect of Covid-19 pandemic response on intrapartum care, stillbirth and neonatal mortality. Outcomes in Nepal: a prospective observational study. Lancet 2020; 8(10): e 1275-e 1281.

26. Khalil A, Von Dadelszen P, Draycott T, Ugwumadu A, O'Brien P, Magee L. Change in the incidence of stillbirth andpreterm delivery during the covid-19 pandemic. JAMA. 2020;324(7):705-6.
27. Kumar M, Puri M, Yadav R, Biswas R, Singh M, Chaudhary V, et al. Stillbirth and the covid-19 pandemic: looking beyond SARS-COV 2 infection. Int J Gynecol Obstet. 2021;00:1-7.

LONG QUESTIONS

1. Describe the challenges faced in reducing PNMR in developing and developed countries.
2. Discuss the methods to improve the surveillance and evaluation of perinatal deaths.
3. Discuss the steps of perinatal death surveillance response.

SHORT QUESTIONS

1. Define perinatal mortality rate and list causes of perinatal death.
2. Describe the modifiable factors associated with perinatal death.
3. What is social autopsy?

MULTIPLE CHOICE QUESTIONS

1. Perinatal mortality rate is:
   a. Number of deaths in fetus >28 weeks of gestation weighing >1000 g up to 7 completed days postdelivery per 1,000 total (live and still births)
   b. Number of deaths in fetus >28 weeks of gestation weighing >1,000 g up to 7 completed days postdelivery per 1,000 total live births
   c. Number of deaths in fetus >28 weeks of gestation up to 28 completed days postdelivery per 1,000 total (live and still births)
   d. Number of deaths in fetus >28 weeks of gestation weighing more than 500 g up to 7 completed days postdelivery per 1,000 total (live and still births)

2. The WHO application of ICD-10 to deaths during the perinatal period is known as:
   a. ICD-SM
   b. ICD-PM
   c. ICD-MM
   d. ICD-LM

3. Solutions provided after audit meets must be SMART. It includes all, except:
   a. Specific
   b. Monitored
   c. Appropriate
   d. Relevant
   e. Time-bound

4. Social autopsy helps in exploring information about cause of perinatal death about all, except:
   a. Social
   b. Cultural
   c. Behavioral
   d. Maternal

5. Delay model for modifiable factors include all, except:
   a. Delay in decision to seek care
   b. Delay in accepting care
   c. Delay in reaching care
   d. Delay in receiving care

6. Absence of fetal heart sound at the time of presentation of pregnant lady at facility not in labor. What is the probable timing of death?
   a. Intrapartum
   b. Antepartum
   c. Unknown timing
   d. Both b or c

7. Aim of perinatal mortality audits is to achieve sustainable development goals both neonatal and stillbirth rates to be less than:
   a. 10 per 1,000/total births
   b. 11 per 1,000/total births
   c. 12 per 1,000 /total births
   d. 14 per 1,000/total births

Answers

1. a 2. b 3. b 4. d 5. b 6. d
7. c

11.2 SAFE MOTHERHOOD INITIATIVE

Alka Pandey

INTRODUCTION

Motherhood is a blessing bestowed on women by the almighty but it becomes a curse when they lose their life while giving birth to a new life. This has profound effects on their family and community. Maternal mortality indicates the quality of healthcare delivery system of a country. There are more than 300,000 maternal deaths worldwide.[1] More than 200 million women wish to avoid, delay, or end child bearing but are not using contraception.[2] Pregnancy and child birth are leading cause of adolescent (15–19 years) deaths.[3] Most sad part of the story is 75% deaths are preventable. 30 million women deliver yearly without the care of a skilled birth attendant.[4]

The overall maternal mortality rate (MMR) in developing regions is 239 (229–275), 20 times higher than that of developed regions where it is just 12 (11–14). Sub-Saharan Africa has a high MMR of 546. Developing regions accounted for 99% of estimated global deaths in 2015.[5] India and Nigeria together accounted for over one third of all global deaths in 2015.[5]

About 50–70% maternal deaths occur in postpartum period of which 45% occur in the first 24 hours and more than two thirds during the first week. Between 11 and 17% of deaths occur during child birth itself.[6]

Maternal death: The death of a woman while pregnant or within 42 days of termination of pregnancy, irrespective of the duration and site of the pregnancy, from any cause related to or aggravated by the pregnancy or its management but not from accidental or incidental causes [10th revision of the International Statistical Classification of Diseases and Related Health Problems, by the World Health Organization (ICD-10, WHO)].

Maternal mortality ratio: The number of maternal deaths during given time period per 100,000 live births during same period.

Maternal mortality rate: It is the number of maternal deaths in given time period per 100,000 women of reproductive age of 15 to 49 years. It is 120 in India and 0.5 in United States.

WHO CLASSIFICATION OF MATERNAL DEATH (FIG. 1)

Direct obstetric deaths: It results from obstetric complications of pregnancy, labor, delivery or postpartum conditions up to 42 days of delivery, e.g., obstetric hemorrhage, preeclampsia, eclampsia, and puerperal sepsis.

Indirect obstetric deaths: It results from pre-existing disease or a new disease that develops during pregnancy and is unrelated to pregnancy but was aggravated by physiological effects of pregnancy, e.g., cardiac disease, anemia, and viral hepatitis.

Unanticipated complications of management: These are deaths resulting from interventions, omissions, incorrect treatment or from chain of events resulting from any of the above during pregnancy, child birth, or puerperium up to 42 days.[7]

Unknown: Not attributable to either direct or indirect causes; deaths from unrelated causes which happen to occur in pregnancy or puerperium such as road traffic accident.

Maternal near miss (MNM): A woman who nearly died but survived a complication that occurred during pregnancy, child birth or within 42 days of termination of pregnancy.[8] For diagnosis of MNM, the patient should meet minimum three criteria one each from the three areas:
1. Clinical (symptoms/sign), e.g., Oliguria urine output < 30 mL per hour
2. Investigations, e.g., SPO_2 < 90%
3. Intervention: Intensive care unit (ICU) admission needing BT > 5 units

or

Any single criterion that signifies cardiorespiratory collapse.[9]

When used in practice, MNM helps in evaluating and improving obstetric care, thus reducing maternal death.

One woman in 150 dies of pregnancy-related complications in developing nation compared to 1 in 49,000 in developed nations. For one maternal death, 16 more suffer from severe morbidities **(Box 1)**.

The analysis of number and causes of maternal deaths help in taking corrective measures.

Data of maternal death can be obtained from the following sources:

Civil registration system: Routine registration of birth and death with medical certificate. This has been made compulsory by parliament in 1969.

Sample registration system (SRS): The SRS is a dual record system consisting of continuous enumeration of birth and death by an enumerator and an independent survey every 6 months by an investigator. From 2000 onward, RHIME

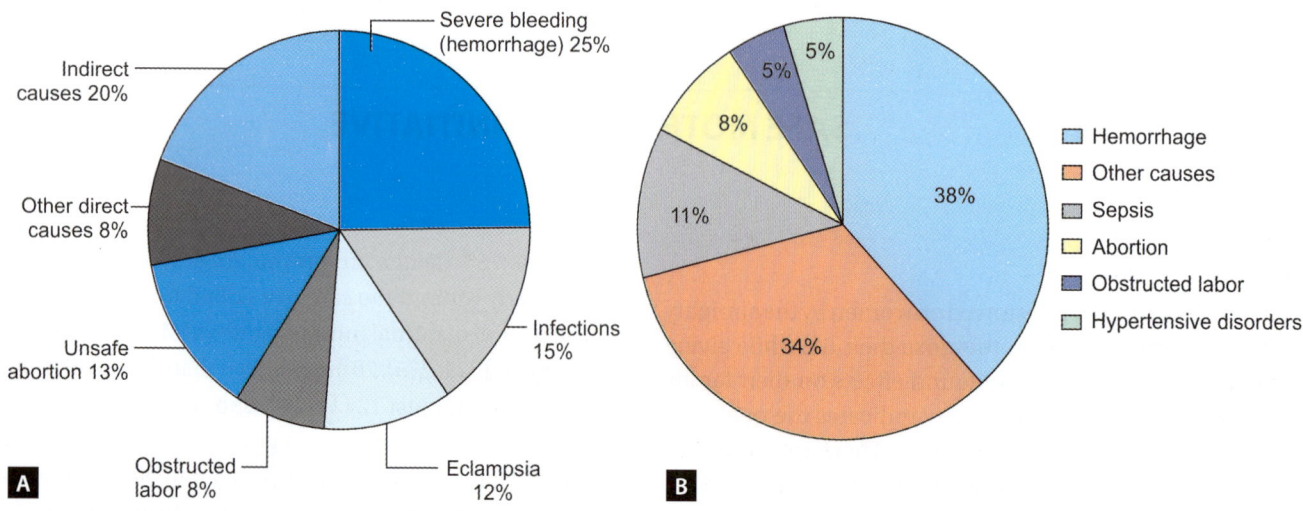

Figs. 1A and B: (A) Causes of maternal mortality worldwide; (B) Causes of maternal mortality in India (2003).
Source: MoHFW, New Delhi. Annual Report 2012–13. [online] Available from: https://main.mohfw.gov.in/documents/publication/publication-archives. [Last accessed November, 2021].

> **BOX 1:** Risk factors associated with maternal mortality.
>
> - Pregnancy at extremes of age carries a higher risk of death
> - Grand multipara are three times more prone, as malpresentation, rupture uterus, and PPH are more common
> - Women of low socioeconomic status have higher MMR
> - Repeated pregnancy, childbirth, and unsafe abortions
> - Lack of transport facilities
> - Lack of ANC, skilled birth attendant during delivery, appropriate referral system, and EMOC

(ANC: antenatal care; EMOC: emergency obstetric care; MMR: maternal mortality rate; PPH: postpartum hemorrhage)

TABLE 1: National Sociodemographic Goals (2030) (SDG) National Population Policy, National Health Mission (NHM)

Parameters	2030 goals
Total fertility rate	<2.1
Maternal mortality ratio (per 100,000 live births)	<70
Infant morality	<12
Antenatal care (%)	100
Institutional deliveries	80
Deliveries by skilled personnel (%)	100

(Representative, Resampled, Routine household interview of mortality and medical reevaluation) is being promoted. This is an enhanced form of verbal autopsy which is the key feature of a prospective study of 1 million deaths within the SRS.[10]

Maternal death surveillance and response: It is an important method to know where things went wrong and what can be done to prevent recurrence. Information of maternal death can be derived from:

- *Community-based approach*: It consists of interview of family members, neighbors, and TBA for deaths which have occurred outside or in the hospital.
- *Facility-based approach*: Detailed enquiry of the cause of facility-based deaths.

Confidential enquiry into maternal deaths: Confidential enquiry gives knowledge of each maternal death and compilation of these records can point toward the main problem and highlight the key areas requiring interventions. It was found that there are three delays which play an important role in causing maternal deaths.

The three delays are:
1. *Delay in seeking professional care:* The attending physician must be capable to recognize the underlying condition and provide necessary interventions and treatment at once.
2. *Delay in reaching the appropriate health facility:* Effective prehospital care is necessary.
3. *Delay in receiving care at facility:* When the pregnant woman reaches the facility, appropriate care is not provided; there may be delay in transferring her to the next facility and there also she might not get appropriate care in time.[11]

Safe motherhood is a basic human right of every woman. Safe motherhood means that the woman is enabled to choose whether she will be pregnant and if she opts for it, she should have access to emergency obstetric care for prevention and treatment of pregnancy complications, receives postnatal care. It is a continuum of care.

Safe motherhood initiative was conceptualized by World Bank, WHO, and United Nations Population Fund (UNFPA) and launched in 1987at the safe motherhood conference in Nairobi, Kenya with an aim to half the maternal mortality and maternal morbidity by 2000.[1] The initiative formulated three key strategies, strengthening of community-level care, upgrading referral-level facilities and ensuring transport from community to referral level. The pillars of safe motherhood are family planning, antenatal care (ANC), obstetrical care, postnatal care, postabortion care, and sexually transmitted diseases (STI)/human deficiency virus (HIV) control.

Though the initial aims of this initiative were not achieved by 2000, it paved the way for introduction of more targeted efforts in reducing MMR.

Millennium Development Goals (MDG) were initiated by the WHO, UNICEF, UNFPA, World Bank, and other organizations (2000–2015) to reduce MMR by 75% and infant mortality rate (IMR) below 30 per 1,000 live births by 2015. The target of MDG-5a was to reduce maternal mortality by 75% and 5b was to promote universal access to reproductive health. Global MMR came down from 385 per 100,000 live births to 216 per 100,000 live births -44% reduction. The annual reduction of MMR was 2.3% much lower than expected target of 5.5%.

In 2014, in Bangkok, the focus shifted from Safe motherhood initiative to "Ending Preventable maternal mortality" addressing social, economic, and political determinants of maternal survival and health.

Respectful maternity care is the basic right of child-bearing women. The WHO in 2014[12] has highlighted the prevention and elimination of disrespect and abuse during facility based child birth. Bad behavior with the women is one of the biggest barriers to women seeking care.

The *MDG* (December, 2015) came to end of their term and was followed by Sustainable Development Goals (SDG) till 2030. By 2030, the goal of SDG is to achieve the parameters mentioned in **Table 1**.

The key five strategies toward ending preventable maternal mortality (EPMM) by 2030 are :
1. To address inequities (WHO 2015) in access to quality of sexual, reproductive, maternal, and newborn healthcare services.
2. To ensure universal and comprehensive healthcare for sexual, reproductive, maternal, and newborn health.
3. To address all causes of maternal mortality, morbidities and related disabilities.

4. To strengthen health system for the needs and priorities of women and girls.
5. To ensure accountability to improve quality care and equity.

GLOBAL SCENARIO

In 2015, one woman in 41, in low-income countries, died of maternal causes.[13]

In resource-poor settings, fertility rates are higher and the risks of dying in labor are greater.[13]

The risk of maternal death can be reduced through better access to modern methods of contraception and by ensuring that women have access to high-quality care before, during, and after childbirth.

Globally, coverage of deliveries by a skilled birth attendant ranges from 59% to over 90%.

The MMR is reduced significantly in women who delivered under supervision of Skilled birth attendant (SBA).

Skilled birth attendant is an accredited health professional, midwife, doctor, or nurse who is trained in managing normal pregnancy, labor, and puerperium, to identify complication in women and new born and organize referrals **(Table 2)**.

In 2018, there were an estimated 12.8 million births among adolescent girls aged 15–19 years.[14] These face higher risks of eclampsia and other complications during childbirth.

Many initiatives and programs have been launched by government of India to reduce maternal morbidity and mortality **(Table 3)**.

India is the first country to declare National Safe Motherhood Day on 11th of April, 2003 which is the birthday of Kasturba Gandhi. This day is celebrated due to the initiative of *White Ribbon Alliance India* to make women aware of various healthcare programs.

The International Conference on Population and Development in Cairo recommended in 1995 implementation of unified Reproduction and Child Health (RCH) Program.

The RCH Program first phase in 1997 and second phase in 2005 focused on essential ANC, emergency obstetric care, referral services, and universal immunization.

New initiatives in RCH were training of MBBS doctors in life-saving anesthetic skills for obstetric emergency care. Provision of adequate and timely EMOC has been recognized as the most important intervention for saving mothers who may develop complications during pregnancy and child birth.

RMNCH+A (Reproductive Maternal Newborn Child Health and Adolescent) Strategy launched in 2013 addresses the following health issues:

TABLE 2: Maternal mortality ratio, deliveries conducted by skilled personnel, antenatal care coverage and lifetime risk of maternal deaths in some developing and developed countries.

Country	Antenatal care coverage (%) 2010–2015 At least once	At least four times	Deliveries conducted by skilled personnel (%) 2010–2015	Lifetime risk maternal death (one in) 2015	Maternal mortality ratio (per 100,000 live births) 2015
India	74	45	52	220	130 (2014-16)
Bangladesh	64	31	42	240	176
Bhutan	98	85	75	310	148
Indonesia	95	84	87	320	126
Myanmar	83	73	71	260	178
Nepal	68	60	56	150	258
Thailand	98	93	100	3,600	20
Sri Lanka	99	93	99	1,580	30
Pakistan	73	37	52	140	178
China	96	–	100	2,400	27
Japan	100	100	100	13,400	5
Singapore	100	100	100	8,200	10
UK	–	–	99	5,800	9
USA	–	97	99	3,800	14
World	85	58	75	180	216

Source: World Health Organization. (2015). Trends in maternal mortality: 1990 to 2015. Estimates by WHO, UNICEF, UNFPA, World Bank Group and the United Nations Population Division. [online] Available from: https://www.who.int/reproductivehealth/publications/monitoring/maternal-mortality2015/en/. [Last accessed November, 2021].
Park K. Park's Textbook of Preventive and Social Medicine, 25th edition. Jabalpur: Bhanot Publishers; 2017. p. 612.

TABLE 3: Evolution of maternal and child health programs in India

Year	Milestones
1952	Family planning program adopted by Government of India (GOI)
1961	Department of Family Planning created in Ministry of Health
1971	Medical Termination of Pregnancy Act (MTP Act) 1971
1977	Renaming of Family Planning to Family Welfare
1978	Expanded Program on Immunization (EPI)
1985	Universal Immunization Program (UIP) + National Oral Rehydration Therapy (ORT) Program
1992	Child Survival and Safe Motherhood Program (CSSM)
1996	Target-free approach
1997	Reproductive and Child Health Program-1 (RCH-1)
2005	Reproductive and Child Health Program-1 (RCH-2)
2005	National Rural Health Mission
2013	RMNCH+A Strategy
2013	National Health Mission
2014	India Newborn Action Plan (INAP)

Source: World Health Organization. (2015). Trends in maternal mortality: 1990 to 2015. Estimates by WHO, UNICEF, UNFPA, World Bank Group and the United Nations Population Division. [online] Available from: https://www.who.int/reproductivehealth/publications/monitoring/maternal-mortality-2015/en/. [Last accessed November, 2021]. Park K. Park's Textbook of Preventive and Social Medicine, 25th edition. Jabalpur: Bhanot Publishers; 2017. p. 610

Reproductive Health

- Focus on spacing methods, particularly postpartum intrauterine contraceptive device (PPIUCD), interval IUCD, home delivery of contraceptives by Accredited Social Health Activist (ASHA), access to pregnancy testing kits, and provide comprehensive abortion care services. It also offered quality sterilization services.

Maternal Health

- Early registration of pregnancy and full ANC.
- Recognition of high-risk pregnancies and their appropriate management.
- Health facilities should have highly trained professionals to ensure provision of EMOC services.
- Audit of maternal, infant, and child deaths for corrective actions.
- Distribution of misoprostol to women in 8th month of pregnancy for consumption during third stage of labor.
- Incentives to ANMs for home deliveries.

Adolescent Health

- Addresses teenage pregnancy, and increase in contraceptive prevalence in adolescents.
- Adolescent Reproductive and Sexual Health clinics (ARSH) should be setup.
- Iron folic acid supplementation should be given weekly.
- Promotion of awareness of menstrual hygiene, access to sanitary pads and their proper disposal.

National Health Mission (NHM) (2013): The targets under NHM are as follows:

- Institutional delivery is to be promoted.
- Training of healthcare providers in basic and comprehensive obstetric care.
- To make subcenters, primary health centers (PHCs), community health centers, and district hospitals functional for providing 24 × 7 basic and comprehensive obstetric care services.
- Name-based web enabled tracking of pregnant women to ensure antenatal, intranatal, and postnatal care.
- Mother and child protection card.
- Antenatal, intranatal, and postnatal care including iron and folic acid supplementation to pregnant and lactating women for prevention and treatment of anemia and health education.
- *Janani Shishu Suraksha Karyakram by government of India* was launched in June 2011. It entitles all pregnant women delivering in public health institutions to absolutely free and no expense delivery including cesarean section, free blood transfusion if required and free transport.
- *Janani Suraksha Yojana (JSY):* The National Maternity Benefit scheme has been modified into a new scheme called JSY. It was launched on 12th April, 2005 for reducing maternal and neonatal mortality through encouraging institutional delivery by giving financial assistance.

The JSY scheme has a provision to hire the services of private practitioners to conduct or manage obstetrical complications. It provides benefit to more than One Crore beneficiaries every year **(Table 4)**.

Impact of JSY: Increase in institutional deliveries which have gone up from 47% (District-Level Household Survey-III, 2007–08) to 78.9% [National Family Health Survey (NFHS-4), 2015–16]

Maternal Mortality Ratio declined from 254 maternal deaths per 100,000 live births in 2004–06 to 130 maternal deaths per 100,000 live births during 2014–16.

Infant mortality rate has declined from 58 per 1,000 live births in 2005 to 34 per 1,000 live births in 2017.

The neonatal mortality rate has declined from 37 per 1,000 live births in 2006 to 24 per 1,000 live births in 2016.

ASHA: Accredited Social Health Activist is the link person between the beneficiary at village level and ANM or doctor of FRU.

- *Safe abortion services:* Abortion is a matter of concern as it may lead to serious complications. 8% (2001–03 SRS) of maternal deaths in India are attributed to unsafe

TABLE 4: Financial incentives in NHM for safe motherhood.

Category	Rural area			Urban area		
	Mother's package	ASHA's package	Total Rs.	Mother's package	ASHA's package	Total Rs.
LPS	1400	600	2000	1000	400	1400
HPS	700	600	1300	600	400	1000

(LPS: low-performing states; HPS: high-performing states)

abortions. Many Medical Officers have been trained in Comprehensive Abortion care.
- *Medical abortion*: Early pregnancy can be terminated with two drugs—mifepristone followed by misoprostol. Currently its use in India is recommended up to 7 weeks of amenorrhea. It should be done in a place where there are facilities of performing safe abortion and blood transfusion.
- *Manual vacuum aspiration*: It can be used in primary health centers as it is safe and simple and does not require electricity.
- Maternal death audit.

Emergency Obstetric Care

Most obstetric deaths are preventable. The barriers to reduce maternal mortality are given in **Box 2**. Importance of EMOC in preventing maternal mortality has been universally accepted. The key strategies of the Government of India are mentioned in **Box 3**. In 2006, the Federation of Obstetric and Gynaecological Societies of India/Indian College of Obstetricians and Gynaecologists (FOGSI/ICOG) in association with Government of India launched a program of EMOC where 16 weeks training of handling emergency obstetric cases was given to MBBS doctors working in PHCs.

Emergency obstetric care is often discussed in terms of basic and comprehensive care that is provided to a woman with obstetric complications.

Basic EMOC has Seven Key Functions: In basic EMOC facility, skilled birth attendant should be able to administer parenteral antibiotics, oxytocic drugs, anticonvulsants for preeclampsia and eclampsia, perform manual removal of placenta and retained products, manual vacuum aspiration and assisted vaginal delivery.

Comprehensive EMOC: The doctors on duty should be able to perform all the functions of basic EMOC and in addition, they should be able to perform emergency cesarean section. Facilities of blood transfusion and anesthesia should also be available.

Pradhan Mantri Surakshit Matritva Abhiyan: The Pradhan Mantri Surakshit Matritva Abhiyan has been launched by the Ministry of Health and Family Welfare (MoHFW), Government of India, in 2016.

BOX 2: Barriers to reduce maternal mortality.

The main factors that prevent women from receiving or seeking care during pregnancy and childbirth are:
- Lack of money and resources
- Long distance to hospitals
- Lack of awareness
- Poor medical services
- Cultural beliefs and practices

BOX 3: Key strategies of Government of India (GOI) for accelerating the pace of decline in maternal mortality rate (MMR).

- Janani Suraksha Yojana
- Janani Shishu Suraksha Karyakram
- Maternal Death Review
- Comprehensive abortion care
- Screening and care for sexually transmitted infections and reproductive tract infections
- Capacity building of health providers
- Prevention of postpartum hemorrhage (PPH) through community-based distribution of misoprostol by Accredited Social Health Activists (ASHAs)
- Setting up of skill labs for different training programs.
- Pradhan Mantri Surakshit Matritva Abhiyan
- Rashtriya Kishor Swasthya Karyakram—launched in January 2014.
- LaQshya program
- Midwifery initiative: 18 months' training is to be provided to GNM/BSc nurses having 2 years' experience in conducting deliveries so that they can conduct deliveries, especially in the rural areas. This initiative was launched in December, 2018

Pradhan Mantri Surakshit Matritva Abhiyan envisages to improve the quality and coverage of ANC including diagnostic and counseling services as part of the Reproductive Maternal Neonatal Child and Adolescent Health (RMNCH+A) Strategy.

The Abhiyan also involves private sector healthcare providers as volunteers to provide specialist care in government facilities.

LaQshya: The Union Health Ministry announced the launch of LaQshya on 16th March 2018, a program aimed at improving quality of care in labor room, maternity operation theater, high-dependency unit (HDU), and obstetric ICU.

Professional Bodies in Reducing MMR

Manyata: The FOGSI in partnership with MSD for Mothers, MacArthur Foundation and Jhpiego (an affiliate of Johns

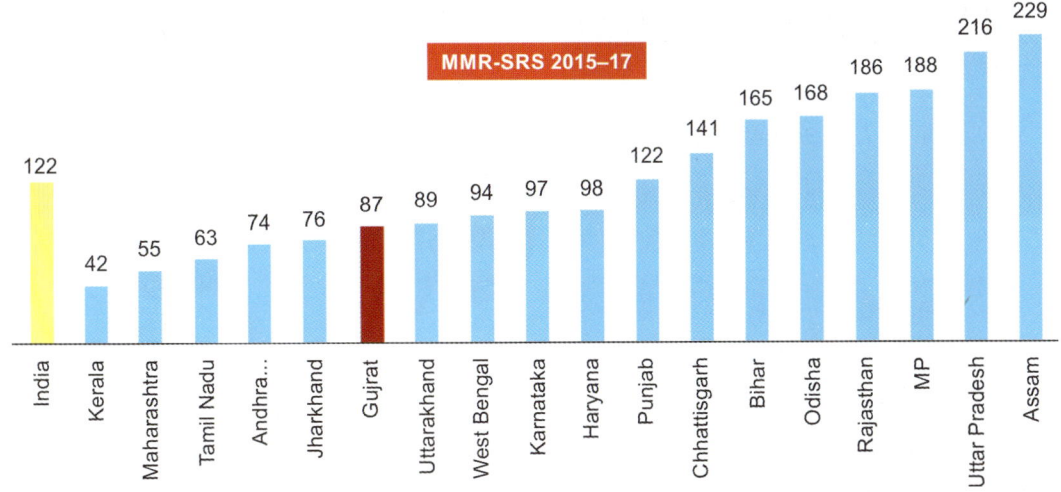

Fig. 2: Institutional deliveries in India have risen sharply from 47% in 2007–08 to over 78.9% in 2015-16 National Family Health Survey (NFHS-4).

Hopkins University), launched "Manyata"—a nationwide movement urging the need for quality care for mothers during and immediately after childbirth when risks of life-threatening complications are the highest.

The Aim of Manyata is to provide best care to mothers by ensuring excellence in maternity care services at small private healthcare facilities in India.

Quality improvement approaches/interventions that have been adopted by many countries to reduce maternal and neonatal mortality:

- Training of healthcare professionals in clinical quality
- Confidential enquiries of maternal deaths
- Financial incentives for beneficiaries
- Rewards for performance
- Provision of proper and adequate supervision
- Involvement of community
- Collaborative efforts public-private partnership.

Causes of Reduction of MMR in India: In 1990, the MMR of India was 556 per 100,000 live births. The global MMR was much lower at 385. Now the MMR is 122 (SRS 2015–17). The MMR in the country has declined against a global MMR of 216 (2015). The annual rate of decline of MMR during the period 2014–16 is 8.01%.

Three states have already met the SDG target for MMR of 70 per 100,000; these are Kerala, Maharashtra and Tamil Nadu. The decline in MMR has been most significant in Empowered Action Group (EAG) States and Assam **(Fig. 2)**.

INNOVATIONS TO REDUCE MATERNAL MORTALITY

- *Brass V drape* **(Fig. 3)**: It estimates blood loss four times more accurately than visual estimation so as to institute timely intervention for saving the life of the mother.
- *Uterine balloon tamponade* **(Fig. 4)**: It is a minimally invasive intervention that involves inserting a condom

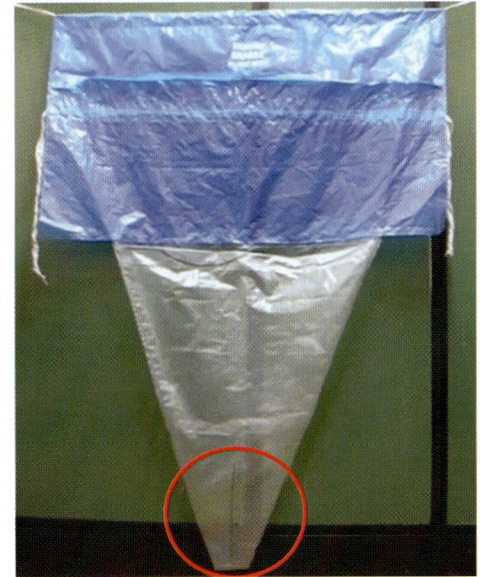

Fig. 3: Brass V drape.

mounted on a catheter in to the uterus and filling it with fluid which applies pressure to the uterine walls until bleeding stops.
- *Nonpneumatic antishock garment* (*NASG*) **(Fig. 5)** studies have shown that NASG can decrease obstetric hemorrhage and stabilize the patient until proper medical treatment is available. It functions by providing circumferential counter pressure to the lower body in order to shunt blood from lower extremities and abdomen to heart, lungs, and brain.
- *HDU* **(Fig. 6)**: Pregnant women can develop life-threatening complications and they need to be transferred to critical care facilities that can manage the problem. HDU are wards for women who need more intensive observation, treatment, and nursing care that is not possible in a routine ward. It is slightly less than ICU. Ratio of nurses to the patients is 2:1.

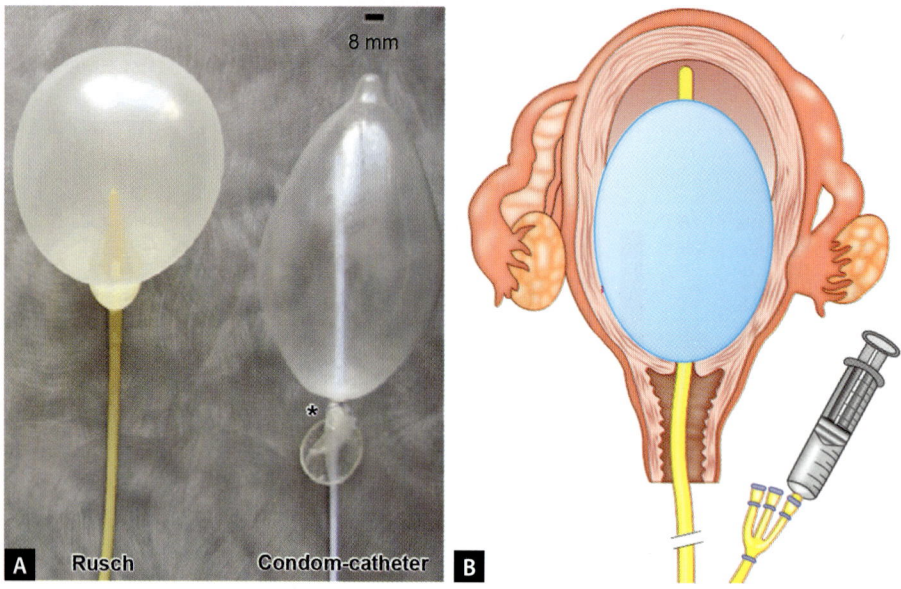

Figs. 4A and B: Uterine balloon tamponade.

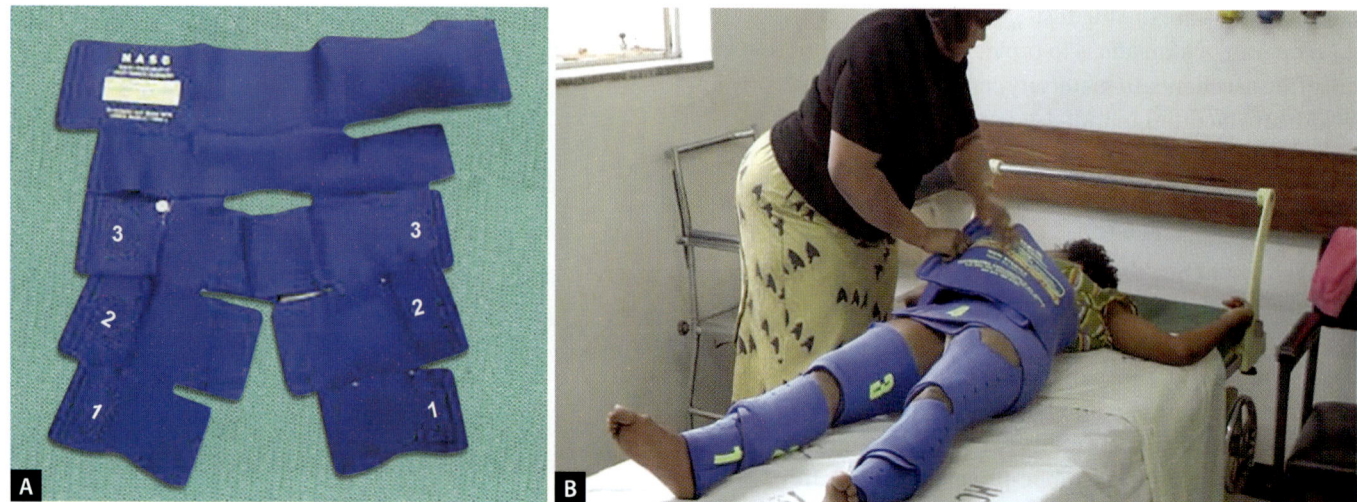

Figs. 5A and B: Nonpneumatic antishock garment.

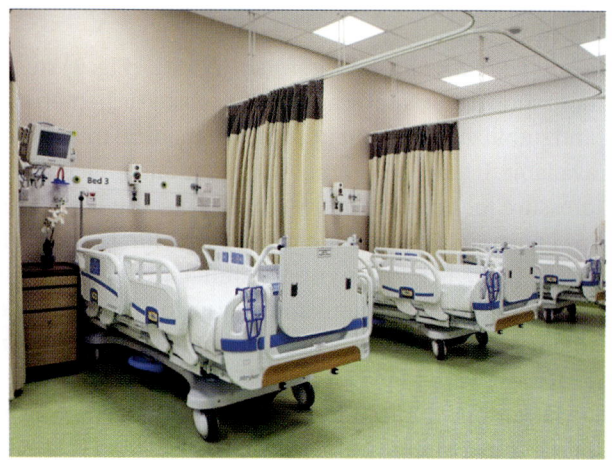

Fig. 6: High-dependency unit.

CONCLUSION

The National Rural Health Mission launched in 2005 has rejuvenated the public health system in the country. To meet the SDG goals, India has to keep the momentum and continue prioritizing the maternal and reproductive healthcare services.

Focused ANC, birth preparedness and complication readiness, skilled attendance at birth care within the first 7 days, access to health information, and contraception to prevent unintended pregnancies are required for safe motherhoods. Healthcare for all can help in reducing maternal mortality.

Women should be drivers of their own health not mere passive recipient of care.

REFERENCES

1. World Health Organization (WHO); United Nations Children's Fund (UNICEF); United Nations Population Fund (UNFPA); World Bank Group; United Nations Population Division. (2015). Trends in Maternal Mortality: 1990 to 2015: Estimates by WHO, UNICEF, UNFPA, World Bank Group and the United Nations Population Division.. [online] Available from: http://www.who.int/reproductivehealth/publications/monitoring/maternal-mortality-2015/en/. [Last accessed November, 2021].
2. United Nations Population Fund (UNFPA). (2017).Investing in Family Planning Is a Best Buy. [online] Available from: https://www.unfpa.org/resources/investing-family-planning-best-buy. [Last accessed November, 2021].
3. World Health Organization. (2018). Adolescent pregnancy. website. [online] Available from: http://www.who.int/news-room/fact-sheets/detail/adolescent-pregnancy. [Last accessed November, 2021].
4. UNICEF. (2018). Millions of births occur annually without any assistance from a skilled attendant despite recent progress. [online] Available from: https://data.unicef.org/topic/maternal-health/delivery-care/. [Last accessed November, 2021].
5. World Health Organization. (2015). Trends in maternal mortality: 1990 to 2015. Estimates by WHO, UNICEF, UNFPA, World Bank Group and the United Nations Population Division. [online] Available from: https://www.who.int/reproductivehealth/publications/monitoring/maternal-mortality-2015/en/. [Last accessed November, 2021].
6. WHO, UNICEF, World Bank. (2010). Trends in Maternal Mortality: 1990 to 2008, Estimates developed by WHO, UNICEF, UNFPA and the World Bank. https://www.who.int/reproductivehealth/publications/monitoring/9789241500265/en/. [Last accessed November, 2021].
7. PHFI, AIIMS and SC-State of India's Newborn (SOIN) 2014- a report. In: Zodpey S, Paul VK (Eds). Public Health Foundation of India. All India Institute of Medical Sciences and Save the Children. New Delhi, India.
8. Say L, Souza JP, Pattinson RC, Maternal Near Miss—towards as standard tool for monitoring quality of maternal health care. Best Pract Res Clin Obstet Gynaecol. 2009;23:287-96.
9. Dutta DC, Konar H. In: Konar H (ed). D.C. Dutta's Textbook of Obstetrics, 9th edition. New Delhi: Jaypee Medical Brothers (P) Ltd.; 2014.
10. Park K. Park's Textbook of Preventive and Social Medicine, 25th edition. Jabalpur: Bhanot Publishers; 2017. p. 904.
11. Thaddeus S, Maine D. Too far to walk maternal mortality in context. Soc Sci Med. 1994;38(8):1091-110.
12. World Health Organization. (2015).The prevention and elimination of Disrespect and abuse during facility based childbirth. [online] Available from: https://apps.who.int/iris/bitstream/handle/10665/134588/WHO_RHR_14.23_eng.pdf. [[Last accessed November, 2021].
13. Zimicki S. The relationship between fertility and maternal mortality. In: Parnell A (ed), Contraceptive use and controlled fertility: Health issues for women and children (background papers). Washington DC: National Research Council (US), National Academies Press (US); 1989
14. Ganchimeg T, Ota E, Morisaki N, Laopaiboon M, Lumbiganon P, Zhang J, et al. Pregnancy and childbirth outcomes among adolescent mothers: a World Health Organization multicountry study. BJOG. 2014;121:40-8.

LONG QUESTION

1. Discuss the strategies adopted by GOI for reducing MMR.

SHORT QUESTION

1. Write notes on:
   a. Janani Suraksha Yojana
   b. Direct maternal deaths
   c. ASHA
   d. Sociodemographic goals for reducing MMR
   e. LaQshya Karyakram

MULTIPLE CHOICE QUESTIONS

1. MMR of India in 2015–17 is:
   a. 178
   b. 196
   c. 138
   d. 144
   e. 122
2. Financial assistance in JSY to mothers in low-performing states in rural areas is:
   a. Rs. 1200/-
   a. Rs. 900/-
   b. Rs. 700/-
   c. Rs. 1400/-
3. Millennium Development Goals extended from:
   a. 2005–2010
   b. 2008–2012
   c. 2000–2015
   d. 2000–2012
4. Which state of India has the lowest MMR:
   a. Assam
   b. Haryana
   c. Kerala
   d. Telangana
5. Where was Safe Motherhood initiative launched?
   a. Netherlands
   b. Cambodia
   c. Geneva
   d. Kenya

Answers
1. e   2. d   3. c   4. c   5. d

11.3 MATERNAL DEATH: SURVEILLANCE AND RESPONSE

Jayam Kannan

INTRODUCTION

Maternal death is mortality of a pregnant woman or within 42 days of termination of pregnancy, irrespective of the site and period of, gestation of pregnancy, from causes, aggravated or related by the pregnancy, or, its management, but not from incidental or accidental causes. Maternal mortality ratio

(MMR) of India has decreased by 8 points from 130/100,000 live births in 2014–16 to 122/100,000 live births in 2015–17 (6.2% decline). Total annual deaths have decreased from 32,000 in 2015 to 30,000 maternal deaths in 2017.[1] Worldwide, 295,000 pregnant or delivered mothers had died in 2017. However, between 2000 and 2017, there is a 38% decrease in maternal mortality ratio worldwide.[2] Sustainable Development Goals[3] (SDG) have a target of reducing MMR to <70 per 100,000 births globally, by 2030. For achieving this target, the World Health Organization (WHO) has united the countries to develop strategy and increase research evidence, provide evidence-based guidance, technical support, and setting standards to Member States.

ZERO Preventable Deaths, are not just a number—it is our mission in order to improve the quality of obstetric care and decrease MMR; the Maternal Death Review (MDR) was initiated by government of India in the year 2010. This program faced various problems such as varying degree of reporting, lack of quality in review, and delayed translation of finding to actions. Based on this drawback, the Government of India in line with the WHO adapted the Maternal Death and Surveillance and Response (MDSR) guidelines **(Fig. 1)**. The MDSR system is a continuous cycle of identification, notification, and review of maternal deaths, followed by actions to improve quality of care and prevent future deaths. The goal of MDSR is to improve reporting, analysis and action to incorporate, confidential review and not to punish the healthcare providers based on the review.[3]

The state of Kerala, in India, was the pioneer in Confidential Review of maternal deaths. With that experience, we learnt that the cause and circumstances of death are revealed only when anonymity of the healthcare provider and not blaming them for the same. The principle "No name, no blame" was used.[4]

The goal of MDSR is to decrease maternal mortality, by obtaining and utilizing that information to guide health actions and monitor their results.

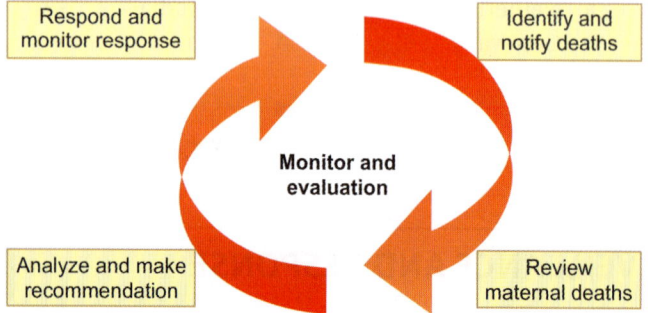

Fig. 1: Maternal Death Surveillance and Response (MDSR) system: A continuous-action cycle.
Source: World Health Organization. (2013). Maternal death surveillance and response: Technical guidance information for action to prevent maternal deaths. [online] Available from: https://www.who.int/publications/i/item/9789241506083. [Last accessed November, 2021].

Objectives of MDSR:[5]

- To collect data on maternal deaths, including (cause, number, contributing factors, facility records, and verbal autopsies)
- Analyze and interpret the collected data (trends and demographic characters, risk factors, and causes contributing to death and avoid preventable deaths)
- Based on the collected data, to provide evidence recommendations, such as community education timely referral, access to services and training of healthcare providers and providing regulations and policy
- To notify the findings and recommendations to society, policy makers and healthcare providers
- To ensure that the recommended actions have been implemented
- To give feedback about the effectiveness of interventions and their impact on maternal mortality
- To allocate the resources properly
- To increase the accountability of maternal health
- To improve statistics and implement civil registration/vital statistics records
- Prioritize research based on maternal mortality.

In India, the process of MDR, is done at two levels: (1) the community-based MDSR and (2) facility-based MDSR. In community-based MDSR, they identify the personal, family, or community factors that contribute to death of women, in reproductive age group by interviewing the patient's family members and neighbors. Interview is done by verbal autopsy format (Form 5). The primary informant will be The Accredited Social Health Activist (ASHA) or Auxiliary Nurse Midwife (ANM) who will report to the block Medical Officer (BMO) or the District Nodal Officer (DNO).[4] Other important members of the village are also encouraged to inform about the women's death. The ASHA worker is expected to report in Form 1 any reproductive age women deaths within 24 hours and an investigation will be done by ANM/urban health worker, whether the deaths are related to, pregnancy and childbirth and that will be submitted to BMO. The BMO will form a three-member team and investigate the maternal death within 3 weeks and prepare a case summary (Form 6). All the case summary and forms should be sent to DNO every month and a confidential review will be conducted by Chief Medical Officer and in few cases, by the District Collector **(Fig. 2)**.

Facility-based MDSR is done at Government teaching hospitals, referral and secondary level hospitals; such as Corporation, Railway, and ESIC; district hospital; subdistrict; and community health centers (CHCs) conducting, >1000 deliveries/year. The facility nodal officer will collect the details from the medical officer, who attended the patient and report the death to DNO who will, in turn, report to State Nodal officer. Community-based review is also done for patients, who died at facility. In case of migrant death, it is also notified to the respective district or state nodal officers in order to facilitate community-based review.

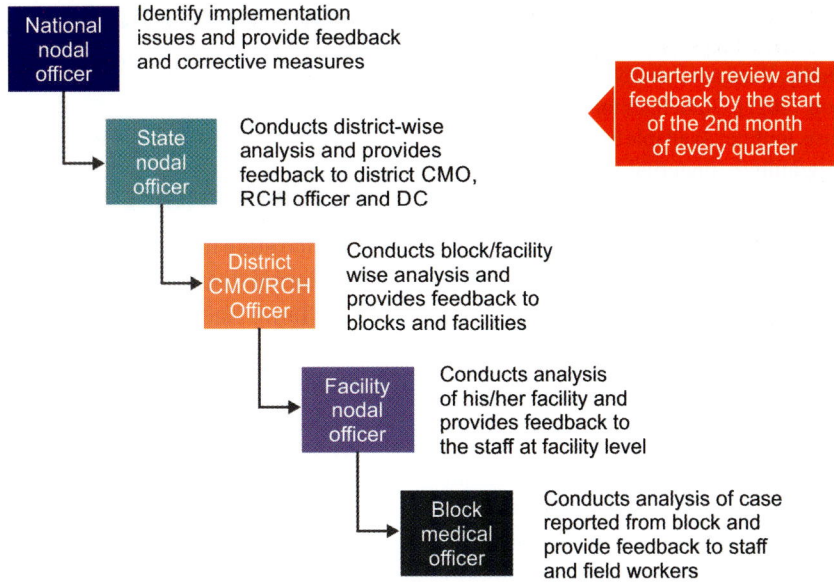

Fig. 2: Nodal persons for implementing MDSR at different levels.[4] (MDSR: Maternal Death and Surveillance and Response)

The recommendation in facility is to classify the deaths based on ICD 10 (International Classification of Diseases, Tenth Revision):

- *M01:* Pregnancies with abortive outcome (maternal death: direct)
- *M02:* Hypertensive disorders in pregnancy, childbirth, and puerperium (maternal death: direct)
- *M03:* Obstetric hemorrhage (maternal death: direct)
- *M04:* Pregnancy-related infections (maternal death: direct)
- *M05:* Other obstetric complications (maternal death: direct)
- *M06:* Unanticipated complications of management (maternal death: direct)
- *M07:* Nonobstetric complications (maternal death: indirect)
- *M08:* Unknown/undetermined (maternal death: unspecified)
- *M09:* Coincidental causes.

OBSTETRIC TRANSITION

The phenomenon called "Obstetric Transition" is introduced, which is a change, in the causes of maternal deaths, as countries gradually shift from high maternal mortality to low maternal mortality. Based on this obstetric transition, the states are classified as high MMR, moderate MMR, and low MMR and different strategies are implemented in different states based on the classifications.

States with high MMR will focus on basic management, timely detection of complication, and referral with assured transport; focus on increasing institutional deliveries, and skilled worker at the time of birth; establish labor room protocols and adhering to the protocols; focus on availability of Comprehensive Emergency Obstetric and Newborn Care (CEmOC) services and action on social determinants leading to complications in pregnancy; and ensure the availability of postpartum intrauterine contraceptive device (PPIUCD) and other contraceptive methods.

States with moderate MMR will focus more on, noncommunicable diseases and other indirect causes of poor health. Along with the above methods, the states with low MMR will focus on maternal near miss at tertiary and district hospitals and implement MDSR.

Implementation of MDSR, its review and monitoring and action is, a difficult job which needs team work, involving clinical staff, program managers, administrators, community mobilizers and workers, and bureaucrats, etc. So, the training need and design will differ. All the program providers are trained by the national-level trainers based on guidelines.

Multiple factors, which affects the proper implementation of MDSR, includes lack of knowledge and awareness of principle and purpose of MDSR, inadequately trained staff and existing blame culture, and lack of, financial resources.[6] The successful implementation of MDSR depends on the strong government commitment, involvement of professional organizations, and legal frame work.[7]

Obstetric safety focuses on improving the quality of care for delivered to soon-to-be mothers. The goal is to improve the early recognition, readiness, and responsiveness of healthcare professionals treating these women to achieve. MDSR is an important strategy adopted by the Government of India. Proper implementation will reduce maternal mortality and morbidity.

REFERENCES

1. UNICEF India. Maternal health: UNICEF's concerted action to increase access to quality maternal health services. [online] Available from: www.unicef.org>india>what-we-do>maternal-health. [Last accessed November, 2021].

2. World Health Organization. (2019). Maternal mortality. [online] Available from: https://www.who.int/news-room/fact-sheets/detail/maternal-mortality. [Last accessed November, 2021].
3. National Health Mission. (2017). Guidelines for Maternal Death Surveillance & Response. [online] Available from: https://nhm.gov.in/images/pdf/programmes/maternal-health/guidelines/Guideline_for_MDSR.pdf. [Last accessed November, 2021].
4. Kansal A, Garg S, Sharma M. Moving from maternal death review to surveillance and response: a paradigm shift. Indian J Public Health. 2018;62:299-301.
5. World Health Organization. (2013). Maternal death surveillance and response: Technical guidance information for action to prevent maternal deaths. [online] Available from: https://www.who.int/publications/i/item/9789241506083. [Last accessed November, 2021].
6. Hadush A, Dagnaw F, Getachew T, Bailey PE, Lawley R, Ruano AL. Triangulating data sources for further learning from and about the MDSR in Ethiopia: a cross-sectional review of facility based maternal death data from EmONC assessment and MDSR system. BMC Pregnancy and Childbirth. 2020;20:206.
7. Smith H, Ameh C, Roos N, van den Broek N. Implementing maternal death surveillance and response: a review of lessons from country case studies. BMC Pregnancy and Childbirth. 2017;17:233.

■ LONG QUESTION

1. Explain how maternal death surveillance and response will help in reducing the maternal mortality.

■ SHORT QUESTIONS

1. What are the objectives of maternal death surveillance and response?
2. Explain the two levels of maternal death review.

■ MULTIPLE CHOICE QUESTIONS

1. Which state in India is pioneer in Confidential Review of maternal deaths?
   a. Tamil Nadu   b. Kerala
   c. Uttar Pradesh   d. Punjab
2. Sustainable Development Goals 3 (SDG) have a target of reducing MMR to <......... per 100,000 births globally by 2030.
   a. 70   b. 80
   c. 60   d. 90
3. In India, the process of maternal death review is done at how many levels?
   a. 2   b. 3
   c. 1   d. 4
4. In community based MDSR the primary informant is:
   a. DMO   b. ASHA worker
   c. BMO   d. Nodal officer

Answers
1. b   2. a   3. a   4. b

11.4 ROLE OF MIDWIFERY IN OBSTETRICS

Evita Fernandez

■ INTRODUCTION

For many women with high-risk pregnancies, obstetric care is vital and may be life-saving. However, obstetric practice with its risk-oriented approach and reliance on technology is associated with an increasing number of interventions, which may not necessarily be beneficial. On the contrary, midwifery highlights the normalcy of pregnancy, labor and childbirth, and focuses on the importance of providing relationship-based respectful care; this is the need of the hour, especially for the vast majority of women whose pregnancies and labors are uncomplicated.

■ THE LANCET SERIES ON MIDWIFERY

This four-paper series on midwifery, which focuses on essential maternal and newborn needs from the woman's perspective, is a landmark in the history of midwifery care. The combined evidence from the series shows the extensive reach and scale of the impact of midwifery and the work of professional midwives on the survival, health, and well-being of women and infants. The salient findings are summarized in **Table 1**.

TABLE 1: Brief summary of the findings from the 2014 Lancet Series on Midwifery

Paper	Conclusion
Midwifery and quality care[1]	• Midwifery care could improve more than 50 outcomes • Provision of the QMNC framework for planning, monitoring, regulation and education
Scaling up midwifery[2]	Universal provision of midwifery could reduce maternal mortality by more than 80%
Country experience of strengthening health systems through midwifery[3]	Focus should not be on numerical coverage but on provision of quality, respectful care
Improvement of maternal and newborn health through midwifery[4]	Midwives are crucial to achievement of national and international goals and targets

The first paper in the Series[1] begins with a definition of the practice of midwifery as: "skilled, knowledgeable, and compassionate care for childbearing women, newborn infants,

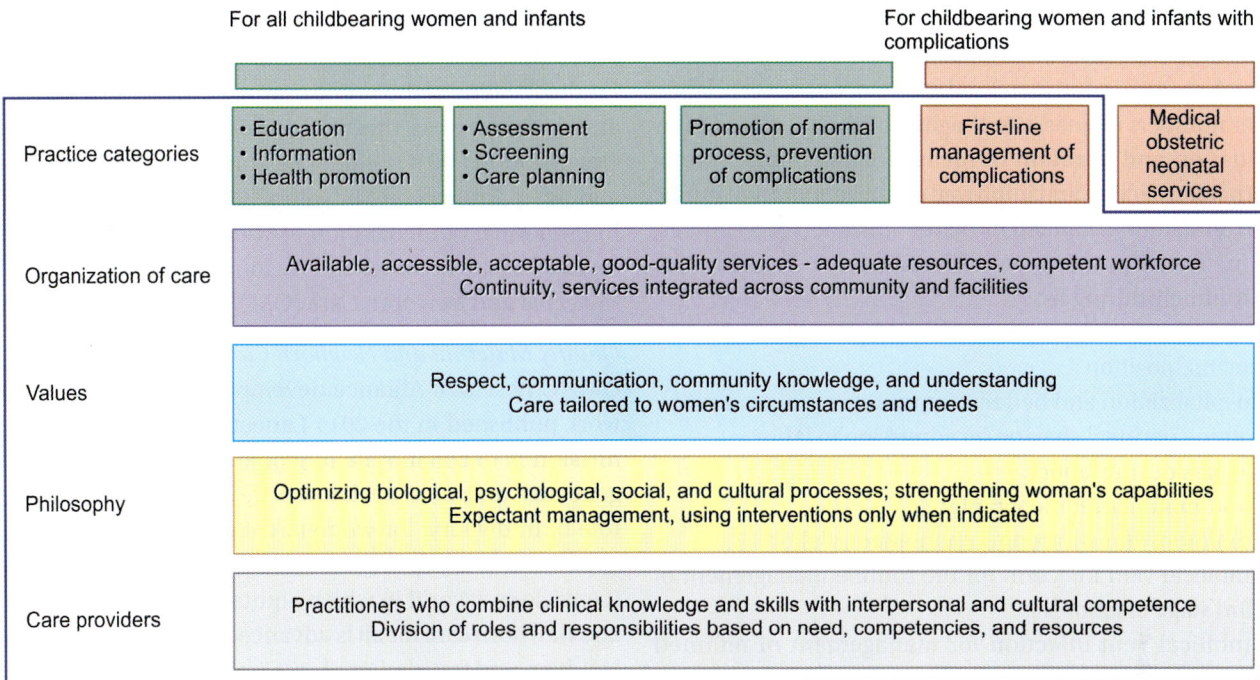

Fig. 1: The framework for quality maternal and newborn care[1] adapted show the scope of midwifery within the blue line.

and families across the continuum throughout prepregnancy, pregnancy, birth, postpartum, and the early weeks of life. Core characteristics include optimizing normal biological, psychological, social, and cultural processes of reproduction and early life; timely prevention and management of complications; consultation with and referral to other services; respect for women's individual circumstances and views; and working in partnership with women to strengthen women's own capabilities to care for themselves and their families."

Women with high-risk pregnancies constitute a minority and it is vital that skilled care be provided not only to them but also to the vast majority with uncomplicated pregnancies. The components of the framework for Quality Maternal and Newborn Care (QMNC) **(Fig. 1)** are enlisted here:

Practices needed by all childbearing women and babies:
- *Education, information, health promotion:* Examples include information about maternal nutrition, family planning services, and breastfeeding promotion.
- *Assessment, screening, and care planning:* Examples include transfer criteria, screening for sexually transmitted diseases, diabetes, HIV, pre-eclampsia assessing labor progress and mental health problems.
- *Promotion of normal processes and prevention of complications:* Examples include prevention of mother-to-child transmission of HIV, encouraging mobility in labor, clinical, emotional, and psychosocial care during uncomplicated labor and birth, immediate care of the newborn, skin-to-skin contact, and support for breastfeeding.

Additional practices needed by women and babies with complications:
- First-line management of complications include treatment of infections in pregnancy, anti-D administration in pregnancy for rhesus-negative women, external cephalic version for breech presentation, and basic and emergency obstetric and newborn care such as management of preeclampsia, postpartum iron deficiency anemia, and postpartum hemorrhage.
- Medical, obstetric, and neonatal services to manage serious complications include elective and emergency cesarean section, blood transfusion, care for women with multiple births and medical complications such as HIV and diabetes, and services for preterm, small for gestational age, and sick neonates.

The other categories in the quality framework **(Fig. 1)** delineate the *organization of care* and the need for competent workers; highlight the *values of* respectful personalized care; spell out the *philosophy* of informed choice and empowerment of women; and emphasize the need for *care providers* who are not only proficient clinically but also able to interact effectively with people of different cultures. *Except when medical practices become necessary for the management of complicated pregnancies, midwives are capable of providing quality care in all other situations relevant to the clinical and cultural context; therefore, their contribution to quality maternal and newborn care is paramount.*

Midwifery practices led to an improvement in as many as 56 outcomes, which include reduced maternal and newborn mortality, reduced stillbirth, reduced perineal trauma, reduced instrumental birth, reduced intrapartum analgesia or anesthesia, less severe blood loss, fewer preterm births, fewer newborn infants with a low birth weight, and less hypothermia. The analyses also found increased spontaneous onset of labor, greater numbers of unassisted vaginal births, increased rates of initiation and duration of breastfeeding, higher rate of maternal satisfaction and improved organizational and public health outcomes facilitated by better utilization of resources. Nine ineffective practices were identified that should not be used routinely during labor:

- Hands and knees posture in late pregnancy or labor for fetal malposition
- Hospitalization and bed rest for multiple pregnancy
- Routine perineal shaving on admission in labor
- Enemas during labor
- Continuous cardiotocography
- Amniotomy for shortening spontaneous labor
- Umbilical vein injection for the routine management of third stage of labor
- Umbilical vein injection for management of retained placenta
- Restricted pacifier use in breastfeeding term infants for increasing duration of breastfeeding.

More than 95% of the maternal and neonatal mortality worldwide is accounted for by 78 low-and middle-income countries. The second paper in the Lancet Series[2] dwells on the results that can be achieved by increasing the extent of midwifery in these nations. Maternal and perinatal mortality can be reduced by 50-75% by including contraceptive services in the scope of midwifery, with an additional 10-20% reduction when linked to specialist care. *Thus, comprehensive midwifery care could potentially prevent a total of 83% of all maternal deaths, stillbirths, and newborn deaths.*

The third paper in the Series[3] focuses on four countries that successfully deployed midwives to reduce maternal mortality: Burkina Faso, Cambodia, Indonesia, and Morocco. The experiences of these countries also signify the need to address quality of care by promoting respectful women-centered care and preventing over medicalization of labor and birth.

The fourth paper in the Series[4] identifies the proactive and pragmatic changes that are needed to ensure provision of universal quality maternal and newborn care. The authors focus on research priorities and conclude that an investment in midwifery is pivotal in achieving national and international health targets. The provision of quality care closer to women and communities has many benefits: identification of students from rural locations who will be retained in that community is crucial.

Evidence from the Series can be used for: education, curriculum development; professional development; advocacy with government or senior decision-makers; policy/strategy development; interprofessional working; standards and guideline development; research program development; monitoring standards and quality indicators; program development and implementation; and donor decisions on funding.[5] Some of the prime examples of its use for advocacy and action across the world include: The World Health Organization (WHO) guidelines on antenatal, intrapartum, and postpartum care; Midwifery Services Framework by the International Confederation of Midwives (ICM); planning of services at the national and regional levels; and the Quality Maternal and Newborn Care (QMNC) Research Alliance.

Quality Maternal and Newborn Care Research Alliance[6]: The QMNC Research Alliance developed out of the pioneering work published in the 2014 Lancet Series on Midwifery. Its mission is to collaborate in global research that promotes, generates, and translates knowledge, particularly of the integral role of midwifery, for women, childbearing people, and all childbearing families to survive, thrive, and transform lives. It envisions a world in which equitable and quality maternal and newborn care for all is advanced through the promotion, conduct, and translation of research that underpins optimal QNMC and that examines the integral role of midwifery.

MATERNAL NEWBORN AND CHILD HEALTH GOALS

According to the latest United Nations Children's Fund (UNICEF) data, >800 women die daily from causes related to pregnancy and childbirth; 6,700 newborn deaths are recorded everyday and almost 2 million babies are stillborn every year.[7] Despite advances in health care, the much slower rate of reduction in Maternal Mortality Ratio (MMR) in lower-income countries compared to higher-income countries has resulted in MMR being the greatest disparity in any mortality between these two groups.[8]

Moller et al. reviewed the progress in monitoring of maternal and newborn health outcomes and identified the gaps and inequities within and between countries.[9] Millenium Development Goals 4 and 5 focused on maternal and child health. Subsequently, the 17 Sustainable Development Goals (SDGs) were launched in September 2015 to provide a framework for universal health coverage until 2030 with SDG 3 addressing health and well-being for all at all ages.[10] The Every Newborn Action Plan (ENAP) and Ending Preventable Maternal Mortality (EPMM) initiatives were launched to guide the SDG agenda on Maternal Newborn and Child Health (MNCH).

The ENAP target is for all countries to reach a stillbirth rate of 12 or lower by 2030. The SDG targets of global MMR<70 and global Neonatal Mortality Rate of <12 pose a formidable challenge. Midwifery care can have an impact not only on SDG 3 (Good Health and Well-being) but also contribute to achieving other SDGs such as: Zero Hunger (SDG 2), Gender Equality (SDG 5), Reducing Inequality (SDG 10), and Sustainable Cities and Communities (SDG 11). Midwifery is central to the reduction of avoidable maternal and newborn mortality and morbidity, and midwife-led continuity models of care are recommended by the WHO.[11]

RESPECTFUL MATERNITY CARE

Respectful maternity care is a fundamental human right and an essential component of safe motherhood. Disrespect and abuse in childbirth can vary from verbal insults to physical assault and may range from neglect to nonconsented interventions. This indicates apathy and a lack of quality and accountability in the health system; putting up with disrespect and abuse belittles the value of women and is itself one of the underlying causes of a slow reduction in MMR.[12] Respect for basic human rights and courteous treatment are important determinants of maternal satisfaction and may be perceived as more important than technical competence of providers. In the quest for a reduction in mortality and morbidity and the ensuing interventions, quality of care must not take a backseat but rather be at the forefront.

Just as lack of availability of services and inadequate access to maternal and newborn care constitute poor quality care, so does the routine use of unindicated interventions in healthy women and newborns with its consequent adverse effects. Used appropriately, interventions can be life-saving procedures. However, unnecessary interventions cause more harm than good: Every intervention carries an inherent risk and unintended consequences can have a cascading effect leading to more interventions resulting in untoward effects.[13] These effects are not limited to the immediate iatrogenic morbidity but have long-lasting consequences that have been linked to autoimmune diseases and lifestyle disorders.[14] Inappropriate use of interventions also has a long-term economic impact on communities and countries.

McCourt describes how women who received caseload midwifery care (and developed a trust-based relationship) were more positive about their birth experience and less dissatisfied with interventions because of better support and communication than were women who received other models of care.[15] The Cochrane review on midwife-led continuity models of care endorsed these findings and concluded that these women had lesser likelihood of amniotomy, regional analgesia, instrumental vaginal birth, preterm birth, and fetal loss plus neonatal death, and a slightly increased probability of a spontaneous vaginal birth.[16]

WHO IS A MIDWIFE?

"The midwife is recognized as a responsible and accountable professional who works in partnership with women to give the necessary support, care, and advice during pregnancy, labor and the postpartum period, to conduct births on the midwife's own responsibility and to provide care for the newborn and the infant. This care includes preventative measures, the promotion of normal birth, the detection of complications in mother and child, the accessing of medical care or other appropriate assistance, and the carrying out of emergency measures. The midwife has an important task in health counseling and education, not only for the woman, but also within the family and the community. This work should involve antenatal education and preparation for parenthood and may extend to women's health, sexual or reproductive health, and childcare. A midwife may practice in any setting including the home, community, hospitals, clinics, or health units."[17]

The International Confederation of Midwives (ICM) defines a midwife as "a person who has successfully completed a midwifery education program that is duly recognized in the country where it is located and that is based on the ICM Essential Competencies for Basic Midwifery Practice and the framework of the ICM Global Standards for Midwifery Education; who has acquired the requisite qualifications to be registered and legally licensed to practice midwifery and use the title 'midwife,' and who demonstrates competency in the practice of midwifery."[17]

PHILOSOPHY OF CARE[18]

Obstetrics can instill fear in women and their families because it tends to focus on the identification and assessment of pathology. Midwifery, on the other hand, views women as healthy individuals, and pregnancy and childbirth as normal physiologic processes. Respecting a woman and supporting her to give birth safely with dignity is at the heart of midwifery care.

Midwife translated as "being with the woman" describes a professional companion, and *it is this concept of companionship that is unique to midwifery*. Midwifery care is shaped by five basic principles:
1. Continuity of care (or carer)
2. Informed choice
3. Community based
4. Choice of birth setting
5. Evidence-informed practice

The motto of midwifery is to humanize birth by being sensitive to the needs of women. The midwifery approach represents a paradigm shift: Childbirth is not an illness to be managed but a momentous occasion in the life of the woman which the care provider is privileged to be a part of.

SCOPE OF PRACTICE[18]

A midwife ought to take on the role of lead professional for all women with low-risk pregnancies and provide antenatal, intrapartum, and postpartum care. *Even if the situation demands an obstetrician to take over as the lead professional, the midwife must continue coordinating care. The midwife-led unit (MLU) model emphasizes normality of birth for women with an uncomplicated pregnancy.* It seeks to provide respectful maternity care and curtail unnecessary intrapartum interventions. Midwives encourage freedom of thought and expression, and facilitate informed decision-making by the woman and her partner by providing relevant information.

They promote practices that will assist natural birth such as maintaining upright positions and actively mobilizing in labor.

Midwives were traditionally community based but can offer services in hospitals, standalone units or alongside birth centers. An alongside birth center is located in a hospital with obstetric services either in a different part of the same building or a separate building on the same site. The midwives' ability to practice in the community and offer care in the place where the woman is comfortable facilitates bonding and a deviation from the medicalized model of care. Central to the midwifery model of care is the freedom of choice with regard to the place of birth. Advocates of hospital birth argue that women should birth in hospitals because of the potential for unforeseen complications while supporters of home birth declare that the greatest likelihood of a normal birth is at home under the care of a competent midwife. The researchers of the Birthplace in England study reported fewer interventions with no deleterious effect on perinatal outcomes in women planning birth in a midwifery unit or at home compared with those opting to birth in an obstetric unit.[19] The National Institute for Health and Care Excellence (NICE) and the Australian guidelines recommend that women may be free to choose any birth setting and should be helped to make an informed choice. This is not feasible in the present Indian context as the Government has mandated institutional births.

Midwives must be committed to constantly updating knowledge, maintaining skills and sharing evidence-based midwifery practices. Clinical decision-making must consider factors such as healthcare resources, clinical condition, the midwife's expertise and experience, and the woman's preferences.

■ SPECIALIZED SKILLS OF THE MIDWIFE

Clinicians

In order to promote the physiologic birth process, midwives must acquire and master the requisite clinical skills. They must be good listeners, perceive nonverbal cues, and demonstrate cultural competence. Also important is an ability to discern the need for transfer of care, especially in those settings in which access to other providers and services might not be easy.

Educators

Translating clinical evidence into lay language and enabling informed decision-making can be achieved by individualized or group discussions or information sessions.

Companions

Midwives are companions on the journey through pregnancy, labor and birth, and immediate postpartum, providing supportive, compassionate care to the women they serve.

Promoters of Health and Well-being

Well-being includes both physical and emotional aspects of health, and is a condition of being content, confident, and hopeful. Midwives promote the well-being of women by supporting physiologic processes and optimizing maternity care.

Interprofessional Collaboration[20]

All those working in maternity care have a specific role to play and are uniquely equipped to carry out their duties. Every cadre of care provider has its strengths and limitations, but each is invaluable to the provision of optimal care. The collaborative practice must include the woman as the key player in the healthcare team. Obstetricians' willingness to learn from midwifery colleagues and allowing them to take the lead when appropriate, is critical to establishing collaborative models of care and reducing unnecessary intrapartum interventions.

International Confederation of Midwives[17]

The ICM is the international midwifery association that has representatives from 124 countries constituting 143 Midwives' Associations. It is a nongovernmental organization that works closely with the WHO, United Nations Population Fund, UNICEF, and other organizations worldwide. The ICM envisions a world where every childbearing woman has access to a midwife's care for herself and her newborn. Its mission is to strengthen Midwives' Associations and to advance the profession of midwifery globally by promoting autonomous midwives as the most appropriate caregivers for childbearing women and in keeping birth normal, in order to enhance the reproductive health of women, their newborns and their families".

The ICM Code of Ethics for Midwives "acknowledges women as persons with human rights, seeks justice for all people and equity in access to health care, and is based on mutual relationships of respect, trust, and the dignity of all members of society". The Code also states that midwives should act in nondiscriminatory ways to promote the health and well-being of women, and addresses the issues of midwifery relationships, practice of midwifery, professional responsibilities of midwives, and the advancement of midwifery.

■ STATE OF THE WORLD'S MIDWIFERY (SoWMy)[21]

Midwives and nurses play a key role in the global progress towards the "Health For All" goal of the WHO. In recognition of their contribution, the year 2020 was designated as the International Year of the Nurse and the Year of the Midwife by the 72nd World Health Assembly. However, the roles played by midwives, obstetricians, nurses, traditional birth attendants, and other health workers in maternity care are not clearly defined in many countries. There exist differences in the way maternity services are set up—predominantly obstetric-led care (as in North America) or midwifery models and collaborative care pathways (as in New Zealand and the Netherlands).

In order to achieve the targets of the health-related SDGs, there needs to be an adequate number of skilled and motivated healthcare workers who are distributed equally in different settings. *The health workers trained in midwifery can provide almost 90% of the essential healthcare services to women and their newborn babies. They must be taught to achieve proficiency as per international standards and supervised to ensure that they maintain the same.* But midwives constitute only just over a third of the maternity care workforce.[22] The State of the World's Midwifery (SoWMy) 2014 report from 73 low- and middle-income countries states that only 22% of countries have enough qualified midwives. As estimated by the WHO, SDG 3 will be attainable by 2030 globally if there are at least an additional 9 million nurses and midwives. An up-to-date evidence of the progress made in extending quality midwifery services, as well as an analysis of the barriers to midwifery will be provided by the SoWMy2021.

MIDWIFERY IN INDIA

India is a prime example of countries with simultaneous excessive and insufficient use of interventions. Social, economic, educational, and gender differences continue to determine India's maternal health inequalities. Certified independent midwives are needed to provide one-to-one optimal care for women. India has over two million nurses and nearly 9,00,000 Auxiliary Nurses. Both these professional nursing streams are certified also as midwives, but do NOT meet the universally accepted definition of a midwife as outlined by the ICM. In addition to the already existing workforce, the Government of India has committed to an additional 85,000 midwives by 2023.[23] Midwives have not received the recognition as qualified health professionals in India. Unless midwifery is viewed as a distinct profession with a scope of practice, it will always be a part of nursing and an addendum to obstetrics.

After several unsuccessful attempts at the introduction of midwives into India's health system, an in-house Professional Midwifery Education and Training program was launched in 2011 at Fernandez Hospital, Hyderabad, Telangana. The year 2017 witnessed the emergence of a public–private partnership between the State Government, UNICEF and Fernandez hospital, wherein an 18-month course based on ICM competencies was rolled out to train nursing students in midwifery. In December 2018, the Government of India acknowledged the urgent need to consider midwifery training separate to nursing and has developed the Guidelines on Midwifery Services in India.[24] Accomplished instructors are essential to create this cadre of Nurse Practitioner in Midwifery (NPM) and Fernandez Foundation is now a recognized National Midwifery Training Institute (NMTI) for midwifery educators in India.

CONCLUSION

The vast majority of low-risk women with uncomplicated pregnancies have a potential to birth naturally. However, over-medicalization in modern-day obstetrics can adversely affect the progress of labor due to inappropriate use of interventions. Midwifery focuses on individualized, respectful, holistic, and woman-centered care, minimizing technological intervention and improving maternal satisfaction. *Integrating high-quality midwifery care into the health system is a cost-effective way to enable all women and children's rights.*

REFERENCES

1. Renfrew MJ, McFadden A, Bastos MH, et al. Midwifery and quality care: findings from a new evidence-informed framework for maternal and newborn care. Lancet. 2014;384(9948):1129-45.
2. Homer CSE, Friberg IK, Bastos Dias MA, et al. The projected effect of scaling up midwifery. Lancet. 2014;384(9948):1146-57.
3. Van Lerberghe W, Matthews Z, Achadi E, et al. Country experience with strengthening of healthy systems and deployment of midwives in countries with high maternal mortality. Lancet. 2014;384(9949):1215-25.
4. ten Hoope-Bender P, de Bernis L, Campbell J, et al. Improvement of maternal and newborn health through midwifery. Lancet. 2014;384(9949):1226-35.
5. McFadden A. The Lancet Series on Midwifery: what impact has it had and what are the next steps? Available from: http://www.maternityandmidwifery.co.uk/events/wp-downloads/mmb-edinburgh-2017/presentations/MMB_Edinburgh_2017_Presentation_Alison_McFadden.pdf [Last accessed December, 2020].
6. Quality Maternal and Newborn Care. Available from: https://www.qmnc.org/qmnc-research-alliance/[Last accessed December 2020].
7. UNICEF data. Available from: https://data.unicef.org/[Last accessed December 2020].
8. Loudon I. Maternal mortality in the past and its relevance to developing countries today. Am J Clin Nutr. 2000;72(1 Suppl):241S-6S.
9. Moller A-B, Patten JH, Hanson C, et al. Monitoring maternal and newborn health outcomes globally: a brief history of key events and initiatives. Trop Med Int Health. 2019;24(12):1342-68.
10. United Nations. Department of Economic and Social Affairs. Sustainable Development. Available from: https://sdgs.un.org/goals [Last accessed December 2020].
11. WHO recommendations on antenatal care for a positive pregnancy experience. World Health Organization, 2016: 152. Available from: http://apps.who.int/iris/bitstream/10665/250796/1/9789241549912-eng.pdf?ua=1. [Last accessed December 2020].
12. Freedman LP, Kruk ME. Disrespect and abuse of women in childbirth: challenging the global quality and accountability agendas. Lancet. 2014;384(9948):e42-4.
13. Jansen L, Gibson M, Bowles BC, Leach J. First do no harm: interventions during childbirth. J Perinat Educ. 2013 Spring;22(2):83-92.
14. Downe S. Reducing routine interventions during labour and birth: first, do no harm. Cad Saude Publica. 2014;30 Suppl 1:S21-2.

15. McCourt C. Technologies of birth and models of midwifery care. Rev Esc Enferm USP. 2014;48(spec), 168-77.
16. Sandall J, Soltani H, Gates S, Shennan A, Devane D. Midwife-led continuity models versus other models of care for childbearing women. Cochrane Database Syst Rev. 2016;CD004667.
17. International Federation of Gynaecology and Obstetrics (FIGO). Definition of the Midwife, The Netherlands: International Confederation of Midwives. 2005. Available from: http://www.internationalmidwives.org [Last accessed December 2020].
18. Comprehensive Midwifery: the role of the midwife in health care practice, education, and research. Available from: https://ecampusontario.pressbooks.pub/cmroleofmidwifery/front-matter/introduction/[Last accessed December 2020].
19. Birthplace in England Collaborative Group. Brocklehurst P, Hardy P, Hollowell J, Linsell L, Macfarlane A, McCourt C, et al. Perinatal and maternal outcomes by planned place of birth for healthy women with low risk pregnancies: the Birthplace in England national prospective cohort study. BMJ. 2011;343:d7400.
20. Shamian J. Interprofessional collaboration, the only way to Save Every Woman and Every Child. Lancet. 2014;384(9948):e41-2.
21. The State of the World's Midwifery 2021 Concept Note August 2019. Available from: https://www.internationalmidwives.org/assets/files/general-files/2020/06/sowmy2021-concept-note_2020.pdf [Last accessed December 2020].
22. Chou D, Daelmans B, Jolivet RR, et al. Ending preventable maternal and newborn mortality and stillbirths. BMJ. 2015; 351:h4255.
23. World Health Organization. Midwives – central to providing quality care to mothers and newborns during COVID-19 pandemic and beyond. Available from: https://www.who.int/india/news/photo-story/detail/midwives--central-to-providing-quality-care-to-mothers-and-newborns-during-covid-19-pandemic-and-beyond [Last accessed December 2020].
24. Guidelines on Midwifery Services in India, 2018. Available from: https://nhm.gov.in/New_Updates_2018/NHM_Components/RMNCHA/MH/Guidelines/Guidelines_on_Midwifery_Services_in_India.pdf [Last accessed January 2020].

■ LONG QUESTION

1. Describe in detail the evidence in favor of midwife-led care. What is India's current stand on midwifery care?

■ SHORT QUESTION

1. What are the components of respectful maternity care? Discuss in brief.

■ MULTIPLE CHOICE QUESTIONS

1. All of the following are true of midwifery care, except:
   a. Increased vaginal births
   b. Less severe blood loss
   c. More preterm births
   d. Higher rate of maternal satisfaction
2. All the following practices should not be routinely used in labor, except:
   a. Continuous cardiotocography
   b. Active mobilization
   c. Perineal shaving on admission in labor
   d. Amniotomy for women in spontaneous labor
3. All the following services can be offered by midwives, except:
   a. Family planning services
   b. Cesarean section
   c. Screening for sexually transmitted diseases
   d. Health education
4. The SDG target for global MMR by the year 2030 is:
   a. ≤60
   b. ≤50
   c. ≤100
   d. ≤70
5. Disrespectful maternity care is:
   a. Overuse of medical interventions
   b. Abandonment of care
   c. Underuse of medical interventions
   d. All of the above
6. Which of the following statements is false?
   a. Midwives are autonomous primary care providers
   b. Midwives, rather than obstetricians should be the lead professionals for the majority of pregnant women
   c. Midwives do not have a role to play in the care of women with high-risk pregnancies
   d. Midwives must take an active part in research on the provision of optimal maternity care
7. Which year was declared the Year of the Midwife?
   a. 2014
   b. 2000
   c. 2020
   d. 2004
8. A midwife practices:
   a. In the community
   b. In the hospital
   c. In the birth center
   d. All of the above
9. Select the true statement:
   a. Midwifery care can avert more than 80% of maternal and newborn deaths and stillbirths
   b. Technical competence of care providers is more important than dignity of care
   c. Midwifery care involves the intrapartum period while the antenatal and postpartum care is provided by the obstetrician
   d. Midwives cannot offer care in a standalone unit but must always be attached to a maternity hospital and be governed by obstetric care protocols
10. A young primigravida has been referred at 35 weeks of gestation in latent labor with a BP recording of 150/104 mm Hg. Which of the following is appropriate?
    a. Home BP monitoring until active labor sets in
    b. Admission and standard obstetric care
    c. Admission and midwife-led care
    d. Admission and collaborative care

Answers
1. c 2. b 3. b 4. d 5. d 6. c
7. c 8. d 9. a 10. d

SECTION 12

Critical Care in Obstetrics

12.1 ROLE OF HDU/ICU IN OBSTETRICS

Pratima Mittal, Rekha Bharti

INTRODUCTION

Availability of dedicated obstetrics critical care units plays an important role in reducing the maternal severe morbidity and mortality. Critical care of pregnant women is different from other patients as pregnancy may modify the disease state and pharmacokinetics of many drugs. Also, physiological changes during pregnancy need to be considered when managing a critically ill woman. Dedicated critical care units have the advantage of providing onsite critical care facilities and these units have concurrent availability of the fetal monitoring, expert obstetricians, and intensive care specialists. Women requiring invasive monitoring or a single organ support can be managed at high-dependency units (HDUs) whereas, those requiring advanced respiratory support alone or basic respiratory support along with at least one additional organ support need intensive care unit (ICU) care.

Women are the supporting pillars of family, society, and hence the nation. Promoting their health by providing quality services and at the same time protecting their right to safe maternity is of vital importance.

Safe motherhood means that all women receive a certain level of care to remain healthy and safe throughout pregnancy and childbirth. According to the World Health Organization (WHO) fact sheet 2019, in 2017, 810 women died each day due to pregnancy and childbirth complications. It is also estimated that 94% of these deaths occurred in low-resource setting and around one fifth of these maternal deaths were in southern Asia.[1] Although, worldwide maternal mortality was reduced by 38% from 2010 to 2017, drop in maternal mortality ratio (MMR) in southern Asia was around 60%, from 384 to 157 per 100,000 live births.[2] Based on the UN Inter–Agency Expert Groups, MMR estimates in the publication *"Trends in Maternal Mortality: 1990 to 2015"*, it was estimated that Nigeria and India reported around one third of all maternal deaths worldwide in 2015, 19% and 15%, respectively.[3]

According to Millennium Development Goal (MDG), between 1990 and 2015, India was to reduce the Maternal Mortality Ratio (MMR) by three quarters. Taking a baseline of 556 per 100,000 live births in 1990, the target was to achieve MMR of 139 per 100,000 live births by the year 2015. However, the MMR declined by 68.7% and came down 174 in 2015.[4] India's MMR declined much faster than the global MMR during the period 1990 to 2010, 5.6% and 2.4%, respectively. The States of Kerala, Maharashtra, and Tamil Nadu and have achieved the MMR level of below 100, 66, 87, and 90 per 100,000 live births, respectively.[5] But still it is higher than the MMR in most of the developed countries, 11–14/100,000 live births.[3]

Availability of critical care units in developed countries has played an important role in reducing their maternal mortality. Worldwide, there has been an increase in ICU admissions which has led to development of separate ICUs for various specialties such as cardiac, neurosurgery, respiratory medicine, and neonatology, but dedicated ICUs for obstetric women are not yet widely available in most developing countries.[6,7]

Women can die of either complications developed during pregnancy, childbirth, and postpartum, or due to preexisting chronic diseases. Conditions that account for three fourths of the maternal deaths include: Antepartum or postpartum hemorrhage (PPH), sepsis, hypertensive disorders, labor complications, and septic abortions.[8] Most of these maternal complications can be treated and maternal mortality can be prevented.[2]

A systematic review of maternal morbidity and mortality by the WHO estimated that 4–8% of pregnant women delivering at hospitals in resource-poor settings suffer SAMM (severe acute maternal morbidity) and need urgent medical intervention to prevent maternal death.[9] It is estimated that in developed countries, approximately 1–10 obstetric patients per 1,000 deliveries required admission to ICU.[10] In Western India, the incidence of ICU utilization by obstetric patients is reported to be 5.4 per 1,000 deliveries.[11] A study from rural central India reported 9.89% admission rate to ICU and HDU and 11.9% of these women who required intensive care needed admission to ICU. This study by Tayade et al. also found that the majority (68.42%) of admissions in HDU were solely due to obstetric complications, while 31.57% women required HDU for preexisting medical diseases. The most common obstetric indications for which critical care was required were septicemia (35.08%), PPH (29.08%), and hypertension (21.05%).[12] Similarly, according to a report from the Intensive Care National Audit and Research Centre (ICNARC), 72% pregnant or recently pregnant women in England, Wales, and Northern Ireland were admitted to critical care units for obstetric reason.[13]

Although, pregnancy and labor are considered physiological processes but catastrophic complications can develop without any warning, anytime during pregnancy, childbirth, or postpartum period.[14] Throughout pregnancy and childbirth, women need access to care by skilled providers who can be obstetricians or Emergency Obstetric Care (EmOC)-trained providers. However, women who have single or multiple organ involvements/dysfunctions need multidisciplinary care by superspecialists at HDUs or ICUs.[15]

To strengthen the critical care, Obstetrics in India, Ministry of Health and Family Welfare launched LaQshya (Labor Room Quality Improvement Initiative) program with an aim of improving quality of care in labor rooms and maternity operation theaters. The program also intends to operationalize dedicated Obstetric ICUs at Medical College Hospital level and Obstetric HDUs at District Hospital level. This will benefit pregnant women and newborns delivering at public health institutions.[16]

■ NEED FOR DEDICATED OBSTETRIC HDU/ICU

In obstetrics, when things go wrong, they go wrong fast—"they fall off a cliff".[15] Increased cardiac output can lead to rapid loss of large volumes of blood, especially from the uterus which receives 10% of cardiac output at term.[13] Therefore, the survival of women during obstetrics emergencies often requires rapid response.

Also, critical care of pregnant women is different from other patients. Pregnancy may modify the disease state and pharmacokinetics of many drugs. The drugs given to the mother may affect the placental perfusion and growing fetus.[10,15] Physiological changes during pregnancy should be considered when managing a critically ill woman.

Diaphragmatic splinting changes lung function and also due to increased oxygen demand during pregnancy, the pregnant women can rapidly develop hypoxia. The intubations are difficult during pregnancy due to laryngeal edema. To avoid risk of aspiration during intubation, effective cricoids pressure and the prophylactic use of H2 antagonists and antacids are required. Aortocaval compression by gravid uterus significantly reduces cardiac output after 20 weeks of gestation; this significantly reduces the efficacy of chest compressions during resuscitation. During resuscitation of pregnant women, who are >20 weeks' gestation, left lateral tilt should be routinely practiced for manual displacement of the uterus to relieve pressure of the gravid uterus from the inferior vena cava and aorta. In women who fail to respond to cardiopulmonary resuscitation (CPR), to assist maternal resuscitation, delivery should be achieved within 5 minutes.[17]

Dedicated critical care units have the advantage of providing onsite critical care facilities to obstetric patients without the need to shift them to medical/surgical ICU. These units also have the advantage of concurrent availability of fetal monitoring, expert obstetricians, and intensive care specialists. Many critically ill obstetric patients have medical disorders complicating pregnancy or involvement of multiple organs that require multidisciplinary approach along with care by the intensivists.[11,12,18]

Level of critical care required by the patient depends on the number of organs involved in the disease process. The term was first defined in Intensive Care Society's "Level of Care" document and updated in 2009.[19]

- *Level 0*: Patients whose needs can be met through normal ward care.
- *Level 1*: Patients at risk of their condition deteriorating and needing a higher level of observation or those recently relocated from higher levels of care.
- *Level 2*: Patients requiring invasive monitoring/intervention that include support for a single failing organ system (excluding advanced respiratory support).
- *Level 3*: Patients requiring advanced respiratory support (mechanical ventilation) alone or basic respiratory support along with support of at least one additional organ (**Fig. 1**).

■ TYPES OF SPECIALIZED CARE UNITS[20]

The specialized care units include HDUs, ICUs, and Hybrid Model.

Intensive Care Unit

Intensive care unit is a specialized area in a hospital or healthcare facility that is specifically designed to provide intensive care. It has skilled staff, is located near the critical areas, and is specially designed, equipped, and dedicated to provide care to critically sick patients. Patients with multiorgan involvement are admitted to ICU and care to the admitted patients is to be provided by a team consisting of superspecialists such as nephrologists, cardiologists, neurologists, and pulmonologists and is led by intensivists. It is a department with dedicated medical, nursing, and allied staff trained in critical care.

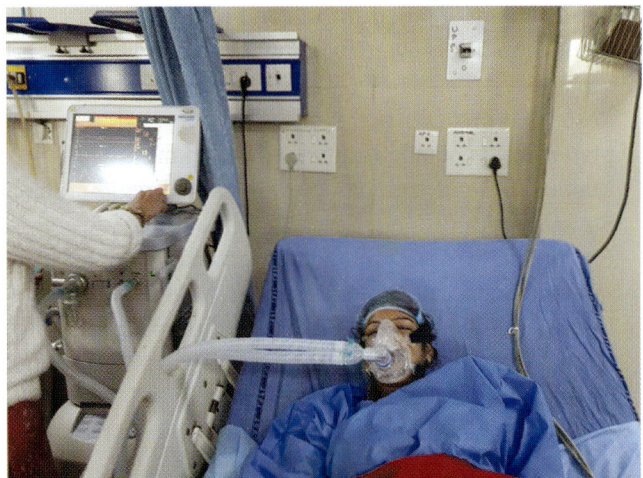

Fig. 1: Mechanical ventilation by CPAP in ICU.
(CPAP: continuous positive airway pressure; ICU: intensive care unit)

TABLE 1: Criteria for admission to obstetric HDU/ICU.	
Obstetric HDU admission	**Obstetric ICU admission**
Systolic blood pressure (SBP) <90 and >160 mm Hg	RR < 8 and > 35 breaths/minute
	Heart rate < 50 and > 140 beats/minute
Diastolic BP <50 and >110 mm Hg	SBP < 80 mm Hg, or 30 mm Hg below patient's usual BP
Mean arterial BP < 60 mm of Hg	Urine output <400 mL in 24 hours, or <160 mL in 8 hours and client unresponsive to simple routine measures
Heart Rate >110 and <60 beats/minute	
Respiratory rate: >25 breaths/minute	GCS < 8 in the context of nontraumatic coma
Urine > 0.5mL/kg/h (>30 mL/h)	Any unarousable patient
	Serum sodium outside the range 110–160 mmol/L
Any single organ dysfunction	Serum potassium outside the range 2.0–7.0 mmol/L
	pH outside the range 7.1–7.7
	PaO_2 < 6.6 kPa and/or $PaCO_2$ > 8.0 kPa
	SaO_2 < 90% on supplemental oxygen
	Need for advanced respiratory support
	Inotropic support
	DIC
	ARDS
	Multiorgan failure

(ARDS: acute respiratory distress syndrome; DIC: disseminated intravascular coagulation; GCS: Glasgow Coma scale; HDU: high-dependency unit; ICU: intensive care unit; RR: respiratory rate)

Obstetric Intensive Care Unit

Obstetric ICU is an area dedicated to the management of obstetric patients who develop obstetric, medical, or surgical complications leading to multiorgan involvement or failure. The care in these units is provided by the staff oriented to physiological changes during pregnancy and management of pathology related to obstetrics.

High-dependency Unit

High-dependency unit is a specialized area of the hospital which is located close to ICU. The care provided in HDU is more extensive than ward care but not to the extent of care provided at ICU. These are intermediate units between hospital wards and ICU. Patients admitted in ICU that show improvement are shifted to HDU before being transferred to hospital wards (step down) and patients admitted in HDU may deteriorate and require shifting to ICU (step up).

Obstetric High-dependency Unit

Obstetric patients that need intensive monitoring can be admitted to HDU dedicated to obstetric patients. These HDUs are equipped with teams that can provide antenatal, intrapartum, and postnatal care. Most antenatal and postpartum women admitted in the ICU do not require life-saving interventions but need only intensive monitoring that can be provided in the HDUs.[10] It reduces the need for ICU admissions and risk of hospital-acquired infections is less in HDU as compared to ICU. Also, the cost of care is much less in HDU. Obstetric HDU can be established in obstetric units in a room which can be equipped with equipments to provide intensive monitoring.[20]

Hybrid Model (Obstetric ICU and Obstetric HDU)

A hybrid model has both ICU and HDU beds and a team dedicated to the management of critically ill obstetric patients.

Criteria for Admission to Obstetric HDU/ICU

The decision for transfer of patient to obstetric ICU or HDU is taken on the basis of bedside evaluation of certain parameters. Mhyre et al. suggested Maternal Early Warning Criteria from the National Partnership for Maternal Safety.[21] Guidelines for Obstetric HDU and ICU by Ministry of Health and Family Welfare (MOHFW), Government of India recommend following criteria for admission to HDU/ICU[15] **(Table 1)**.

Triaging Policy

Women admitted to obstetric HDU/ICU may be shifted directly from the emergency room or may have been admitted to the ward after deteriorating condition that requires intensive care. They may also have been transferred from the operation room due to surgical or medical risks. The decision for shifting to HDU or ICU depends on the level of care needed.

Number of Beds in HDU/ICU

In United States, there are around 20 ICU beds per 100,000 population.[10,22] According to MOHFW, Government of India recommendations, calculation of critical care beds is done on the basis of delivery load in the Obstetric units.[15]

Number of deliveries	Number of HDU beds required
Up to 250	4
250–500	8
>500	No of beds can be increased proportionately
501–1000	8 bed Hybrid ICU (6 HDU+2 ICU)
>1,000 deliveries/month	4 bed ICU + 8 bed HDU

It is also recommended to designate one room of 150 sq ft with a separate entry, at the end of obstetric HDU as Isolation Room for management of mothers with infections requiring isolation (such as pregnant women with H1N1, HBsAg, Chicken Pox, etc.).

Infrastructure

It is recommended that at least 100–120 sq feet space per bed should be there for HDU and 120–140 sq feet for ICU.[15] Extra space of 100–120% is needed for the nursing station/storage/patient movement area/equipment area, patient toilet, and to maneuver equipment, beds and trolleys, etc.

For patient privacy, each bed should be separated by fixed partitions or curtains **(Fig. 2)**. The ceiling should be leak proof and free of lines or wires.

Nursing Station

The nursing station should have adequate space for central monitoring and computers, a scrub area, and facility for keeping records and emergency medicines.

Staff Required

The staff requirement is according to the number of beds in HDU/ICU.

Number of HDU/ICU beds	Staff required
8-bedded HDU	4 dedicated nurses and 2 EmOC/MOs
4-bedded HDU	2 dedicated nurses and 1 EmOC/ MO
4-bedded obstetric ICU	4 dedicated nurses and 1 intensivist

Human Resource Requirement for Obstetric ICU/HDU

Anesthetists/Intensivists are not required in HDUs. The staff required for HDU/ICU is given in **Table 2**.

Protocols and checklists are placed that ensure and encourage appropriate and immediate responses to critical situations and should include initial assessment of maternal and fetal condition, immediately resuscitation, baseline and specific investigations as indicated and treatment of primary condition (e.g., severe preeclampsia, hemorrhage, sepsis). Involvement of appropriate clinicians from relevant specialties may also be required.

List of protocols for Obstetrics Critical Care Unit:
- Admission and discharge criteria to/from HDU
- Management of major hemorrhage
- Management of preeclampsia and eclampsia
- Management of severe hypotension/hypertension/DM/sepsis
- Resuscitation of the pregnant patient
- Management of failed/difficult intubation
- Management of regional anesthesia and regional block for analgesia
- Management of postdural puncture headache
- Management of postoperative pain
- Management of patients on thromboprophylaxis
- Antacid prophylaxis, fasting policies and Oral intake during labor and delivery.

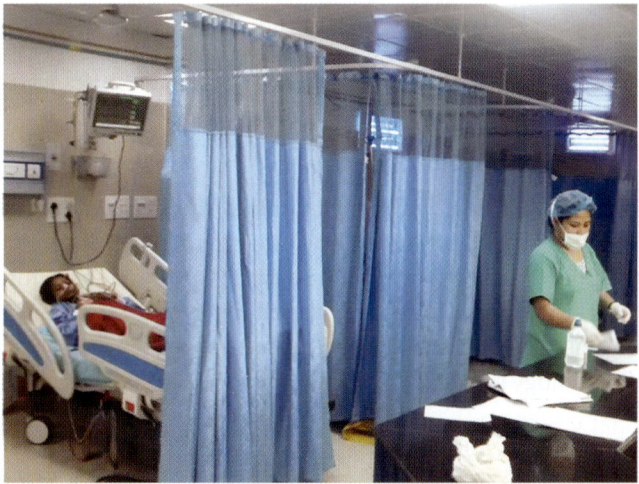

Fig. 2: Use of curtains to ensure privacy in critical care unit.

TABLE 2: Conditions requiring HDU/ICU admission.	
Obstetric complications	**Pregnancy with medical complications**
Pregnancy/labor pain with severe anemia (<7 g%) and its complications	Pregnancy with gestational diabetes
Accidental hemorrhage placental abruption, couvelaire uterus	Pregnancy with diabetic ketoacidosis
Postpartum hemorrhage	Pregnancy with cardiac diseases
Placenta previa	Pregnancy with jaundice
Adherent placenta and other placental abnormalities	Pregnancy with thyrotoxicosis
Obstetric hysterectomy	Pregnancy with thyroid storm
Severe preeclampsia/hypertensive crisis	Pregnancy with pheochromocytoma
Eclampsia	Pregnancy with other endocrine crisis like Addison's disease, etc.
Broad ligament hematoma	Postoperative ARF and other renal problems
HELLP syndrome	Leukemia and other hemolytic disorders

Contd...

Contd...

Obstetric complications	Pregnancy with medical complications
Perforation during abortion	Pregnancy with dengue
Sepsis and systemic inflammatory response syndrome (SIRS)	Pregnancy with complications of malaria
Pregnancy with thrombophilia	Pregnancy with asthma and other respiratory problems
Multiple gestation with complications	Pregnancy with OHSS (ovarian hyperstimulation syndrome)
Pregnancy with complications due to uterine anomaly and pathologies	Pregnancy with appendectomy or any other surgical emergency
Hydatidiform mole	Pregnancy with trauma/burns/cancer/poisoning
Ruptured ectopic	Pregnancy with DIC
Postoperative patients requiring hemodynamic monitoring or intensive nursing care	Pulmonary edema due to perioperative fluid overload, CCF, complication of severe pre-eclampsia, or tocolytic therapy with agonists, etc

(ARF: acute renal failure; HDU: high-dependency unit; HELLP: hemolysis, elevated liver enzymes, low platelet count; ICU: intensive care unit)

TABLE 3: Human resource requirement for obstetric ICU/HDU.

Cadre	Obstetric HDU	Obstetric ICU
Anesthetist/Intensivist	Not required	1 per unit (new or existing)
Medical Officer	1 per shift per unit	1 per shift per unit
Staff nurses	1 per two bed per shift	1 per bed per shift
M and E Assistant - cum DEO	Existing LR DEO/1 common for LR and ICU	Existing LR DEO/1 common for LR and ICU
Cleaning staff	As per requirement	As per requirement
Guard	As per requirement	As per requirement

(LR DEO: data entry operator; HDU: high-dependency unit; ICU: intensive care unit; LR: labor room; M and E assistant: monitoring and evaluation assistant)

Lactation Support

Facilities for breastfeeding should be available to all postnatal mothers in obstetric HDU. Babies are usually not allowed in obstetric ICU, but breast pump facilities should be made available.

Conditions that require HDU admissions include the following: Obstetric patients with hemodynamic instability, respiratory dysfunction, neurologic complications, and acute kidney injury or hematological complications may require admission in obstetric HDU[15] **(Table 3)**.

HEALTH MANAGEMENT AND INFORMATION SYSTEM

Health management and information system should be available for data collection, storage, processing, and analysis. This will help in regular audits and will improve the health-care services.

REFERENCES

1. World Health Organization. (2019). Trends in maternal mortality: 2000 to 2017: Estimates by WHO, UNICEF, UNFPA, World Bank Group and the United Nations Population Division. [online] Available from: https://apps.who.int/iris/bitstream/handle/10665/327596/WHO-RHR-19.23-eng.pdf?sequence=13&isAllowed=y . [Last accessed November, 2021].
2. World Health Organization. (2019). Maternal mortality. [online] Available from: https://www.who.int/news-room/fact-sheets/detail/maternal-mortality. [Last accessed November, 2021].
3. World Health Organization. (2015). Trends in maternal mortality: 1990 to 2015: Estimates by WHO, UNICEF, UNFPA, World Bank Group and the United Nations Population Division. [online] Available from: http://apps.who.int/iris/bitstream/handle/10665/194254/9789241565141_eng.pdf?sequence=1. [Last accessed November, 2021].
4. Ministry of Health and Family Welfare. Annual Report 2013-14: Maternal & Adolescent Healthcare. [online] Available from https://main.mohfw.gov.in/sites/default/files/03Chapter.pdf. [Last accessed November, 2021].
5. Ministry of Health and Family Welfare. Annual Report 2013-14: Maternal Health Programme. [online] Available from: https://main.mohfw.gov.in/sites/default/files/Chapter415.pdf. [Last accessed November, 2021].
6. Gupta S, Naithani U, Doshi V, Bhargava V, Vijay BS. Obstetric critical care: a prospective analysis of clinical characteristics, predictability, and fetomaternal outcome in a new dedicated obstetric intensive care unit. Indian J Anaesth. 2011;55:146-53.
7. Osinaike B, Amanor-Boadu S, Sanusi A. Obstetric intensive care: a developing country experience. Internet J Anesthesiol. 2006;10(2):1-5.
8. Say L, Chou D, Gemmill A, Tunçalp Ö, Moller AB, Daniels JD, et al. Global causes of maternal death: a WHO systematic analysis. Lancet Global Health. 2014;2(6):e323-3.
9. Say L, Pattinson RC, Gülmezoglu AM. WHO systematic review of maternal morbidity and mortality: the prevalence of severe acute maternal morbidity (near miss). Reprod Health. 2004;1:3.
10. Critical care in pregnancy. ACOG Practice Bulletin No. 211. American College of Obstetricians and Gynecologists. Obstet Gynecol 2019;133:e303-19.
11. Karnad DR, Lapsia V, Krishnan A, Salvi VS. Prognostic factors in obstetric patients admitted to an Indian intensive care unit. Crit Care Med. 2004;32: 1294-9.
12. Tayade S, Gangane N, Shivkumar P, Baswal D, Ratnu A, Bhushan H, et al. Role of obstetric high dependency and intensive care unit in improving pregnancy outcome and reducing maternal mortality-a study in rural central India. Int J Crit Care Emerg Med. 2018;4(2):1-9.
13. RCOG, UK. (2011). Providing equity of critical and maternity care for the critically ill pregnant or recently pregnant woman. https://www.oaa-anaes.ac.uk/assets/_managed/cms/files/Maternal_Critical_Care.pdf. [Last accessed November, 2021].

14. Ministry of Health and Family Welfare. (2016). Pradhan Mantri Surakshit Matritva Abhiyan. [online] Available from: http://www.nrhmhp.gov.in/sites/default/files/files/PMSMA-Guidelines.pdf. [Last accessed November, 2021].
15. Maternal Health Division, Ministry of Health and Family Welfare, Government of India. (2016). Guidelines for Obstetric HDU and ICU. [online] Available from: https://nhm.gov.in/images/pdf/programmes/maternal-health/guidelines/Operational_Guidelines_for_Obstetric_ICUs_and_HDUs.pdf. [Last accessed November, 2021].
16. National Health Mission, MOHFW. (2017). LaQshya (Labour Room Quality Improvement Initiative) [online] Available from: http://nhsrcindia.org/sites/default/files/LaQshya-%20Labour%20Room%20Quality%20Improvement%20Initiative%20Guideline.pdf. [Last accessed November, 2021].
17. Royal College of Anaesthetists. (2018). Care of the critically ill woman in childbirth; enhanced maternal care. [online] Available from: https://www.rcoa.ac.uk/sites/default/files/documents/2020-06/EMC-Guidelines2018.pdf. [Last accessed November, 2021].
18. Ryan M, Hamilton V, Bowen M, McKenna P. The role of a high-dependency unit in a regional obstetric hospital. Anaesthesia. 2000;55:1155-8.
19. Intensive Care Society. (2009). Levels of Critical Care for Adult Patients. Standards and Guidelines. [online] Available from: https://icmwk.com/wp-content/uploads/2014/02/Revised-Levels-of-Care-21-12-09.pdf. [Last accessed November, 2021].
20. Ministry of Health and Family Welfare, Government of India. (2016). Operational guidelines for Obstetrics ICUs and HDUs. [online] Available from: https://nhm.gov.in/images/pdf/programmes/maternal-health/guidelines/Operational_Guidelines_for_Obstetric_ICUs_and_HDUs.pdf. [Last accessed November, 2021].
21. Mhyre JM, D'Oria R, Hameed AB, Lappen JR, Holley SL, Hunter SK, et al. The maternal early warning criteria: a proposal from the national partnership for maternal safety. Obstet Gynecol. 2014;124:782-6.
22. Murthy S, Wunsch H. Clinical review: international comparisons in critical care—lessons learned. Crit Care. 2012;16:218.

LONG QUESTIONS

1. Elaborate on obstetric critical care unit functioning.
2. Define maternal mortality rate. What is the current maternal mortality rate in India? How well has India served in reducing maternal mortality rates over the past few decades?
3. What are the types of specialized care units? Elaborate on each one of them in detail.
4. Explain in detail the criteria for admission to obstetric intensive care units (ICUs) and the high dependency unit (HDU).
5. What are the infrastructure and manpower standards for establishing an obstetric critical unit in India?

SHORT QUESTIONS

1. What are the guiding principles for resuscitating a pregnant woman?
2. Write a short note on the obstetric critical care aspect of the LaQshya initiative.
3. Define Obstetric High Dependency Unit (HDU). How do you differentiate an obstetric Intensive Care Unit from a HDU?
4. Write a short note on the indications of obstetric critical care unit admissions.
5. Give a short description of human resource requirements for obstetric critical care units.

MULTIPLE CHOICE QUESTIONS

1. Criteria for obstetric HDU admission include:
   a. SBP <90 mm Hg, DBP <50 mm Hg, Mean arterial pressure <65 mm Hg
   b. Urine output > 30 mL/h
   c. Respiratory rate >28 breaths/min
   d. Heart rate >120 bpm
2. Admission criteria for obstetric ICU admissions include all, except:
   a. Need for advanced respiratory support
   b. Heart rate <50 or 140 bpm
   c. SaO$_2$ < 90% on supplemental oxygen
   d. GCS < 6 in nontraumatic coma
3. Regarding 'Level of care' defined by Intensive Care Society in 2009, true statement is:
   a. Level 1 includes patients who require normal ward care
   b. Level 1 includes patients with deteriorating conditions and those who require a higher level of care
   c. Level 2 includes patients requiring invasive monitoring/failing organ support for two organs
   d. Level 3 includes patients requiring advanced/basic respiratory support with the support of at least three organs
4. Which of the following statements is correct regarding obstetric ICU and HDU?
   a. HDU and ICU are synonymous with each other regarding the level of care provided
   b. LaQshya initiative strives to operationalize obstetric ICU at medical college and District hospital levels
   c. HDU is an intermediate unit between the obstetric ward and obstetric ICU
   d. The hybrid model incorporates obstetric ward, HDU, and ICU under the same roof in the same setting
5. Requirement of an obstetrical critical care unit for a facility conducting 250 deliveries should be:
   a. 4 HDU beds
   b. 6 HDU + 2 ICU +beds
   c. 8 HDU beds +4 ICU beds
   d. No need for HDU/ICU
6. Minimum space requirement for each bed in an obstetrical critical care unit should be:
   a. 60–80 Sq ft space/bed for HDU and 80–100 Sq ft space for ICU

b. 200–220 Sq ft space/bed for HDU and 220–240 Sq ft space for ICU
   c. 100–120 Sq ft space/bed for HDU and 120–140 Sq ft space for ICU
   d. Space requirement is as per obstetrician's discretion
7. In cardiopulmonary resuscitation of a pregnant woman:
   a. Tracheal intubation can be difficult in pregnant females and should be tried with a wider endotracheal tube
   b. Chest compression to rescue breath ratio should be 30:2
   c. Effective cricoid pressure and the use of H_2 antagonists and antacids reduce the risk of aspiration
   d. Chest compliance increases in pregnancy due to ribs flaring and diaphragm splinting
8. True statement regarding indications of obstetric Intensive care unit admissions:
   a. Systolic blood pressure 20 mm Hg below patient's usual blood pressure
   b. Urine output <160 mL in 8 hours
   c. PaO_2 <7.6 kPa and/or $PaCO_2$ >10 kPa
   d. Serum sodium 115 mmol/L
9. Human resource requirement for obstetric ICU/HDU includes:
   a. 1 intensivist per 4 beds in HDU
   b. 1 medical officer per shift per unit
   c. 2 staff nurses per two beds per shift for HDU
   d. 2 staff nurses per one bed per shift for ICU
10. Which among them is true regarding the LaQshya program?
    a. LaQshya stands for Labor Related Quality Improvement Services
    b. Launched by the Ministry of Child and Women Development, Government of India, in 2017
    c. Aims to improve quality of care in labor rooms and maternity operation theater
    d. All government and private medical college hospitals to have an operational dedicated obstetric ICU

Answers										
1.	b	2.	d	3.	a	4.	c	5.	a	6. c
7.	b	8.	c	9.	b	10.	c			

12.2 MONITORING IN OBSTETRIC HDU AND ICU

Nuzhat Aziz, Siri Yerubandi, Ananth K

INTRODUCTION

Obstetrics is a specialty, which deals with one physiological aspect of the life cycle of a woman. Majority of women go through pregnancy without any complication, but few develop complications which are life-threatening. The evolution of critical care in obstetrics has been responsible for improving outcomes through integration of principles of intensive critical care medicine with obstetric plans. High-dependency unit (HDU) and intensive care unit (ICU) in an obstetric service allow the care to be stratified based on the severity of the conditions and should have well-defined criteria for admission **(Table 1)**.[1] Monitoring in these units has to be appropriate, relevant with optimal utilization of resources. The monitoring must be designed with a scope of early identification of disease worsening. This chapter is designed to give an overview to postgraduates, to understand, and to design an obstetric monitoring system.

PHYSIOLOGICAL CHANGES OF PREGNANCY

Physiological adaptations of pregnancy affect all the organ systems and bring about a change in the normal accepted range of all monitoring parameters, from vital signs to electrocardiography (ECG) to laboratory tests. It is essential to differentiate these physiological changes from pathological causes.[2] The first step towards monitoring of critically ill pregnant women is to summarize the physiological change in parameters commonly used in ICU and HDU in comparison to nonpregnant values **(Table 2)**.

ASSESSMENT AT ADMISSION AND PROGNOSTICATION

Admission scores need to be used at admission to prognosticate and predict mortality, and the most commonly used ones are Acute Physiology and Chronic Health Evaluation (APACHE) II, Simplified Acute Physiology Score (SAPS) II, Sequential Organ Failure Assessment (SOFA), and Multiple Organ Dysfunction Score (MODS).[3] The modified SOFA score is another commonly used scoring system to predict and counsel morbidity and mortality **(Table 3)**. All these systems have multiple parameters and need to be scored on paper or electronically. The shock index is a valuable indicator of shock based on ratio of pulse rate to systolic BP. Normal range is 0.7–0.9 in obstetrics, and any value > 1 signifies significant volume loss.

The quick SOFA (sepsis-related organ function assessment) score is rapid bedside assessment in sepsis, and has only three variables: (1) Change in mental status, (2) respiratory rate > 22 per min and (3) systolic BP < 100 mm Hg **(Table 4)**. Each of these is scored as 1 if present and a combined score of 2 or more predicts ICU stay and mortality. Studies showed that

TABLE 1: Criteria for admission into Obstetric HDU and ICU.[1]

HDU Admission	ICU Admission
☐ **Hemorrhage**	
☐ PPH ☐ Placenta Previa ☐ Abruption ☐ Others	☐ Obstetric hemorrhage with any organ involvement
☐ **Hypertensive disorders**	
☐ Preeclampsia, severe features ☐ Eclampsia ☐ HELLP syndrome	☐ Eclampsia with neurological signs ☐ Status eclampticus
☐ **Sepsis**	
Pregnancy with febrile conditions ☐ Dengue ☐ Malaria ☐ Swine flu ☐ Others	☐ Septic shock
☐ **Renal dysfunction**	
☐ S Creatinine > 1.2 mg/dL ☐ Decreased urine output	☐ Urine output <400 mL in 24 hours, or <160 mL in 8 hours and client unresponsive to simple routine measures
☐ **Jaundice in pregnancy**	☐ **Multiorgan dysfunction**
☐ AFLP ☐ Infective ☐ Others	☐ Two or more organ involvement ☐ Combined SOFA score > 4 ☐ SOFA score > 2 for individual organ
☐ **Coagulation system**	
☐ Thrombocytopenia	☐ Disseminated intravascular coagulation
☐ **Abnormal vitals**	
☐ Any deviation from normal requiring surveillance and observation	☐ GCS <8 (non traumatic coma) ☐ RR <8 and >35 breaths/minute ☐ Heart rate <50 and >140 beats/min ☐ Systolic BP <80 mm Hg, or 30 mm Hg ☐ Systolic BP below patient's usual BP ☐ SaO$_2$ <90% on supplemental oxygen
☐ **ABG abnormalities**	
☐ Any deviation from normal	☐ pH outside the range 7.3 to 7.7 ☐ PaO$_2$ < 6.6 kPa (< 50 mm Hg) ☐ PaCO$_2$ >8.0 kPa (>50 mmHg)
☐ **Electrolyte disturbances**	
☐ Any deviation from normal	☐ S. Sodium outside the range of 110–160 mmol/L ☐ S. potassium outside the range 2.5–5.5 mmol/L
☐ **Medical disorders**	
☐ Neurological ☐ Cardiac diseases ☐ Respiratory ☐ Thromboembolism ☐ Trauma ☐ Poisoning	☐ Any individual organ SOFA score > 2
☐ **Others**	

(ABG: arterial blood gases; AFLP: acute fatty liver of pregnancy; BP: blood pressure; GCS: Glasgow Coma scale; HDU: high-dependency unit; HELLP: hemolysis, elevated liver enzymes, low platelet count; ICU: intensive care unit; PPH: postpartum hemorrhage; RR: respiratory rate; S: serum; SOFA: sequential organ failure assessment)

24% of infected patients with 2 or 3 qSOFA points accounted for 70% of deaths.

DEFINITION OF MONITORING AND ITS ROLE IN OBSTETRICS

Serial or continuous measurements of parameters such as heart rate, respiratory rate, blood pressure, oxygen saturation, and body temperature along with urinary output have been used to assess a person's well-being. These vital signs have been grouped together to give monitoring systems that are better than individual parameters for assessment. The monitoring is also needed for management decisions, to introduce therapeutic interventions, and to assess the impact of these interventions. The monitoring systems in obstetrics differ from the other specialties as there is a fetus with special

TABLE 2: Normal values in pregnancy.		
	Pregnant range	**Nonpregnant**
Vital signs		
Heart rate	60–110	60–100
Systolic blood pressure	90–140	90–140
Diastolic blood pressure	60–90	60–90
Respiratory rate	15–24	12–20
SpO$_2$	95–100	95–100
Temperature	96–99.2	97.1–99.1
Full blood count		
Hemoglobin (g/dL)	10.5–14	12–15
WBC	6000–16,000	4000–11,000
Platelets	150,000–400,000	150,000–400,000
Indices	No change	
Renal function		
Serum creatinine (mg/dL)	0.6–0.9	0.7–1.1
Serum potassium (mmol/L)	3.3–4.1	3.5–5.0
Serum sodium (mmol/L)	130–140	135–145
24 hours proteinuria (g)	<0.3	<0.15
Protein creatinine ratio (mg/mg)	<0.3	<0.3
Liver function tests		
Serum bilirubin (mg/dL)	0–1	0–1
Total protein (g/dL)	4.8–6.4	6.4–8.6
Albumin (g/dL)	2.8–3.7	3.5–4.6
AST (IU/L)	11–30	7–40
Bile acids (µmol/L)	0–14	0–14
Thyroid function tests		
TSH (mU/L)	0.1–4.0	0.3–4.2
fT4 (pmol/L)	10–16	9–26
fT3 (pmol/L)	3–7	2.6–5.7
Respiratory function		
pH	7.40–7.47	7.35–7.45
pO$_2$, mm Hg (kPa)	≤30 (3.6–4.3)	35–40 (4.7–6.0)
pCO$_2$, mm Hg (kPa)	100–104 (12.6–14.0)	90–100 (10.6–14.0)
Base excess	No change	+2 to –2
Bicarbonate (mmol/L)	18–22	20–28
Lactate (mmol/L)	Same cutoffs	<2
Coagulation profile	No change	
Serum electrolytes	No change	

needs. The fetus gets affected by the maternal condition and must be monitored with tools entirely different from the ones used for maternal monitoring. Early warning systems should identify the change from normal to abnormal, from mild to severe sickness and from stable to an unstable state.[4] HDU has those women who are in need of surveillance, who are hemodynamically stable, and not in need of organ support or invasive monitoring. The early warning systems apply very well to women in HDU. The ICU monitoring systems are based on the same principles but require additional parameters to intensively assess organ function or need for organ support.

EARLY WARNING SYSTEMS IN OBSTETRICS AS A MONITORING TOOL IN HDU

The modified obstetric early warning system from the Royal College of Obstetricians and Gynaecologists (MEOWS) was advocated in 2007 **(Fig. 1)**. The alerts were defined, color coded as red and yellow; triggers were one red and two yellow to call for a doctor's review **(Table 5)**. The MEOWS chart was widely used, studied, and adapted to various needs. This system had good sensitivity but a low specificity resulting in overload of triggers in many units. Maternal Early Warning Criteria and Maternal Early Warning Trigger Tool were designed with the aim of decreasing the rate of false alarms, improving specificity for disease worsening and maternal morbidity. The triggers were refined, validated, and the concept of repeat assessment was introduced **(Table 6)**.[5] The aim of monitoring was to improve the prediction of disease worsening and improve outcomes through earlier, prompt identification, and timely appropriate response **(Fig. 2)**. The obstetric team leads the HDU with support from other specialties.

A trigger system should have designed pathways and responses which covers most of the maternal morbidity. The major conditions that have been responsible for maternal morbidity or mortality are hemorrhage, sepsis, hypertension, labor complications, and cardiorespiratory disease. Each of these triggers needs a pathway, which should be evidence based and validated to improve the clinically meaningful outcomes. The Maternal Early Warning Trigger Tool has pathways for an appropriate response to triggers and has shown an effect on decreasing morbidity **(Figs. 3 and 4)**.

All monitoring systems are based on monitoring of vital signs: Level of alertness, heart rate, respiratory rate, blood pressure, temperature, and oxygen saturation. It is important to understand that obstetric early warning scores complement review by senior clinicians, and neither should be used in isolation.

THE VITAL SIGNS

The vital signs have been used traditionally for assessment and monitoring of condition by nurses and doctors; they were only four to start with: (1) pulse, (2) blood pressure,

TABLE 3: Modified Sequential Organ Failure Assessment (SOFA) score.

	0	1	2	3	4
Respiratory* PaO_2/FiO_2	>400	≤400	≤315	≤235	≤150
Liver	No scleral icterus or jaundice			Scleral icterus or jaundice	
Cardiovascular, hypotension	No hypotension	MAP < 70 mm Hg	dopamine≤5 or dobutamine any dose	Dopamine >5 epinephrine ≤0.1 norepinephrine ≤0.1	Dopamine >15 epinephrine >0.1 norepinephrine >0.1
CNS, Glasgow Coma Score	15	13–14	10–12	6–9	<6
Renal, Creatinine mg/dL	<1.2	1.2–1.9	2.0–3.4	3.5–4.9	>5.0

TABLE 4: Quick sepsis-related organ function assessment (qSOFA).

Parameter	Score
Systolic blood pressure < 100 mm Hg	1
Respiratory rate > 22 breaths per minute	1
Altered mental status	1
qSOFA score of 2 or more than 2 warrants ICU admission.	

(3) temperature, and (4) respiratory rate. Oxygen saturation was suggested as a vital sign in 2008; level of consciousness was added to make them six. As the demographics were changing and the concepts of care were evolving, two more parameters were added: (1) pain and (2) urinary output for better assessment and monitoring.[6] The multiparameter monitors usually capture and display the readings and it is important that we all understand the display and significance of recordings **(Fig. 5)**.

Alertness, Pain Scores, and Monitoring of Level of Consciousness

Sick patients can have altered consciousness, unconscious, be in severe pain, or may have been under drug effect. The importance of assessment, monitoring and early detection of worsening cannot be more emphasized. The abbreviated coma scale—AVPU mnemonic is used for primary survey, rapid assessment of state of consciousness. The mnemonic describes the alertness states of A: Alert, V: responsive to verbal commands, P: responsive to painful commands and U: unresponsive.[7] This is the most used assessment tool for all inpatient monitoring. The Glasgow Coma Scale (GCS) is used in ICU for assessment at admission to ICU, prognostication, monitoring over time to assess improvement or worsening. Glasgow Coma scale has four steps: (1) CHECK, (2) OBSERVE, (3) STIMULATE and (4) RATE. Check any factors that may influence assessment, such as sedation, muscle relaxant, or drug effect. Observe spontaneous behavior in the three GCS segments: Eye opening, verbal response, and motor response. Stimulation may be needed sometimes to assess the response; it can be a verbal or pain stimuli. Scoring is done as given in **Table 7**. GCS-P is a modification where the pupillary reaction to light was added. Both pupils unresponsive (2), one pupil unresponsive (1) and both responsive to light (0) was subtracted from the total GSC score to give GCS – P score **(Table 8)**.[8] GCS is scored out of 14 and written as GCS 14, M5, V5, E4 (M for Motor response, V for Verbal response, and E for Eye opening response). All obstetricians must be able to score and assess the state of consciousness.

Pain is usually a subjective complaint. Monitoring over a period may require grading of pain. Pain scores vary from easy one such as Wong-Baker pain scale, numerical pain score to categorical pain score to very elaborate ones such as McGill scale. The smiley based pictorial scale of Wong-Baker is commonly used in awake responsive patients **(Fig. 6)**.[9] In ICU monitoring, different pain scales may be needed for the critically ill may not be able to subjectively assess their pain.

Temperature Monitoring

Monitoring and maintenance of temperature is an important aspect of care of critically ill parturient. Hyperthermia and hypothermia are both important from the perspective of prognosis and care. Peripheral body temperature or core body temperature can be measured, later being more accurate representation but it is invasive. Normal core body temperature range is 97.88–100.4°F (36.6–38°C). Oral and axillary temperature is lower than core body temperature. Axillary temperature is most used, noninvasive, subjected to variations due to sweating, poor placement, and inadequate time. The instrument must be calibrated, be used correctly and the user should be aware of temperature difference between a peripheral measuring site and core body. Temperature of more than 38.3°C (101°F) is called as hyperthermia and <35°C (95°F) is referred to as hypothermia (mild, moderate, and severe). Axillary temperature is lower and rectal temperature

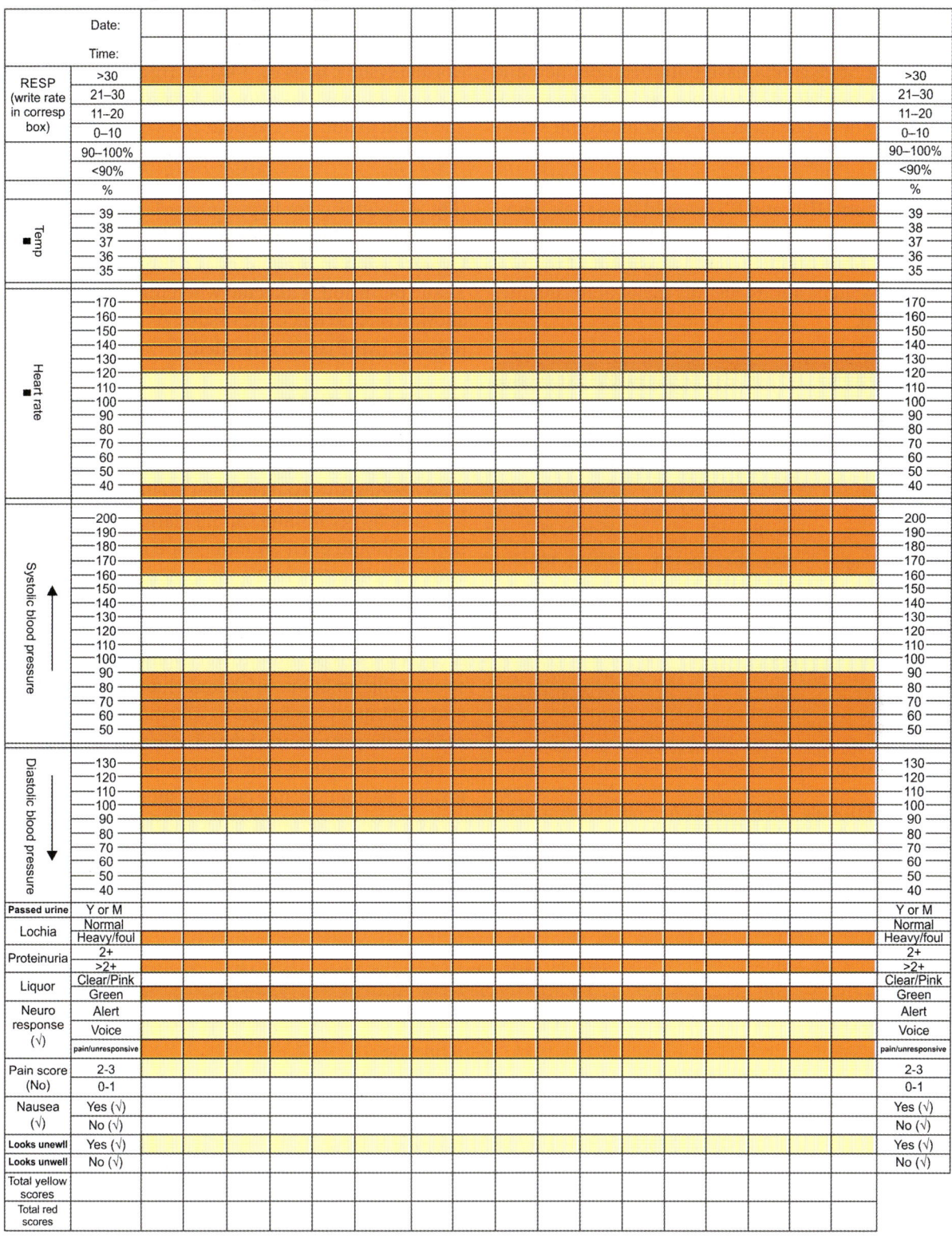

Fig. 1: Early Obstetrics Warning Score.*
*MEOWS chart by Stirling Royal Infirmary, Dr Fiona McIlveney and recommended by CEMACH.

is higher than oral temperature. Rectal temperature is a better reflector of core body temperature.[10] Hypothermia can be due to lower environmental temperature or decreased perfusion or shock. Hyperthermia causes vary from infection to drugs to central nervous system (CNS lesions), which needs to be explored.

Heart Rate

Pulse rate is a clinical measurement and monitoring of pulse, is very much dependent on training and has a high scope of error. Heart rate has almost replaced measuring the pulse rate, as it is more accurate and less prone to human errors. Tachycardia and bradycardia have both been defined and the cutoffs were described for response. The triggers for tachycardia have been placed at 110 per minute and severe trigger response at 130 per minute. Bradycardia is defined as <60 but trigger was placed at <50 per minute for evaluation and response. Every HDU and ICU should have their teams agree on triggers and create alerting systems. Rate cannot be measured without simultaneous assessment of rhythm. Obstetricians should be able to identify major abnormalities of cardiac rhythm.

TABLE 5: Modified early obstetric warning system (MEOWS).

Physiological parameters	Yellow alert	Red alert
Respiration rate	21–30	< 10 or > 30
Oxygen saturation		< 95
Temperature	35–36	< 35 or > 38
Systolic blood pressure	150–160 or 90–100	< 90 or > 160
Diastolic blood pressure	90–100	>100
Heart rate	100–120 or 40–50	>120 or < 40
Pain score	2–3	
Neurological response*	Voice	Unresponsive, pain

Note: Respiration rate (breaths per minute); oxygen saturation (%); temperature (°C); systolic blood pressure (mm Hg); heart rate (beats per minute); level of consciousness is based on the Alert Voice Pain Unresponsive (AVPU) scale which assesses four possible outcomes to measure and record a patient's level of consciousness; pain scores (0 = no pain, 1 = slight pain on movement, 2 = intermittent pain at rest/moderate pain on movement). A single red score or two yellow scores triggers an evaluation.

Blood Pressure

Blood pressure (BP) is the measurement of pressure exerted by the flowing blood against the arterial walls. Noninvasive BP is commonly used in HDU and ICU, but critically ill pregnant women may need invasive arterial BP monitoring. Normal systolic BP is 90–140 mm Hg and normal diastolic BP is accepted as 60–90 mm Hg. Severe triggers for evaluation and rapid action were kept at 160 systolic and 110 diastolic. The evaluation of the abnormal trigger must be made into pathways, as given in the maternal early warning trigger tool (**Fig. 4**—pathway for hypertension). Hypotension is defined across all warning systems as systolic pressure of <90 mm Hg. Hypertension in pregnancy is defined as >140/90 mm Hg. Tissue perfusion is affected when the pressure is not able to allow oxygen to reach the tissues. A minimum mean arterial pressure (MAP) of 65 is needed.

Respiratory Rate

Of all the vital signs, respiratory rate is a marker which is altered by many pathways including acidosis. It is also the most forgotten, missed vital sign in clinical practice. Any value >24 breaths per minute should alarm and any value >30 per minute should elicit an immediate response for evaluation and correction. There is good concurrence in these limits of alarm across most of the early warning systems. Respiratory rate on a ventilated patient may reflect settings. Normal range is 15–24 breaths per minute. Tachypnea may be due to anxiety, stress, inflammation, infection, changes in pH, and cardiac and respiratory dysfunction. Decreased respiratory rate of <15 breaths per minute defined as bradypnea is usually a sign of central nervous system depression or magnesium sulfate toxicity. Respiratory rate changes should always be correlated with clinical background, SpO_2 and if necessary arterial blood gas (ABG). As an example, a woman with severe preeclampsia showing a respiratory rate of 28/min and SpO_2 of 93% would immediately make us suspect pulmonary edema as a possible

TABLE 6: Maternal Early Warning Trigger (MEWT) tool.[5]

	Triggers	Severe triggers
Systolic blood pressure	< 80 or 156–160 mm Hg	
Diastolic blood pressure	< 45 or 106–110 mm Hg	
Heart rate	<50 or 111–130 beats per minute	>130 beats per minute
Respiratory rate	<12 or 25–30 breaths per minute	>30 breaths per minute
Temperature	≤36°C	
Oxygen saturation	90–93 % in room air	<90 %
Altered mental status		
Mean arterial pressure (MAP)		< 55 mm Hg
Nursing clinically uncomfortable with patient status		Yes

Note: A single red trigger or two yellow triggers requires evaluation by provider. Abnormal vital signs must be sustained over at least 20 minutes to be considered triggers.

SECTION 12: Critical Care in Obstetrics

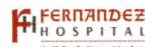

Early warning chart																
Name:				MR No:				☐ Unit	☐ BG HG			☐ Chart No:				
	Date															
	Time															
	Monitoring frequency															
Respiration rate/min –x–	30 or more															
	24–30															
	13–23															
	<12															
O_2 Saturation in % –x–	94 or more															
	93–91															
	90 or less															
Temperature Fahrenheit _G_	105 or more															
	104															
	103															
	102															
	101															
	100															
	99															
	98															
	97 or less															
Pulse rate rate/min _X_	130 or less															
	120															
	110															
	100															
	90															
	70-80															
	60															
	<50															
Systolic BP mm Hg ↑	170 or more															
	160															
	150															
	140															
	130															
	120															
	110															
	100															
	90															
	80 or less															
Diastolic BP mm Hg ↓	120 or more															
	110															
	100															
	90															
	80															
	70															
	60															
	50 of less															
Consciousness wake up the patient if need be –X–	Alert															
	Voice															
	Pain															
	Unresponsive															
Pain socre																
Total intake, mL																
Urine outpurt, mL																
Proteinuria																
Mat weight, kg																
FHR, bpm																
Nurse signature name																

Yellow is alert, Red is for doctors review, Purple is rapid emergency response

Fig. 2: Fernandez Hospital Early Warning Chart (based on MEWT triggers).
(BP: blood pressure; bpm: beats per minute; FHR: fetal heart rate)

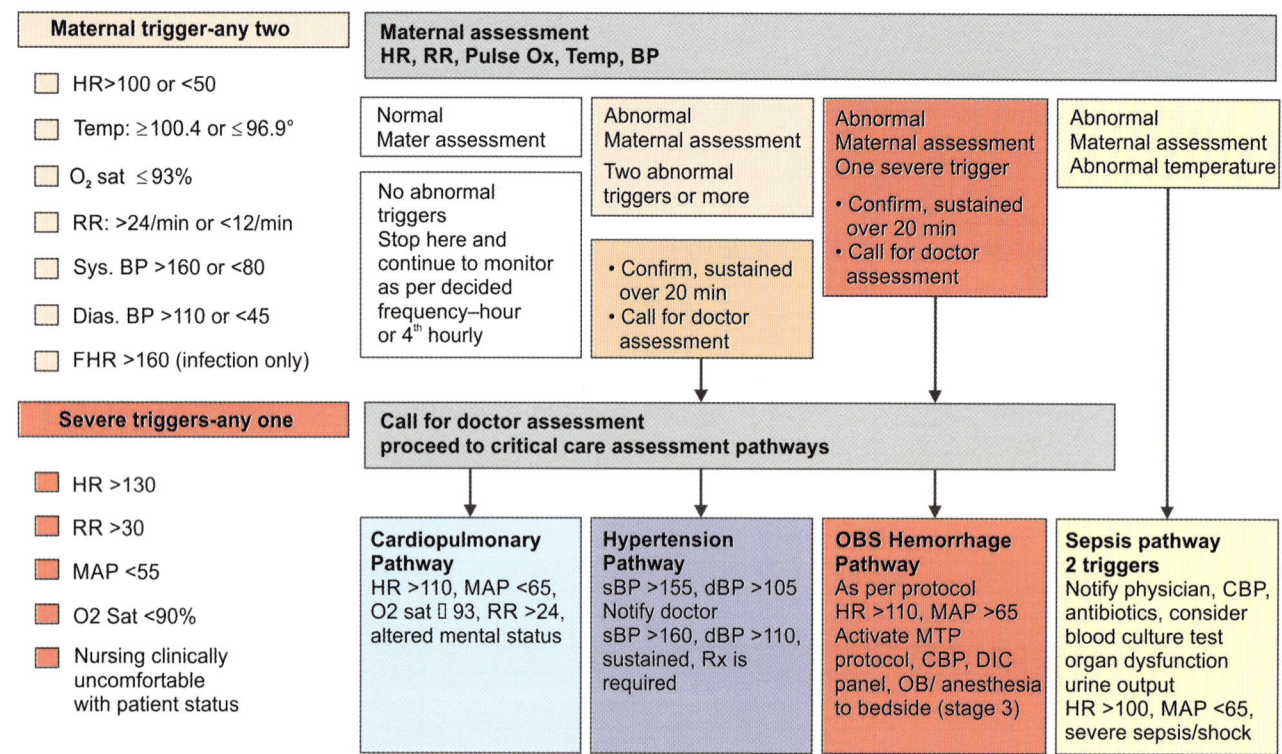

Fig. 3: Maternal Monitoring, Pathways based on Maternal Early Warning Trigger Tool.[5]
(BP: blood pressure; dBP: diastolic BP; CBC: complete blood count; DIC: disseminated intravascular coagulation; ECG: electrocardiography; Echo: echocardiography; HR: heart rate; HTN: hypertension; ICU: intensive care unit; IM: intramuscular; IV: intravenous; LFT: liver function test; MAP: mean arterial pressure; NIBP: noninvasive BP; Ox: oxygen; PPH: postpartum hemorrhage; RR: respiratory rate; sBP: systolic BP)

diagnosis. Associated increased $PaCO_2$ would reflect drug effect or increased intracranial pressure or respiratory failure.

Pulse Oximetry

Noninvasive peripheral oxygen saturations, SpO_2 are extremely useful clinical tool to guide further management and to monitor the respiratory function, or tissue perfusion. It is affected by many external factors and this knowledge is mandatory to prevent false or inappropriate alarms. All hospital in-patient monitoring should include SpO_2, which means that automated machines, which are calibrated and used as first-line monitoring tool. Coronavirus disease 2019 (COVID-19) pandemic has increased the importance of this measurement. Value >95% is regarded as normal. <95% is a trigger and <90% is a severe trigger, warranting rapid response.

Urine Output

Urine output is a very essential bedside monitoring tool in the ICU. It should be monitored with respect to weight and the minimum normal should be 0.5 mL per kg/min. Urine output measurement per hour requires an indwelling catheter and an urometer which has gradings to measure minimum of 5–10 mL. The Urobag alone cannot accurately measure and hence a urometer should be requested for hourly measurement. Decreased urine output should alert us to possible decreased cardiac output, decreased blood volume (prerenal) or renal impairment or post renal injury. Intake output chart should be meticulously maintained. Urine color is also an important monitoring tool in critically ill. Hematuria, hemoglobinuria, and bilirubinemia all have significant and characteristic color changes **(Fig. 7)**.

MONITORING IN THE OBSTETRIC ICU

Monitoring in the critically unwell obstetric patient is to ensure adequate perfusion of oxygen-containing blood to organs and tissues throughout the body including the placenta and the fetus. The Obstetric ICU patient is best managed by a multidisciplinary team (MDT) approach consisting senior clinicians including an intensivist, obstetrician, midwife, neonatologist, and physician with a 1:1 nurse to patient ratio **(Fig. 8)**. The critical care teams lead the ICU, with support from other specialties. The Obstetric ICU patient needs organ support and consequently requires close monitoring of her airway, breathing, circulation, and disability ("ABCD").

The Tools of ICU Monitoring

Tools and options for monitoring in ICU are innumerable, and can be broadly categorized as invasive/noninvasive, less sensitive/more sensitive, less errors/more errors. The best tool would be noninvasive, most accurate, most sensitive, and least scope of errors.[11] Example is pulse oximetry versus pulmonary catheter placement to know the oxygenation

Fernandez Hospital maternal assessment protocol and pathways

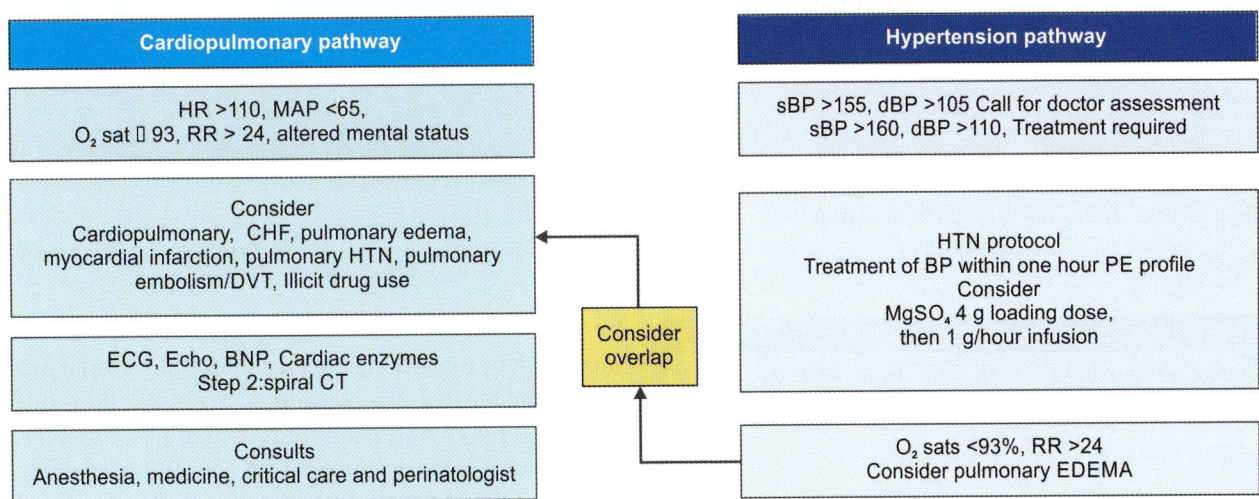

Fernandez hospital maternal assessment protocol and pathways

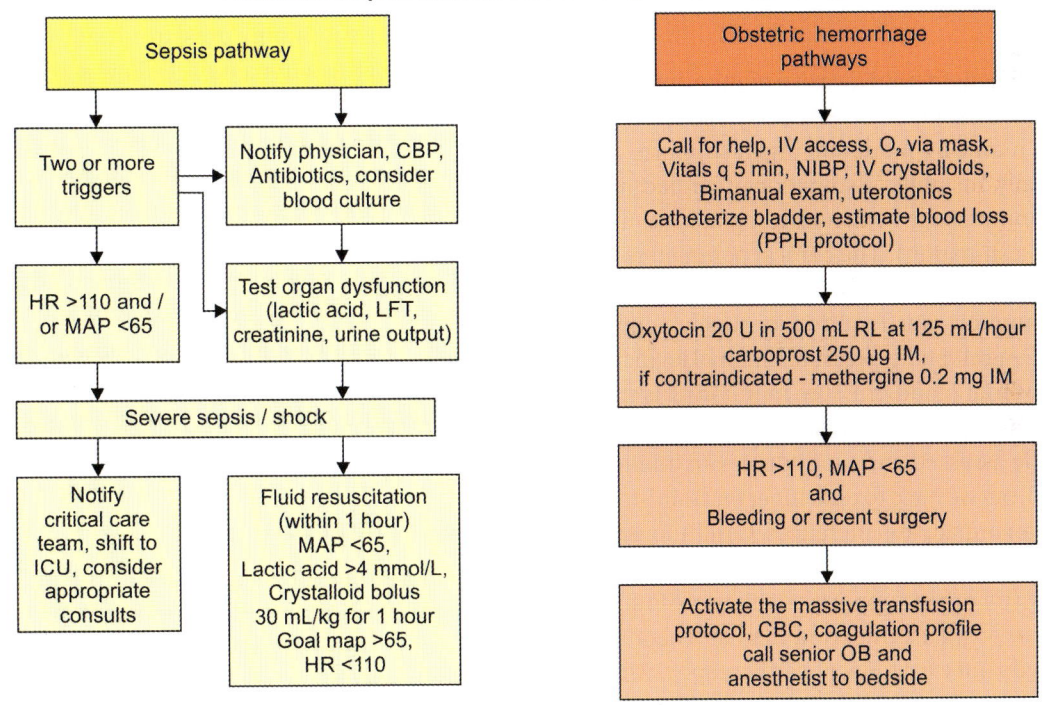

Fig. 4: Response pathways based on MEWT.[5]

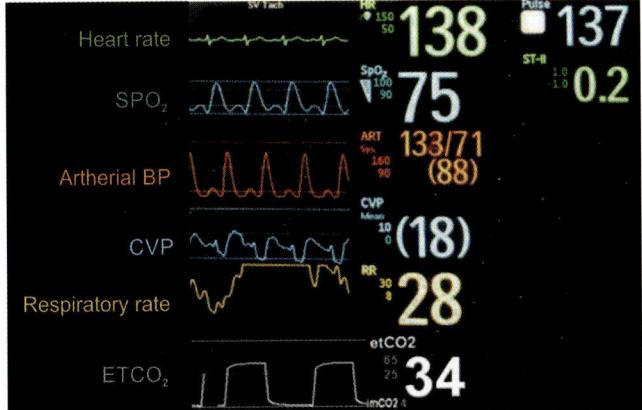

Fig. 5: Learning to interpret the multiparameter monitor. (BP: blood pressure; CVP: central venous pressure)

status of an individual. The measurements are continuous real time and need appropriate display with alarms and graphical display to alert the teams appropriately. The best monitor is the caregiver who amalgamates the information from various monitors, alerts, cutoffs, and clinical condition of the patient to create an appropriate response.

Monitoring and Maintenance of Circulation

The circulation must be monitored at frequent and clinically appropriate intervals by detection of the arterial pulse, ECG display, and measurement of the blood pressure as baseline. Continuous monitoring with the eight vital signs is the noninvasive baseline monitoring for the circulatory system. The noninvasive monitoring helps in identifying

TABLE 7: Glasgow Coma Scale.

	1	2	3	4	5	6
Eyes	Does not open eyes	Opens eyes to painful stimulus	Opens eyes in response voice	Opens eyes spontaneously	N/A	N/A
Verbal	Makes no sounds	Incomprehensible sounds	Inappropriate words	Confused, disoriented	Oriented	N/A
Motor	Makes no movement	Extension to pain	Abnormal flexion to pain	Flexion or withdrawal to pain	Localizes painful stimulus	Obeys commands

TABLE 8: Pupil Reactivity Score (PRS).

Pupils unreactive to light	Pupil reactivity score
Both pupils	2
One pupil	1
Neither pupil	0

GCS-P = GCS − PRS
(GCS: Glasgow Coma Scale; GCS: GCS Pupils Score)

women, who will benefit from invasive monitoring. Critically ill parturient benefit from invasive hemodynamic monitoring when they are requiring moderate organ supports and are hemodynamically unstable.[12] Estimation of cardiac output in ICU is done noninvasively by Echocardiography and $ETCO_2$ (End Tidal CO_2 estimation). The clinical parameters are not helpful when rapid cardiovascular circulation changes occur, and invasive monitoring is required for timely appropriate interventions. Central venous pressure (internal jugular) along with invasive arterial blood pressure monitoring is the most useful in monitoring and guiding decisions. Blood volume depletion can be assessed and monitored with inferior vena cava ultrasound, but we need to remember that third-trimester gravid uterus can impact the inferences. Continuous cardiac output monitoring devices are available and can be used if she is requiring stiff organ supports and they are found to be more effective in postpartum period than antenatal period. The drawbacks do not exist for echocardiography, which can give good information, irrespective of the gravid status.[13]

Arterial Invasive BP Monitoring

The need for continuous measurement of arterial pressure and frequent laboratory testing (especially of ABG) are the primary indications for arterial cannulation. Invasive (intra-arterial) blood pressure (IBP) monitoring is a commonly used technique in the ICU and the operating theater.[14] It involves the insertion of a catheter into a suitable artery under strict asepsis, using a stiff saline-filled tubing to connect to a transducer and then displaying the measured pressure wave on a monitor. Radial artery is most commonly cannulated and brachial artery should be avoided as occlusion of the brachial artery will result in loss of blood supply to the lower arm.

A pressure transducer is attached to give systolic, diastolic, and the MAP. Calculation of MAP is done either by using the formula of diastolic pressure + one-third pulse pressure or measured by integrating the area under the arterial pressure waveform. MAP of 65 is considered a resuscitation end point to ensure tissue perfusion, but MAP of 55 or less leads to hypoxia and acidosis. Invasive BP is useful in patients who are likely to display sudden changes in blood pressure (cardiac arrhythmia), in whom close control of blood pressure is required (e.g., preeclampsia), or in patients receiving drugs to maintain the blood pressure (e.g., patients receiving inotropes such as adrenaline). It allows accurate measurement of blood pressure at low pressures. Validated techniques (in the nonobstetric population) allow intravascular volume status and cardiac output to be estimated from the shape of the arterial pressure trace through the attachment of a specific device, e.g., a pulse contour analysis system. It is extremely helpful in patients with gross peripheral edema or morbidly obese patients, where noninvasive BP measurement is not feasible. The risks of invasive BP monitoring are infection, thrombus, or embolism. It is important to label this port as ARTERIAL line and not for injecting drugs.

Central Venous Pressure and Pulmonary Artery Pressure Monitoring

Central venous pressure (CVP) and pulmonary artery pressure (PAP) monitoring are useful in the management of patients with hemodynamic compromise in the ICU.[15] Treatment decisions are based on being able to distinguish between preload, afterload, and contractility, as per the Starling's forces.[16] CVP is the pressure within the intrathoracic venae cavae measured by the insertion of a catheter using a landmark or an ultrasound-guided approach. The internal jugular or subclavian veins are cannulated with maintenance of strict asepsis and in the presence of skilled assistance. CVP is normally equal to the right atrial pressure (mean right atrial pressure = 3–8 mm Hg). This pressure varies with the cardiac cycle, with breathing, and on change of position between upright and recumbent. PAP is measured by insertion of a flotation catheter, usually via an internal jugular or subclavian vein, not commonly used in obstetrics.

Benefits of central venous line is good IV access, administration of medications that require central access, e.g., amiodarone, inotropes, high concentration electrolytes (e.g., potassium) is possible via the central venous catheter.

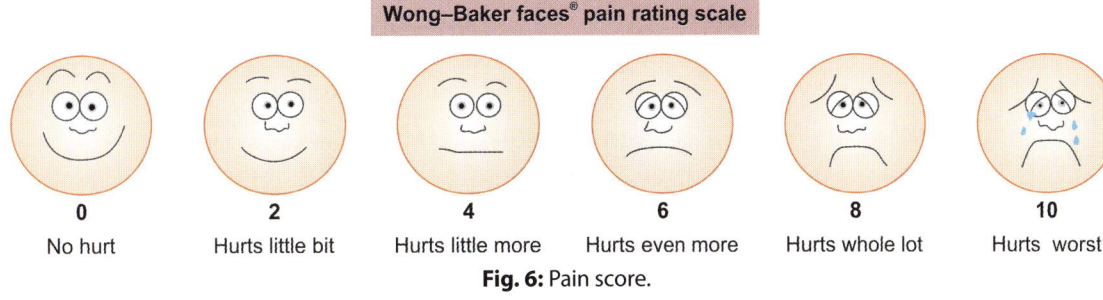

Fig. 6: Pain score.

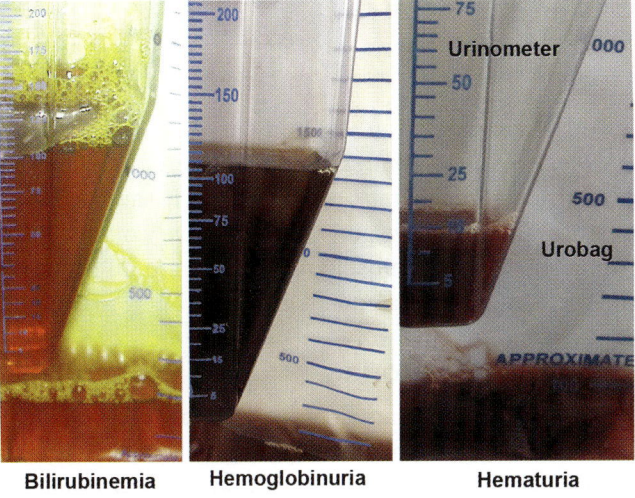

Fig. 7: Monitoring the color of urine.

Fluid balance can be monitored with CVP and PAP as indirect measures of cardiovascular filling.

Risks associated with invasive monitoring are blood vessel injury (internal carotid artery, subclavian artery, or aortic arch), local hematoma, hemothorax, cardiac tamponade, cerebral ischemia, or upper limb ischemia. Very rarely dysrhythmias, nerve injury, pneumothorax, cardiac chamber perforation, valve injury, infection and thrombotic complications must be monitored as possible complications of this catheter.[17,18]

Tissue Perfusion Assessment and Monitoring

Tissue perfusion is the end point of the circulatory organ function, failure of tissue perfusion leads to accumulation of toxic metabolites, cellular dysfunction, tissue injury, organ injury and cardiac failure.[19] Pulse oximetry is a noninvasive means of checking peripheral oxygenation, but gets affected by lot of external factors. Serial monitoring of the blood gases, lactate, mixed and central venous oxygenation saturations, CO_2 gap are few ways of assessing adequacy of tissue perfusion. Lactate is an end product of anaerobic metabolism and is a good marker of cellular hypoxia and tissue hypoperfusion. Cutoff values of 2 mmol/L and 4 mmol/L have been used as a marker for prognosis. Improvement in lactate levels over time has been proven to be associated with improved prognosis. Lactate is also used as near miss criteria and in many prognostic scoring systems.

Monitoring Respiratory Function

The physiological vital signs do direct toward an abnormality in the respiratory function. SpO_2 is regarded as the fifth vital sign but it reflects oxygenation and not ventilation. Any deviation of these vital signs requires ABG to estimate the functioning of gas exchange process in the body. ABG sample can be obtained easily and analyzed very rapidly; basic analyzer gives the PaO_2, $PaCO_2$, pH, HCO_3, base deficit **(Fig. 9)**. The PaO_2/FiO_2 ratio determines the extent of acute lung injury and can be calculated from these measurements; a value <200 signifying poor gas exchange. This ratio has also become a part of definitions for acute lung injury (ALI <300) and acute respiratory distress syndrome (ARDS < 200). PaO_2/FiO_2 ratio calculation is shown in **Figure 10**.

■ MONITORING THE RENAL FUNCTION

Laboratory monitoring of renal function is done through timed measurement of serum creatinine, blood urea, blood urea nitrogen (BUN), serum electrolytes; with ABG providing the acid–base monitoring. Many other parameters may be used in specific cases, but these tests should be available as part of baseline monitoring.

Monitoring of Glycemia

Studies have shown that critically ill patients have fluctuating glycemic control and hyperglycemia and hypoglycemia has been shown to be prognosticators for mortality. Intensive glucose control versus nonintensive control has been debated over the past few years. The frequency of glucose monitoring is required depending on the condition of the patient and glycemic stability. The use of bedside glucometers may not be the best way of assessment but is least invasive in a patient who has not got invasive monitoring lines. Arterial line sample would be the best if there are invasive monitoring catheters in place. Special precautions to be remembered about flush solution and prevention of infection. The range of 70–180 mg/dL is accepted as the recommended standard.

Monitoring of Nutrition

Patients admitted after injury or infection to ICU show a phase of ebb where the nutritional requirement lowers for a period of 48 hours followed by a flow phase where the needs are

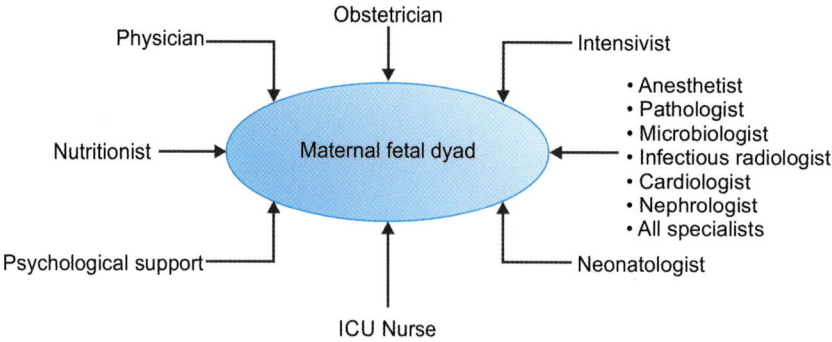

Fig. 8: Monitoring in ICU is a multidisciplinary team effort.
(ICU: intensive care unit)

Normal values we must know in ABG

37.0°C		Normal
pH	7.081	7.40 to 7.74
PCO₂	29.7 mm Hg	≤30
PO₂	113 mm Hg	100 to 104
BEecf	–21 mmol/L	+2 to –2
HCO₃	8.8 mmol/L	18 to 22
TCO₂	10 mmol/L	
sO₂	96 %	95 to 100
Lac	1.68 mmol/L	<2

Fig. 9: Normal values of ABG in pregnancy.
(ABG: arterial blood gases)

P divided by F = P/F Ratio
"P" is PaO₂ (arterial pO₂) From ABG
"F" is the FiO₂ – the fraction of inspired oxygen
Expressed as a decimal; example 40% oxygen = FiO₂ of 0.040

Room air has 21% oxygen – FiO₂ 0.21%
Each liter adds 4% of oxygen
FiO₂ When on 5 liters of O₂ = 21% + 20% = 41% = 0.41

Example 1: ABG show PaO₂ of 90, on room air (FiO₂ 0.21)
P/F ratio is 90/0.21 = 428
Example 1: ABG PaO₂ of 90 on 6 liters of O₂ (0.21+0.24)
P/F ratio is 90/0.45 = 200

Fig. 10: Calculation of PaO₂/FiO₂ Ratio.
(ABG: arterial blood gases)

increased. If the patient does not recover and come out of ICU, the catabolism deters the exit. Many studies have shown focus on nutritional needs help in preventing catabolic states and allow for faster ICU and post ICU care.

Physical Examination

Physical examination has an important role in ICU and should never be missed. Peripheral edema and rapid weight gain signifies cardiac failure, hypoproteinemia, decreased oncotic pressure, or altered capillary permeability. Weight measurement may be difficult in sick patients on organ support. Capillary refill time is also a reflection of perfusion of peripheries and will be reduced when there is decreased blood flow or vasoconstriction. Assessment of alertness, psyche, neurological assessment, skin temperature, oral hygiene, eye care, auscultation of lungs, pressure areas for any redness or pressure effect, invasive port sites, operative wounds, gastric distension, and calf muscle tenderness are all important aspects of monitoring a patient in ICU.

Laboratory Monitoring

Various laboratory parameters are used to monitor critically ill patients. ABG, serum electrolytes, and lactate are used for monitoring the oxygen exchange and acid–base balance. Organ function assessments with hemogram, renal function, liver function tests, ammonia levels, and coagulation tests are ordered almost daily in women with organ failure. Glycemic control and nutritional status monitoring are also needed and should not be neglected. Evaluation and control of infection may require cultures to be done, as per the condition or as per the needs of invasive testing and organ supports.

Fetal Monitoring

Maternal resuscitation and monitoring is the priority in a sick or a critically ill parturient. Fetal monitoring is done by handheld Doppler and a nonstress test, if the fetus is beyond the period of viability. Ultrasound can be done for fetal assessment, which aids in appropriate counseling and decision-making.

Psychological Monitoring

Admission to an ICU has a powerful psychological impact on the women and her family. This impact is profound if the woman experiences pregnancy loss. The ICU environment was found to be stressful as they experience pain, interventions, lack of privacy, inability to communicate, loneliness, and fear of death. Psychological support would be an added help to patient, their families and to the ICU staff. The assessment should include underlying disorders, depression, anxiety, panic episodes, nightmares, flashback, and support to prevent psychological morbidity which aid recovery in critical care units.

Monitoring Charts

High-dependency unit has patients which require intermittent monitoring depending on the indication for admission. Early warning charts can be continued for HDU care since the patients do not have multiorgan failure or need invasive monitoring (*see* **Fig. 1**). ICU monitoring sheets have many additional scales to be assessed and hence need different monitoring charts. The capturing of data is now moving into electronic medical records either by manual entry or by direct connection of the monitor to capture the details.

■ CONCLUSION

Meticulous monitoring of critically ill and prompt and timely intervention is most important for survival. Assessment and monitoring must be regular, frequent, and should be plotted on a chart or be real time on a monitor. Frequency of monitoring depends on severity of illness and organ failure. Monitoring is essential for data capture, documentation, early warning of adverse trends, assessment of effect of interventions, and most importantly, this data is valuable for integration into patient management and care. The monitoring is best possible when every member of the team is well versed with protocols and monitoring algorithms. It will be complete only when staffing is adequate and appropriate. Teaching and training should be an integral part of any ICU team. Importance of measurement cannot be more emphasized; data gathering, and analysis is crucial.

■ REFERENCES

1. National Health Mission. (2017). Operational Guidelines for Obstetric ICUs and HDUs. [online] Available from: https://nhm.gov.in/images/pdf/programmes/maternal-health/guidelines/Operational_Guidelines_for_Obstetric_ICUs_and_HDUs.pdf. [Last accessed November, 2021].
2. Soma-Pillay P, Nelson-Piercy C, Tolppanen H, Mebazaa A. Physiological changes in pregnancy. Cardiovasc J Afr. 2016;27(2):89-94.
3. Aarvold ABR, Ryan HM, Magee LA, von Dadelszen P, Fjell C, Walley KR. Multiple organ dysfunction score is superior to the obstetric-specific sepsis in obstetrics score in predicting mortality in septic obstetric patients. Crit Care Med. 2017;45(1):e49-57.
4. Royal College of Anaesthetists. (2018).Care of the critically ill woman in childbirth; enhanced maternal care [online] Available from: https://www.rcoa.ac.uk/sites/default/files/documents/2019-09/EMC-Guidelines2018.pdf. [Last accessed November, 2021].
5. Shields LE, Wiesner S, Klein C, et. Use of maternal early warning trigger tool reduces maternal morbidity. Am J Obstet Gynecol 2016;214:527.e1-6.
6. Elliott M, Coventry A. Critical care: the eight vital signs of patient monitoring. Br J Nurs. 2012;21(10):621-5.
7. Romanelli D, Farrell MW. AVPU Score. Treasure Island (FL): StatPearls Publishing; 2020.
8. Brennan PM, Murray GD, Teasdale GM. Simplifying the use of prognostic information in traumatic brain injury. Part 1: The GCS-Pupils score: an extended index of clinical severity J Neurosurg. 2018;128:1612-20.
9. Hockenberry MJ, Wilson D (eds). Pain Assessment and Management. Wong's nursing care of infants and children, 10th edition. Mosby.
10. Lefrant JY, Muller L, de La Coussaye JE, Benbabaali M, Lebris C, Zeitoun N, et al. Temperature measurement in intensive care patients: Comparison of urinary bladder, oesophageal, rectal, axillary, and inguinal methods versus pulmonary artery core method. Intensive Care Med. 2003;29:414-8.
11. Vincent JL, Rhodes A, Perel A, Martin GS, Della Rocca G, Vallet B, et al. Clinical review : Update on hemodynamic monitoring - a consensus of 16. Crit Care. 2011;15:229.
12. Invasive hemodynamic monitoring in obstetrics and gynecology. ACOG Technical Bulletin Number 175 - December 1992. Int J Gynaecol Obstet. 1993;42:199-205.
13. Karim HM, Mitra JK, Bhattacharyya P, Roy J. Significance of hemodynamic monitoring in perioperative and critical care management in obstetric practice. Astrocyte. 2015;1:295-300.
14. Gupta B. (2012). Invasive blood pressure monitoring. Update in Anaesthesia. [online] Available from: https://www.wfsahq.org/components/com_virtual_library/media/81574a863feeed2ee3ac5c8c824ab4e0-35c06d5dc14372e5d743d057a889ab42-Invasive-Blood-Pressure-Monitoring--Update-28-2012-.pdf. [Last accessed November, 2021].
15. Pandya ST, Mangalampally K. Critical care in obstetrics. Indian J Anaesth. 2018;62(9):724-33.
16. Gilbert M. Central venous pressure and pulmonary artery pressure monitoring. Anaesth. Intensive Care Med. 2018;19(4): 189-93.
17. Shah MR, Hasselblad V, Stevenson LW, Binanay C, O'Connor CM, Sopko G, et al. Impact of the pulmonary artery catheter in critically ill patients: meta-analysis of randomized clinical trials. JAMA. 2005;294:1664-70.
18. Harvey S, Harrison DA, Singer M, Ashcroft J, Jones CM, Elbourne D, et al. Assessment of the clinical effectiveness of pulmonary artery catheters in management of patients in intensive care (PAC-Man): a randomised controlled trial. Lancet. 2005;366:472-7.
19. Hasanin A, Mukhtar A, Nassar, H. Perfusion indices revisited. J Intensive Care. 2017;4:24.

■ LONG QUESTIONS

1. Explain the monitoring of obstetric patient in HDU.
2. Discuss the monitoring of obstetric patient in ICU.
3. What are the indications for HDU and ICU admissions in obstetrics?

■ SHORT QUESTIONS

1. Mention the vital signs.
2. What is Quick SOFA score?
3. What is shock index?
4. Explain invasive hemodynamic monitoring in obstetrics along with its advantages and complications.
5. What are early warning obstetric systems?

MULTIPLE CHOICE QUESTIONS

1. Severe hypertension in pregnancy is defined as:
   a. Systolic BP of 140 mm Hg
   b. Systolic BP of 160 mm Hg
   c. Diastolic BP of 90 mm Hg
   d. None of the above
2. Which is not a vital sign?
   a. Heart rate
   b. Temperature
   c. Mean arterial pressure
   d. Respiratory rate
3. Which one of the following is criterion for admission into ICU?
   a. Respiratory rate >35 breaths per minute
   b. Systolic BP <80 mm Hg
   c. Urine output <400 mL in 24 hours
   d. All of the above
4. Which of the following is a parameter of qSOFA score?
   a. Glasgow Coma scale
   b. Creatinine
   c. Icterus
   d. Altered mental status
5. Which of the following is not normal in ABG analysis?
   a. pH: 7.4–7.47
   b. HCO$_3$ – 18–22
   c. Lactate >4
   d. None of the above

Answers
1. b 2. c 3. d 4. d 5. c

12.3 FLUID AND BLOOD THERAPY IN OBSTETRIC SHOCK

Jyotsna Suri, Divya Pandey

INTRODUCTION

Shock is an emergent clinical condition of circulatory collapse leading to impaired tissue oxygenation eventually leading to cellular dysfunction or death if there is no intervention. Treating shock in pregnancy is very challenging because of the physiological changes of pregnancy, which make the interpretation of the clinical picture difficult, and also changes the goals of treatment. Moreover, rapid response to shock is very crucial for preventing not only maternal morbidity and mortality but also fetal mortality.

PHYSIOLOGICAL CHANGES DURING PREGNANCY

There are certain physiological changes in maternal hemodynamics. Cardiac output (CO) and blood volume increases while systemic vascular resistance (SVR) and blood pressure reduces.[1] The impact of these changes in relation to shock and its management is shown in **Table 1**.

SHOCK AND ITS PATHOPHYSIOLOGY

"*Shock*" is an emergency clinical condition characterized by failure of circulation causing diminished tissue oxygenation and eventually dysfunction at cellular level often leading to death.

To understand the pathophysiology, it is important to know the concept of oxygen delivery. Oxygen delivery (DO$_2$) is calculated using the following equation

$$DO_2 (mL\ O_2/min) = Cardiac\ output\ (L/min) \times Hb\ (g/L) \times 1.34\ (mL\ O_2/g\ Hb) \times \%\ Oxygen\ saturation$$

Thus, DO$_2$ is directly proportional to cardiac output (stroke volume × Heart rate), hemoglobin concentration (Hb) and oxygen saturation. This can help in comprehending the actual pathophysiology behind all kinds of shock, which remains, "diminished tissue oxygenation." This understanding will help in better shock management. **Figure 1** depicts different classes, the pathophysiology behind, and causes of shock.

FLUID THERAPY IN SHOCK

Fluid Resuscitation

Fluid resuscitation refers to rapid fluid administration (in form of intravenous bolus) to patient with unstable hemodynamics. Conventionally, Mean Arterial Pressure (MAP) <60 mm Hg or Central Venous Pressure (CVP) <8 mm Hg without cardiogenic pulmonary edema is indication for immediate fluid administration. The *therapeutic aim of fluid resuscitation* is to increase preload or the stressed venous volume leading to improvement in stroke volume hence cardiac output. Fluid resuscitation is indicated in hypovolemic and septic shock in obstetric patient (**Flowchart 1**).

Estimation of Fluid Responsiveness

Fluid responsiveness has been defined as a 10% or greater increase in stroke volume in response to rapid infusion of 500 mL of fluid over 10–15 minutes.[2]

Fluid load leading to stroke volume change (dynamic parameter) can precisely tell about fluid responsiveness as compared to static parameters such as CVP and MAP.[2]

Many recent studies have advocated Passive Leg Raise (PLR) maneuver to assess volume/fluid responsiveness. In fact,

TABLE 1: Physiological and anatomical changes in the cardiovascular system during pregnancy and postpartum and its impact on shock.

Parameter	Change	Antenatal period	Labor	Postpartum	Clinical implication
Plasma volume	Increase 50%	Increases from 6 weeks, peaks 30–32 weeks	Remains same	There is fall due to blood loss	Signs of shock may not appear till almost 25% of blood loss
Stroke volume	Increase 20%	Increases from early pregnancy Peaks at 20 weeks, gradually falls	During straining in second stage (Valsalva) there is a fall	Normal in 6 weeks	
Heart rate	Increase 15–20 bpm	Rise more in second half	Further rise seen	Prelabor level by 1 hour; normal in 6–12 weeks	Interpretation of early signs of shock is difficult
Arterial blood pressure*	Decrease 10–15%	Declines by 5–10 mm Hg in second T, normal values in 3rd T	Rise by 10–25% during contractions	Normal values	Interpretation of hemodynamic changes in shock is challenging
Cardiac output†	Increase 40%	Increases from 8 weeks, peaks at 32 weeks	Further increase by 25–50%	Immediate postpartum rise by 80%†; prelabor level in 1 hour; Normal by 6–12 weeks	Interpretation of hemodynamic changes in shock is challenging
Uterine blood flow	~10% of Cardiac output at term	–	–	–	APH and PPH can exsanguinate a patient within 1–2 hours
Colloid oncotic pressure	Falls in pregnancy	–	–	Reaches a nadir in 6–16 hours and becomes normal after 24 hours	More susceptible to fluid overload and pulmonary edema in pregnancy and postpartum and more so in preeclampsia

*The decrease in blood pressure during pregnancy is mainly secondary to a fall in the diastolic component which in turn is due to decrease in systemic vascular resistance due to progesterone, and the development of the placenta, a low resistance vascular bed.
†The increased cardiac output that develops in pregnancy is further augmented during the third stage of labor as a result of autotransfusion of blood from the uteroplacental to maternal circulation as the uterus contracts
(APH: antepartum hemorrhage; PPH: postpartum hemorrhage)

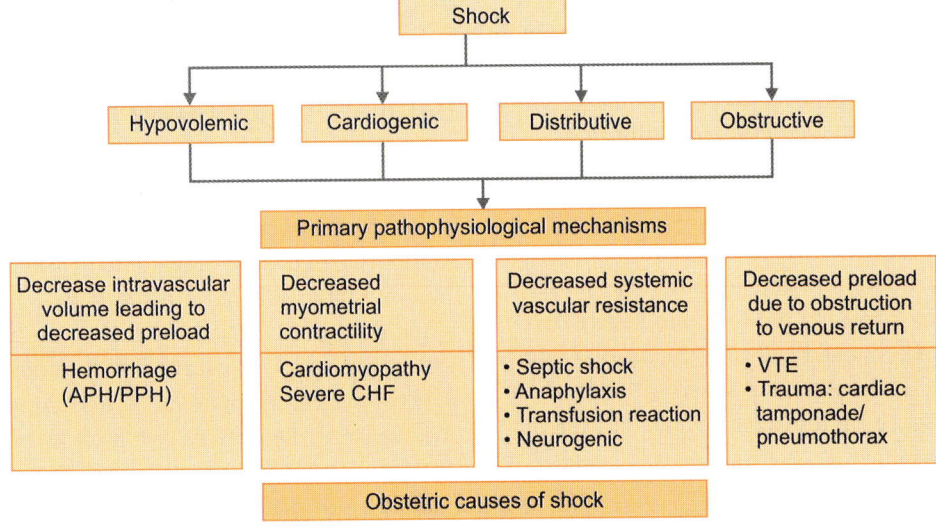

Flowchart 1: Classification of shock, with the primary pathophysiological mechanism, and different causes of obstetric shock.

(APH: antepartum hemorrhage; CHF: congestive heart failure; PPH: postpartum hemorrhage; VTE: venous thromboembolism)

PLR is the best tool to predict volume and fluid responsiveness in a spontaneously breathing patient.[3,4]

In PLR test, fluid load (challenge) is given by shifting venous blood (about 300 mL) from lower extremities to right side of the heart. Thus, it can predict whether cardiac output can improve after volume expansion. And since the hemodynamic response so obtained is quickly reversible, it practically negates the risk associated with fluid overload.[5,6]

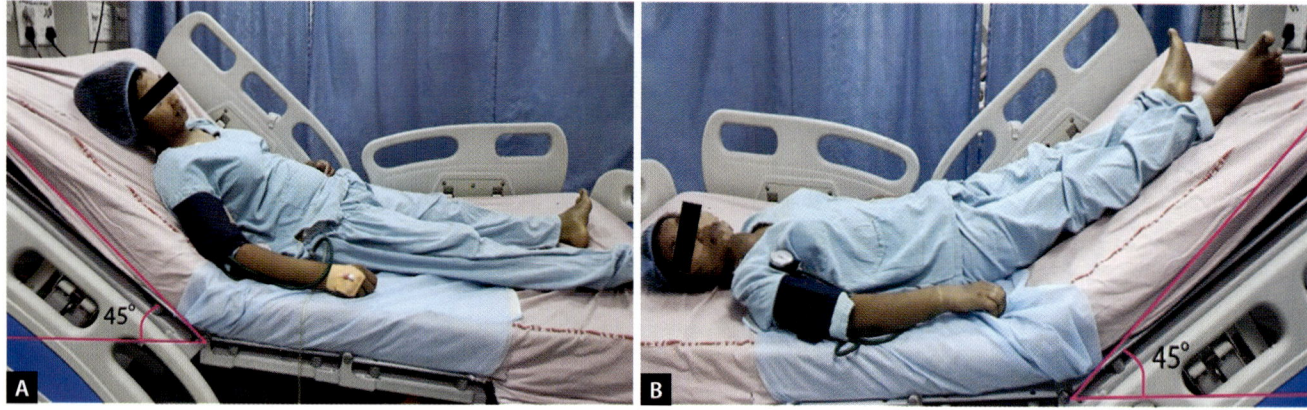

Figs. 1A and B: Demonstration of passive leg raising test.

Ultrasonographic assessment of collapsibility of inferior vena cava during inspiration, using an ECHO (echocardiography) probe is another dynamic noninvasive bedside test to assess fluid responsiveness.[3]

How is PLR test done?
This dynamic bedside clinical test with high sensitivity and specificity is very simple. The patient is kept in 45° head up posture and BP is checked. This is followed by posture change to 45° leg up position. BP is checked again after 5 minutes in this position. More than 9% difference in *pulse pressure* (Diastolic BP-Systolic BP) indicates that the patient is fluid responsive and will benefit from fluid resuscitation **(Fig. 1)**. The test is repeated after every volume infusion to check whether additional volume will be helpful without posing risk of pulmonary edema.[6]

Estimation of Blood Loss in Hypovolemic Shock

The blood loss estimation in order to replace it adequately by fluid and blood products remains the cornerstone of the treatment strategy. The various clinical parameters which reflect the amount of blood loss are given in **Table 2**.

Types of Resuscitative Fluids

Crystalloids and colloids are the main resuscitative fluids available. The main differences and types of these fluids are mentioned in **Tables 3 to 5**. In moderate-to-severe degree of hemorrhagic shock, packed cells are the fluid of choice **(Table 2)**. However, in shock due to sepsis or hemorrhage, crystalloids should be used as resuscitative fluid till availability of the blood components.

Choice between Crystalloids and Colloids for Fluid Resuscitation

Colloids have no benefit over crystalloids for fluid resuscitation. In fact, they may exacerbate dilution coagulopathy due to fibrin polymerization and platelet aggregation.[7,8] Colloids should not be used as initial management of shock due to sepsis or hemorrhage.[9] Moreover, colloids may lead to mortality due to anaphylaxis, coagulopathy, and acute renal injury (especially by HES). In fact, HES is contraindicated in septic shock due to risk of acute renal injury and sometimes even mortality.[10,11] The solutes in the colloids have tendency to enter the interstitial space, causing third space loss which in turn leads to low intravascular volume.

Normal saline (NS) and Ringer lactate (RL) are the crystalloids fluid of choice but have a minimal risk of normal anion gap metabolic acidosis of uncertain significance in the event of transfusion of a very large amount. Owing to its physiologic resemblance to plasma, RL is an excellent resuscitative fluid. It is relatively contraindicated in hyperkalemia. Due to binding tendency of calcium in RL, with citrate in blood, it should not be given along with blood transfusion. Dextrose 5% is although isotonic, yet after its infusion, the glucose metabolizes to form free water and makes it hypotonic. Thus, its large volume transfusion can lead to cellular edema. Thus, it should never be used as a resuscitative fluid.

Optimal Dosing of Fluid Therapy

Resuscitative fluids are administered in boluses. Central or peripheral venous line maintained with 14 or 16-G cannula is used for fluid resuscitation. In absence of Congestive Heart Failure (CHF) or End-Stage Renal Disease (ESRD), One-two liters of fluid can be administered to a patient in shock. The initial fluid bolus dose is 30 mL/kg body weight in patients with septic shock. However, the fluid bolus dose adjustment may vary as per the patients' status. For mild CHF or ESRD, it is decreased to 500 to 1 liter while for women with severe CHF; the bolus has to be decreased to 250–500 mL. After each bolus, reassessment of the clinical parameters is a must. For balanced management of shock without fluid overload risk, the fluid responsiveness can be gauged by PLR test after every bolus.

End Point of Fluid Resuscitation

The end point of fluid resuscitation can be assessed by the following parameters: (1) Mean arterial pressure ≥ 65 mm Hg,

TABLE 2: Estimation of blood loss by clinical parameters.

Parameters	Compensation	Mild	Moderate	Severe
Blood loss	15%	15–30%	30–40%	>40%
Nonpregnant (mL)	750	1,000	1,500	2,000
Pregnant (mL)	<1000	1,000–2,000	2,000–2,700	>2,700
Respiratory rate (per min)	14–20	20–30	30–40	>40
Heart rate (per min)	<100	>100	>120	>140
SBP (systolic blood pressure)	No change	Minor (postural) fall (80–100 mm Hg)	Marked fall (70–80 mm Hg)	Profound fall (<70 mm Hg)
DBP (diastolic blood pressure)	No change	Increased	Decreased	Decreased
Mental status	Anxious	Anxious	Restless/confused/agitate	Lethargic
Urine (mL/h)	>30	20–30	5–15	Negligible
Fluid of choice	crystalloid	Crystalloid/Blood products	Blood products	Blood products

TABLE 3: Properties of crystalloids and colloids.

Crystalloids	Colloids
Small solute molecules which exert low oncotic pressure	Large solute molecules hence exert considerable oncotic pressure
These fluids have low tendency to stay intravascular (about 30 minutes)	These have high tendency to remain intravascular (for 24 hours)
Administered in the ratio of 1:3	Administered in the ratio of 1:1
Used in immediate fluid resuscitation of lost volume.	Can be used in situation of massive blood loss till blood products are available or in severe hypovolemia
For example: Ringer lactate Normal saline Dextrose 5%	For example: Natural colloids Human albumin Synthetic Dextran Hydroxyethyl starch

TABLE 4: Composition of different crystalloids and their properties.

Fluid	pH	Na$^+$ mEq/L	Cl$^-$ mEq/L	K$^+$ mEq/L	Ca^{2+} mEq/L	Other	mOsm/L	Comments
0.9%NaCl NS	5.5	154	154	0	0	0	308	Choice replacement fluid, hypercholeremic acidosis to be watched for
Ringer lactate (RL)	6.5	130	109	4	3	Lactate 28 Eq/L	275	Choice replacement fluid
Dextrose 5% (D5%)	4.5	0	0	0	0	Dextrose 50 g/L	285	Free water hypotonic
D5%RL	5	130	109	4	3	Dextrose 50 g/L	275	Initial postoperative replacement
D5%NS	4	154	154	0	0	Dextrose 50 g/L	308	Initial postoperative replacement
D5%NS 0.45%	4	77	77	0	0	Dextrose 50 g/L	154 + 285	Hypotonic
D5%NS2.5%	4	34	34	0	0	Dextrose 50 g/L	68+285	Hypotonic

TABLE 5: Composition of different colloids and their properties.

Fluid	pH	Average molecular weight (kD)	Oncotic pressure (mm Hg)	Initial volume expansion (%)	Duration of volume expansion
4–5% Albumin	6.9	69	20–30	70–100	12–24
25% Albumin	6.9	69	70–100	300–500	12–24
Dextran 40	4.5	40	20–60	100–200	1–2
6% Hydroxyethyl starch (Hestar, HES)	5.5	450	25030	100–200	8–36

(2) urine output ≥ 0.5 mL/kg/h, (3) central venous pressure 8–12 mm Hg, (4) normalization of lactate levels, and (5) improvement of mental state.

BLOOD AND COMPONENT THERAPY

The World Health Organization (WHO) strategy stresses upon decreasing unnecessary transfusions. This inappropriate blood transfusion rate is around 15–45%. This is attributed to improper timing of transfusion (very early or very late) or even unindicated transfusions. Thus, judicious use of blood component therapy is the need of the hour.

Aims of blood component therapy are: (1) restoration of intravascular volume; (2) restoration and enhancement of the oxygen carrying capacity by red blood cells replacement; (3) replacement of clotting factor; and (4) anemia correction.

Significant blood loss resulting in symptomatic reduced oxygen-carrying capacity is an indication of blood transfusion. In acute blood loss, the indications of blood transfusion are: (1) Moderate-to-severe shock, (2) diastolic blood pressure < 60 mm Hg (3) fall of systolic blood pressure by >30 mm Hg (4) oliguria/anuria suggestive of acute renal failure; (5) tachycardia (>100 beats/min) (6) altered mentation, (7) shortness of breath, light-headedness or dizziness with mild exertion.

Concept of Component Therapy

In modern practice, blood component therapy is recommended and the practice of whole blood use in hypovolemic shock has been condemned. Whole blood has a short shelf-life of only 7 days due to inactivation of platelets, factor V, and factor VIII after 24 hours. Moreover with segregation of blood into its components, one unit of blood can help many patients. Even the storage requirement of different components varies. Whole blood needs to be stored at 4–6°C, red cells at 4°C, platelets at 22–24°C, fresh frozen plasma (FFP) at –30 to –40°C, cryoprecipitate at –30 to –40°C. Moreover, the shelf-life of different components is different. It is 35–40 days for red blood cells, 1 year for FFP/cryoprecipitate while for platelets and white blood cells, it is 5 days and 2 days, respectively. Thus, it is seen that when whole blood is transfused, FFP and cryoprecipitate have already lost its function and there is wastage of FFP and cryoprecipitate, which could have been used for other patient. The transfusion of extra volume should also be avoided. Precisely, plasma expanders are required for correction of hypovolemia, packed cells are required for increasing oxygen-carrying capacity, FFP and cryoprecipitate for clotting factors and platelets for correction of thrombocytopenia.

Massive Transfusion Protocol

Massive transfusion has been conventionally defined as transfusion of 10 units of red cells in 24 hours, due to uncontrolled hemorrhage. In modern practice, alternative definitions are three units of packed cells' transfusion over 1 hour or any four blood components' transfusion in 30 minutes. Massive transfusion protocol is used for managing massive obstetric hemorrhage by the use of blood component therapy. In patients who need massive transfusion, resuscitation must start at the earliest for prevention of dilutional coagulopathy, with rule of 4. As per this protocol, transfusion is done in a ratio of four units packed cells: 4 units of FFP: Four units of platelets and four units of cryoprecipitate. Two intravenous lines should be placed; through first-line packed cells transfusions should be given and through second one cryoprecipitate, platelets and FFP should be given. The risks of massive transfusion include hypothermia and hyperkalemia. Hypothermia can be prevented by infusing blood through blood warmer, whereas hyperkalemia can be prevented by using blood less than 10 days old and also by washing the red cells to remove the extracellular potassium prior to transfusion.

BLOOD TRANSFUSION IN SPECIAL CONDITIONS

- *Postoperative period:* In hemodynamically stable patients, transfusion should be considered if Hb ≤ 8 g/dL or in presence of symptoms of insufficient oxygen delivery (chest pain of cardiac origin, orthostatic hypotension or tachycardia unresponsive to fluid resuscitation or congestive heart failure).[12]
- *Patients in the intensive care unit and with sepsis:* In critically ill, normovolemic patients, transfusion is considered at an Hb level of ≤7 mg/dL with a target of 7–9 g/dL.[13]
- During the early stage of severe sepsis, in presence of evidence of inadequate tissue perfusion, blood transfusion is considered to achieve a target Hb of 9–10 g/dL.
- In the later stages of severe sepsis, the recommendations are similar as for critically ill patients with target Hb of 7–9 g/dL.
- Blood transfusion (BT) should not be used to assist weaning from mechanical ventilation if the Hb is >7 g/dL.

Key Features of Various Blood Products

Whole Blood

With 350 mL volume, one whole blood unit raises hemoglobin by 1 g/dL and hematocrit by 3%. It must be used where packed red blood concentrates (PRBCs) are not available. Whole blood transfusion must not be used to stop bleeding due to coagulopathies. Transfusion must be initiated within 30 minutes of removal from refrigerator. The transfusion rate should be 150–200 mL/h and it must complete within 4 hours (unit to be discarded if this period has exceeded). ABO and Rh compatibility and cross-matching are a must. However, in an emergency, till compatible blood availability, O negative blood can be used.

Packed Red Blood Cell Concentrates (PRBCs)/Packed Cell Volume (PCV)/Red Cell Concentrates (RCC)/Plasma Reduced Blood (PRB)

One unit of PRBC, with 200 mL volume, increases hemoglobin by 1 g/dL and hematocrit by 3%.[14] The indications of its use are severe decompensated maternal anemia during pregnancy, severe acute blood loss after vaginal or cesarean delivery, intrapartum Hb <7 g%, replacement of acute blood loss in obstetric hemorrhage along with other components and postpartum anemia with signs of shock. It has to be used within 30 minutes of removal from refrigerator and should be transfused within 4 hours (unit to be discarded if this period has exceeded). The transfusion rate must be between 150–200 mL/h. The target Hb to be achieved is 7–9 g/dL. ABO and Rh compatibility and cross-matching must be done prior. In clinical emergency, till compatible blood availability, O negative blood can be used.

Platelet-rich Plasma (FFP)

One platelet-rich plasma (PRP) unit has 50–70 mL volume and increases platelet count by $5-8 \times 10^9$/L. One platelet apheresis unit increases platelet by $40-50x \times 0^9$/L. It is indicated in bleeding due to thrombocytopenia, with count $<50 \times 10^9$/L where surgery or delivery is anticipated and cases where platelet count is $<20 \times 10^9$/L. The rate of transfusion must be between 50 and 150 mL/h. PRP unit must be transfused immediately and should be completed within 30 minutes of removal from optimal storage condition. The target platelet count to be attained is 50×10^9/L. ABO and Rh compatibility is needed.[14]

Fresh Frozen Plasma

One unit of FFP has 50–70 mL volume and 1 mL of FFP contains 1 unit of coagulation factor activity.[14] It is indicated for replacement of multiple coagulation factors, Disseminated Intravascular Coagulation (DIC), repletion of coagulation factors in massive blood transfusions and warfarin overdose. The dose of FFP is 12–15 mL/kg. The rate of transfusion is kept between 150–300 mL/h. The transfusion must start as soon as possible, or maximum within 6 hours of thawing but must be completed within 30 minutes. The transfusion goal is to attain target prothrombin time (PT) and activated partial thromboplastin time (APTT), international normalized ratio (INR) <1.5. ABO compatibility is needed; however cross-matching is not required. If an Rh-negative woman has received Rh-positive FFP, Anti-D prophylaxis is not needed.

Cryoprecipitate

It is indicated in correction of microvascular bleeding in massively transfused patients with hypofibrinogenemia. This is specifically needed in patients who seek fluid restriction. The rate of transfusion is kept between 150 and 300 mL/h. The transfusion must start as soon as possible, or maximum within 6 hours of thawing but must be completed within 30 minutes. The target is to attain fibrinogen level >150 mg/dL. Though ABO compatibility is preferred, it is not essential. One unit/10 kg body weight raises plasma fibrinogen by 50 mg/dL. Anti-D prophylaxis is not required, if Rh-negative women receive Rh-positive cryoprecipitate.

Recombinant Factor VIIa

It is a promising new alternative to blood component therapy. The mechanism of action is to enhance the intrinsic clotting pathway by binding with tissue factor and directly activating factors IX and X. Its use may be considered as a treatment for unremitting life-threatening postpartum hemorrhage (PPH) at a dose of 50–100 μg/kg intravenously every 2 hours until hemostasis is attained, with majority of patients needing only one dose.[15] It is essential to maintain adequate platelets' and clotting factors' level because recombinant factor VIIa (rFVIIa) increases clotting by acting on these subtrates.[16] As the drug is derived from recombinant technology, there is no risk of viral transmission. The serious side effect of thromboembolism limits its use in clinical practice.

Checklist for Blood Transfusion[16,17]

- Informed consent should be taken. Reason for transfusion and signature of the person administering should be clearly mentioned in case sheet.
- Verification of patient/component compatibility and identity should be done by two people, at least one of whom should be a doctor or registered nurse. Donation number on blood bag label should match the accompanying document.
- Check blood bag for signs of hemolysis, clotting, or contamination
- Check for any leaks/seal/discoloration. BT SET: must be new (170–200 μ filter). Change the set at least 12 hourly during BT or after every four units of blood.
- Record the volume and type of blood products transfused, unique donation number of all products transfused, blood group, time of start and completion of transfusion and any adverse effect.
- Use slow infusion through 21–25-G cannulas; for rapid infusion, use large-bore cannulas, e.g., 14 G.
- Platelets should be administered before *red cell concentrate* (RCC) with same set and if it is to be used after RCC transfusion, use a separate BT set.
- Before the start of BT, record baseline observations: General condition, temperature, pulse rate, blood pressure, respiratory rate, and fluid balance (intake/output charting).
- Monitoring is continued 15 minutes after starting transfusion, at least every hour during transfusion and on completion of transfusion and 4 hours after completion of transfusion.

- There is no evidence of benefit of warming blood, when transfusion is slow. Keeping patient warm is more important than warming the blood. Warmed blood is needed for large-volume rapid transfusion in adults > 50 mL/kg/hr.
- Routine use of premedication is not recommended.
- Use separate IV line for fluids or IV drugs.
- If a patient needs more than three units of blood within 24 hours, then calcium must be administered.

Transfusion Reactions

Acute transfusion reactions must be recognized and managed efficiently. The severity of the reactions can be categorized as mild, moderate, and severe category.

Category 1: Mild—The earliest sign is urticarial rash leading to pruritus due to hypersensitivity reaction. On recognition, the transfusion should be slowed and antihistamine should be administered intramuscularly. If there is no improvement within 30 minutes or there is worsening, treat as moderate category.

Category 2: Moderately severe—Presents with flushing, urticaria, rigors, fever, restlessness and tachycardia. Patient complains of anxiety, pruritus, palpitations, mild breathlessness, and headache. Transfusion should be stopped immediately. This is due to hypersensitivity or febrile-nonhemolytic transfusion reaction. Airway should be managed and oxygen administered. The blood unit with BT set, freshly collected urine, and new blood sample (plain and EDTA vial) should be returned to the blood bank. Antihistamine, IV corticosteroid, and bronchodilators (if bronchospasm) should be given. If there is clinical improvement, restart the transfusion slowly with new blood unit. However, if there is no clinical improvement within 15 minutes or there is worsening, treat as category 3. Collect urine for next 24 hours for evidence of hemolysis. If available, WBC filter may be used in repeated transfusion.

Category 3: Life-Threatening—Rigors, fever, restlessness, hypotension, tachycardia, hemoglobinuria and unexplained bleeding [disseminated intravascular coagulation (DIC)]. The patient may complain of anxiety, chest pain, pain along transfusion line, respiratory difficulty, loin/back pain, and headache. The reason for severe reaction may be acute intravascular hemolysis, bacterial contamination, septic shock, fluid overload, anaphylaxis, or transfusion-related acute lung injury (TRALI). On recognition of this category, stop transfusion and manage as in category 2. Adrenaline (1:1,000) can be given in the dose of 0.01 mg/kg body weight, as slow intramuscular injection. Senior doctor must be notified. New blood sample should be sent. 24-hour urine sampling should be done and intake output monitoring to be done. Bleeding from puncture sites and wounds should be assessed to rule out DIC. If patient is hypotensive, crystalloids and/or inotropes should be given. Acute renal failure (ARF) and bacteremia should be managed (if present).

In all cases of reactions:
- Report all BT reactions to blood bank and doctor responsible for the patient.
- Record, type of transfusion, time between start of transfusion and reaction; volume transfused and bag number.
- Immediately take blood sample from different site for—repeat ABO/Rh/antibody screen and cross-match, complete blood count (CBC), coagulation screen, urea and creatinine, electrolyte.
- Return to blood bank: Blood bag and BT set, blood culture in blood culture bottle, first specimen of patient's urine following reaction and completed transfusion reaction form.

KEY MESSAGES

- Dynamic tests passive leg raising test and inferior vena cava collapsibility by ECHO are preferred over static tests [central venous pressure(CVP)] to determine fluid responsiveness.
- IV fluids should be administered in discrete boluses through a wide-bore short cannula.
- Initial fluid replacement should be with an isotonic crystalloid solution (Grade 1A).
- Lactated Ringer or normal saline are fluids of choice for resuscitation in shock and are almost comparable.
- D5 W should never be used as a resuscitative fluid.
- For patients with severe hemorrhagic hypovolemia, red blood cell transfusions are an appropriate choice for initial volume resuscitation.
- Component therapy is far superior to administering whole blood.
- Massive blood transfusion uses the rule of 4 to prevent dilution coagulopathy. This entails transfusion of packed RBC, FFP, and PRP in a ratio of 4:4:4 units.
- The risks of massive blood transfusion includes hypothermia and hyperkalemia.
- Blood should be transfused after informed consent and a checklist should be followed strictly.
- Transfusion reactions should be identified and managed aggressively.

REFERENCES

1. Tomlinson M, Cotton D. Fluid management in the complicated obstetric patient. Globlibr Women's Med. 2008.
2. Assadi F. Passive leg raising: simple and reliable technique to prevent fluid overload in critically ill patients. Int J Prev Med. 2017;8:48.
3. Mackenzie DC, Noble VE. Assessing volume status and fluid responsiveness in the emergency department. Clin Exp Emerg Med. 2014;1(2):67-77.

4. Marik PE, Levitov A, Young A, Andrews L. The use of bioreactance and carotid Doppler to determine volume responsiveness and blood flow redistribution following passive leg raising in hemodynamically unstable patients. Chest. 2013;143(2):364-70
5. Jabot J, Teboul JL, Richard C, Monnet X. Passive leg raising for predicting fluid responsiveness: importance of the postural change. Intensive Care Med. 2009;35(1):85-90.
6. Monnet X, Teboul JL. Passive leg raising: Five rules, not a drop of fluid! Crit care. 2015;19(1):18.
7. Haase N, Perner A, Hennings LI, Siegemund M, Lauridsen B, Wetterslev M, et al. Hydroxyethyl starch 130/0.38-0.45 versus crystalloid or albumin in patients with sepsis: systematic review with meta-analysis and trial sequential analysis. BMJ. 2013;346:f839.
8. Lewis SR, Pritchard MW, Evans DJ, Butler AR, Alderson P, Smith AF, et al. Colloids versus crystalloids for fluid resuscitation in critically ill people. Cochrane Database Syst Rev. 2018;8:CD000567.
9. Muñoz M, Stensballe J, Ducloy-Bouthors A-S, Bonnet M-P, De Robertis E, InoFornet, et al. Patient blood management in Obstetrics: Prevention and treatment of post partum hemorrhage. A NATA Consensus statement. Blood Transfus. 2019;17:112-36.
10. Young P, Bailey M, Beasley R, Henderson S, Mackle D, McArthur C, et al. Effect of a buffered crystalloid solution versus saline on acute kidney injury among patients in Intensive care Unit: The SPLIT randomised clinical trial. JAMA. 2015;314(16):1701-10.
11. Allen SJ. Fluid therapy and outcome: balance is best. J Extra Corpor Technol. 2014;46(1):28-32.
12. Carson JL, Grossman BJ, Kleinman S, Tinmouth AT, Marques MB, Fung MK, et al. Red blood cell transfusion: a clinical practice guideline from the AABB. Ann Intern Med. 2012;157(1):49-58.
13. Retter A, Wyncoll D, Pearse R, Carson D, McKechnie S, Stanworth S, et al. Guidelines on the management of anaemia and red cell transfusion in adult critically ill patients. Br J Haematol. 2013;160:445-64.
14. Blood Transfusion in Obstetrics. Green-top Guideline No. 47. (2015). [online] Available from: https://www.rcog.org.uk/globalassets/documents/guidelines/gtg-47.pdf. [Last accessed November, 2021].
15. Fuller AJ, Bucklin B. Blood component therapy on Obstetrics. Obstetrics and Gynecology Clinics of North America. 2007; 34:443-58.
16. World Health Organization; Blood Transfusion Safety. The Clinical Use of Blood. [online] Available from: https://www.who.int/bloodsafety/clinical_use/en/Handbook_EN.pdf. [Last accessed November, 2021].
17. Padhi S, Kemmis-Betty S, Rajesh S, Hill J, Murphy MF. Guideline Development Group. Blood transfusion: summary of NICE guidance. BMJ. 2015;351.

LONG QUESTIONS

1. Write the pathophysiology of Obstetric Shock and outline the principle of its management?
2. What are the indications of different blood components?
3. What is transfusion reaction and how it is managed?

SHORT QUESTIONS

Write short notes on
1. Classification of Shock
2. Fluid responsiveness
3. Crystalloids and colloids
4. Fluid resuscitation
5. Massive blood transfusion

MULTIPLE CHOICE QUESTIONS

1. All of the following are crystalloids, except:
    a. 0.9% Normal saline   b. Ringer lactate
    c. 5% Albumin   d. Dextrose 5%
2. The adequacy of fluid resuscitation can be assessed reliably by all, except:
    a. MAP >65 mm Hg
    b. Urine output >0.5 mL/kg/hr
    c. Normalization of lactate levels
    d. Heart rate
3. Which of the following is true?
    a. Dextrose 5% should never be used as a resuscitative fluid
    b. Dextrose 5% is preferred fluid in pre-eclamptics
    c. RL can be given with blood transfusion
    d. Normal saline does not cause abnormal anion gap metabolic acidosis
4. What is false for colloids?
    a. Colloids can lead to anaphylaxis
    b. There may be aggravation of coagulation abnormalities
    c. They have low tendency to stay intravascular (about 30 minutes)
    d. Crystalloids have better safety profile over colloids
5. Which is the incorrect match?
    Blood component—shelf life
    a. Packed cells—40 days
    b. Platelets—30 days
    c. FFP—1 year
    d. Cryoprecipitate—1 year
6. Which is correct for massive transfusion protocol?
    a. PRBC:FFP:PRP—4:4:4
    b. PRBC:FFP:PRP—6:4:4
    c. PRBC:FFP:PRP—4:8:8
    d. PRBC:FFP:PRP—1:4:4
7. Which is the incorrect match?
    Blood component—storage temperature
    a. Whole blood—4-6°C
    b. FFP—-30 to -40°C
    c. Platelets—4 to 6°C
    d. Cryoprecipitate—-30 to -40°C
8. Which of the following is not a colloid?
    a. RL   b. Albumin
    c. Dextran   d. Hestar

9. What is not correct about Ringer lactate solution?
   a. Ph—6.5
   b. Sodium—130 mEq/L
   c. Lactate—28 mEq/L
   d. Potassium—10 mEq/L
10. What is shock index?
    a. HR × DBP
    b. HR × SBP
    c. SBP/MAP
    d. HR/SBP

Answers										
1. c	2. d	3. a	4. c	5. b	6. a
7. c	8. a	9. d	10. d

12.4 SUDDEN OBSTETRIC COLLAPSE

Alpesh Gandhi, Amita Gandhi

■ INTRODUCTION

Maternal collapse is a rare but life-threatening event with a wide range of etiology. The outcome for the mother and also for the fetus depends on prompt and effective resuscitation. Maternal collapse is defined as an acute event involving the cardiorespiratory system and/or brain resulting in a reduced or absent conscious level (and potentially death) at any stage in pregnancy and up to 6 weeks after delivery. The incidence of maternal collapse or severe maternal morbidity is unknown as morbidity data are not routinely collected. A recent publication from Dublin showed a severe maternal morbidity rate of 3.2/1,000 (320/100,000) births. In the last triennium in the UK, the maternal mortality rate was 14/100,000 births, but again not all maternal deaths are preceded by maternal collapse. The true rate of maternal collapse lies between 0.14 and 6/1000 (14 and 600/100,000) births.[1] Cardiac arrest in pregnancy is rarely encountered and considered to occur in 1:30,000 births.[2] Cardiopulmonary arrest in the pregnant woman triggers highly emotional reactions and can put the parturient at risk. There are four different levels of care to which the obstetric patient can be taken depending on her condition:

1. *Level 0:* Normal ward care
2. *Level 1:* Patients whose condition is at risk of deteriorating
3. *Level 2:* Patients requiring invasive monitoring/intervention or single organ failure support
4. *Level 3:* Patients requiring advanced respiratory support with support of more than one organ.

Patients requiring care at level 2 and level 3 are likely to develop sudden collapse, but any pregnant woman can develop sudden collapse at any time during the pregnancy.

■ CLINICAL CAUSES

There are many causes of sudden obstetric collapse, which may be pregnancy related or result from condiotions not related to pregnancy and possibly existing before pregnancy. Inclusion of all causes of the obstetric collapse is beyond the scope of the chapter, but the common causes of maternal collapse are discussed in the following text.

Hemorrhage

Hemorrhage is one of the most common causes of maternal collapse and is responsible for most maternal deaths. Causes of major obstetric hemorrhage are postpartum hemorrhage (PPH) and antepartum hemorrhage (APH) from placenta previa/accreta, placental abruption, uterine rupture and ectopic pregnancy. In most cases of massive hemorrhage leading to collapse, the cause is obvious, but the concealed hemorrhage should not be forgotten, including following cesarean section and ruptured ectopic pregnancy. Other rare causes of concealed hemorrhage include splenic rupture and hepatic rupture. Acute inversion of the uterus may also be a cause following improper conduct of the third stage of labor. Resuscitation includes establishment of respiration and restoration of blood volume deficit and arrest of the source of hemorrhage.

Eclampsia

Eclampsia as a cause of maternal collapse is usually obvious in patient settings; often the diagnosis of preeclampsia has already been made when the seizure occurs. Epilepsy should also always be considered in cases of maternal collapse associated with seizure activity. Resuscitation includes correction of airway, control of seizures and blood pressure, and delivery.

Amniotic Fluid Embolism

Amniotic fluid embolism (AFE) presents as collapse during labor, delivery or within 30 minutes of delivery in the form of acute hypotension, respiratory distress, and acute hypoxia. Seizures and cardiac arrest may occur. Pulmonary hypertension may develop secondary to vascular occlusion, by both debris or vasoconstriction followed by left ventricular failure and often giving rise to massive PPH. If AFE occurs prior to delivery, profound fetal distress develops acutely. Speedy resuscitation with oxygen administration, positive-pressure ventilation, intravenous fluids, vasopressors and, if the fetus is undelivered, immediate delivery should be undertaken. In case of hemorrhage, replacement with red cells, platelets, fresh frozen plasma, cryoprecipitate or fibrinogen is done according to the need.

Pulmonary Thromboembolism

Women with a clinical suspicion of deep vein thrombosis may develop release of thrombus. Pulmonary embolism occurs due to a thrombus blocking a pulmonary artery, which causes sudden onset of dyspnea, chest pain, and features of collapse. Prompt resuscitation and antithrombotic therapy must be started immediately.

Sepsis

Sepsis has been recognized for centuries as a significant cause of maternal morbidity and mortality. Bacteremia, which may be present even in the absence of pyrexia or a raised white cell count, can progress rapidly to severe septic shock, leading to collapse. Management includes resuscitation, broad-spectrum antibiotic coverage and removal of septic foci.

Cardiac Disease

The majority of deaths secondary to cardiac causes occur in women with no previous history. The main causes of death are myocardial infarction, aortic dissection, and cardiomyopathy.

Intracranial Hemorrhage

Intracranial hemorrhage is a significant complication of uncontrolled systolic hypertension with severe headache followed by maternal collapse.

Anaphylaxis

Anaphylaxis is a severely, life-threatening, generalized or systemic reaction resulting in respiratory, cutaneous and circulatory changes and possibly gastrointestinal disturbances and collapse. Prompt resuscitation with arrest of anaphylaxis is the key to management.

Drug Toxicity and Overdoses

Drug toxicity and overdoses should be considered in all cases of obstetric collapse; and illicit drug overdose should be considered as a potential cause of collapse in the hospital, as should magnesium sulfate in the presence of renal impairment or local anesthetic agents injected intravenously by accident.

PHYSIOLOGICAL CHANGES IN PREGNANCY AFFECT RESUSCITATION

There are a number of reasons why the processes of cardiopulmonary resuscitation (CPR) are more difficult to perform and may be less effective in the pregnant compared with the nonpregnant population. Gradually increasing uterus size compromises resuscitative efforts. This may be the case from 20 weeks onward but will be more marked as the mother approaches term.

Cardiac Output

Cardiac output increases by as much as 50% by 32 weeks' gestation. At 20 weeks, significant aortocaval compression compromises venous return, and at 30 weeks' gestation, the woman has a significant drop in blood pressure when lying supine.

Vena Caval occlusion

After 20 weeks' gestation, the pregnant woman's uterus can compress the inferior vena cava and the aorta, impeding venous return, cardiac output, and uterine perfusion. The vena cava is completely occluded in 90% of term pregnant women lying supine and the stroke volume may be only 30% of that of a nonpregnant woman. Therefore, in late pregnancy, cardiac output can be increased by as much as 25–30% simply by moving the patient in a left lateral decubitus position.[3] Delivery of the fetus during cardiac arrest will reduce the oxygen demands on the mother, empty the uterus, and thus also increase the venous return to the heart, making it more probable that resuscitation will be successful.

Changes in Lung Function

The pregnant uterus and increased breast size lead to a 20% decrease in functional residual capacity and 45% decrease in chest compliance. With such limited reserve and 20% increased oxygen consumption, there can be a rapid decline in oxygen saturation following hypoventilation.

The presence of mucosal edema and friability, increased secretions and weight gain, all contribute to a more difficult airway intubation. There is also a greater risk of aspiration due to the relaxation of the esophageal sphincter. Passive regurgitation of stomach contents is a very real concern as it is greater in volume and more acidic during pregnancy and, therefore, more likely to lead to damaging acid aspiration into the lungs. It is imperative that experienced staff provide a protected airway and adequate ventilation as quickly as possible following cardiac arrest.

Management

Cardiac arrest management has four main steps:
1. Immediate resuscitation.

2. Supportive management is undertaken immediately once CPR is effective and mother is resuscitated. Move the patient to obstetric ICU.
3. Try to undertake a differential diagnosis to determine the cause of the sudden collapse once supportive management is started.
4. Continuing management: Correct the reversible causes for the sudden collapse.

IMMEDIATE RESUSCITATION

Resuscitation is conducted according to different guidelines. The American Heart Association (AHA) has issued guidelines for basic life support (BLS), adult advanced life support (ALS), and automated external defibrillation (AED) including algorithms and recommendations.[4] The 2010 AHA guidelines were updated in 2015, and are now used widely in the resuscitation of the pregnant woman worldwide. It is recognized that the divisions into BLS and ALS are somewhat arbitrary in the hospital setting. In the community setting, BLS should be administered and rapid transfer arranged, unless appropriate personnel and equipments are available.

Cardiopulmonary resuscitation should be started immediately and should be the same whether the patient is pregnant or not, though with few modifications, if she is pregnant owing to the physiological alterations occurring during pregnancy. The following modifications are necessary for managing cardiac arrest in pregnancy:
1. Left lateral displacement of the uterus if gestational age is >20 weeks
2. Earlier definitive airway control
3. The removal of the fetal monitor to avoid electrical arcing during defibrillation
4. The defibrillation pads may be positioned in anterior and posterior on the left side of the chest if it is difficult to apply the apical pad in left tilted position of the patient
5. Consideration of an early cesarean delivery.

Basic Life Support and Adult Advanced Life Support for Obstetric Patient

As per the latest recommendations, emergency management is CAB (circulation, airway, and breathing) (not ABC). If defibrillation is available immediately, then this may take precedence over BLS.[5] Make sure the patient, any bystanders, and you are safe before performing CPR. The most important prerequisite is that anyone performing CPR should be very much alert as their confidence and presence of mind will determine the outcome for the patient.

Adult Basic Life Support for Obstetric Patient[4]

- Immediately call for the help. The adult BLS algorithm has been modified to reflect the fact that rescuers can activate an emergency response (i.e., through use of a mobile telephone) without leaving the victim's side.
- Do not waste precious time before starting resuscitation and do not wait for help to arrive or to know the cause for sudden obstetric collapse. Immediately start resuscitation because management speed makes the difference. A delay of 1 minute may decrease survival chance by 10%.
- *Check responsiveness (shake and shout):* To confirm whether she is responsive to verbal commands and stimulation. This step is omitted if patient is under anesthesia.
- Turn the patient onto her back.
- *Left uterine displacement:* The gravid uterus at >20 weeks may compress the inferior vena cava and aorta which limits the effectiveness of chest compressions. Shift the uterus a minimum 1.5 inches away from the midline toward the left side. This may be accomplished manually. One person should be dedicated to manually displacing the uterus toward the left to relieve the aortocaval compression known as left uterine displacement (LUD). If rescuer is on patient's left side, then pull the uterus with two hands. If rescuer is on patient's right side, push the uterus with the one hand.[6] (Do not tilt the woman on left side as that would decrease the performance and effectiveness of chest compressions and vascular access.) This will preserve supine positioning for optimal chest compressions, minimize aortocaval compression, optimize venous return (preload), generate adequate stroke volume during CPR, improve airway and intravenous access, access for defibrillation (**Fig. 1**).
- Check breathing and simultaneously check for the carotid pulse (within the first 10 seconds).
  - If there is no normal breathing and the patient as a pulse, then provide rescue breathing at the rate of one breath at every 5–6 seconds, or about 10–12 breaths/min. Continue rescue breathing and check pulse at every 2 minutes. If there is no pulse, begin CPR as below.
  - If there are no breathing movements or only gasping and no pulse, proceed immediately to high-quality compressions. Absence of breathing in the presence of a clear airway is now used as a sign of the absence of circulation. Agonal gasps are present in up to 40% of cardiac arrest victims. Agonal gasps can occur commonly within the first few minutes after sudden cardiac arrest; they are an indication for starting CPR immediately and should not be confused with normal breathing. If the victim is unresponsive with absent or abnormal breathing, the rescuer should assume that the victim is in cardiac arrest. Rescue breathing to be started only after starting compressions.

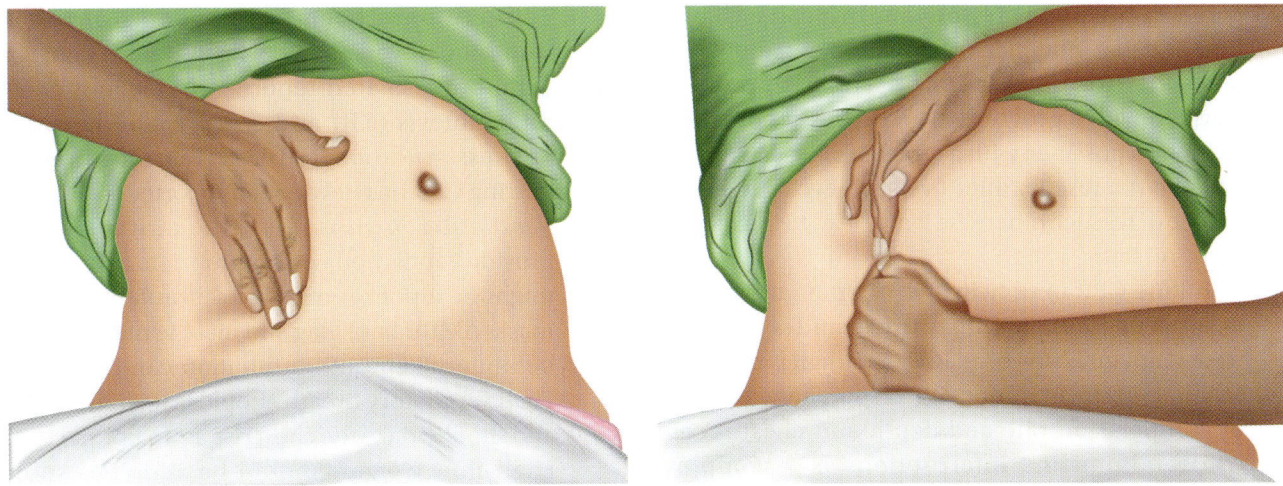

Fig. 1: Left uterine displacement.[6]

- Immediately start good-quality chest compressions. There should be continued emphasis on the characteristics of high-quality CPR: Compressing the chest at an adequate rate and depth, allowing complete chest recoil after each compression, minimizing interruptions in compressions, and avoiding excessive ventilation.
  - Put the victim on the flat surface.
  - Position yourself on the side of the victim and above the patient's chest.
  - Do not remove her underclothes.
  - The gravid uterus at >20 weeks limits the effectiveness of chest compressions. It may be shifted away from the inferior vena cava and aorta manually by left uterine displacement.
  - Perform 100–120 chest compressions/minute. The compression rate has recently been modified from 100/min to a range of 100–120/min. The number of chest compressions delivered per minute during CPR is an important determinant of return of spontaneous circulation (ROSC) and survival with good neurologic function. Provision of adequate chest compressions requires an emphasis not only on an adequate compression rate but also on minimizing interruptions to this critical component of CPR. The upper limits of recommended compression rate and compression depth are based on preliminary data suggesting that excessive compression rate and depth adversely affect outcomes as do inadequate compression depth.[4]
  - The compression: Breath ratio is 30:Two (considered as one cycle).
  - The person undertaking the CPR should keep their arms straight; elbows should not be bent while performing chest compressions; doing so will deliver weak, ineffective chest compression.
  - Compression should be given at the lower border of the sternum between the nipples with heel of the hand.
  - Place the heel of one hand there, with the heel of the other hand on the first hand. Interlock the fingers of both the hands and lift the fingers.

  Principle of the chest compression is "Push the chest hard and fast." Press down on the sternum to depress it at least by 5–6 cm. Compression depth for adults is modified to at least 2 inches (5 cm) but should not exceed 2.4 inches (6 cm). Compressions create blood flow primarily by increasing intrathoracic pressure and directly compressing the heart, which in turn results in critical blood flow and oxygen delivery to the heart and brain. While a compression depth of at least 2 inches (5 cm) is recommended, the 2015 Guidelines Update incorporates new evidence about the potential for an upper threshold of compression depth [>2.4 inches (6 cm)], beyond which complications may occur. Compression depth may be difficult to judge without use of feedback devices, and identification of upper limits of compression depth may be challenging.[4]
  - Give time for chest to recoil in between chest compressions. To allow full chest wall recoil after each compression, rescuers must avoid leaning on the chest between compressions. It will allow full chest wall to recoil in cardiac arrest. Rescuers should allow complete recoil of the chest after each compression, to allow the heart to fill completely before the next compression. Full chest wall recoil occurs when the sternum returns to its natural position during the decompression phase of CPR. Chest wall recoil creates a relative negative intrathoracic pressure that promotes venous return and cardiopulmonary blood flow. Leaning on the chest wall between compressions precludes full chest wall recoil. Incomplete recoil raises intrathoracic pressure and reduces venous return,

coronary perfusion pressure, and myocardial blood flow and can influence resuscitation outcomes.[4]
- One criterion for minimizing interruptions is clarified with a goal of chest compression fraction as high as possible, with a target of at least 60%.[4]
- Change the rescuer after five such cycles to avoid fatigue of rescuer, otherwise it may lead to ineffective compressions.
- Continue CPR until help arrives or an automated external defibrillator (AED) arrives and is ready for use or patient is moved to ICU or patient is revived.[4]
- Maintaining focus during CPR on the characteristics of compression rate and depth and chest recoil while minimizing interruptions is a complex challenge even for highly trained professionals. It may be reasonable to use audiovisual feedback devices during CPR for real-time optimization of CPR performance and to improve the quality of CPR in actual resuscitations **(Fig. 2)**.

■ *Breathing:*
- *Mouth-to-mouth breathing:* Ensuring head tilt and chin lift. Close the soft part of the patient's nose with your thumb and index finger. Open her mouth a little but maintain chin lift. Take a breath and place your lips around her mouth, making sure that you have good seal. Blow steadily into her mouth over 1 second and watching for her chest to rise. Maintaining head tilt and chin lift, take your mouth away from the patient and watch for her chest to fall as the air comes out. Take another breath and repeat the sequence to give another effective breath. Give two effective breaths with use of barrier devices if available to provide ventilation such as pocket mask, face shield, and bag valve mask. Return to chest compressions quickly.

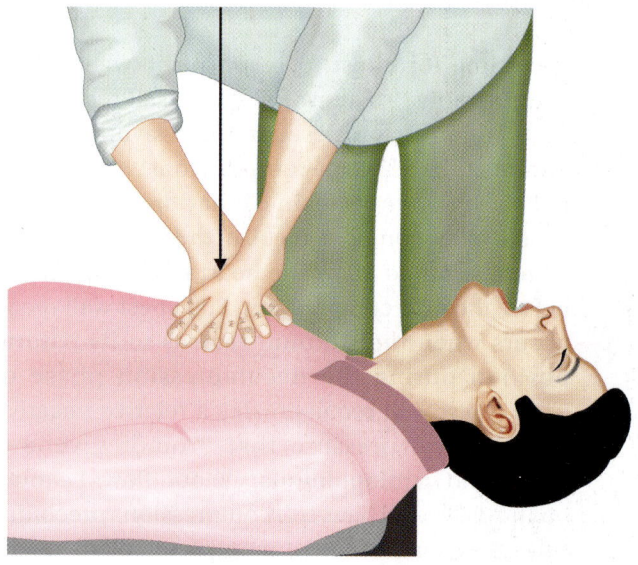

Fig. 2: Chest compressions.

There have been few incidents of rescuers suffering adverse effects from undertaking CPR, with only isolated reports of infections such as tuberculosis (TB) and severe acute respiratory distress syndrome (SARS). Transmission of HIV during CPR has never been reported.
- *Ventilation breaths:* Keep the airway open and provide ventilation with appropriate adjuncts. This might be a pocket mask or self-inflating bag with mask (AMBU bag). Bag and mask ventilation should be undertaken until intubation can be achieved. Each ventilatory breath should last about 1 second and should make the chest rise as if a normal breath. High-flow oxygen should be added as soon as possible.
- *Intubated ventilation:* Tracheal intubation is the most effective way of providing adequate ventilation and should be performed as soon as a trained member of staff is available. Apply continuous cricoids pressure during ventilation and intubation due to the risk of regurgitation. Early intubation is mandatory, with attention to the use of an endotracheal tube (ETT) 0.5–1 mm smaller in internal diameter than that which would be used for a nonpregnant woman because the airway may be narrowed from edema. Avoid nasal intubation because of the increased mucosal friability during pregnancy. A laryngoscope with a shorter handle is useful as the presence of large breasts may interfere with access. Once the patient is intubated, ventilation should continue at 10 breaths/min but does not need to be synchronized with chest compressions. It should then be uninterrupted. For patients with ongoing CPR and an advanced airway in place, a simplified ventilation rate of 1 breath every 6 seconds (10 breaths per minute) is recommended. During pregnancy, there is increased oxygen requirements and rapid onset of hypoxia, and therefore, it is important to ensure optimal oxygen delivery by high-flow 100% oxygen to whatever method of ventilation is being employed.

If circulation is present but no breathing (respiratory arrest), continue rescue breathing and bag and mask ventilation at a rate of 10 breaths/min and a tidal volume large enough to raise the chest.

It must be noted that hyperventilation is harmful and should be avoided.[7] If the patient starts to breathe on her own but remains unconscious, turn her into the recovery position and apply oxygen at the rate of 15 L/min. Check her condition and be ready to turn her back to start rescue breathing if she stops breathing.
■ *Defibrillation:* If AED is available, attach it, analyze the rhythm, and defibrillate the patient. In majority of these

types of cases, ventricular fibrillation or flutter is the dying rhythm of heart. In this case, defibrillation with defibrillator is the definitive treatment. Defibrillate the victim using standard advanced cardiac life support (ACLS) defibrillation doses. The most frequent initial rhythm in the context of sudden collapse is ventricular fibrillation (VF). The AED allows for early defibrillation by lesser-trained personnel as it performs rhythm analysis and gives information by voice or visual display, and the delivery of the shock is then delivered automatically. The 2010 Guidelines recommended the establishment of AED programs in public locations where there is a relatively high likelihood of witnessed cardiac arrest (e.g., airports, casinos, sports facilities, etc.). There is clear and consistent evidence of improved survival from cardiac arrest when a bystander performs CPR and rapidly uses an AED. For witnessed adult cardiac arrest when an AED is immediately available, it is reasonable that the defibrillator be used as soon as possible. For adults with unmonitored cardiac arrest or for whom an AED is not immediately available, it is reasonable that CPR be initiated while the defibrillator equipment is being retrieved and applied and that defibrillation, if indicated, be attempted as soon as the device is ready for use. With in-hospital sudden cardiac arrest, there is insufficient evidence to support or refute CPR before defibrillation. However, in monitored patients, the time from VF to shock delivery should be under 3 minutes, and CPR should be performed while the defibrillator is readied. CPR should be provided while the AED pads are applied and until the AED is ready to analyze the rhythm. If an AED is not available, manage with immediate ECG, if possible to differentiate the shockable and nonshockable rhythm and plan defibrillation as follows:

Shockable rhythms: There is no evidence that shocks from a direct current defibrillator have adverse effects on the heart of the fetus. If fetal or uterine monitors are in place, remove them before delivering shocks.

Shockable rhythms are treated with a shock. It is followed by immediate continuation of CPR without stopping for a rhythm or pulse check. Every 2 minutes, the rhythm is assessed and if necessary a further shock is delivered. Injection adrenaline (epinephrine) 1 mg IV is given immediately before the third and every subsequent alternate shock, i.e., approximately every 4 min. Amiodarone 300 mg IV is given before the fourth shock.

Defibrillator safety management: The patient should not be near inflammable fluids, fumes, or chemicals that could ignite.

If paddles are used rather than the pads: Keep paddles pressed firmly on the patient's chest—failure to do so may result in a flash arc. The defibrillation paddles should be placed back in the appropriate containers as soon as the shocks have ended. Do not discharge the paddles in the air.[8] The operator's hands should be dry prior to applying a shock; the operator must check that nobody has direct or indirect contact with the patient. Advise all bystanders and personnel to "stand clear" **(Fig. 3)**.

Nonshockable rhythms: In case of the nonshockable rhythm, i.e., pulseless electrical activity or asystole, adrenaline (epinephrine) 1 mg should be given intravenously immediately. Atropine 3 mg IV may be given once for asystole or slow rate, i.e., <60 bpm. This will minimize any vagal tone if present. The combined use of vasopressin and epinephrine offers no advantage to using standard-dose epinephrine in cardiac arrest. Also, vasopressin does not offer an advantage over the use of epinephrine alone. Therefore, to simplify the algorithm, vasopressin has been

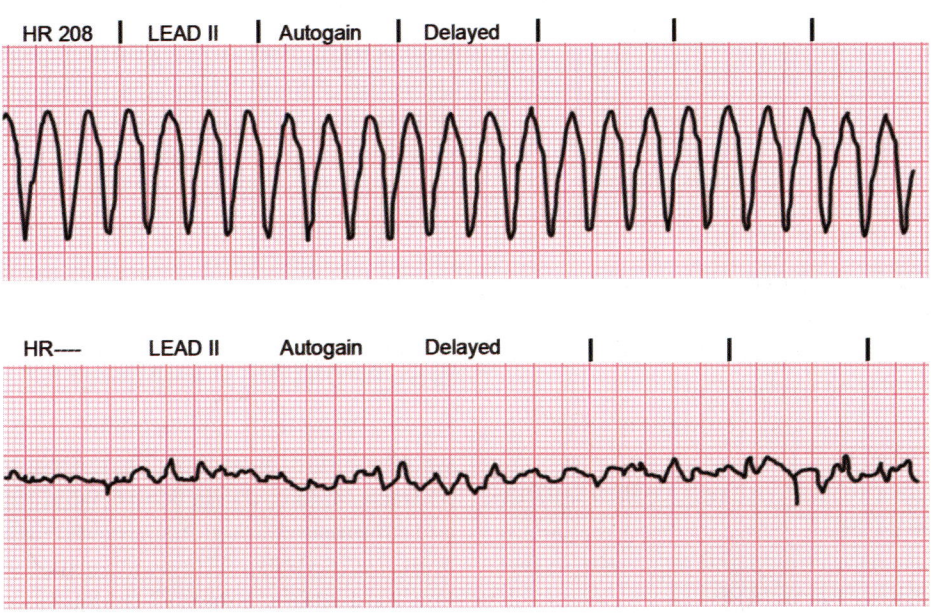

Fig. 3: Cardiac rhythms: Ventricular flutter and fibrillation.

removed from the Adult Cardiac Arrest Algorithm–2015 Update. It may be reasonable to administer epinephrine as soon as feasible after the onset of cardiac arrest due to an initial nonshockable rhythm.

Steroids may provide some benefit when bundled with vasopressin and epinephrine in treating an in-hospital cardiac arrest (IHCA). While routine use is not recommended pending follow-up studies, it would be reasonable for a provider to administer the bundle for IHCA. When rapidly implemented, *extracorporeal cardiopulmonary resuscitation* (ECPR) can prolong viability, as it may provide time to treat potentially reversible conditions or arrange for cardiac transplantation for patients who are not resuscitated by conventional CPR **(Flowchart 1 and Fig. 4)**.

- *Resuscitative cesarean section delivery* [Also called perimortem cesarean delivery) (PMCD)]: It is important to remember that both, mother and infant may die if the provider cannot restore blood flow to the mother's heart. At gestational age > 22 weeks and if CPR is not effective, consider the need for an emergency cesarean delivery which requires delivery to begin about 3–4 minutes after cardiac arrest. It will also facilitate effectiveness of CPR. Perimortem *cesarean section packs are available* on resuscitation trolleys in all areas where maternal collapse may occur.[5]
  - PMCD needs to be initiated within 3–4 minutes of cardiac arrest and is essentially done to save the mother, irrespective of whether fetus is alive or dead.
  - Perimortem cesarean section should be performed where resuscitation is taking place. The principle of successful cesarean delivery is rapid incision, rapid delivery, and rapid closure.
  - It is best obtained with large vertical abdominal incision and closure of the uterus and then the abdomen with large running sutures in a single layer.
  - There is no need to scrub the abdomen.
  - No need to administer anesthesia, as patient is not responsive.
  - Cesarean delivery will be relatively bloodless, since there is no circulation and cardiac output.
  - Immediately deliver the baby and handover to neonatologist.
  - The placenta should be delivered manually.
  - The best survival rate for infants >28 weeks occurs when delivery of infant occurs in <5 minutes after the mother's heart stops beating.
  - Chest compressions and ventilation should be continued during PMCD.
  - Emptying of the uterus will also facilitate effectiveness of CPR.
  - If the mother is resuscitated and pulse returns then immediately move her to ICU.
  - Start broad-spectrum antibiotics.
  - If the patient has sudden collapse during cesarean delivery, chest compressions and ventilation should be started immediately. The baby should be delivered immediately and the uterus emptied. The principle again here for successful resuscitation is "Rapid incision, Rapid delivery and Rapid closure." The placenta should be removed manually, and the abdomen closed with large running sutures in a single layer.
  - Document the procedure in the patient's record.
  - All patients who progress to brain death or circulatory death after initial cardiac arrest should be considered potential organ donors.

A study was conducted Katz *et al.*[9] of cases from 1985 to 2004 identified 38 cases of PMCD; 34 infants survived (three sets of twins, one set of triplets). Of the 34 infants (25–42 weeks' gestation), time of delivery after maternal cardiac arrest was available for 25. Eleven infants were delivered within 5 minutes, four in from 6 to 10 minutes, two in 11 to 15 minutes, and seven in more than 15 minutes. Of 20 PMCD deliveries with potentially resuscitatable causes, 13 mothers were resuscitated and discharged from the hospital in good condition. One other mother was successfully resuscitated after the delivery, but died within 24 hours from complications related to AFE. In 12 of 18 reports that documented hemodynamic status, cesarean delivery preceded return of maternal pulse and blood pressure, often in a dramatic fashion. Eight other cases noted improvement in maternal status. Importantly, in no case was there deterioration of the maternal condition with the cesarean delivery.[9] Cesarean delivery might be necessary to accomplish a successful resuscitation even if the fetus has died.[7]

Laparoscopic Patient

Bradycardia may occur during laparoscopic surgeries because of insufflating gas which may compress the inferior vena cava and reduce the venous return. If bradycardia is not managed quickly, it may lead to asystole. Immediately releasing the insufflating gas usually restores venous return and improves the heart rate. Injection atropine or glycopyrrolate may be given to improve the heart rate.

■ SUPPORTIVE MANAGEMENT

Studies of patients after cardiac arrest have found that a systolic blood pressure <90 mm Hg or a mean arterial pressure of <65 mm Hg is associated with higher mortality and diminished functional recovery, while systolic arterial pressures of >100 mm Hg are associated with better recovery. The 2015 AHA Guidelines Update recommendations for postcardiac arrest care recommended identification and

SECTION 12: Critical Care in Obstetrics

Flowchart 1: Basic life support (BLS) healthcare provider adult cardiac arrest algorithm–2015.

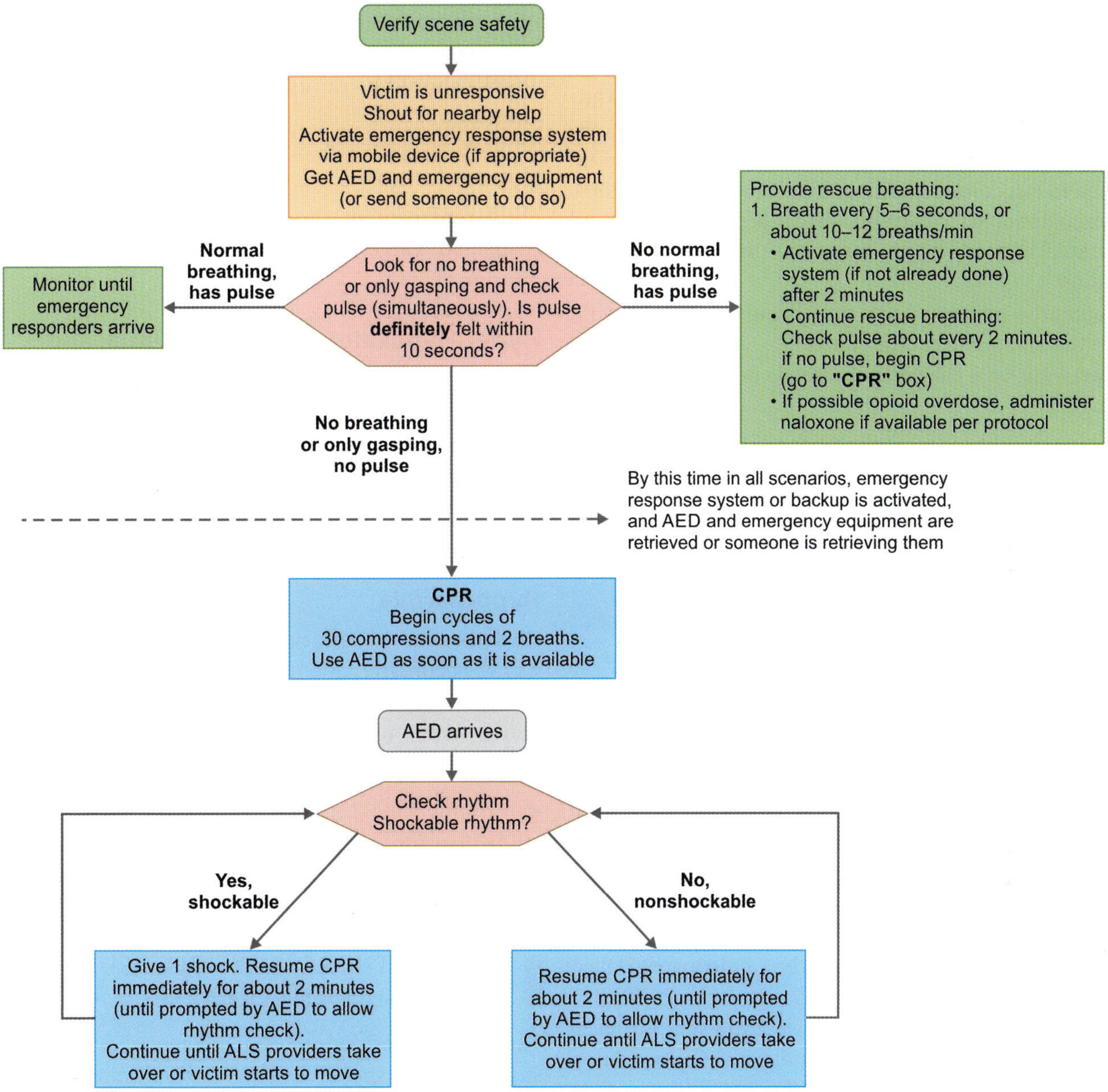

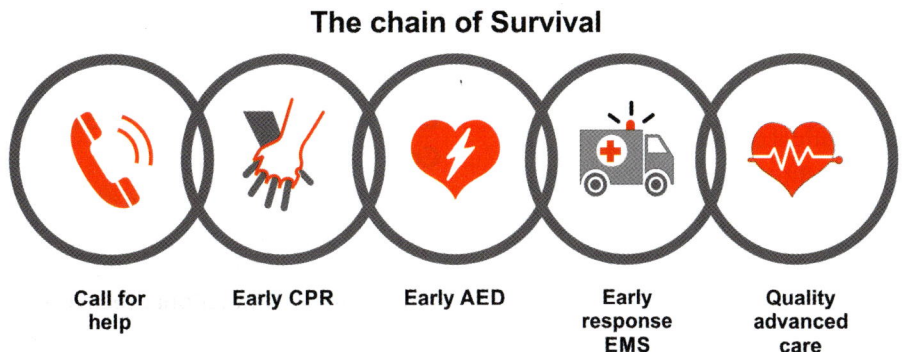

(AED: automated external defibrillation; ALS: advanced life support; CPR: cardiopulmonary resuscitation)
Source: American Heart Association,[4] with permission.

Fig. 4: Basic life support algorithm.[4]
(AED: automated external defibrillation; CPR: cardiopulmonary resuscitation; EMS: emergency medical service)

correction of hypotension in the immediate postcardiac arrest period.[4] After ROSC, fluids and vasoactive infusions should be used to maintain a systolic blood pressure above the fifth centile for age. Early, rapid IV administration of isotonic fluids is widely accepted as a cornerstone of therapy. After ROSC, normoxemia should be targeted. When the necessary equipment is available, oxygen administration should be weaned to target an oxyhemoglobin saturation of 94–99%. Hypoxemia should be strictly avoided. Ideally, oxygen should be titrated to a value appropriate to the specific patient condition.

Supportive management is started immediately after CPR is effective and mother resuscitated:
- Two wide-bore cannulas should be inserted as early as possible.
- There should be an aggressive approach to volume. Fluids—isotonic normal saline, Ringer's lactate or plasmalyte A—are given rapidly in bolus as per an individual case. Caution must be exercised in the case of severe preeclampsia and eclampsia to avoid pulmonary edema owing to fluid overload.
- Oxygen administration is continued to prevent hypoxia.
- Catheterization should be done.
- Broad-spectrum antibiotics should be started.
- If required, should be managed for blood transfusion.
- The patient should be examined for resuscitation related injuries, e.g., rib fractures.
- Immediately the patient should be moved to obstetric ICU. The patient should be accompanied by qualified personnel during transportation to obstetric ICU.
- Senior experienced staff should be involved at an early stage.
- The patient should be supervised by an adequately skilled team.
- Blood samples should be collected and sent for basic initial laboratory investigations during initial resuscitation mainly complete blood count (CBC), blood sugar, liver function test (LFT), renal function test, bleeding and coagulation profile, pH, bicarbonate, etc.
- Abdominal ultrasound by a skilled operator can assist in the diagnosis of concealed hemorrhage and to know the condition of a fetus. The interpretation of fetal well-being by external electronic monitoring may be of utmost importance.
- Multidisciplinary teamwork is involved as per the requirement of an individual case.
- Along with CPR, correct the reversible causes of cardiac arrest 4 Hs and 4 Ts:

Four Hs:
- Hypoxia
- Hypovolemia (hemorrhage or sepsis)
- Hyperkalemia and other metabolic disorders
- Hypothermia.

Hypoxia
Effective ventilation and supplementation is ensured with 100% oxygen delivery as soon as possible. Regular checks should be done to ensure adequate airway and ventilation.

Hypovolemia
Fluid replacement should be given if hypovolemia is suspected. Large-bore cannula is inserted to allow rapid infusion of fluids.[10]

Hyper/Hypokalemia, Hypocalcemia, and Metabolic Disorders
Electrolyte imbalance may lead to cardiac arrest—it should be confirmed or ruled out with arterial blood gases and serum electrolytes analysis. Electrocardiography (ECG) monitoring and baseline blood tests should be done for urea and electrolytes at regular interval.

Hypothermia
Hypothermia is defined when the core temperature is <35°C. Record the patient's temperature as soon as possible after a cardiac arrest. In case of hypothermia, consider active warming with warm blankets.

Four Ts:
- Thromboembolism
- Toxicity (drugs associated)
- Tension pneumothorax
- Cardiac tamponade.

IDENTIFY THE RESPONSIBLE CAUSE FOR THE SUDDEN COLLAPSE

The spot diagnosis of probable differential diagnosis for the sudden collapse should be undertaken as further management depends on the responsible cause for the situation. It is imperative to identify reversible causes of cardiac arrest. The gestational age should be quickly established in order to determine fetal viability. Abdominal ultrasound examination can be performed for this purpose, but it should not delay the resuscitation procedures. The etiology can also be classified into anesthesia-related causes and/or nonanesthesia-related causes.

Differential Diagnosis of Sudden Collapse in Pregnancy
Is it APH or PPH or inversion of uterus? If not, then consider for nonhemorrhagic causes.

History of and Probable Diagnosis
Obstetric or medical causes:
- History of hypertension in pregnancy and convulsions—*eclampsia*

- History of grand multipara or previous uterine scar or instrumental delivery—*rupture of the uterus*
- History of mismanaged third stage of labor, short cord, or manual removal of placenta (MRP)—*inversion of uterus*
- History of previous cardiac problems, complaints of acute left-sided chest pain, anxiety, hypotension—*maternal cardiac problems*, mainly *myocardial infarction*
- History of vehicular accidents or domiciliary violence—*trauma*
- History of collapse after administration of drugs, signs, and symptoms of allergic reactions—*drug reaction or overdose*
- History of painful stimuli, injections, etc.,—*anaphylactic reaction*
- History of collapse immediately after delivery, mainly in multipara or in precipitate labor and no obvious cause or in any case always consider the possibility of *AFE*
- History of sudden onset of unexplained dyspnea and tachypnea, especially in western countries because of venous stasis and hypercoagulability of blood—*pulmonary thromboembolism.*

Anesthesia-related causes:
- History of spinal anesthesia (SA) in higher position, difficult SA during surgery, complaints of heaviness in the chest, anxiety, breathlessness within few minutes of SA—*high spinal anesthesia*
- History of vomiting under anesthesia and problem starts within few hours—*Mendelson's syndrome*
- History of fall in the blood pressure within few minutes after SA—*supine spinal shock*
- Mortality related to airway problems during extubation of the trachea has increased with spinal anesthesia-related mortality.[11,12] Of all maternal deaths due to anesthesia, 27% occurred among obese women, whereas 24% occurred among overweight women.

CONTINUING THERAPY: CORRECT THE REVERSIBLE CAUSES FOR THE SUDDEN COLLAPSE

Continuing therapy can be directed toward the specific cause of the caused sudden collapse in a pregnant woman to optimize the outcome and continued in an obstetric ICU. Management of each individual cause is not within the scope of this chapter. Decisions should not be delayed if surgical intervention is required.

PREARM TO PERFORM

Drugs Used in Adult Cardiac Arrest

Adrenaline

Adrenaline causes vasoconstriction and increases perfusion to myocardium and cerebrum.[13] The usually prescribed dosage of adrenaline is 1 mg IV (1 mL of 1:1,000 or 10 mL of 1:10,000). Ventricular fibrillation/pulseless ventricular tachycardia (VF/pulseless VT) after initial counter shocks have failed (after second shock and then after every second cycle). Asystole and pulseless electrical activity in initial cycle (and then every second cycle). Do not interrupt CPR to administer medications.

Adverse effects include tachyarrhythmias and hypertension after the person is resuscitated.

Amiodarone

Amiodarone is an antiarrhythmic drug. It is given for VF/pulseless VT (between the third and fourth shock when refractory to defibrillator shocks and a vasopressor). If there have been three unsuccessful defibrillation shocks for VF/pulseless VT, the adult bolus dose of 300 mg (5 mg/kg) of amiodarone IV should be given. An additional bolus of 150 mg could be considered. This may be followed by an infusion of 15 mg/kg over 24 h. Major side effects include bradycardia, heart block and hypotension.

Lignocaine and amiodarone should not be given together.[14,15]

Vasopressor

Epinephrine may reasonably be administered as soon as feasible after the onset of cardiac arrest due to an initial nonshockable rhythm.[4]

Vasopressin in combination with epinephrine offers no advantage as a substitute for standard-dose epinephrine in cardiac arrest.[4]

Intravenous Lipid Emulsion

It may be reasonable to administer intravenous lipid emulsion, concomitant with standard resuscitative care, to patients who have premonitory neurotoxicity or cardiac arrest due to local anesthetic toxicity.

Sodium Bicarbonate

Sodium bicarbonate is given in the dose of 50 mmol IV to patients when arrest is associated with hyperkalemia. It is also given in response to severe acidosis when pH is <7.1, usually in cases of septicemia and diabetic ketoacidosis. It should be used with caution, because rapid correction of maternal acidosis can reduce the compensatory hyperventilation.[16]

Calcium Chloride

A dose of 10 mL 10% calcium chloride (6.8 mmol Ca^{2+}) IV can be used if it is thought that pulseless electrical activity (PEA) is caused by hyperkalemia, hypocalcemia, overdose of calcium channel blocking drugs or overdose of magnesium sulfate (for treatment of preeclampsia).

Inotropic Agent

Dopamine: Initial intravenous infusion of 2–5 µg/kg/min and increase up to 5–10 µg/kg/min as needed.

Dobutamine: Intravenous infusion of 2–40 µg/kg/min.

Noradrenaline: 2–4 µg/kg/min dose depending upon blood pressure.

Intra-arrest and Postarrest Prognostic Factors

Low end-tidal carbon dioxide ($ETCO_2$) in intubated patients after 20 minutes of CPR is associated with a very low likelihood of resuscitation. While this parameter should not be used in isolation for decision making, providers may consider low $ETCO_2$ after 20 minutes of CPR in combination with other factors to help determine when to terminate resuscitation.

Multiple factors should be considered when trying to predict outcomes of cardiac arrest. Multiple factors play a role in the decision to continue or to terminate resuscitative efforts during cardiac arrest and in the estimation of potential for recovery after cardiac arrest. No single intra-arrest or postcardiac arrest variable has been found that reliably predicts favorable or poor outcomes.

Communication

Wherever possible, senior personnel from the obstetric, anesthesia and midwifery should communicate properly. Ensure that the family is looked after and kept informed about patient's conditions and management undertaken. All interventions should be documented accurately with timings.

To improve outcomes for maternal collapse in future:
- Always be set up ready to tackle such cases. All obstetric units must be ready to tackle the unpredictable.
- Form a permanent team which should include the cardiac arrest team, a senior obstetrician, an obstetric anesthetist a senior midwife.
- Develop systems that assemble more staff.
- Plan regular training of the staff.
- Plan and perform regular practice drills for medical and paramedical staff.
- Review, revise and audit each such event and update the protocol as and when required.
- Identify and treat the patient in response to early signs of demise may prevent deterioration of situation to cardiac arrest. An early warning sign score (EWS) can help to identify deteriorating patients and can be given attention to prevent cardiac arrest.

CONCLUSION

Cardiopulmonary resuscitation in the pregnant patient with cardiac arrest should be performed with consideration of the physiological changes associated with pregnancy. The standard algorithm should be followed according to BLS and ALS protocols, with few exceptions. Attention should be given to lateral displacement of the uterus, to secure early airway, aggressive airway management, and early consideration of emergency cesarean delivery which are major modifications in the management of maternal sudden cardiac arrest. Immediate cesarean delivery not only improves survival of infant but also facilitates maternal resuscitation. CPR drill should be performed regularly for medical and paramedical staff.

KEY MESSAGES

- Maternal collapse is defined as an acute event involving the cardiorespiratory system and/or brain resulting in a reduced or absent conscious level (and potentially death) at any stage in pregnancy and up to 6 weeks after delivery.
- There are many causes of sudden obstetric collapse, which may be pregnancy related or result from conditions not related to pregnancy and possibly existing before pregnancy.
- Hemorrhage is one of the most common causes of maternal collapse and is responsible for most maternal deaths.
- CPR is more difficult to perform and may be less effective in the pregnant compared with the nonpregnant population.
- Emergency management is CAB (circulation, airway and breathing) (not ABC).
- The 2015 AHA Guidelines Update recommendations for postcardiac arrest care recommended identification and correction of hypotension in the immediate postcardiac arrest period.
- Along with CPR, the reversible causes of cardiac arrest the 4 Hs and 4 Ts should be corrected.
- Continuing therapy can be directed toward the specific cause of the caused sudden collapse in a pregnant woman to optimize the outcome and continued in an obstetric ICU.
- Decisions should not be delayed if surgical intervention is required.
- CPR drill should be performed regularly for medical and paramedical staff.

REFERENCES

1. Maternal collapse in pregnancy and the puerperium. Green-top Guideline No. 56. RCOG. 2011;1:24.
2. Morris S, Stacey M. Resuscitation in pregnancy. BMJ 2003;327:1277-9.
3. Lapinsky SE, Kruczynski K, Slutsky AS. Critical care in the pregnant patient. Am J Respir Crit Care Med. 1995;152:427-55.
4. American Heart Association. Highlights of the 2015 American Heart Association Guidelines Update for CPR and ECC. 2015 Available from: https://eccguidelines.heart.org/wp-content/uploads/2015/10/2015-AHA-Guidelines-Highlights-English.pdf. [Last accessed November, 2021].
5. Women and Newborn Health Services, King Edward Memorial Hospital. Clinical Guidelines-Obstetrics & Gynaecology, Advanced Life Support. Government of Western Australia Department of Health. [online] Available from: https://www.kemh.health.wa.gov.au/For-health-professionals/Clinical-guidelines/OG. [Last accessed November, 2021].
6. Sinz E, Lavonas EJ, Jeejeebhoy FM. American Heart Association Guidelines for Cardiopulmonary Resuscitation and Emergency Cardiovascular Care. Part 12: cardiac arrest in special situations. Circulation 2010;122:S829-61.
7. Ezri T, Lurie S, Weiniger C, Golan A, Evron S. Cardiopulmonary resuscitation in the pregnant woman – an update. IMAJ 2011; 13:306-10.

8. Defibrillation theory and practice. In: Moule P, Albarran J (eds). Practical resuscitation recognition and response. Melbourne: Blackwell Publishing, 2005;151-76.
9. Katz V, Balderston K, DeFreest M. Perimortem caesarean delivery: were our assumptions correct? Am J Obstet Gynecol 2005;192:1916-20; discussion.
10. Australian Resuscitation Council. Guideline 11.2 protocols for adult advanced life support Dec 2010: ARC/NZRC. (2010). [online] Available from: http://www.resus.org.au/policy/guidelines/section_11/guideline-11-7dec10.pdf. [Last accessed November, 2021].
11. Arendt KW. Present and emerging strategies for reducing anesthesia-related maternal morbidity and mortality. Curr Opin Anaesthesiol. 2009;22:330-5.
12. Mhyre JM, Riesner MN, Polley LS, Naughton NN. A series of anesthesia-related maternal deaths in Michigan, 1985-2003 A.nesthesiology. 2007;106:1096-104.
13. Gillimore D. Understanding the drugs used during cardiac arrest response. Nurs Times. 2006;102:24.
14. Thomas J (ed.) APP Guide. Australian prescription products guide. Melbourne: Australian Pharmaceutical Publishing Company Ltd.; 2006.
15. Atta E, Gardner M. Cardiopulmonary resuscitation in pregnancy. Obstet Gynecol Clin North Am. 2007;34:585-97.
16. Australian Resuscitation Council, New Zealand Resuscitation Council. (2010) Guideline 11.7: post-resuscitation therapy in adult advanced life support: Australian Resuscitation Council. [online] Available from: http://www.resus.org.au/policy/guidelines/section_11/guideline-11-7dec10.pdf. [Last accessed November, 2021].

LONG QUESTIONS

1. Discuss in detail about the management of cardiac arrest in pregnancy.
2. What should be the supportive therapy after return of spontaneous circulation (ROSC) in a pregnant woman, who had a cardiac arrest?
3. Define maternal collapse. What are the important causes of maternal collapse? How will you identify the cause responsible for the sudden maternal collapse?

SHORT QUESTIONS

1. What are the physiological changes in pregnancy? Which can affect resuscitation in a pregnant woman?
2. Write short note on resuscitative cesarean section (perimortem cesarean section).
3. Write short note on drugs used in maternal cardiac arrest.
4. Role of defibrillation in maternal collapse.
5. How should resuscitation be modified for a pregnant patient?

MULTIPLE CHOICE QUESTIONS

1. The most important difference in CPR in pregnancy from general population is:
    a. Right uterine displacement
    b. Left uterine displacement
    c. Number of compressions is more
    d. Defibrillator should not be used
2. Perimortem CS is done primarily to save the baby:
    a. True   b. False
3. PMCD should ideally be performed by:
    a. 5 mins of cardiac arrest   b. 3 mins of arrest
    c. 10 mins of arrest   d. 30 mins of arrest
4. The commonest cause of maternal collapse in India is:
    a. Hemorrhage   b. Thromboembolism
    c. High blood pressure d. Rupture uterus
5. The 4 H for causes of collapse does not include:
    a. Hypertension   b. Hypothermia
    c. Hemorrhage   d. Hyperkalemia
6. Cardiopulmonary resuscitation is less effective in women:
    a. <12 weeks   b. >12 weeks
    c. >20 weeks   d. <20 weeks
7. CPR should be performed with:
    a. 30 chest compression with 5 rescue breaths
    b. 20 chest compression with 2 rescue breaths
    c. 30 chest compression with 2 rescue breaths
    d. 30 chest compression with 3 rescue breaths
8. As per AHA 2015 guidelines the chest compression is to press down on the sternum to depress it by 5 cm. Upper threshold of compression depth, beyond which complications may occur is?
    a. 10 cm   b. 6 cm
    c. 5 cm   d. 4 cm
9. During CPR, compression: breath ratio is 30 : 2 (considered as 1 cycle). A rescuer doing chest compressions should be changed after every:
    a. 10 cycles   b. 5 cycles
    c. 2 cycles   d. No need to change
10. After the onset of cardiac arrest due to an initial non-shockable rhythm. It may be reasonable to administer:
    a. Epinephrine as soon as feasible
    b. Corticosteroids as soon as feasible
    c. Vasopressin as soon as feasible
    d. Atropine as soon as feasible

Answers
1. b   2. b   3. a   4. a   5. a   6. c
7. c   8. b   9. b   10. a

Acknowledgment: Some of the material in this chapter has also been appeared in FIGO—*The Continuous Textbook of Women's Medicine Series* published by GLOWM.com

Index

Page numbers followed by *b* refer to box, *f* refer to figure, *fc* refer to flowchart, and *t* refer to table.

A

Abatacept 313
Abdomen 306
　causes of acute 428, 429, 432*t*
　surgical 428
Abdominal closure 615
Abdominal contour 556*f*
Abdominal examination 92, 556, 565
Abdominal fat, excessive 350
Abdominal organs 176
Abdominal pain 99, 304, 306, 439
　acute 428
Abdominal situs 175, 176
Abdominal tenderness 430
Abdominal tilt, maternal 437
Abdominal trauma 544
Abdominal wall 630
Abortion 193, 201
　classification 193
　clinical grading of 196*t*
　complete 193, 195
　etiology of 194
　first-trimester 194, 197
　incidence 193
　incomplete 193, 195, 292
　induced 194, 197
　inevitable 193, 195, 195*f*
　medical 730
　missed 193, 195
　pathology of 194
　recurrent spontaneous 544
　second-trimester 194, 197
　spontaneous 193, 201, 461
　threatened 193, 194
　unsafe 198
Abruptio placenta 154, 267, 522, 524*f*, 526*f*, 653
　complications of 524*t*
Abruption 227, 688
Abscess 667
　epidural 625
Absent end-diastolic volume 492
Absolute lymphocyte count 394
Acardiac twin 464
Accredited Social Health Activist 729, 734
Acetaminophen 444
　poisoning 444
Acetylcholine esterase inhibitors 313, 404
Acetylsalicylic acid 252
Acid-base
　balance 107
　changes 108*t*
　equilibrium 82
　monitoring 759
Acid-fast bacilli 321
Acidosis 154, 297, 697
Acid-suppressing drugs 305
Acne vulgaris 336
Acquired immunodeficiency
　disease 367
　syndrome 367

Acquired thrombophilia 227, 543
Acrania 75
Acrosome reaction 54
Act of violence 51
Actim® Partus kit 505*f*
Actinomycin 206
Activated charcoal 444
Activated partial thromboplastin time 252, 311
Acupressure 622
Acupuncture 622
Acute kidney injury 292, 293, 293*t*, 294
Acute respiratory distress syndrome 324, 524, 745
　pregnancy-specific 324
　severe 774
Acute seizure
　differential diagnosis of 328*f*
　intrapartum management of 331*fc*
Adalimumab 313
Addison disease 267
Adenocarcinoma 295
Adhesion 57
Adipocytes 259
Adipokines 348
Adnexal torsion 364
Adrenal hyperplasia, congenital 715
Adrenal tumor 235
Adrenaline 779
Adult advanced life support 772
Adult basic life support 772
Advance fetal echocardiography 175
Advanced cardiac
　life support 775
　support 437
Advanced magnetic resonance techniques 701
Agalactia 631
Airborne transmission 387
Airway 756
Ajit Rawal method 647, 648*f*
Alanine
　aminotransferase 401, 408
　transaminase 302
Albumin infusions 296
Alcohol 97
　abuse, chronic 447
　poisoning 447
　use screening tools 342*t*
Alcoholic liver disease 418
Alkali denaturation tests 286
Alkalosis 324
Alleles 114
Allergic rhinitis 336
Allograft function 303
Alloimmune factors 194
Alloimmunization 158
Alpha-fetoprotein 135
Alpha-thalassemia 279, 284, 285, 540
　minor 285

Aluminum containing antacids 305
Alveolar glands 38
Ambiguous genitalia 715, 718
Ambu bag 691
Amenorrhea 417
Amikacin 667
Amino acids 259, 302, 304
　salicylic 306, 315
Aminoglycosides 323, 390
Amiodarone 779
　use of 267
Ammonia 304
Amniocentesis 135, 149, 152, 186, 191, 282, 297, 461, 505
　advantages of 152
　gestational age 149
　procedure of 150
　tests 150
Amnioinfusion 472, 473, 593
Amnion 459
Amnionitis 154
Amniotic cavity, microbial infection of 484, 505*f*
Amniotic fluid 144, 321, 470, 514*f*, 546
　abnormal levels of 472*t*
　amount of 162
　embolism 325, 522, 770
　index 472, 486, 488, 490, 496
　pocket 471*f*
　resorption of 470
　samples 284
　sludge 504
　water, circulation of 470*f*
Amniotic fluid volume 401, 470*f*
　abnormalities of 470
　assessment of 158, 471
　dynamics of 470
　sonographic assessment of 158
Amniotomy 582, 739
Amoxicillin 305, 515
Amphetamines 342
Ampicillin 515
Anaemia Mukt Bharat 380
Anakinra 313
Anal agenesis 715
Anal epithelium 639
Analgesia 621
　during labor, indications of 624
Analgesics 282, 674
Anaphylactic reaction 779
Anaphylaxis 771
Ancylostoma duodenale 380
Androgenetic complete hydatidiform mole 211
Anecdotal herbal galactagogues 677
Anemia 273, 279, 320, 461
　causes of 274
　correction of 275
　cycle 274*fc*
　eradication of 277
　mild 286
　moderate-to-severe 277
　postpartum 275, 276

prevention of 297
severe 544
severity of 273t
tests to diagnose 274
treatment of 276, 297
Anencephaly 74, 147, 147f, 542f
Anesthesia 150, 531, 621, 779
Aneuploidy 114, 120, 194, 298, 542
markers 129
screening 95, 128
ultrasonography for 129
Angelman syndrome 68, 117
Angiogenesis 358
Angiotensin-converting enzyme inhibitors 244, 295, 310, 325
Angiotensin-receptor blockers 310
Anisocytes 286
Ankyloglossia 671
Anomaly scan 230
Antacids 305
Antenatal anti-D immunoglobulin 95
Antenatal care 89, 97, 236, 302, 499, 727
components of 94t
contacts 89, 90t
model 89
package 92
pyramids 128f
utilization of 96
Antenatal complications 461, 508
Antenatal exercises 425
Antenatal information 632
Antenatal management 330
Antenatal pharmacologic therapy 425
Antenatal protocols 230
Antenatal screening 95, 330
Antenatal steroid
role of 240
trial 34
Antenatal wellbeing tests 698
Antepartum fetal
assessment 158
methods of 158
surveillance tests 157, 410, 537
Antepartum management 245
Anterior diaphragmatic defects 78
Anthelmintic treatment, preventive 95
Anthropoid 45
Antiangiogenic drugs 358
Antiarrhythmic drugs 253t
Antiarrhythmic therapy 253
Antibiotic 6, 150, 315, 389, 505, 514
intravenous 197
prophylaxis 247t, 297
therapy 667
Antibody
loss of 374
phospholipid-dependent 311
Anticardiolipin 311
antibody 199, 235
positive for 311
Anticholinergics 304
Anticoagulants 253, 395
prophylaxis 252
Anticonvulsants 194
Anti-D immunoglobulin 437
Anti-D immunoprophylaxis 633
Antiemetics 99
Antiendomysial antibodies 68
Antiepileptic drug 327, 329t, 331

Antiestrogenic hormonal therapy 358
Antihistamines 99
Antihypertensive agents 238
Antihypertensive medications 240
Antimalarials, use of 317
Antimicrobials, role of 506
Antimicrosomal antibody 235, 267
Antineutrophil cytoplasmic antibody 315
Antinuclear antibody 198, 235
Antiobesity 353
Antiperoxidase 267
Antiphospholipid
antibody syndrome 230, 303, 309, 485
autoantibody 311
syndrome 158, 194, 201, 311, 541, 543
Antiretroviral drugs 368, 369t
classes of 368t
Antiretroviral therapy 367, 371b, 384
Anti-Rh immunoglobulin 546
Anti-rheumatic drugs, disease-modifying 312
Antisepsis 6
Antithyroglobulin 267
Antithyroid medications 269, 314
Anti-tumor necrosis factor, use of 313
Anti-vascular endothelial growth factor 358
Anxiety 341, 779, 768
generalized 340
Aorta
coarctation of 235
diseases of 255
posterior wall of 180f
size index 249, 250
Aorta-gonad-mesonephros 76
Aortic arch 184f
transverse 183f
Aortic dissection 255
Aortic isthmus 168f
Aortic origin 177
Aortic regurgitation 251
Aortic stenosis 251
causes of 251
Aortic valve 180f, 251
Aplastic crisis 281
Appendages 336
Appendicitis 306, 388
Appendix 306
Arabin cervical pessary 508f
Areola 81f
Arginine butyrate infusions 282
Arnold-Chiari malformation 75
Arrhythmia 253, 287
Arterial blood gas 318t, 322, 331, 443, 754, 760
estimation of 330
Arterial blood pressure 85
Arterial hypertension 348
Arterial invasive blood pressure monitoring 758
Arterial perfusion sequence, twin reverse 464, 542
Arterial pressure, shape of 758
Arteriovenous malformation 331, 610
Arthralgia 310
Arthrogryposis multiplex congenita 496
Arthropathy 323
Artificial intelligence 26
Ascaris lumbricoides 380
Ascites 304, 401
Aseptic bone necrosis 281
Asherman syndrome 194
Aspartate aminotransferase 408, 412

Aspartate transaminase 302, 401
Asphyxia 463, 697
laboratory evaluation of 699
Aspirin 238, 296, 403
low-dose 230, 312, 491
Asplenia, functional 281
Assisted breech delivery 559, 561
Assisted reproductive technology 135, 228, 256, 457, 460, 512
Asthma 321, 336
acute severe 322
clinical features of 321
during labor, management of 322
exacerbation, acute 322
triggers 321
control of 321
uncontrolled 321
Asymptomatic bacteriuria 95, 283
Ataxia 344
Atelectasis 283
Atenolol 237
Atopic dermatitis develops 336
Atosiban 506, 507
Atria 175
Atrial septal defect 247, 248, 254
Attention-deficit disorder 68, 274, 344
Auditory nerve agenesis 303
Autism attention-deficit hyperactivity disorder 350
Autoimmune
defects 194, 230, 270, 544
diseases 739
disorders 68, 308, 311
number of 308
hepatitis 417
vasculitis 314
Automated external defibrillation 772, 774, 777
Autosomal dominant disorders 116b
Autosomal recessive disorders 116b, 288
Auxiliary nurse midwife 734
Avascular necrosis 281
Axilla, management of 361
Axillary lymph node dissection 361
Azathioprine 296, 303, 314, 315, 317, 418
Azithromycin 323, 505
Azoospermic factor C deletion 68
Azygous system 301

B

Baby's heart rate 689
Back pressure 473
Bacteria 451
Bacterial contamination 768
Bacterial infections 380, 385, 451
Bacterial respiratory infections 323
Bacterial vaginosis 94, 375, 387, 504, 512
Bacteroides 387, 504
Bakri balloon 646
Balanced chromosomal structural rearrangements 120
Balloon occlusion catheters 532
Bariatric surgery 306, 354
Barkers hypothesis 414
Bartholin's glands 38, 38f
Basal pneumonia 430
Basic fetal echocardiography 175
Basic life support 777fc
Battledore placenta 482

Beau's lines 336
Bedside clot observation test 525
Bell's palsy 332
Benson and Durfee cerclage 201
Benzene 194
Benzodiazepines 342, 448
   poisoning 444
Beta hemolytic streptococci, group B 384
Beta-1 glycoprotein 110
Beta-adrenergic receptors agonists 507
Beta-blockers 237
Beta-cell function 119
Beta-human chorionic gonadotropin 134, 135, 170, 297
Beta-lactamase-resistant penicillins 674
Betamethasone 505
Beta-thalassemia 279, 284, 286
  hallmark of 286
  major 286, 286f, 287
  minor 286
Bicornuate uterus 194
Bicuspid aortic valve 256
Biguanide 261
Bilaminar germ disk, formation of 70f
Bilateral renal
  agenesis 472
  dysplasia 472
Bile acids, accumulation of 410
Biliary cholangitis, primary 416
Biliary cirrhosis, primary 416
Bilirubin levels 410
Bilirubinemia 756
Bilobate placenta 478
Binovular twins 457
Biochemical parameters 357
Biochemical screening 133
Biochemical test 133, 461
Biophysical profile 157, 161, 488, 490, 492
  interpretation of 161t
  modified 157, 161, 410
  reliability of 162
  score 161t
Biopsy 320, 360
Biparental complete hydatidiform mole 211, 212, 213f
Biparental familial recurrent mole 213f
Biparietal diameter 140f
  measurement of 486
Bird's modifications 599
Birth
  asphyxia 227
  canal 629
  defects, types of 66
  preparedness 96
  timing of 489
Birth injuries 704
  classification 705
  ranges, spectrum of 704
  risk factors 704
Bishop's score 578, 585, 579fc, 580fc
  modified 578, 578t
Bladder 235
  care 569, 632
  dissected down 658f
  dissection of 658
  exstrophy 78
  identification of 655f
  overdistension 473
  rupture 473
  sharp dissection, dissection of 658f

Blastocyst 57
Blastulation 69f
Bleeding 655, 778
  amount of 520t
  causes of 438
  cessation of 649
  diathesis 703
  disorder 718
  severe 222
Bleomycin 320
Block feeding 675
Blood 628, 766
  and blood products 525t
  borne transmission 387
  changes 104t
    in cellular composition of 83t
  collection of 38
  conservation technique 531
  culture 197
  gases, implications for 318
  glucose monitoring 264
  group incompatibility 194
  hypercoagulability of 779
  hypercoagulable state of 325
  products 766
  therapy 762
  transfusion 6, 282, 287, 766, 767
Blood coagulation factors 105
  changes in 105t
Blood loss 644
  estimation of 764, 765t
  large amount of 646
Blood pressure 233, 234f, 235, 240, 331, 398, 400, 628, 754, 756, 757f
  control of 304, 412
  measurement
    apparatus 233f
    method 241
  reduces 762
  systolic 296, 756 756
Blood sugar
  level 421
  postprandial 106
  raised postprandial 258
Blood urea 759
  nitrogen 235, 759
Blood volume 82, 400
  loss of 644
Bloody nipple discharge 675
Blunt trauma 439
B-lynch suture 648, 649f
Body cavity, formation of 77
Body fluids 715
Body mass index 260, 349
  elevated 303
Boerhaave syndrome 99
Bone marrow 282
  micronormoblastic reaction 286
  transplant 287
Bone morphogenetic protein 74
  activity of 74
Bony pelvis 44, 44t
  classification of 44t
Bowel care 632
Bowel injury 196f
Brachial plexus injury 607, 708
Bradycardia 154, 590, 754, 776
Brain injury 697
  classic patterns of 698t
  neurologic markers of 700

Brain iron concentrations 277
Brain natriuretic peptide 105
Brass V drape 731f
Breast 81, 348, 630, 671
  care 632
  conserving surgery 360
  crawl 686
  emptying 674
  engorgement 631, 671, 711, 711f
  examination of 92
  infections 673
  lump, differential diagnosis of 360b
  mass, evaluation of 360
  support garment 674
  tumor 332
Breast abscess 667, 673, 674f
  risk of 360
Breast cancer
  early stage 361fc
  late stage 361fc
  pregnancy after 362
  pregnancy-associated 359
Breast milk
  and colostrum, composition of 630t
  jaundice 675
Breastfeeding 264, 321, 359, 368, 371, 454, 632
  advantages of 676
  care 633
  contraindications for 631
  preparation for 631
  preterm 678
  techniques 676
Breath holding spells 274
Breathing 436, 622, 756, 774
Breathlessness 394
Breech and transverse lie, diagnosis of 500t
Breech delivery, spontaneous 559
Breech extraction 559
  partial 559
Breech presentation 176f, 501b, 562
Broad ligament, anterior part of 40
Bromocriptine 253, 547
Bronchiectasis 323
Bronchopneumonia 395
Bronchoscopy 320
Brow presentation 566, 566f
Brown adipose tissue 682
Budd-Chiari syndrome 303, 417
Bullous lesions 337
Bullous pemphigoid 338
Buprenorphine 448
Buttonhole tear 638

C

Cabergoline 547
Calcineurin inhibitors 296
Calcium 239, 296
  binding tendency of 764
  channel blockers 238, 506
  chloride 779
  metabolism 107, 108t
  supplements 94
Campylobacter fetus 451
Cancer 356
  management of 356, 358t
Candida albicans 671
Candidiasis 375
Cannabis 342
Capillary hemangiomas 76

Capillary refill time 760
Captopril 237
Caput succedaneum 705, 705f, 711, 711f
Carbamazepine 329
Carbetocin 644
Carbohydrate 82
    metabolism 105, 258
Carboprost, dosage of 645
Carboxyhemoglobinemia 279
Carcinoma ovary 28
Cardiac arrest 437, 624, 772
    in-hospital 776
Cardiac arrhythmia 758
Cardiac disease 244, 245b, 771
Cardiac disorders 256
Cardiac evaluation 235, 700
Cardiac failure 269, 270
Cardiac lesions 252t
Cardiac malformations 177f, 178
    rate of 176
Cardiac markers 105
Cardiac organs 176
Cardiac outflow tracts 144
Cardiac output 85, 771
    reduced 254
Cardiac rhythm 775f
    abnormalities of 754
Cardiac situs 144
Cardiac systole, peak velocity during 167
Cardiac transplantation 256
Cardiac valve surgery 256
Cardiff method 158
Cardiff's chart 158f
Cardinal ligaments 659f
Cardiomyopathy 252, 283, 287
Cardiopulmonary adaptation 682
Cardiopulmonary blood flow 773
Cardiopulmonary resuscitation 437, 744, 772, 777
Cardiorespiratory diseases 485
Cardiotocograph trace features 574t
Cardiotocography 27, 490, 492, 573, 579, 580
    components of 590
    continuous 438, 573
    role of 487
Cardiovascular anomalies 68
Cardiovascular changes 83f, 435
Cardiovascular system 83, 85, 92
    development of 76
Carneous mole 196
Carnett's sign 431
Carpal tunnel syndrome 102, 336
Casirivimab 395
Cataracts 68
Category B medication 261
Cauda equina syndrome 624
Caudal dysgenesis 72
Caudal regression sequence 72
Cavum septum pellucidum 142f
Cefotaxime 323, 667
Ceftriaxone 323
Celiac disease 267, 306
Cell
    adhesion molecules 57
    culture artifact 116
    division 54
    fail 280
    free deoxyribonucleic acid 135, 186, 188f, 461, 495

salvage 532
size of 57
Central nervous system 74, 87, 222, 253, 327, 384
    effects on 274
    infections 327
Central pontine myelinolysis 304
Central venous pressure 757f, 758, 762, 768
Cephalhematoma 712f
Cephalic version, external 501
Cephalocele 75
Cephalohematoma 705, 706f, 712
Cephalopelvic disproportion 353, 577, 588, 588t
    borderline 596
Cephalosporins 323, 390, 667
Cerclage, abdominal 201
Cerebellar diameter 144
Cerebral aneurysm 610
Cerebral artery, middle 162, 163f, 167, 490
Cerebral palsy 515
Cerebral tumors 327, 332
    clinical features 332
    imaging status 332
    laboratory findings 332
Cerebral venous thrombosis 283, 327, 331
Cerebral ventricles 144
Cerebroplacental ratio 168, 490
Cerebrospinal fluid 75, 332, 386, 718
Cerebrovascular disease 405
Cerebrovascular disorders 327, 330
Certolizumab 313
Cervical
    conization 362
    dilatation 618
    dystocia 353
    encerclage 200
    index 200
    insufficiency, signs of 200
    smears, abnormal 362
    status 581
Cervical cancer 362
    diagnostic evaluation of 362
    management of 362, 363fc
    screening 28
    severe hemorrhage in 5
    treatment of 7
Cervical incompetence 194, 199
    complications 201
    contraindications 201
    diagnosis 200
    etiology of 200, 200t
    management of 200
    pathogenesis 200
Cervical length 504
    measurement 462
Cervix 40, 81, 629
    effacement of 578
    evaluation of 578
    funneling of 504f
    length of 504f
Cesarean delivery 405, 490
    high incidence of 610
    indications of 610
    surgical techniques for 612
    uterine incisions for 613f
Cesarean hysterectomy
    specimen 532f
    technique of 531

Cesarean radical hysterectomy 363
Cesarean scar 529
    pregnancy 529
Cesarean section 201, 247, 322, 372, 454, 492, 521, 562, 585, 609, 617
    anesthesia for 611
    complications of 588
    consent for 611
    epidemiology of 610
    indications of 611t
    packs 776
    surgical techniques 614
Chagas disease 387
Chelation therapy 282, 287
Chemical pleurodesis 320
Chemoprophylaxis 218
Chemotherapy 219, 357, 361, 365
    administration of 357
    drugs, dose of 357
    indications of 219, 220t
Cherney incision 612
Chest compressions 689, 691, 774f
Chest
    pain 283, 394, 768
        acute left-sided 779
    syndrome, acute 281-283
    X-ray of 216f
Chicken pox 123
Chlamydia trachomatis 385
Chloasma 102
Chlorpromazine 304
Chlorpropamide 426
Cholangitis 388
Cholecystectomy 288
Cholecystitis 281, 306
Cholelithiasis 281, 287, 348
Cholestasis 227, 302t
Cholestatic hepatosis 409
Chordin 74
Chorioamnionitis 387, 484
Chorioangioma 480
Choriocarcinoma 215, 215f, 332, 337
    histology 216f
Chorionic sac 459
Chorionic villus sampling 135, 149, 151, 152, 154, 186, 282, 285, 297
    advantages of 152
    disadvantages of 152
    gestational age 151
    techniques 151
Chorionicity 458, 458t
Choroid plexus cyst 144, 145, 146f
Chromatin 114
Chromosomal aberrations 133, 174
Chromosomal abnormalities 67, 119, 123, 128, 129, 153, 174f
Chromosomal anomalies 198
Chromosomal defect 66
Chromosomal disorders 114, 118
Chromosomal markers 144
Chromosomal microarray 117, 118, 120, 124
Chromosomal mosaicism 116
Chromosomal theory 66
Chromosomal translocation 194
Chromosome 53, 113, 114f
    analysis 150
    extra set of 118
    ploidy status, determination of 188f
    segment of 114

Chronic disease, anemia of 288
Chronic hypertension, investigations for 235*t*
Chronic inflammatory disease 305
Chronic medical disorders 228
Chronic obstructive pulmonary disease 237
Churg-Strauss syndrome 315
Circumvallate placenta 479
Cirrhosis 287, 418
Cisterna magna 142*f*, 144
Civil registration system 726
Clamping upper pedicles 657*f*
Clarithromycin 305, 323
Classical cesarean section 654*f*
Classical uterine
    incision 532*f*
    scar 585
Clavicle 707
Clavicular fracture 607, 707, 707*f*
Cleft palate 117
Clitoris 37
Cloacal exstrophy 78
Clogged milk ducts 672
Clonidine 238
Clostridium 387
    welchii 547
Cloxacillin 674
Clubfoot 716*f*
Clubfoot-congenital talipes equinovarus 716
Coagulation disorders 642
Coagulation profile 197, 778
Coagulopathy 304
Cocaine 342
Coccygeus muscles 41
Coenzymes 350
Cognitive behavioral therapy 344
Cognitive performance, impaired 274
Collagen vascular diseases 235, 295, 337
Collapse, postpartum 522
Colloid 764, 765*t*
    properties of 765*t*
Colonoscopy 305
Color Doppler 165, 166, 171*f*
    assisted ductus venosus 171*f*
    examination 172
    ultrasound 540*f*
Colposcopic biopsy 362
Columnar epithelium dips 40
Combined oral contraceptives 219, 240, 283
Common bacterial infections 384*t*
Communication 10, 16, 17
    barriers of 14, 14*t*, 14*b*
    categories of 12*t*
    formal 13
    informal 13
    methods of 12
    nonverbal 12, 13*t*
    one-way 12*t*
    physical nonverbal 12
    skills 11
    social behavior change 14
    two-way 12*t*
    verbal 13*t*
Community acquired pneumonia 322
Complete blood count 68, 331, 401, 411, 665, 756, 778
Conception
    products of 193*f*
    types of 487

Condom 454
    catheter 646
Condylomata acuminate grows 336
Congenital adrenal hyperplasia, types of 715
Congenital anomalies 463, 684
    higher incidence of 319
    incidence of 349
Congenital high airway obstruction syndrome 475
Congenital malformation 66*t*, 329, 522
    higher risk of 124
    severe 703
Congestive cardiac failure 251, 267, 404, 718
Congestive heart failure 763, 764
Congo red dot test 403
Conjoint twins 464, 464*f*
Connective tissue diseases 255
Constipation 100, 305
    etiology 100
    treatment 100
Contact dermatitis 338, 712, 712*f*
Continuous fetal monitoring 602
Continuous intrapartum fetal monitoring 473
Continuous positive airway pressure 745, 745*f*
Contraception 240, 240*t*, 248, 264, 372, 633
    counseling 303
    field of 7
Contraceptive advice 633
Contracted pelvis 564
Contraction stress test 157, 160, 262
    advantages of 161
    disadvantages of 161
Convulsive disorder 406
Cooley's anemia 287
Coombs test, indirect 495
Cooper's ligament 674
Cord 227, 483*t*
    abnormality of 478, 542
    blood glucose evaluation 713
    clamping, delayed 684
    complications 522
    entanglement 464*f*
    hematoma 154, 543, 543*f*
    insertion
        abdominal 144
        abnormalities 482
    length, antenatal determination of 482
    round neck 564
    vessel
        number of 144
        thrombosis 496
Cordocentesis 135, 152, 476
    complications of 154
Coronary artery disease 255, 348
Coronavirus disease 2019 (COVID-19) 201, 323, 393, 455, 665, 756
    infection 396
        moderate 395
        severe 395
    pandemic 28, 583, 723
    risk markers in 394*t*
    RT-PCR 583
    vaccination against 396
    vaccine 34
Corpus callosum, agenesis of 75
Cortical necrosis, acute 292
Cortical reaction 54, 55
Corticosteroids 314, 505, 506, 513
    use of 508

Cortisol 259
    production of 258
Cosmetic distress 335
Costochondral junction 546
Cotrimoxazole 371
Cotrimoxazole preventive therapy 372
Cough 319
    pain test 430
Couvelaire uterus 526*f*
Cow's milk 630*t*
    disadvantages of 631
Cradle cap 713
Cranial fractures 708
Cranial nerves, disorders of 327
Cranial neuropore, closure of 74
Cranial ultrasound 700
Craniofacial defects 76
C-reactive protein 235, 305, 322, 545
    levels of 348
Cri du chat syndrome 68
Crichton's method 572
Crohn disease 305
Crown-rump length 76, 91, 129, 130*f*
Cryoprecipitate 644, 767
Crystalloids 765*t*
    fluid 764
    properties of 765*t*
Culdocentesis 205
Cushing syndrome 235
Cutaneous lupus erythematosus 310*f*
Cyanosis 715, 715*f*
Cyanotic heart disease 244
    complex 703
Cyclooxygenase 313
Cyclophosphamide 312, 314, 315, 317
Cyclosporine 303, 316, 317
Cylindrical helix 482
Cyst adenoid malformation 476
Cystic fibrosis 323
Cytokines 57, 504
Cytomegalovirus 123, 194, 302, 381, 384, 389, 414, 542, 678
    infection 452

D

Dactylitis 281
Dalteparin 230
Dandy-Walker malformation 75
Decidual bleeding 523
Deep tendon reflexes 708
Deep transverse arrest 557
Deep vein thrombosis 283, 304, 336, 522
    pregnancy-related 325
    risk of 632
Deferasirox 282, 287
Deferiprone 282, 287
Deferoxamine 282, 287
Defibrillation 774
Defibrillator safety management 775
Deflexion, severe degree of 556
Delivery
    in breech, mechanism of 559
    of buttocks, mechanism of 559
    of head, mechanism of 559
    of shoulder, mechanism of 559
    timing of 239, 404, 491, 531, 536
Delivery room 684
    management 701
Delta hepatitis 415

Dengue 430
  virus 383
Deoxyribonucleic acid 53, 113f, 114f, 187f, 189f
  analysis 287
  determination of fetal 187
  direct 150
  sequences 113
Depot-medroxy-progesterone acetate 240
Depression 341
Depressive disorder 341t
Dermatological disorders 335
Desferrioxamine 446
Dexamethasone 303, 505
  administration of 514
Dextrocardia 177, 177f
Dextroposition 177
Dextrose 304, 444
Diabetes insipidus 475
Diabetes mellitus 158, 201, 258, 259b, 264, 296, 404, 405, 420, 421t, 543, 578
  classification 258
  global emergency 421f
  pregestational 258
  type 1 267, 308
  type 2 348
  uncontrolled 198
Diabetic ketoacidosis 426
Diabetic mother, management of infant of 263t
Diabetic nephropathy 295
Diabetic pregnancy, infant born from 263
Diabetogenic pregnancy 258, 422f
Dialysis 297
Diamorphine 622, 623
Diaphragm 78
Diaphragmatic hernia 78
  congenital 476
Diarrhea 717
Diastolic blood pressure 296, 756
Diazepam 444
Dichlorophenolindophenol 287
Dichorionic diamniotic placenta 467f
Dichorionic twins 459f, 542f
Dicloxacillin 674
Dicyclomine 304
Diet 94, 632
DiGeorge syndrome 117
Digestive tract defects 350
Dihydrocodeine 622
Dilation and curettage 204, 205
Dipeptidyl-peptidase 4 262
Diploid 66
Direct obstetric deaths 726
Discharge per vaginum 362
Disseminated intravascular coagulation 302, 411, 518, 522, 524, 525, 545, 653, 668, 745, 756, 767, 768
Diuretics 238, 325, 404
Dizygotic twins 457
Dobutamine 779
Doderlein's bacilli 38
Dolicocephalic head 564
Dolutegravir 368, 369
Domestic violence and abuse 440
Domperidone 304, 676
Dopamine 779
  agonists 547
Doppler cerebroplacental ratio 487

Doppler effect 166
Doppler flow indices 167, 167f
Doppler flow velocimetry waveform analysis, abnormal 311
Doppler velocimetry 158, 162, 262, 495
Dorsal mesentery 77
Double marker test 67
Down syndrome 67, 114, 129, 133, 134t, 135t, 150, 186
  phenotype features of 67f
  prediction of 67
Doxylamine 99
Drip-drop feeding 678f
Drug
  ionization of 357
  of abuse, poisoning of 447
  toxicity 771
  use of 618
Ductal arch 184, 184f
Ductus venosus 134, 167, 168f, 490, 492
Duodenal atresia 474f, 475
Dysfunctional labor 554
Dysgerminomas 364
Dysmaturity syndrome 684
Dyspareunia 638
Dyspepsia 305, 462
Dysphagia 316
Dysplasia 123
Dyspnea 318, 319
Dysrhythmias 174
Dystocia 555
Dysuria 430

E

Early amniocentesis 150
Early obstetric warning
  score 753f
  system, modified 754t
Early pregnancy 259
  complications 193
Ebola 384
Ebstein anomaly 254
Echocardiography 245, 756
  timing for 175
Echogenic bowel 145, 145f
Echogenic cardiac focus 144
Eclampsia 35, 267, 311, 398, 404, 406, 411, 541, 543, 770
  anticonvulsants for 730
  management of 746
  prevention of 404
  vigilance for 405
Ectoderm 74
  development 74f
Ectodermal derivatives 74
Ectodermal dysplasia syndromes 155
Ectopia cordis 78
Ectopic hydatidiform mole 215
Ectopic implantation, site of 203f
Ectopic kidney 473
Ectopic mass 205f
Ectopic pregnancy 70, 198, 202, 206fc
  clinical features 203
  diagnosis 204
  differential diagnosis 205
  evolution of 202
  incidence 202
  location of 70

management of 206
  methotrexate treatment for 207t
  risk factors for 202, 203t
  ultrasound features of 205t
Eculizumab, administration of 294
Eczema 336
Edema, severe 296
Edward's syndrome 67, 114, 129, 150, 186
Efavirenz 369
Ehlers-Danlos syndrome 255, 337
Eisenmenger syndrome 247, 254
Ejection fraction 249
Elective cesarean section, indications of 559
Electrical injuries 440
Electrocardiography 689, 692, 756
Electroencephalogram 328, 331
Electrolyte 702
  imbalance 305
  panel 197
Electronic fetal
  heart rate monitoring 577
  monitoring 27, 405, 590
Electronic health
  informatics, advantages of 26
  record, components of 27, 27f
Electronic partograph 575
Elemental iron 276
Elevated cardiac troponin 700
Elevated liver enzymes 239, 413, 747
Embryo, implantation of 53
Embryoblast 69
Embryo-endometrial interaction 57
Embryogenesis, timeline of 65f
Embryonic stem cells 69
Emergency cesarean section 521
  risk of 154
Emergency medical service 777
Emergency obstetric care 727, 730, 744
Emerging infectious diseases 455
Emesis, pregnancy unique quantification of 100t
Encephalocele 75
Encephalopathy 294, 304
End-diastolic flow velocity 163f, 167
Endocardial cushion 76
Endocrine
  disorders 485
  system 84
Endodermal derivatives 77
Endodermal development 77f
Endodermal sinus tumors 364
Endoglin concentrations 402
Endometrial neoplasms 348
Endometritis 387
Endometrium 40, 57
  thickness of 40f
Endoscopy 305
  field of 7
Endothelial dysfunction 400
Endotoxin mediated injury 294
Endotracheal intubation, indications of 691
Endotracheal tube 774
Enema 568
Energy sources 274
Enoxaparin 230
  prophylactic dose of 395
Enterobius vermicularis 380
Enteroviruses 384
Entonox 622

Enzyme
    inducing drugs 329
    inhibitors 57
    linked immunosorbent assay 311
Eosinophilic hyalinization 217f
Epidermal growth factor 57
Epidermal melanocytes, number of 335
Epidermis 74
Epidermolysis bullosa 155
Epidural analgesia 560, 623
Epidural anesthesia 611
Epidural hematoma 707f
Epigastric pain, symptoms of 305
Epigenetic regulations 405
Epilepsy 327, 328, 544
    effects of 328
    incidence of 327
    maternal implications of 328
    treatment of 328
Epileptic seizures 327
Epinephrine 693, 779
Episiotomy 605, 607, 635, 636t
    collections 667
    complications 637
    indications 635
    late 638
    median 636t
    mediolateral 636t
    postoperative care 637
    types of 636
Epithelial ovarian tumors 364
Epithelioid trophoblastic tumor 211, 216, 217f, 223
Epithelium leading, erosion of 306
Epoprostenol 254
Epstein-Bar virus 414
Erb's Duchenne palsy 708, 708f, 713, 713f
Ergometrine 615, 645
    use of 247
Erythema multiforme 337, 338
Erythrocytapheresis 282
Erythrocyte
    porphyrin levels 287
    sedimentation rate 235, 282, 320
Erythroid hyperplasia 282, 286
Erythromycin 323, 505, 674
Erythropoiesis, augmentation of 287
Escherichia coli 380, 674
Esophageal atresia 474, 474f
Esophageal cancer 57
Estriol 258
Estrogen 98, 111, 335
    role of 409
Etanercept 313
Etymology 610
Euploid pregnancy loss, rate of 348
Exacerbations 321
Exercise 237, 261
Exome 114
Exons 113, 120
External cephalic version, complications of 501, 502b
Extracardiac malformations 174
Extracorporeal cardiopulmonary resuscitation 776
Extracranial injuries 705
Extraembryonic mesoderm, formation of 71f
Extramedullary hematopoiesis 287

Extrapulmonary tuberculosis 321
    diagnosis of 321
    treatment of 321

F

Face presentation 564
    causes of 564
Facial injury 706
Facial lesions 76
Facial nerve injury 708
Facial palsy 709f
Fallopian tube 41, 70, 207f, 657f
    ampulla of 53
Falx cerebri 142f
Family planning 727
Fascia of Scarpa's, blunt dissection of 613
Fasciitis, necrotizing 638
Fasting glucose 68
Fasting plasma glucose 421
Fat metabolism 82
Fatty acid 410, 683
Fatty infiltration, evidence of 304
Fatty lever, acute 292, 293, 301, 304, 408, 410, 411b
Fatty metamorphosis, acute 304
Feasible prediction policy 402
Febrile seizures 274
Feet, edema of 325
Femur 708
    length 141f
Fentanyl 622
Ferric carboxy maltose, intravenous 276
Fertilization 53, 55f
    defects in 56
    process of 54
Fetal abdomen 142f
Fetal abnormality 122, 123, 130f
    etiology 122, 123
    pathophysiology 122
    prevention 124
    treatment 124
Fetal adaptive immune responses 451
Fetal alcohol syndrome 344
Fetal anatomy
    look for in 139
    survey 140
Fetal anemia 123, 153, 168, 169f, 522
Fetal aneuploidy 169, 186, 188, 188f
    prenatal diagnosis of 186
    risk, estimation of 28
Fetal anomalies, assessment of 169
Fetal ascites 496
Fetal asphyxia 561
Fetal assessment 438
Fetal autopsy 229, 544
Fetal biometry 401
Fetal bladder tapping 154
Fetal blood
    loss 688
    sampling 152, 591, 592
        technical aspects of 153t
Fetal bradycardia 688
Fetal brain 259
    damage 465
    development 267
Fetal cardiac anatomy 170f
Fetal cells
    chromosomal analysis of 186
    direct analysis of 186

Fetal cephalic presentation 176, 176f
Fetal chromosomal abnormality 540
Fetal circulation 63, 697f
    normal 696
Fetal complications 269, 380, 450, 463, 501b
Fetal condition 572
Fetal congenital malformations, diagnosis of 113
Fetal consequences, long-term 463
Fetal crown rump length, measurement of 170
Fetal death 154, 194, 227, 244, 440
    etiology of 540
Fetal defects 73t
Fetal defense 379
Fetal demise 442, 466
    diagnosis of 539
Fetal development 61
    effects on 329
    normal process of 122
Fetal diagnosis, invasive tests for 149
Fetal distress 303, 439, 588
    consequences of 267
    risk factors for 589
Fetal echocardiography 174, 175, 184
    advantages of 184f
    analysis 592
    indications of 174
Fetal face 142f
Fetal fibronectin 504
Fetal fraction, percentage of 135
Fetal gender, evaluation of 459
Fetal genetics 229
Fetal growth 63
    and development 62
    monitoring 230
    ultrasonographic assessment of 236
Fetal growth restriction 118, 158, 167, 267, 287, 303, 319, 384, 387, 400, 410, 463, 485, 490, 492, 542, 684
    diagnosis 486
    etiology 485
    management principles 487
    monitoring 487
    pathophysiological progression 487
    recent advances 491
    screening for 486
    severe 541f
    ultrasonographic biometry 486
Fetal head 561
    delivery of 552
    expulsion of 552
    hyper extended 502
    molding of 572t
    rotation of 552
Fetal heart 142f, 540f, 562
    monitoring 593
    screening 175
    sound 320, 556
Fetal heart rate 159, 590f-592f, 694, 755f
    deceleration of 688
    management of abnormal 591
    mean of 590
    monitoring, minimal duration of 159
Fetal hydantoin syndrome 329
Fetal hydrops 153, 475, 495, 540f, 543, 607, 688
Fetal hyperinsulinemia, complications of 259fc
Fetal hypoxia, marker of 167

Fetal infections 154, 388, 450, 540
Fetal inflammation 505f
Fetal inflammatory response syndrome 388
Fetal lungs 476
Fetal macrosomia 323, 349, 354, 588
   pathogenesis of 349
   risk of 349
Fetal malformations 119, 323, 358
Fetal malposition, effects of 554
Fetal markers 129
Fetal membranes, inflammation of 505f
Fetal metabolism 421
Fetal middle cerebral artery 168f
Fetal monitoring 262, 262t, 438, 760
Fetal morbidity 408
Fetal mortality 408
Fetal movement 476, 590f
   count 158, 158f
   loss of 439
Fetal neural tube defects 149
Fetal neuroprotection 240
Fetal nutrition 63
Fetal origin 485
   anemia of 540
Fetal pancreatic insulin secretion 259
Fetal pelvis 143f
Fetal period 62
Fetal phase 65
Fetal physiology 61, 259, 688
Fetal position 562
Fetal presentation, abnormal 704
Fetal programming 423f
Fetal pulse oximetry 592
Fetal red cells 279
Fetal reduction, selective 461
Fetal renal tract, abnormalities in 472
Fetal scalp
   lactate 592
   stimulation 592
Fetal screening, biochemical test for 133
Fetal situs 139, 139t
   normal 139
Fetal skull 552
   transverse section of 141f, 142f
Fetal spinal vertebra 143f
Fetal spine 143f
Fetal stage 61
Fetal status, nonreassuring 439
Fetal structural malformations 230
Fetal surveillance 236, 283, 401, 425, 426
   indications of 158
Fetal tachyarrhythmias 497
Fetal tachycardia 591
Fetal therapy 154
Fetal thrombocytopenia, diagnosis of 153
Fetal thrombotic vasculopathy 484
Fetal tissue
   biopsy 135, 155
   internal 546
Fetal ultrasonography, indications of 95t
Fetal urine 155t
Fetofetal transfusion syndrome 475, 542
Fetomaternal bleed, amount of 546
Fetomaternal organ 478
Fetoscope 155f
Fetoscopic endotracheal occlusion 78
Fetus 542f, 704
   and placenta, inspection of 544
   exposure of 123
   head of 552
   papyraceous 467f
   sonogram of 473f
Fever 310, 718
   causes of 388t
   postpartum 387
Fibrinogen, large amounts of 523
Fibroblast growth factor 74
Fibromyoma 194
Fine needle aspiration cytology 360
First-trimester 91, 126, 260, 306
   body mass index 267
   recurrent pregnancy loss 198
   screening 134
Fist percussion test 431
Flexible fiberoptic bronchoscopy 320
Flow velocity waveforms 163f
Flucloxacillin 674
Fludrocortisone 715
Fluid 762
   color of 150
   management 100t, 405, 702
   overload 305
   responsiveness, estimation of 762
   restriction 324
Fluid resuscitation 762
   colloids for 764
   end point of 764
Fluid therapy 762
   dosing of 764
Flumazenil 444
Fluorescence in situ hybridization 120, 150
Fluoroscopy 320
Focal nodular hyperplasia 417
Folate, neurological deficiency of 306
Foley's catheter 582, 646
Folic acid 288, 330, 371
   supplementation 34, 315, 729
Folinic acid regimen 221
Follicle stimulating hormone 298
Folliculitis, infectious 339
Follistatin 74
Food poisoning 447
Foodborne transmission 387
Footling presentation 558f
Forceps 595
   contraindications 596
   functions of 596
   indications 596
   parts of 596f
   types of 595
Formaldehyde 194
Foul lochia 387
Fracture 707
   risk factors for 708
Fragile sites 68
Fragile X syndrome 68
Fragmentation defects 70
Frank breech 558f
Fraternal twins 457
Free androgens, large amount of 348
Free fatty acids 258
Fresh frozen plasma 644, 767
Friedman's curve 569f
Fulcrum 552
Full fetal echocardiography 246
Functional menstrual disorders 198
Fundal grip 562
Fundoscopy 401
Fundus 39
Fungal dermatitis 712
Fungal infections 380
Funipuncture 152
Furosemide 237, 247
Fusion of gametes 54

G

Gadolinium contrast 356
Gadolinium-enhanced magnetic resonance angiography 235
Galactagogues, role of 676
Galactocele 631, 672
   management 673
   ultrasonography 673f
Galactokinesis 630
Galactopoiesis 630
Galactosialidosis 496
Galen malformations 169
Gallbladder 141, 142f
   disease 306
Gallium scans 432
Gametes, abnormal 68
Gamma-glutamyl transferase 302, 410
Gardnerella vaginalis 504
Gas exchange, impaired 697
Gaskin's maneuver 606, 607f
Gastric peristalsis 305
Gastric pressure 305
Gastroenteritis 305
Gastroesophageal reflux 304, 322
   and heartburn 100
   disease 319
Gastroesophageal rupture 99
Gastrointestinal conditions 305, 412, 473
   pregnancy-specific 304
Gastrointestinal disease 301
Gastrointestinal tract 84, 221, 628
   anatomy of 304
   physiology of 304
Gastroschisis 78, 473
   risk of 350
Gastroscopy 305
Gaucher disease 496
Gel electrophoresis 282
General anesthesia 625
Genes 113, 119, 405
   therapy 287
Genetic abnormalities 229
Genetic counseling 230, 282, 288
   post-test 188
Genetic disorder 114
   suspicion of 230
   types of 114, 115fc
Genetic information 191
Genetic syndromes 473
Genetic tests 152, 230, 282
   types of 119
Genital tract disorders 518
Genitalia, female external 37f
Genitourinary system 430
Genitourinary tract conditions 412
Genome 113
   editing techniques 288
Genomic disorders 117
Genotype 68, 114
Germ cell tumors 364
Gestation trophoblastic disease 325
Gestation, length of 71

Gestational ages 471*t*
    large for 349, 420, 422
        parameter of 470*f*
        small for 167, 275, 294, 414, 490, 492, 714
Gestational anemia 275
Gestational carcinoma 211
Gestational choriocarcinoma 215
Gestational diabetes mellitus 105, 117, 119, 258, 267, 349, 350, 420, 475
    diagnosis of 422
    epidemiology 420
    management of 424
    screening tests for 106*t*
Gestational epilepsy 328
Gestational hypertension 398, 404
Gestational pemphigoid 337
Gestational transient thyrotoxicosis 269, 270
Gestational trophoblastic disease 198, 210, 217, 223, 269
Gestational trophoblastic neoplasia 211, 216*f*, 219, 220, 220*t*, 222, 222*t*
    diagnosis of 219
    high-risk 221
    low risk 221
    postmolar 219
Gestosis score 398, 402*t*, 420
    enigma of 405
    significance of 402
Glasgow coma scale 745, 752, 758, 758*t*
Glibenclamide 261
Globin chain
    composition 284
    synthesis, quantitative disorders of 279
Glomerular disease 293
Glomerular endotheliosis 293
Glomerular filtration rate 84, 291
Glomerulonephritis 295
Glucocorticoids, administration of 294
Glucometer 260*f*
Glucose 63
    metabolism 63, 422*f*
    monitoring, frequency of 759
    transport 63
Glucose-6-phosphate dehydrogenase deficiency 390
Glutamic acid
    beta-chain substitution of 284
    lysine for 284
Gluten sensitive enteropathy 306
Glyburide therapy 426
Glycemia monitoring 264, 759
Glycemic control 261
Glycerol trinitrate 501
Glycoprotein 311
Glycosylated fibronectin 403
Golimumab 313
Gonadal mosaicism 116
Gonadotropins 348
Gonorrhea 375
Gram-negative enteric bacilli 281
Grand multipara 779
Granular cytoplasmic bodies 286
Granulocyte colony stimulating factors 357
Granulomatosis 315
Granulomatous inflammatory disease, chronic 305
Graves' disease 268, 269, 271, 313, 314
    risk of 338
Graves' hyperthyroidism 269

Gravid uterus 301
Greater vestibular glands 38
Growth 61
    centile chart of fetal demise 541*f*
    factor beta, transforming 110
    factors 357
Guillain-Barré syndrome 316, 327
Gynecoid 45

H

H1N1 virus 323, 380
Haemophilus influenza 281, 323, 380
Hair changes 336
Haploid chromosomes 113
Hartmann's sign 71
Hashimoto thyroiditis 314
Head
    and neck masses 475
    circumference 486
    deflexion of 556
Headache 304, 623
Health and well-being, promoters of 740
Health care, communication in 15
Health communication, applications of 14
Health impacts, severe 266
Health management and information system 747
Health system interventions 96
Healthcare personnel 682
    violence 48*t*
Healthcare seeking behavior 721
Healthcare system 10
Heart
    axis 144
    chambers of 178*f*
    connections of 175*t*
    defects, congenital 117, 254, 350, 710
    disease 243, 244*t*, 245, 246*t*, 544
        functional class of 246
    failure 270
    function 180
    rate 331, 754, 756
    septum 76
    size 178
    valves of 183*f*
Heat loss, prevention of 684
Heavy metal absorption 274
Hectic fevers 664
Heinz bodies 286
Helicobacter pylori 305
Hellin-Zeleny's law 457
HELLP syndrome 239, 293, 301, 303, 408, 410, 413, 525
Hemangioendothelioma 496
Hemangiomas 336
Hematological changes 82, 104, 435
Hematoma 523, 667
Hematopoiesis, stage of 287
Hematopoietic stem cells 287
Hematuria 292, 310, 756
Hemoconcentration, severe 411
Hemodynamic adaptation 349
Hemodynamic status 204*t*
Hemoglobin 104, 279, 403, 531
    Bart disease 286*f*
    C 284
    concentration 762
    deficit, basis of 276
    disorders 279

    E 284
    electrophoresis 286
        report, normal 287*f*
    gamma genes of 122
    level, normal 273*t*
    structural variants of 279
    synthesis, inherited disorders of 279
Hemoglobinopathy 153, 279, 284
    classification of 279
    clinical features 280
    pathophysiology 280
    unstable 280
Hemoglobinuria 756, 768
Hemogram 433
Hemolysis 239, 293, 302*t*, 411, 413, 747
    signs of 767
Hemolytic crises 281
Hemolytic reaction, delayed 283
Hemolytic uremic syndrome 292
Hemoperitoneum 207*f*
Hemopoietic cell transplantation 282
Hemorrhage 223*f*, 255, 430, 438, 546*f*, 746, 770
    accidental 522
    antepartum 292, 462, 518, 527, 694, 743, 763, 770
        causes of 518, 518*t*
    epidural 706
    fetomaternal 154, 496
    intracerebral 328
    intracranial 771
    intraventricular 707
    mild 525
    obstetric, causes of 770
    postpartum 267, 292, 349, 405, 522, 547, 607, 608, 641, 644*t*, 645*fc*, 646, 665, 727, 743, 756, 763, 770
        causes of 642
        etiology of 647*f*
        preventing 405
        severe 675
        surgical management of 645
    subarachnoid 328, 331, 707
        causes of 331
    subchorionic 194
    subgaleal 706
    unavoidable 518
Hemorrhoids 101, 101*f*, 306
    develop 306
    etiology 101
    symptoms 101
    treatment 101
    veins develop 336
Hemostasis, special care for 654
Heparin, unfractionated 252
Hepatic adenoma 417
Hepatic dysfunction 411, 412
Hepatic failure 445
Hepatic system 408
Hepatitis 382, 414, 415*f*
    A 95, 414
        prevention of 414
        virus 414
    B 89, 95, 408, 414, 453
        acute 415
        surface antigen 149
    C 89, 408, 414, 415
        virus 94, 149
    D 408, 414, 415
    E 414, 416

infective 408
  viral serology 411
  viruses 413t
Hepatobiliary iminodiacetic acid 432
Hepatobiliary system 430
Hepatocellular carcinoma 418
Hepatocytes 259, 304
Hepatolenticular degeneration 416
Hereditary anemias 279
Hereditary renal disease 295
Hereditary thrombophilias 541, 543
Heritable thoracic aortic disease 249
Hernia, inguinal 716
Herpes gestationis 337
Herpes simplex 194, 452, 671, 678
  virus 375, 381
    infections 452
Herpes zoster 671, 678
  lesions 671
Heterozygosity, absence of 120
High dependency unit 411
High fetal middle cerebral artery 169f
Hirsutisim 336
Home uterine activity monitoring 504
Homozygous 211, 280, 410
Hormonal abnormalities 339
Hormonal therapy 357
Hormones 677
  enzymes 350
Human attitude 8
Human chorionic gonadotropin 70, 84, 85f, 98, 109, 110f, 134, 204, 206, 211, 217, 220, 224, 266, 304, 715
  abnormal 198
Human chorionic thyrotropin 266
Human chromosome
  packaging of 113f
  structure of 113f
Human deficiency virus control 727
Human genome project 113
Human growth hormone 259
Human immunodeficiency virus 89, 124, 149, 194, 321, 323, 367, 370, 382, 454, 678
  infection 367, 369, 370
  laboratory diagnosis of 368
  low prevalence of 368
  management of 372
  mother-to-child transmission of 737
  prevalence 367
  transmission 454
  types of 367
Human leukocyte antigen 270
Human milk 630t, 674
Human papilloma virus 375
  exacerbates 336
Human placental
  alpha macroglobulin 504
  lactogen 105, 110, 259, 486
  lipids 335
Humerus, fracture of 607
Hydatidiform mole 211, 337, 466
  complete 211, 212, 214, 214f, 215t
  diagnosis of 217
  genetics of 211
  management of 218
  partial 118, 211, 212f, 214, 215t
Hydatidiform pregnancy, benign 325
Hydralazine 238, 296, 310
Hydramnios 324, 461

Hydration 474
Hydrocortisone 357, 715
Hydronephrosis 473
Hydrops 476, 495f
  fetalis 475f
Hydroquinones 335
Hydroureter 473
Hydroxychloroquine sulfate 310
Hymen 38
Hyperactivity disorder 68
Hyperbilirubinemia, congenital 302t
Hyperechoic bowel 144
Hyperemesis gravidarum 98, 269, 270, 304, 413
Hypergalactia 675
Hyperglycemia 260, 420
  clinical clues for 421
Hyperintense heterogeneous placenta 530f
Hyperkalemia 294, 297, 715, 778
Hyperlactation 675
Hypermetabolic state 270
Hyperosmolar glucose 206
Hyperprolactinemia 198
Hypertension 194, 233, 296, 401, 523, 754, 756
  chronic 158, 233-236, 240t, 398, 405, 485, 541, 543
  control of 237
  degree of 237
  essential 234
  management of 296
  masked effect 234
  mild 233
  pathway for 754
  portal 418
  pregnancy 158, 292, 303, 461
  resistant 237
  secondary causes of chronic 234t
  severe 233
    chronic 239
  transient 234, 235
  treatment of chronic 236
Hypertensive disorders 158, 398, 420, 485, 541, 543, 547, 743
  clinical classification of 399
  diagnosis 400
  incidence of 398
  spectrum of 411
Hyperthyroidism 268, 270
  causes of 268
  clinical features of 268
  effects of 267, 269
  essential of diagnosis 268
  manifestations of 269
  subclinical 268, 270
  temporary 270
  treatment of 269
Hypertonicity 344
Hypertrophic cardiomyopathy 253
Hypertrophic obstructive cardiomyopathy 253
Hyperviscosity 684
Hypocalcemia 297, 684, 778
Hypoglycemia 683, 684
  clinical 264
  prevention of neonatal 264
Hypokalemia 778
Hyponatremia 304, 715
Hypoplastic kidney 473
Hypoplastic umbilical artery 482

Hypoproteinemia 296
Hypospadias 329, 718
Hypotension 754
  management of severe 746
  severe 623, 624
Hypothalamic receptors, regulation of 348
Hypothalamic-pituitary-ovarian axis 348
Hypothermia 683, 684, 778
Hypothyroid
  state 270
  treatment of 268
Hypothyroidism 267, 405
  causes of 267
  complicated pregnancy 271
  consequences of 267
  diagnostic criteria of 267
  encountered, types of 267
  management of 266, 267
  permanent 270
  prevalence of 266
  risk factors for 266
  severity of 267
  temporary 270
Hypotonic saline 474
Hypovolemia 591, 778
  acute maternal 473
Hypovolemic shock 764
Hypoxemia, progressive 158
Hypoxia 154, 778
  chronic 244
  prevent 778
Hypoxic ischemic encephalopathy
  classification of 700t
  risk factor for 697
  treatment of 701
Hysterectomy 215f, 219f, 223f, 647
Hysterotomy 197
  resuscitative 438

I

Ichthyotic disorders 155
Icterus gravidarum 409
Iliac crest, right 306
Iliac vessels, external 171
Iliopsoas test 430
Illness, self-limiting 332
Imatinib 358
Imdevimab 395
Imipenem 323
Immune
  complexes 485
  fetal hydrops 495
    diagnosis 495
    management 495
  status, impaired 274
  system 104
    changes 450
Immunization 95, 451, 633
Immunoglobulin 302, 309
  G 268, 311, 667
Immunologic techniques 389
Immunology 399
Immunosuppressive agents 296
Impetigo herpetiformis 337
Implantation failure 58
Imprinting disorders 117
In situ publication bias 25
In utero hypoxia 688

Index

In vitro fertilization 212
　　embryos 69
Inadequate placental perfusion 399
Indomethacin 297, 473, 476
Infant feeding policy 632
Infections 194, 227, 336, 378, 379t, 388, 504, 637
　　categories of 379t
　　chronic 485
　　congenital 388
　　control policy 615
　　effects of 388
　　prevention of 390
　　types of 389
Infectious disease screening 89
Infective endocarditis 247
　　prevention of 247t
Infertility 28, 267, 348
Inflammation, intensity of 484
Inflammatory bowel disease 305, 315
Infliximab 313
Influenza 323
　　A 380
　　vaccination 323
　　vaccine 95
　　virus 414
Inherited anemias 153
Inotropic agent 779
Insect-borne transmission 387
Instrument, parts of 595, 599
Instrumental birth, reduced 737
Instrumental delivery
　　frequency of 610
　　high 596
　　incidence of 595
Instrumental vaginal delivery 595
　　classification of 596t
　　complications 598
Insulin 6, 426
　　binding of 259
　　free 259
　　resistance 422f
　　　　obesity related 349
　　secretion 258
　　therapy 261, 425
Insulin-like growth factor 76
　　binding protein, levels of 348
Intensive care unit 349, 411, 743-745, 745f, 747, 749, 756, 760, 766
Intensive critical care medicine, principles of 749
Intensive multi-modality therapy 222
Interglandular tissue 40
Interleukin 348
Internal capsule, posterior limb of 700
Internal iliac artery 42, 648f
　　anterior division of 43f
　　branches of 43f
　　ligation 532
　　ligation of 649f
Interstitial nephritis 295
Intertwin membrane thickness 460
Interventional chest procedures 319
Intestine 430
Intimate partner violence 89, 437
Intra-amniotic infections 505
Intracardiac echogenic focus 146f
Intracranial injuries 706, 706f
Intracranial translucency 130
Intractable heart failure, acute 247

Intraembryonic mesoderm
　　formation of 72f
　　migration of 73f
Intrapartum analgesia, reduced 737
Intrapartum care 240, 396, 476, 586
　　routine 567
Intrapartum complication 368, 463
Intrapartum fetal heart rate monitoring 573
　　methods of 573fc
Intrapartum fetal monitoring 405
Intrapartum loss 230
Intrapartum management 330, 404, 426, 507, 593
Intrapartum periods, management of 418
Intrapartum surveillance, methods of 589
Intrapartum tests 567
Intrathoracic masses 475
Intrauterine death 292
　　late 118
Intrauterine device 240, 303
　　failure 194
Intrauterine fetal death 230, 545, 578, 583
　　causes for 542
Intrauterine fetal demise 267, 539
　　evaluation of 544
Intrauterine gestational sac 126f
Intrauterine growth
　　restriction 227, 283, 442, 522, 524, 540, 578, 694, 713, 714f
　　retardation 384
Intrauterine infection 504
　　stages of 505f
Intrauterine system 240
Intrauterine transfusion 476
Introns 113
Invasive disease 362
　　early stage 362
Invasive mole 215
Invasive monitoring, methods of 644
Invasive squamous cell 217f
Inverted nipple 631
Iodine insufficiency, moderate-to-severe 266
Iron 633
　　absorption
　　　　enhancers of 276
　　　　inhibitors of 276
　　chelators 282, 287
　　deficiency 274, 286
　　　　anemia 274, 287, 288
　　　　consequences of 274
　　deposition 286
　　indices 286
　　intoxication, acute 446
　　metabolism 82
　　sucrose
　　　　complex therapy 276
　　　　intravenous 276
　　supplementation 94, 729
Ischemia 688
Ischemic heart disease 255, 405
Ischemic stroke 327, 330
Ischial spine 624
Isochromosome 116
Isoniazid 321
　　prophylaxis 321
　　indications of 321t
Isotonic crystalloid solution 768
Isotonic saline 474

J

Jacobs syndrome 186
Jacquemier's maneuver 606, 607f
Janani Shishu Suraksha Karyakram 729
Janani Suraksha Yojana 729
Janus kinase inhibitors 313
Japanese encephalitis 384
Jaundice 91, 287, 302, 302t, 430, 714, 714f
　　causes of 302t
　　physiological 714
　　recurrent 409
Jehovah's witnesses 532
Joel-Cohen incision 612
Joint replacement 312
Jugular venous pressure 325

K

Kangaroo mother care 676, 684
Karyotype, abnormal 542
Kasabach Merritt syndrome 496
Kayser-Fleischer ring 416
Kerr incision 613
Ketones 258, 259
Ketonuria, quantification of 414
Ketosis, signs of 414
Kidney 235, 281, 473, 496
　　biopsy 294
　　damage 473
　　disease 405
　　　　chronic 294, 295, 298
　　donors 298
　　dysfunction, stage of 295
　　function 291
　　　　assessment of 296
　　　　measurement of 293
　　injury, postrenal acute 293
Kielland forceps 598, 598f
Klebsiella 380
Kleihauer test 546
Kleihauer-Betke test 437
Klinefelter syndrome 67, 133, 150, 186
Klumpke's palsy 708

L

Labetalol 237, 296
Labia
　　majora 37
　　minora 37
Labor 550, 555
　　active management of 573
　　analgesia 621
　　clinical correlation 551
　　clinical course of 563
　　complications 743
　　course of 556
　　elective induction of 583
　　first stage of 586
　　general management of 247
　　induction of 405, 537, 577, 579, 580t, 582, 582t
　　initiation of 550fc
　　malpresentations in 558
　　management of 565
　　　　first stage of 568
　　　　fourth stage of 574
　　　　second stage of 573
　　mechanism of 553, 554, 556, 559, 565

poor progress of 586
preparation for 567
progress of 568, 569, 572
prolonged second stage of 588t
room nurse 371
second stage of 586, 588
stage of 560
third stage of 353, 522, 574, 643
Labor and delivery 246, 319, 353
    management of 283
Lacerations 704, 705
Lactate dehydrogenase 401, 403
Lactation 305, 547, 630
    management 454
    mastitis 387
    physiology of 630
    preparation for 631
    support 747
    suppression of 631
Lactation failure 675, 677fc
    management of 676
    secondary 675
Lactogenesis 630
Lactogenic diet 677
Lamivudine 368, 369
Language impairment, risk of 264
Laparoscopic surgery 206, 357
Laparoscopy 205
Laparotomy 206, 668
Large-bore cannula 778
Laryngeal mask airway 436
Laryngeal nerve injury 709
Laryngeal papilloma 336
Lassa fever 384
Latching pain 671
Late pregnancy
    complications 499
    loss 229t
        maternal evaluation for 228t
Laxatives 639
Lead poisoning 288, 446
    chronic 447
Leaving placenta in situ 532
Lecithin 150
Leflunomide 312
Left tubal ectopic pregnancy 207f
Left uterine displacement 772, 773f
Left ventricular ejection fraction 248
Left ventricular failure 398
Left ventricular outflow tract 140, 175, 177, 180, 180f
Leopald's maneuver 93f
Leprosy 337
Leptin 98
Leptospirosis 385
Lethal multiple pterygium 496
Leukocytes 83, 104
Leukopenia 310
Levator ani 41
    muscle 38, 552
Levetiracetam 330, 702
Levonorgestrel 240
Levothyroxine sodium 267
Leydig cell testosterone secretion 348
Life-threatening postpartum hemorrhage 767
Ligament 655
    broad 657f
    ligation of 660
    portion of broad 657f

Lignocaine 779
Limb
    defects 350
        reduction 123, 123f
    shortening 144
Linea nigra 102f
Lipid emulsion, intravenous 779
Lipid metabolism 106
    changes in 106t
Lipid profile 68
Lipid solubility 357, 678
Lipolysis 683
Liquid based cytology 28
Liquid chromatography 282
Liquor amnii 572
Listeria monocytogenes 451
Listeriosis 388
    monocytogenes 542
Lithium 267, 475
Litzmann obliquity 551
Liver
    anatomy of 301
    biopsy 304, 410, 411
    conditions 301
    enzymes 68, 401
    functions of 301
    hematoma 304
    metastases 222
    oxidize ketones 259
    parameters 665
    physiology of 301
    spleen scans 432
    test 235
    volume 78
Liver disease 301, 302, 408
    chronic 416
    classification of 409t
    end-stage 416
    nonpregnancy-related 409
    pregnancy-related 409
Liver disorders
    classification of 408
    evaluation of 418
Liver function test 106, 107t, 197, 218, 302, 303, 310, 331, 384, 403, 408, 409, 433, 443, 756, 778
    abnormal 408
    physiological changes in 408t
Liver transplant 418
    recipient 303
Local anesthesia 624
Lochia 629
    alba 629
    rubra 629
    serosa 629
Long forgotten disease 453
Loop diuretics 237
Loss of weight 628
Lovset's maneuver 561, 562f
Low birth weight babies 678, 683
Low end-tidal carbon dioxide 780
Low intelligence quotient 267
Low molecular weight heparin 252, 283, 296, 312, 325, 395, 491
Low platelet count 747
Low serum alpha-fetoprotein 133
Lower esophageal
    pressure 304
    sphincter tone, reduced 305

Lower segment cesarean section 197, 230, 384, 577, 580, 582, 586f, 718
Lower urinary tract 654
    obstruction 154, 473
Lower uterine segment 613
    cesarean section 353
    measurement of 619
Lump, abdominal 430
Lung
    diseases, infiltrative 324, 324t
    injury, acute 320, 768
    tumor 332
Lung-to-head ratio 78
Lupus anticoagulant 199, 311
Lupus nephritis 297
Luteal phase defects 198
Luteinizing hormone 298
Lyme disease 386
Lymphadenopathy 310
Lymphatic abnormalities 496
Lymphedema, congenital 496
Lymphocyte abnormalities 270
Lymphocytic hypophysitis 271

M

Macerated fetus 195f
Mackenrodt's ligaments 40
Macrolide 323, 390
Macrosomia 353, 420, 704
Macular pigmentation 335
Magnesium sulfate 324, 506, 515
    role of 240
Magpie trial 35
Maladaptation, risk of 683
Malar rash 310f
Malaria 194, 386
    abdominal 430
    parasite 411
    prevention intermittent 95
    prophylaxis 282
Malformation 66, 450, 542
Mallory-Weiss tear 98
Malpresentations 462, 499, 522
    diagnosis 499
    differential diagnosis 499
    investigations 500
    management 499
Mammary gland 74
Mammogenesis 630
Manual uterine displacement 437
Manual vacuum aspiration 730
Marfan syndrome 255
Marijuana 342
Marshall burn's technique 560
Mass media method 14
Massive blood transfusion 768
    risk of 768
Massive hemoperitoneum 207f
Massive perivillous fibrin deposition 483
Massive transfusion protocol 766
Mastectomy 360
    therapeutic equivalence of 360
Mastitis 388, 673, 674f, 711
    causes of 673
    infectious 673
Maternal adaptations 80
Maternal anatomy uterus 144
Maternal anemia 295

Index 795

Maternal blood
glucose levels 349
supply, development of 59f
Maternal cancers 190
Maternal cardiac disease 243, 610
effects of 244
Maternal cardiovascular risk 248
classification of 249t
Maternal circulation, glucagon in 259
Maternal cyanotic heart disease 158
Maternal death 405, 726, 727, 733, 734
audit 730
causes of 726
classification of 726
surveillance 734f
Maternal defenses 378
Maternal depression 405
Maternal dietary supplementation 489
Maternal disorders 199
Maternal early warning criteria 751
Maternal human leukocyte antigen 312
Maternal hydration 473, 474
Maternal hyperglycemia 422, 423f
Maternal hyperthyroidism, poorly controlled 158
Maternal hypothyroidism 271
Maternal hypoxemia, severe 254
Maternal infection 123, 199, 388, 450, 451, 678
routes of 387
Maternal injury, risk of 608
Maternal morbidity 583, 762
severe acute 349, 743
Maternal mortality 255, 725
rate 725-727
ratio 726, 728t, 729, 738, 743
reduce 731
Maternal nutritional deficiency 123
Maternal obesity 350, 354, 705
Maternal organs 400
Maternal plasma 186, 495
Maternal polycythemia 244
Maternal preeclampsia, screening for 171
Maternal pulmonary disease 610
Maternal serum biochemical markers, abnormal 523
Maternal syndrome 400
Maternal syphilis 374
Maternal trauma 541
Maternal ultrasonography 401
Maternal uterine vasculature 84
Maternal varicella infection 123f
Maternal vascular
diseases 158
malperfusion 483
Mauriceau-Smellie-Veit technique 561f
Maylard incision 612
McDonald's operation 200
McFonald's suture, placement of 201f
McRobert's maneuver 605, 606, 606f, 607
Mean corpuscular hemoglobin 282
concentration 104
Mean corpuscular volume 282
Mechanical ventilation 745f
Meckel Gruber syndrome 473
Meconium aspiration syndrome 349, 683, 684, 710
Meconium passage 688
Meconium-stained
amniotic fluid 694
liquor 593, 693

Mediastinal adenopathy 321
Medical disorders, prevalence of 610
Medical nutritional therapy 425
Medical simulation technology 27
Medical termination of pregnancy 194
indications of 271
role of 271
Medical therapy, maximal 251
Megacystis 473
microcolon 473
Meiosis 66f
Melanocyte stimulating hormone 335
Melanoma 337
Melena 430
Melisma, exacerbations of 335
Membrane 483t
rupture of
artificial 579, 580
prelabor 463, 721
premature 154, 578, 694
prolonged 524
Memory, impaired 405
Mendelson's syndrome 779
Meningeal sac, herniation of 75
Meningocele 147f
Meningomyelocele 716, 716f
Menstrual irregularities 348
Menstrual losses 275
Menstrual period 71
Menstruation 629
Mental health
impact of 340, 343
issues 340, 341, 345
problem 341, 343
management strategies for 343
Mental retardation 344, 450
genetic cause of 133
Mentzer index 286
Mercury sphygmomanometers 241
Meropenem 323
Mesoderm 75
development 75f
Metabolic acidosis 222, 667, 715
refractory 294
Metabolic adaptation 683
Metabolic control 260
Metabolic disorder 258, 303, 778
Metabolism, inborn errors of 496
Metalloproteinase, tissue inhibitors of 57
Metastatic cerebral tumors 332
Metastatic disease 223
Metastatic tumors 481
Metformin 261, 677
therapy 425
Methadone 448
Methamphetamine 543
Methemoglobinemia 279
Methicillin-resistant *Staphylococcus aureus* 323, 675
Methimazole 269
Methotrexate 206, 221, 312, 314, 315, 317
therapy 207t, 315
use of 533
Methyldopa 238, 296, 404
Methylene dioxymethamphetamine 342
Methylergometrine 405
Methylprednisolone 357
Metoclopramide 305, 676
Metronidazole 305, 390, 505, 667

Microarray analysis 542
Microinvasive disease 362
Micronized progesterone 462
Microvesicular fatty infiltration 304
Microvesicular steatosis 304
Mid face hypoplasia 344
Midpelvis 44
Midwifery services framework 738
Mifepristone 197
combination of 547
Migraine headache 327
Milia 718
Milk
blisters 671, 672
fever 671
fistula 360
insufficiency syndrome, secondary 675
rejection sign 360
stasis 673
Millennium development goals 693, 727
Miller-Dieker syndrome 68
Mineral metabolism 82
Mineralocorticoids 715
Miscarriage 198
rates of 294
recurrent 198, 199t, 417
risk of 135, 244
spontaneous 117
Misoprostol 197, 305, 579, 580, 615
Mitigate violence 48, 49t
Mitochondrial fatty acid oxidation 410
Mitosis 66f
Mitral regurgitation 251
etiologies of 251
Mitral stenosis 248
Mitral valve 180f, 248
Mitral valvotomy, closed 251
Mityvac cup 599f
Mityvac vacuum 599
Mobilization 568
Mode of delivery 405, 497, 676, 705
Molar pregnancy 98, 118, 218f
clinical presentation of 217
Mole-focal hydropic degeneration, partial 214f
Mongolian blue spots 718
Monoamniotic twins 458, 459f, 463, 464f
Monochorionic twin 459f, 460f, 464
complications 172
gestation 475
Monoclonal antibodies 395
Monogenic disorders 116
Mononuclear cells 339
Monosomy X 189
Monotherapy, antihypertensive for 237
Monozygotic twinning 457, 458, 458t, 463
etiology of 460
rate of 457
testing in 190
Mons pubis 37
Mood disorders 340
symptoms of 341
Moro's biceps 708
Moro's reflex 707
Morphine 444
Morphological growth 62
Morphological left atrium 178
Morphological right ventricle 178

Mortality
    maternal 731
    neonatal 731
Morula stage embryo 57f
Morulation 69f
Mosaicism 66
Motor vehicle collision 439
Mouth ulcers 306
Mouth-to-mouth breathing 774
Mucolipidoses 496
Mucopolysaccharidoses 496
Mucus, passage of 305
Mucus-secreting tubule, pair of 38
Müllerian anomalies 194
Müllerian defect 194
Multicystic dysplastic kidney, bilateral 472
Multidisciplinary team
    approach 288
    care 530
    involvement of 395
Multifactorial disorders 117
Multifetal gestation
    diagnosis of 461
    mechanism of 457
Multiorgan failure 222
Multiparity 564
Multiple births, incidence of 457
Multiple café-au-lait spots 337
Multiple gestation 154, 227, 324, 475, 523, 684
Multiple organ dysfunction score 749
Multiple pregnancy 154, 194, 304, 457, 519, 540
    complications of 544
    incidence 457
    screening in 135
    testing in 190
Multiple sclerosis 316, 327, 332
Multiple soft markers 146
Multiplex ligation-dependent probe
        amplification 120
Multisystem disorders 684
Mumps 384
Murphy's sign 430
Muscle
    cells 274
    fibers 216f
    spasm 316
Musculoskeletal dysplasia 129
Musculoskeletal injuries 441
Musculoskeletal system 87
Music and aroma therapy 622
Myasthenia gravis 313, 332
Mycobacteria 674
Mycobacterium tuberculosis 321, 385, 451
Mycophenolate 314
    mofetil 317, 418
Mycoplasma hominis 504
    colonization 512
Myeloid leukemia, positive chronic 358
Myelomeningocele 75
Myelosuppression 222
Myocardial infarction
    acute 255t
    risk of 240
Myoma uterus 194
Myomectomy scar 197
Myometrial scar thickness, role of 583
Myometrium 223f
Myotonic dystrophy 333, 496

N

N acetyl-P-benzoquinone imine 445f
N-acetylcysteine 444, 445f
Naegele's s obliquity 551
Nail growth 336
Naloxone 444, 448, 693
    administration of 444
Narrow palpebral fissures 344
Nasal bone 134
Nasal septal dislocation 706
National AIDS Control Organization
        guidelines 369
National Center of Health Statistics 720
National Family Health Survey 686
National Health Mission 729
National Infant Feeding Guideline 372
National Institute for Health and Care
        Excellence 237, 740
National Institutes of Health 514
    database 248
National Maternity Benefit Scheme 729
National Medical Commission 28
National Midwifery Training Institute 741
National Partnership for Maternal Safety 745
National Program 368
National Registries 28
National Safe Motherhood 728
National Technical Advisory Group on
        Immunization 95
Nausea 98, 99, 412f
    and vomiting, form of 413
    complication 98
    examination 99
    excessive 461
    investigations 99
    treatment 99
Navirapine, single dose 368
Navjaat Shishu Suraksha Karyakram 693
Necator americanus 380
Necrotizing enterocolitis 683
    risk of 515
Neisseria gonorrheae 384, 512
Neoglucogenic substrate 259
Neonatal abstinence syndrome 344, 345, 448
Neonatal alloimmune thrombocytopenia 153
Neonatal care 263
Neonatal coagulopathy 329
Neonatal complications 244
Neonatal encephalopathy 700
Neonatal hypothyroidism 267
Neonatal infection 388
Neonatal intensive care unit 168
Neonatal iron biology 277
Neonatal mortality 319
Neonatal resuscitation 688
    program 689
Neonatal screening 124
Neonatal sepsis 349
Neonatal transport 686
Neonate develops respiratory depression 623
Neonates born 277
Nephrotic syndrome 295
Nerve
    grafting 708
    injuries 624, 708
Neu-laxova 496
Neural crest cells 74
Neural tube defects 74, 117, 147, 329
Neurofibromatosis 337

Neurological conditions, classification 327
Neurological disorders 327, 412
Neurological disruption 475
Neuromuscular junction blocker 330
Neuromusculoskeletal problems 633
Neuronal discharge, abnormal 327
Neuronal trauma 697
Neuroplasty 708
Neuroprotective strategies 702
Neutrophil lymphocyte ratio 394
Newborn care corner 684
Newborn mortality 737
Nifedipine 238, 296, 404, 501, 506
Nimesulide 473, 476
Nipple
    bite 671
    fissuring of 336
    pain 671
Nitric oxide 254
    donors 507
    inhaled 282
    synthesis 349
Nitrous oxide 622
Nonalcoholic hepatitis 418
Non-breastfeeding infants 454
Nonimmune fetal hydrops 118, 227, 495, 496
    diagnosis 496
    etiology 496
    management 497
Noninvasive continuous positive airway
        pressure 395
Noninvasive peripheral oxygen saturations 756
Noninvasive prenatal testing 186, 187
    accuracy of 188, 189t
    principle of 187f
Nonnucleoside reverse-transcriptase
        inhibitors 368
Nonopioid analgesics 622
Nonpersonal violence 47
Nonpharmacologic lifestyle interventions 236
Nonpneumatic antishock garment 731, 732f
Nonreactive nonstress test 160f
Nonretractable prepuce 718
Nonshockable rhythms 775
Nonsteroidal anti-inflammatory drug 246,
        282, 305, 310, 321, 615, 622
Nonstress test 157-159
    advantages of 160
    disadvantages of 160
    twice weekly 263
Nonsurgical scar 529
Nontraumatic liver rupture 304
Nontubal ectopic pregnancy 206, 208t
Noonan syndrome 255
Noradrenaline 779
Nordic obstetric surveillance study 529
Normal pregnancy, hyperlipidemia of 106
Normal puerperium 628
    anatomical changes 629
    physiological changes 628
Nuchal arms 502
Nuchal cord 143f
Nuchal fold 144
    thickness 144, 145f
Nuchal translucency 130f, 133, 134
    levels 297
Nucleic acid 413
Nucleotide 113
    polymorphism, single 189f

Nutrition
    monitoring of 759
    supplementation 371
Nutritional deficiency 485
Nutritional interventions 94
Nystagmus 68

O

O'lLeary method 648f
Obese pregnant patients 348
Obesity 267, 318, 347, 348, 543
    effects of 348
    management of 350
    paradox 348
    postpartum 353t
    prevention of 354
Obsessive compulsive disorder 340, 341
Obstetric care 297
Obstetric cholestasis 303, 409, 541, 543
Obstetric deaths, indirect 726
Obstetric emergency 619
Obstetric examination 92
Obstetric formula, terminology for 92t
Obstetric high-dependency unit 745
Obstetric hysterectomy 652, 655f
    complications of 652t
    decision of 652
    indications of 653
    technique of 647
Obstetric intensive care unit 745
Obstetric management 444, 546
Obstetric shock 598, 762, 763fc
Obstetric transition 735
Obstetrical care 727
Obstetrical complications 292, 348
Obstetrical emergency 304
Obstetrical neuropathy 633
Obstructed labor 618
Obstructive sleep apnea 348
Obturator test 431
Occipital cortex 557
Occipital frontal circumference 706
Occipitoposterior position, diagnosis of 556
Occult blood 433
Occulta 147
Ocular injuries 706
Oculocutaneous albinism 155
Odon device 602
Oligohydramnios 158, 162f, 287, 311, 472, 475
    causes 472
    etiology of 472, 472t
    incidence 472
    pathogenesis 472
    sequence 472
Oligomenorrhea 417
Omissions 726
Omphalocele 78
Ondansetron 304
Oocyte
    denudation 56f
    maturation 54
Operations, types of 595
Operative deliveries, risk of 420
Operative vaginal delivery 602, 618, 705
Opioid 282, 622
    diagnostic of 444
    poisoning, chronic 448
Opium poisoning 448
Oral anticoagulant 250

Oral cavity 91
Oral contraceptive pills, use of 460
Oral glucose challenge test 105, 230, 263, 545
Oral heart failure therapy 253
Oral hygiene 102, 760
Oral hypoglycemic agents 158, 261, 262, 262t
Oral iron 276
Oral steroids, indications of 394
Organ function assessment
    quick sepsis-related 752t
    sepsis-related 749
Organ systems, range of 405
Organogenesis 73
Orofacial clefts 329
Oseltamivir 323
Osmotic fragility 282, 286
Osmotic laxatives 305
Osteomyelitis 281
Osteonecrosis 281
Osteoporosis 306
Outflow tracts 142f
Ovarian artery ligation 647, 648f
Ovarian cancer 363
    clinical presentation 363
    management 364
Ovarian cystectomy 364
Ovarian follicle grows 53
Ovarian function 315
Ovarian germ cell tumors 364
Ovarian hyperstimulation syndrome 256
Ovarian ligament 657f
Ovarian torsion 198
Ovarian tumors, malignant 364
Ovary corpus luteum 85
Overwhelming post splenectomy infection 281
Ovular phase 65, 69
Ovulation 629
Ovum
    plasma membrane of 53
    transport 54
Oxygen
    administration 778
    affinity, altered 279
    consumption 84
    delivery 762
        concept of 762
    saturation 752, 762
    toxicity 717
Oxytocic drugs 730
    use of 615
Oxytocin 247, 581, 588, 615, 645
    contraindications for 644
    drip 579
    infusion 602
    nasal spray 677

P

P-450 enzyme 321
Packed cell volume 767
Packed red blood cell concentrates 767
Pain 101
    changes, location of 306
    etiology 101
    medication 282
    relief 569
    score 759f
    treatment 101
    types 101

Palatal anomalies 671
Pallor 91
    severe degree of 430
Palmar edema 102
Palmar erythema 335
Palpable tender liver 325
Pancreatitis, acute 411, 430
Panel tests 190
Papillary necrosis, acute 281
Paracentesis, abdominal 432
Paracentric inversion 114, 115f
Paracetamol 622
Paralysis 316
Parasites 380, 451
Parasitic twin, external 464
Parathyroid glands 85
Paraxial mesoderm 76
Parenteral antiemetic therapy 304
Parenteral steroids, indications of 394
Parietal fascia 42
Paroxysmal disorder 327
Partogram 569
    components of 572
Parvovirus B_{19} 123, 381, 542
    infection 123
Passive leg raise maneuver 762
Patau syndrome 67, 116, 129, 150, 186
Patent ductus arteriosus 247, 248, 254, 507, 683
Patwardhan's maneuver 589f, 614
Peak systolic velocity 169f
Pedal edema 102, 102f, 461
Pedicles 655
    ligation of 658
Pelvic
    anatomy 37, 604
    architecture, influence of 553
    assessment 230
    brim 572
    collections 667
    diaphragm 41
    fascia 42
    floor muscle 39f
        rehabilitation 639
    grip 562
    hematoma 38
    infection, acute 428
    inlet 44
    kidneys 170f
    musculature 630
    organs 629
    outlet 45
    region, muscles of 41
    shape 555
    ureters 43
Pelvis, abnormal 588
Pemphigoid gestationis 337
Pena-Shokeir syndromes 496
Penicillin 323
    G benzathine 374
Peptic ulcer
    disease 305
    perforation of 430
Per vaginal examination, procedure of 568b
Perfusion 702
Pericardial effusions 496
Pericarditis 294
Pericentric inversion 114, 115f
Periconceptional folic acid supplementation 74

Perimortem cesarean
   delivery 776
   section 247, 438
Perinatal asphyxia 684, 696-698, 698fc, 699
   causes of 696, 697t
   neonatal signs of 698t
   postpartum screening for 699
   risk of 699
      developing 683
   screening tests for 699
Perinatal death 284, 720, 721
   causes of 721b
   classification of 721, 721b
   majority of 720
   notification of 724
   surveillance 721, 722
Perinatal infection 73t
Perinatal management 701
Perinatal mortality
   rate 720
   risk increases 544
Perinatal transmission
   estimated risk of 367
   rate of 367
   with intervention, risk of 367t
   without intervention, risk of 367t
Perineal muscles 639
Perineal skin 639
Perineal tears 638
   classification 638
   management 639
   risk factors 638
Perineal trauma 635
   reduced 737
Periodic fevers 664
Peripartum cardiomyopathy 252, 325
Peripheral fat 348
Peripheral nerve injury 708
Peripheral nervous system 74
Peripheral neuropathy 327
Peripheral smear 275f, 286, 411
Peripheral vascular resistance 85, 233
Peripheral vasodilators 238
Peristaltic sounds 431
Peritoneal closure 614
Peritoneum 40, 630
   reflections of 39f
Peritonitis, complications of 430
Pethidine 622
Pfannenstiel incision 612
Phenothiazines 304
Phenotype 114
Phenytoin 329
Pheochromocytoma 235
Phosphoenolpyruvate carboxykinase,
      activation of 683
Phosphorylated insulin 504
Phrenic nerve injury 709
Physiological adaptation 80, 85t, 266, 762
Pinard's maneuver 562f
Piper's forceps 560
Piperacillin 323
Pituitary gland 74, 84
Placenta 63, 69, 143f, 144, 227, 410, 478, 483t
   abnormality 475, 478, 542
   accrete spectrum, incidence of 169
   delivery of 643
   development of 58, 59f
   diffusa 480

   gross examination of 480f
   increta 520, 532f
   lacks 167
   low lying 519
   manual removal of 779
   normal 478
   percreta 520, 530f
   posterior 152f
   processing of 484b
   removal of 730
   shape, abnormalities of 478
   single 459
   size, abnormalities of 480
   triangular projection of 459f
Placenta accreta 520, 530f
   spectrum disorders 528, 529t
      diagnosis 530
      epidemiology 529
      management 530, 534fc
Placenta previa 227, 502, 519, 520, 577, 653,
      653f
   accreta 529
   diagnosis of 519f
   incidence of 519
   lateral 519
   marginal 519
   partial 519
   previous 519
   total 519
   woman with 522
Placental abruption 283, 439
   chance of 438
   classification 524
   clinical picture 523
   complications 524
   incidence 522
   management 524
   pathophysiology 522
   previous 523
   risk factors 523
Placental adherent syndrome 653
Placental block 546
Placental chorioangioma 496
Placental circulation 60f
Placental development 53, 59
Placental evaluation 483
Placental examination 229
Placental gene expression changes 405
Placental growth 58
   hormone 98
Placental insufficiency 472, 541, 543, 715
Placental location 401
Placental morphology 401
Placental site trophoblastic tumor 211, 216,
      223
Placental transfusion 715
Placental tropism 388
Placental tumors 480
Plaques 338, 338f
Plasma
   reduced blood 767
   volume 104
Plasma protein
   A, pregnancy-associated 134, 170
   changes 106t
   levels of pregnancy-associated 186
Plasmodium falciparum 388
Plate mesoderm, lateral 76
Platelet-rich plasma 767

Pleonasm 610
Pleural effusion 321, 401, 496
Pleuritic pain 310
Plotting partogram 572
Plugged ducts, management 672
Pneumococcal vaccine 95
Pneumocystis jirovecii 321
Pneumonia 282, 322, 380, 388, 430, 668, 710
   bacteriology of 322
   causative organisms for 323t
   severity of 323t
Pneumothorax 710
Poikilocytes 286
Point-of-care
   quality improvement methodology 723
   test 374
Poison 442, 443, 448
Poisoning
   diagnosis of 443
   effects of 443
   fetal effects of 445
   high risk factors for 443t
   management of 444
   medicolegal aspects of 444, 444b
Polar bodies, abnormal 68
Policeman tip appearance 708
Polyangiitis 315
   microscopic 315
Polyarteritis nodosa 295, 315
Polycystic kidney 295
   disease 472
Polycystic ovary syndrome 348, 420, 677
Polycythemia 684, 715
Polydipsia 304
Polygenic cardiac disease 244
Polygenic disorders 117
Polyhydramnios 158, 174, 474, 475, 475f, 496, 523
   causes of 475
   development of acute 462
   etiology 474
   fetal causes 474
   incidence 474
   mild 476
   pathogenesis of 474
   relief of 476
   severe 476
Polymastia 631
Polymerase chain reaction 284, 384, 386, 387, 389
Polymicrobial infections 380
Polymorphic eruption 337, 338, 338f
Polypeptide chains 286
Polyploidy 114
Polythelia 631
Polyuria 304
Ponderal index 486
Portal vein thrombosis 418
Positive antinuclear antibody 309
Postabortion care 727
Postarrest prognostic factors 780
Post-cesarean analgesia 625
Postdural puncture headache, management
      of 746
Postmolar gestational trophoblastic neoplasia,
      diagnosis of 220t
Postpartum complication 463, 522
Postpartum convulsions 400
Postpartum hemorrhage, risk factors for 643t
Postpartum management 330, 353
Postpartum periods, management of 418

Postpartum pyrexia 663
   clinical monitoring 666
   complications 668
   etiopathogenesis 664
   history 664
   investigations 665
   management 667
   physical examination 665
   prevention 668
   prognosis 668
   risk factors 664
Postpartum surveillance 270
Postprocedural fetal loss rates 151, 154
Postresuscitation care 693
Post-term pregnancy 158, 473, 535
   etiology 536
   incidence 535
   management 536
   pathogenesis 536
   prevention 537
Post-traumatic stress disorder 230, 340
Potassium chloride 206
Prader-Willi syndrome 68, 117
Pradhan Mantri Surakshit Matritva Abhiyan 730
Prazosin 237
Precipitate labor 573
Pre-conception and Pre-natal Diagnostic Techniques Act 320
Preconception care 88, 97
Preconception clinic 124
Preconception screening 124
Preconceptional counseling 88, 123, 245, 260, 269, 329
Predelivery, risk factors in 664t
Prednisolone 303, 315, 357
Prednisone 296, 332
Predominant bacterial organism 665t
Preeclampsia 109, 117, 119, 255, 267, 283, 293, 304, 310, 319, 324, 398, 399f, 406, 411, 412b, 541, 543, 758
   anticonvulsants for 730
   early-onset 399, 400
   epidemiology of 398
   etiopathology of 399
   late-onset 399, 400
   management of 403fc, 746
   mild 403, 404
   pathogenesis of 241
   prevention of 296, 403
   screening for 241
   severe 239t, 292, 399, 404, 404t, 746
   sign of 406
   superimposed 239, 398
Pre-existing morbidities, pregnancy with 233
Pregnancy
   abnormal 301
   autoimmune disorders of 308
   causes of 293t
   complications 283, 461
   continuation of 362
   dating of 536
   dermatoses of 337
   effects of 243, 295, 310, 312, 336
   failure 127t
   first half of 428
   high-risk 737
   intrahepatic cholestasis of 118, 409
   management 350
   morbidity 311
   normal 53, 106
   obesity 352t
   progression, abnormal 174
   research 33
   second half of 428
   stage of 539
   treatment of 267, 294, 360
   underlying risk of 256
   vomiting of 412b
Pregnancy after previous fetal loss 227
   etiology 227
   evaluation of fetal death 228
   management strategies 229
   maternal evaluation 228
   postnatal follow-up 229
   risk assessment 228
Pregnancy loss 227, 312, 348
   recurrent 67, 118, 199f, 348
   second-trimester 199
Pregnant women, resuscitation of 744
Preimplantation genetic
   screening 282
   testing 298
Preinvasive disease 362
Premarital screening 124
Premature labor 324
Prenatal genetic screening test, timing of 135
Prenatal screening 330
Prenatal testing 190
Prepartum management 426
Prepregnancy
   care 350
   counseling 305
   immunization 89
Preterm baby 713
Preterm birth 462
   prediction of 508
Preterm delivery 294
Preterm infant 683
Preterm labor 154, 440, 503, 522
   complications 507
   diagnosis of 504
   incidence of 350
   management of 505, 506t, 507
   predictors 504
   prevention of 505
   risk factors 503
   treatment of 462
Preterm premature rupture of membranes 158, 389, 512, 516
   complications 513
   diagnosing 513
   etiology 512
   infections 512
   management of 513
   prediction of 513
Prevent circulatory collapse 437
Previous cesarean
   delivery 582
   section 519, 617, 617f
Primary health centers 729
Primary lactation failure 675
Primary milk insufficiency syndrome 675
Primi paternity, concept of 399
Primidone 329
Primitive chorionic villi 62
Proctosigmoidoscopy 432
Progesterone 98, 110, 258, 259, 291, 335, 505
   only pills 240

Progressive familial intrahepatic cholestasis 409
Proinflammatory cytokines 504
Prolactin 98, 259
   levels 298
Prolapse piles leads 306
Proliferated columnar endocervical glands, extension of 81f
Promethazine 304
Pronucleus, abnormal 68
Prophylactic forceps 599
   concept of 599
Propranolol 237
Propylthiouracil 269, 270
Prostaglandin 206, 254, 547, 579, 643, 645
   inhibitors 476, 506
Prosthetic heart valve 251, 252
Protein
   binding 357
   capacity 678
   metabolism 82
   synthesis 301
Proteinuria 109, 293, 401
   hypertension without 643
   management of 296
Proton pump inhibitor 305
Protozoal infections 380, 386t
Prune Belly syndrome 473
Pruritic folliculitis 337, 339
Pruritic uricarial pappules 338, 338f
Pruritus 102, 623
   gravidarum 335
   severe 335
Pseudomonas 380
Pseudoseizures 328
Psoriasis 316, 336, 671
Psychiatric medications 344
Psychogenic nonepileptic seizures 328
Psychological monitoring 760
Psychosis 341
Psychotherapeutic drugs 345t
Psychotropic drugs 345
Ptosis 344
Pubic symphysis 93f
Pubocervical ligaments 40
Pudendal block 624
Puerperal fever 663
Puerperal pyrexia 663
   causes of 664, 664t, 666t
Puerperal sepsis 292, 663
   delivery for 664t
   labor for 664t
Pulmonary arterial hypertension 324
Pulmonary arterioles 688
Pulmonary artery 182f
   bifurcation 182f
   pressure 254
      monitoring 758
   right 182
Pulmonary edema 294, 324, 325
   causes of 405
Pulmonary emboli, acute 255
Pulmonary embolism 282, 325
Pulmonary fluid secretion 472
Pulmonary function tests 318
Pulmonary hypertension 270, 281, 282, 324, 325, 507
   consequences of 254
   persistent 683, 684
   primary 255
   severe forms of 247

Index

Pulmonary hypoplasia 465
Pulmonary infarction 282
Pulmonary stenosis 248, 251
    etiology of 251
Pulmonary thromboembolic disease 254, 325
Pulmonary thromboembolism 771, 779
Pulmonary veins 179f
Pulsatility index 171f, 490
Pulse 628
    oximetry 322, 756
Pupil
    reactivity score 758t
    score 758
Purandare's system 646f
Pus, aspiration of 674
Push technique 588
Pustules 714, 714f
Pyelectasis 144
    mild 146, 146f
Pyelonephritis 283
    acute 430
Pyloric sphincter competence 305
Pyloric stenosis 475

Q

Q fever 380
Quadruple test 134
Quantitative defect 279
Quantitative fluorescent polymerase chain reaction 120
Quiescent gestational trophoblastic disease 224
Quotidian 664

R

Radial aplasia 329
Radiation 6, 194
    therapy 359, 361
Radical cesarean hysterectomy 363
Radical hysterectomy 363
Radical trachelectomy 363
Radiculopathy 624
Radiocolloid, dose of 356
Radionuclide scans 432
Ramipril 237
Range of movements 313
Rational emotive behavior therapy 344
Raynaud's phenomenon 671
Reactive nonstress test 159f, 160
Recombinant human erythropoietin 282
Rectal bleeding 430
Rectal examination 639
Rectovaginal fistula 638
Recurrent abortion 194, 198
    causes 198
    diagnosis 199
    etiology 199
    treatment 199
Recurrent pregnancy loss, causes of 200
Red blood cell 104
Red cell concentrate 767
Reflection and echoing 15
Reflux
    esophagitis 305
    nephropathy 295
Refractory hypoxemia 254
Refractory neoplasia 222
Refuting misconception 676

Regional analgesia 623, 739
Regional anesthesia 353
Regress postpartum 336
Regular fetal antepartum testing 158
Regular perinatal death audits 723
Rehydration 304
Remdesivir 395
Remifentanil 622, 623
Renal agenesis 473f
Renal anomalies 68, 473
Renal causes, signs of 401
Renal disease 227, 291, 293, 295
    chronic 194, 199
    end-stage 295, 297, 764
    pregnancy of 294
Renal evaluation 700
Renal failure 283
    acute 98, 403, 747, 764, 768
    anemia of 288
    chronic 281
Renal function 155t
    monitoring 759
    parameters 108t
    test 68, 107, 197, 218, 235, 403, 433, 443, 778
Renal impairment 304
Renal insufficiency 293
    degree of 294
Renal parameters 665
Renal parenchyma 401
Renal pathology 235
Renal plasma flow 84
Renal system 84, 233
Renal transplantation, pregnancy after 298
Renal ultrasonography 68
Renal ultrasound 294
Replacement feeding 371
Reproductive autonomy 190
Reproductive capacity 298
Reproductive cloning 69
Reproductive health 729
Reproductive system 80
Reproductive tract, internal 39f
Rescue cerclage 200
Respectful maternity care 739
Respiratory arrest 304
Respiratory autogenic training 622
Respiratory changes 435
Respiratory depression 623
Respiratory disorders, management of 318
Respiratory distress 267, 476, 710
    syndrome 683, 710
Respiratory function, monitoring 759
Respiratory physiology 318
Respiratory rate 430, 745, 754, 756
Respiratory signs 319
Respiratory symptoms 319
Respiratory system 92
Respiratory tract 84
Responsive feeding 632
Rest and exercise 632
Resuscitation 685, 688
Resuscitative cesarean section delivery 776
Resuscitative fluids, types of 764
Reticulocyte count 282
Retinal detachment 281
Retinal hemorrhage 707
Retinoids 335
Retinopathy of prematurity 683, 716, 717
    examination for 716

Retinopathy, progressive 281
Retracted nipple 673f
Retroperitoneal adenopathy 321
Retroplacental bleeding 523
Retroplacental hematoma 524f
Rh
    alloimmunization 150
    immune globulin 149
    incompatibility 518, 540
Rheumatoid arthritis 267, 308, 312
    effects of 312
Rh-negative blood 694
Rhythm, assessment of 754
Ribonucleic acid 187f
Rickettsiae 380
Rifampicin 321, 371
Right umbilical vein, persistent 482
Right ventricular outflow tract 140, 175, 177, 180, 181
Ring chromosome 116
Ringer's lactate 304, 694, 764, 778
Ripening cervix, process of 579
Ritodrine 324, 507
Robertsonian translocation 115, 115f, 116
Robotic cerclage 201
Robotic surgery, form of 8
Root-cause analysis 722
Rosacral ligaments 40
Routine antenatal care 88
Rubella 94, 123, 194, 381, 451, 452, 542
Rubeola virus 384
Rubin's maneuver 606, 606f
Rupture uterus 616, 779
    diagnosis 618
    management 619
    risk factors 617
Ruptured berry aneurysm 331
Ruptured ectopic pregnancy 207f
Rusty pipe syndrome 675

S

Sacral agenesis 72
Sacrococcygeal teratoma 72, 169, 496
Safe abortion services 729
Safe motherhood
    initiative 725, 727
    pillars of 727
Salicylate poisoning 445
Salivary estriol 504
    surge, detection of 504
Salmonella 674
    typhosa 451
Salpingectomy 207f
Salt restriction 237
Sampson's artery 657
    branches of 654
Saphenous, varicosities of 336
Scalp electrode injuries 706
Scar
    ectopic pregnancy 208f
    endometriosis 638
    integrity of 582
Schizophrenia 341, 343
Schlusskoagulum 71
Scleroderma 295, 313
Sclerosing cholangitis, primary 416
Seborrheic dermatitis 713
Sedation 150

Index

Seizure 304, 344
  absence of 327
  activity 328
  causes of 327
  disorder 327, 328
  persist 330
Selective estrogen receptor modulators 362
Selective serotonin reuptake inhibitors 72
Self-inflating bag 691
Sengstaken-Blakemore tube 646f
Sensory abnormalities 316
Sensory epithelium of ear 74
Sentinel node procedure 356
Sepsis 387, 743, 746, 766, 771
  stage of severe 766
  syndrome 283
Septate uterus 194
  partial 199f
Septic abortion 194, 196, 196f, 201, 387, 743
  management 197
  pathology 196
  surgery in 197
Septic shock 197, 768
Septicemia 194, 222, 430
Septostomy 461
Sequential organ failure assessment 388, 749, 752t
Serology 373
Sertoli cell function leading 348
Serum
  alpha-fetoprotein, measurement of 134
  beta-human chorionic gonadotropin measurement 204, 205
  bilirubin 401, 714
  complement levels 294
  creatinine 294, 296
  electrolytes 218, 443, 759
  ferritin 274
  human chorionic gonadotropin level 109t
  lactate levels 107
  tumor markers 364
Severe acute respiratory syndrome 455
  conronavirus 383
Sex chromosome 68
  anomalies 150
  monosomy 133
Sex cord-stromal tumors 364
Sex hormone-binding globulin, levels of 348
Sexually transmitted disease 386, 727
Sexually transmitted infections 89, 367, 372
  effects of 375t
Sheehan's syndrome 675
Shirodkar operation, modified 200
Shock 683, 762, 763t
  classification of 763fc
  maternal 440
  moderate-to-severe 766
Shockable rhythms 775
Short obstetric forceps 596f
Shoulder
  delivery of 553, 560
  disimpaction, anterior 607
  neglected 563, 563f
  posterior 606f
Shoulder dystocia 604, 605, 605t, 608
  complications 607
  incidence 604
  management 605
  risk factors 604

Shunt
  right-to-left 254
  vesicoamniotic 474
Sialidosis 496
Sickle cell
  anemia 279, 280
  C disease 280
  crisis 255
  D disease 280
  disease 158, 279, 280, 283, 288
  disorders 279
  E disease 280
  syndrome 282
  thalassemia disease 280
  trait 280, 284
Sickling process, stages in 280f
Sickling solubility test 282
Sickling test 282
Sideroblastic anemia 286, 288
Silastic vacuum cup 599f
Sildenafil citrate 474
Silent stroke 281
Simpson's long forceps 596
Single gene 116
  defects 153
  deletion 285
  disease 124
  disorders, diagnosis of 298
Singleton pregnancy 461, 463
Sinusitis 321
Sinusoidal pattern 591, 592f
Sirenomelia 72
Situs inversus 72, 176
Situs solitus 176
Skeletal defects 329
Skeletal system 107
Skilled birth attendant 728, 730
  supervision of 728
Skilled manpower 28
Skin 81
  changes 102
  contact, direct 387
  edema 496
  incision 612
  lesions 310
  suturing 637
Skin-to-skin contact 686, 737
Skull 708
  base 140
  bones, overlapping of 540f
Sleep 632
  pattern, abnormal 344
  wake cycles 701
Sloping pelvic floor 552
Small cortical cysts 473
Smith-Lemli-Opitz syndrome 473
Sneezing 344
Sodium
  bicarbonate 305, 779
  deficiency 715
  dithionite, solution-like 282
  nitroprusside 238
Soft markers, absence of 146
Soft tissues
  injury 705
  swelling of 705
Somite differentiation 76
Sonoembryology 126
Spalding sign 540f

Special poisoning syndromes 444
Sperm
  acrosome reaction 55f
  oocyte binding 55
  plasma membrane of 53
  transport 54
Sphingomyelin 150
Spider nevi 335
Spina bifida 75, 147, 147f
Spinal anesthesia 611
  high 779
Spinal cord
  disorders 327
  injuries 704, 709
Spinal epidural hematoma 624
Splanchnopleuric mesoderms 77
Splenectomy 288
Splenic sequestration crisis 281
Spontaneous labor, risk of rupture in 618
Spot urine protein 401
Squamous cell carcinoma 363f
Staphylococcus aureus 671
Static intensity 319
Static pulmonary function tests 318, 318t
Statins 244
Status epilepticus 330
Steal phenomenon 701
Stem cell transplant 287
Stenotic lesion 248
Sterile water injections 622
Sternal defects 78
Sternocleidomastoid muscle, spasm of 564
Steroid 394, 776
  and immunosuppressive therapy 294
  hormone 291
    production 110
  therapy 304
  treatment 335
Stillbirth 319, 463
  recommendation 548b
  reduced 737
  trends of 539
Stomach 142f
Stool culture 305
Streptococcus pneumonia 281, 323, 380
Streptomycin 321
Striae gravidarum 102f, 335
Striking basophilic stippling 286
Stroke 281
Strongyloides stercoralis 380
Structural chromosomal abnormalities 120, 298
Structural valve deterioration 251
Strychnine 444
Subcapsular hematoma 401
Subcutaneous fat necrosis 705
Subdural hematoma 707f
Subdural hemorrhage 706
Subfertility 348, 417
Subsequent pregnancy, management of 230, 639
Substance abuse 447, 543, 678
  assessment 89
Substance use, management strategies for 344
Substantial blood loss 362
Subtotal obstetric hysterectomy 659f
Suburethral nodule 216f
Succenturiate placenta 479f
Suckling promotes 631
Sucralfate 305
Sudden collapse 778

Index

Sudden obstetric collapse 770
    clinical causes 770
        supportive management 776
Sudden tumor collapse 220
Suicide 343
Sulfasalazine 313, 315, 317
Sulfonamides 390
Sulpiride 676
Supplementary therapy, role of 241
Supralevator hematoma 38
Suprapubic pressure 606, 606f, 607
Supraventricular tachyarrhythmia 253
Surgical scar, direct 529
Suturing muscles 637
Swansea criteria 304
Swansea diagnostic criteria 411b
Sweating 344
Symphysiotomy 607
Symphysis-fundal height, measurement of 93f
Symptomatic systemic
    bacterial infection 703
    congenital viral infection 703
Syndrome of inappropriate antidiuretic hormone 702
Syphilis 89, 94, 124, 373, 375, 374t, 376t, 384, 388, 451, 542
    congenital 375, 376b, 453
    pappules 374f
Syrup
    navirapine, dose of 370
    zidovudine 370
Systematic analysis 178
Systemic absorption 323
Systemic diseases 194
Systemic lupus erythematosus 71, 124, 158, 199, 227, 235, 267, 308-310, 337, 541, 544
    effects of 310
    management of 310
Systemic vascular resistance 85, 762

T

T sign 460f
Tachycardia 320, 387, 590, 718, 768
Tachypnea, transient 683
Tachysystole 581
Tacrolimus 303, 317, 418
Tactile stimulation 689
Takayasu arteritis 314
Talipes equinovarus, congenital 716f
Tazobactam 323
Tear drop cells 286
Teeth, enamel of 74
Telangiectasia 335
Telemedicine 28
    practice guidelines 28
Tenderness, site of 431t
Tennessee classification 413
Tenofovir 368, 369
    regimen of 369
Teratogen exposure, effects of 65f
Teratogenesis 71
Teratogenic drug 297
    defects 73t
Teratomas, immature 364
Teratospermia 68
Terbutaline 324
Term breech trial 35

Terminal ileum 305
Termination of pregnancy 198, 201, 362
Tetanus toxoid 95
    injection 197
Tetracyclines 320, 323, 390
Tetralogy of Fallot 254
Thalassemia 284, 287, 288
    major 286f, 288f
    mild 287
    minor 284, 286
    severe forms of 284
    types of 284
Theca lutein cysts 218f
Therapeutic hypothermia 702
Thermal adaptation 682
Thermal injury 440
Thermoneutral environment 684, 685f
Thermoregulatory imbalance 345
Thiamine deficiency 99
Thiazides 237, 238
Thionamides 269
Third stage bleeding 247
Third-trimester 260, 460
Thoracic abnormalities 496
Thoracic cavity 78
Thoracoscopy 320
Thoracotomy tube 437
Thrombocytopenia 153, 309
Thromboembolism 252, 283, 328, 405
    side effect of 767
Thrombophilia 523, 544
    inherited 198
Thromboplastin 523
Thromboprophylaxis 282, 296
Thrombotic microangiopathy 293, 294
Thrombotic thrombocytopenic purpura, clinical syndromes of 293
Thumb technique 691
Thyroglobulin, proteolytic destruction of 270
Thyroid
    antibodies 267
    autoimmune disorders of 313
    binding globulin 85f
        production of 266
    cancer 365
    disease, screening for 266
    disorder 201, 266, 271
        treatment of 269, 269fc
    dysfunction 198
    function test 218, 751
        levels of 107t
    gland 84
        functioning 266
    hormone 267
        physiology 266, 266t
    peroxidase antibodies 270
    physiology 106, 107t
    stimulating hormone 68, 266, 268fc, 268t
    storm 269, 270
        treatment of 270, 270fc
Thyroiditis 270
    postpartum 270, 314
Thyroid-stimulating antibody, formation of 268
Thyrotoxicosis 269
    destruction-induced 270
Thyrotropin, inhibition of 266
Thyroxine 266
    myocardial effects of 270

Tissue
    oxygenation 762
    thromboplastin 523
Tocilizumab 395
Tocolysis 150, 297, 501, 506, 593
    short-term 515, 463
Tocolytic agents 246t, 324
Tocolytic pulmonary edema 324
Tocolytic therapy 515
Tolbutamide 426
Tongue tie 671, 718
Topical bleaching creams 335
TORCH infections 59, 452
Total breech extraction 559
Total obstetric hysterectomy 654f, 660f
Touch technology 47
Toxic compounds
    formation of 445f
    pathophysiology of 445f
Toxic doses, radiation in 194
Toxic effects 303
Toxicologic analysis 443
Toxins, environmental 194
Toxoplasma gondii 451
Toxoplasmosis 123, 386, 452
T-piece resuscitator 691
Tracheal occlusion 78
Tranexamic acid 531
Tranquilizer poisoning 446
Transabdominal technique 151
Transcerebellar diameter 141f
Transcervical technique 151
Transcutaneous electrical nerve stimulation 622
Transfusion reactions 768
    life-threatening 768
    mild 768
    moderately severe 768
Transient diabetes insipidus 411
Transplacental passage 453
Transplacental therapy, monitoring of 154
Transvaginal chorionic villus 151
Transvaginal scan 200, 204
Transvaginal sonography 519
Transvaginal ultrasonography 204
Transverse grooves 336
Transverse lie 502, 562, 563f, 577
Transverse section 143f
Trauma 434, 436, 439, 523
    assessment of 436
    causes of 436, 439
    complications of 441
    management of 436, 438
    penetrating 440
    signs of 438b
    symptoms of 438b
    types of 436
Trendelenburg position 685
Treponema 123, 373
    infection 123
    tests 374
Treponema pallidum 451, 453
    hemagglutination 374
    particle agglutination 374
Triaging policy 745
Trichomoniasis 336, 375, 386, 512
Trichuris trichiura 380
Tricuspid regurgitation 134, 251
Triglyceride 258
Triiodothyronine 266

Index

Trimethadione 329
Trinucleotide repeats 120
Triple drug therapy 368
Triple X syndrome 186
Trisomy 67, 114, 129, 133, 135, 186, 189
    screening for 230
    sonological marker in 134*t*
Trophoblast 69, 213*f*
    hyperplasia of 214*f*
    normal 212
Trophoblastic disease 211
    management of 222
Trophoblastic disorder 337
Trophoblastic invasion, second wave of 485
Trophoblastic lesions, pathology of 214
Trophoblastic tumor cells 217*f*
True knot 483
Trypanosoma cruzi 451
Tubal ectopic pregnancy, ruptured left 207*f*
Tuberculin skin test 320
Tuberculosis 124, 320, 321, 678
Tuberculous ulcer 430
Tubular necrosis, acute 292
Tumor 496
    borderline 364
    collapse 222
    necrosis factor 512
Turner syndrome 68, 150, 186, 255, 256
    phenotype features of 68*f*
Turtle sign 605, 605*f*
Twin anemia polycythemia
    sequence 466, 496
    syndrome 465
Twin fetuses, discordant growth of 466
Twin molar pregnancy 466
Twin pregnancy 158, 172*t*, 194, 224, 224*f*, 461
Twin delivery 462
Twin-to-twin transfusion syndrome 170, 463, 465, 465*f*, 476, 496
Typhoid 388
    ulcer 430
Tyrosinase, upregulation of 335
Tyrosine kinase inhibitor 358

U

Ulcerative colitis 305
Ultrasound
    basic steps of 140*f*
    biometry 95
Umbilical artery 162, 167, 482, 490
    perivesical 170*f*
    single 482
Umbilical artery Doppler
    fallacy of 487
    measurements, abnormal 689
    serial worsening of 168*f*
    velocimetry 592
    waveforms 488*f*
Umbilical blood sampling, percutaneous 152
Umbilical cord 166*f*, 481
    abnormalities of 481*t*
    bleeding 154
    clamping of 689
        timing of 684
    contents of 481
    cyst 483
    four vessel 482
    normal 143*f*
    segment 546

Umbilical granuloma 714, 715
Umbilical venous catheter 690
Undescended testis 715, 715*f*
Unicornuate uterus, inversion of 654*f*
Unilateral salpingo-oophorectomy 364
Uniovular twins 457
Uniparental disomy 116, 117
United Nations Children's Fund 670, 738
United Nations Population Fund 727
Universal vaccination 414
Unstable hemoglobin variants 279
Upper pedicles 658*f*
Upper respiratory tract infection 321
Ureaplasma urealyticum 504, 512
Uremic organ dysfunction 294
Ureter 43*t*, 235
Ureteric injury 662
Ureterovaginal fistula 652
Urethral obstruction 472
Urgent exploratory laparotomy 432
Uric acid 304
Urinalysis 197, 292, 293, 433
Urinary albumin 109
Urinary bladder 143*f*
Urinary casts 310
Urinary components 155*t*
Urinary dipstick method 401
Urinary infection 84
Urinary protein 108, 311, 401
Urinary sepsis, suspicion of 667
Urinary symptoms 99
Urinary tract 496, 628
    infection 259, 380, 386, 389, 512, 652
    obstruction, congenital 472
    tumors of 295
Urine 628
    albumin 401
    analysis 107, 235, 282, 443
    monitoring color of 759*f*
    output 756
    retention of 101
    tests, rapid qualitative 443
Urine sample 109*t*
    chemical examination of 109*t*
    physical examination of 108*t*
    types of 108*t*
Urogenital defects 329
Ursodeoxycholic acid 303, 410
Uterine activity 551, 554
    classification of abnormal 554
Uterine anomalies 529
Uterine artery 164, 172*f*
    blood flows, normal 172*f*
    embolization 648, 649
        retrograde 649*f*
    ligation of 647, 648*f*
        bilateral 647
Uterine atony 642
    refractory 653
Uterine balloon tamponade 731, 732*f*
Uterine blood flow 85
Uterine closure 614
Uterine compression techniques 648
Uterine contractions 439
    assessment of 438
Uterine dehiscence 617, 617*f*, 619*fc*
Uterine discharge 634
Uterine dysfunction 561
Uterine endometrium 53

Uterine evacuation 668
Uterine exteriorization 614
Uterine incisions 613
Uterine malformations, congenital 618
Uterine manipulation maneuvers 618
Uterine massage 643
Uterine pathology
    primary 529*t*
    secondary 529*t*
Uterine pedicles 659*f*
Uterine rupture 541, 583, 586*f*, 617*f*, 618, 619, 619*fc*
    complete 617
    effects of 620*t*
    incomplete 617
    previous 585
    risk factors for 617*t*
    risk of 617*t*
    types of 617
Uterine scar
    extension of 585
    rupture, clinical features of 586
Uterine surgery 617
    previous 585
Uterine vessels 658*f*
    clamping of 662
Utero-ovarian ligament 531
Uteroplacental blood flow 81
Uteroplacental circulation, spasm of 543
Uteroplacental insufficiency 410, 440
Uterovesical interface evaluation 171*f*
Uterus 39, 80
    appearance of 223*f*
    brace suturing of 649*f*
    dropsy of 211
    enlarged 80*f*, 305
    inversion of 779
    involution of 629, 629*f*
    layers of 40
    ligaments of 40
    lower segment of 39
    myometrial wall of 647
    parts of 39
    relations of 40
    round ligaments of 40
    section of 223*f*
    sub-involution of 633

V

Vacuum cup 600*f*
Vacuum extractor 599
    complications 601
    contraindications 600
    over forceps, advantages of 601
    principles of traction 600
    steps of operation 600
Vagina 38
    posteriorly 38
Vaginal birth 585
    after cesarean
        delivery 585
        section 585, 618
    spontaneous 739
Vaginal bleeding 216*f*, 439, 520, 523, 525, 712, 712*f*
Vaginal breech delivery, modes of 559
Vaginal candidiasis 101
    etiology 101
    incidence 101
    treatment 101

Index

Vaginal cerclage 200
Vaginal clindamycin 505
Vaginal delivery 247, 416, 578t
Vaginal discharge 712, 712f
Vaginal examination 92, 372, 438, 562, 581
Vaginal infection 505f
Vaginal insertion 462
Vaginal lacerations 607
Vaginal mucosa 639
    suturing of 637
Vaginal swabbing 661
Vaginal vault 662f
Valproate 329
Vanillylmandelic acid 235
Varicella 123, 388, 542
    zoster 382
        virus 336
Varicose veins 102
    etiology 102
    treatment 102
Variola 194
Vasa previa 483, 526, 577
    classification 526
    clinical presentation 526
    diagnosis 527
    incidence 526
    management 527
Vascular anastomosis 464
Vascular Ehlers-Danlos syndrome 256
Vascular endothelial damage 485
Vascular endothelium 349
Vascular thrombosis 311, 353
Vasculitis 314
Vasoconstriction secondary 400
Vaso-occlusive crises 281, 282
Vasopressin 779
Vasopressor support 324
Vasorelaxing agents 253
Velamentous cord insertion 482
Vena cava
    compression of inferior 357
    inferior 301, 320, 776
    occlusion 771
    superior 182f
Venous stasis 306
Venous system 163
Venous thromboembolism 283, 395, 522, 763
Ventilation 701
    breaths 774
    lack of 693
    positive-pressure 690, 692
Ventral body wall defects 78
Ventricles 175
Ventricular fibrillation 775
Ventricular septal defect 77, 247, 248, 254
Verbal communication 12, 12t
Vermian agenesis 75
Vertical skin incision 532f
Vertical transmission, risk of 408

Vesicovaginal fistula 652
Vesiculobullous lesions 338
Vessel number 482
Vestibule 37
    bulbs of 38
Vibroacoustic stimulation test 591
Vice versa 235
Vicious circle 523
Vigilant fetal monitoring 230
Vigorous suctioning 689
Villous dysmaturity 484
Villous invasion, depth of 529
Violence
    effects of 48
    incidents of 48
    types of 47, 47f
Viral hepatitis 302t, 418
    acute 414
Viral infections 194, 379, 381t, 451
Viral load test 369
Virus 451
Viscera herniate, abdominal 78
Visceral fascia 42
Visceral injuries 709
Visceral layer 76
Visceral situs 177
Visual aids 14
Visual disturbances 304
Vital signs 751
    abnormal 754
    physiological 759
    unstable 430
Vitamin 633
    A supplements 94
    B_{12} 99
    B_6 99
    C 288
    D_3 296
    K 330
        deficiency 99
    supplementation 304
Vitreous hemorrhages 281
Voluntary muscles, movement of 539
Vomiting 98, 99, 304, 430, 717
    complication 98
    examination 99
    excessive 461
    investigations 99
    treatment 99
Vulval hematoma 38, 637
Vulval lacerations 607

W

Waiter's tip deformity 713
Wandering method 599
Warfarin 244, 252
    overdose 767
Warm stool smears 433

Warm water immersion 622
Water intoxication, risk of 645
Water metabolism 82
Waterborne transmission 387
Weak cry 688
Wegener granulomatosis 315
Weight gain 82
    range of 92t
Weight loss 237
Weight management 237
Wernicke's encephalopathy 99
Wheezing 283
White blood cell count 431
White coat hypertension 234
Whole blood 766
    finger prick test 371
Whole exome sequencing 120
Whole genome sequencing 120
Widal test 666
Wilson's disease 416
Witch's milk 711
Woman's dating ultrasound scan 190
Woman's death 5
Wood's screw maneuver 606, 606f
Wound dehiscence, incidence of 638
Wound infection 387
Wurm's stitch 201

X

X chromosome 67, 114
X-linked dominant disorders 117b
X-linked recessive disorders 117b

Y

Y chromosomal microdeletion 68
Yellow atrophy, acute 304, 410
Yolk sac, secondary 70

Z

Zanamivir 323
Zarate 262
Zavanelli maneuver 607, 608f
Zidovudine therapy 454
Zika 123
    virus 383, 542
Zinc 282
Zona pellucida 57
    glycoprotein of 53
    penetration of 55, 56f
Zona reaction 54, 56
Zona thinning 70
Zoonotic disease 380
Zoonotic transmission 387
ZPP test 287
Zygosity 458, 458t
Zygote 53
    division of 69, 458, 458t